KHAN'S
Treatment Planning in Radiation Oncology

FIFTH EDITION

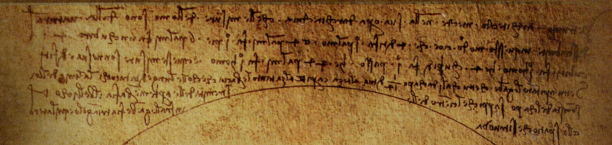

KHAN'S
Treatment Planning
in Radiation Oncology

FIFTH EDITION

EDITORS

Paul W. Sperduto, MD, MPP, FASTRO

Radiation Oncologist
Minneapolis Radiation Oncology
Minneapolis, Minnesota

John P. Gibbons, PhD

Chief Medical Physicist
Department of Radiation Oncology
Ochsner Health System
New Orleans, Louisiana

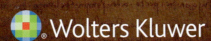

. Wolters Kluwer

Philadelphia • Baltimore • New York • London
Buenos Aires • Hong Kong • Sydney • Tokyo

Acquisitions Editor: Nicole Dernoski
Development Editor: Ariel S. Winter
Editorial Coordinator: Vinodhini Varadharajalu
Editorial Assistant: Maribeth Wood
Marketing Manager: Kirsten Watrud
Production Project Manager: Barton Dudlick
Design Coordinator: Stephen Druding
Manufacturing Coordinator: Beth Welsh
Prepress Vendor: Lumina Datamatics

5th edition
Copyright © 2022 Wolters Kluwer

9 8 7 6 5 4 3 2 1

Printed in Mexico

Library of Congress Cataloging-in-Publication Data
Names: Sperduto, Paul W., editor. | Gibbons, John P., Jr., editor.
Title: Khan's treatment planning in radiation oncology / editors, Paul
  Sperduto, MD, MPP, FASTRO, Radiation Oncologist, Minneapolis Radiation
  Oncology, Minneapolis, Minnesota, John Gibbons, PhD, Chief Medical
  Physicist, Department of Radiation Oncology, Ochsner Health System, New
  Orleans, Louisiana.
Other titles: Treatment planning in radiation oncology.
Description: Fifth edition. | Philadelphia, PA : Wolters Kluwer, [2022] |
  Includes bibliographical references and index.
Identifiers: LCCN 2021038919 | ISBN 9781975162016 (hardback) | ISBN
  9781975162047 (ebook)
Subjects: LCSH: Cancer--Radiotherapy--Planning--Computer programs. | BISAC:
  MEDICAL / Oncology / General | MEDICAL / Radiology, Radiotherapy &
  Nuclear Medicine
Classification: LCC RC271.R3 T74 2022 | DDC 616.99/40642--dc23
LC record available at https://lccn.loc.gov/2021038919

shop.LWW.com

QUADM1021

To Teddi Dawn, my sister who had Down Syndrome, who inspired my interest in science and sadly died from COVID-19 during the writing of this book. I am forever grateful for your joy and mischief and forever saddened that I could not be with you or help you understand.

—Paul W. Sperduto

To my children Valerie, Britton, Jay, Madison, Jack, and Vivienne who have brought much joy to my life

—John P. Gibbons

Contributors

Judith Adams, CMD
Proton Training and Development Specialist
Radiation Oncology
Massachusetts General Hospital
Boston, Massachusetts

Karthik Adapa, MBBS, MPP, MPH
Doctoral Candidate
Department of Radiation Oncology
School of Medicine
University of North Carolina
Chapel Hill, North Carolina

Alison N. Amos, PhD
Clinical Assistant Professor
Department of Radiation Oncology
Division of Healthcare Engineering
University of North Carolina
Chapel Hill, North Carolina

John A. Antolak, PhD
Associate Professor & Consultant
Department of Radiation Oncology
Mayo Clinic
Rochester, Minnesota

Elizabeth H. Baldini, MD
Radiation Oncology Director, Sarcoma Center
Radiation Oncology
Dana-Farber Cancer Institute/Brigham and Women's
    Hospital
Boston, Massachusetts

James M. Balter, PhD, FAAPM
Professor and Director of Physics Research
Department of Radiation Oncology
University of Michigan
Ann Arbor, Michigan

Christopher Beltran, PhD
Chair, Medical Physics
Department of Radiation Oncology
Mayo Clinic
Jacksonville, Florida

Rachel C. Blitzblau, PhD
Associate Professor
Radiation Oncology
Duke University
Durham, North Carolina

Stefan Both, PhD
Professor & Head of Medical Physics
Department of Radiation Oncology
University Medical Center Groningen
Groningen, the Netherlands

Frank J. Bova, PhD
Professor
Neurosurgery
University of Florida
Gainesville, Florida

Andrew Brandmaier, MD, PhD
Assistant Professor
Department of Radiation Oncology
Weill Cornell Medicine
New York, New York

David Carpenter, MD, MHSc
Resident Physician
Duke Cancer Institute
Department of Radiation Oncology
Durham, North Carolina

Robert L. Carver, PhD
Physicist
Mary Bird Perkins Cancer Centre
Baton Rouge, Louisiana

Colin E. Champ, MD, CSCS
Associate Professor
Department of Radiation Oncology
Duke University Medical Center
Durham, North Carolina

Albert Chang, MD, PhD
Associate Professor and Director of Brachytherapy
Radiation Oncology
University of California, Los Angeles
Los Angeles, California

Zhe (Jay) Chen, PhD
Professor
Department of Therapeutic Radiology
Yale University School of Medicine
Yale-New Haven Hospital
New Haven, Connecticut

Yen-Lin Chen, MD
Assistant Radiation Oncologist
Department of Radiation Oncologist
Massachusetts General Hospital
Boston, Massachusetts

Bhisham Chera, MD
Associate Professor
Associate Chair of Clinical Operations & Improvement
Director of Patient Safety and Quality
Department of Radiation Oncology
University of North Carolina School of Medicine
Chapel Hill, North Carolina

James C. L. Chow, PhD
Medical Physicist/Associate Professor
Radiation Medicine Program/Department of Radiation
    Oncology
Princess Margaret Cancer Centre, University Health
    Network/University of Toronto
Toronto, Ontario, Canada

Benjamin M. Clasie, PhD
Department of Radiation Oncology
Massachusetts General Hospital & Harvard Medical
    School
Boston, Massachusetts

Brian G. Czito, MD
Professor
Duke Cancer Institute
Department of Radiation Oncology
Durham, North Carolina

Shiva Das, PhD
Professor
Department of Radiation Oncology
University of North Carolina at Chapel Hill
Chapel Hill, North Carolina

Thomas F. DeLaney, MD
Andres Soriano Professor of Radiation Oncology
Massachusetts General Hospital
Boston, Massachusetts

Nicolas Depauw, PhD, DABR
Physics Proton Treatment Planning Lead
Radiation Oncology
Massachusetts General Hospital
Boston, Massachusetts

Lei Dong, PhD
Professor and Director of Medical Physics
Department of Radiation Oncology
Hospital of the Friedman University of Pennsylvania
Philadelphia, Pennsylvania

Robert L. Foote, MD
Hitachi Professor of Radiation Oncology Research
Radiation Oncology
Mayo Clinic College of Medicine and Science
Rochester, Minnesota

William A. Friedman, MD
Professor
Neurosurgery
University of Florida
Gainesville, Florida

Yolanda I. Garces, MS, MD
Associate Professor
Radiation Oncology
Mayo Clinic
Northfield, Minnesota

John P. Gibbons, PhD
Chief Medical Physicist
Department of Radiation Oncology
Ochsner Health System
New Orleans, Louisiana

Andrew Godley, PhD
Director of Clinical Physics
Department of Radiation Oncology
UT Southwestern Medical Center
Dallas, Texas

Vinai Gondi, MD
Co-Director, Brain and Spine Tumor Center
Director of Research and Education
Northwestern Medicine Cancer Center Warrenville
Warrenville, Illinois

Deen Gu, MHA
Operations Manager
Radiation Oncology
University of North Carolina
Chapel Hill, North Carolina

Kenneth R. Hogstrom, PhD
Professor Emeritus and Senior Medical Physics Advisor
Department of Physics and Astronomy, Louisiana State
    University
Radiation Oncology, Mary Bird Perkins Cancer Center
Baton Rouge, Louisiana

Myrsini Ioakeim–Ioannidou, MD
Post-doctoral Research Fellow
Radiation Oncology
Massachusetts General Hospital
Boston, Massachusetts

Andrew Jackson, PhD
Attending Medical Physicist
Department of Medical Physics
Memorial Sloan-Kettering Cancer Center
New York, New York

James A. Kavanaugh, PhD
Assistant Professor
Radiation Oncology
Washington University School of Medicine
St. Louis, Missouri

Paul J. Keall, PhD
Professor and Director, ACRF Image X Institute
Faculty of Medicine and Health
University of Sydney
Sydney, Australia

Faiz M. Khan, PhD
Professor Emeritus
Department of Radiation Oncology
University of Minnesota Medical School
Minneapolis, Minnesota

Jonathan P. S. Knisely, MD
Assistant Professor Interim
Department of Radiation Oncology
Weill Cornell Medicine and New York Presbyterian
    Hospital
New York, New York

Hanne M. Kooy, PhD
Associate Professor
Radiation Oncology
Massachusetts General Brigham & Harvard Medical
    School
Boston, Massachusetts

Rupesh Kotecha, MD
Chief of Radiosurgery
Department of Radiation Oncology
Miami Cancer Institute, Baptist Health South Florida
Miami, Florida

Gerald J. Kutcher, PhD
Professor of History
Institution, Department of History
Binghamton University
Binghamton, New York

Guang Li, PhD
Associate Attending Physicist
Department of Medical Physics
Memorial Sloan Kettering Cancer Center
New York, New York

Jonathan G. Li, PhD
Professor
Radiation Oncology
University of Florida
Gainesville, Florida

Andrew S. Lim, MD, FRCPC
Radiation Oncologist
University of California, Los Angeles
Los Angeles, California

Mu-Han Lin, PhD
Director of Treatment Planning
Radiation Oncology
UT Southwestern Medical Center
Dallas, Texas

Shannon M. MacDonald, MD
Associate Professor of Radiation Oncology
Massachusetts General Hospital
Boston, Massachusetts

Gig S. Mageras, PhD
Emeritus
Medical Physics
Memorial Sloan Kettering Cancer Center
New York, New York

Lawrence B. Marks, MD
Dr. Sidney K. Simon Distinguished Professor of
    Oncology Research
Professor and Chair, Department of Radiation Oncology
Lineberger Cancer Center
University of North Carolina
Chapel Hill, North Carolina

Jyoti Mayadev, MD
Associate Professor of Radiation Medicine and Applied
    Sciences
UC San Diego
San Diego, California

Charles Mayo, PhD
Professor
Radiation Oncology
University of Michigan
Ann Arbor, Michigan

Lukasz M. Mazur, PhD
Associated Professor and Director of Division of
    Healthcare Engineering
Department of Radiation Oncology
University of North Carolina
Chapel Hill, North Carolina

Susan G.R. McDuff, MD, PhD
Assistant Professor
Department of Radiation Oncology
Duke Cancer Center
Durham, North Carolina

Ross McGurk, PhD
Assistant Clinical Professor
Radiation Oncology
University of North Carolina
Chapel Hill, North Carolina

Todd R. McNutt, PhD
Associate Professor Radiation Oncology and Molecular
    Radiation Sciences
Johns Hopkins Medicine
Baltimore, Maryland

Minesh P. Mehta, MD
Medical Doctor
Deputy Director and Chief of Radiation Oncology
Radiation Oncology
Miami Cancer Institute
Miami, Florida

Loren K. Mell, MD
Tenured Professor and Vice chair
Radiation Medicine and Applied Science
UC San Diego
San Diego, California

Dimitris N. Mihailidis, PhD
Associate Professor
Radiation Oncology
University of Pennsylvania Perelman School of Medicine
Philadelphia, Pennsylvania

Jessica Miller, PhD, DABR
Associate Professor
Department of Human Oncology
School of Medicine & Public Health
University of Wisconsin
Madison, Wisconsin

Radhe Mohan, PhD
Professor
Department of Radiation Physics
The University of Texas MD Anderson Cancer Center
Houston, Texas

Dominic H. Moon, MD
Assistant Professor
Department of Radiation Oncology
UT Southwestern Medical Center
Dallas, Texas

Arno J. Mundt, MD
Professor and Chair
Radiation Medicine and Applied Sciences
UC San Deigo
La Jolla, California

Himanshu Nagar, MD
Weill Cornell Medicine
New York, New York

Colin Orton, PhD
Professor Emeritus
Wayne State University
Detroit, Michigan

Niko Papanikolaou, PhD
Professor and Director
University of Texas UTHSCSA: The University of Texas
    Health Science Center at San Antonio
Medical Physics
San Antonio, Texas

Ima Paydar, MD
Department of Radiation Oncology
University of Pennsylvania
Philadelphia, Pennsylvania

Garrett M. Pitcher, PhD
Academic Medical Physicist
Mary Bird Perkins Cancer Center
Baton Rouge, Louisiana

John P. Plastaras, MD, PhD
Professor
Department of Radiation Oncology
University of Pennsylvania
Philadelphia, Pennsylvania

Dominique Rash, MD
Assistant Clinical Professor
Radiation Medicine and Health Sciences
University of California, San Diego
San Diego, California

Francisco J. Reynoso, PhD
Assistant Professor
Department of Radiation Oncology
Washington University in St. Louis
St. Louis, Missouri

Susan Richardson, PhD
Medical Physicist
Radiation Oncology
Swedish Cancer Institute
Seattle, Washington, DC

Mark J. Rivard, PhD, FAAPM
Professor of Radiation Oncology
Department of Radiation Oncology
Brown University
Providence, Rhode Island

Kilian E. Salerno, MD
Radiation Oncologist
National Cancer Institute
Radiation Oncology Branch
Bethesda, Maryland

Bret Shultz, MHA
Research Project Manager
Department of Radiation Oncology
University of North Carolina
Chapel Hill, North Carolina

Aaron B. Simon, MD, PhD
Assistant Professor
Radiation Oncology
University of California Irvine
Orange, California

Daniel R. Simpson, MD
Assistant Professor
Department of Radiation Medicine and Applied Sciences
Moores Cancer Center
UCSD School of Medicine
La Jolla, California

Paul W. Sperduto, MD, MPP, FASTRO
Medical Director, Minneapolis Radiation Oncology
Co-Director, University of Minnesota Gamma Knife
  Center
Minneapolis, Minnesota

Kevin L. Stephans, MD
Assistant Professor
Department of Radiation Oncology
Taussig Cancer Institute, Cleveland Clinic
Cleveland, Ohio

Kenneth R. Stevens Jr., MD
Former Chair and Professor Emeritus
Radiation Medicine Department
Oregon Health & Sciences University
Portland, Oregon

Alexander Sun, MD, FRCPC
Associate Professor
Department of Radiation Oncology
University of Toronto
Staff Radiation Oncologist
Princess Margaret Cancer Centre
Toronto, Ontario, Canada

Nancy J. Tarbell, MD, FASTRO
CC Wang Professor of Radiation Oncology
Massachusetts General Hospital/Harvard Medical School
Francis H. Burr Proton Therapy Center
Boston, Massachusetts

Bruce R. Thomadsen, PhD
Professor
Medical Physics
University of Wisconsin
Madison, Wisconsin

Robert D. Timmerman, MD
Professor, Vice Chair
Department of Radiation Oncology
University of Texas Southwestern Medical Center
Dallas, Texas

Jordan Torok, MD
Assistant Professor
Radiation Oncology
UPMC Saint Clair Hospital Cancer Center
Pittsburgh, Pennsylvania

Jan Unkelbach, PhD
Assistant Professor of Medical Physics
Radiation Oncology
University Hospital Zurich
Zurich, Switzerland

Raj Varadhan, PhD, DABR, DABMP
Director of Physics/Technology
Minneapolis Radiation Oncology
Edina, Minnesota

Gregory M.M. Videtic, MD, CM, FRPC, FACR, FASTRO
Professor of Medicine
Cleveland Clinic Lerner College of Medicine
Staff Physician
Department of Radiation Oncology, Taussig Cancer
  Center
Cleveland Clinic
Cleveland, Ohio

Kenneth J. Weeks, PhD
Medical Physicist
Federal Medical Center
Butner, North Carolina

Christopher G. Willett, MD, FASTRO
Professor and Chairman
Department of Radiation Oncology
Duke University
Durham, North Carolina

Neil M. Woody, MD, MS
Department of Radiation Oncology
Taussig Cancer Institute, Cleveland Clinic
Cleveland, Ohio

Binbin Wu, PhD
Senior Medical Physicist
Radiation Oncology & Molecular Radiation Sciences
Johns Hopkins University
Baltimore, Maryland

Poonam Yadav, PhD, DABR
Associate Professor, Lead MR Linac Program
Department of Radiation Oncology
Northwestern Memorial Hospital
Northwestern University Feinberg School of Medicine
Chicago, Illinois

Yun Yang, PhD, DABR
Assistant Professor of Radiation Oncology
Department of Radiation Oncology
Brown University Alpert School of Medicine
Rhode Island Hospital
Providence, Rhode Island

Catheryn M. Yashar, MD
Professor and Vice Chair Clinical Affairs
Department of Radiation Medicine and Applied Science
University of California San Diego
La Jolla, California

Fang-Fang Yin, PhD
Professor Department of Radiation Oncology
Duke Clinics
Durham, North Carolina

Sua Yoo, PhD
Associate Professor
Department of Radiation Oncology
Duke University Medical Center
Durham, North Carolina

Stephanie M. Yoon, MD
Physician
Department of Radiation Oncology
University of California
Los Angeles, California

Ellen D. Yorke, PhD
Attending Physicist
Memorial Sloan Kettering Cancer Center
Department of Medical Physics
New York, New York

Preface

This edition includes new chapters and updates of prior chapters designed to keep pace with the many exciting innovations in radiation oncology. It is our hope that this edition will bring readers from yesterday's standard of care to today's state of the art and provide a peek over the horizon at the dawn of a new era in which the science and the art of radiation oncology come together as never before. The science includes new understanding of the potential lurking within discoveries in physics, biology, and technology. The art is the integrated clinical application of those discoveries, in concert with advances in systemic therapies. For example, there is a new chapter on the treatment planning implications of combined immunotherapy and radiation. This and other chapters hold clues that may lead us beyond local control of an individual tumor to a future in which a systemic response may be ignited by the application of modern radiation techniques and systemic therapies in proper sequence and intensity. In addition, there is a re-focus on the patient, beginning with a new chapter on treatment planning and patient safety.

As in previous editions, this textbook provides a comprehensive discussion of the clinical, physical, and biological aspects of treatment planning. Because of its primary focus on treatment planning, it covers this subject in more depth than other books dedicated purely to medical physics or clinical radiation oncology. This book is written for the entire treatment planning team, namely the radiation oncologist, medical physicist, dosimetrist, and radiation therapist. In addition, we keep the students in focus by including key points and study questions at the end of each chapter.

We are immensely grateful for the time and expertise of the chapter authors and acknowledge them as world-renowned experts on their respective topics. We also acknowledge Anne Malcolm, Senior Managing Editor, Ariel Winter, Development Editor, and the other editorial staff of Wolters Kluwer for their support and patience in the development and production of this book.

Most importantly, we are deeply indebted to Faiz Khan for his passion for excellence, joy for teaching, youthful curiosity, and warm friendship which continue to inspire us both personally and professionally.

Paul W. Sperduto
John P. Gibbons

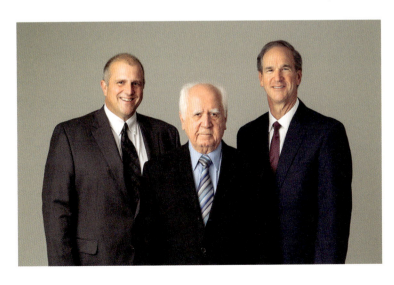

Preface to First Edition

Traditionally, treatment planning has been thought of as a way of devising beam arrangements that will result in an acceptable isodose pattern within a patient's external contour. With the advent of computer technology and medical imaging, treatment planning has developed into a sophisticated process whereby imaging scanners are used to define target volume, simulators are used to outline treatment volume, and computers are used to select optimal beam arrangements for treatment. The results are displayed as isodose curves overlaid on multiple body cross-sections or as isodose surfaces in three dimensions. The intent of the book is to review these methodologies and present a modern version of the treatment planning process. The emphasis is not on what is new and glamorous, but rather on techniques and procedures that are considered to be the state of the art in providing the best possible care for cancer patients.

Treatment Planning in Radiation Oncology provides a comprehensive discussion of the clinical, physical, and technical aspects of treatment planning. We focus on the application of physical and clinical concepts of treatment planning to solve treatment planning problems routinely encountered in the clinic. Since basic physics and basic radiation oncology are covered adequately in other textbooks, they are not included in this book.

This book is written for radiation oncologists, physicists, and dosimetrists and will be useful to both the novice and those experienced in the practice of radiation oncology. Ample references are provided for those who would like to explore the subject in greater detail.

We greatly appreciate the assistance of Sally Humphreys in managing this lengthy project. She has been responsible for keeping the communication channels open among the editors, the contributors, and the publisher.

Faiz M. Khan
Roger A. Potish

Contents

Treatment Planning: Safety and Biological Principles

1 Patient Safety

Lukasz M. Mazur, Lawrence B. Marks, Shiva Das, Ross McGurk, Karthik Adapa, Alison N. Amos, Deen Gu, Bret Shultz, and Bhisham Chera

INTRODUCTION

The concept of patient safety in health care is long-standing. The ethical standard of *first do no harm* was given to us by Hippocrates in the 5th century BC[1] and further commanded as a first principle in medical practice by Florence Nightingale in the late 19th century.[2] However, the sad truth is that patients often suffer harm from medical errors. In 1999, the Institute of Medicine (IOM) reported that 44,000 to 98,000 people die each year in the United States as a result of preventable medical errors, which roughly equates to three jumbo jet crashes every 2 days.[1] A more recent estimate was even more sobering: 200,000 to 400,000.[3]

Radiation oncology (RO) is a modest-sized field with ≈4,000 practicing radiation oncologists in the United States (out of ≈1 million physicians overall). Nevertheless, the clinical impact of radiation therapy (RT) is large. Cancer is one of the most common diseases, with approximately 1.5 million new diagnoses per year in the United States, with approximately 60% of these patients receiving radiation as part of their therapy. Cancer is also a leading cause of death accounting for approximately 600,000 deaths per year.[4] Further, the number of cancer survivors in the United States who have been treated with RT is approximately 3 million,[4] and this is expected to rapidly increase over the next several years. Thus, the practice of RO has a large and meaningful impact on our society.

Radiation is a potent agent with an ability to cure cancer, but can also cause meaningful acute and late normal tissue toxicity. Thus, assuring its accurate delivery is critical. Further, many in our society have a profound fear of radiation, and thus even "small errors" (i.e., those without any expected meaningful change in overall outcome or normal tissue risks) can cause distress and need to be avoided. Fortunately, RT is generally very safe, largely because of the decades-long recognition of its risks. This is a tribute to the founding members of our field, who recognized the risks of RT and who instilled within the very fabric of our field the need for careful oversight and clinical observation. Further, physicists, engineers, and other technical- and quantitative-minded individuals, integral to our practice, have brought an objective and systematic approach to quality assurance (QA). Our professional societies (e.g., American Association of Physicists in Medicine [AAPM], American Society for Radiation Oncology [ASTRO], European Society for Radiotherapy and Oncology [ESTRO]) have done an excellent job generating guidance documents to facilitate the safe practice of RO.

However, over approximately the past 10 to 20 years, there appears to have been an *increase* in safety challenges within our field related, at least in part, to the increased complexity of advanced technologies and techniques (discussed in detail in Section 2). While some might suggest that this renewed focus on safety merely reflects the uncovering of decades-old issues, we believe that this is not entirely the case. Rather, we believe that *there are ongoing fundamental changes in our practice* leading to new challenges that need to be acknowledged and addressed. Public awareness of radiation delivery errors increased after a number of a *New York Times* articles.[5–10] Our professional societies responded by publishing numerous quality and safety publications, such as the ASTRO-sponsored *Safety Is no Accident*, and have held several safety-focused meetings.[11] Serious accidents were also reported in the 1990s in the United Kingdom, triggering a strong response by the National Health Service (NHS). One result was the publication of the report titled "Organization with a Memory."[12] Along the same lines, the Radiation Oncology Safety Information System (ROSIS) project started in the early 2000s to promote safety through systematic incident reporting and analysis.[13]

The content of this chapter is based on our previous contributions, including: Marks LM and Mazur LM, with contributions from Chera B and Adams R. *Engineering Patient Safety in Radiation Oncology*, in CRC Press: Taylor and Francis Group. 2015; Chera B, Mazur LM, Mosaly P, Marks LM. Error Avoidance, In: *Principles and Practice of Radiation Oncology*, 7th edition. 2018. Chapter 102, 44 pages; Mazur LM, Keefe M, and Adams R. Culture of Safety, In: *Principles and Practice of Radiation Therapy*, 4th edition. Chapter 18, pp. 350–365, 2014.

The chapter is organized into five sections:

- **Section 1** summarizes the key definitions and terms in safety and provides an overview of event rates in RO and a theoretical approach to understand why events occur in RO.
- **Section 2** reviews factors that we believe have led to the apparent increase in safety challenges within our field.
- **Section 3** summarizes the strategies that can be used to improve safety within RO.
- **Section 4** provides a brief summary of technically focused initiatives.
- **Section 5** provides a brief summary and concluding remarks.

SECTION 1: ERROR RATES
Terminology and Definitions

There are numerous overlapping terms to describe safety-related issues, and confusion often occurs because the same term is used with different meanings. Thus, before we discuss the error rates, we must establish some key terminology:

- **Event**: A generic term used as a general descriptor that includes both near-misses and incidents.[14]
- **Near-miss**: An event or situation that *could* have resulted in an incident but did not either by chance or through timely intervention.[15] Though *near-miss* is a commonly used term, other equivalent terms such as *close call*,[16] *near hit*,[17] *good catch*,[18] or *near-error*[19] are also often used.
- **Incidents**: *An event that reached the patient, whether or not there was harm involved.*[20] Within RO, it is often challenging to identify whether an incident has or has not caused harm since small treatment deviations may not cause harm for many years (e.g., complication or recurrence).[21–23] Incidents can be further divided into the following:

  - *Never event* refers to a particularly serious medical incident, such as wrong-site surgery or treatment.[24]
  - *Sentinel event* is a term used by the Joint Commission (JC) in the United States that indicates the presence of an incident with grave injury (or risk of grave injury) and the need for immediate investigation and response.[25]
  - *Adverse event* refers to injury from medical care, which may be the result of a known side effect, a medical error, or some combination.[26]
  - *Reportable event* refers to incidents that are reportable to regulatory bodies. In this review, the focus is not on reportable events but on voluntary reporting, that is, incidents, near-misses, and other events that do not necessarily rise to the level of being reportable to a regulatory body.

- *Failure* refers to a single, specific, isolated, and discrete omission of expected or required action.

Event Rates in Radiation Oncology

Single-institutional studies show differing rates of events because of different definitions and assessment methods. The characteristics and findings from multiple single institutional reports are summarized in Table 1.1. These reports are from diverse centers located in 4 continents (North America = 23, Asia = 3, Europe = 3, Australia = 2), and 7 countries (United States = 20, Canada = 3, Australia = 2, Italy = 2, Pakistan = 2, China = 1, Sweden = 1). As shown, there is much variation in the reported event rates per patient (e.g., from 0.07[27] to 1[28] per patient), and per fraction (e.g., from 0.01%[29] to 4%[30,31] per fraction). Since patients often receive multiple fractions of radiation, the reported rate can vary widely if reported on *per fraction* versus *per patient* basis. Some reports have even reported event rate *per field* treated, and since there are often multiple fields per fraction the apparent incidence can be even lower. Also, the threshold for being included as an event also impacts the reported rate. Studies that include near-misses and incidents generally report higher rates of events than those including *only* incidents on either a per-patient basis (e.g., 0.3 vs. 0.069 per patient) or a per-fraction basis (e.g., 0.79 vs. 0.020 per fraction).

Reporting Near-Misses in Radiation Oncology

It is widely reported and understood that most errors in medicine in general, and in RO in particular, are minor in nature. Thus, much can be learned from recognizing and studying these minor events/near-misses. They represent opportunities for *free lessons*[28,30,32,33] (or sometimes termed *weak signals*) that can inform efforts aimed at improving clinical practice, processes, and thus prevent more serious safety events (that lead to patient/staff harm).[34] In RO studies reporting both near-misses and incidents (i.e., events that reach the patient), the ratio of near-misses to incidents is often high (see Table 1.2). Reporting near-misses is vitally important to prevent the more serious, fatal, and catastrophic incidents that are less frequent but far more harmful than other safety-related events.

Why Do Events Occur? Understanding How Our Processes and Systems Interact and Behave

Although errors are often attributed to human error, the root causes of error is often poor system and organizational design.[35] When all components of system function well together, they serve collectively as a set of barriers (or system of defenses) to prevent events. However, when weaknesses or vulnerabilities exist within these components they can interact in random and unforeseen ways. Usually, errors resulting from a

TABLE 1.1 Event rates in RO

First author	Year of publication	Reporting years	Number of years	Country of the first author	Name of institution	Event Type	Total number of events	Events/ patients	Events/ fraction
Valli[31]	1994	1994	0.2	Italy	St. Anna Hospital	Incidents	155	46.0%	4.10%
Calandrino[36]	1997	1991–1996	5.2	Italy	San Raffaele Hospital	Incidents	217	4.3%	NR
Fraass[37]	1998	1996–1997	1.3	USA	University of Michigan, Ann Arbor	Incidents	152	12.0%	0.44%
Macklis[38]	1998	1995	1	USA	Cleveland Clinic, Cleveland	Incidents	59	3.1%	0.06%
Holmberg[34]	2002	1998–2001	3	Sweden	St. Lukes, Dublin/Malmo Hospital	Incidents & near-misses	568	2.5%	NR
Patton[39]	2003	1999–2000	1	USA	Northwest Cancer Specialists, Portland	Incidents	38	2.2%	0.17%
Huang[40]	2005	1997–2003	6	Canada	Princess Margaret Hospital, Toronto	Incidents	555	2.0%	0.23%
Yeung[41]	2005	1992–2002	10	Canada	NE Ontario Regional CC, Sudbury	Incidents & near-misses	624	4.7%	0.26%
Marks[42]	2007	2003–2006	4	USA	Duke University, Durham	Incidents	88	NR	0.08%
Ur-Rahman[43]	2008	2005–2006	1.5	Pakistan	NORI, Islamabad	Incidents	105	13.1%	NR
Konski[27]	2009	2003	1	USA	Fox Chase Cancer Center, Philadelphia	Incidents	25	NR	0.07%
Arnold[28]	2010	2004–2007	3	Australia	Wollongong Hospital, Sydney	Incidents & near-misses	688	14.3%	1.00%
Clark[33]	2010	2007–2010	3	Canada	Ottawa Cancer Center, Ottawa	Incidents & near-misses	1808	10.1%	0.89%
Bissonnette[44]	2010	2001–2007	7	Canada	Princess Margaret Hospital, Toronto	Incidents & near-misses	1063	2.0%	NR
Mutic[32]	2010	2008–2009	2	USA	Washington University, St. Louis	Incidents & near-misses	2870	65.2%	NR
Margalit[45]	2011	2004–2009	5.5	USA	Brigham and Womens Hospital/ Dana Farber Cancer Institute, Boston	Incidents	155	NR	0.06%
Olson[29]*	2012	2006–2010	4	USA	University of Pittsburgh, Pittsburgh	NR	75	NR	0.01%
Hunt[46]**	2012	2001–2011	10	USA	Memorial Sloan-Kettering Cancer Center, New York	NR	284	NR	0.05%
Kalapurakal[47]	2013	2001–2011	10.6	USA	Northwestern University, Chicago	Incidents	256	NR	0.10%

Study	Year		Country	Institution	Event definition	Number		
Das[48]	2013	3.9	USA	MD Anderson Cancer Center, Houston	Incidents & near-misses	188	0.7%	0.03%
Clark[49]	2013	5	Canada	Ottawa Cancer Center, Ottawa	Incidents & near-misses	2506	8.4%	0.17%
Chang[50]	2014	10.4	Australia	Peter McCullum Cancer Center, Melbourne	Incidents & near-misses	1726	3.8%	NR
Rahn[51]	2014	2.4	USA	University of California, San Diego	Incidents & near-misses	108	3.4%	0.18%
Yang[52]	2014	2	China	Peking University	Incidents & near-misses	33	2.6%	NR
Gabriel[53]***	2015	3.8	USA	University of Pennsylvania, Philadelphia	Condition	8504	112.0%	3.90%
Nyflot[30]	2015	2	USA	University of Washington, Seattle	Incidents & near-misses	1897	99.8%	4.10%
Deraniyagala[54]	2015	1.3	USA	University of Florida, Gainesville	Incidents	194	NR	NR
Dominello[55]	2015	11	USA	Wayne State University, Detroit	Incidents	461	NR	0.18%
Hossain[56]	2017	1.1	USA	Unity Point Health Trinity Cancer Center, Moline, Illinois	Incidents, near-misses and unsafe conditions	299	45.0%	NR
Hussain[57]	2018	10	Canada	Aga Khan University Hospital, Pakistan	Unusual occurrences	501	NR	NR
Schubert[58]	2018	~2	USA	University of Colorado, Aurora, USA	Therapeutic radiation incidents, near-misses, operational issues, unsafe conditions	1125	NR	NR

*Used "error" term rather than events; developed Clinical Radiotherapy Error Severity Scale to rank the severity of errors and potential errors
**Used events but haven't categorized them into incidents/near-misses
***Used term "condition" instead of event
NR- not reported

Notes: Event rate (per patient or per fraction) has been included based on the information provided.

TABLE 1.2   Studies reporting both incidents and near-misses

First author	Name of institution	Total number of events	Number of incidents	Number of near-misses	Ratio of near-misses to incidents
Yeung[41]	NE Ontario Regional CC, Sudbury	624	*24*	*600*	25
Ur-Rahman[43]	NORI, Islamabad	105	28	77	3
Arnold[28]	Wollongong Hospital, Sydney	688	155	533	3
Clark[33]	Wollongong Hospital, Sydney	1808	*263*	*1545*	6
Bissonnette[44]	Princess Margaret Hospital, Toronto	1063	*13*	*1050*	81
Mutic[32]	Washington University, St. Louis	2870	*130*	*2740*	21
Das[48]	MD Anderson Cancer Center, Houston	188	38	150	4
Clark[49]	Ottawa Cancer Center, Ottawa	2506	*49*	*2457*	50
Chang[50]	Peter McCullum Cancer Center, Melbourne	1726	104	1378	13
Rahn[51]	University of California, San Diego	108	*27*	*81*	3
Yang[52]	Peking University, China	33	5	28	6
Nyflot[30]	University of Washington, Seattle	1897	322	1575	5
*Schubert[58]	University of Colorado, Aurora, USA	1125	*101*	*146*	1.4

Numbers in italics are not explicitly reported but estimated from available data in the report.

*Report includes four types of events based on RO-ILS definitions.

weakness in one component are caught (or corrected) by another component that can be functioning in parallel or that is downstream to where the error originates. This is why most errors do not lead to harm and why the number of near-misses is far larger than the number of serious incidents (that reach the patient). However, sometimes (and fortunately not that often) weaknesses within components align, and errors overlap (or even reinforce each other), leading to serious incidents and causing harm. This concept has been described as the *Swiss Cheese Model* (SCM) of accident causation, made popular by James Reason[59–62] (see Fig. 1.1), with weaknesses illustrated as "holes."

From the SCM's perspective, peoples' actions are influenced by upstream *latent failure* pathways (contributory factors that may lie dormant for long periods of time) at the administrative (e.g., culture, management), workplace (e.g., workplace design, policies), and people levels (e.g., schedules, workflows, training, perceptions). The worker's action that is linked to the incident (e.g., forgetting to do something) is often referred to as the *active failure*. Often during root cause analyses, too much emphasis is placed on the person's active failures and not enough attention to the upstream layers of the SCM (see Fig. 1.2). In other words, people do not perform tasks in a vacuum.

From this discussion, it is clear that Murphy's law (i.e., that everything that can go wrong will go wrong) is *not* correct. Indeed, everything that can go wrong usually *does not* go wrong; that is, we are often *fortunate*. RO practice relies on an interdisciplinary team's ability to repeatedly perform diverse tasks in a reliable and accurate manner. Major events in RO more likely occur due to evolution in practice over time, and often involve several people and broader contributory factors. For instance, a change in a treatment planning system without corresponding changes to other procedures may result in error when several events converge months later. Thus, the SCM provides a practical approach to understanding why errors occur in RO. By understanding *why* errors occur, systems and strategies can be put into place to minimize error frequency and maximize their detection before harm occurs.[63]

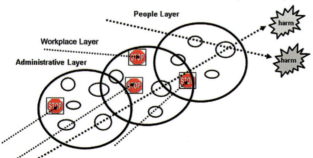

FIGURE 1.1. The *Swiss Cheese* Model of Accident Causation.

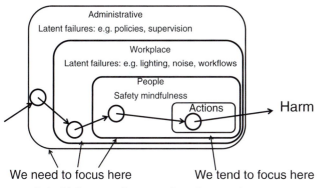

We need to focus here   We tend to focus here

Latent failures predispose us to make errors!

FIGURE 1.2. Adaptation of Reason's Swiss Cheese Model to radiation oncology practice.

SECTION 2 – HOW WE GOT HERE: FACTORS CONTRIBUTING TO ERRORS IN RADIATION ONCOLOGY

A. The way it used to be is as follows:
For many decades (from roughly the 1950s through the 1980s), the practice of RO was largely straightforward:

- Targeted tissues were defined by physical exam, surface anatomy and imaging, and the likely pattern of spread of the tumor. Targets were generally large (often encompassing an anatomic region).
- Treatment beams were relatively simple, and were largely in the axial plane; for example, anterior–posterior, laterals, and only occasionally obliques. Since radiation oncologists were indeed a subset of diagnostic radiologists, beams were oriented to be in the directions used for diagnostic imaging (the physicians best understood the relative location of the various organs from those directions).
- Beam-on times were largely based on simple calculations of dose to a single point.
- The accuracy of beam placement could be readily checked by viewing the light field on the patient's skin and via simple portal films (analogous to a diagnostic image demonstrating the irradiated tissues).
- Curative treatments were often given in multiple relatively small fractions.

These approaches were not perfect or necessarily accurate. For example, the extent of tumor spread was likely often underappreciated due to the lack of modern imaging of internal anatomy (e.g., with Computerized Tomography [CT], Magnetic Resonance Imaging [MRI], Positron Emission Tomog-raphy [PET]), which led to the use of large fields covering anatomic regions. Similarly, there were undoubtedly errors in the daily patient setup (particularly on non-portal-film day); but again, the use of relatively large fields would tend to minimize these effects. Gross errors in beam design were readily detected by the review of the light field and portal films, and the use of multiple small daily fractions afforded the opportunity to modify the treatment early during the course of therapy (e.g., if an error was detected on a portal film). The point doses calculated did not necessarily reflect the dose throughout the targeted volume, but the calculation was simple and easy to check. Thus, while these approaches were not elegant, they were simple.

Further, the introduction of fluoroscopic simulators and later CT-based three-dimensional treatment planning altered the manner in which beams were *planned*, but really did not alter the manner in which treatment was *delivered*. Physicians largely obtained the needed skills for 3D planning (e.g., to segment 3D images) and our physics/computer colleagues defined robust ways to transfer data (and monitor that data transfer). Beams remained largely axial, the clinical reasonableness of a beam/plan could still be verified by the light field and portal images, and conventional fractionation remained common.

B. Evolving changes largely specific to RO
The broad embrace of advanced technologies may promote an underappreciation of the limitations of our systems. As with many things electronic, there is an underlying presumption that the information is correct (call it a societal/human-nature bias). Thus, technology and automation (while very powerful and useful approaches to assure safety) often promote complacency and might inadvertently reduce safety mindfulness. Further, the electronic environment displays much more information (compared to the paper chart), and it is often not practical to realistically verify all of the critical components. Diligence, checklists, reminders, and so on are often needed to assist with these verification tasks.

Within RO, the broad concept of a therapist reviewing the chart for correctness is not as fervently emphasized in today's training programs compared to therapists' training 15 to 25 years ago. Their review to make sure that things *make sense from a clinical perspective* is more challenging with many modern techniques compared to the 2D/3D era. On the other hand, therapists are taking on an increasing role in the review of pretreatment images, and often make decisions regarding the adequacy of setup, and the necessary shifts to improve localization. Following is a list of factors contributing to the evolving changes largely specific to RO:

- **Rapid application of newer technologies:** The recent rapid introduction of intensity-modulated radiation therapy (IMRT) and stereotactic radiosurgery (SRS)/stereotactic body radiotherapy (SBRT) has presented a fundamental change in the way that RT is planned and delivered. For example, the light field and portal films are necessarily not as useful today as an "end of the line check" of the accuracy of the upstream work. The number of monitor units for a beam/arc/plan is no longer readily intuitive or clinically meaningful. Additionally, the use of fewer fractions, with higher-doses-per-fraction (e.g., with SBRT/SRS), makes it critical to *get it right the first time.*

- **Greater time demands, handoffs, and associated challenges:** These newer technologies require increased efforts for many members of the RO team, whose tasks include image segmentation, iterative dose calculations, patient-specific QA, image acquisition/review, treatment delivery, and machine and multi-leaf collimator (MLC) maintenance/repair. Individual tasks are more interdependent, with more handoffs, thus increasing opportunities for delay and suboptimal information transfer; for example, dosimetrist image segmentation → MD image segmentation and specification of dose/volume constraint → dosimetrist planning → MD review → dosimetrist replan → iterate → etc. The time pressures on all involved are increased. The need for unambiguous communication and for easy-to-use tools is increased. For example, IMRT planning and treatment initiation requires approximately 54 discrete tasks to be performed by physicians, dosimetrists, physicists, and therapists (with about 15 handoffs).[9] At the same time, many health systems have expanded to include multiple locations, and providers (including physicians, physicists, and dosimetrists) may have fewer opportunities for face-to-face interactions, making these multiple handoffs challenging and potentially hindering the smooth application of these advanced approaches.

- **Managing expectations:** Care providers, referring physicians, patients, and administrators have been accustomed to our historic ability to proceed with consultation, simulation, and treatment in relatively rapid succession. With advanced technologies, this is less practical. Patient volumes have largely remained constant or increased (due to the increasing incidence of cancer related to the aging population), yet the work-per-case has (on average) increased.

- **Evolving role of the radiation therapists:** Most incidents ultimately manifest at the treatment machine, where the therapists deliver the actual treatment. Often, these end-of-the-line staff are blamed for errors even if there are multiple contributing factors (e.g., latent failures and their associated pathways), and/or if the error occurred further upstream (e.g., a calculation error in dosimetry, or an ambiguous directive from the physician). The critical role that "end-of-the-line" therapists play emphasizes the importance of discussing the impact of the technological evolution (from 2D to 3D to IMRT) on the therapist's role.

- **Training:** More senior radiation therapists (i.e., trained >15 years ago) learned on older linear accelerators (LINACs) and were taught and required to think about the correct field size (that they manually set), gantry position for the treatment fields (also manually set), and field shapes (determined by blocks that they manually placed onto the machine). Historically, therapists routinely assessed the correctness of the patient setup by looking at the actual light field, field size, gantry angle, and block patterns on the skin; and then comparing these parameters with the printed (or written) information from dosimetry, and considering if it made sense from a clinical perspective (e.g., was the light field shining on the location of the target?). Therapists instinctively knew the approximate number of monitor units typically used for various beams. The introduction of IMRT and SRS/SBRT has made such training and intuition somewhat obsolete due to the increasing complexities of such treatments and changing workflows, as discussed next.

- **Workflows:** Changing technologies have altered workflows and made some of these traditional QA tools less useful. For example, review of the light field on the patient's skin and review of portal films, both long-standing QA procedures in traditional RT, are less applicable in the era of IMRT and image-guided radiation therapy (IGRT). Computer/remote control of the gantry and table and the use of MLCs to shape the fields (rather than cerrobend blocks) obviate the need for the therapists to even enter the treatment room between fields. This makes review of the light fields cumbersome and almost quaintly old-fashioned. Currently, radiation therapists are trained to retrieve electronic information about a patient on a computer screen, and review this for accuracy (see Fig. 1.3).

C. **Changes and traditions beyond RO that can challenge safety**

The practice of medicine has become more complex, and it is rapidly changing. Errors can occur due to unforeseen complex interactions between various components of our organizations. Within RO, our field's long-standing QA-/safety-based initiatives/approaches, that have served us well for so long, have

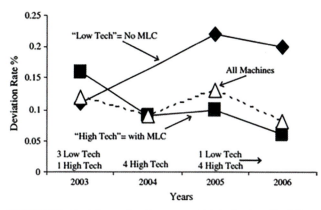

FIGURE 1.4. Deviations rate of *low* versus *high* technology. Deviations rates during time of transition from low to high technology machines[42]

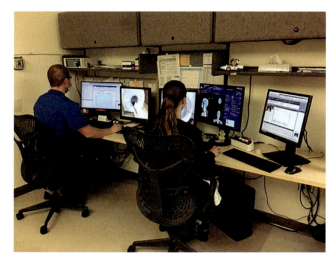

FIGURE 1.3. Treatment delivery station at UNC.

been somewhat strained by these various factors. As we have moved to better address these challenges, there are some broader factors that have hindered the development of a safety culture in medicine.

- **Societal demands, change, and complexity:** Changes in the United States with regard to insurance (e.g., leading to increasing requirements for pre-authorization, that can take time, leading to delays and subsequent rushing), increasing/changing regulatory burdens (e.g., related to documentation, and billing compliance), and increasing demands on providers (e.g., related to the electronic medical record) can increase workload and strain our existing systems. Further, all forms of change, both within RO and more broadly in medicine/society, can strain systems and increase the risks of error. As stated by Hatlie and Youngberg,[12] "change is creating new paths for failure and new demands on workers … revising their understanding of these paths is an important aspect of work on safety … missing the side effects of change is the most common form of failure for organizations and individuals." For example, within RO, Marks and colleagues[42] prospectively monitored the rate of RT delivery deviations during a time of technology upgrade. In January 2003, their department had three *low-technology* accelerators (defined as without MLC). In 2003 to 2004, they upgraded to five *high-technology* accelerators (i.e., with MLC, and associated advanced capabilities). The upgrade appeared to be associated with an *increase* in the deviation rates on the low-technology machines ($p = 0.05$). At first, the deviation rate on the high-technology machines was a tad higher than the older machines (as perhaps might be expected with new technologies), but this appeared to decline over time ($p = 0.15$), as might be expected

with increasing familiarity with the new technology. The persistently elevated increase in deviations on the low-technology machines emphasizes the need for continued diligence during times of change (see Fig. 1.4).

- **Culture:** Traditional medical training has promoted a culture with a powerful tenet that patient safety is the personal responsibility of providers. All of us—physicians, nurses, dosimetrists, physicists, and therapists—are taught that if we work and study hard enough, we won't make errors. Thus, many of us believe that patient safety improvements are a personal endeavor to be conducted in our autonomous microsystem. That is wrong! This credence does not allow for a system-based perspective and naturally leads to a suboptimal safety culture. We are taught to strive for an error-free practice, and that mistakes are unacceptable, and thus condition ourselves to be infallible. We are motivated to not commit errors, in part, for fear of punishment via social/peer disapproval, and for personal self-esteem. Often, errors are seen as character flaws or as someone's fault, and blame is used to encourage proper performance. This desire to be infallible may result in burnout, and in people choosing not to report errors. Also, as errors are not discussed, potential lessons that could be learned are not identified or shared, and the underlying processes and systems are not improved. Dr. Lucian Leape has stated, "The single greatest impediment to error prevention is … that we punish people for making mistakes."[3]
- **Failure to recognize the system's nature of our operations:** Medicine does not consistently understand that physicians and other providers are humans performing in imperfect systems. While the proximate error is often deemed to be *human error*, the root causes of the error is often poor system and organizational design (see discussion of the SCM mentioned earlier). As a result, investigations of errors are often somewhat superficial, focus on downstream factors, and lead

to *focal solutions* aimed at preventing specific individuals from repeating the error. This approach may temporarily prevent that specific error, but often fails to address the deeper/upstream factors that might lead to a variety of different errors. This superficial approach often leads to a patchwork of workarounds that each address (often in different ways) some upstream shortcoming.

- **Lack of physician involvement:** Physicians are generally leaders in most clinical settings. However, they tend to have little training, or interest, in quality improvement, and thus tend not to participate in such efforts. As leaders, this current arrangement will not support the culture needed to build robust and sustainable systems. Physicians have unique clinical perspectives that are needed during continuous quality improvement (CQI) initiatives and as leaders they must be actively involved to motivate others and build an optimal culture to support this work.[64]

SECTION 3: PATH FORWARD: REVIEW OF PHILOSOPHIES, METHODS, AND TOOLS FOR FACILITATING IMPROVEMENTS IN PATIENT SAFETY AND SAFETY CULTURE

Error-free performance is simply unachievable, and the mentality of infallibility will inevitably result in system failure. Expecting errors to occur and realizing that they are part of everyday practice allows us to practice in a no-blame culture focusing on the underlying root causes of system failures. Industries have grappled with these issues for decades, and in the following section we outline several concepts from various resultant quality/safety philosophies. As these philosophies have been developed largely in industry, none are perfectly applicable to health care. However, *many* of the concepts can be, and have been, successfully applied to medicine, and examples are provided in the following section.

A. **High-Reliability Organizations**
   Psychologists and engineers have studied organizations that have managed to operate in complex, high-hazard domains for extended periods largely without catastrophic events (e.g., airlines, manufacturing, railroads, nuclear power), and have termed these as *highly reliable organizations* (HROs).[65,66] They found that HROs maintain a commitment to safety at all levels from frontline workers to top executive leaders. The concept of high reliability is attractive for RO, due to the complexity of operations and the risk of significant and even potentially catastrophic events. The key features of a culture in HROs are as follows:

   - **Preoccupation with failure:** HROs do not ignore any "weak" signals, no matter how small, because

any deviation from the expected result can snowball into tragedy. HROs aim to address them immediately and completely.
   - **Reluctance to simplify:** HROs do not simplify too much or too quickly; some complex problems require complex solutions.
   - **Sensitivity to operations:** HROs believe that every voice matters. HROs are committed to *safety walks* (leaders having a presence at the workplace) and providing feedback on all concerns that are voiced.
   - **Commitment to resilience:** HROs believe in rapid recovery when the unexpected occurs. HROs adapt continuously. HROs foster resilience and cross-functional collaboration.
   - **Deference to expertise:** HROs believe and defer to expertise, and *not authority*.

In non–health care HROs, the safety of workers themselves is typically the focus of the safety culture. In health care, a culture of safety is usually focused on the patient (and hence the term *patient safety culture*), but worker safety is a concern as well. Assessing the safety culture in an organization can be challenging. The Agency for Healthcare Research & Quality (AHRQ) administers a patient safety culture survey that is generally regarded as a reasonable measure.[67]

Interestingly, there are some data, albeit limited, to support the notion that centers with better safety culture scores, as assessed by their own staff, have lower rates of severe adverse events.[68]

B. **Culture within aviation industry**
   The following are a few of the key components of the safety culture within commercial aviation.[65,69]

   - **Training:** Most commercial airline carriers encourage, reward, and pay staff to attend required quality/safety training. If an employee misses or fails training/proficiency checks, they usually face restrictions until their underperformance has been rectified. Training focuses on the inevitability of errors and the importance of culture, teamwork, and communication in avoiding errors as well as containing their spread and mitigating their effects before they lead to serious or catastrophic harm.
   - **Policies and procedures that enforce safe operations:** There must always be two physiologically and psychologically sound pilots to fly a plane. This minimum safety requirement *always* applies. No exceptions are granted. This is often audited by random drug and alcohol tests. Further, during the safety-critical phases of a flight such as flying below an altitude of 10,000 feet, the pilots and cabin crew must adhere to strict standard operating procedures and refrain from all nonessential activities (e.g., reading newspapers or chatting idly). This safety requirement is known as the *sterile cockpit rule*. Crew members are taught how to call, without awkwardness,

for implementation of the sterile cockpit rule at additional times when particular concentration becomes necessary. The entire crew is informed about the enforced rule through warnings or alert systems. Adoption of comparable policies in RO centers would be controversial, but they might better ensure patient safety.

- **Flight recorders:** These recorders, also known as *black boxes*, monitor key flight parameters throughout each flight. This data is analyzed by computers after every flight. Readings outside of predetermined acceptable ranges trigger warning signals that can initiate an investigation. The full exploration of flight recording is conducted only in catastrophic circumstances, but pilots and staff know that all of their actions are being monitored and that everything they do and say is being recorded.
- **Error reporting:** All employees are encouraged to report errors. Pilots' contracts (endorsed by the airline, the union, and the Federal Aviation Association [FAA]) stipulate that *there will be no retribution for reporting errors* unless they involve drugs, criminal behavior, or purposeful violation of workflows/policy. In other words, the leadership are saying to their pilots, "We know that you are human and that you will make errors, please tell us about them." Indeed, workers who fail to report errors that they have witnessed or were involved with can face serious penalty.

C. Applying HROs' cultural principles to RO:
So, how do we build an infrastructure to support a culture of safety in RO centers? Where do we start? Perhaps, not with flight recorders right away. In our clinic (UNC-Chapel Hill) we developed and continue to maintain a high level of urgency toward change and innovation to improve patient safety using the following initiatives:[70]

- **Incident learning systems (ILS):** Incident learning refers to the process of reporting incidents and near-misses, analyzing these in detail, and developing interventions to prevent future events.[14,71] ILS represent a *nonpunitive* approach to learning and improvement[19] (i.e., analogous to that described earlier for the pilots). Reporting can be done anonymously, if desired, if people are reluctant/anxious about reporting. In our clinic, reporting is encouraged and celebrated; the person(s) reporting the "best" good catches each month is publicly celebrated with their names and pictures posted in several places throughout the department (see Fig. 1.5). We also ask the good catch award recipients to sign a basketball, which is proudly displayed in the depatment's "trophy" shelves.

Many clinics have implemented similar ILS, and several publications (including from us) suggest that incident learning broadly improves quality and safety.[19]

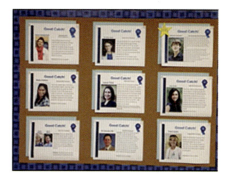
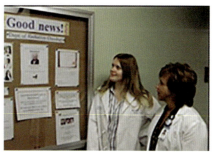
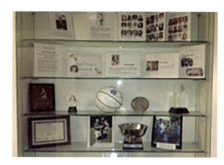

FIGURE 1.5. Examples of recognition boards.

There are also several national and international ILS sponsored by our professional groups: Radiation Oncology Incident Learning System[72] (RO-ILS sponsored by ASTRO, AAPM), Radiation Oncology Safety Education and Information System[73] (ROSEIS sponsored by ESTRO), and Safety in Radiation Oncology[74] (SAFRON sponsored by International Atomic Energy Agency [IAEA]). As of quarter 4 of 2018, there were 7,968 events reported to RO-ILS, and at the time of writing this chapter 550 facilities across the United States have joined RO-ILS.[72,75] The mission of RO-ILS is to facilitate safer and higher-quality care in RO by providing a mechanism for shared learning in a secure and nonpunitive environment. Participation in RO-ILS is free. RO-ILS provides U.S.-based practices access to a secure, web-based portal and the ability to send data to a federally listed *patient safety organization* (Clarity PSO). The events are triaged and prioritized for review by members of the Radiation Oncology Health Advisory Committee (RO-HAC), a multidisciplinary group of RO professionals (e.g., therapists, dosimetrists, physicists, physicians). The RO-HAC produces regular educational work products in the forms of aggregate data reports, case reports, safety notices, and scientific publications (e.g., a recent review noted that common error pathways included things such as planning on the wrong CT images set, and desired isocenter shifts being misdirected or misapplied).[23]

- **Safety rounds:** Our departmental leaders speak with frontline employees about their work; for example, "What is good, what can be better, how we can improve things for them, do they have the tools they need to work safety, efficiently and reliably?"[76] *These discussions occur at their workstations, not in a conference room or office*, as a sign of respect for the workers, and so leadership can better appreciate the issues being discussed (see Fig. 1.6). The goal is to improve performance of the overall system, empower workers to think about how they can make improvements, and help build a culture of respect and improvement.
- **Huddles:** Suboptimal communication is one of the most common factors implicated in root cause analyses of critical incidents. Huddles, brief meetings among various members of work teams, held at regularly scheduled times, are an approach attempting to improve communication.[77] For example, in our clinic, we ask our teams (e.g., nurses, residents, and faculty) to briefly huddle at the start of a clinic day to review the schedule and identify any anticipated challenges (e.g., conflicts, double-bookings) that may be mitigated or accommodated.

We also have a daily department-wide huddle where that day's planned clinical work is reviewed, again to identify and plan for anticipated challenges (see Fig. 1.7). The daily list of patients due for treatment planning and CT simulation are reviewed. Staff have the opportunity to seek clarifications regarding ambiguities in any of the directives and the names of the doctor, resident, physicist, and dosimetrist "of the day" are reviewed. It is a time for announcements, introductions of visitors, and brief discussions of any items of broad interest or concern. These daily

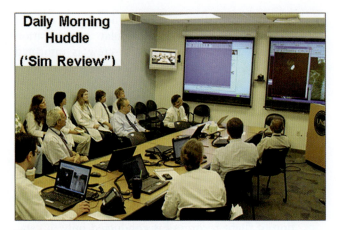

FIGURE 1.7. Daily morning huddle.

departmental huddles serve a social function, help improve interpersonal and organizational communication, and break down unnecessary hierarchies.[76–78] The concepts and power of routine huddles have been demonstrated by others.[78]

- **Peer review:** Peer review can be loosely defined as the process whereby providers evaluate the quality of their colleagues' work to ensure that prevailing care standards are met.[79,80] Typically, peer review is most valuable for the somewhat subjective aspects of work that are not readily amenable to objective assessment. In medicine, this is often done retrospectively through chart review after patients complete their treatment. This retrospective approach can be helpful to detect shortcomings that can be addressed or to reinforce positive actions to improve care for future patients. Obviously, from an individual patient's perspective, peer review done *prior* to therapy or early during the course of therapy is better than peer review done later or after therapy is completed. Peer review in RO appears to be a useful tool to improve patient care[81–83] and has been strongly endorsed by several national and international organizations.[79] Indeed, radiation treatment plans that deviate from standard protocols are associated with inferior patient outcomes (i.e., cancer control and survival) and prospective peer review holds promise to improve patient outcomes.[84,85] We have a daily peer review session (typically linked to our daily huddles) where the image segmentations for patients about to undergo IMRT or 3D planning are reviewed *prior* to planning. Our data suggests that out of 1,271 patient cases that underwent peer review, 326 (26%) received peer-based recommendations. Of 356 recommendations, 37% were minor, 36% were moderate, and 27% were major. Overall compliance to recommendations was 59% (95% confidence interval, 54%–64%).[86]

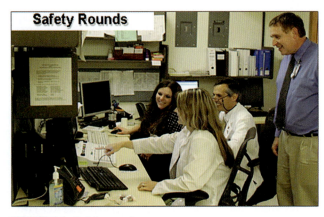

FIGURE 1.6. Safety rounds.

Innovative work along these lines has been done by Dr. Potters et al. at Long Island Jewish Hospital.[87] Out of the total of 11,843 treatment plans from 7,854 patients they reviewed using the prospective peer review evaluation system, 28% ($n = 3,303$) required modifications before treatment planning commenced. This approach is not practical for small centers or solo-practitioners. However, with teleconferencing, interinstitutional peer review is possible. For example, chart rounds is a national program where radiation oncologists can discuss interesting/challenging cases with peers and disease-specific experts.[88] This approach has proven to be valuable and has been implemented internationally as well. In a review of multiple chart rounds sessions, ≈≥80% of participants responding to a survey rated the sessions as high or very high quality and a good use of their time, and 67% agreed that the sessions will result in a change in their practice.[89]

- **Time-outs:** These are formal standardized methods to help review the most crucial aspects of the radiation planning and delivery process (similar to a pre surgery checklist in an operating room).[90] Our dosimetrists and physicians perform a time-out at the time of signing the treatment plan and prescription to review the dose per fraction, number of fractions, treatment site, and the presence or absence of receipt of prior radiation that aids in identifying possible overlap issues (see Fig. 1.8). Our radiation therapists perform a similar time-out on the first day of a patient setup on the treatment machine, and a slightly different time-out on each day prior to treatment.[91]

- **Hierarchy of effectiveness and automated QA tools:** We endorse the concept (common in industrial engineering) of the Hierarchy of Effectiveness; that is, a range of strategies provide different levels of reliability (Fig. 1.9). In brief, higher reliability

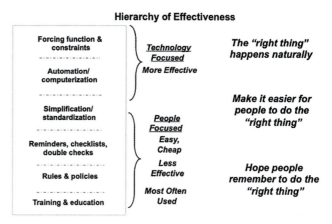

FIGURE 1.9. Hierarchy of effectiveness.

results from making it "as easy as possible" to do the right thing, or better yet make the right thing happen automatically.

Thus, the most effective way to facilitate reliability is to hardwire actions into processes. For example, some light fixtures are wired to illuminate only when, for example, the door to that space is open (e.g., a closet) or the light is linked to a motion sensor to detect if anyone is in a certain space. In an airplane lavatory, the lights usually automatically become illuminated when you lock the door. These are examples of "forcing" the desired outcome. Thus, to the degree possible, we try to apply these principles in our RO clinic. Thus, we automate wherever able. For example, we use an IMRT goal sheet highlighting pass/fail conditions for certain plan objectives (Fig. 1.10; goal sheet). We use standard logic-driven systems for simulation and treatment planning directives/orders (hardwired into the commercial software where able), and use software to reduce planning variability.[80] Similar approaches have been successfully implemented by others.[92,93] For example, providers at the Princess Margaret hospital have largely automated treatment planning for breast cancer,[94] and providers at Johns Hopkins have used experiences from prior patients to automatically assess plan quality in subsequent patients.[95] Further, apart from routine pretreatment QA tests for IMRT delivery, automated QA tools are being implemented to verify integrity of data transfer from the treatment planning system to the oncology information system (OIS), especially those occurring between different vendor systems.[96] Finally, real-time checks of delivered treatments using machine log files and/or real-time imaging using existing on-board equipment have been commercialized and have the potential to detect differences between the planned and delivered treatment fields.[97]

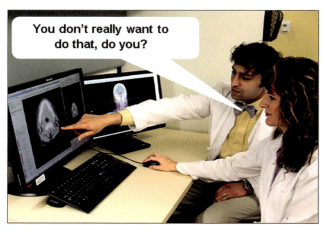

FIGURE 1.8. Time-out between dosimetrist and physician.

Priority	Dose	ROI/POI	Clinical goal	Value	Result	% outside grid
	Plan dose: UnknownPrimary+Necks_IMRT...	Brain+3mm	At most 6000 cGy dose at 0.10 cm³ volume	4996 cGy	✓	0%
	Plan dose: UnknownPrimary+Necks_IMRT...	Brainstem+3mm	At most 6000 cGy dose at 0.10 cm³ volume	3503 cGy	✓	0%
	Plan dose: UnknownPrimary+Necks_IMRT...	Cochlea_Lt+3mm	At most 4500 cGy average dose	2284 cGy	✓	0%
	Plan dose: UnknownPrimary+Necks_IMRT...	Cochlea_Rt+3mm	At most 4500 cGy average dose	2065 cGy	✓	0%
	Plan dose: UnknownPrimary+Necks_IMRT...	Constrictors+3mm	At most 5000 cGy average dose	5445 cGy	!	0%
	Plan dose: UnknownPrimary+Necks_IMRT...	Cord+3mm	At most 5000 cGy dose at 0.10 cm³ volume	3086 cGy	✓	0%
	Plan dose: UnknownPrimary+Necks_IMRT...	Esophagus+3mm	At most 5500 cGy dose at 67.00 % volume	153 cGy	✓	0%
	Plan dose: UnknownPrimary+Necks_IMRT...	Esophagus+3mm	At most 6500 cGy dose at 33.00 % volume	2732 cGy	✓	0%
	Plan dose: UnknownPrimary+Necks_IMRT...	External ROI	At most 6600 cGy dose at 0.00 cm³ volume	6440 cGy	✓	0%
	Plan dose: UnknownPrimary+Necks_IMRT...	Larynx	At most 4100 cGy average dose	3844 cGy	✓	0%
	Plan dose: UnknownPrimary+Necks_IMRT...	Larynx+3mm	At most 4100 cGy average dose	4055 cGy	✓	0%
	Plan dose: UnknownPrimary+Necks_IMRT...	Larynx+3mm	At most 6000 cGy dose at 24.00 % volume	5391 cGy	✓	0%
	Plan dose: UnknownPrimary+Necks_IMRT...	Oral_Cavity+3mm	At most 3900 cGy average dose	2585 cGy	✓	0%
	Plan dose: UnknownPrimary+Necks_IMRT...	Parotid_Lt+3mm	At most 2600 cGy average dose	3900 cGy	!	0%
	Plan dose: UnknownPrimary+Necks_IMRT...	Parotid_Lt+3mm	At most 3000 cGy dose at 50.00 % volume	3811 cGy	!	0%
	Plan dose: UnknownPrimary+Necks_IMRT...	Parotid_Rt+3mm	At most 2600 cGy average dose	2254 cGy	✓	0%
	Plan dose: UnknownPrimary+Necks_IMRT...	Parotid_Rt+3mm	At most 3000 cGy dose at 50.00 % volume	1859 cGy	✓	0%
	Plan dose: UnknownPrimary+Necks_IMRT...	PTV_HR_inSkin	At least 95.00 % volume at 6000 cGy dose	96.28 %	✓	0%
	Plan dose: UnknownPrimary+Necks_IMRT...	PTV_HR_inSkin	At least 99.00 % volume at 5580 cGy dose	99.90 %	✓	0%
	Plan dose: UnknownPrimary+Necks_IMRT...	PTV_HR_inSkin	At least a conformity index of 0.75 at 6000 cGy isodose	0.53	✓	0%
	Plan dose: UnknownPrimary+Necks_IMRT...	PTV_SR_inSkin	At least 95.00 % volume at 5400 cGy dose	96.30 %	✓	0%
	Plan dose: UnknownPrimary+Necks_IMRT...	PTV_SR_inSkin	At least 99.00 % volume at 5022 cGy dose	99.75 %	✓	0%
	Plan dose: UnknownPrimary+Necks_IMRT...	PTV_SR_inSkin	At least a conformity index of 0.75 at 5400 cGy isodose	0.91	✓	0%
	Plan dose: UnknownPrimary+Necks_IMRT...	Submandibular_Lt+3mm	At most 3500 cGy average dose	6012 cGy	!	0%
	Plan dose: UnknownPrimary+Necks_IMRT...	Submandibular_Rt+3mm	At most 3500 cGy average dose	4057 cGy	!	0%

FIGURE 1.10. IMRT goal sheet.

Thus, wherever possible, we should strive to (preferably) automate and standardize the work to increase reliability. Automation is preferred (as noted above). For items that cannot be easily automated, we embrace peer review to assure quality (as noted above). There are many examples of similar initiatives along these lines (e.g., ASTRO-sponsored contouring atlases). The Michigan Radiation Oncology Quality Consortium (MROQC), established in 2011, is a particularly notable initiative that should be celebrated. Providers across Michigan have been pooling data to create a comprehensive clinical data registry (e.g., techniques and outcomes) of patients receiving radiation treatment for several diseases to help guide therapy and improve quality statewide.

- **No-fly safety culture:** Ensuring the timely planning/delivery of radiotherapy can be challenging (e.g., due to multiple steps/handoffs), and delays along the care pathway can be difficult to manage, and lead to errors and rework. To address this issue, Potters and colleagues at North Shore-LIJ Health System implemented a—some would consider radical—no-fly policy, whereby patient care could not proceed (i.e., a hard stop) unless needed prior steps were completed (as tracked within the record and verify system).[91] Over time, the no-fly policy helped mitigate risk from expedited care, convert reactive to proactive delays, and created a checklist, process-driven, and variance-reducing culture in a large, multicenter department. This policy did lead to some patients having treatment delays (mean of 2 days, maximum of 4), but there were no reported adverse events.
- **Practice accreditation:** Obtaining practice accreditation through (for example) ASTRO's Accreditation Program for Excellence (APEx) and/or American College of Radiation Oncology (ACRO) accreditation programs is a global way of obtaining objective, external review of quality and safety of one's clinical program.[98] The accreditation process is time con-suming and labor intensive; however, there is significant value in having an external review and can help guide centers' changes to their policies, procedures, and processes.

D. **Normal accident theory (NAT):** Substantial work in non–health care settings has been performed to better understand the causes of accidents and investigate potential mitigation strategies. One of the nation's leading theorists in the area of safety, Dr. Charles Perrow, coined the term (NAT, see Fig. 1.11).[99] He argues that failures in systems occur often and are indeed expected and part of the normal operations (hence the name *normal*). He categorizes systems based on how these failures interact within the larger system and lead to major accidents. Systems in which failures propagate and interact predictably

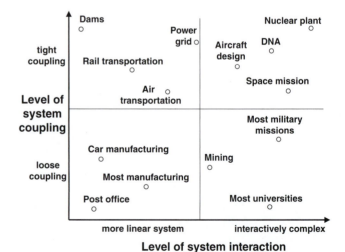

FIGURE 1.11. Normal accident theory concepts of loose versus tight coupling (*y*-axis) and linear versus interactively complex (*x*-axis). Adapted from Perrow C. Normal accidents: living with high-risk technologies. *Princeton Paperbacks.* Princeton, NJ: Princeton University Press; 1999:451 p.

are considered *linear* and those where failures behave unpredictably are *interactively complex*. He further categorizes systems in their ability to detect and respond to failures. Systems that are relatively slow with more opportunity to detect and respond to failures are termed *loosely coupled*, while those that are fast with less opportunity to detect and respond to failures are termed *tightly coupled*. For example, the post office is linear (failures have predictable consequences) and is loosely coupled (failures are largely corrected and most of the mail ultimately gets delivered). Dams are also linear, but are tightly coupled. A dam breach will likely lead to a flood because the time scale required to fix the breach is too long to mitigate the (literally) downstream effects. Universities are interactively complex because events in their varied components (multiple departments, schools, social events, athletics, etc.) interact in unforeseen ways. Perrow argues that systems that are both interactively complex and tightly coupled have a particular propensity for catastrophic failure. Failures in these subsystems are assuredly going to occur and, because these will propagate in unforeseen ways that cannot be mitigated, major global system failures are probable. In other words, complex systems cannot be fully understood and their behavior will always have some element of chaos. He argues that only a change in their structure (e.g., reducing coupling, or reducing interactive complexity) can help reduce the probability of a catastrophic event.

E. **Applying NAT constructs to RO:** For the most part, our processes are largely linear and failures typically propagate forward in an orderly (likely predictable) manner from one step to the next. However, there are many nonlinear components (e.g., iterations in the treatment planning process, and the repeats in the treatment management). With some of the newer technologies (e.g., adaptive therapy, IGRT), information flows in the reverse direction, causing some procedures to be repeated, essentially introducing non-linearity and interactive complexity. Further, some of the processes are long, with many steps (e.g., IMRT planning and delivery), thus increasing the possibility of unexpected interactions of different failures. Is RO coupled or uncoupled? Broadly speaking, most RO processes are modestly coupled. The pace of the work is generally slow enough for unexpected interactions between failures to be evident. For example, suboptimal decisions about patient positioning and immobilization are typically evident early in the course of therapy and can be addressed. In many areas of RO, as well as other areas of medicine, the relatively slow pace tends to soften the impact of failure (i.e., reduce their clinical impact). Are there parts of our practice that are tightly coupled? Yes. Consider intraoperative radiotherapy, brachy-

therapy, and radiosurgery settings where the entire procedure is often compressed into a few hours. In these instances, some steps have near-immediate impacts on other steps. Further, portions of our routine processes are *very* fast. Consider the setup and delivery steps for each individual fraction of radiation: for example, patient identification, setup, image verification, and treatment delivery. This sequence of steps occurs rapidly, which leaves the potential for errors to reach the patient. Also, failures in some processes can be difficult to detect and may affect many treatments or patients downstream (e.g., system commissioning), and thus may be considered tightly coupled. As we introduce more components to the processes (such as combined chemo-radiotherapy and adaptive therapy), the number of steps, and people involved, increases. Interactions become more complex (unusual interactions between failures become more likely), coupling may become tighter, and it may become more difficult to detect and address these failures. So, what is the relevance of this discussion? Can we use these constructs to guide QA strategies in RO? Safety experts suggest there are global optimal QA strategies applicable to all types of systems (e.g., leadership-driven safety mindfulness, the application of automation and forcing functions wherever able, etc.). However, there are particular QA considerations for different systems depending where they lie on this paradigm of linear versus interactively complex and loosely coupled versus tightly coupled. For example, a course of conventionally fractionated external RT (mostly linear, modestly coupled, and generally slow) might be amenable to employee-based CQI strategies. For interactively complex systems that are loosely coupled, their behavior is less predictable than the linear systems. Failures and their interactive effects can be detected, but corrective actions often have further unforeseen effects. Thus, to assure quality, a strategy of continuous comprehensive monitoring (perhaps with forcing functions) is best. Any changes or interventions need to be carefully considered as they may result in unexpected consequences. CQI-based improvement cycles may be useful in some areas but may be more challenging because there are more stakeholders and interactive effects can be difficult to predict.[100] Thus, these systems may appear to be sometimes chaotic, as leadership responds to continual iterations. Since their pace is somewhat slow observers have the luxury to analyze system behavior retrospectively and to second-guess previous actions (since interactions may seem obvious in hindsight). Processes that are both interactively complex and tightly coupled can be unpredictable. Failures and their interactive effects are often not detected until they manifest as a catastrophic event given that their character may be unknown (e.g., it is hard to monitor and thus detect an unforeseen type of failure). Even if failure effects are detected, human-based corrections are unreliable as system behavior is interactively complex. Thus, quality is best assured by rather strict adherence to process standardization in all areas. System performance needs to be comprehensively monitored because the nature or type of a failure cannot be reliably predicted. Ideally this monitoring process should be automated to assure compliance; human intervention is too slow and often misguided. Vigilant testing and verification are needed before any changes in the system or its processes are made. Within RO, the adoption of automation and forcing functions (where possible), end-to-end testing, strict QA, and redundant checks for IMRT planning, brachytherapy, and system commissioning reflects our field's recognition that these systems are interactively complex and tightly coupled. These processes are made safe for clinical use through these aggressive QA initiatives.

F. **Continuous improvement:** Even if systems were "perfect" at one instance in time, they will assuredly drift toward imperfection as workflows change. Further, given the complexities of these systems, changes in processes may have unforeseen consequences. For these reasons, it is generally understood that *continuous* incremental improvements are needed to adapt to evolving systems and to carefully evaluate the consequences of any changes as well as minimize the risk of unforeseen problems. A cornerstone of CQI work is improvement cycles with ongoing monitoring informing additional cycles in a never-ending iterative manner.[101] This approach continually drives change forward and ensures that proposed improvements are implemented, sustained, and modified (as needed) over time. Often this cycle is referred to as *plan do study act*, or PDSA. RO departments are entities that require numerous subsets of employees working simultaneously to achieve the common goal of treating patients safely, effectively, and efficiently. Within these groups are numerous opportunities to improve workflow and outcomes. While any improvement may have a positive effect within its specific group, there is a real possibility that other groups will develop unforeseen problems as a result of changes made in order to achieve that improvement. The PDSA cycle, when correctly implemented, takes into account the complexity of the interrelationships between these groups and considers the unintended consequences that suggested improvements might have on the system as a whole instead of just one part. The major steps in the PDSA cycle are as follows:

- **Plan:** This is the start of the cycle. In the planning stage, a problem within the system is identified and described in detail so that a set of goals and expected outcomes can be determined. During this phase, it

is crucial to grasp the current state of the perceived problem. After the issue is described in detail both quantitatively and qualitatively and issues are identified, the next step is to perform a root cause analysis (RCA). The RCA is completed simply by asking *why* approximatly five times. Once a root cause that is measurable and actionable a countermeasure that solves for the root cause is developed. The creation of an implementation and follow-up plan completes the plan phase of problem-solving. Most of the problem-solving effort and time should be spent in the planning step. A common error is moving to the Do-step in a rush without truly understanding what problem needs to be solved.

- **Do:** This is the initial implementation stage. Countermeasures developed in the *Plan* step are implemented and data that relate to the efficacy of these corrections are collected. Change is not easy and formal change management skills usually need to be applied in this phase. People are often reluctant to change; they may perceive that *others* need to change and do not have a full understanding of their own role in the prior or modified workflows.

- **Study:** Here, the data collected in the previous step are analyzed to assess how well everything is working. The planned and implemented changes are compared, and the expected and actual outcomes from the changes are compared. Analyses completed here are carried forward to the next step.

- **Act:** This is sometimes considered the *adjust* phase of the cycle. The focus is to assess the analyses from the study phase and determine what adjustments can, or should, be made in order to better address the identified problem. It is also important in this step to determine how to communicate the change. What was learned? Who else can benefit from the change? If the change was unsuccessful in generating the expected outcomes, there must be a clear and honest discussion, and with a focus on determining *why* the change was unsuccessful. If people did not change their workflow as desired, rather than blaming and finger-pointing, there is a need to understand *why*.

G. **Lean approach to PDSA:** Lean is a management philosophy derived from the Toyota Production System.[102,103] The heart of Lean is preserving value with less work by the identification and elimination of *waste* and developing highly reliable processes. This is performed in a context of connectedness, respect for people, and growth of all employees who are trained to identify waste and errors and suggest possibilities for improvements that will be tested using scientific methods. Categories of waste include defects, overproduction, waiting, overprocessing, excessive inventory and motion, and (most damaging) failure to use employees to their highest potential. Waste reduction results in quality improvement and reduction in time and cost. The Institute for Healthcare Improvement (IHI) believes that Lean principles can be, and are being, successfully applied to the delivery of health care.[101] Hence, it makes sense to take a closer look at Toyota to learn how they have developed their processes. A few of the more common process engineering practices are as follows:

- **Just-in-time:** Producing only what is needed, when it is needed, and in only the necessary quantities; reducing work-in-process inventory. This concept might be particularly challenging to apply in medicine since the workload is not always predictable (e.g., motor vehicle accidents and heart attacks are not scheduled).
- **Kanban:** A card that signals production of a set quantity of goods once that number of goods has been used by a customer process.
- **Production leveling (or *heijunka*):** Spreading production evenly over time; reducing batch sizes to one.
- **Setup time reduction:** Reducing the time to changeover between producing different products; required to make production more even.
- **Standardized work:** Documented and detailed work procedures strictly followed by everyone doing the job such that the work is performed the same way every time.
- **Multiskilled workers:** Workers trained in multiple job tasks, so work can be assigned flexibly to balance the line dynamically.
- **Gemba:** The real place where the work is done. Gemba walks are done to observe processes.
- **Kaizen:** An activity with a purpose to remove the waste ("muda") and to humanize the workplace by eliminating overly hard work ("muri").

At the operational level, Lean is equipped with two basic tools *Value Stream Mapping*[104] and the *A3 problem-solving tool*.[105,106] Value stream maps graphically represent key people, material, and information required to deliver a product or service (see example in Fig. 1.12). They Value stream maps are designed to distinguish value-adding from non-value-adding steps.

A3s are a problem-solving tool where the user documents the problem area, current state, RCA of the problem, target condition, countermeasures, implementation plan (who, what , when, outcome, metrics), and follow-up plan (30, 60, 90 days' assessment) on a sheet of paper (the name *A3* is derived from the paper size). These basic tools are often used during Kaizen events, which are usually one- to four-day activities where employees engage in small cycles of improvement that promote Lean thinking and behavior. Kaizen events are a critical component in implementing Lean because they directly eliminate

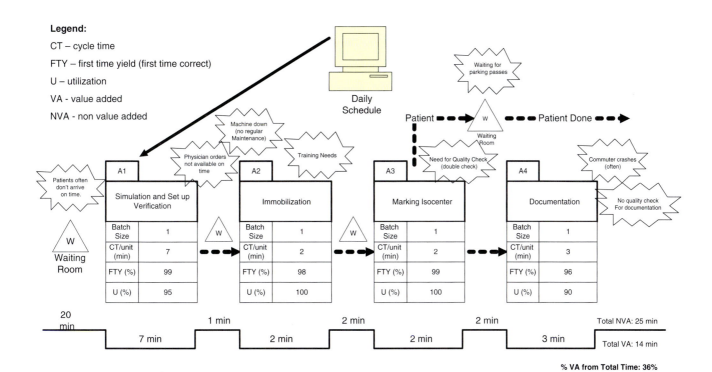

FIGURE 1.12. Example of value stream mapping.

unnecessary waste and bring the organization closer to desired performance outputs.

H. A3 thinking: A3 thinking is a scientific problem-solving process using one sheet of paper as a medium to document the problem-solving effort. This type of thinking aligns seamlessly with the PDSA cycle described earlier. Thus, the text in the following section somewhat mirrors the PDSA cycle described earlier. Here, we highlight some key tips to enhance the A3 problem-solving process.

- The first steps in A3 thinking are to truly understand what is the actual problem that needs to be solved, describe the process to be improved, who is the customer of the process, and what is the waste preventing the process from delivering the desired outcome. Care must be taken not to include a solution in the problem statement. It is important to define the scope, what is included in the project, and what is excluded.
- The next step is to define the current state and how the process is performing now. This is achieved by collecting qualitative and quantitative data. A common misstep is relying on automatic reports and aggregated data. To understand a problem, it must be observed. This is done by completing *Gemba walks* at the point of occurrence. Once the process has been observed, it can be mapped out using a value stream map or a process map. Completing the map of the process and documenting the waste on the map helps identify the areas in which to concentrate the problem-solving efforts. The map also highlights the connections and handoffs.
- The problem analysis then follows by reviewing the map and completing an RCA for the identified waste, as well as completing the "five whys" as mentioned in the PDSA description to arrive at an actionable and measurable root cause.
- The solution approach in A3 thinking requires hypothesis testing; that is, utilizing the phrase "If want to do 'x,' then we expect 'y.'" This is another step that is often skipped in conventional problem-solving. The goal of A3 thinking is not only to solve the problem but also to develop problem-solving thinkers while solving problems. Now that the hypotheses have been created, it is time to develop countermeasures that solve for the root causes. When developing the countermeasures, it is sometimes helpful to predict how much improvement will result from the change. This is not a true scientific way to do this. We often tell teams to *halve the bad, and double the good*. Implementation of the countermeasures is the next step. It is important to develop a plan that details, who, what, when, where, and how the countermeasures will be carried out. As mentioned in the PDSA description, there will be a need for change management in the step.

- Now that the countermeasures are in place it is necessary to confirm the hypotheses and measure the improvement. This is done by collecting process and outcome metric data (e.g., at 30, 60, and 90 days) and comparing this to the predicted outcomes. Once the predicted outcomes have been sustained (e.g., for 90 days), the A3 can be closed after the team reflection is completed. This is done simply by asking, "What did we learn? Any "aha" moments? What went well? What hindered? What could be improved in our problem-solving processes?"

I. Six-Sigma approach to improvement: Six-Sigma is a business management philosophy for quality improvement that originated in the U.S. manufacturing industry. It seeks to improve efficiency and reliability of processes by identifying and removing the causes of failures and minimizing process variability.[107] The approach is heavily dependent on quantitative data; thus, the process can take many months to quantitatively assess the multiple components of the current state, design an improvement plan, and assess its impact. The term Six-Sigma reflects the desire for critical errors to occur at a rate approximating six standard deviations away from the desired performance. Six-Sigma approaches require experts in data generation, analysis, and associated statistical knowledge. It uses the DMAIC process (define, measure, analyze, improve, and control) to conduct improvement projects:

- **Define:** To clearly articulate the problem under investigation, while focusing on the voice of the customer (VOC) and critical to quality (CTQs) drivers. In addition, to establish project goal, potential resources, project scope, and project timeline and milestones.
- **Measure:** To collect data to objectively establish process performance baselines prior to the improvement effort.
- **Analyze:** To identify, validate, and select root causes for elimination.
- **Improve:** To identify, test, and implement a solution to the problem; in part or in whole. Lean and Six-Sigma are often combined at this step, especially when the goal is to reduce operational waste.
- **Control:** To sustain gains and monitor improvements to ensure continued and sustainable success. Control charts are often used during this stage to assess the stability of the improvements over time.

Compared to Lean, there is relatively little empirical research on the utility of Six-Sigma to effectively improve quality and safety, other than "best practice" studies by consultants or practitioners. Further, Six-Sigma is a more time-consuming and complicated process compared to Lean-based approaches. When applied to complex systems within health care, Six-

Sigma can be particularly challenging since quantitative data may be needed from *many* interactive areas, thus complicating analyses. In practice, the length and difficulty of this approach can make physicians and other stakeholders cynical with, and resistant to, improvement work. Nevertheless, this ultra-data-driven approach can be very helpful in settings where the simpler Lean-based approaches cannot be applied. This may include settings where iterative trial-and-error approaches are not safe (e.g., where any failure can be catastrophic such as with nuclear power plants) and where such detailed multifaceted data are needed to even understand the current state.

J. **Risk analysis:** Failure mode and effect analysis (FMEA) is a prospective way to conduct failure analysis based on trying to predict where failures will occur.[92,93,108] The FMEA technique is a well-established and widely used tool for safety and improvement in many industries,[93] including health care[109–111] and, specifically, RT.[112,113] The FMEA technique consists of three steps. First, it requires generating or selecting process steps for analysis. Second, it lists all possible failure modes for each process step. Third, a numeric value is assigned for each failure mode based on (a) likelihood of occurrence, (b) likelihood of detection, and (c) potential severity. The numeric values usually range from 1 to 10, with 1 meaning "very unlikely to occur/detect" and 10 meaning "very likely to occur/detect." Finally, a risk priority number (RPN) for each failure mode is calculated by multiplying the three scores. The lowest possible score can be 1 ($1 \times 1 \times 1$) and the highest 1,000 ($10 \times 10 \times 10$). Identifying the failure modes with highest RPNs should help improvement teams prioritize improvement opportunities. Ford et al. applied this FMEA approach to processes within their RO clinic.[108] Only approximately 50% of the actual incidents occurring in their clinic were predicted by the formal FMEA analysis. This observation highlights the complex nature of our systems; that is, failure modes cannot always be predicted as there are often unforeseen failures and failure interactions.

K. **Human factors analysis and classification system (HFACS):** From a system-thinking perspective, it is critical to analyze both the active and latent failure pathways to fully understand root causes of patient harm. The HFACS is perhaps the most widely used applied improvement model, having been used in civil and military aviation,[114,115] helicopter maintenance,[116] coal mining,[117] rail transportation,[118] maritime,[119] construction,[120] health care,[121] and road transportation.[122] HFACS was developed by Shappell and Wiegmann,[114] based on Reason's SCM. HFACS investigates events using 4 main levels of failure and 12 additional sublevels (see Fig. 1.13).[61] Below the 12 sublevels, there are further *nano-codes*, which are tags identifying specific reasons for an incident occurring. To classify an event into the various categories of the HFACS model, a user starts at the first level (unsafe act, mandatory to select), then proceeds to the corresponding sublevels (e.g., unintended vs. intended violation), followed by the nano-codes (e.g. unintended violation: skill-based vs. decision-based vs. perceptual; intended violation: routine violation vs. exceptional violation). While these categorizations are somewhat arbitrary and inexact, they can help drive improvement work by providing a framework to better analyze and understand errors and system behaviors.

SECTION 4: TECHNICAL CONSIDERATIONS

Our field is highly technical, and errors can result from technical failures. Within the multidisciplinary RO team, medical physicists play a unique role in ensuring RO patient safety. Due to their training and position, medical physicists are generally charged with assessing the capabilities and limitations of hardware and software used for treatment. In support of this role, there are many published guidance documents and practice standards aimed at assuring *technical accuracy* in our practice. A brief summary of some of these are provided here.

- **Commissioning and** QA **of RO hardware, software, and processes:** Many guidance documents address the commissioning CT units for patient simulations,[123] undertaking commissioning measurements on linear accelerators,[124] implementation of treatment planning software,[112,113] and ongoing machine QA.[125,126] Other guidance documents exist for special procedures or equipment such as brachytherapy,[127–131] IMRT,[132] and LINAC-based and robotic SRS/SBRT.[133–135]
- **Standard naming conventions:** The AAPM has generated a recommendation for naming of anatomic structures (TG 263) that facilitates the application of software to manipulate/extract/analyze such data in a reliable fashion.[136] In addition to providing a clear standard across vendors and clinics, clinical trials and other informatics research can be accelerated by reducing the time spent "cleaning" data prior to analysis.
- **Standard prescription:** The AAPM, ASTRO, AAMD, and ASRT have endorsed a standard formulation for radiation prescriptions to reduce ambiguity and increase system reliability (e.g., [Dose per fraction] × [Number of fractions] = [Total dose]).[136] In addition, standards have been proposed for the radiation treatment summary.[137] Such standards can be integrated into a patient's electronic medical record for reference by health care providers, including RO professions contemplating further radiation and/or understanding post-RT effects.

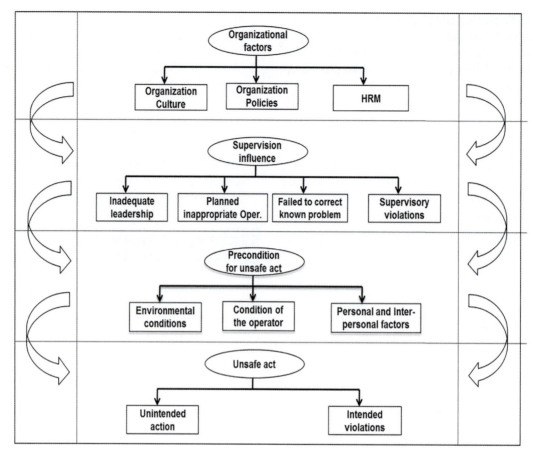

FIGURE 1.13. HFACS Model with categories, subcategories and hierarchy. Reproduced with permission from Mosaly P, Mazur LM, Burkhardt K, et al. Application of Human Factors and Classification System (HFACS) model to event analysis in radiation oncology. *Pract Radiat Oncol.* 2014;5(2):113–119. doi:10.1016/j.prro.2014.05.010

- **Initiatives for improving interoperability between vendors:** Integrating the Healthcare Enterprise-Radiation Oncology (IHE-RO) is an initiative of health care and industry professionals, sponsored by ASTRO/AAPM,[138] that aims to coordinate the standards that enable the transfer of health care information between different vendors. *Connectathons* are an important aspect in their collaborative work, where users test the ability of various vendors' products to accurately communicate and transfer information (patient identifiers, machine, dose, imaging, etc.) between each other. Fidelity in imaging data is obviously crucial for the RO treatment planning and delivery processes.
- **Vendor-access infrastructure for automation:** Many vendors now offer access to an application-programming-interface (API) to allow integration between external software increasing the functionality of existing products. Examples include automated tasks where a script is run on a patient plan to check a variety of parameters are within established baseline values. Such work has been shown to improve the reliability of checks done upstream to patient delivery.[36–38] However, such tools require extensive customization for each

clinic and thus have limited applications across different clinics that use different configurations of hardware and software. We believe efforts to improve interoperability and deploy such tools more broadly could result in thousands of hours of work saved each year if automation is applied to appropriate tasks (with appropriate supervision by medical physicists, computer scientists, and other health information technology specialists who develop and monitor their use).

These technical considerations are complementary to the culture/industrial engineering–focused items that most of this chapter addresses. We chose to do this purposefully since the technical factors are generally accepted as being critical, but the culture/industrial engineering–related items (we believe) are often less-often appreciated (see Fig. 1.14). Nevertheless, we recognize that these are synergistic. To promote these synergies, we have our Division of Healthcare Engineering (DHE) located *within* our clinical department. Division members include multiple improvement coaches as well as several PhD faculty members (e.g., with degrees in industrial and biomedical engineering). This elevates the stature of improvement work and sends a strong message that the departmental leadership embraces their work.

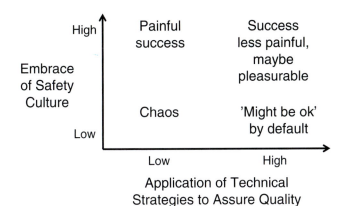

FIGURE 1.14. Chaos versus Success.

SECTION 5: CONCLUDING REMARKS

Our field is highly technical and errors can result from technical failures and improvement efforts aimed at these technical issues are critical. However, the practice of RO is largely a human endeavor and most errors are strongly linked to human-based aspects (e.g., workflows, communication, human–machine interactions). Our systems currently behave somewhat unpredictably (due to many interactive variables) and the resulting complexity requires an ongoing robust embrace of continuous improvement; there are no easy fixes. Our field can achieve very high levels of reliability only if we acknowledge these complexities and our challenges as human beings working in a complex system. We need to embrace a culture of safety in which leaders and workers together openly identify existing waste or shortcomings and generate improved systems that are more reliable and efficient.[39] A greater understanding of the multifaceted causes of errors is needed, and we must systematically and openly discuss and address our latent failures. They occur all around us and are currently tolerated given they largely do not lead to major problems (except when they do). The many strategies outlined in this chapter, proven successful in many industries, can be more broadly applied in our field to reduce the risks of errors. We owe this to our patients and to ourselves.

KEY POINTS

- RT is generally very safe, largely because of the decades-long recognition of its risks.

- Maintaining patient safety is not the responsibility of a single person.

- Maintaining patient safety in our increasingly complex environment requires all stakeholders to work in a coordinated manner to define optimal workflows, monitor performance, speak openly about errors, and refine systems as needed to improve our systems, environment, and workflows.

- We must develop highly reliable systems and nurture our safety culture; physicians, as leaders, play a critical role in this process.

REVIEW QUESTIONS

1. The field of radiation oncology is rapidly evolving mostly due to:
   A. Cultural changes
   B. Training requirements
   C. Technological advancements
   D. Accreditation requirements

2. Which of the following elements are crucial in creating an organization-wide transformation to a culture of safety?
   1. Leadership
   2. Higher-level technology
   3. Culture of safety
   4. Improvement cycles

   A. 1,2,3
   B. 1,2,4
   C. 1,3,4
   D. All of the above

3. Which of these strategies is the *most* effective in providing reliable system performance?
   A. Automation
   B. Standard procedures
   C. Check lists
   D. Education

4. Which of these strategies is the *least* effective in providing reliable system performance?
   A. Automation
   B. Standard procedures
   C. Check lists
   D. Education

5. The goal of safety rounds in a radiation oncology practice is to assure that
   A. Workers have the needed tools and support
   B. Workers can learn about organizational goals
   C. Workers can perform higher-level physics QA
   D. Workers have a chance to practice continuing education

6. What is the PDSA cycle?
   A. Plan, Do, Safety, Act
   B. Plan, Do, Study, Act
   C. Prepare, Do, Study, Act
   D. Perform, Discuss, Simplify, Accept

ANSWERS

1. C   Technological advancements
2. C   1,3,4
3. A   Automation
4. D   Education
5. A   Workers have the needed tools and support
6. B   Plan, Do, Study, Act

REFERENCES

1. Kohn L, Corrigan J, Donaldson M. *To Err is Human: Building a Safer Health System.* Vol 6. Washington DC: National Academy Press; 2000.
2. Leape LL. Error in medicine. *JAMA.* 1994;272(23):1851–1857.
3. James JT. A new, evidence-based estimate of patient harms associated with hospital care. *J Patient Saf.* 2013;9(3):122–128. doi:10.1097/PTS.0b013e3182948a69
4. Bryant AK, Banegas MP, Martinez ME, Mell LK, Murphy JD. Trends in radiation therapyamong cancer survivors in the United States, 2000–2030. *Cancer Epidemiol Biomarkers Prev.* 2017;26(6):963–970. doi:10.1158/1055-9965.EPI-16-1023
5. World Health Organization. Radiotherapy Risk Profile, Technical Manual. 2008.
6. Bogadanich W. Safety features planned for radiation machines. *New York Times.* 2010.
7. Bogadanich W. VA is fined over errors in radiation at hospital. *New York Times.* 2010.
8. Bogadanich W. Radiation errors reported in Missouri. *New York Times.* 2010.
9. Bogadanich W. Radiation offers new cures and ways to do harm. *New York Times.* 2010.
10. Peiffert D, Simon JM, Eschwege F. [Epinal radiotherapy accident: passed, present, future]. *Cancer Radiother.* 2007;11(6–7):309–312. doi:10.1016/j.canrad.2007.09.004
11. ASTRO. Safety is no accident: A framework for quality radiaiton oncology and care. 2012.
12. NHS Department of Health Expert Group (Chairman CMO. An organization with a memory. Report of an expert group on learning fromadverse events in the NHS. 2000:92.
13. Cunningham J, Coffey M, Knöös T, Holmberg O. Radiation Oncology Safety Information System (ROSIS)–profiles of participants and the first 1074 incident reports. *Radiother Oncol.* 2010;97(3):601–607. doi:10.1016/j.radonc.2010.10.023
14. Ford EC, Fong de Los Santos L, Pawlicki T, Sutlief S, Dunscombe P. Consensus recommendations for incident learning database structures in radiation oncology. *Med Phys.* 2012;39(12):7272–7290. doi:10.1118/1.4764914
15. Fletcher M, Jakob R, Koss R, Lewalle P. *Report on the Results of the Web-Based Modified DelphiSurvey of the International Classification for Patient Safety Overview.* World Health Organization; 2007.
16. Near-Miss/Close Call Incident Reporting Form | Environmental Health & Safety | Nebraska. https://ehs.unl.edu/near-missclose-call-incident-reporting-form. Accessed April 24, 2020.
17. Safety pros: Should the term "near miss" replaced by a different term, such as "near hit"? | 2016-09-21 | Safety+Health Magazine. https://www.safetyandhealthmagazine.com/articles/14711-safety-pros-should-the-term-near-miss-replaced-by-a-different-term-such-as-near-hit. Accessed April 24, 2020.
18. Chera BS, Mazur L, Buchanan I, et al. Improving patient safety in clinical oncology: applying lessons from normal accident theory. *JAMA Oncol.* 2015;1(7):958–964.doi:10.1001/jamaoncol.2015.0891
19. Ford EC, Evans SB. Incident learning in radiation oncology: A review. *Med Phys.* 2018;45(5):e100–e119. doi:10.1002/mp.12800
20. Common Formats | AHRQ Patient Safety Organization Program. https://www.pso.ahrq.gov/common. Accessed February 28, 2020.
21. Hoopes DJ, Dicker AP, Eads NL, et al. RO-ILS: Radiation Oncology Incident Learning System: a report from the first year of experience. *Pract Radiat Oncol.* 2015;5(5):312–318. doi:10.1016/j.prro.2015.06.009
22. Novak A, Nyflot MJ, Ermoian RP, et al. Targeting safety improvements through identification of incident origination and detection in a near-miss incident learning system. *Med Phys.* 2016;43(5):2053–2062. doi:10.1118/1.4944739
23. Ezzell G, Chera B, Dicker A, et al. Common error pathways seen in the RO-ILS data that demonstrate opportunities for improving treatment safety. *Pract Radiat Oncol.* 2018;8(2):123–132. doi:10.1016/j.prro.2017.10.007
24. Never Events. https://psnet.ahrq.gov/primer/never-events. Accessed March 19, 2020.
25. The Joint Commission. Sentinel Event. https://www.jointcommission.org/resources/patient-safety-topics/sentinel-event/. Accessed October 8, 2020.
26. Committee on Patient Safety and Health Information Technology, Institute of Medicine. *Health IT and Patient Safety: Building Safer Systems for Better Care.* Washington (DC): National Academies Press (US); 2011. doi:10.17226/13269
27. Konski A, Movsas B, Konopka M, Ma C, Price R, Pollack A. Developing a radiation error scoring system to monitor quality control events in a radiation oncology department. *J Am Coll Radiol.* 2009;6(1):45–50. doi:10.1016/j.jacr.2008.07.009
28. Arnold A, Delaney GP, Cassapi L, Barton M. The use of categorized time-trend reporting of radiation oncology incidents: a proactive analytical approach to improving quality and safety over time. *Int J Radiat Oncol Biol Phys.* 2010;78(5):1548–1554. doi:10.1016/j.ijrobp.2010.02.029
29. Olson AC, Wegner RE, Scicutella C, et al. Quality assurance analysis of a large multicenter practice: does increased complexity of intensity-modulated radiotherapy lead to increased error frequency? *Int J Radiat Oncol Biol Phys.* 2012;82(1):e77–82. doi:10.1016/j.ijrobp.2011.01.033
30. Nyflot MJ, Zeng J, Kusano AS, et al. Metrics of success: measuring impact of a departmental near-miss incident learning system. *Pract Radiat Oncol.* 2015;5(5):e409–16. doi:10.1016/j.prro.2015.05.009

31. Valli MC, Prina M, Bossi A, et al. Evaluation of most frequent errors in daily compilation and use of a radiation treatment chart. *Radiother Oncol.* 1994;32(1):87–89. doi:10.1016/0167-8140(94)90453-7

32. Mutic S, Brame RS, Oddiraju S, et al. Event (error and near-miss) reporting and learning system for process improvement in radiation oncology. *Med Phys.* 2010;37(9):5027–5036. doi:10.1118/1.3471377

33. Clark BG, Brown RJ, Ploquin JL, Kind AL, Grimard L. The management of radiation treatment error through incident learning. *Radiother Oncol.* 2010;95(3):344–349. doi:10.1016/j.radonc.2010.03.022

34. Holmberg O, McClean B. Preventing treatment errors in radiotherapy by identifying and evaluating near misses and actual incidents. *J Radiother Pract.* 2002;3(1):13–25. doi:10.1017/S1460396902000122

35. Chera BS, Mazur L, Adams RD, Kim HJ, Milowsky MI, Marks LB. Creating a culture of safety within an institution: walking the walk. *J Oncol Pract.* 2016;12(10):880–883. doi:10.1200/JOP.2016.012864

36. Calandrino R, Cattaneo GM, Fiorino C, Longobardi B, Mangili P, Signorotto P. Detection of systematic errors in external radiotherapy before treatment delivery. *Radiother Oncol.* 1997;45(3):271–274. doi:10.1016/s0167-8140(97)00095-9

37. Fraass BA, Lash KL, Matrone GM, et al. The impact of treatment complexity and computer-control delivery technology on treatment delivery errors. *Int J Radiat Oncol Biol Phys.* 1998;42(3):651–659. doi:10.1016/s0360-3016(98)00244-2

38. Macklis RM, Meier T, Weinhous MS. Error rates in clinical radiotherapy. *J Clin Oncol.* 1998;16(2):551–556. doi:10.1200/JCO.1998.16.2.551

39. Patton GA, Gaffney DK, Moeller JH. Facilitation of radiotherapeutic error by computerized record and verify systems. *Int J Radiat Oncol Biol Phys.* 2003;56(1):50–57. doi:10.1016/s0360-3016(02)04418-8

40. Huang G, Medlam G, Lee J, et al. Error in the delivery of radiation therapy: results of a quality assurance review. *Int J Radiat Oncol Biol Phys.* 2005;61(5):1590–1595. doi:10.1016/j.ijrobp.2004.10.017

41. Yeung TK, Bortolotto K, Cosby S, Hoar M, Lederer E. Quality assurance in radiotherapy: evaluation of errors and incidents recorded over a 10 year period. *Radiother Oncol.* 2005;74(3):283–291. doi:10.1016/j.radonc.2004.12.003

42. Marks LB, Light KL, Hubbs JL, et al. The impact of advanced technologies on treatment deviations in radiation treatment delivery. *Int J Radiat Oncol Biol Phys.* 2007;69(5):1579–1586. doi:10.1016/j.ijrobp.2007.08.017

43. Ur-Rahman S, Matiullah, Faaruq S. Investigation of the occurrence of human errors in treatment of cancer patients with external beam radiotherapy. *J Med Imaging Radiat Sci.* 2008;39(4):179–182. doi:10.1016/j.jmir.2008.08.002

44. Bissonnette J-P, Medlam G. Trend analysis of radiation therapy incidents over seven years. *Radiother Oncol.* 2010;96(1):139–144. doi:10.1016/j.radonc.2010.05.002

45. Margalit DN, Chen Y-H, Catalano PJ, et al. Technological advancements and error rates in radiation therapy delivery. *Int J Radiat Oncol Biol Phys.* 2011;81(4):e673–9. doi:10.1016/j.ijrobp.2011.04.036

46. Hunt MA, Pastrana G, Amols HI, Killen A, Alektiar K. The impact of new technologies on radiation oncology events and trends in the past decade: an institutional experience. *Int J Radiat Oncol Biol Phys.* 2012;84(4):925–931. doi:10.1016/j.ijrobp.2012.01.042

47. Kalapurakal JA, Zafirovski A, Smith J, et al. A comprehensive quality assurance program for personnel and procedures in radiation oncology: value of voluntary error reporting and checklists. *Int J Radiat Oncol Biol Phys.* 2013;86(2):241–248. doi:10.1016/j.ijrobp.2013.02.003

48. Das P, Johnson J, Hayden SE, et al. Rate of radiation therapy events in a large academic institution. *J Am Coll Radiol.* 2013;10(6):452–455. doi:10.1016/j.jacr.2012.12.010

49. Clark BG, Brown RJ, Ploquin J, Dunscombe P. Patient safety improvements in radiation treatment through 5 years of incident learning. *Pract Radiat Oncol.* 2013;3(3):157–163. doi:10.1016/j.prro.2012.08.001

50. Chang DW, Cheetham L, te Marvelde L, et al. Risk factors for radiotherapy incidents and impact of an online electronic reporting system. *Radiother Oncol.* 2014;112(2):199–204. doi:10.1016/j.radonc.2014.07.011

51. Rahn DA, Kim G-Y, Mundt AJ, Pawlicki T. A real-time safety and quality reporting system: assessment of clinical data and staff participation. *Int J Radiat Oncol Biol Phys.* 2014;90(5):1202–1207. doi:10.1016/j.ijrobp.2014.08.332

52. Yang R, Wang J, Zhang X, et al. Implementation of incident learning in the safety and quality management of radiotherapy: the primary experience in a new established program with advanced technology. *Biomed Res Int.* 2014;2014:392596. doi:10.1155/2014/392596

53. Gabriel PE, Volz E, Bergendahl HW, et al. Incident learning in pursuit of high reliability: implementing a comprehensive, low-threshold reporting program in a large, multisite radiation oncology department. *Jt Comm J Qual Patient Saf.* 2015;41(4):160–168. doi:10.1016/s1553-7250(15)41021-9

54. Deraniyagala R, Liu C, Mittauer K, Greenwalt J, Morris CG, Yeung AR. Implementing an electronic event-reporting system in a radiation oncology department: the effect on safety culture and near-miss prevention. *J Am Coll Radiol.* 2015;12(11):1191–1195. doi:10.1016/j.jacr.2015.04.014

55. Dominello MM, Paximadis PA, Zaki M, et al. Ten-year trends in safe radiation therapy delivery and results of a radiation therapy quality assurance intervention. *Int J Radiat Oncol Biol Phys.* 2015;93(3):E501–E502.doi:10.1016/j.ijrobp.2015.07.1828

56. Hossain M, Papalia NM, Stoffel TJ, Carpenter HE, Sharis CM. A simple incident learning system for radiation oncology in a community hospital. *J Am Coll Radiol.* 2017;14(7):952–955. doi:10.1016/j.jacr.2017.01.055

57. Hussain A, Khan Y, Ali N, et al. Unusual occurrence reporting system: sharing a ten years experience from a tertiary care JCIA accredited university hospital. *Cancer Radiother.* 2018;22(3):248–254. doi:10.1016/j.canrad.2017.09.011

58. Schubert L, Petit J, Vinogradskiy Y, et al. Implementation and operation of incident learning across a newly-created health system. *J Appl Clin Med Phys.* 2018;19(6):298–305.doi:10.1002/acm2.12447

59. Reason JT, Carthey J, de Leval MR. Diagnosing "vulnerable system syndrome": an essential prerequisite to effective risk management. *Qual Health Care.* 2001;10 Suppl 2:ii21–5.

60. Reason J. Human error: models and management. *BMJ.* 2000;320(7237):768–770. doi:10.1136/bmj.320.7237.768

61. Reason J. *Human Error.* 1st ed. Cambridge [England]: Cambridge University Press; 1990:320.

62. Reason J. Understanding adverse events: human factors. *Qual Health Care.* 1995;4(2):80–89. doi:10.1136/qshc.4.2.80

63. Mazur LM, Mosaly PR, Jackson M, et al. Quantitative assessment of workload and stressors in clinical radiation oncology. *Int J Radiat Oncol Biol Phys.* 2012;83(5):e571–6. doi:10.1016/j.ijrobp.2012.01.063

64. Marks LB, Rose CM, Hayman JA, Williams TR. The need for physician leadership in creating a culture of safety. *Int J Radiat Oncol Biol Phys.* 2011;79(5):1287–1289. doi:10.1016/j.ijrobp.2010.12.004

65. Roberts KH. Some characteristics of one type of high reliability organization. *Organ. Sci.* 1990;1(2):160–176. doi:10.1287/orsc.1.2.160

66. Roberts KH, Bea R, Bartles DL. Must accidents happen? Lessons from high-reliability organizations. *Acad Manag Exec.* 2001;15(3):70–78.

67. Agency for Healthcare Research and Quality. Surveys on Patient Safety Culture. http://www.ahrq.gov/professionals/quality-patient-safety/patientsafetyculture/index.html. Published 2015.

68. Mardon RE, Khanna K, Sorra J, Dyer N, Famolaro T. Exploring relationships between hospital patient safety culture and adverse events. *J Patient Saf.* 2010;6(4):226–232. doi:10.1097/PTS.0b013e3181fd1a00

69. Chassin MR, Loeb JM. The ongoing quality improvement journey: next stop, high reliability. *Health Aff (Millwood).* 2011;30(4):559–568. doi:10.1377/hlthaff.2011.0076

70. Marks L, Mazur L, Chera B, Adams R. *Engineering Patient Safety in Radiation Oncology.* 1st ed. Boca Raton: Taylor & Francis Group; 2015.

71. Evans SB. Patient safety across disciplines: radiation oncology incident learning system. *J Oncol Pract.* 2015;11(3):202–203. doi:10.1200/JOP.2015.004341

72. American Society for Radiation Oncology. RO-ILS- American Society for Radiation Oncology (ASTRO) - American Society for Radiation Oncology (ASTRO). https://www.astro.org/Patient-Care-and-Research/Patient-Safety/RO-ILS. Accessed October 19, 2020.

73. European Society for Radiotherapy and Oncology. ESTRO-Radiation Oncology Safety Education and Information System. https://www.estro.org/Advocacy/ROSEIS. Accessed October 19, 2020.

74. International Atomic Energy Agency. Safety in Radiation Oncology (SAFRON). https://www.iaea.org/resources/rpop/resources/databases-and-learning-systems/safron. Accessed July 27, 2020.

75. American Society for Radiation Oncology. RO-ILS Education. https://www.astro.org/Patient-Care-and-Research/Patient-Safety/RO-ILS/RO-ILS-Education. Accessed October 19, 2020.

76. Frankel A, Grillo SP, Pittman M, et al. Revealing and resolving patient safety defects: the impact of leadership WalkRounds on frontline caregiver assessments of patient safety. *Health Serv Res.* 2008;43(6):2050–2066. doi:10.1111/j.1475-6773.2008.00878.x

77. Provost SM, Lanham HJ, Leykum LK, McDaniel RR, Pugh J. Health care huddles: managing complexity to achieve high reliability. *Health Care Manage Rev.* 2015;40(1):2–12. doi:10.1097/HMR.0000000000000009

78. Marks LB, Adams RD, Pawlicki T, et al. Enhancing the role of case-oriented peer review to improve quality and safety in radiation oncology: executive summary. *Pract Radiat Oncol.* 2013;3(3):149–156. doi:10.1016/j.prro.2012.11.010

79. Adams RD, Marks LB, Pawlicki T, Hayman J, Church J. The new radiation therapy clinical practice: the emerging role of clinical peer review for radiation therapists and medical dosimetrists. *Med Dosim.* 2010;35(4):320–323. doi:10.1016/j.meddos.2010.09.002

80. Brundage MD, Dixon PF, Mackillop WJ, et al. A real-time audit of radiation therapy in a regional cancer center. *Int J Radiat Oncol Biol Phys.* 1999;43(1):115–24.

81. Shakespeare TP, Mukherjee RK, Lu JJ, Lee KM, Back MF. Evaluation of an audit with feedback continuing medical education program for radiation oncologists. *J Cancer Educ.* 2005;20(4):216–221. doi:10.1207/s15430154jce2004_9

82. Boxer M, Forstner D, Kneebone A, et al. Impact of a real-time peer review audit on patient management in a radiation oncology department. *J Med Imaging Radiat Oncol.* 2009;53(4):405–411. doi:10.1111/j.1754-9485.2009.02096.x

83. Ohri N, Shen X, Dicker AP, Doyle LA, Harrison AS, Showalter TN. Radiotherapy protocol deviations and clinical outcomes: a meta-analysis of cooperative group clinical trials. *J Natl Cancer Inst.* 2013;105(6):387–393. doi:10.1093/jnci/djt001

84. Peters LJ, O'Sullivan B, Giralt J, et al. Critical impact of radiotherapy protocol compliance and quality in the treatment of advanced head and neck cancer: results from TROG 02.02. *J Clin Oncol.* 2010;28(18):2996–3001. doi:10.1200/JCO.2009.27.4498

85. Robin TP, Grover S, Reddy Palkonda VA, et al. Utilization of a web-based conferencing platform to improve global radiation oncology education and quality-proof of principle through implementation in India. *Int J Radiat Oncol Biol Phys.* 2019;103(1):276–280. doi:10.1016/j.ijrobp.2018.07.2003

86. Berlinger N, Dietz E. Time-out: the professional and organizational ethics of speaking up in the OR. *AMA J Ethics.* 2016;18(9):925–932. doi:10.1001/journalofethics.2016.18.9.stas1-1609

87. Gawande A. *The Checklist Manifesto: How To Get Things Right.* 1st ed. New York: Metropolitan Books; 2009:224.

88. Purdie TG, Dinniwell RE, Fyles A, Sharpe MB. Automation and intensity modulated radiation therapy for individualized high-quality tangent breast treatment plans. *Int J Radiat Oncol Biol Phys.* 2014;90(3):688–695. doi:10.1016/j.ijrobp.2014.06.056

89. Noel CE, Gutti V, Bosch W, et al. Quality assurance with plan veto: reincarnation of a record and verify system and its potential value. *Int J Radiat Oncol Biol Phys.* 2014;88(5):1161–1166. doi:10.1016/j.ijrobp.2013.12.044

90. Sun B, Rangaraj D, Palaniswaamy G, et al. Initial experience with TrueBeam trajectory log files for radiation therapy delivery verification. *Pract Radiat Oncol.* 2013;3(4):e199–208. doi:10.1016/j.prro.2012.11.013

91. Potters L, Kapur A. Implementation of a "No Fly" safety culture in a multicenter radiation medicine department. *Pract Radiat Oncol.* 2012;2(1):18–26. doi:10.1016/j.prro.2011.04.010

92. Wetterneck TB, Skibinski KA, Roberts TL, et al. Using failure mode and effects analysis to plan implementation of smart i. v. pump technology. *Am J Health Syst Pharm.* 2006;63(16):1528–1538. doi:10.2146/ajhp050515

93. Shappel SA, Wiegmann DA. *The Human Factors Analysis and Classification System--HFACS.* US Federal Aviation Administration, Office of Aviation Medicine; 2000.

94. American College of Radiation Oncology. Accreditation. http://www.acro.org/accreditation/. Accessed October 19, 2020.

95. Grimes AJ, Perrow C. Normal accidents: living with high risk technologies. *Acad Manage Rev.* 1985;10(2):366. doi:10.2307/257982

96. Huq Z, Martin TN. Workforce cultural factors in TQM/CQI implementation in hospitals. *Health Care Manage Rev.* 2000;25(3):80–93. doi:10.1097/00004010-200007000-00009

97. Institute of Healthcare Improvement. *Going Lean in Health Care: IHI Innovation Series White Paper.* Cambridge, MA: Institute of Healthcare Improvement; 2005.

98. Ohno T. *Toyota Production System: Beyond Large-scale Production.* 1st ed. Cambridge, Mass: Productivity Press; 1988:152.

99. Shah R, Ward PT. Defining and developing measures of lean production. *J Oper Manag.* 2007;25(4):785–805. doi:10.1016/j.jom.2007.01.019

100. Mazur LM, Chen S-J (Gary). Understanding and reducing the medication delivery waste via systems mapping and analysis. *Health Care Manag Sci.* 2008;11(1):55–65. doi:10.1007/s10729-007-9024-9

101. Mazur LM, Chen S-J (Gary). Evaluation of industrial engineering students' competencies for process improvement in hospitals. *J Ind Eng Manag.* December 2010.

102. Mazur LM, Chen S-J (Gary), Prescott B. Pragmatic evaluation of the Toyota Production System (TPS) analysis procedure for problem solving with entry-level nurses. *JIEM.* 2008;1(2). doi:10.3926/jiem.2008.v1n2.p240-268

103. Antony J, Palsuk P, Gupta S, Mishra D, Barach P. Six Sigma in healthcare: a systematic review of the literature. *Int J Qual & Reliability Mgmt.* 2018;35(5):1075–1092. doi:10.1108/IJQRM-02-2017-0027

104. Ford EC, Gaudette R, Myers L, et al. Evaluation of safety in a radiation oncology setting using failure mode and effects analysis. *Int J Radiat Oncol Biol Phys.* 2009;74(3):852–858. doi:10.1016/j.ijrobp.2008.10.038

105. Huq MS, Fraass BA, Dunscombe PB, et al. A method for evaluating quality assurance needs in radiation therapy. *Int J Radiat Oncol Biol Phys.* 2008;71(1 Suppl):S170-3. doi:10.1016/j.ijrobp.2007.06.081

106. Stamatis DH. *Failure Mode and Effect Analysis: Fmea from Theory to Execution.* Revised. Milwaukee, Wisc: Asq Pr; 2003:300.

107. Sheridan-Leos N, Schulmeister L, Hartranft S. Failure mode and effect analysis (TM): a technique to prevent chemotherapy errors. *Clin J Oncol Nurs.* 2006;10(3):393.

108. Duwe B, Fuchs BD, Hansen-Flaschen J. Failure mode and effects analysis application to critical care medicine. *Crit Care Clin.* 2005;21(1):21–30.

109. Portaluri M, Fucilli FI, Bambace S, et al. Incidents analysis in radiation therapy: application of the human factors analysis and classification system. *Ann Ist Super Sanita.* 2008;45(2):128–133.

110. Rashid HSJ, Place CS, Braithwaite GR. Helicopter maintenance error analysis: beyond the third order of the HFACS-ME. *Int J Ind Ergon.* 2010;40(6):636–647.

111. Patterson JM, Shappell SA. Operator error and system deficiencies: analysis of 508 mining incidents and accidents from Queensland, Australia using HFACS. *Accid Anal Prev.* 2010;42(4):1379–1385.

112. Rivard MJ, Butler WM, DeWerd LA, et al. Erratum: "Supplement to the 2004 update of the AAPM Task Group No. 43 Report" [Med. Phys. 34, 2187–2205 (2007)]. *Med Phys.* 2010;37(5):2396–2396. doi:10.1118/1.3388848

113. Rivard MJ, Butler WM, DeWerd LA, et al. Supplement to the 2004 update of the AAPM Task Group No. 43 Report. *Med Phys.* 2007;34(6):2187–2205. doi:10.1118/1.2736790

114. Baysari MT, McIntosh AS, Wilson JR. Understanding the human factors contribution to railway accidents and incidents in Australia. *Accid Anal Prev.* 2008;40(5):1750–1757.

115. Celik M, Cebi S. Analytical HFACS for investigating human errors in shipping accidents. *Accid Anal Prev.* 2009;41(1):66–75.

116. Walker D. Applying the Human Factors Analysis and Classification System (HFACS) to incidents in the UK construction industry. 2007.

117. ElBardissi AW, Wiegmann DA, Dearani JA, Daly RC, Sundt TM. Application of the human factors analysis and classification system methodology to the cardiovascular surgery operating room. *Ann Thorac Surg.* 2007;83(4):1412–8; discussion 1418. doi:10.1016/j.athoracsur.2006.11.002

118. Iden R, Shappell SA. A human error analysis of US fatal highway crashes 1990–2004. In: Vol 50. Sage Publications; 2006:2000–2003.

119. Mutic S, Palta JR, Butker EK, et al. Quality assurance for computed-tomography simulators and the computed-tomography-simulation process: report of the AAPM Radiation Therapy Committee Task Group No. 66. *Med Phys.* 2003;30(10):2762–2792. doi:10.1118/1.1609271

120. Das IJ, Cheng C-W, Watts RJ, et al. Accelerator beam data commissioning equipment and procedures: report of the TG-106 of the therapy physics committee of the AAPM. *Med Phys.* 2008;35(9):4186–4215. doi:10.1118/1.2969070

121. Smilowitz JB, Das IJ, Feygelman V, et al. AAPM Medical Physics Practice Guideline 5.a.: commissioning and QA of treatment planning dose calculations - megavoltage photon and electron beams. *J Appl Clin Med Phys.* 2015;16(5):14–34. doi:10.1120/jacmp.v16i5.5768

122. Fraass B, Doppke K, Hunt M, et al. American Association of Physicists in Medicine Radiation Therapy Committee Task Group 53: quality assurance for clinical radiotherapy treatment planning. *Med Phys.* 1998;25(10):1773–1829. doi:10.1118/1.598373

123. Smith K, Balter P, Duhon J, et al. AAPM Medical Physics Practice Guideline 8.a.: linear accelerator performance tests. *J Appl Clin Med Phys.* 2017;18(4):23–39. doi:10.1002/acm2.12080

124. Klein EE, Hanley J, Bayouth J, et al. Task Group 142 report: quality assurance of medical accelerators. *Med Phys.* 2009;36(9):4197–4212. doi:10.1118/1.3190392

125. Rivard MJ, Coursey BM, DeWerd LA, et al. Update of AAPM Task Group No. 43 Report: a revised AAPM protocol for brachytherapy dose calculations. *Med Phys.* 2004;31(3):633–674. doi:10.1118/1.1646040

126. Kubo HD, Glasgow GP, Pethel TD, Thomadsen BR, Williamson JF. High dose-rate brachytherapy treatment delivery: report of the AAPM Radiation Therapy Committee Task Group No. 59. *Med Phys.* 1998;25(4):375–403. doi:10.1118/1.598232

127. Nath R, Bice WS, Butler WM, et al. AAPM recommendations on dose prescription and reporting methods for permanent interstitial brachytherapy for prostate cancer: report of Task Group 137. *Med Phys.* 2009;36(11):5310–5322. doi:10.1118/1.3246613

128. Moran JM, Dempsey M, Eisbruch A, et al. Safety considerations for IMRT: executive summary. *Pract Radiat Oncol.* 2011;1(3):190–195. doi:10.1016/j.prro.2011.04.008

129. Benedict SH, Yenice KM, Followill D, et al. Stereotactic body radiation therapy: the report of AAPM Task Group 101. *Med Phys.* 2010;37(8):4078–4101. doi:10.1118/1.3438081

130. Halvorsen PH, Cirino E, Das IJ, et al. AAPM-RSS Medical Physics Practice Guideline 9.a. for SRS-SBRT. *J Appl Clin Med Phys.* 2017;18(5):10–21. doi:10.1002/acm2.12146

131. Dieterich S, Cavedon C, Chuang CF, et al. Report of AAPM TG 135: quality assurance for robotic radiosurgery. *Med Phys.* 2011;38(6):2914–2936. doi:10.1118/1.3579139

132. Mayo id Fuller Ellen D. Yorke Jatinder R. Palta Peter C, Moran J, Bosch W, et al. *Standardizing Nomenclatures in Radiation Oncology.* American Association of Physicists in Medicine; 2018. doi:10.37206/171

133. Christodouleas JP, Anderson N, Gabriel P, et al. A multidisciplinary consensus recommendation on a synoptic radiation treatment summary: a commission on cancer workgroup report. *Pract Radiat Oncol.* January 2020. doi:10.1016/j.prro.2020.01.002

134. Walz-Flannigan A, Weiser J, Goode A, et al. *Interoperability Assessment for the Commissioning of Medical Imaging Acquisition Systems.* American Association of Physicists in Medicine; 2019. doi:10.37206/180

135. Liu S, Bush KK, Bertini J, et al. Optimizing efficiency and safety in external beam radiotherapy using automated plan check (APC) tool and six sigma methodology. *J Appl Clin Med Phys.* 2019;20(8):56–64. doi:10.1002/acm2.12678

136. Hadley SW, Kessler ML, Litzenberg DW, et al. SafetyNet: streamlining and automating QA in radiotherapy. *J Appl Clin Med Phys.* 2016;17(1):387–395. doi:10.1120/jacmp.v17i1.5920

137. Yang D, Wu Y, Brame RS, et al. Technical note: electronic chart checks in a paperless radiation therapy clinic. *Med Phys.* 2012;39(8):4726–4732. doi:10.1118/1.4736825

138. Mazur L, McCreery J, Chen S-J. Quality improvement in hospitals: identifying and understanding behaviors. *J Healthc Eng.* 2012;3(4):621–648. doi:10.1260/2040-2295.3.4.621

2 Normal Tissue Tolerance

Dominic H. Moon and Robert D. Timmerman

INTRODUCTION

The more-than-a-century-old field of radiation oncology has enjoyed a recent dramatic technological advancement since the transition from two-dimensional (2D) to three-dimensional (3D) treatment planning in the late 1980s and early 1990s. Modulation of photon beam intensity in conjunction with inverse planning allowed for intensity-modulated radiotherapy with improved sparing of organs at risk. With more conformal treatments, the need to account for geometric uncertainties increased, leading to image-guided radiotherapy incorporating on-board imaging and real-time tracking. Prior to these technological improvements, conventionally fractionated radiotherapy treated most patient presentations to normal tissue tolerance given that normal tissue compartments were dose limiting and often treated to high doses intended for tumor. More recently, stereotactic ablative radiotherapy (SABR), also known as stereotactic body radiotherapy (SBRT), has enabled delivery of large doses of radiation per fraction with precise targeting of tumor volume and sharp dose gradients leading to biologically ablative doses to the tumor while sparing adjacent normal tissues. For decades prior to the technological renaissance, large daily doses of radiation treatment were taboo due to the inability to geometrically avoid nearby critical structures. Indeed, this long-endured limitation was nearly the entire biological basis justifying the inconvenience and increased cost of conventionally fractionated radiotherapy. Collectively, the technological improvements and clearer appreciation of normal tissue tolerance have allowed a forward leap in achieving tolerable tumor control while greatly expanding the indications for radiotherapy.

NORMAL TISSUE TOLERANCE OF CONVENTIONALLY FRACTIONATED RADIOTHERAPY

In the early days of the 3D era in radiation oncology, a task force was created as part of a National Cancer Institute contract to comprehensively review available data on normal tissue tolerance to radiotherapy. Commonly known as the "Emami paper", the manuscript published in 1991 combined limited available data with expert opinion of the task force members to delineate organ tolerance, divided into one-third, two-third, and whole-organ volumes.[1] This is an example of what has been termed an eminence-based directive where experienced and knowledgeable experts determine practice. In the subsequent two decades, data addressing the dose–volume parameters of 3D treatment plans and their relationship to normal tissue outcomes accumulated. As a result, an update termed "Quantitative Analyses of Normal Tissue Effects in the Clinic" (QUANTEC) was published in 2010 to summarize the accrued information in a clinically useful manner.[2] More data-driven QUANTEC is an example of an evidence-based directive. Despite its limitations due to pooling of data presented in different formats and constraint recommendations pertaining only to clinical situations with adequate data, QUANTEC continues to provide valuable and practical normal tissue dose parameters for conventionally fractionated radiotherapy (Table 2.1). In addition to QUANTEC and constraints used in published clinical trials, the Department of Radiation Oncology at UT Southwestern Medical Center incorporates maximum point dose and volume dose parameters (shown in Table 2.2) as safety checks for all conventionally fractionated radiotherapy cases.

NEW PERSPECTIVE ON NORMAL TISSUE TOLERANCE IN THE ERA OF STEREOTACTIC ABLATIVE RADIOTHERAPY

Traditionally, radiation oncology as a field has been primarily risk averse to causing practically any normal tissue injury. For many decades since its first use in the clinical setting and prior to recent technological advancements, radiation was generally delivered with large fields bathing large volumes of normal tissue

TABLE 2.1   QUANTEC Normal Tissue Dose Guidelines for Conventional Fractionation

Organ	Endpoint	D_{max} (Gy)	D_{mean} (Gy)	Dose–Volume Parameters	Rate (%)
Brain	Symptomatic necrosis	<60 72			<3 5
Brainstem	Permanent cranial neuropathy or necrosis	<64 Point (<<1 cc) <54		D1–10 cc ≤59 Gy	<5
Spinal cord	Myelopathy	50 60			0.2 6
Optic nerve and chiasm	Optic neuropathy	<55 55–60 >60			<3 3–7 >7
Cochlea	Sensory neural hearing loss		≤45		<30
Parotid (unilateral)	Salivary function reduction to <25%		<20		<20
Parotid (bilateral)	Salivary function reduction to <25%		<25		<20
Pharyngeal constrictors	Symptomatic dysphagia and aspiration		<50		<20
Larynx	Edema		<44	V50 <27%	<20
	Aspiration		<50		<30
Lung	Symptomatic pneumonitis		 7 13 20 24 27	V20 ≤30%	<20 5 10 20 30 40
Esophagus	Grade ≥2 esophagitis			V35 <50% V50 <40% V70 <20%	<30
	Grade ≥3 esophagitis		<34		5–20
Heart	Pericarditis		<26	V30 <46%	<15
	Long-term cardiac mortality			V25 <10%	<1
Liver	Classic RILD, normal liver		<30–32		<5
	Classic RILD, liver disease		<28		<5
Kidney (bilateral)	Clinical renal dysfunction		<15–18	V12 <55% V20 <32% V23 <30% V28 <20%	<5
Stomach	Ulceration			D100 <45 Gy	<7
Small bowel	Grade ≥3 acute toxicity			V15 <120 cc	<10
Rectum	Grade ≥2/≥3 late toxicity			V50 <50% V60 <35% V65 <25% V70 <20% V75 <15%	<15/<10

(continued)

TABLE 2.1   QUANTEC Normal Tissue Dose Guidelines for Conventional Fractionation (*Continued*)

Organ	Endpoint	D_{max} (Gy)	D_{mean} (Gy)	Dose–Volume Parameters	Rate (%)
Bladder	Grade ≥3 late toxicity		<65	V65 ≤50%* V70 ≤35%* V75 ≤25%* V80 ≤15%*	<6
Penile bulb	Severe erectile dysfunction		<50	D90 <50 Gy D60–70 <70 Gy	<35

D_{max}, maximum dose; D_{mean}, mean dose; DX, minimum dose received by X% of the organ; RILD, radiation induced liver disease; VX, volume of the organ receiving ≥X Gy.
*Per RTOG 0415 recommendations

TABLE 2.2   UT Southwestern Normal Tissue Dose Guidelines for Conventional Fractionation

Organ	Volume/Parameter	Volume Maximum/Parameter Dose (Gy)	Max Point Dose (Gy)	Endpoint (≥Grade 3)
Serial Tissue				
Optic pathway	<0.5 cc	44 Gy	52 Gy	Neuritis
Eye (retina)	Mean dose	<38 Gy	45 Gy	Retinitis
Lens			10 Gy	Cataract
Eyelid—meibomian glands (one side)			32 Gy	Dry eye syndrome
Lacrimal gland (one side)	<1 cc	20 Gy	36 Gy	Lack of tears
Cochlea	<0.5 cc	36 Gy	40 Gy	Hearing loss
Brainstem (not medulla)	<5 cc	52 Gy	60 Gy	Cranial neuropathy
Spinal cord	<5 cc	47.4 Gy	52.8 Gy	Myelitis
Salivary gland (one side)	<7 cc Mean dose	20 Gy <26 Gy	32 Gy	Xerostomia
Larynx	<3 cc	39 Gy	63 Gy	Necrosis/edema
Temporomandibular joint	<1 cc	60 Gy	65 Gy	Inflammation
Cauda equina	<5 cc	50 Gy	60 Gy	Neuritis
Sacral plexus	<5 cc	50 Gy	60 Gy	Neuropathy
Esophagus	<5 cc	51 Gy	60 Gy	Esophagitis
Brachial plexus	<3 cc	62 Gy	66 Gy	Neuropathy
Heart/pericardium	<15 cc <20% of total heart volume	60 Gy 40 Gy	68 Gy	Pericarditis
Great vessels	<10 cc	60 Gy	76 Gy	Aneurysm
Trachea and large bronchus	<5 cc	60 Gy	69 Gy	Impairment of pulmonary toilet
Skin	<10 cc	70 Gy	76 Gy	Ulceration
Stomach	<50 cc	45 Gy	60 Gy	Ulceration/fistula
Duodenum	<5 cc	45 Gy	60 Gy	Ulceration
Jejunum/ileum	<120 cc	45 Gy	54 Gy	Enteritis/obstruction

(continued)

TABLE 2.2	UT Southwestern Normal Tissue Dose Guidelines for Conventional Fractionation *(Continued)*			
Organ	**Volume/Parameter**	**Volume Maximum/Parameter Dose (Gy)**	**Max Point Dose (Gy)**	**Endpoint (≥Grade 3)**
Renal hilum/vascular trunk	15 cc	42 Gy		Malignant hypertension
Colon	<20 cc	54 Gy	70 Gy	Colitis/fistula
Rectum (including stool)	<10 cc	75 Gy	79 Gy	Proctitis/fistula
	<20 cc	70 Gy		
	<30 cc	65 Gy		
	<40 cc	60 Gy		
Bladder (with urine)	<90 cc	70 Gy	79 Gy	Cystitis/fistula
	<125 cc	65 Gy		
Bladder (suprapubic wall)	<5 cc	30 Gy	60 Gy	Dysuria
Penile bulb	<3 cc	48 Gy	56 Gy	Impotence
Femoral heads	<10 cc	48 Gy	56 Gy	Necrosis
Growth plate				
Parallel Tissue				
Lung (right and left) minus GTV	1500 cc (male), 950 cc (female)*	18 Gy		Basic lung function
Lung (right and left) minus GTV	V20 Gy	<37%		Pneumonitis
Liver minus GTV	700 cc*	36 Gy		Basic liver function
Renal cortex (right and left)	200 cc*	27 Gy		Basic renal function

GTV, gross tumor volume.
*Or one third of the "native" total organ volume (prior to any resection or volume reducing disease), whichever is greater.

with prescription dose. As a result, priority was given to safety versus efficacy based on the concept of "first do no harm," even if tumor control with this priority may be low. This perspective continues to be prevalent, as evidenced by the target rate of toxicity less than 5% to 10% in a majority of the endpoints presented in QUANTEC and the widely used term "dose constraints" to normal tissue, implying a limit or hard stop. "Dose guidelines" is a more apt descriptor of the parameters since there are numerous clinical scenarios where required treatments may exceed the constraint values depending on the risk–benefit calculation. As the field embraces another leap in potential by incorporating SABR into the treatment of various cancers, a shift in perception regarding normal tissue injury will be necessary.

Radiation oncologists can learn from the surgeon's perspective when operating on a patient with cancer. During a curative oncologic surgery, a surgeon has a clear priority to obtain a gross total resection of the tumor to maximize the chance of eradicating the disease

with the understanding that normal tissue injury is part of the overall treatment calculus. Through training and experience, surgeons have insight into how, when, and to what extent normal tissue injury occurs for a particular surgical approach. Importantly, they also appreciate, through experience and study, the likelihood of healing or recovery. This discussion is integrated into the patient consent process prior to the operation. In surgery, expected perioperative morbidity is not routinely classified as "toxicity" of the treatment. Surgery has the highest rate of cure for cancer as a single modality among all available treatments in part due to the acceptance of a relatively high risk of injury and even complications. Similarly, radiation therapy may be able to increase its potential cure rate with a concomitant acceptance of appropriate risk of normal tissue injury and, importantly, a new or better understanding of tissue repair after focal ablative injury.

Ablation from a radiotherapy perspective is providing dose intensity great enough to both suspend cellular proliferation (e.g., stop a tumor from growing) and disrupt cellular and tissue function. While all normal tissues provide a necessary function, most tumors do not (with rare exceptions such as a functioning pituitary adenoma). The required dose potency to disrupt function is considerably greater than that for stopping proliferation. Delivering such doses, then, will have higher probability of controlling tumor growth even up to the range of surgical success. While this is a much-desired effect, the user should be reminded that normal tissues receiving ablative range dose may not function either temporarily or permanently. With focal ablative dose deposition, the injury to normal tissue structure and function may be severe, as is seen with many surgeries. Yet it is no accident that the overall therapeutic ratio comparing benefit to harm for SABR is on par with and often exceeds that of surgery. The ablative potential of SABR warrants special consideration not derived or modeled from less impactful conventionally fractionated radiotherapy.

Acceptable level of risk depends on the specified harm. For a catastrophic toxicity such as a permanent spinal cord injury, 1% risk in 10 years may be suitable. For damage to a limited part of an organ unlikely to have clinically apparent consequences, the acceptable risk will be much higher. Acceptable level of risk also depends on various factors including patient characteristics, intent of therapy (e.g., curative versus palliative), expected natural history of the disease, and the time frame of injury being considered. Acceptable risk for an otherwise healthy patient with an aggressive malignancy receiving treatment with curative intent may be vastly different from that for a frail patient with an indolent tumor receiving palliative therapy. The level of risk is, thus, an individualized assessment for the patient and treatment being planned.

When tumor ablation is the primary goal, the treatment cannot, and should not, always be "safe." The previous historical context of conventionally fractionated radiotherapy did not allow for injury. But to maximize the chance to eradicate disease, a significant risk of normal tissue injury must be a part of the equation. Radiation oncologists often view injury to the patient as treatment failure as it is harm caused directly by the treatment delivered. A recurrence, on the other hand, is often considered an inevitable possibility of the cancer diagnosis and intrinsic to the disease itself. In reality, recurrence of cancer, or failure to cure, can be a much larger threat to the patient's well-being and cause of ongoing morbidity than a possible injury from radiation treatment that is successful in eradicating the disease. Two questions need to be considered when delivering radiotherapy: (1) Will the radiation dose/fractionation kill the tumor? (2) To what extent will the dose/fractionation irreversibly damage normal tissue (i.e., if injuries occur, will they subsequently heal)? A better understanding of how and how likely normal tissue injury and repair occur can facilitate risk assessment of debilitating or permanent injury in relation to a chance for cure.

FACTORS AFFECTING TISSUE INJURY AND HEALING

Multiple factors affect normal tissue tolerance to radiotherapy. Total dose and fraction size are well-recognized factors. Patient characteristics including age and comorbid conditions such as diabetes and smoking status also determine the tissue's ability to withstand or heal from radiation injury. More recently, studies have investigated the role of genetic profiles to determine an individual patient's radiosensitivity, which has the potential to personalize treatment while minimizing the probability of toxicity.[3] Concurrent therapy such as antiangiogenic or immunosuppressive agents may also impact the ability of injured tissues to repair. Lastly, the structure and organization of the specific organ being injured is a critical determinant of normal tissue damage.

STRUCTURAL ORGANIZATION AND REGENERATIVE POTENTIAL OF TISSUE AND THEIR RELATIONSHIP TO RADIATION INJURY

Organs have been described as being composed of functional subunits consisting of a large population of well-differentiated functional cells and a smaller population of clonogenic cells.[4] This formalism describes two types of functional subunits, namely, structurally defined with discrete anatomical architecture and structurally undefined with monotonous architecture without anatomical boundaries. Lung is an example of a structurally defined organ with the alveolus/capillary complex as its smallest functional subunit responsible for exchanging oxygen with carbon dioxide. In this setting, clonogens can generally migrate within a functional subunit but not between subunits due to anatomic barriers (e.g., basement membranes).[5] Esophagus is an example of a structurally undefined organ with the entire organ acting as a conduit for nutrients. In such organs, clonogens can freely migrate along the entire length of the structure, only limited by the physical distance.[5] Tissues made up of predominantly structurally defined functional subunits are called parallel functioning tissues, characterized by independent redundancy (peripheral lung, liver, kidney, etc.), whereas tissues made up of predominantly structurally undefined functional subunits are called serial functioning tissues, characterized by a "chain" of function (gastrointestinal tract, spinal cord, etc.). An organ can have both a parallel and a serial functioning component. Lung, kidney, liver, and breast all have large conduits (e.g., bronchi, duct), splitting into smaller conduits (e.g., bronchioles, ductules), ending in terminal structures (e.g., alveoli, acini). In such branching tubular structure, the larger conduits can behave like serial tissue, while the terminal structures behave like parallel tissue. Linear tubular structures such as the bowel tend to behave like a serial tissue throughout. Radiation organ damage is closely related to the cumulative damage of the constituent functional subunits.

For parallel tissues, radiation-induced toxicity is volume related, where each functional subunit is damaged at a relatively low dose and damage is mostly an all-or-none phenomenon. As a result, overall toxicity is determined by the number of units damaged, not the degree of damage to each unit, and metrics such as V20 (the volume getting 20 Gy or more) become relevant. Clinically, the most critical component is the tissue volume outside the threshold dose (remaining functional tissue). This is because, for many of the parallel organs, such as the lung, liver, or kidney, there is intrinsic functional reserve. How much tissue can sustain a permanent injury while maintaining adequate organ function? This is the underlying question behind the critical volume model.[6,7] An absolute volume of parallel organ must be spared to avoid dysfunction.[8] Evidence comes from surgical series elucidating the amount of healthy organ required to preserve function (e.g., volume of lung or liver left after resection). When treating tumors within or near parallel tissues, the key is to deliver higher tumor doses by going to extreme measures to limit the volume of normal tissue exposed to a threshold dose that disables the constituent functional subunits. This is the reason why technology can dramatically improve outcomes for parallel tissues as high targeting accuracy and smaller irradiated volumes can prevent reaching a critical volume of normal tissue beyond which unrepaired toxicity ensues.

For serial tissues, on the other hand, toxicity is mostly dose related. Damage to a section of a serial organ can render the entire downstream organ dysfunctional, and metrics such as maximum dose, or "critical dose", become relevant. The spinal cord is a prime example, where the maximum point dose has been shown to be the most significant factor associated with myelopathy after SABR.[9] When treating tumors within or near serial functioning tissues, the key is to limit the organ from exposure to the critical dose, and the delivery of higher tumor doses generally requires fractionation. As a result, technology may only modestly improve outcomes as steeper gradients and smaller margins can help avoid injury to nearby critical structures but cannot avoid damage to critical structures directly adjacent to or within the target.

The ability of the organ to regenerate also plays a key role in estimating tissue tolerance to ablative doses.[10]

For example, mucosal injury to the rectum, a serial organ, can undergo repair through stem cell repopulation. The ability to repair depends on the extent of the mucosal and vascular damage. If there are sufficient neighboring viable stem cells that can migrate to the sites of damage, as well as adequate functional vasculature and stroma to promote effective angiogenesis and recruitment of immune mediators, permanent damage can be avoided. Unlike surgery, where a part of an organ can be removed and continuity restored by reconstruction, radiation cannot reestablish continuity of tissue. As such, even in tissues that may be amenable to repair, it is critical to avoid circumferential irradiation of tubular structures to allow for sparing of nearby clonogens. For regenerating serial tissue, critical volume or circumferential length of tissue leading to injury beyond repair may be clinically relevant parameters, in addition to the classic critical dose.[10] Interestingly, the degree of circumferential length is not a parameter routinely mined from a dose–volume histogram (DVH), the source medical physicists and radiation oncologists routinely use for safety assessments. For SABR repair considerations, the radiation oncologist must make assessments beyond DVH analysis.

Liver is a good example of a parallel organ with regenerative potential. After radiation-induced injury, the remaining functional liver can slowly undergo hyperplasia to compensate for the lost reserve. Dose–volume relationship and the importance of sparing enough volume of functional liver is well recognized for both conventionally fractionated radiotherapy and SABR.[11,12] For regenerating parallel tissue such as the liver, the critical volume needing to be spared may be lower relative to a much slower-to-regenerate parallel tissue such as the lung parenchyma. It is important to consider the complexity of the organ architecture, as even in a regenerating parallel organ such as the liver, increased dose to the central biliary tract, a serial tissue within the confines of the liver, may be associated with increased risk of toxicity to SABR.[13]

CURRENT UNDERSTANDING OF NORMAL TISSUE TOLERANCE TO STEREOTACTIC ABLATIVE RADIOTHERAPY

The linear quadratic model has been a useful tool for estimating normal tissue effects of conventionally fractionated radiotherapy. However, the parameters for the linear quadratic model were derived from data of conventional fractionation, and therefore may not be generalizable to ablative doses used in SABR. The model predicts a continuously bending curve between dose and the log of the proportion of surviving cells, when in fact, experimental data suggest a less damaging linear relationship in the high-dose range. As a result, the linear quadratic model tends to overestimate the effects of radiation in the high doses commonly use in SABR. This, in part, led to a cautious approach to the study of SABR in its infancy, often leading to a failure to control tumors within a viable therapeutic window.

To address the discrepancy in the model to describe SABR treatment, Park and colleagues introduced a novel survival curve that hybridizes the linear quadratic model for the low-dose range and the multitarget model asymptote for the high-dose range called the universal survival curve.[14] The model has been validated using published parameters of the linear quadratic and multitarget models to better represent the experimentally derived in vitro data of survival in ablative ranges.[14] Although it is yet to be determined whether the universal survival curve is superior to the linear quadratic model in reflecting real world clinical outcomes,[15] it has allowed for clinically plausible predictions of normal tissue tolerance as well as direct comparisons of SABR fractionation schemes. Moreover, it has provided predictive insight navigating clinical trials, pushing the limits of both dose and clinical indications such as the many important cooperative group studies (e.g., RTOG and NRG) that guide clinical care.

Ideally, normal tissue tolerance dose parameters should be derived based on outcomes data from well-designed prospective studies with valid statistical assessment. Unfortunately, these data are not available for the vast majority of clinical scenarios, and as a result, interpolation of data using models such as the universal survival curve is incorporated in practice. An overview of hypofractionation published in 2008 with accompanying dose guidelines formulated at UT Southwestern Medical Center as a starting point has been cited by more than 250 articles and used as a reference in many clinical trials.[16] As data continue to accumulate on the outcomes associated with SABR treatments, dose–response modeling of commonly encountered normal tissues has been attempted.[17–26] In addition, the American Association of Physicists in Medicine (AAPM) has created a working group on the biological effects of hypofractionated radiotherapy/SABR akin to QUAN-TEC for conventionally fractionated radiotherapy. The project, named HyTEC (Hypofractionated Treatment Effects in the Clinic), is an ongoing process with reports published regarding normal tissue tolerance of the optic pathway, lung, liver, and spinal cord, with plans for additional organs in the near future.[12,27–29] At UT Southwestern Medical Center, the dose guidelines originally published in 2008 have been continuously updated with accumulated clinical experience. Based on the best estimation of single fraction treatment toxicity (from animal studies and intra-operative radiotherapy data), conventional fractionation toxicity, and available data of SABR treatment toxicity, dose

parameters to organs at risk have been generated for each fraction number. Normal tissue dose guidelines for SABR and hypofractionated radiotherapy are presented in Tables 2.3 and 2.4, respectively. The dose parameters for a select group of normal tissues are discussed below.

Spinal Cord

The spinal cord is a classic non-regenerating serial organ with injury closely linked to a critical dose irrespective of volume that is irradiated. In a recent review of the literature on outcomes of de novo SABR delivered in 1 to 5 fractions, the following spinal cord point maximum doses (D_{max}) were estimated to be associated with a 1% to 5% risk of radiation myelopathy: 12.4 to 14.0 Gy in 1 fraction, 17.0 Gy in 2 fractions, 20.3 Gy in 3 fractions, 23.0 Gy in 4 fractions, and 25.3 Gy in 5 fractions.[29] These values are slightly less than point D_{max} used at UT Southwestern Medical Center: 14 Gy in 1 fraction, 18.3 Gy in 2 fractions, 22.5 Gy in 3 fractions, 25.6 Gy in 4 fractions, and 28 Gy in 5 fractions. In the same review, outcomes in patients with prior history of radiation were analyzed. Factors associated with a lower risk of radiation myelopathy from re-irradiation SABR included cumulative thecal sac equivalent doses in 2 Gy fractions with an alpha/beta of 2 (EQD2$_2$) $D_{max} \leq 70$ Gy, SABR thecal sac EQD2$_2$ $D_{max} \leq 25$ Gy, thecal sac SABR EQD2$_2$ D_{max} to cumulative EQD2$_2$ D_{max} ratio of ≤ 0.5, and a minimum time interval to reirradiation of ≥ 5 months.[29]

Optic Structures

Similar to the spinal cord, optic structures are considered a non-regenerating serial organ. A pooled analysis of 34 studies including 1,578 patients showed that D_{max} of 10 Gy in 1 fraction, 20 Gy in 3 fractions, and 25 Gy in 5 fractions yield less than a 1% chance of radiation-induced optic nerve or chiasm neuropathy.[27] As expected, prior irradiation to the area was associated with an increase in the risk of neuropathy, estimated to be approximately 10-fold. In a normal tissue complication probability modeling study of 262 patients not included in the previously mentioned pooled analysis, the D_{max} limits were similar: 12.7 Gy in 1 fraction, 17.5 Gy for 2 fractions, 20.9 Gy in 3 fractions, 23.7 Gy in 4 fractions, and 26.1 Gy in 5 fractions.[17] Point D_{max} used at UT Southwestern Medical Center is slightly more conservative: 10 Gy in 1 fraction, 17.4 Gy in 3 fractions, and 25 Gy in 5 fractions.

Rectum

Rectum is considered a serial regenerating organ in regard to mucosal injury. Both the extent of the depletion of viable stem cells and the destruction of vasculature and

TABLE 2.3 UT Southwestern Normal Tissue Dose Guidelines for Stereotactic Ablative Radiotherapy/Stereotactic Body Radiotherapy

Number of Fractions		One Fraction		Two Fractions		Three Fractions		Four Fractions		Five Fractions		Endpoint (≥Grade 3)
Organ	Volume/Parameter	Volume Max (Gy)	Max Point Dose (Gy)**	Volume Max (Gy)	Max Point Dose (Gy)**	Volume Max (Gy)	Max Point Dose (Gy)**	Volume Max (Gy)	Max Point Dose (Gy)**	Volume Max (Gy)	Max Point Dose (Gy)**	
Serial Tissue												
Optic pathway	<0.2 cc	8 Gy	10 Gy	11.7 Gy	13.7 Gy	15.3 Gy	17.4 Gy	19.2 Gy	21.2 Gy	23 Gy	25 Gy	Neuritis
Cochlea			9 Gy		11.7 Gy		14.4 Gy		18 Gy		22 Gy	Hearing loss
Brainstem (not medulla)	<0.5 cc	10 Gy	15 Gy	13 Gy	19.1 Gy	15.9 Gy	23.1 Gy	20.8 Gy	27.2 Gy	23 Gy	31 Gy	Cranial neuropathy
Spinal cord and medulla	<0.35 cc	10 Gy	14 Gy	13 Gy	18.3 Gy	15.9 Gy	22.5 Gy	18 Gy	25.6 Gy	22 Gy	28 Gy	Myelitis
Cauda equina	<5 cc	14 Gy	16 Gy	18 Gy	20.8 Gy	21.9 Gy	25.5 Gy	26 Gy	28.8 Gy	30 Gy	31.5 Gy	Neuritis
Sacral plexus	<5 cc	14.4 Gy	16 Gy	18.5 Gy	20.8 Gy	22.5 Gy	25.5 Gy	26 Gy	28.8 Gy	30 Gy	32 Gy	Neuropathy
Esophagus*	<5 cc	20 Gy	24 Gy	24.3 Gy	28.3 Gy	27.9 Gy	32.4 Gy	30.4 Gy	35.6 Gy	32.5 Gy	38 Gy	Esophagitis
Brachial plexus	<3 cc	13.6 Gy	16.4 Gy	17.8 Gy	21.2 Gy	22 Gy	26 Gy	24.8 Gy	29.6 Gy	27 Gy	32.5 Gy	Neuropathy
Peripheral (named) nerve	<2 cm length	16 Gy	20 Gy	21 Gy	25.5 Gy	25.5 Gy	30.6 Gy	28.8 Gy	34.8 Gy	31.5 Gy	38 Gy	Neuropathy
Heart/pericardium	<15 cc	16 Gy	22 Gy	20 Gy	26 Gy	24 Gy	30 Gy	28 Gy	34 Gy	32 Gy	38 Gy	Pericarditis
Great vessels	<10 cc	31 Gy	37 Gy	35 Gy	41 Gy	39 Gy	45 Gy	43 Gy	49 Gy	47 Gy	53 Gy	Aneurysm
Trachea and large bronchus*	<4 cc	27.5 Gy	30 Gy	34.5 Gy	38 Gy	39 Gy	43 Gy	42.4 Gy	47 Gy	45 Gy	50 Gy	Impairment of pulmonary toilet
Bronchus-smaller airways	<0.5 cc	17.4 Gy	20.2 Gy	21.6 Gy	25.1 Gy	25.8 Gy	30 Gy	28.8 Gy	34.8 Gy	32 Gy	40 Gy	Stenosis with atelectasis
Rib	<5 cc	28 Gy	33 Gy	34 Gy	41.5 Gy	40 Gy	50 Gy	43 Gy	54 Gy	45 Gy	57 Gy	Pain or fracture
Skin	<10 cc	25.5 Gy	27.5 Gy	28.3 Gy	30.3 Gy	31 Gy	33 Gy	33.6 Gy	36 Gy	36.5 Gy	38.5 Gy	Ulceration
Stomach	<5 cc	17.4 Gy	22 Gy	20 Gy	26 Gy	22.5 Gy	30 Gy	25 Gy	33.2 Gy	26.5 Gy	35 Gy	Ulceration/fistula
Bile duct			30 Gy		33 Gy		36 Gy		38.4 Gy		41 Gy	Stenosis
Duodenum*	<5 cc	17.4 Gy	22 Gy	20 Gy	26 Gy	22.5 Gy	30 Gy	25 Gy	33.2 Gy	26.5 Gy	35 Gy	Ulceration
Jejunum/ileum*	<30 cc	17.6 Gy	20 Gy	19.2 Gy	24 Gy	20.7 Gy	28.5 Gy	22.4 Gy	31.6 Gy	24 Gy	34.5 Gy	Enteritis/obstruction

(continued)

TABLE 2.3   UT Southwestern Normal Tissue Dose Guidelines for Stereotactic Ablative Radiotherapy/Stereotactic Body Radiotherapy *(Continued)*

Number of Fractions	One Fraction	Two Fractions	Three Fractions	Four Fractions	Five Fractions	Endpoint (≥Grade 3)
Colon*	<20 cc	20.5 Gy	25.8 Gy	28.8 Gy	30.8 Gy	32.5 Gy	Colitis/fistula
		31 Gy	39 Gy	45 Gy	48.5 Gy	52.5 Gy	
Rectum*	<3.5 cc	30 Gy	38 Gy	43 Gy	47.2 Gy	50 Gy	Proctitis/fistula
	<20 cc	33.7 Gy	41.3 Gy	47 Gy	51.6 Gy	55 Gy	
		23 Gy	26.7 Gy	30.3 Gy	34 Gy	37.5 Gy	
Ureter		35 Gy	37.5 Gy	40 Gy	43 Gy	45 Gy	Stenosis
Bladder wall	<15 cc	12 Gy	14.5 Gy	17 Gy	18.5 Gy	20 Gy	Cystitis/fistula
		25 Gy	29 Gy	33 Gy	35.6 Gy	38 Gy	
Penile bulb	<3 cc	16 Gy	20.5 Gy	25 Gy	27 Gy	30 Gy	Impotence
Femoral heads	<10 cc	15 Gy	19.5 Gy	24 Gy	27 Gy	30 Gy	Necrosis
Renal hilum/vascular trunk	15 cc	14 Gy	16.8 Gy	19.5 Gy	21.5 Gy	23 Gy	Malignant hypertension
Parallel Tissue							
Lung (right and left)	1500 cc (male), 950 cc (female)***	7.2 Gy	9.4 Gy	10.8 Gy	12 Gy	12.5 Gy	Basic lung function
Lung (right and left)	Other parameter	V8Gy <37%	V10 Gy <37%	V11.4 Gy<37%	V12.8 Gy<37%	V13.5 Gy<37%	Pneumonitis
Liver	700 cc***	11.6 Gy	15.1 Gy	17.7 Gy	19.6 Gy	21.5 Gy	Basic liver function
Renal cortex (right and left)	200 cc***	9.5 Gy	12.5 Gy	14.7 Gy	16 Gy	17.5 Gy	Basic renal function

*Avoid circumferential irradiation.
**"Point" defined as 0.035 cc or less.
***Or one third of the "native" total organ volume (prior to any resection or volume reducing disease), whichever is greater.

| TABLE 2.4 | | UT Southwestern Normal Tissue Dose Guidelines for Hypofractionated Radiotherapy | | | | | | |

Number of Fractions		Ten Fractions		Fifteen Fractions		Twenty Fractions		Endpoint (≥Grade 3)
Organ	Volume/ Parameter	Volume Max (Gy)	Max Point Dose (Gy)	Volume Max (Gy)	Max Point Dose (Gy)	Volume Max (Gy)	Max Point Dose (Gy)	
Serial Tissue								
Optic pathway	<0.5 cc	30.6 Gy	33.1 Gy	39 Gy	42 Gy	42 Gy	48 Gy	Neuritis
Eye (retina)	Mean dose	<26 Gy	30 Gy	<33 Gy	37.5 Gy	<36 Gy	42 Gy	Retinitis
Lens		7 Gy		9 Gy		10 Gy		Cataract
Eyelid—meibomian glands (one side)		21.3 Gy		27 Gy		30 Gy		Dry eye syndrome
Lacrimal gland (one side)	<1 cc	14.1 Gy	23.6 Gy	18 Gy	30 Gy	18 Gy	32 Gy	Lack of tears
Cochlea	<0.5 cc	25 Gy	27 Gy	30 Gy	33 Gy	32 Gy	36 Gy	Hearing loss
Brainstem (not medulla)	<5 cc	32 Gy	38 Gy	40 Gy	44 Gy	44 Gy	50 Gy	Cranial neuropathy
Spinal cord	<5 cc	31 Gy	36 Gy	39 Gy	42.0 Gy	42 Gy	46 Gy	Myelitis
Salivary gland (one side)	<7 cc Mean dose	14.1 Gy <17.7 Gy	21.3 Gy	18 Gy <22.5 Gy	27 Gy	18 Gy <24 Gy	30 Gy	Xerostomia
Larynx	<3 cc	30 Gy	45 Gy	34.5 Gy	52.5 Gy	36 Gy	58 Gy	Necrosis/edema
Temporomandibular joint	<1 cc	37.7 Gy	41.4 Gy	48 Gy	52.5 Gy	52 Gy	58 Gy	Inflammation
Cauda equina	<5 cc	35 Gy	41 Gy	40.5 Gy	48 Gy	44 Gy	52 Gy	Neuritis
Sacral plexus	<5 cc	35 Gy	41 Gy	40.5 Gy	48 Gy	44 Gy	52 Gy	Neuropathy
Esophagus	<5 cc	40 Gy	48 Gy	45 Gy	54 Gy	48 Gy	58 Gy	Esophagitis
Brachial plexus	<3 cc	37 Gy	43 Gy	48 Gy	52.5 Gy	54 Gy	58 Gy	Neuropathy
Heart/pericardium	<15 cc	36.6 Gy	42.5 Gy	42 Gy	48.9 Gy	46 Gy	52 Gy	Pericarditis
Great vessels	<10 cc	55.7 Gy	62.9 Gy	57 Gy	65 Gy	60 Gy	70 Gy	Aneurysm
Trachea and large bronchus	<5 cc	52 Gy	59 Gy	55.5 Gy	63 Gy	58 Gy	66 Gy	Impairment of pulmonary toilet
Skin	<10 cc	46.3 Gy	48.9 Gy	54 Gy	57 Gy	60 Gy	64 Gy	Ulceration
Stomach	<50 cc	33.9 Gy	45 Gy	39 Gy	51 Gy	42 Gy	54 Gy	Ulceration/fistula
Duodenum	<5 cc	33.9 Gy	45 Gy	39 Gy	51 Gy	42 Gy	54 Gy	Ulceration
Jejunum/ileum	<120 cc	33.9 Gy	41 Gy	39 Gy	46.5 Gy	42 Gy	50 Gy	Enteritis/ obstruction
Renal hilum/vascular trunk	15 cc	30.7 Gy		37.5 Gy		40 Gy		Malignant hypertension
Colon	<20 cc	47 Gy	60 Gy	47 Gy	64.5 Gy	50 Gy	66 Gy	Colitis/fistula
Rectum (including stool)	<10 cc <20 cc <30 cc <40 cc	52 Gy 49 Gy 46 Gy 43 Gy	65 Gy	60 Gy 57 Gy 52.5 Gy 49.5 Gy	70.5 Gy	66 Gy 62 Gy 58 Gy 54 Gy	74 Gy	Proctitis/fistula
Bladder (with urine)	<90 cc <125 cc	48 Gy 45 Gy	53 Gy	55.5 Gy 52.5 Gy	61.5 Gy	60 Gy 56 Gy	66 Gy	Cystitis/fistula
Bladder (suprapubic wall)	<5 cc	23 Gy	42 Gy	26 Gy	48 Gy	28 Gy	52 Gy	Dysuria

(continued)

TABLE 2.4	UT Southwestern Normal Tissue Dose Guidelines for Hypofractionated Radiotherapy (*Continued*)						
Number of Fractions		**Ten Fractions**		**Fifteen Fractions**	**Twenty Fractions**		**Endpoint (≥Grade 3)**
Penile bulb	<3 cc	38 Gy	44 Gy	42 Gy	48 Gy	44 Gy	52 Gy	Impotence
Femoral Heads	<10 cc	38 Gy	43.5 Gy	40 Gy	46.5 Gy	44 Gy	50 Gy	Necrosis
Parallel Tissue							
Lung (right and left) minus GTV	1500 cc (male), 950 cc (female)*	15 Gy		16.5 Gy		18 Gy		Basic lung function
Lung (right and left) minus GTV	Other parameter	V16 Gy <37%		V18 Gy <37%		V19 Gy <37%		Pneumonitis
Liver minus GTV	700 cc*	27 Gy		30 Gy		32 Gy		Basic liver function
Renal cortex (right and left)	200 cc*	21 Gy		24 Gy		26 Gy		Basic renal function

GTV, gross tumor volume.
*Or one third of the "native" total organ volume (prior to any resection or volume reducing disease), whichever is greater.

stroma are relevant to the ability of the tissue to regenerate. In an analysis of early-phase trials of SABR for localized prostate cancer treated to 45 to 50 Gy in 5 fractions at UT Southwestern Medical Center, >3 cc receiving 50 Gy or more and >35% circumference of the rectal wall receiving 39 Gy or more were strongly correlated with grade 3+ rectal toxicity.[30] The trials were designed to spare the adjacent lateral and posterior rectal wall to allow for clonal stem cells to migrate into sites of damage in the anterior wall. The 39-Gy constraint to the third of the circumference of the rectum may represent the stem cell depleting dose and the distance requirement of adjacent stem cells to be able to migrate into the site of injury. The 50-Gy constraint to a critical volume may represent the dose sufficient to devitalize the tissue (i.e., destroy the vasculature and/or stroma) to prevent any repair. Current 5-fraction parameters for rectum at UT Southwestern Medical Center are V37.5 Gy < 20 cc and V50 Gy < 3.5 cc.

Lung

Lung is an extremely slowly regenerating parallel organ. In a pooled analysis of 97 studies, radiation-induced lung toxicity including radiation pneumonitis and pulmonary fibrosis was associated with size and location of tumor. As a general guideline, studies reported safe treatment with acceptable rates of symptomatic lung toxicity (10%–15%) after lung SABR when the mean lung dose of the bilateral lungs was kept ≤8 Gy in 3 to 5 fractions and V20 < 10% to 15%.[28] At UT Southwestern Medical Center, mean dose is not considered a meaningful parameter in evaluating risk to all but very small organs. Instead, residual viable lung tissue (i.e., lung kept below a threshold dose leading to toxicity) is deemed critical. For example, dose to at least 1,500 cc (male)/950 cc (female) or a third, whichever is greater, of normal lung is kept at or below 10.8 Gy and 12.5 Gy for 3- and 5-fraction SABRs, respectively. In addition, the plan aims to keep V11.4 Gy and V13.5 Gy <37% of the lung volume for 3- and 5-fraction treatments, respectively.

Liver

Liver is a regenerating parallel organ. The QUANTEC liver report recommends mean liver dose <13 Gy in 3 fractions and <18 Gy in 6 fractions for primary disease and <15 Gy in 3 fractions and <20 Gy in 6 fractions for metastatic lesions.[31] Again, at UT Southwestern Medical Center, critical volume dose parameters are considered in favor of mean dose limits. The recommended dose–volume parameter for the liver per QUATENC is ≥700 mL of normal liver receiving ≤15 Gy in 3 to 5 fractions for ≤5% risk of radiation-induced liver disease.[31] In a recent update with normal tissue complication probability modeling based on 12 studies, QUANTEC recommendations were deemed reasonable with acceptable grade 3 liver enzyme toxicity risk (<20%) for the mean liver dose constraint and ≥grade 3 gastrointestinal toxicity risk (<10%) for the normal liver volume constraint.[12] At UT Southwestern Medical Center, dose to at least 700 cc (or a third, whichever is greater) of normal liver is constrained to 17.7 Gy and 21.5 Gy for 3- and 5-fraction treatments, respectively.

CONCURRENT THERAPY AND ITS EFFECTS ON NORMAL TISSUE TOLERANCE TO RADIOTHERAPY

Concurrent treatments with radiotherapy that can alter the degree of normal tissue injury or repair can have an impact on observed toxicity. An essential component of wound healing is new blood vessel formation, and reports from the surgical literature suggest that agents affecting angiogenesis, such as anti-vascular endothelial growth factor (VEGF) therapy (e.g., bevacizumab) or multi-receptor tyrosine kinase inhibitors (e.g., sorafenib), can lead to an increase in wound complications following tissue injury.[32,33] Similar effects may be at play when these agents are used during or within a few months of SABR. In a series of 74 patients treated with SABR to the abdomen, of whom 20 patients received VEGF inhibitor, the rate of serious bowel injury for those who received VEGF inhibitor therapy within 3 months of SABR was 38% versus 0% for those without VEGF inhibition.[34] Severe gastrointestinal toxicity has also been associated with concurrent sorafenib and SABR to the liver in patients with hepatocellular carcinoma.[35] In addition, possible increase in toxicity has been observed with SABR in conjunction with epidermal growth factor receptor (EGFR) inhibitors such as gefitinib and erlotinib, which have antiangiogenic properties.[36] Interestingly, a significant increase in toxicity has not been found with stereotactic treatments and VEGF inhibitors in non-regenerating organs such as the brain or spinal cord, where angiogenesis and wound repair may not play a major role in normal tissue tolerance.[37,38] Further research is needed to elucidate the precise effects of antiangiogenic and targeted therapies on normal tissue tolerance to SABR, as it may be both site- and agent-specific. In patients receiving or expected to receive such agents, stricter dose recommendations may be required to avoid serious complications.

Conversely, the use of radioprotectors may be a viable strategy to increase the therapeutic ratio of radiotherapy. Most radioprotectors are antioxidants that can mitigate cell damage from free radicals generated by ionizing radiation. The only radioprotector approved by the U.S. Food and Drug Administration for use in patients receiving therapeutic radiotherapy is amifostine, to reduce xerostomia in the setting of head and neck cancer.[39] However, its clinical use has been limited with conflicting data on its benefit in decreasing toxicity such as oral mucositis or esophagitis.[40] Despite decades of research and a myriad of potential candidates including nitroxides, sulfhydryl compounds, vitamins, hormones, DNA binding agents, and cytokines, no other radioprotector has been shown to be of clinical utility to date.[39] One limitation has been achieving high enough concentrations of radioprotector at the time of radiation exposure given the short half-life of free radicals and narrow therapeutic window of some of the agents.

In the setting of SABR, where local control is excellent with sufficient doses delivered, treatment is often constrained by the normal tissue tolerance of nearby serial functioning critical structures. Given the small number of fractions required for SABR versus conventionally fractionated radiotherapy, more invasive methods to deliver or instill radioprotective agents to adjacent normal tissues timed with radiotherapy may enable high-dose ablation.[41]

FUTURE DIRECTIONS

Accurate delineation of normal tissue injury risk from SABR is a work in progress. Currently available data, largely derived from retrospective analyses, have multiple limitations: nonuniform treatment delivery, follow-up, and reporting; selection bias of patients receiving treatment; and variable dose constraints imposed affecting the range of doses delivered to normal tissue. Well-conducted prospective dose-escalation phase I studies with uniform treatment context, patient eligibility, and delivery method are needed to accurately characterize the grade and timing of acute and late toxicities as well as estimate dose–volume parameters. Because such studies are not feasible or practical for many disease sites, uniform reporting standards should be developed and followed for each organ at risk to allow for aggregation of accurate data. Such efforts are currently under way as part of HyTEC. Innovative ways to evaluate and predict radiation-related tissue damage using advanced imaging techniques such as magnetic resonance imaging or virtual endoscopy will also improve our understanding of normal tissue tolerance.[42] More fundamentally, studies to elucidate the radiobiological mechanisms of radiation injury to SABR dose ranges, including the complex interplay between direct damage to the tissue and the vasculature, are urgently needed. Further investigation of the molecular pathways responsible for wound repair and stem cell regeneration, as well as the role of chemical and biological modifiers to radiation damage, will allow for maximizing the curative potential of radiotherapy while minimizing normal tissue toxicity.

CONCLUSIONS

Normal tissue injury is a necessary part of ablative treatments aimed at eradicating disease in the treatment of patients with cancer. A shift in perspective and acceptance of appropriate level of risk may augment the therapeutic potential of radiotherapy, especially in the setting of SABR. A better understanding of the structure and function of organs at risk, mechanisms of normal tissue damage and repair, and modifiers of radiosensitivity and regeneration of tissue will be critical as the field takes another quantum leap of progress.

KEY POINTS

● Technological advancement including intensity-modulated radiotherapy, image-guided radiotherapy, and stereotactic ablative radiotherapy has enabled more precise targeting of tumor and sparing of adjacent normal tissues.

● QUANTEC provides valuable and practical normal tissue dose parameters for conventionally fractionated radiotherapy (Table 2.1).

● A shift in perception is necessary to accept an appropriate level of risk of normal tissue injury from radiotherapy to maximize the potential for cure, especially in the setting of stereotactic ablative radiotherapy.

● A better understanding of normal tissue structural organization, factors affecting the degree of radiation injury and repair, and concurrent treatments altering radiosensitivity will be critical in widening the therapeutic ratio of radiotherapy.

● Normal tissue dose guidelines derived from modeling and available clinical data for stereotactic ablative radiotherapy and hypofractionated radiotherapy at UT Southwestern Medical Center are shown in Tables 2.3 and 2.4, respectively.

REVIEW QUESTIONS

1. Which of the following is false regarding parallel functioning tissues?
   A. Peripheral lung, liver, and kidney are examples of parallel functioning tissues.
   B. Technology to improve accuracy of radiation delivery can dramatically improve normal tissue outcomes.
   C. Radiation-related toxicity is mostly volume dependent (i.e., critical volume spared of a threshold dose is important).
   D. Clonogens capable of rescuing injured tissue can migrate within and between subunits
   E. Organs can have both a parallel functioning component and a serial functioning component.

2. Which of the following is false regarding serial functioning tissues?
   A. Clonogens capable of rescuing injured tissue can migrate along the entire length of the structure, limited only by the physical distance.
   B. Gastrointestinal tract and spinal cord are examples of serial functioning tissues.
   C. Circumferential length of tissue sustaining damage is not relevant for a regenerating serial tissue.
   D. Technology to improve accuracy of radiation delivery may only modestly improve normal tissue outcomes.
   E. Radiation-related toxicity is mostly dose dependent (i.e., critical dose, regardless of volume treated, is important).

3. What is the recommended volume of normal liver receiving ≤15 Gy in 3 to 5 fractions to limit the risk of radiation-induced liver dysfunction to ≤5%?
   A. ≥400 mL
   B. ≥700 mL
   C. ≥1,000 mL
   D. ≥1,200 mL
   E. ≥1,500 mL

4. In reviewing treatment plans for stereotactic ablative radiotherapy to the spine, which combination of spinal cord maximum point doses would be acceptable for treatment in 1, 3, and 5 fractions, respectively, to limit the risk of radiation myelopathy to ≤5%?
   A. 12 Gy, 18 Gy, 25 Gy
   B. 10 Gy, 24 Gy, 29 Gy
   C. 8 Gy, 23 Gy, 26 Gy
   D. 15 Gy, 17 Gy, 22 Gy
   E. 11 Gy, 21 Gy, 30 Gy

5. Which of the following agents, when given in conjunction with radiotherapy, has the potential to decrease radiation toxicity?
   A. Sorafenib
   B. Erlotinib
   C. Cisplatin
   D. Ipilimumab
   E. Amifostine

ANSWERS

1. **D** In parallel functioning tissues, clonogens can generally migrate within subunits but not between subunits due to anatomic barriers such as the basement membrane.[5]

2. **C** In addition to critical dose, circumferential length or critical volume of tissue leading to injury may be clinically important for regenerating serial tissues such as the rectum.[10]

3. **B** According to QUANTEC, ≥700 mL of normal liver should receive ≤15 Gy of stereotactic ablative radiotherapy to minimize the risk of radiation-induced liver disease.[31]

Normal tissue complication probability modeling confirms that the QUANTEC recommendation leads to acceptable gastrointestinal toxicity rates.[12]

4. **A** According to HyTEC, the recommended spinal cord D_{max} for stereotactic ablative radiotherapy in 1, 3, and 5 fractions are 12.4 to 14.0 Gy, 20.3 Gy, and 25.3 Gy, respectively.[29]

5. **E** Amifostine is the only U.S. Food and Drug Administration–approved radioprotector in the clinical setting.[39] Sorafenib, erlotinib, cisplatin, and ipilimumab have all been shown to potentially increase the risk of toxicity when used concurrently with radiotherapy.[35,36]

REFERENCES

1. Emami B, Lyman J, Brown A, et al. Tolerance of normal tissue to therapeutic irradiation. *Int J Radiat Oncol Biol Phys.* 1991; 21:109–122.

2. Marks LB, Yorke ED, Jackson A, et al. Use of normal tissue complication probability models in the clinic. *Int J Radiat Oncol Biol Phys.* 2010;76:S10–S19.

3. Barnett GC, West CML, Dunning AM, et al. Normal tissue reactions to radiotherapy: towards tailoring treatment dose by genotype. *Nat Rev Cancer.* 2009;9:134–142.

4. Wolbarst AB, Chin LM, Svensson GK. Optimization of radiation therapy: integral-response of a model biological system. *Int J Radiat Oncol Biol Phys.* 1982;8:1761–1769.

5. Timmerman R, Bastasch M, Saha D, et al. Stereotactic body radiation therapy: normal tissue and tumor control effects with large dose per fraction. *Front Radiat Ther Oncol.* 2011;43:382–394.

6. Yaes RJ, Kalend A. Local stem cell depletion model for radiation myelitis. *Int J Radiat Oncol Biol Phys.* 1988;14:1247–1259.

7. Niemierko A, Goitein M. Modeling of normal tissue response to radiation: the critical volume model. *Int J Radiat Oncol Biol Phys.* 1993;25:135–145.

8. Ritter TA, Matuszak M, Chetty IJ, et al. Application of critical volume-dose constraints for stereotactic body radiation therapy in NRG radiation therapy trials. *Int J Radiat Oncol Biol Phys.* 2017;98:34–36.

9. Wong CS, Fehlings MG, Sahgal A. Pathobiology of radiation myelopathy and strategies to mitigate injury. *Spinal Cord.* 2015;53:574–580.

10. Kim DWN, Medin PM, Timmerman RD. Emphasis on repair, not just avoidance of injury, facilitates prudent stereotactic ablative radiotherapy. *Semin Radiat Oncol.* 2017;27:378–392.

11. Dawson LA, Ten Haken RK. Partial volume tolerance of the liver to radiation. *Semin Radiat Oncol.* 2005;15:279–283.

12. Miften M, Vinogradskiy Y, Moiseenko V, et al. Radiation dose-volume effects for liver SBRT. *Int J Radiat Oncol Biol Phys.* 2021;110(1):196–205.

13. Toesca DAS, Osmundson EC, Eyben R von, et al. Central liver toxicity after SBRT: an expanded analysis and predictive nomogram. *Radiother Oncol.* 2017;122:130–136.

14. Park C, Papiez L, Zhang S, et al. Universal survival curve and single fraction equivalent dose: useful tools in understanding potency of ablative radiotherapy. *Int J Radiat Oncol Biol Phys.* 2008;70:847–852.

15. Brown JM, Carlson DJ, Brenner DJ. The tumor radiobiology of SRS and SBRT: are more than the 5 Rs involved? *Int J Radiat Oncol Biol Phys.* 2014;88:254–262.

16. Timmerman RD. An overview of hypofractionation and introduction to this issue of seminars in radiation oncology. *Semin Radiat Oncol.* 2008;18:215–222.

17. Hiniker SM, Modlin LA, Choi CY, et al. Dose-response modeling of the visual pathway tolerance to single-fraction and hypofractionated stereotactic radiosurgery. *Semin Radiat Oncol.* 2016;26:97–104.

18. Rashid A, Karam SD, Rashid B, et al. Multisession radiosurgery for hearing preservation. *Semin Radiat Oncol.* 2016;26:105–111.

19. Quan K, Xu KM, Zhang Y, et al. Toxicities following stereotactic ablative radiotherapy treatment of locally-recurrent and previously irradiated head and neck squamous cell carcinoma. *Semin Radiat Oncol.* 2016;26:112–119.

20. Nuyttens JJ, Moiseenko V, McLaughlin M, et al. Esophageal dose tolerance in patients treated with stereotactic body radiation therapy. *Semin Radiat Oncol.* 2016;26:120–128.

21. Kimsey F, McKay J, Gefter J, et al. Dose-response model for chest wall tolerance of stereotactic body radiation therapy. *Semin Radiat Oncol.* 2016;26:129–134.

22. Xue J, Kubicek G, Patel A, et al. Validity of current stereotactic body radiation therapy dose constraints for aorta and major vessels. *Semin Radiat Oncol.* 2016;26:135–139.

23. Duijm M, Schillemans W, Aerts JG, et al. Dose and volume of the irradiated main bronchi and related side effects in the treatment of central lung tumors with stereotactic radiotherapy. *Semin Radiat Oncol.* 2016;26:140–148.

24. Goldsmith C, Price P, Cross T, et al. Dose-volume histogram analysis of stereotactic body radiotherapy treatment of pancreatic cancer: a focus on duodenal dose constraints. *Semin Radiat Oncol.* 2016;26:149–156.

25. LaCouture TA, Xue J, Subedi G, et al. Small bowel dose tolerance for stereotactic body radiation therapy. *Semin Radiat Oncol.* 2016;26:157–164.

26. Grimm J, Sahgal A, Soltys SG, et al. Estimated risk level of unified stereotactic body radiation therapy dose tolerance limits for spinal cord. *Semin Radiat Oncol.* 2016;26:165–171.

27. Milano MT, Grimm J, Soltys SG, et al. Single- and multi-fraction stereotactic radiosurgery dose tolerances of the optic pathways. *Int J Radiat Oncol Biol Phys.* 2021;110(1):87–99.

28. Kong F-MS, Moiseenko V, Zhao J, et al. Organs at risk considerations for thoracic stereotactic body radiation therapy: what is safe for lung parenchyma? *Int J Radiat Oncol Biol Phys.* 2021;110(1):172–187.

29. Sahgal A, Chang JH, Ma L, et al. Spinal cord dose tolerance to stereotactic body radiation therapy. *Int J Radiat Oncol Biol Phys.* 2021;110(1):124–136.

30. Kim DWN, Cho LC, Straka C, et al. Predictors of rectal tolerance observed in a dose-escalated phase 1-2 trial of stereotactic body radiation therapy for prostate cancer. *Int J Radiat Oncol Biol Phys.* 2014;89:509–517.

31. Pan CC, Kavanagh BD, Dawson LA, et al. Radiation-associated liver injury. *Int J Radiat Oncol Biol Phys.* 2010;76:S94–S100.

32. Scappaticci FA, Fehrenbacher L, Cartwright T, et al. Surgical wound healing complications in metastatic colorectal cancer patients treated with bevacizumab. *J Surg Oncol.* 2005;91:173–180.

33. Chapin BF, Delacroix SE, Culp SH, et al. Safety of presurgical targeted therapy in the setting of metastatic renal cell carcinoma. *Eur Urol.* 2011;60:964–971.

34. Barney BM, Markovic SN, Laack NN, et al. Increased bowel toxicity in patients treated with a vascular endothelial growth factor inhibitor (VEGFI) after stereotactic body radiation therapy (SBRT). *Int J Radiat Oncol Biol Phys.* 2013;87:73–80.

35. Brade AM, Ng S, Brierley J, et al. Phase 1 trial of sorafenib and stereotactic body radiation therapy for hepatocellular carcinoma. *Int J Radiat Oncol Biol Phys.* 2016;94:580–587.

36. Iyengar P, Kavanagh BD, Wardak Z, et al. Phase II trial of stereotactic body radiation therapy combined with erlotinib for patients with limited but progressive metastatic non-small-cell lung cancer. *J Clin Oncol.* 2014;32:3824–3830.

37. Cabrera AR, Cuneo KC, Desjardins A, et al. Concurrent stereotactic radiosurgery and bevacizumab in recurrent malignant gliomas: a prospective trial. *Int J Radiat Oncol Biol Phys.* 2013;86:873–879.

38. Miller JA, Balagamwala EH, Angelov L, et al. Spine stereotactic radiosurgery with concurrent tyrosine kinase inhibitors for metastatic renal cell carcinoma. *J Neurosurg Spine.* 2016;25:766–774.

39. Mishra K, Alsbeih G. Appraisal of biochemical classes of radioprotectors: evidence, current status and guidelines for future development. *3 Biotech.* 2017;7:292.

40. Nicolatou-Galitis O, Sarri T, Bowen J, et al. Systematic review of amifostine for the management of oral mucositis in cancer patients. *Support Care Cancer.* 2013;21:357–364.

41. Citrin DE. Radiation modifiers. *Hematol Oncol Clin North Am.* 2019;33:1041–1055.

42. Kazemzadeh N, Modiri A, Samanta S, et al. Virtual bronchoscopy-guided treatment planning to map and mitigate radiation-induced airway injury in lung SAbR. *Int J Radiat Oncol Biol Phys.* 2018;102:210–218.

3 Fractionation: Radiobiologic Principles and Clinical Practice

Colin Orton

INTRODUCTION

Radiotherapy for the treatment of cancer was first started in 1896, but it was not realized until 1932 that fractionation was essential if cancerocidal doses were to be delivered without exceeding normal tissue tolerance. It was then that Henri Coutard published the excellent results he had obtained using fractionated radiotherapy[1] and fractionation was thereafter established as the standard of practice. However, radiobiologic rationales for fractionated radiotherapy were fully understood only many decades later.

RADIOBIOLOGIC PRINCIPLES OF FRACTIONATION

The basic principle of radiotherapy is the destruction of all cancer cells without killing so many normal cells as to exceed tolerance. Thus, cell survival and the shape of cell-survival curves are of utmost importance in radiotherapy.

Cell-Survival Curves

A plot of the fraction of surviving cells as a function of dose for acutely irradiated cells is shown in Figure 3.1. Note that surviving fraction is plotted on a log scale. This is partly because, as we will see later, the shape of the log-linear survival curve for specific cell types tells us something about the important radiobiologic properties of these cells and partly because much of the important information about cell survival is contained within the low- and high-dose extremes of the survival curve (regions A and B in Fig. 3.1). Plotting cell survival on a log scale helps us visualize and study the shape of the survival curve in these regions. Low doses per fraction (region A) are commonly used for fractionated radiotherapy (1–3 Gy/fraction) and, to cure a tumor with typically 10^8 to 10^{10} cells, cell-surviving fractions as low as 10^{-8} to 10^{-12} are required (region B).

Since the shapes of cell-survival curves are so important, it is necessary to have a mathematical model that can predict these shapes. Currently, the model of choice is the linear quadratic (LQ) theory of cell survival.

Linear Quadratic Theory

The basis of the LQ theory is that a cell is inactivated only when both strands of a deoxyribonucleic acid (DNA) molecule are damaged in close proximity. Actually, this is a gross oversimplification of the highly complex chemical and biologic responses triggered by irradiation of cells, but this was the basic assumption made when the LQ model was first devised[2]; therefore, for simplicity, we will adopt this approach here. Readers interested in a more thorough (and accurate) discussion of the complex events that occur when cells are irradiated are referred to an excellent review by Wouters and Begg.[3]

On this simple model, double-strand breaks in close proximity can be produced either during the passage across the cell of a single ionizing particle or by independent interactions by two separate ionizing particles. Such events are random and, because there are large numbers of cells, the probability that any specific DNA molecule will be damaged is extremely low. Under such conditions, the statistics of rare events (Poisson statistics) prevails. According to Poisson statistics, the probability, P_0, of there being no such events is given by the expression[4]

$$P_0 = e^{-p} \tag{3.1}$$

where p is the mean number of hits per target molecule. For single-particle events, p is a linear function of dose, D, so the mean number of lethal events per DNA molecule can be expressed as αD; P_0 represents the probability of there being no single-particle–induced lethal events; that is, it is the surviving fraction of cells, S. Then, Equation 3.1 may be written as

$$S = e^{-\alpha D} \tag{3.2}$$

where α is the average probability per unit dose that such a single-particle event will occur. In order for a single particle to damage both arms of the DNA in its passage across the molecule, it has to be fairly densely ionizing, that is, high linear energy transfer (LET). With photon and electron irradiation, it is only the slow electrons that are responsible for most of these interactions. Conversely, when cells are irradiated with high-LET radiations, such as α-particles and heavy ions, almost all the events will be by single particles, so cell survival will be governed by Equation 3.2 and

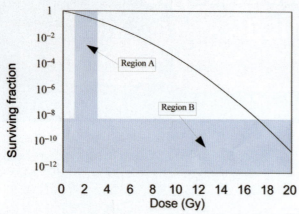

FIGURE 3.1. The surviving fraction of cells (log scale) as a function of dose. The two *shaded areas* represent the regions of most interest in fractionated radiotherapy for which doses per fraction normally range from 1 to 3 Gy (region A); the cell-surviving fraction required to control a typical tumor containing 10^8 to 10^{10} cells must be of the order of 10^{-8} to 10^{-12} (region B). This hypothetical graph has been constructed according to the linear quadratic model with parameters $\alpha = 0.4$ Gy^{-1}, $\alpha/\beta = 10$ Gy.

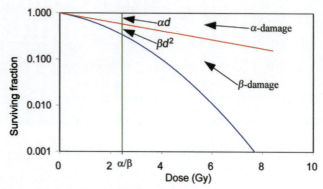

FIGURE 3.2. Linear-quadratic cell-survival curve, with $\alpha = 0.22$ Gy^{-1} and $\alpha/\beta = 2.5$ Gy; d is the dose/fraction. Note that the log cell kill for α-type damage equals that for β-damage at a dose equal to α/β.

be an exponential function of dose so that survival curves plotted on log-linear scales will be practically linear.

For the two separate ionizing particle events of the LQ theory, the mean probability of one particle causing damage in one arm of a DNA molecule in any specific cell is linearly proportional to dose, as also is the mean probability that a second particle will have such an interaction in the adjacent arm of this same DNA molecule. Therefore, unless the damage to the first arm of the DNA is repaired before the damage to the second arm occurs (see section Repair), the mean probability of both arms being damaged at any one time is βD^2, so the probability that no such two-particle events will occur, that is, the surviving fraction S, is given by

$$S = e^{-\beta D^2} \qquad (3.3)$$

where β is the mean probability per unit square of the dose that such complementary events will occur.

The overall LQ equation for cell survival is therefore

$$S = e^{-\alpha D - \beta D^2} \qquad (3.4)$$

This is illustrated in Figure 3.2, which shows how the two components of cell killing, α-damage and β-damage, combine to form the cell-survival curve. It will be shown later that α-damage and β-damage relate to irreparable and repairable damage, respectively. For two-particle events (β-type), if the damage from the second particle occurs before the lesion from the first particle has been repaired, the cell will be inactivated ("killed"). Since cellular repair half-times are of the order of 1 hour, this gives rise to the dose–rate effect: the higher the dose rate, the greater the effect.

Of special interest is the dose at which the log-surviving fraction for α-damage ($e^{-\alpha d}$) equals that for β-damage ($e^{-\beta d^2}$), that is, $\alpha d = \beta d^2$, or $d = \alpha/\beta$. This is also illustrated

in Figure 3.2. This parameter, α/β, represents the curviness of the cell-survival curve. Specifically, the higher the α/β, the straighter the survival curve. A high α/β is characteristic of a type of cell that exhibits considerable irreparable damage and/or little repair (high α and/or low β). In contrast, a low α/β (low α and/or high β) indicates little irreparable damage and/or a high capability of repair. Here lies the major difference between the cells of tumors and those of late-responding normal tissues: α/β values tend to be high for cancers and low for late-reacting normal tissues. For example, typical α/β values determined for cancer cells range from 5 to 20 Gy (mean ~10 Gy), but for late-responding normal tissues the range is 1 to 4 Gy (mean ~2.5 Gy). There appear to be some exceptions, however. For example, the α/β values for prostate and breast cancer cells have been reported to be about 1.5 and 4 Gy, respectively.[5,6]

Figure 3.3 shows typical survival curves for tumor and late-reacting normal cells, superimposed for comparison.

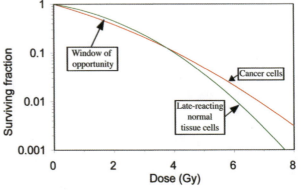

FIGURE 3.3. Typical survival curves for cancer and late-reacting normal tissue cells, superimposed for comparison. Compared with the cancer curve, the normal tissue cell-survival curve has a shallower initial slope (lower α) and is curvier (lower α/β). Note that there is a window of opportunity below ~4 Gy (with the parameters used here) where normal tissue cells exhibit a higher survival than cancer cells. Parameters used to draw these hypothetical curves are as follows: tumor, $\alpha = 0.4$ Gy^{-1}, $\alpha/\beta = 10$ Gy; late-reacting normal tissues, $\alpha = 0.22$ Gy^{-1}, $\alpha/\beta = 2.5$ Gy.

The difference in the shapes of cell-survival curves of cancer and normal cells provides the major rationale for fractionated radiotherapy.

Rationale for Fractionation

Radiotherapy, in general, is governed by the four R's—repair, reoxygenation, repopulation, and redistribution—and so also is fractionation. Following is a discussion of how each of the four R's affects the practice of fractionation.

Repair

Of the four R's, repair is the most important in terms of the rationale for fractionation. As discussed in the preceding section, late-reacting normal tissue cells tend to exhibit a greater propensity for repair than do tumor cells. This is exhibited by their low α/β values and hence their curvier survival curves, as shown in Figure 3.3. In this illustration, the normal tissue and tumor cell curves cross at doses of the order of 4 Gy. At doses below the crossover point, cell survival for late-reacting tissues is greater than that for tumors, and the reverse is true above the crossover. This means that delivery of doses greater than ~4 Gy will be more destructive to normal tissues than to cancer cells. There is essentially a "window of opportunity" centered at ~2 Gy, within which normal cells have a greater survival than cancer cells. However, doses far in excess of 4 Gy are needed to control tumors. There are two ways to safely deliver such high doses. One is to deliver much higher doses to the tumor than to the normal tissues, such as with stereotactic radiosurgery (SRS), intensity-modulated radiation therapy (IMRT), and various other forms of conformal therapy. This will be discussed in detail later. The second option is to fractionate with doses/fraction within the window of opportunity.

If a course of fractionated radiotherapy is delivered with time between fractions sufficient for complete repair (which clinical evidence has shown to be about 6 hours or more), all the cells that have been sublethally (but not lethally) damaged during the first fraction (i.e., only one DNA strand has been damaged or both arms are damaged but the lesions are far apart) will have repaired before the second fraction is delivered, and so on. This relates to the β-type damage in the LQ model. Then, at least to a first approximation, cell-surviving fractions for each successive treatment will be identical and the shape of the survival curve will simply repeat for each fraction. Then, the cell-surviving fraction equation becomes

$$S = e^{-N(\alpha d + \beta d^2)} \qquad (3.5)$$

where N is the number of fractions and d is the dose per fraction. Then, if the dose per fraction is below the crossover point shown in Figure 3.3, the resultant cell-survival

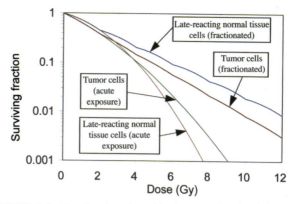

FIGURE 3.4. How fractionation with dose per fraction below the crossover point of the late-responding normal tissue and tumor cell-survival curves in Figure 3.3 results in higher cell survival for the normal tissue cells as the total dose increases.

curves gradually separate, with tumor cells suffering more damage than normal cells, as illustrated in Figure 3.4, which has been derived using Equation 3.5.

At least as far as repair is concerned, the optimal dose per fraction is that which will produce the maximum separation of the two fractionated radiotherapy curves in Figure 3.4. However, the LQ model predicts that this maximum separation occurs with an infinite number of infinitely small dose fractions, each separated by sufficient time for complete repair. Clearly, this is not a realistic fractionation scheme, and in any event it ignores the influence of the other three R's of radiotherapy, especially repopulation (see later discussion). With this in mind, a better definition of the optimal (or at least the most efficient) dose per fraction might be where the rate of increase in separation of the two fractionated radiotherapy curves in Figure 3.4 per unit number of fractions is a maximum. It can be shown that this occurs at the point of maximum separation between the cancer and normal tissue curves shown in Figure 3.3, which turns out to be at exactly 50% of the dose at the crossover point. For the parameters used to plot the survival curves in Figure 3.3, this dose is ~2 Gy. Hence, the optimal dose per fraction is about 2 Gy. If the α and β values for normal tissues and tumor were known for each patient, it would be possible to design patient-specific fractionation regimens but, unfortunately, the technology to do this is not refined enough at present. The alternative is to determine the optimal dose per fraction for specific types of disease for the average patient, and this has been the objective of numerous clinical trials of altered fractionation.[2–17]

The situation is somewhat different for SRS and other types of highly conformal radiotherapy because the effective dose to normal tissues is usually kept well below that to the tumor, where the "effective dose" may be defined as the dose that, if delivered uniformly to the

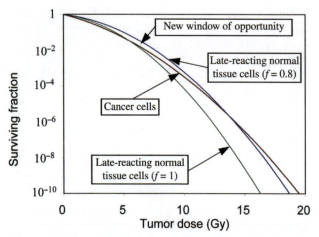

FIGURE 3.5. How the crossover point for single (acute) irradiations shown in Figure 3.3 moves to considerably higher tumor doses if there is even a modest amount of "geometrical sparing" of the normal tissues (the normal tissue curve moves 20% to the right). In this example, a 20% sparing (f = 0.8) causes the crossover point to move from ~4 Gy out to 14 Gy. The same linear quadratic model parameters used for Figure 3.3 are used here.

tissue in question, would result in the same probability of local control or complication as the actual inhomogeneous dose distribution in that tissue. Several methods to determine such effective doses from dose–volume data have been published[18–24] and these are reviewed in Chapter 23. For example, if f (the geometrical sparing factor) is the ratio of the effective dose in normal tissues to effective dose in tumor, even a modest sparing represented by $f = 0.8$ moves the crossover point to considerably higher doses and significantly widens the window of opportunity, as shown in Figure 3.5. In this example, the crossover point moves from 4 Gy all the way out to about 14 Gy, so the optimal tumor dose per fraction becomes ~7 Gy.

For SRS, single doses of the order of 20 Gy are used. It is readily shown that with the parameters used to plot Figures 3.3 to 3.5, this will be optimal if f equals ~0.6, which is not too unlikely, especially for small tumors. For large tumors, f may exceed 0.6, so fractionated radiotherapy might be required.

One concern with SRS and other types of radiotherapy such as IMRT and CyberKnife, for which the time it takes to deliver a treatment session can be of the same order of magnitude as the half-time for cellular repair, is that repair *during* irradiation might reduce the effectiveness of the treatment. Studies have shown that this effect might cause reductions in effective dose by as much as 12% if the time to deliver the treatment is as high as 0.5 hours, with concomitant reductions in tumor control as much as 30%.[25] Fortunately, it is possible that protraction of irradiation time during a treatment might reduce the effect on normal tissues more than on cancers.[26] Hence, it might be possible to increase the total dose sufficiently to offset the effect of

this intrafraction repair without increasing the damage to normal tissues.

All the foregoing discussions, especially the dose per fraction estimates, are, of course, highly dependent on the α and β values assumed. They also totally ignore the effect of the other three R's of radiotherapy.

Reoxygenation and the Oxygen Effect

Oxygen is the most powerful of all radiation sensitizers, so cells deprived of oxygen are relatively resistant to radiation and require approximately three times as much dose as well-oxygenated cells to destroy them. Such doses in a course of radiotherapy will likely exceed normal tissue tolerance unless highly conformal therapy is used. Furthermore, there is evidence that a significant proportion of human cancers contain hypoxic cells.[27–32] For such tumors, it would be expected that, immediately after exposure, the fraction of the surviving cells that are hypoxic should increase because the sensitive, well-oxygenated cells will be killed preferentially. Indeed, this is exactly what has been observed in many animal in vivo experiments. However, in some of these experiments, the hypoxic-cell fraction rapidly returned to the much lower pre-irradiation levels, and this has been interpreted as reoxygenation.[33] In that case, if enough time is allowed for reoxygenation between exposures in a course of fractionated radiotherapy (typically 24 hours is sufficient), the number of hypoxic cells in a tumor gradually decreases. Hence, fractionation takes on added importance when treating tumors with a significant hypoxic-cell fraction. However, because cell kill is reduced during each fraction due to the presence of some resistant hypoxic cells, it is possible that, even with reoxygenation, delivery of a high enough dose to kill all the cancer cells without exceeding normal tissue tolerance might not be possible. For example, several clinical trials have demonstrated that pre-irradiation hypoxia significantly reduces local control even after an extended course of fractionated radiotherapy long enough to ensure reoxygenation.[27–32]

Another aspect of the effect of oxygen on fractionated radiotherapy relates to the effect of LET. When cells are exposed to high-LET radiation, the protective effect of hypoxia is greatly reduced.[33] Hence, in the part of the cell-survival curve where α (i.e., high-LET) damage predominates, at low dose or low dose per fraction (see Fig. 3.2), the effect of hypoxia should be less than where β-damage predominates, which is at high dose or high dose per fraction. This effect of dose or dose per fraction has been demonstrated by cell-survival experiments[34,35] and has been shown to be consistent with clinical data.[30]

The effect of O_2 is represented by the oxygen enhancement ratio (OER), where

$$OER = \frac{\text{Dose under anoxic conditions}}{\text{Dose under aerobic conditions}} \qquad (3.6)$$

to produce the same biologic effect, for example, the cell-surviving fraction. Low OER means that the protective effect of hypoxia on cell survival is low, and high OER means that the effect is great. The potential magnitude of the effect of dose per fraction on the OER can be illustrated using the LQ model in Equation 3.5 and taking the natural logs of both sides, giving

$$-\ln S = Nd(\alpha + \beta d) \qquad (3.7)$$

Then, if subscripts a and h represent aerobic and hypoxic irradiation conditions, respectively, and equating values of $-\ln S$ for N fractions of dose d/fraction for equal biologic effect, we get

$$N_a d(\alpha_a + \beta_a d) = N_h d(\alpha_h + \beta_h d) \qquad (3.8)$$

Then,

$$\text{OER} = \frac{N_h d}{N_a d} = \frac{\alpha_a + \beta_a d}{\alpha_h + \beta_h d} \qquad (3.9)$$

Figure 3.6 shows how OER varies with dose per fraction for prostate cancer using values of α and β that have been shown to fit clinical data[36,37]: $\alpha_a = 0.26$ Gy^{-1}, $\beta_a = 0.0312$ Gy^{-2}, $\alpha_h = 0.149$ Gy^{-1}, and $\beta_h = 0.00293$ Gy^{-2}. Figure 3.6 shows the trend of increasing OER as dose per fraction increases, but it should be realized that the actual numbers depicted here represent just a single study for a single type of cancer. Data from other analyses of clinical results for prostate and other cancers will yield different OER versus dose/fraction curves, but the trend should be as shown in Figure 3.6.

Similar observations of increasing OER with dose/fraction above 1 Gy/fraction have been made using modified versions of the LQ model and different parameters.[38,39] This would indicate that, for the treatment of cancers that might contain significant numbers of hypoxic cells, low dose/fraction techniques, with the order of 1 Gy/fraction, might have an advantage over conventional (about 2 Gy/fraction) and high dose/fraction (>2 Gy/fraction) regimens. The inappropriateness of high dose/fraction

radiotherapy for hypoxic cancers was demonstrated by Carlson et al.,[40] who modified the LQ model to account for the effect of oxygen partial pressure, the change in OER as a function of dose/fraction, and reoxygenation. As illustrated for head-and-neck cancers in Figure 3.7, they showed that cancer-cell survival should increase with increase in dose/fraction, especially above 5 Gy/fraction.

In summary, fractionation is essential for reoxygenation but, even with fractionated radiotherapy, it may not be possible to deliver doses high enough to control cancers without exceeding normal tissue tolerance. Also, with high doses per fraction above about 5 Gy, the OER is high and reoxygenation between fractions is reduced because of the fewer number of fractions, so survival of cells in hypoxic cancers is increased. It would appear that the use of high doses per fraction for hypoxic cancers is contraindicated, but this ignores the effect of the third R of radiotherapy: repopulation.

Repopulation

By their very nature, all cancers contain dividing cells, with viable cancer cells usually dividing much faster than late-reacting normal tissues. Hence, during a course of radiotherapy, there is considerably more repopulation of cancer cells than cells of the late-responding normal tissues, so the longer a course of radiotherapy, the more difficult it becomes to control the tumor without exceeding normal tissue tolerance. Furthermore, some studies show that repopulation of cancer cells might accelerate during a course of fractionated radiotherapy (accelerated repopulation), with the faster rate of division kicking in after the first 2 to 4 weeks of treatment (the so-called kick-in time, T_k).[41] On these grounds, therefore, repopulation appears to dictate that courses of radiotherapy should not be overly protracted and that accelerated repopulation, if it exists—there is some controversy about this[42]—even indicates that optimal schedules of treatment might be as short as 2 to 4 weeks, or even less. However, repopulation is not entirely detrimental. Acutely responding normal tissues need to repopulate during a course of radiotherapy to avoid exceeding acute tolerance. Hence, the length of a course of radiotherapy, and therefore the fractionation, must be controlled so as to not allow too much time for excessive repopulation of tumor cells, at the same time not treating so rapidly that acute tolerance is exceeded.

One problem with shortening the course of therapy is that this probably means increasing the dose/fraction unless multiple fractions are to be delivered each day, which is very inconvenient (see later). But, as shown in the previous section, increasing the dose per fraction will reduce the effectiveness of the treatments if hypoxic cells are present in the tumor (Fig. 3.7). A delicate balance has to be struck between too few fractions (less opportunity for reoxygenation) and too many fractions (increased repopulation of cancer cells). Carlson et al. demonstrated this for the head-and-neck cancers shown in Figure 3.7, and showed that there ought to be an optimal number of

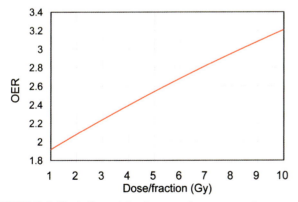

FIGURE 3.6. Illustration of the increase in oxygen enhancement ratio with increase in dose/fraction. Parameters used (see text) are those derived to fit clinical data for the treatment of prostate cancers by Nahum et al.[30]

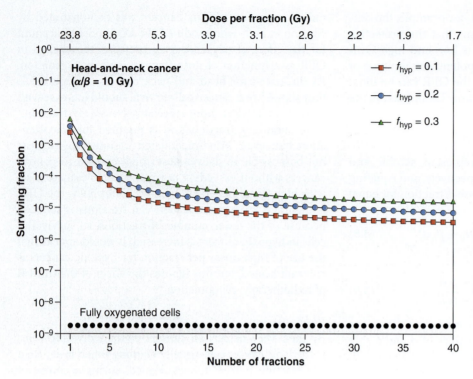

FIGURE 3.7. Surviving fraction of tumor cells as a function of the number of fractions and the dose/fraction to yield equivalent tumor control under normoxic conditions for hypoxic fractions 0.1 (*red*), 0.2 (*blue*), and 0.3 (*green*), assuming daily fractionation, full reoxygenation, and no repopulation. Modified from Carlson DJ, Keall PJ, Loo BW, et al. Hypofractionation results in reduced cell kill compared to conventional fractionation for tumors with regions of hypoxia. *Int J Radiat Oncol Biol Phys.* 2011;79:1188–1195.

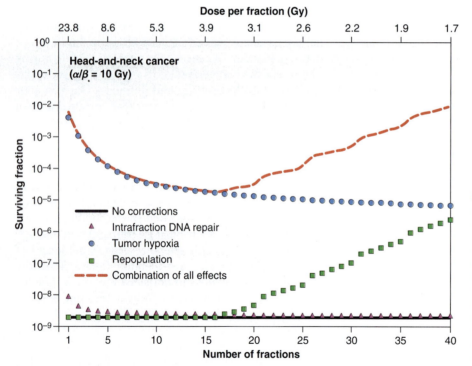

FIGURE 3.8. Surviving fraction of tumor cells as a function of the number of fractions and the dose/fraction at 5 fractions/week to yield equivalent tumor control under normoxic conditions for hypoxic fraction 0.2, including repopulation with a kick-in time T_k of 21 days. Modified from Carlson DJ, Keall PJ, Loo BW, et al. Hypofractionation results in reduced cell kill compared to conventional fractionation for tumors with regions of hypoxia. *Int J Radiat Oncol Biol Phys.* 2011;79:1188–1195.

fractions and dose/fraction,[40] as shown in Figure 3.8. With the parameters used in this study, this occurs at about 15 fractions of 3.7 Gy, but the actual optimal fractionation is highly dependent upon the parameters used and the accuracy of the model. For example, in this study, a kick-in time T_k of 21 days was assumed for 5 fraction/week treatments. Hence, accelerated repopulation kicked in after 15

fractions. But, as shown in Figure 3.7, after 15 fractions, the decrease in surviving fraction of the cancer cells due to OER and reoxygenation effects has practically saturated. Hence, the effect of accelerated repopulation kicking in causes the cell-survival curve to increase suddenly, thus making 15 fractions the apparent optimal fractionation. The optimal fractionation is, therefore, highly dependent upon the value of T_k assumed. For T_k less than 15 days, the optimal number of fractions should be less than 15, and high dose/fraction regimens will not, after all, be contraindicated for hypoxic cancers.

Redistribution

According to the cell cycle effect, cells irradiated during the mitotic (M) phase of the cell cycle are most sensitive, and during late synthesis (late S) they are most resistant, with a second peak of resistance in $G1$ in some cells.[43] For cells irradiated in the M phase, the survival curve is practically linear, indicating minimal repair. In contrast, for cells irradiated in late S, survival curves exhibit the greatest curvature, representing considerable repair. Consequently, when tumors are treated with fractionated radiotherapy, cells surviving the first fraction tend to be partially synchronized, with an overabundance of surviving cells in late S moving into early $G2$ immediately after exposure. If a second exposure is delivered sometime after the first, the number of cells inactivated depends on how far this surviving bolus of cells has traveled around the cell cycle. For example, if they have reached the M phase at the time of the second fraction, they will be most sensitive. It is this radiation-induced partial synchronization of cells that is known as redistribution (or reassortment).

Redistribution can be a benefit in a course of fractionated radiotherapy if the cancer cells can be caught in mitosis after each fraction or detrimental if they have reached a resistant phase of the cell cycle. In theory, it ought to be possible to adjust the interval between fractions so as to gain maximum benefit from redistribution, but to date there has been no evidence that such an advantage can be obtained in practice. Consequently, potential effects of redistribution are generally ignored when designing fractionation strategies.

Fractionation Strategies

The radiobiologic principles discussed in the foregoing sections have been used extensively to guide in the design of numerous clinical trials of altered-fractionation regimens. In this section, the rationale for various fractionation schemes will be presented. Table 3.1 lists a variety of fractionation schemes, their typical parameters, and some brief comments. Following is a detailed description of each of these fractionation schemes.

Conventional Fractionation

The most common fractionation for curative radiotherapy is about 1.8 to 2.2 Gy/fraction delivered at 5 fractions/week. This has evolved as the conventional fractionation regimen because it is convenient (no weekend treatments), efficient (treatment every weekday), and effective (high doses can be delivered without exceeding either acute or chronic normal tissue tolerance). The principal rationale for the prescription of conventional fractionation for a particular patient or disease is that most experience is with this type of fractionation, for which both tumoricidal and tolerance doses are well documented. Unless there is a good reason to change, radiation oncologists are reluctant to deviate from this tried-and-true method of treatment.

Hyperfractionation

A hyperfractionated course of radiotherapy is one in which more than one fraction is delivered each day but the overall treatment time remains similar to that for conventional fractionation. Typically, this means 1.2 to 1.3 Gy/fraction, 2 fractions a day, with an increase in total dose of the order of 20% to account for increased repair at the lower dose per fraction.

The major rationale for hyperfractionation is taking full advantage of the difference in repair capacity of

TABLE 3.1	Fractionation Schemes with Typical Parameters			
Fractionation Scheme	Dose/Fraction (Gy)	Fractions/Week	Total Dose (Gy)	Comments
Conventional	2.2–1.8	5	~60	Used for most patients
Hyperfractionation	1.3–1.2	10	~70	Allows higher dose to tumors without increased late complications
Accelerated fractionation	2.2–2.0	7	~60	Used for rapidly proliferating cancers to obtain increased local control but with the risk of increased acute reactions
	1.6–1.4	10	~54	
	~2.5	5	~50	
Hyperfractionated accelerated radiotherapy	1.5	15 (CHARTWEL) 21 (CHART)	54	Used for rapidly proliferating cancers but with increased risk of severe acute complications
Hypofractionation for palliation	3–10	1–5	10–30	Total dose too low for cure
Hypofractionation for cure	2.5–30	1–5	30–50	Used for cure with highly conformal radiotherapy

CHART, continuous hyperfractionated accelerated radiotherapy; CHARTWEL, CHART weekend less.

late-reacting normal tissues compared with tumors. This was illustrated by the curvier cell-survival curves for these normal tissues (Fig. 3.3) and the concomitantly lower α/β values. If conventional radiotherapy is not producing particularly good clinical results and no obvious reasons for this are evident, perhaps the reason is that the dose per fraction that adequately separates the two fractionated radiotherapy curves in Figure 3.4 is below that used in conventional fractionation. With such a low dose per fraction, more than 1 fraction per day is necessary to keep the course of therapy short enough to avoid the risk of excessive tumor cell repopulation. Such hyperfractionation regimens will have to be delivered at about 1.2 to 1.3 Gy/fraction, 2 fractions a day. To treat with higher than 1.3 Gy/fraction at more than 1 fraction per day may exceed acute tolerance, and to use <1.2 Gy/fraction will require 3 fractions per day in order to not overly increase overall treatment time, with at least 6 hours between fractions required for complete repair, a treatment schedule that would be highly inconvenient.

Another potential advantage of hyperfractionation might be the reduced OER at low dose/fraction compared with that with conventional fractionation (see Fig. 3.6). This could be important for cancers that might be expected to contain significant numbers of hypoxic cells.

Accelerated Fractionation

For rapidly growing tumors with short potential doubling times of the viable cycling cancer cells (T_{pot}), accelerated treatment is desirable.

There are several ways to achieve reduced overall treatment time. The simplest is to treat 6 or 7 days a week instead of the normal 5, keeping the dose per fraction the same as with conventional fractionation. This produces a modest acceleration that may be enough to influence clinical outcome. A more drastic acceleration can be achieved by treating twice a day at 1.4 to 1.6 Gy/fraction but only at the risk of exceeding acute normal tissue tolerance. Such accelerated fractionation regimens have been tried but have usually been unsuccessful because many patients had to be given a rest of 1 to 2 weeks during the course of therapy to allow acute reactions to subside, negating the intent to accelerate the treatments.

Another possibility is to increase the dose per fraction to about 2.5 Gy (often called rapid fractionation), but this risks losing the repair advantage of late-responding normal tissues. Increased late reactions usually occur unless the dose to the normal tissues can be reduced, such as with conformal therapy. Alternatively, for rapidly growing cancers, it is possible to exploit the difference in repair between late-reacting normal tissues and tumors by hyperfractionating while accelerating the course of therapy by treating with 3 fractions per day. Such treatment is known as accelerated hyperfractionation.

Accelerated Hyperfractionation

A major problem with accelerated fractionation is that cancerocidal doses delivered in such short overall times are likely to exceed acute tolerance unless a rest period is included part way through treatment to allow early reactions to subside. One way around this is to complete the treatments in such a short time that the acute reactions reach their peak only after the radiotherapy has been completed. This was the rationale for the development of the continuous hyperfractionated accelerated radiotherapy (CHART) regimen at Mount Vernon Hospital in London.[10] With CHART, treatments 6 hours apart are delivered 3 times a day, 7 days a week. With a dose/fraction of 1.5 Gy, a total dose of 54 Gy can be delivered in 36 fractions over 12 successive treatment days including weekends. With this schedule, patients can complete treatment without a break because peak acute reactions occur approximately 2 weeks after the start of therapy. Although clinical results for the treatment of lung and head-and-neck cancers have been promising with CHART, they have been achieved with considerable trauma to the patients: Many of these patients developed grade 3 or worse acute complications.[44] CHART is also difficult for the staff, since delivery of 3 fractions per day 6 hours apart for 12 successive days, including weekends, is very inconvenient. Some of this inconvenience is reduced with an alternative form of CHART called CHARTWEL (CHART weekend less), wherein the 54 Gy at 1.5 Gy/fraction at 3 fractions per day is delivered over a total of 16 days without the weekend treatments.[13] Clinical trials have shown that CHARTWEL is a viable alternative to CHART.[45]

Hypofractionation

All the fractionation regimens presented previously require the delivery of many fractions over many days. They are costly in terms of resources and are inconvenient for patients. These fractionation schemes were necessitated by the desire to "cure" cancers without exceeding normal tissue tolerance. However, not all radiotherapy is aimed at "cure." For many patients, the aim is to simply palliate, so there is no need to employ the very high doses required for "cure" and hence no need to approach tolerance of normal tissues. For these patients, it is, therefore, possible to design much more convenient and cost-effective treatments, which use far fewer fractions, that is, to employ hypofractionation. Typical hypofractionation schemes used for palliation range from as many as 10 fractions of 3 Gy to as few as a single fraction of about 10 Gy, with anything from 1 to 5 fractions per week.

With conformal radiotherapy, because there is considerable geometrical sparing of normal tissues, the window of opportunity (Fig. 3.5) is widened such that the high doses/fraction needed for hypofractionated treatments can be used for curative radiotherapy. This has led to the development of many clinical trials of hypofractionation, especially for prostate and breast cancers, for which the α/β ratio is lower than the 10 Gy typically assumed for most cancers.[9,14,16,46]

As discussed earlier, potential disadvantages of hypofractionation relate to the increased OER and decreased reoxygenation that might be expected with high dose/fraction schedules (Fig. 3.6). But this disadvantage might be mitigated for rapidly dividing cancers if the hypofractionation allows the course of treatment to be shortened. All this depends significantly on radiobiologic properties of the cancer cells, which are difficult to predict. Hence, it seems prudent to not apply hypofractionation for the treatment of cancers thought to contain significant fractions of hypoxic cells without extensive clinical trials.

One possible advantage of hypofractionation for cancers with a high α/β that might be exploited is the increase in intrafraction repair that takes place with long treatment times, which should benefit late-reacting normal tissues because of their lower α/β (prostate cancer might be an exception). This would require increasing the total dose to account for this increased repair just enough so as to not increase the risk of late complications. This could be determined by, for example, a carefully controlled dose-escalation clinical trial or, maybe, calculation of the appropriate dose using a bioeffect dose model. This exemplifies a major challenge with most modified fractionation regimens for which there is no previous experience: the determination of the appropriate total dose to use. Rather than just guessing, it has been a common practice to use mathematical bioeffect dose models to calculate these doses. The most popular of these is the biologically effective dose (BED) model.

The Biologically Effective Dose Model

The BED model for fractionated radiotherapy can be derived directly from the LQ equation for cell survival for fractionated irradiations presented earlier (Equation 3.7): $-\ln S = Nd (\alpha + \beta d)$

This equation could be used to calculate treatment regimens that are equally effective biologically (constant $-\ln S$) but, to do so, we would need to know the values of the two parameters α and β for each tissue involved. Unfortunately, it is difficult enough to determine a single biologic parameter from clinical data, let alone two. However, it is possible to reduce the number of unknown parameters to one by dividing both sides of Equation 3.7 by α to derive the BED, originally called the extrapolated response dose (ERD)[47,48]:

$$\frac{-\ln S}{\alpha} = \text{BED} = Nd\left(1 + \frac{d}{\alpha/\beta}\right) \quad (3.10)$$

Fractionation schemes for which BEDs are equal will be equally effective biologically. Here, we have just one biologic parameter, α/β, to determine from clinical data for each type of tissue involved where, as we saw earlier, α/β is the dose at which α-type and β-type damages are equal (Fig. 3.2).

Equation 3.10 is derived assuming acute radiation conditions (i.e., no time for repair during each fraction) and complete repair between fractions. This does not always prevail, however, since there may be occasions when the time between fractions is not sufficient for full repair or the time to deliver each fraction is long enough for some repair to occur during irradiation. The former has been observed clinically with some of the early 3 fractions per day patients, for example, when less than 6 hours between fractions was used,[49] and the latter probably occurs for some of the highly conformal therapy techniques such as with SRS, IMRT, Stereotactic Body Radiation Therapy (SBRT), and CyberKnife treatments.[25,26,50] For these situations, a more complex form of the BED equation is needed that takes into account the rate at which cells repair, the rate at which each part of the tissue is irradiated, and the time between fractions. The full BED equation for such fractionated therapy has been published[25,51,52] but it is extremely complicated and outside the scope of this chapter.

Equation 3.10 accounts for repair only, but cells, especially cancer cells, are known to repopulate during a course of therapy. If tumor cell repopulation is assumed to be an exponential function of time, with doubling time for repopulation of the cycling cells T_{pot}, then $\ln S$ will be increased by $(0.693/T_{\text{pot}})T$, so[53]

$$\ln S = N(\alpha d + \beta d^2) + \left(\frac{0.693}{T_{\text{pot}}}\right)T \quad (3.11)$$

and hence the BED equation becomes

$$\frac{\ln S}{\alpha} = \text{BED} = Nd\left(1 + \frac{d}{\alpha/\beta}\right) - \frac{0.693}{\alpha T_{\text{pot}}} \quad (3.12)$$

However, since the two additional biologic parameters T_{pot} and α are very difficult to determine from analysis of clinical data, it is useful to replace $0.693/\alpha T_{\text{pot}}$ by a single repopulation rate parameter, k, estimated from loss of local control when radiotherapy is prolonged.[54] For example, if retrospective analysis of data shows that a patient has a rapidly repopulating type of tumor, a value of $k = 0.6$ BED units/day might be used. At the other extreme, for a slowly proliferating disease like prostate cancer, $k = 0.1$ BED units/day might be more appropriate. Note that it is usual to assume that $k = 0$ for late-responding normal tissues, since little or no repopulation of these cells would be expected to occur during a course of therapy. For acutely responding normal tissues, the value of k is probably in the range of 0.2 to 0.4 BED units/day.[54]

One further refinement of the BED equation is required if cells are believed to exhibit accelerated repopulation after a kick-in time T_k. If it is assumed that repopulation is negligible before T_k and after that proceeds at a rate represented by k BED units/day[54]

$$\text{BED} = Nd\left(1 + \frac{d}{\alpha/\beta}\right) - k(T - T_k) \quad (3.13)$$

where $k = 0$ for $T < T_k$.

A further useful application of the LQ model for comparison of different fractionation regimens is to calculate the equivalent dose at 2 Gy/fraction, because much of the clinical data used to represent tumor control and normal tissue complication probabilities has been published for 2 Gy/fraction treatment schedules.[55-57] This is achieved by equating BEDs. For example, if we ignore repopulation effects, the 2 Gy/fraction total dose, D_2, equivalent to a regimen of D_d Gy delivered at d Gy/fraction, is given by

$$\text{BED} = D_2\left(1 + \frac{2}{\alpha/\beta}\right) = D_d\left(1 + \frac{d}{\alpha/\beta}\right) \quad (3.14)$$

Then,

$$D_2 = D_d\left[\frac{\left(1 + \dfrac{d}{\alpha/\beta}\right)}{\left(1 + \dfrac{2}{\alpha/\beta}\right)}\right] \quad (3.15)$$

Another useful application of the LQ model is to correct for errors in dose/fraction. For example, if the wrong dose/fraction is delivered for the first several fractions, Joiner showed that it is possible (with some obvious exceptions) to use the LQ model to calculate a treatment schedule to complete the course of treatment and achieve the same biologic effects that were originally planned for both tumor and normal tissues, provided repopulation effects can be ignored.[58] He showed that, if the planned total dose was D_p Gy at d_p Gy/fraction but, due to an error, the first D_e Gy was delivered at dose/fraction d_e Gy, the course could be completed with dose D_c delivered at d_c Gy/fraction, where $D_c = D_p - D_e$ and

$$d_c = \frac{D_p d_p - D_e d_e}{D_p - D_e} \quad (3.16)$$

Note that the total dose is unchanged ($D_p = D_e + D_c$) and that the solution is independent of the α/β of the tissues involved, which is why the effects on both tumor and normal tissues are the same as originally planned. Also, although not stated in Joiner's paper,[58] it can be shown that the solution is independent of any geometrical sparing of normal tissues; that is, it is independent of geometrical sparing factor, f.

The Linear Quadratic Model in Clinical Practice

It is important to realize that the LQ model is an approximation. How could such a simple mathematical model account for all the complex changes that occur in tissues and cells when they are irradiated? But, like all models, it can be useful and has been shown to provide an adequate fit to clinical data in many studies. Problems with the model, apart from the over-simplicity of the model itself, include lack of accurate values for the biologic parameters α, α/β, k, T_{pot}, and T_k, and a concern that there may be an upper limit to the dose/fraction above which the model no longer applies.

As far as the biologic parameters are concerned, studies of tumor and normal tissue effects in clinical trials are gradually providing progressively better estimates of their values. Of special interest as far as normal tissues are concerned are the studies being analyzed as part of the Quantitative Analyses of Normal Tissue Effects in the Clinic (QUANTEC) program.[59] Hopefully, this will provide reliable estimates of the parameters for a whole variety of normal tissues.

The problem of a possible upper limit in dose/fraction for the LQ model is a concern for uses of the model for extreme hypofractionation with doses/fraction above about 7 Gy. One concern relates to the shape of cell-survival curves at high doses. Many have claimed that these straighten out at doses above about 7 Gy, whereas the LQ model predicts that they continue to curve downward.[60] This would mean that the LQ model would predict more cell kill than really occurs at high doses; that is, it *overestimates* radiation effects. On the other hand, many claim that the LQ model *underestimates* the effect at high doses above about 10 Gy because it ignores indirect cell death due to vascular damage.[61,62] Perhaps because the LQ model *overestimates* the direct effect on cells but *underestimates* it in tissues, these two "errors" at least partially cancel each other and the LQ model can be used at doses well above 10 Gy. Only carefully designed clinical trials are likely to give us a clear answer to this conundrum. Regardless, the LQ model is always an approximation. It should be applied with caution when designing or modifying fractionation schemes and, if used for patients, it is important to watch out for signs of unexpected tissue reactions or poor tumor control.

The following examples illustrate how these models can be applied to the solution of practical radiotherapy problems.

EXAMPLES

Problem 1: Gap in treatment: A patient with a rapidly growing cancer is planned to receive a course of 70 Gy in 35 fractions in 7 weeks. After 25 fractions, the patient develops a severe acute reaction that necessitates a 2-week rest period. To complete the treatment in 10 more fractions in 2 weeks, what dose per fraction should be delivered?

SOLUTION

Application of the LQ model to problems such as this is complicated since different solutions are possible for different tissues considered and several tissue-specific parameters have to be assumed. For this problem, assume the following parameters for this patient:

   For tumor:

$\alpha/\beta = 10\,\text{Gy}, \quad T_k = 28\,\text{days}, \quad k = 0.6\,\text{BED units/day}$

   For late-responding normal tissues:

$\alpha/\beta = 2.5\,\text{Gy}, \quad k = 0$

Tumor solution: Before the break, the BED is (using Equation 3.13)

$$BED = 50(1 + 0.2) - 0.6(35 - 28) = 55.8$$

After the break this reduces to

$$55.8 - 0.6(14) = 47.4$$

The planned BED was

$$BED = 70(1 + 0.2) - 0.6(49 - 28) = 71.4$$

Therefore, the residual BED that needs to be delivered is

$$71.4 - 47.4 = 24$$

If d is the dose per fraction required to complete the treatment in 10 fractions over 2 weeks

$$24.0 = 10d(1 + 0.1d) - 0.6(14)$$

Therefore,

$$d^2 + 10d - 32.4 = 0$$

Solving this for d gives

$$d = 2.58 \text{ Gy/fraction}$$

Late-responding normal tissue solution: Since no repopulation is assumed for late-responding normal tissues ($k = 0$), the break should have no effect, so the dose to complete the course of therapy should be unchanged. Therefore

$$d = 2.00 \text{ Gy/fraction}$$

If it is assumed that the original course represented the maximum dose that could be delivered safely to this patient then, in order not to increase the risk of late normal tissue injuries, the treatment should be completed in 10 fractions of 2 Gy. However, since the dose per fraction required for the tumor (2.58 Gy) is much higher than this, it might be necessary to compromise in order to not reduce tumor control too much. It might be decided to treat with more than 10 fractions of 2 Gy but less than the number that would be required for the full tumor effect. This illustrates the undesirability of allowing rest periods during the treatment of rapidly proliferating cancers.

Problem 2: Hyperfractionation: A hyperfractionation regimen consisting of 2 fractions per day, 6 hours apart, for a total of 60 fractions in 6 weeks is designed to be equivalent to 60 Gy in 30 fractions in 6 weeks. What dose per fraction is required?

SOLUTION

Assume all the same parameters as in the first problem. However, since the overall time is unchanged, no account need be taken of repopulation.

Tumor solution: Equating the conventional to the hyperfractionated regimens, the dose/fraction d is determined using Equation 3.10:

$$60(1 + 0.2) = 60d(1 + 0.1d)$$

or

$$6d^2 + 60d - 72 = 0$$

Solving for d gives

$$d = 1.08 \text{ Gy/fraction}$$

Late-responding normal tissue solution: Equating the two regimens gives (using Equation 3.10)

$$60\left(1 + \frac{2}{2.5}\right) = 60d\left(1 + \frac{d}{2.5}\right)$$

or

$$24d^2 + 60d - 108 = 0$$

The solution to this is

$$d = 1.21 \text{ Gy/fraction}$$

Note that the late-reacting tissues can tolerate doses much higher than those required for the tumor. This is a consequence of the low dose per fraction and is the major rationale for hyperfractionation. However, even though a course of 60 fractions at 1.21 Gy/fraction in 6 weeks is tolerable as far as late reactions are concerned, the risk of acute reactions might be higher than that for the conventional course of treatment because a total of 2.42 Gy will be delivered each day. But this might not be a problem if the risk of acute injuries is negligible for the conventional course. If these calculations are to be used as the basis for the design of a hyperfractionation regimen for real patients, it might be prudent for the radiation oncologist to develop some experience by treating the first few patients with slightly fewer fractions and, if the acute reactions appear tolerable, to escalate the number of fractions to the required 60. Several national clinical trials of hyperfractionation have been designed using dose escalation in this way.

Problem 3: Accelerated fractionation: An accelerated fractionation scheme consisting of 40 treatments 2 times a day for 4 weeks is to be equivalent to 60 Gy in 30 fractions in 6 weeks. What dose per fraction is required? Assume the same parameters as in Problem 1.

SOLUTION

Tumor solution: The accelerated regimen is completed before the kick-in time for repopulation (28 days); equating BEDs using Equation 3.13 to determine the dose/fraction d

$$60(1 + 0.2) - 0.6(42 - 28) = 40d(1 + 0.1d)$$

or

$$4d^2 + 40d - 63.6 = 0$$

Solving this for d gives

$$d = 1.40 \text{ Gy/fraction}$$

Late-responding normal tissue solution: No repopulation correction is needed, so (using Equation 3.10)

$$60\left(1 + \frac{2}{2.5}\right) = 40d\left(1 + \frac{d}{2.5}\right)$$

or

$$16d^2 + 40d - 108 = 0$$

The solution is

$$d = 1.63\,\text{Gy/fraction}$$

According to these calculations, it would be safe to deliver the treatment at 1.63 Gy/fraction, which means that the effect on the tumor should be greater than that for the conventional fractionation scheme. This is the rationale for accelerated fractionation for such rapidly proliferating cancers. Note that the daily dose for the accelerated regimen is 3.26 Gy, which might not be tolerated acutely. As in the previous problem, it might be prudent to start out using less than the desired 40 fractions of 1.63 Gy/fraction and to dose-escalate with this accelerated radiotherapy schedule, carefully watching out for excessive acute reactions.

Problem 4: Hypofractionation: What is the appropriate dose/fraction required for hypofractionated whole breast irradiation (WBI) in 16 fractions at 5 fractions/week over 22 days in order for this to be equivalent in terms of tumor control to standard radiotherapy with 25 fractions of 2 Gy delivered over 5 weeks, assuming that α/β for breast cancer is 4 Gy, the cancer cells repopulate at an average rate equivalent to a repopulation parameter k of 0.4 BED units/day, and there is no delay time for repopulation, that is, $T_k = 0$?

SOLUTION

Using Equation 3.13, the standard treatment BED is $50(1 + 2/4) - 0.4(35) = 61$. Then, if d Gy is the dose/fraction needed for the hypofractionated treatments,

$$61 = 16d(1 + d/4) - 0.4(22)$$

Therefore,

$$4d^2 + 16d - 69.8 = 0$$

Solving this for d gives

$$d = 2.63\ \text{Gy/fraction}$$

Note that the recommended dose/fraction in the American Society for Radiation Oncology (ASTRO) guidelines for hypofractionated WBI delivered in 16 fractions at 5 fractions/week is about 2.65 Gy.[63]

Problem 5: Correction of treatment error: A patient is planned to receive 30 daily fractions of 1.8 Gy but, due to an error, the first 5 fractions are delivered at 2 Gy/fraction. How can the treatment continue so as to result in the same effects on tumor and normal tissues as originally planned?

SOLUTION

According to Equation 3.16, the remainder of the treatments should be delivered at a dose/fraction d_c given by

$$d_c = \frac{D_p d_p - D_e d_e}{D_p - D_e} = \frac{54 \times 1.8 - 10 \times 2}{54 - 10}$$
$$= 1.75\,\text{Gy}$$

The total dose remains as planned at 54 Gy, so the remaining 44 Gy has to be delivered in 44/1.75 = 25.1 fractions. Since we cannot deliver 0.1 of a fraction, 25 fractions of 44/25 = 1.76 Gy should be used.

Problem 6: Accelerated hyperfractionation: A CHART scheme consisting of 36 treatments 3 times a day for 12 successive days with at least 6 hours between fractions is to be equivalent to 70 Gy in 35 fractions in 49 days as far as tumor control is concerned. What dose per fraction is required? With this treatment regimen, will the effect on late-responding normal tissues exceed that expected from a conventional course of 30 fractions of 2 Gy in 42 days?

SOLUTION

Assume the same parameters as before, except for the repopulation kick-in time for the tumor, which is assumed to be 0 (assume CHART is being tried for these patients because their cancers are rapidly proliferating right from the start of treatment).

For tumor: Equating BEDs, the CHART dose/fraction d is given by (using Equation 3.13)

$$70(1 + 0.2) - 0.6(49) = 36d(1 + 0.1d) - 0.6(12)$$

or

$$3.6d^2 + 36d - 61.8 = 0$$

Solving this for d gives

$$d = 1.49\,\text{Gy/fraction}$$

For late-reacting normal tissues: The BED for the conventional regimen is (using Equation 3.10)

$$\text{BED} = 60(1 + 2/2.5) = 108$$

For the CHART treatments, it is

$$\text{BED} = 36 \times 1.49(1 + 1.49/2.5) = 85.6$$

Hence, the CHART treatments should be far more tolerable as far as late reactions are concerned. One would expect that, compared to conventional therapy with 60 Gy at 2 Gy/fraction, CHART should provide equivalent tumor control without the added risk of severe late reactions. However, because the daily dose is about 4.5 Gy, one would expect acute reactions to be very severe, as clinical results have demonstrated.[13]

SUMMARY

Treatments have been fractionated from the very inception of radiotherapy a century ago, although it was not until the early 1930s that it was generally accepted that curative therapy required fractionation. Recent studies of the radiobiologic principles of cell survival demonstrate that the major reason fractionation is so important is the difference in the capacity of tumor and late-responding normal tissue cells to repair damage at low doses per fraction. Specifically, normal tissue cells are more capable of repair than are tumor cells. This causes their cell-survival curves to be curvier than those for tumors which, according to the LQ model, correspond to a lower value of the α/β ratio.

A second difference between tumor and late-reacting normal cells is repopulation. These normal cells repopulate little, if at all, during a course of fractionated radiotherapy, whereas tumor cells, especially those with a short potential doubling time, exhibit significant repopulation.

These repair and repopulation differences between normal and tumor cells provide the major rationale for clinical trials of several types of modified fractionation schemes, such as hyperfractionation, accelerated fractionation, and accelerated hyperfractionation.

One problem encountered whenever fractionation regimens are modified is how to decide on an appropriate total dose when little prior clinical experience is available. The most common way this has been done is by the use of the BED model. However, it must be realized that this model provides only approximate solutions to clinical problems. It represents a grossly oversimplified view of the extremely complex biologic changes that occur during a course of fractionated radiotherapy. It is useful for demonstration of the effects of fractionation but, if applied to actual patient treatment calculations, it should be used with caution, preferably only when previous clinical experience is not available.

KEY POINTS

- The clinical need to fractionate treatments first became accepted in the 1930s.

- Late-reacting normal tissue cells are better able to repair damage than are cancer cells.

- There is a window of opportunity at low dose and low doses/fraction within which cancers can be controlled without exceeding normal tissue tolerance.

- The window of opportunity widens with geometrical sparing of normal tissues, thus allowing much higher doses/fraction to be used for curative therapy.

- Radiobiologic effects are regulated by the four R's of radiotherapy: repair, reoxygenation, repopulation, and redistribution.

- Different fractionation strategies have been investigated to try to find the best treatment for specific types of cancers.

- The LQ model can be used to compare different fractionation schemes but, because it is an approximation, it has to be used with caution.

REVIEW QUESTIONS

1. The principle radiobiologic rationale for fractionating radiotherapy at low doses/fraction is that
   A. this improves utilization of treatment machines.
   B. cells of late-reacting normal tissues are better able to repair than those of most cancers.
   C. this gives the staff time to rest between treatments.
   D. survival curves for cancer cells are typically curvier than for normal cells.
   E. cancer cells repair faster than normal cells so session times have to be kept short.

2. One reason why the CHART technique might be better for reducing the overall time of a course of treatment than conventional accelerated fractionation is that with CHART
   A. there will be increased probability of reoxygenation of hypoxic cancer cells.
   B. treatments are more convenient to deliver.

   C. there is a comparable risk of severe acute complications with increased tumor control.
   D. there is a reduced risk of severe acute complications.
   E. severe acute reactions peak after the course of radiotherapy has been completed.

3. Hypofractionation might be better than other forms of fractionation because
   A. with fewer fractions, reduced reoxygenation will protect late-reacting normal tissues.
   B. longer treatment times will allow some cancer cells to repair.
   C. fewer fractions will be more cost effective.
   D. shorter courses of radiotherapy will reduce the risk of acute reactions.
   E. shorter courses of radiotherapy will reduce the risk of late complications.

4. The major radiobiologic rationale for hyperfractionation is to take
  A. full advantage of the difference in repair capacity of late-reacting normal tissues compared with tumors.
  B. full advantage of the difference in repair capacity of acutely reacting normal tissues compared with tumors.
  C. advantage of the higher OER for tumors at low dose/fraction.
  D. advantage of the short time between fractions to "catch" the cancer cells in a sensitive phase of the cell cycle.
  E. advantage of the short time between fractions to "catch" the normal tissue cells in a resistant phase of the cell cycle.

5. In the 1930s, it was realized that treatments needed to be fractionated because
  A. repair at low doses/fraction was known to be better for normal tissue cells than for tumor cells.
  B. repair at low doses/fraction was known to be better for tumor cells than for normal tissue cells.
  C. it was known that reoxygenation improved as fractionation was increased.
  D. it was known that the OER of tumor cells was lower for fractionated as opposed to single dose treatments.
  E. clinical experience had demonstrated that only by fractionating could cancerocidal doses be delivered without exceeding normal tissue tolerance.

ANSWERS

1. B   At low doses and doses/fraction, cell survival is greater for late-reacting normal tissue cells than for cancer cells due to their better ability to repair, thus giving rise to the window of opportunity.

2. E   With accelerated radiotherapy regimens, acute reactions tend to reach a peak after about 2 weeks of treatment, and this often makes it impossible to complete the course of therapy without giving the patient a rest period, thus negating the benefit of accelerated treatment desired. With CHART, this peak in acute reactions occurs after the completion of treatment.

3. C   Fewer fractions is clearly more cost effective; the other potential answers either have no significant effect or make the treatments worse.

4. A   At low doses/fraction, the surviving fraction of both late-reacting normal tissue and tumor cells will both be increased but, because the normal tissue cells are better able to repair, the differential advantage will increase. The other potential answers either have no significant effect or make the treatments worse.

5. E   It was the excellent clinical results Coutard published in 1932 that demonstrated that fractionation was needed if cancerocidal doses were to be delivered without exceeding normal tissue tolerance. Answer B is wrong and the rationales given in the A, C, and D are now known to be good reasons to fractionate but they were not understood for several decades after Coutard's results were published.

REFERENCES

1. Coutard H. Roentgen therapy of epitheliomas of tonsillar regions, hypopharynx, and larynx from 1920 to 1926. *Am J Roentgenol.* 1932;28:313–331.
2. Chadwick KH, Leenhouts HP. A molecular theory of cell survival. *Phys Med Biol.* 1973;18:78–87.
3. Wouters BG, Begg AC. Irradiation-induced damage and DNA damage response. In: Joiner M, van der Kogel A, eds. *Basic Clinical Radiobiology.* 4th ed. London: Hodder Arnold; 2009:11–26.
4. Tubiana M, Dutreix J, Wambersie A. *Introduction to Radiobiology.* Bristol, PA: Taylor & Francis; 1990:97–104.
5. Fowler JF. The radiobiology of prostate cancer. *Acta Oncol.* 2005;44:265–276.
6. Thames HD. On the origin of dose fractionation regimens in radiotherapy. *Semin Radiat Oncol.* 1992;2:3–9.
7. Owen JR, Ashton A, Bliss JM, et al. Effect of radiotherapy fraction size on tumour control in patients with early-stage breast cancer after local tumour excision: long-term results of a randomised trial. *Lancet Oncol.* 2006;7:467–471.
8. Cox JD. Clinical perspectives of recent developments in fractionation. *Semin Radiat Oncol.* 1992;2:10–15.
9. Fowler JF. Intercomparisons of new and old schedules in fractionated radiotherapy. *Semin Radiat Oncol.* 1992;2:67–72.
10. Saunders MI, Dische S. Continuous, hyperfractionated, accelerated radiotherapy (CHART). *Semin Radiat Oncol.* 1992;2:41–44.
11. Stuschke M, Thames H. Hyperfractionation: where do we stand? *Radiother Oncol.* 1998;46:131–133.
12. Kaanders J, Van Der Kogel A, Ang KK. Altered fractionation: limited by mucosal reactions? *Radiother Oncol.* 1998;50:247–260.
13. Wilson EM, Williams JF, Lyn BE, et al. Comparison of two dimensional and three dimensional radiotherapy treatment planning in locally advanced non-small cell lung cancer treated with continuous hyperfractionated accelerated radiotherapy weekend less. *Radiother Oncol.* 2005;74:307–314.
14. Khoo VS, Dearnaley DP. Question of dose, fractionation and technique: ingredients for testing hypofractionation in prostate cancer—the CHHiP trial. *Clin Oncol.* 2008;20:12–14.
15. Stuschke M, Thames HD. Hyperfractionated radiotherapy of human tumors: overview of the randomized clinical trials. *Int J Radiat Oncol Phys Biol.* 1997;37:259–267.
16. Miles EF, Lee WR. Hypofractionation for prostate cancer: a critical review. *Semin Radiat Oncol.* 2008;18:41–47.
17. Haviland JS, Owen JR, Dewar JA, et al. The UK standardisation of breast radiotherapy (START) trials of radiotherapy hypofractionation for treatment of early breast cancer: 10-year follow-up results of two randomised controlled trials. *Lancet Oncol.* 2013;14:1086–1094.
18. Lyman JT. Complication probabilities as assessed from dose-volume histograms. *Radiat Res.* 1985;104:S13–S19.
19. Kutcher GJ, Burman C, Brewster L, et al. Histogram reduction method for calculating complication probabilities for three-dimensional treatment planning evaluations. *Int J Radiat Oncol Phys Biol.* 1991;21:137–146.

20. Mohan R, Mageras GS, Baldwin B, et al. Clinically relevant optimization of 3-D conformal treatments. *Med Phys.* 1992;19:933–944.

21. Niemierko A, Goitein M. Calculation of normal tissue complication probability and dose–volume histogram reduction schemes for tissue with a critical element architecture. *Radiother Oncol.* 1991;20:161–176.

22. Niemierko A. Reporting and analyzing dose distributions: a concept of equivalent uniform dose. *Med Phys.* 1997;24:103–110.

23. Kwa S, Theuws J, Wagenaar A, et al. Evaluation of two dose-volume histogram reduction models for the prediction of radiation pneumonitis. *Radiother Oncol.* 1998;48:61–69.

24. Moiseenko V, Battista J, Van Dyk J. Normal tissue complication probabilities: dependence on choice of biological model and dose-volume histogram reduction scheme. *Int J Radiat Oncol Biol Phys.* 2000;46:983–993.

25. Wang JZ, Li XA, D'Souza WD, et al. Impact of prolonged fraction delivery times on tumor control: a note of caution for intensity-modulated radiation therapy (IMRT). *Int J Radiat Oncol Phys Biol.* 2003;57:543–552.

26. Liao Y, Joiner M, Huang Y, et al. Hypofractionation: what does it mean for prostate cancer treatment? *Int J Radiat Oncol Phys Biol.* 2010;76:260–268.

27. Fyles AW, Milosevic M, Wong R, et al. Oxygen predicts radiation response and survival in patients with cervix cancer. *Radiother Oncol.* 1998;48:149–156.

28. Stadler P, Becker A, Feldmann HJ, et al. Influence of the hypoxic subvolume on the survival of patients with head and neck cancer. *Int J Radiat Oncol Biol Phys.* 1999;44:749–754.

29. Brizel DM, Dodge RK, Clough RW, et al. Oxygenation of head and neck cancer: changes during radiotherapy and impact on treatment outcome. *Radiother Oncol.* 1999;53:113–117.

30. Nahum AE, Movsas B, Horwitz EM, et al. Incorporating clinical measurements of hypoxia into tumor local control modeling of prostate cancer: implications for the α/β ratio. *Int J Radiat Oncol Biol Phys.* 2003;57:391–401.

31. Nordsmark M, Bentzen SM, Rudat V, et al. Prognostic value of tumor oxygenation in 397 head and neck tumors after primary radiation therapy: an international multi-center study. *Radiother Oncol.* 2005;77:18–24.

32. Movsas B, Chapman JD, Hanlon AL, et al. A hypoxic ratio of prostate pO₂/muscle pO₂ predicts for biochemical failure in prostate cancer patients. *Urology.* 2002;60:634–639.

33. Hall EJ. *Radiobiology for the Radiologist.* 5th ed. Philadelphia, PA: Lippincott Williams & Wilkins; 2000:112–123.

34. Chapman JD, Gillespie CJ, Reuvers AP, et al. The inactivation of Chinese hamster cells by x-rays: the effects of chemical modifiers on single- and double-events. *Rad Res.* 1975;64:365–375.

35. Palcic B, Skarsgard LD. Reduced oxygen enhancement ratio at low doses of radiation. *Rad Res.* 1984;100:328–329.

36. Orton C. In regard to Nahum et al. (*Int J Radiat Oncol Biol Phys.* 2003;57:391–401): incorporating clinical measurements of hypoxia into tumor control modeling of prostate cancer: implications for the α/β ratio. *Int J Radiat Oncol Biol Phys.* 2004;58:1637.

37. Nahum AE, Chapman JD. In response to Dr. Orton. *Int J Radiat Oncol Biol Phys.* 2004;58:1637–1639.

38. Daşu A, Denekamp J. New insights into factors influencing the clinically relevant oxygen enhancement ratio. *Radiother Oncol.* 1998;46:269–277.

39. Daşu A, Denekamp J. Superfractionation as a potential hypoxic cell radiosensitizer: prediction of an optimal dose per fraction. *Int J Radiat Oncol Biol Phys.* 1999;43:1083–1094.

40. Carlson DJ, Keall PJ, Loo BW, et al. Hypofractionation results in reduced cell kill compared to conventional fractionation for tumors with regions of hypoxia. *Int J Radiat Oncol Biol Phys.* 2011;79:1188–1195.

41. Withers HR, Taylor JM, Maciejewski B. The hazard of accelerated tumor clonogen repopulation during radiation therapy. *Acta Oncol.* 1988;27:131–146.

42. Bentzen S, Thames HD. Clinical evidence for tumor clonogen regeneration: interpretations of the data. *Radiother Oncol.* 1991;22:161–166.

43. Hall EJ. *Radiobiology for the Radiologist.* 5th ed. Philadelphia, PA: Lippincott Williams & Wilkins; 2000:51–66.

44. Bentzen SM, Saunders MI, Dische S, et al. Radiotherapy-related early morbidity in head and neck cancer: quantitative clinical radiobiology as deduced from the CHART trial. *Radiother Oncol.* 2001;60:123–135.

45. Saunders MI, Rojas A, Lyn BE, et al. Experience with dose escalation using CHARTWEL (continuous hyperfractionated accelerated radiotherapy weekend less) in non-small cell lung cancer. *Br J Cancer.* 1998;78:1323–1328.

46. Fowler JF, Ritter MA, Chappell RJ, et al. What hypofractionated protocols should be tested for prostate cancer? *Int J Radiat Oncol Biol Phys.* 2003;56:1093–1104.

47. Barendsen GW. Dose fractionation, dose-rate and isoeffect relationships for normal tissue responses. *Int J Radiat Oncol Biol Phys.* 1982;8:1981–1997.

48. Dale RG. The application of the linear-quadratic dose-effect equation to fractionated and protracted radiotherapy. *Br J Radiol.* 1985;58:515–528.

49. Bentzen SM, Ruifrok ACC, Thames HD. Repair capacity and kinetics for human mucosa and epithelial tumors in the head and neck: clinical data on the effect of changing the time interval between multiple fractions per day in radiotherapy. *Radiother Oncol.* 1996;38:89–101.

50. Murphy MJ, Peck-Sun L. Intra-fraction dose delivery timing during stereotactic radiotherapy can influence the radiobiological effect. *Med Phys.* 2007;34:481–484.

51. Narayana V, Orton C. Pulsed brachytherapy: a formalism to account for the variation in dose rate of the stepping source. *Med Phys.* 1999;26:161–165.

52. Manning MA, Zwicker RD, Arthur DW, et al. Biologic treatment planning for high-dose-rate brachytherapy. *Int J Radiat Oncol Biol Phys.* 2001;49:839–845.

53. Fowler JF. Brief summary of radiobiological principles in fractionated radiotherapy. *Semin Radiat Oncol.* 1992;2:16–21.

54. Orton CG. Recent developments in time–dose modeling. *Austral Phys Eng Sci Med.* 1991;14:57–64.

55. Emami B, Lyman J, Brown A, et al. Tolerance of normal tissue to therapeutic irradiation. *Int J Radiat Oncol Biol Phys.* 1991;21:109–122.

56. Marks LB, Yorke ED, Jackson A, et al. Use of normal tissue complication models in the clinic. *Int J Radiat Oncol Biol Phys.* 2010;76:S10–S19.

57. Kirkpatrick JP, Van Der Kogel AJ, Schultheiss TE. Radiation dose-volume effects in the spinal cord. *Int J Radiat Oncol Biol Phys.* 2010;76:S42–S49.

58. Joiner MC. A simple α/β-independent method to derive fully isoeffective schedules following changes in dose per fraction. *Int J Radiat Oncol Biol Phys.* 2004;58:871–875.

59. Marks LB, TenHaken RK, Martel MK. Guest editor's introduction to QUANTEC: a user's guide. *Int J Radiat Oncol Biol Phys.* 2010;76:S1–S2.

60. Astrahan M. Some implications of linear-quadratic-linear radiation dose-response with regard to hypofractionation. *Med Phys.* 2008;35:4161–4172.

61. Song CW, Mi-Sook K, Cho C, et al. Radiobiological basis of SBRT and SRS. *Int J Clin Oncol.* 2014;19:570–578.

62. Kirkpatrick J, Meyer J, Marks L. The linear-quadratic model is inappropriate to model high-dose per fraction effects. *Semin Radiat Oncol.* 2008;18:240–243.

63. Smith BD. Radiation therapy for the whole breast: executive summary of an American Society for Radiation Oncology (ASTRO) evidenced-based guideline. *Practical Rad Oncol.* 2018;8:145–152.

4 Immunologic Principles of Treatment Planning: Radiation as In Situ Vaccine and Dose Fractionation in the Immunotherapy Era

Andrew Brandmaier

INTRODUCTION

The rise of immunotherapy is transforming traditional cancer treatment paradigms. Immunotherapeutics for cancer represent a broad category of agents that modulate the immune system to elicit antitumor responses. Oncology practice has historically relied on various combinations of tumor reductive or cytotoxic modalities: surgery, chemotherapy, and radiation therapy. The expanding utilization of immunotherapy is part of a broader shift toward biologics that strategically target molecular pathways to modulate cellular phenotypes to achieve tumor destruction. Clinical trials continue to establish new indications for immune checkpoint inhibitors across a broad spectrum of malignancies, including melanoma, lung cancer, bladder cancer, renal cell carcinoma, and breast cancer. Checkpoint inhibitors are drugs that block regulatory molecules on T cells, such as PD-1 and CTLA-4, to enhance their activation and lower the threshold for an antitumor immune response. Evidence from in vivo tumor models and clinical trials has highlighted the therapeutic benefit of potent antitumor T cell immune responses against cancer. Developing protocols that reliably generate these responses in tumors is an ongoing area of investigation.

Radiation therapy stands apart as a modality capable of noninvasively targeting tumors with anatomic precision. The ability to deliver a volumetric cytotoxic therapy has complemented surgery and chemotherapy as an effective and reliable treatment for cancer patients. New discoveries in cancer biology, including enhanced characterization of the tumor microenvironment, have uncovered ways that radiation may also complement T cell immunity. Considerable evidence shows that successfully merging radiation and immunotherapy has the potential to elicit antitumor responses and improve therapeutic outcomes. This chapter will survey the role of T cells in tumor immunity, the pro-immunogenic and immunosuppressive effects of radiation on the tumor microenvironment, and preclinical data supporting synergy between radiation and immunotherapy as well as translational applications for treating cancer.

RADIATION DAMAGE AND INNATE IMMUNITY

Tumor radiation releases a constellation of molecular and cellular debris within the microenvironment, which broadens the effect of treatment beyond tumor killing into the realm of innate signaling of the immune system (Fig. 4.1). Cellular damage induced by radiation effectively activates pathways that sense danger and elicit immunity. Polly Matzinger conceptualized this general phenomenon as the "danger model" of immunity.[1] In the danger paradigm, immune activation is driven by the composite of damage and pathogen-related substrates detected by innate immune cells of the host. The framework of danger underlies how the immune system, in the correct context, can sense and destroy tumor cells. Damage-associated molecular patterns (DAMPs) are a subset of molecules released from dead and dying cells that are recognized by innate immune receptors.[2] Engagement of these receptors promotes downstream signaling cascades and activation of transcriptional programs that promote maturation of antigen-presenting cells (APCs), such as dendritic cells (DCs) and macrophages. Radiation has been found to release DAMPs that contribute to APC activation within tumors and promote antitumor immunity.

Radiation therapy produces free radicals in tissue that damage atomic bonds within deoxyribonucleic acid (DNA) and create chromatin breaks. One component of this damage was characterized decades ago with electron microscopy studies demonstrating the presence of perinuclear chromosome fragments persisting in cells after

Promotion of Anti-Tumor Activity

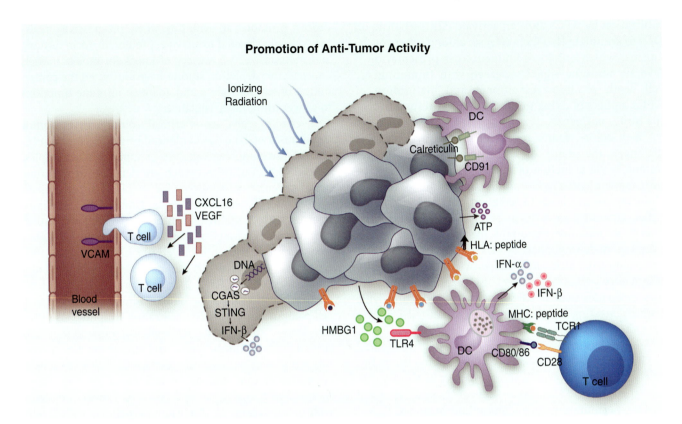

FIGURE 4.1. Ionizing radiation releases immune stimulatory signals in the tumor microenvironment. Induction of immunogenic cell death leads to externalization of calreticulin which promotes engulfment by professional APCs for processing and presentation of tumor antigens. Release of ATP and HMGB1 from dying cells stimulates maturation of APCs leading to antigen cross-presentation and priming of anti-tumor T cells. Perinuclear DNA fragments from radiation activate the cGAS-STING signaling cascade which stimulates production of cytokines and chemokines such as type I IFN and CXCL16 which, respectively, promote APC activation and recruitment of immune effector cells.

radiation. These chromosome pieces are encased in a nuclear envelope with lamina and nuclear pores and have the appearance of "micronuclei."[3] The innate immune pattern recognition receptor, cyclic GMP–AMP synthase (cGAS), is able to detect cytoplasmic DNA fragments, which serves as a key defensive mechanism against viral pathogens. When cGAS binds double-stranded DNA, it is activated to catalyze the synthesis of the second messenger cycle guanosine monophosphate GMP-adenosine monophosphate (cGAMP). cGAMP binds to the molecule STING (stimulator of interferon genes), a dimer on the endoplasmic reticulum membrane. Following this activation process, STING activates tank binding kinase 1 (TBK1), which phosphorylates interferon regulatory factor 3 (IRF3), a transcription factor that promotes gene expression of multiple proinflammatory mediators, including type I interferon, which promote adaptive immune processes.[4] Harding and colleagues demonstrated that micronuclei are produced when radiated cells undergo mitosis and linked that process with tumor expression of inflammatory cytokines, including interferon beta, interferon gamma, and chemokine ligand.[5] Thus, radiation promotes immune activation with downstream cytokine release by damaging chromatin and launching the cGAS signaling cascade.

An important connection between radiation, immune activation, and antitumor responses was illuminated in the work of Zitvogel and Kroemer, who framed the "immunogenic cell death" (ICD) paradigm.[6] Cell death occurs through a variety of programs, broadly classified as apoptotic, necrotic, and autophagic.[7] In the context of cancer treatment, radiation and certain classes of chemotherapy can trigger a mode of cell death that releases DAMPs and triggers innate immune receptors and maturation of APCs to activate antitumor immunity. Three hallmark DAMPs associated with ICD are calreticulin, HGMB2, and ATP. Calreticulin is an endoplasmic reticulum protein that relocates to the outer surface of the plasma membrane during ICD. DCs and macrophages recognize calreticulum via the CD91 receptor. This promotes phagocytosis of the cell and presentation of its associated tumor antigens to T cells.[8] HMGB1 (high mobility group box 1) functions as a chromatin-binding factor in the nucleus; it is released during ICD and binds the toll-like receptor 4 (TLR4) on DCs to promote their maturation. These activated DCs upregulate surface costimulatory molecules as well as endocytose tumor debris and cross-present associated antigens to prime antitumor CD8[+] T cells.[9] Adenosine triphosphate (ATP) recruits infiltration by APCs and can activate P2X receptors on DCs to stimulate IL-1-beta release, among other mechanisms, which enhances antigen cross-presentation.[10] Overall, immune signals released with immunogenic cell death promote recruitment and maturation of APCs, uptake of dying tumor cells, and presentation of the tumor antigens.

Furthermore, tumor treatment models in mice have illustrated the ability of radiation to promote cancer immunity via induction of cGAS–STING signaling. The pathway is initiated by the production of double stranded DNA breaks and leads to secretion of type I interferon, which promotes maturation of DCs. DCs matured by interferon mobilize important mechanisms for T cell priming, including phagocytosis of dead cells, cross-presentation of associated antigens, and production of stimulatory cytokines. They also express costimulatory molecules such as CD80 and CD86, which provide critical activating signals to naive and exhausted T cells to promote their function and proliferation.[11]

Studies in a mouse breast cancer model highlighted the importance of activated DCs in mediating the radiation immune response. Cohorts of mice with two distantly engrafted TSA breast cancer tumors received various permutations of radiation and/or anti-CTLA-4 therapy. Combination therapy with radiation to a single tumor of 8 Gy × 3 and anti-CTLA-4 achieved significant regression of the unirradiated (abscopal) tumor. This was shown to be mediated by cGAS–STING associated production of the cytokine IFN-beta, which activated BATF-3 dependent DCs. Importantly, high doses of radiation above 15 Gy per fraction upregulated an exonuclease, TREX1, which degraded double strand fragments produced by radiation and consequently attenuated cGAS activation and diminished the antitumor immune response.[12] These findings demonstrated the clinical utility of combination radiation with immunotherapy and illustrated that radiation dose needs to be calibrated for combinatorial applications.

IMMUNE SURVEILLANCE AND T CELLS

Malignantly transformed cells are often detected and eliminated by the host immune system prior to forming clinically apparent cancers. Paul Ehrlich first predicted a role for immune protection from tumors in the early 1900s, and this concept was subsequently validated by mouse genetic studies that demonstrated the tumor immunosurveillance phenomenon.[13] An equilibrium state exists between malignant cells and the host immune system; disease progression occurs when malignant clones ultimately evolve a sufficient profile of mutations to evade immune recognition altogether. This "immunoediting"

process promotes an evolution where progressively resistant cells are selected to survive, proliferate, form tumors, and metastasize.[14] A variety of knockout mouse models and selective depletion studies have illustrated the contribution of several innate and adaptive immune functions to cancer immunosurveillance.

T effector cells are a critical component of tumor immunosurveillance, as evidenced by findings from multiple mouse models and analysis of human tumor samples. RAG-2 knockout mice, which are deficient in a recombination enzyme required for V(D)J rearrangement, lack mature T cells and B cells. Notably, RAG-2' mice injected with 2'-methylcholanthrene (MCA), a chemical carcinogen, developed sarcomas more quickly, at higher frequency, and with lower levels of carcinogen than wild-type mice.[15] Spontaneous tumors were also observed at a higher frequency in RAG-2$^{-/-}$ mice compared to wild-type cohorts. Furthermore, in human tumor samples, the T cell composition of tumor-infiltrating lymphocytes (TIL) was shown to correlate with clinical outcomes across several different tumor types. An increase in CD8$^+$ T cells was associated with favorable survival in patients with colorectal cancer, and dense infiltration of TIL corresponded with longer survival in a large cohort of patients with breast cancer.[16,17] Additionally, patients with locally advanced esophageal squamous cell carcinoma with low levels of TIL were found to have inferior survival outcomes relative to those with higher levels.[18] In patients with oral cancer, the presence of zeta chain–deficient T cells, which corresponds with effector dysfunction, were found to have a worse survival.[19] The evidence suggests that functional T effector cells within tumors are a critical component of cancer immunity.

RADIATION AND T CELL IMMUNITY

Alpha–beta T cells play a key role in adaptive immune responses, including antitumor immunity. Every T cell clone expresses an alpha–beta T cell receptor with a randomly generated variable receptor subunit that has a high specificity for recognizing a specific major histocompatibility complex (MHC) associated with a peptide antigen. A human T cell repertoire also has a broad range of antigen recognition with an estimated 10^{10} unique clonotypes.[20] CD8$^+$ T cells that recognize tumor-associated antigenic peptides presented on MHC class I molecules can respond by secreting cytokines, such as IFN-gamma and TNF-alpha, and releasing granules with cytotoxic perforin and granzyme molecules to lyse tumor cells.[21] CD4$^+$ T helper cells usually adopt various phenotypic subtypes with characteristic cytokine profiles. When activated by tumor peptides presented on MHC class II molecule, helper T cells can amplify an antitumor immune response.[22] For example, the T_h1 subtype secretes IL-12, which stimulates cytotoxic CD8$^+$ T cells; IL-2, which is a T cell growth factor; and IFN-gamma, which promotes macrophage activation. Helper T cells and cytotoxic T cells work together at the center of cellular immune responses to attack antigen-bearing cells.

As previously described, radiation creates potent danger signals within tumors and promotes maturation of APCs, which is a critical first step in activating antitumor T cells. Activated DCs can endocytose dying tumor cells or debris, process the material, and cross-present tumor-associated peptides to CD8$^+$ T cells. Amplified display of tumor antigens coupled with co-stimulation increases the likelihood of activating the desired clones to mediate tumor destruction. Reits et al. showed that radiation of human melanoma cells increased expression of MHC class I molecules.[23] Also, Newcomb et al. examined a vaccination therapy for the murine glioblastoma, GL261; whole brain radiation increased tumor

expression of MHC-I molecules and enhanced the efficacy of the vaccine.[24] Taken together, the multitude of danger signals released by radiation and the corresponding activation of local APCs to co-stimulate and cross-prime tumor-specific T cells make radiotherapy a potent immune adjuvant to elicit an in situ vaccine within the treated tumor.

IMMUNE REGULATION WITHIN TUMORS

The tumor microenvironment varies among patients and cancer histologies but is often conditioned to actively suppress host antitumor immune responses. The composition of stroma and infiltrating immune cells plays a pivotal role in maintaining the health and growth of the tumor (Fig. 4.2). A characteristic milieu of chemokines

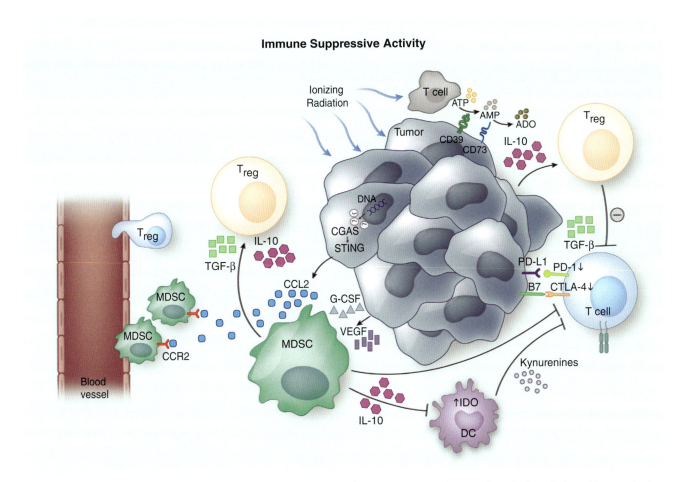

Immune Suppressive Activity

FIGURE 4.2. Immune regulatory effects from radiation can dampen anti-tumor responses. Increased production of chemokines and cytokines, such as CCL2 and VEGF, promotes recruitment of suppressive myeloid cells and T$_{regs}$ to the tumor. IL-10 and TGF-b promote T$_{reg}$ cell functions and suppress activation of effector T cells. Enzymes such as IDO, CD39, and CD73 are also upregulated and metabolize immune suppressive substrates. IDO promotes degradation of tryptophan into kynurenines. CD39 and CD73 sequentially dephosphorylate ATP into ADP and AMP.

and growth factors such as GM-CSF, VEGF, and CCL2 attract immature myeloid cells and sustain angiogenesis. Fibroblasts, vascular endothelial cells, myeloid-derived suppressor cells (MDSCs), M2 macrophages, and T regulatory cells (T$_{regs}$) form an immunosuppressive network that sustains tumor integrity and blocks T cell entry and priming.[25]

MDSCs, M2 macrophages, T$_{regs}$, and even some tumor cells secrete regulatory cytokines such as TGF-beta and IL-10. TGF-beta has multiple effects on growth, differentiation, and immunity and is potently immunosuppressive; it promotes expansion of the T$_{reg}$ compartment and suppresses cytolytic activity of CD8$^+$ T cells and also induces them to undergo apoptosis.[26,27] IL-10 inhibits maturation of DCs and reduces macrophage expression of co-stimulatory molecules and MHC class II expression.[28] MDSCs and tumor macrophages also synthesize reactive oxygen species, which impair effector function of CD8$^+$ T cells by reducing levels of T cell receptor (TCR) zeta chain and increase their proclivity for apoptosis by downregulating BCL-2.[29] MDSCs also modulate immunity through metabolic processes. They express indoleamine oxygenase (IDO), an enzyme that converts tryptophan to kyurenines, which promote conversion of naive CD4$^+$ T cells to T$_{regs}$. The depletion of tryptophan also sensitizes T cells to apoptosis.[30] Notably, high levels of tumor MDSCs in patients have been correlated with progression of disease and poor prognosis.[31]

Tumor mesenchymal cells, including fibroblasts and endothelium, also modulate local immunity. Fibroblasts form structural barriers by laying a collagen matrix around the tumor periphery to obstruct the entry of T cells. Furthermore, they have the ability to cross-present tumor antigens to CD8$^+$ T cells while concomitantly engaging them with PD-L2 and Fas ligand (FAS-L) to mediate their deletion.[32] Tumor endothelial cells are exposed to elevated levels of hypoxia inducible factor (HIF1-alpha) and VEGF, which upregulates FAS-L expression on their luminal surface. FAS-L can engage approaching CD8$^+$ T cells and induce apoptosis before they even extravasate into the tumor.[33] Overall, the constitutive cells of the tumor microenvironment deploy a broad spectrum of mechanisms to block T cell activity.

While radiation initiates immune activation through release of DAMPs, it also potentiates immunoregulatory processes within the microenvironment. For example, reoxygenation that occurs following radiation stabilizes HIF-1 and enhances gene expression of its targets. Reactive oxygen species from radiation also promote release of the active form of TGB-beta by causing a conformation change in the latency-associated peptide.[34,35] Additionally, activation of the cGAS–STING axis by radiation leads to upregulation of chemokines, such as CCL2, that attract MDSCs, macrophages, and T$_{regs}$ into the tumor. The impact of these mechanisms has been demonstrated with various in vivo tumor challenge studies. For example, two in vivo models of breast carcinoma challenged mice with a primary flank tumor and evaluated abscopal progression (lung metastases in 4T1 and a contralateral flank tumor in TSA), which demonstrated the impact of TGF-beta on immune suppression. In both models, radiation of the primary flank tumor combined with anti-TGF-beta blockade resulted in tumor infiltration with activated DCs and reduction of metastatic tumor burden.[36] In another in vivo study, Liang et al. showed that radiation resulted in increased tumor infiltration by MDSCs in a STING-dependent manner via the chemokine receptor 2 (CCR) axis. The combination of CCR2 blockade with tumor radiation in mice facilitated CD8$^+$ T cell–mediated tumor rejection, which could not be achieved with radiation alone.[37] These studies showed that radiation induces immune suppressive pathways. Rationally combining targeted immunotherapy with radiation could achieve synergistic therapeutic effects.

COMBINATION RADIATION THERAPY AND CHECKPOINT INHIBITION

The host immune system interacts closely with tumors, and T cells that recognize tumor antigens play a key role in eliminating neoplastic cells to prevent tumor growth. However, malignant cells can utilize the previously described immune regulatory mechanisms to create a tumor microenvironment that suppresses APCs and T cells and ultimately neutralizes antitumor immunity. The advent of immunotherapy has shown that targeting key immune regulatory mechanisms can effectively reinvigorate antitumor immune activity with clinically meaningful responses. Numerous clinical trials with immune checkpoint inhibitors such as anti-PD-1 and anti-CTLA-4 have demonstrated this phenomenon across a variety of tumor types.

Radiation therapy produces multiple innate immune signals that activate APCs, which have the potential to prime T cells and initiate antitumor immune responses. However, off-target tumor regression following radiation monotherapy is uncommon and only documented in limited case reports, likely due to the high barrier posed by homeostatic immune regulatory processes. Several preclinical models have demonstrated therapeutic efficacy by combining tumor radiation with immune checkpoint inhibition. Demaria and colleagues challenged mice with 4T1 breast carcinoma, a poorly immunogenic tumor, and showed that monotherapy with either anti-CTLA-4 or radiation was individually ineffective. However, combinatorial therapy employing radiation of cutaneous 4T1 tumors with concomitant administration of anti-CTLA-4 improved survival and decreased the number of lung metastases.[38] Minn and colleagues treated B16 melanoma in mice with dual checkpoint inhibition of anti-PD-1 and anti-CTLA-4. A cohort of mice that received dual checkpoint inhibition as well as tumor radiation achieved the highest efficacy of the various treatment groups, and each therapy contributed nonredundant immune activation. The conclusion was that dual checkpoint inhibition decreased T_{regs} and reinvigorated exhausted $CD8^+$ T cells, which increased the $CD8^+/T_{reg}$ ratio and tipped the overall homeostatic balance toward immune activation.[39] Additionally, radiation therapy increased antitumor TCR repertoire diversity, further amplifying the potential of an immune response. Rudqvist and colleagues have separately reported that treating tumor-challenged mice with combination radiation and anti-CTLA-4 therapy expanded the T cell repertoire, with an increase in diversity of TCR variable region motifs.[40] Combining the immune-priming activity of radiation with antiregulatory stimulation from checkpoint inhibitors has the potential to manifest an in situ vaccine effect within tumors.

Translating combinations of radiation and checkpoint immunotherapy into successful clinical protocols requires synergistic regimens. Dose, fractionation, sequencing, and target selection are key radiation variables to be optimized as this strategy evolves. Most case reports detailing examples of patients experiencing off-target tumor regression following radiation and immunotherapy involved hypofractionated courses (five or fewer fractions of treatment).[39,41,42] There is no consensus framework for optimally immunogenic radiation prescriptions; however, ongoing clinical trials have adopted key principles from preclinical data. Vanpouille-Box and colleagues demonstrated the nuances associated with dose and fractionation in an in vivo breast cancer model, where mice were challenged with bilateral flank tumors. They showed that tumor radiation of 8 Gy × 3 daily fractions potently induced cGAS–STING signaling and, when given together with anti-CTLA-4 therapy, led to significant contralateral abscopal tumor regression.[12] Lower doses of radiation, such as a single fraction of 8 Gy × 1, were ineffective at inducing cGAS–STING. Moreover, higher ablative doses, such as 20 Gy × 1, were counterproductive due to induction of the exonuclease TREX1, which degraded dsDNA produced by radiation and thereby attenuated cGAS activation and abscopal tumor response. A separate model of 67NR (mouse mammary carcinoma) showed that combination of single fraction radiation with FLT3 ligand, a growth factor that stimulates DCs, was able to generate an abscopal response.[43] Primary flank tumor radiation with a dose as low as 2 Gy demonstrated abscopal growth attenuation of a contralateral flank tumor with equivalent efficacy to a comparison cohort that received 6 Gy. Furthermore, these models illustrate that complex biologic factors impact the selection of immunogenic radiation doses. An optimal radiation prescription will balance tumor killing with innate immune signaling to activate systemic antitumor immunity.

Clinical trials of immunotherapy coupled with various radiation dose and fractionation regimens will continue to accrue until a solid framework of best principles is established. To this end, multiple early phase clinical trials are actively under way, and some have already reported preliminary findings. Luke and colleagues administered combination pembrolizumab and stereotactic body radiation therapy (SBRT) with doses ranging from 30 to 50 Gy in a phase I clinical trial for patients with progressing solid tumor metastases. The objective response rate of 13.2% and overall survival of 3.1 months was similar to that of an unselected cohort receiving pembrolizumab monotherapy.[44] A phase II trial from the Netherlands Cancer Institute randomized patients with metastatic non-small cell lung cancer (NSCLC) to pembrolizumab plus upfront radiation of 8 Gy × 3 to a single metastatic lesion versus pembrolizumab alone. The combined treatment cohort achieved an objective response rate of 41% versus 19% in the control cohort and a median progression-free survival (PFS) of 6.4 versus 1.8 months, respectively.[45] This finding bolsters approaches utilizing intermediate, fractionated SBRT doses that align with the Vanpouille-Box preclinical data. Other clinical trials are incorporating checkpoint immunotherapy with more conventional fractionated radiation protocols. The PACIFIC trial for patients with stage III NSCLC is the most prominent example. Patients who received adjuvant anti-PD-L1 therapy following conventional chemoradiation with 54 to 66 Gy achieved a superior PFS compared to the placebo group, establishing a new standard of care. Clinical trials for diseases where fractionated radiation is part of the traditional treatment paradigm, such as stage III NSCLC, will likely incorporate checkpoint immunotherapy with the conventional radiation prescriptions. Conversely, clinical trials in the metastatic setting will be at the forefront of testing immunogenicity of various dose and fractionation regimens.

Radiation therapy of metastatic cancer has traditionally utilized prescriptions with modest a biologically effective dose (BED) for palliative purposes, such as pain relief and focal preservation of function. However, the paradigm for oligometastatic disease is evolving with evidence pointing toward objective benefits from comprehensive ablation. The SABR-COMET trial provided phase II evidence that treating patients harboring five or fewer metastases with stereotactic ablative radiation improved PFS and overall survival compared to standard palliative doses.[46] Subsequent phase III trials are proceeding to validate these findings. Widespread adoption of SBRT for metastases should complement efforts to integrate immune checkpoint inhibitors with radiotherapy. A key question is whether an abscopal approach targeting a subset of lesions for immunogenic activation versus comprehensive maximum tumor ablation would best synergize with immune checkpoint blockade. As previously described, high dose per fraction above 10 Gy may attenuate cGAS–STING signaling and consequently reduce DC activation. However, maximum ablative doses would more effectively reduce the patient's tumor burden. Higher tumor bulk leads to chronic antigen overexposure of tumor-specific T cells, resulting in an exhausted phenotype, similar to that seen in chronic viral infections.[47] Ablative radiation doses that reduce tumor burden to a microscopic level may establish a more favorable environment for antitumor T cells to destroy the residual disease. Huang and colleagues studied the impact of tumor burden on a cohort of metastatic melanoma patients receiving anti-PD-1 therapy. Patients with higher tumor burden at the outset had weaker clinical responses with a corresponding inability to reinvigorate exhausted CD8$^+$ T cells.[48] Newer clinical trials are emerging to test SABR-COMET radiation regimens together with checkpoint inhibition.

RADIATION TARGETING FOR ANTITUMOR IMMUNITY

Target selection is another complex variable still evolving in immunotherapy protocols. Most of the initial clinical trials combining radiation and checkpoint inhibitors have prescribed radiation to a single lesion and monitored response in nonradiated abscopal lesions. Given the diverse presentation of metastases in terms of number and location, a variety of approaches could impact treatment response. Studies have shown that metastases in different organs may have varying levels of immune response to radiation. For example, data from a phase I study suggested that radiation of liver metastases was more immunogenic than pulmonary metastases based on measurements of increase in peripheral CD8$^+$ T cells and T cell expression of activation markers.[49] A phase III study for patients with prostate cancer assessed efficacy of radiating bone metastases followed by anti-CTLA-4 versus placebo. There was no significant improvement in outcome with addition of immunotherapy, though the trial protocol administered immunotherapy following radiation, which may have been suboptimal.[50] Jiao et al. showed in a separate study that bone metastases produce high levels of TGF-beta which skews the phenotype of infiltrating CD4$^+$ helper T cells away from the IFN-gamma-producing T$_h$1 subtype. These findings are hypothesis generating, and no ranking of organ immunogenicity has been established.

Another variable of target selection is the number of lesions receiving radiation. For oligometastatic disease, integrating the SABR-COMET approach of comprehensive tumor targeting and adding checkpoint therapy would expand the scope of in situ vaccination. Instead of activating immunity against a single tumor, global abscopal responses across the spectrum of metastases could potentially be generated. A growing literature has characterized the phenomenon of heterogeneity within tumor microenvironments and also between metastatic tumors

and their primary tumor.[51,52] Distinct genetic mutations among different metastases may create unique neoantigen profiles. Therefore, directly activating immune priming within multiple, potentially heterogenous metastases should provide more comprehensive antitumor T cell activation. Nonetheless, targeting every metastasis with high-dose radiation is not feasible for patients with widespread disease due to practical limitations such as delivery time and volumetric limitations of organs at risk. However, some evidence suggests that even lower doses of radiation can enhance immune responses within tumors, so a hybrid approach could potentially emerge employing SBRT for a predetermined number of lesions and conventional dosing for additional areas. An alternative strategy to achieve spatial diversity would target at least one tumor within each different organ site with metastases. At this time, target selection in the metastatic setting is largely subject to clinical judgment for the individual patient.

Various sequences combining radiation and checkpoint inhibitors have been evaluated preclinically and from retrospective patient data. Preclinical findings favor starting the immunotherapy just prior to or at the beginning of radiation. For example, checkpoint inhibition with anti-CTLA-4 given the week prior to radiation demonstrated superior efficacy to other sequences in a model of murine colon carcinoma. The results showed how anti-CTLA-4 therapy depleted T$_{regs}$, and upfront administration facilitated maximum priming of CD8$^+$ T cells at the time of radiation.[53] Clinical data from melanoma patients with brain metastases demonstrated that dual checkpoint inhibition with anti-PD-1 and anti-CTLA-4 followed by stereotactic radiosurgery achieved the greatest reduction in tumor volume if the therapies were given within 4 weeks of each other.[54] Additionally, in the Pacific Trial, a post-hoc analysis showed that administration of anti-PD-L1 within 2 weeks of completion of chemoradiation was associated with improved PFS compared to a lapse of greater than 2 weeks.[55] Overall, evidence favors initiation of checkpoint inhibitor therapy just prior to or at the start of radiation, and most clinical trials follow this precedent.

An additional factor for radiation planning with concomitant immunotherapy is exposure of the lymphocyte population. T cells are highly sensitive to radiation with a D$_{50}$ (dose inactivating 50% of cells) of approximately 2 Gy. Radiotherapy plans that encompass tumor-draining lymph nodes in the target field or expose a significant proportion of the peripheral blood pool through protracted fractionation can deplete the lymphocyte population and potentially diminish antitumor immunity. Notably, for combination regimens with radiation and immunotherapy, the absolute lymphocyte count is predictive of abscopal response and patient outcomes.[56] A study of patients receiving various courses of palliative radiation showed that more than 5 treatment fractions was associated with greater reductions in absolute lymphocyte count. Severe lymphopenia at the onset of immunotherapy was also associated with increased mortality.[57] Yovino and colleagues analyzed glioblastoma radiation plans and modeled the dose to circulating cells. Based on the model, a single fraction from a typical plan exposed 5% of circulating cells to 0.5 Gy, whereas a 30-fraction course exposed 99% of circulating cells to 0.5 Gy. This underscores an advantage of hypofractionated radiation, which limits cumulative exposure of circulating lymphocytes, relative to protracted courses. Exposure of tumor-draining lymph nodes, a rich reservoir of antitumor T cells, also impacts radiation immunity. Marciscano evaluated a mouse model where subjects were challenged with flank tumors and treated with 12 Gy of radiation together with a checkpoint inhibition. Two cohorts were treated with different radiation plans, with one directly targeting just the tumor and the other targeting the tumor and the draining lymph nodes. The addition of nodal radiation resulted in reduced immune cell infiltration of tumors and reduced overall survival.[58] Thus, for combinatorial regimens of radiation and immunotherapy, radiation planning should avoid lymphocyte reservoirs in the nodes and circulating blood.

SUMMARY

Radiation therapy has a substantial impact on the tumor microenvironment. The direct cytocidal elimination of tumor is accompanied by release of an array of damage molecules that trigger innate immune receptors on professional APCs. This leads to increased processing and presentation of tumor antigens with the potential to prime antitumor T cells. Radiation also elicits homeostatic immune regulatory cells and cytokines that suppress APC function and T cell activation. The addition of immunotherapy drugs, such as checkpoint inhibitors, to radiation has demonstrated promising results in preclinical tumor models by eliciting systemic antitumor immune activity with measurable abscopal tumor destruction.

Therapeutic strategies combining radiation and immunotherapy are actively being explored in clinical trials. Utilization of hypofractionation radiation regimens for metastatic disease is rapidly expanding and provides a rich opportunity for testing combination protocols with checkpoint immunotherapy. When using anti-CTLA-4 and anti-PD-1 checkpoint inhibitors, optimal results are obtained from immunotherapy administration just prior to or concurrently with tumor radiation. Additional variables such as tumor target selection and whether to use ablative doses or intermediate doses remain a matter of investigation. However, evidence does support hypofractionated regimens that spare radiation exposure of the peripheral lymphocyte blood pool and tumor-draining lymph nodes. As ongoing clinical trials mature, new data will inform strategies to integrate radiation and immunotherapy in ways that achieve greater efficacy against tumors.

KEY POINTS

- Tumor radiation releases damage-associated molecular patterns (DAMPS), which are sensed by innate receptors of the immune system. In this way, radiation triggers immune activation within the tumor microenvironment.

- Calreticulin, HGMB2, and ATP are three characteristic molecules released during immunogenic cell death. dsDNA fragments produced from radiation damage also activate cGAS-STING signaling, which upregulates type I interferon production. These molecules facilitate innate immune activation, including maturation of antigen-presenting cells. This enables them to take up tumor antigens and prime antitumor T cells with co-stimulation.

- The tumor microenvironment is usually immuno-suppressive with a population of regulatory T cells and myeloid cells and a milieu of modulatory cytokines such as TGF-β and IL-10. Radiation of tumors upregulates secretion of chemokines that recruit myeloid suppressor cells which counteracts T cell priming and effector functions.

- Combinations of radiation and checkpoint immunotherapy can synergize to stimulate immune activation of the tumor microenvironment. A preclinical model demonstrated that 8 Gy × 3 effectively promoted type I interferon release and, together with anti-CTLA-4, mediated abscopal tumor destruction.

- Various immunogenic radiation protocols are being studied in clinical trials. Common features include hypofractionated prescriptions and conformal targeting. In combination regimens with immunotherapy, checkpoint inhibitors are typically administered prior to or concurrent with the start of radiation.

REVIEW QUESTIONS

1. Which of the following are immune-stimulating danger signals released in the tumor microenvironment following radiation?
   A. HMGB1, p53, HIF1-α
   B. HIF1-α, VEGF, TREX1
   C. Calreticulin, p53, ATP
   D. Calreticulin, ATP, HMGB1

2. What process initiated by radiation leads to production of type I interferon?
   A. Reactive oxygen species deplete the coenzyme NAD^+.
   B. dsDNA breaks form fragments that activate cGAS.
   C. Free radical formation triggers innate immune receptors on T cells.
   D. dsDNA breaks form fragments that activate HIF1-α

3. How does type I interferon promote antitumor immunity
   A. It promotes maturation of dendritic cells.
   B. It promotes apoptosis of infiltrating T_{reg} cells.
   C. It promotes apoptosis of myeloid suppressor cells.
   D. It activates the cGAS-STING signaling pathway.

4. Which of the following effects of radiation promotes antitumor immunity when combined with checkpoint inhibition?
   A. Activation of M2 macrophages
   B. Increased T cell receptor clonal diversity
   C. Inhibition of PD-1 signaling
   D. Upregulation of tumor expression of MHC class II

5. Which radiation regimen has been shown in preclinical studies to maximally induce synthesis of the DNA exonuclease, TREX1?
   A. 8 Gy $\times$ 1
   B. 8 Gy $\times$ 3
   C. 30 Gy $\times$ 1
   D. 10 Gy $\times$ 2

ANSWERS

1. D   HMGB1, ATP, and calreticulin are molecules released from cells during immunogenic death. These DAMPS collectively signal pattern receptors on neighboring immune cells, which triggers innate activation that can prime antitumor immunity.[6–10]

2. B   Radiation induces double-stranded DNA breaks, which leads to formation of dsDNA fragments that accumulate in micronuclei. cGAS detects these DNA fragments and catalyzes synthesis of second messenger cycle guanosine monophosphate (GMP) adenosine monophosphate (cGAMP). cGAMP binds STING (stimulator of interferon genes) which initiates a signaling cascade leading to transcriptional activation of type I interferon expression.[4,5]

3. A   Type I interferons bind to the IFN-α receptor on the surface of antigen presenting cells. IFN-α signaling promotes differentiation of dendritic cells from precursor blood cells. It induces maturation of dendritic cells with increased expression of co-stimulatory molecules such as CD80 and CD86 and increased processing and presentation of MHC class II antigen complexes. Additionally, IFN-α signaling upregulates dendritic cell cross-presentation of antigens. In the tumor microenvironment, this enhances endocytosis and processing of tumor antigens to prime cytotoxic $CD8^+$ T cells.[11,12]

4. B   Tumor radiation increases T cell receptor diversity. Minn and colleagues treated B_{16} melanoma in mice with dual checkpoint inhibition of anti-PD-1 and anti-CTLA-4. The addition of radiation therapy increased antitumor TCR repertoire diversity.[39] Rudqvist and colleagues have separately reported that treating tumor-challenged mice with combination radiation and anti-CTLA-4 therapy expanded the T cell repertoire with an increase in diversity of TCR variable region motifs.[40]

5. C   In a preclinical study of combinatorial radiation and checkpoint inhibition, it was shown that 8 Gy $\times$ 3 fractions effectively produced dsDNA fragments and activated cGAS-STING leading to antitumor immunity. However, high doses of radiation above 15 Gy per fraction upregulated an exonuclease, TREX1, which degraded double-strand fragments produced by radiation and consequently attenuated cGAS activation and diminished the antitumor immune response.[12]

REFERENCES

1. Matzinger P. The danger model: a renewed sense of self. *Science.* 2002;296(5566):301–305. doi:10.1126/science.1071059
2. Gong T, Liu L, Jiang W, Zhou R. DAMP-sensing receptors in sterile inflammation and inflammatory diseases. *Nat Rev Immunol.* 2019;20(2):95–112. doi:10.1038/s41577-019-0215-7
3. Géraud G, Laquerriere F, Masson C, Arnoult J, Labidi B, Hernandez-Verdun D. Three-dimensional organization of micronuclei induced by colchicine in PtK1 cells. *Exp Cell Res.* 1989; 181(1):27–39. doi:10.1016/0014-4827(89)90179-1
4. Barber GN. STING: infection, inflammation and cancer. *Nat Rev Immunol.* 2015;15(12):760–770. doi:10.1038/nri3921
5. Harding SM, Benci JL, Irianto J, Discher DE, Minn AJ, Greenberg RA. Mitotic progression following DNA damage enables pattern recognition within micronuclei. *Nature.* 2017; 548(7668):466–470. doi:10.1038/nature23470
6. Kepp O, Senovilla L, Vitale I, et al. Consensus guidelines for the detection of immunogenic cell death. *Oncoimmunology.* 2014:e955691vol. 9.
7. Green D, Llambi F. Cell death signaling. *Cold Spring Harb Perspect Biol.* 2015;7(12):a006080. doi:10.1101/cshperspect.a006080
8. Wiersma VR, Michalak M, Abdullah TM, Bremer E, Eggleton P. Mechanisms of translocation of ER chaperones to the cell surface and immunomodulatory roles in cancer and autoimmunity. *Front Oncol.* 2015;5:7. doi:10.3389/fonc.2015.00007
9. Pathak SK, Skold AE, Mohanram V, Persson C, Johansson U, Spetz AL. Activated apoptotic cells induce dendritic cell maturation via engagement of Toll-like receptor 4 (TLR4), dendritic cell-specific intercellular adhesion molecule 3 (ICAM-3)-grabbing nonintegrin (DC-SIGN), and beta2 integrins. *J Biol Chem.* 2012; 287(17):13731–13742. doi:10.1074/jbc.M111.336545
10. Englezou E, Rothwell S, Ainscough J, et al. P2X7R activation drives distinct IL-1 responses in dendritic cells compared to macrophages. *Cytokine.* 2015;74(2):293–304. doi:10.1016/j.cyto.2015.05.013
11. Larsen C, Ritchie S, Pearson T, Linsley P, Lowry R. Functional expression of the costimulatory molecule, B7/BB1, on murine dendritic cell populations. *J Exp Med.* 1992;176(4):1215–1220. doi:10.1084/jem.176.4.1215.
12. Vanpouille-Box C, Alard A, Aryankalayil MJ, et al. DNA exonuclease Trex1 regulates radiotherapy-induced tumour immunogenicity. *Nat Commun.* 2017;8:15618. doi:10.1038/ncomms15618
13. Smyth M, Godfrey D, Trapani J. A fresh look at tumor immunosurveillance and immunotherapy. *Nat Immunol.* 2001;2(4):293–299. doi:10.1038/86297
14. Dunn G, Bruce A, Ikeda H, Old L, Schreiber R. Cancer immunoediting: from immunosurveillance to tumor escape. *Nat Immunol.* 2002;3(11):991–998. doi:10.1038/ni1102-991
15. Shankaran V, Ikeda H, Bruce A, et al. IFNgamma and lymphocytes prevent primary tumour development and shape tumour immunogenicity. *Nature.* 2001;410(6832):1107–1111. doi:10.1038/35074122
16. Naito Y, Saito K, Shiiba K, et al. CD8+ T cells infiltrated within cancer cell nests as a prognostic factor in human colorectal cancer. *Cancer Res.* 1998;58(16):3491–3494.
17. Yoshimoto M, Sakamoto G, Ohashi Y. Time dependency of the influence of prognostic factors on relapse in breast cancer. *Cancer.* 1993;72(10):2993–3001. doi:10.1002/1097-0142(19931115) 72:10<2993::aid-cncr2820721022>3.0.co;2-6
18. Yasunaga M, Tabira Y, Nakano K, et al. Accelerated growth signals and low tumor-infiltrating lymphocyte levels predict poor outcome in T4 esophageal squamous cell carcinoma. *Ann Thorac Surg.* 2000;70(5):1634–1640. doi:10.1016/s0003-4975(00)01915-9
19. Reichert T, Day R, Wagner E, Whiteside T. Absent or low expression of the zeta chain in T cells at the tumor site correlates with poor survival in patients with oral carcinoma. *Cancer Res.* 1998;58(23):5344–5347.
20. Lythe G, Callard RE, Hoare RL, Molina-París C. How many TCR clonotypes does a body maintain? *J Theor Biol.* 2016:214–224.
21. Zhang N, Bevan MJ. CD8(+) T cells: foot soldiers of the immune system. *Immunity.* 2011;35(2):161–168. doi:10.1016/j.immuni.2011.07.010
22. Borst J, Ahrends T, Babala N, Melief CJM, Kastenmuller W. CD4(+) T cell help in cancer immunology and immunotherapy. *Nat Rev Immunol.* 2018;18(10):635–647. doi:10.1038/s41577-018-0044-0
23. Reits EA, Hodge JW, Herberts CA, et al. Radiation modulates the peptide repertoire, enhances MHC class I expression, and induces successful antitumor immunotherapy. *J Exp Med.* 2006;203(5):1259–1271. doi:10.1084/jem.20052494
24. Newcomb EW, Demaria S, Lukyanov Y, et al. The combination of ionizing radiation and peripheral vaccination produces long-term survival of mice bearing established invasive GL261 gliomas. *Clin Cancer Res.* 2006;12(15):4730–4737. doi:10.1158/1078-0432.ccr-06-0593
25. Joyce JA, Fearon DT. T cell exclusion, immune privilege, and the tumor microenvironment. *Science.* 2015;348(6230):74–80. doi:10.1126/science.aaa6204
26. Massagué J. TGFβ in cancer. *Cell.* 2008;134(2):215–230. doi:10.1016/j.cell.2008.07.001
27. Travis MA, Sheppard D. TGF-beta activation and function in immunity. *Annu Rev Immunol.* 2014;32:51–82. doi:10.1146/annurev-immunol-032713-120257
28. Sanjabi S, Zenewicz L, Kamanaka M, Flavell R. Anti-inflammatory and pro-inflammatory roles of TGF-beta, IL-10, and IL-22 in immunity and autoimmunity. *Curr Opin Pharmacol.* 2009;9(4):447–453. doi:10.1016/j.coph.2009.04.008
29. Ezernitchi AV, Vaknin I, Cohen-Daniel L, et al. TCR zeta down-regulation under chronic inflammation is mediated by myeloid suppressor cells differentially distributed between various lymphatic organs. *J Immunol.* 2006;177(7):4763–4772.
30. Marvel D, Gabrilovich DI. Myeloid-derived suppressor cells in the tumor microenvironment: expect the unexpected. *J Clin Invest.* 2015;125(9):3356–3364. doi:10.1172/jci80005
31. Weide B, Martens A, Zelba H, et al. Myeloid-derived suppressor cells predict survival of patients with advanced melanoma: comparison with regulatory T cells and NY-ESO-1- or melan-A-specific T cells. *Clin Cancer Res.* 2014;20(6):1601–1609. doi:10.1158/1078-0432.ccr-13-2508
32. Lakins M, Ghorani E, Munir H, Martins C, Shields J. Cancer-associated fibroblasts induce antigen-specific deletion of CD8+ T Cells to protect tumour cells. *Nat Commun.* 2018;9(1):1–9. doi:10.1038/s41467-018-03347-0
33. Motz GT, Santoro SP, Wang LP, et al. Tumor endothelium FasL establishes a selective immune barrier promoting tolerance in tumors. *Nat Med.* 2014;20(6):607–615. doi:10.1038/nm.3541
34. Jobling M, Mott J, Finnegan M, et al. Isoform-specific activation of latent transforming growth factor beta (LTGF-beta) by reactive oxygen species. *Radiat Res.* 2006;166(6):839–848. doi:10.1667/RR0695.1
35. Barcellos-Hoff M, Derynck R, Tsang M, Weatherbee J. Transforming growth factor-beta activation in irradiated murine mammary gland. *J Clin Investig.* 1994;93(2):892–899. doi:10.1172/JCI117045
36. Vanpouille-Box C, Diamond JM, Pilones KA, et al. TGFbeta is a master regulator of radiation therapy-induced antitumor immunity. *Cancer Res.* 2015;75(11):2232–2242. doi:10.1158/0008-5472.can-14-3511
37. Liang H, Deng L, Hou Y, et al. Host STING-dependent MDSC mobilization drives extrinsic radiation resistance. *Nat Commun.* 2017;8(1):1736. doi:10.1038/s41467-017-01566-5
38. Demaria S, Kawashima N, Yang AM, et al. Immune-mediated inhibition of metastases after treatment with local radiation and CTLA-4 blockade in a mouse model of breast cancer. *Clin Cancer Res.* 2005;11(2 Pt 1):728–734.
39. Twyman-Saint Victor C, Rech AJ, Maity A, et al. Radiation and dual checkpoint blockade activate non-redundant immune mechanisms in cancer. *Nature.* 2015;520(7547):373–377. doi:10.1038/nature14292
40. Rudqvist NP, Pilones KA, Lhuillier C, et al. Radiotherapy and CTLA-4 blockade shape the TCR repertoire of tumor-infiltrating T cells. *Cancer Immunol Res.* 2018;6(2):139–150. doi:10.1158/2326-6066.cir-17-0134

41. Postow MA, Callahan MK, Barker CA, et al. Immunologic correlates of the abscopal effect in a patient with melanoma. *N Engl J Med.* 2012;366(10):925–931. doi:10.1056/NEJMoa1112824

42. Xu MJ, Wu S, Daud AI, Yu SS, Yom SS. In-field and abscopal response after short-course radiation therapy in patients with metastatic Merkel cell carcinoma progressing on PD-1 checkpoint blockade: a case series. *J Immunother Cancer.* 2018;6(1):43. doi:10.1186/s40425-018-0352-8

43. Demaria S, Ng B, Devitt ML, et al. Ionizing radiation inhibition of distant untreated tumors (abscopal effect) is immune mediated. *Int J Radiat Oncol Biol Phys.* 2004;58(3):862–870. doi:10.1016/j.ijrobp.2003.09.012a

44. Luke JJ, Lemons JM, Karrison TG, et al. Safety and clinical activity of pembrolizumab and multisite stereotactic body radiotherapy in patients with advanced solid tumors. *J Clin Oncol.* 2018;36(16):1611–1618. doi:10.1200/jco.2017.76.2229

45. Theelen W, Peulen HMU, Lalezari F, et al. Effect of pembrolizumab after stereotactic body radiotherapy vs pembrolizumab alone on tumor response in patients with advanced non-small cell Lung cancer: results of the PEMBRO-RT phase 2 randomized clinical trial. *JAMA Oncol.* 2019;5(9):1276–1282. doi:10.1001/jamaoncol.2019.1478

46. Palma D, Olson R, Harrow S, et al. Stereotactic ablative radiotherapy versus standard of care palliative treatment in patients with oligometastatic cancers (SABR-COMET): a randomised, phase 2, open-label trial. *Lancet.* 2019;393(10185):2051–2058. doi:10.1016/S0140-6736(18)32487-5

47. Bordon Y. TOX for tired T cells. *Nat Rev Immunol.* 2019;19(8):476. doi:10.1038/s41577-019-0193-9

48. Huang A, Postow M, Orlowski R, et al. T-cell invigoration to tumour burden ratio associated with anti-PD-1 response. *Nature.* 2017;545(7652):60–65. doi:10.1038/nature22079

49. Tang C, Welsh J, de Groot P, et al. Ipilimumab with stereotactic ablative radiation therapy: phase I results and immunologic correlates from peripheral T cells. *Clin Cancer Res.* 2017;23(6):1388–1396. doi:10.1158/1078-0432.CCR-16-1432

50. Kwon E, Drake C, Scher H, et al. Ipilimumab versus placebo after radiotherapy in patients with metastatic castration-resistant prostate cancer that had progressed after docetaxel chemotherapy (CA184-043): a multicentre, randomised, double-blind, phase 3 trial. *Lancet Oncol.* 2014;15(7):700–712. doi:10.1016/S1470-2045(14)70189-5

51. Angus L, Smid M, Wilting S, et al. The genomic landscape of metastatic breast cancer highlights changes in mutation and signature frequencies. *Nature Genetics.* 2019;51(10). doi:10.1038/s41588-019-0507-7

52. Easwaran H, Tsai H, Baylin S. Cancer epigenetics: tumor heterogeneity, plasticity of stem-like states, and drug resistance. *Molecular Cell.* 2014;54(5):716–727. doi:10.1016/j.molcel.2014.05.015

53. Young KH, Baird JR, Savage T, et al. Optimizing timing of immunotherapy improves control of tumors by hypofractionated radiation therapy. *PLoS One.* 2016;11(6):e0157164. doi:10.1371/journal.pone.0157164

54. Qian JM, Yu JB, Kluger HM, Chiang VL. Timing and type of immune checkpoint therapy affect the early radiographic response of melanoma brain metastases to stereotactic radiosurgery. *Cancer.* 2016;122(19):3051–3058. doi:10.1002/cncr.30138

55. Wang Y, Deng W, Li N, et al. Combining immunotherapy and radiotherapy for cancer treatment: current challenges and future directions. *Front Pharmacol.* 2018;9:185. doi:10.3389/fphar.2018.00185

56. Absolute lymphocyte count predicts abscopal responses and outcomes in patients receiving combined immunotherapy and radiation therapy: analysis of 3 phase 1/2 trials. *Int J Radiat Oncol Biol Phys.* 2020;108:196–203. doi:10.1016/j.ijrobp.2020.01.032

57. Pike L, Bang A, Mahal B, et al. The impact of radiation therapy on lymphocyte count and survival in metastatic cancer patients receiving PD-1 immune checkpoint inhibitors. *Int J Radiat Oncol Biol Phys.* 2019;103(1):142–151. doi:10.1016/j.ijrobp.2018.09.010

58. Marciscano AE, Ghasemzadeh A, Nirschl TR, et al. Elective nodal irradiation attenuates the combinatorial efficacy of stereotactic radiation therapy and immunotherapy. *Clin Cancer Res.* 2018;24(20):5058–5071. doi:10.1158/1078-0432.ccr-17-3427

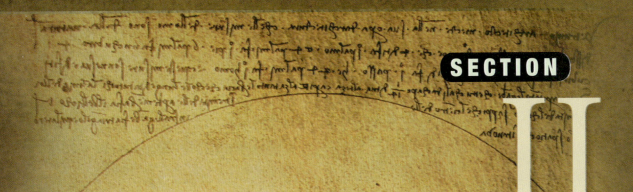

Treatment Planning: Site-Specific Cancers

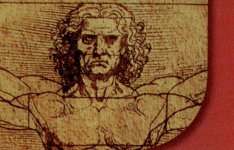

5 Cancers of the Central Nervous System

Vinai Gondi, Paul W. Sperduto, and Minesh P. Mehta

INTRODUCTION

The central nervous system (CNS) comprises the brain, the spinal cord, and their coverings. Patients with benign lesions may live out their natural life span, whereas the survival of those with malignant tumors is frequently measured in months to years. Radiotherapy has a major role to play in a substantial majority of these tumors, and treatment-related complications can occur in various anatomic and physiologic compartments. The optimal radiation therapy technique should maximize tumor control and minimize potential toxicities.

EPIDEMIOLOGY

Primary Central Nervous System Tumors

Annually, an estimated 79,000 new cases of primary non-malignant and malignant CNS tumors are diagnosed in the United States with an estimated 15,000 deaths.[1,2] The incidence of all primary nonmalignant and malignant brain and CNS tumors is 23.03 cases per 100,000 person-years. In the United States, the rate is slightly higher in females (24.31 per 100,000 person-years) than males (20.59 per 100,000 person-years).[2] The incidence rates are higher in more developed countries than in less-developed countries.[8] The incidence rate of childhood primary nonmalignant and malignant brain and CNS tumors is 5.94 cases per 100,000 person-years.[2]

The majority of primary CNS tumors are located within the frontal, temporal, parietal, and occipital lobes of the brain. Just under two thirds (61%) of gliomas occur in these lobes. Tumors in other locations in the cerebrum account for another 5%. Only a small minority of tumors, 2%, 3%, and 4%, are found in the ventricles, cerebellum, and brain stem, respectively. The pituitary and craniopharyngeal duct account for 16% of tumors. Tumors of the meninges represent 37% of all tumors.[2]

The overall incidence of primary spinal cord and cauda equina tumors is approximately 3% of all primary CNS tumors.[3] Schwannomas and meningiomas account for 61% of primary spinal tumors, with meningiomas being more frequent; adults are affected far more commonly than children. The frequency of individual spinal cord tumor types is substantially different from their histopathologic counterparts in the brain. For example, gliomas constitute 46% of primary intracranial tumors but only 23% of spinal tumors. The incidence ratios of intracranial to intraspinal astrocytomas, ependymomas, and meningiomas are approximately 10:1, 3:1, and 18:1, respectively.[4] Finally, the incidence ratio of intracranial to intraspinal tumors is up to four times higher in pediatric patients than in adults.

Table 5.1 shows the current WHO pathologic classification system of common primary CNS tumors.[5] The most frequently reported histology is meningioma, which accounts for over 36% of all tumors, followed closely by glioblastoma and astrocytoma.[2] The predominately benign nerve sheath tumors account for 8% of all tumors, of which 54% are acoustic neuromas. Gliomas account for 28% of all primary brain and CNS tumors and 80% of malignant tumors.[2] The most common spinal cord intramedullary tumors are derived from glial precursors (astrocytes, ependymal cells, and oligodendrocytes).[6]

Tumors Metastatic to the Central Nervous System

Metastatic brain tumors are the most common intracranial neoplasm in adults, about 10 times more common than primary intracranial tumors. In a population-based study, brain metastases were diagnosed in >10% of patients for small cell lung cancer, non-small cell lung cancer at diagnosis. In the context of metastatic disease, >10% of patients with melanoma, small cell and non-small cell lung cancer, and renal cell carcinoma are found to have brain metastases.[7,8]

With the exception of a primary paraspinal or neuraxis tumor, spinal cord tumors occur most often in the setting of disseminated disease from a distant primary tumor site. The spine is the most common site of bony metastases, with a reported incidence of 40% in patients with cancer.[9] Of patients with spine metastases, 10% to 20% develop malignant spinal cord compression (MSCC), accounting for 14,100 to 28,200 cases annually.[10–12] MSCC from epidural metastases occurs in 5% to 10% of all patients with cancer and ultimately in up to 40% of patients with

TABLE 5.1   WHO Grades of CNS Tumors

Astrocytic tumours	I	II	III	IV		Central neurocytoma	I	II	III	IV
Subependymal giant cell astrocytoma	•					Central neurocytoma		•		
Pilocytic astrocytoma	•					Extraventricular neurocytoma		•		
Pilomyxoid astrocytoma		•				Cerebellar liponeurocytoma		•		
Diffuse astrocytoma		•				Paraganglioma of the spinal cord	•			
Pleomorphic xanthoastrocytoma		•				Papillary glioneuronal tumour	•			
Anaplastic astrocytoma			•			Rosette-forming glioneuronal tumour of the fourth ventricle	•			
Glioblastoma				•						
Giant cell glioblastoma				•		**Pineal tumours**				
Gliosarcoma				•		Pineocytoma	•			
						Pineal parenchymal tumour of intermediate differentiation		•	•	
Oligodendroglial tumours						Pineoblastoma				•
Oligodendroglioma		•				Papillary tumour of the pineal region		•	•	
Anaplastic oligodendroglioma			•							
						Embryonal tumours				
Oligoastrocytic tumours						Medulloblastoma				•
Oligoastrocytoma		•				CNS primitive neuroectodermal tumour (PNET)				•
Anaplastic oligoastrocytoma			•			Atypical teratoid / rhabdoid tumour				•
Ependymal tumours						**Tumours of the cranial and paraspinal nerves**				
Subependymoma	•					Schwannoma	•			
Myxopapillary ependymoma	•					Neurofibroma	•			
Ependymoma		•				Perineurioma	•	•	•	
Anaplastic ependymoma			•			Malignant peripheral nerve sheath tumour (MPNST)		•	•	•
Choroid plexus tumours						**Meningeal tumours**				
Choroid plexus papilloma	•					Meningioma	•			
Atypical choroid plexus papilloma		•				Atypical meningioma		•		
Choroid plexus carcinoma			•			Anaplastic / malignant meningioma			•	
						Haemangiopericytoma		•		
Other neuroepithelial tumours						Anaplastic haemangiopericytoma			•	
Angiocentric glioma	•					Haemangioblastoma	•			
Chordoid glioma of the third ventricle		•								
						Tumours of the sellar region				
Neuronal and mixed neuronal-glial tumours						Craniopharyngioma	•			
Gangliocytoma	•					Granular cell tumour of the neurohypophysis	•			
Ganglioglioma	•					Pituicytoma	•			
Anaplastic ganglioglioma			•			Spindle cell oncocytoma of the adenohypophysis	•			
Desmoplastic infantile astrocytoma and ganglioglioma	•									
Dysembryoplastic neuroepithelial tumour	•									

non-spinal bone metastases.[9,13–15] MSCC may involve the spinal cord at any level, and symptoms depend on the location. The incidence of MSCC by vertebral levels is 10% to 16% cervical, 35% to 40% from T1-6, 44% to 55% from T7-12, and 20% in the lumbar spine.[16–18] In 10% to 38% of cases, metastatic lesions are initially found at multiple, noncontiguous levels.[16,19,20]

The most common malignancies that metastasize to the spine are breast, lung, and prostate cancers, accounting for approximately half of all cases.[1,9] Approximately 25% of all patients with MSCC have breast cancer, 15% have lung cancer, and 10% have prostate carcinomas. Overall, 5.5% of patients with breast cancer, 2.6% of patients with lung cancer, 7.2% of patients with prostate cancer, and 0.8% of patients with colorectal cancer experience MSCC.[11] Other commonly reported histologic diagnoses in adults include, in the order of cumulative incidence, multiple myeloma, nasopharynx, renal cell, melanoma, small cell lung, lymphoma, and cervix.[9,11,21]

WORKUP AND STAGING

For both benign and malignant CNS tumors, magnetic resonance imaging (MRI) is the gold standard.[22,23] Table 5.2 provides suggested/recommended MR sequences for imaging brain metastases.[22]

The preferred MRI slice thickness is ≤5 mm with ≤2.5 mm slice sampling; 1.25 mm slice thickness, routinely found on newer MRI volumetric sequences, permits even more detailed visualization and is recommended if available. T1-weighted images with contrast provide excellent visualization of contrast-enhancing tumors, such as meningiomas, glioblastoma, and brain metastases. T2-weighted images generally demonstrate the areas of edema, and T1-weighted fluid-attenuated inversion recovery (FLAIR) images better delineate infiltration by low- or high-grade gliomas. MRI registration with the treatment-planning computed tomography (CT) scan is essential for target delineation. Additional imaging studies can reflect the biologic characteristics of CNS tumors, such as tumor metabolism, proliferation, oxygenation, blood flow, and the function of surrounding normal brain; these include MR spectroscopy, diffusion and perfusion MR, BOLD MR, fMRI, amino acid positron-emission tomography (PET), and single-photon emission computed tomography (SPECT) scans.[24–26] After radiation therapy, PET scans and MRI spectroscopy may assist in differentiating active tumor versus radionecrosis, although the discriminatory power is still lower than clinically desirable.

MRI of the entire neural axis along with cerebrospinal fluid (CSF) cytology is required for staging of tumors with a high propensity for spread within the CNS by involvement of the CSF, periventricular space, leptomeninges, or spinal cord. Examples include medulloblastomas,

primitive neuroectodermal tumors (PNETs), anaplastic ependymomas, choroid plexus carcinomas, pineoblastomas, germ cell tumors, and lymphomas.

In patients who present for urgent symptom management, CT scan can be obtained rapidly, providing information on ventricular obstruction, hemorrhage, or edema. Owing to the risk of herniation and death, lumbar puncture should be avoided, if at all possible, until the intracranial pressure has normalized. The most important modality in the workup of suspected MSCC is gadolinium-enhanced MRI of the entire spinal axis. In the initial evaluation of a patient with suspected metastatic spinal cord compression, it is critical to image the entire spine, as 25% of these patients have spinal cord compression verified at multiple levels by MRI, and approximately two thirds of these have involvement of different regions of the spine.[27] In addition, a sensory level present on patient evaluation may be two or more levels different from the actual lesion on MRI in 28% of patients and four or more levels distant in 21% of patients.[27]

GENERAL MANAGEMENT

Multimodality therapy for CNS tumors may consist of medical therapy, surgical resection, radiation therapy, or some combination of these treatments.

Medical Therapy

Medical treatment generally consists of steroids with or without mannitol.[28] Patients who present with emergent symptoms are typically treated with dexamethasone. Response to therapy is usually noted within minutes to hours of administration, and over 80% of patients show dramatic improvement by 3 to 4 days after initiation of steroids.[29,30] A common regimen in patients receiving radiation therapy is high-dose dexamethasone (10–25 mg IV or po) followed by maintenance on oral steroids (4–6 mg three or four times a day), with tapering initiated upon stabilization of symptoms and initiation of therapy, usually over 1 to 2 months.[28,31,32] However, once daily dosing is pharmacologically sufficient and might in fact produce fewer symptoms; additionally, whether an initial large dose is better delivered intravenously or orally remains controversial. In the setting of MSCC from solid tumors, dexamethasone has been shown to improve rates of surviving with intact gait function.[33,34] High-dose dexamethasone has numerous side effects. Consequences of intermediate- to long-term steroid use may include hyperglycemia, insomnia, emotional lability, thrush, gastric irritation, ulceration and possibly perforation, proximal muscle wasting, weight gain and adiposity (moon facies, buffalo hump, and centripetal obesity), osteoporotic

| TABLE 5.2 | Recommended MR Imaging Sequences for Patients with Brain Metastases |

	3T MRI (Preferred)				1.5T MRI			
	3D T1 Pre[a]	3D T1 Post[b]	Ax 2D T2/FLAIR[c,d]	Ax 2D T2[c]	3D T1 Pre[a]	3D T1 Post[b]	Ax 2D T2/FLAIR[c,d]	Ax 2D T2[c]
Sequence	IR-GRE[e]	IR-GRE[e]	TSE[f]	TSE[f]	IR-GRE[e]	IR-GRE[e]	TSE[f]	TSE[f]
Plane	Sagittal or axial	Sagittal or axial	Axial	Axial	Sagittal or axial	Sagittal or axial	Axial	Axial
Mode	3D	3D	2D	2D	3D	3D	2D	2D
TR (ms)	2100[g]	2100[g]	>6000	>2500	2100[g]	2100[g]	>6000	>3500
TE (ms)	Min	Min	100–140	80–120	Min	Min	100–140	80–120
TI (ms)	1100[h]	1100[h]	2000–2500[i]		1100[h]	1100[h]	2000–2500[i]	
Flip angle	10°–15°	10°–15°	90°/≥160°	90°/≥160°	10°–15°	10°–15°	90°/≥160°	90°/≥160°
Frequency	256	256	≥256	≥256	≥172	≥172	≥256	≥256
Phase	256	256	≥256	≥256	≥172	≥172	≥256	≥256
NEX	≥1	≥1	≥1	≥1	≥1	≥1	≥1	≥1
FOV	256 mm	256 mm	240 mm	240 mm	256 mm	256 mm	240 mm	240 mm
Slice thickness	1 mm	1 mm	3 mm	3 mm	≤1.5 mm	≤1.5 mm	≤4 mm	≤4 mm
Gap/spacing	0	0	0	0	0	0	0	0
Other options								
Parallel imaging	Up to 3x	Up to 3x	Up to 2x	Up to 2x	Up to 2x	Up to 2x	Up to 2x	Up to 2x

FOV, field of view; NEX, number of excitations; TE, echo time; TI, inversion time; TR, repetition time.

[a] Pre-contrast T1 imaging is required and strongly encouraged to be acquired as a 3D imaging sequence with equivalent parameters to the 3D post-contrast T1 imaging.

[b] 3D post-contrast T1 imaging is required.

[c] Axial T2/FLAIR or T2 sequence is required. Axial T2/FLAIR is strongly preferred.

[d] 3D FLAIR is an optional alternative to 2D FLAIR with sequence parameters as follows per the EORTC guidelines: 3D TSE/FSE acquisition; TE = 90–140 ms; TR = 6000–10,000 ms; TI = 2000–2500 ms (chosen based on vendor recommendations for optimized protocol and field strength); GRAPPA ≤2; fat suppression; slice thickness ≤1.5 mm; orientation: sagittal or axial; FOV ≤250 mm × 250 mm; Matrix ≥244 × 244.

[e] IR-GRE: inversion-recovery gradient-recalled echo sequence is equivalent to magnetization prepared rapid gradient echo (MPRAGE; Siemens & Hitachi), and the inversion recovery spoiled gradient echo (IR-SPGR or FAST SPGR with inversion activated or BRAVO; GE), 3D turbo field echo (TFE; Philips), or 3D fast field echo (3D Fast FE; Toshiba). A 3D acquisition without inversion preparation will result in different contrasts compared with MPRAGE or another IR-prepped 3D T1-weighted sequences and therefore should be avoided.

[f] TSE (turbo spin echo; Siemens & Philips) is equivalent to FSE (fast spin echo; Hitachi, Toshiba).

[g] For Siemens and Hitachi scanners. GE, Philips, and Toshiba scanners should use a TR = 5–15 ms for similar contrast.

[h] For Siemens and Hitachi scanners. GE, Philips, and Toshiba scanners should use a TI = 400–450 ms for similar contrast.

[i] Choice of TI should be chosen based on the magnetic field strength of the system (e.g., TI = 2000 ms for 1.5T and TI = 2500 ms for 3T).

Modified from Kaufmann TJ, Smits M, Boxerman J, et al. Consensus recommendations for a standardized brain tumor imaging protocol for clinical trials in brain metastases. *Neuro-Oncol.* 2020;22(6);757–772.

compression fractures, arthralgias with withdrawal, aseptic necrosis of the hip joints, increased susceptibility to infections, and prolonged lymphopenia.[35] Some of these side effects persist even after steroid withdrawal. Owing to the incidence of steroid-induced complications with dosing longer than 21 days in duration, higher doses and longer tapering schedules should be based on the physician's assessment of symptom severity and response.[34,36,37] Steroid tapering has to be individualized and closely monitored. Asymptomatic patients generally do not require corticosteroids, and routine use of corticosteroids during radiation therapy in asymptomatic patients should be avoided. Select patients with MSCC may not receive steroids during treatment if they are at high risk of complications due to underlying medical comorbidities, such as peptic ulcer disease, uncontrolled diabetes, or other medical problems, that may cause severe or life-threatening problems if exacerbated by steroids.[38] Dexamethasone and mannitol decrease peritumoral brain edema by different mechanisms of action, and mannitol is therefore sometimes used in steroid-refractory patients.[39] A common regimen of mannitol is a 20% to 25% solution given intravenously over 30 minutes, dosed at 0.5 to 2.0 g/kg.[45]

Stabilization of the patient in status epilepticus is critical. After securing the airway and stabilizing the patient, seizure activity must be terminated as rapidly as possible, especially, as failure to control seizures can potentially lead to physical injuries, airway compromise, secondary brain hypoxia/injury, or coma.[40,41] Rapid onset/short acting benzodiazepines and phenytoin are commonly used. Recommended initial regimens include 0.1 mg/kg at 2 mg/min of lorazepam or diazepam at 0.2 mg/kg at 5 mg/min. Phenytoin infusion of 15 to 20 mg/kg at <50 mg/min in adults is indicated for seizure activity refractory to benzodiazepines or after truncation of seizures with diazepam.[41] There is no clear evidence to support the prophylactic use of anticonvulsants in patients diagnosed with a brain tumor in the absence of documented seizures.[42,43]

Surgical Therapy

Surgical resection and/or placement of a shunt are often required for emergent management of tumors causing life-threatening hydrocephalus, mass effect (herniation), or profound neurologic impairment. This may relieve symptoms so that other treatment modalities can be initiated safely. Symptoms are usually related to mass effect, so resection and/or debulking are often the only logical choices if medical therapy fails to provide improvement in neurologic symptoms. Rapid surgical decompression is the treatment of choice for such problems when surgery can be safely performed based on the patient performance status or tumor location.

Two randomized trials comparing radiotherapy with or without resection in the management of a solitary brain metastasis have documented a survival advantage with the addition of surgery to radiation.[44,45] However, a third randomized trial was negative.[46] There is no level I evidence demonstrating any survival benefit from operating on patients with multiple metastases. However, patients with severe neurologic symptoms from one or more dominant metastases who are unresponsive to medical therapy may benefit from a craniotomy. An improvement in the patient's performance status can then be followed by other therapeutic options.

Many patients with spinal cord compression are not candidates for laminectomy and are treated with steroids and radiation therapy. Most series in the literature show no difference in outcomes when comparing laminectomy-treated patients to those managed with radiation therapy alone.[9,18,47,48] However, a randomized trial evaluating the benefit of adding surgical decompression to the radiotherapeutic management of symptomatic metastatic spinal cord compression showed that ambulatory patients who underwent decompressive surgery had a significantly improved median time of gait retention and ability to regain gait function, albeit without affecting overall survival.[49] Therefore, all patients presenting with MSCC of short duration should be evaluated by an experienced spine surgeon for emergent decompression before initiating radiation therapy.

GENERAL CONCEPTS OF RADIATION THERAPY

Multimodality Imaging for Simulation, Treatment Planning, and Dose Delivery

The success of modern radiation therapy can be attributed to the development and availability of various novel imaging techniques that help to (1) better delineate targets and regions of avoidance, (2) better understand the dosimetrically relevant composition of the tissue in the path of the radiation, (3) lower the setup uncertainty of the patient, (4) verify the location of the target during dose delivery, and (5) assess the location of the deposited dose, as well as the development of advanced immobilization techniques, on-board imaging for setup verification with consequential reduction of uncertainty margin expansions, and advanced conformal delivery techniques to decrease the dose to organs at risk (OARs).

A high-resolution CT scan acquired at the time of treatment-planning simulation provides a three-dimensional (3D) voxel grid of the patient. In each voxel, the CT software calculates the linear attenuation coefficient of the matter contained within it. Based on this, each voxel is assigned a shade of gray (for visualization purposes) and a CT number, the Hounsfield unit, which is translated into physical density in the treatment-planning software for dose calculation purposes. Since CT has poor soft tissue discrimination, iodine-based intravenous contrast agents are often utilized to better visualize vessels or tumor. Images with sub-millimeter voxel dimensions can be acquired with only a minute or two scanning time.

MRI does not involve ionizing radiation, and because of exquisite soft tissue visualization, it is widely used in providing anatomic contouring detail for radiotherapy planning. The two most commonly used sequences are the T1- and T2-weighted sequences, where T1 and T2 are the longitudinal and transverse relaxation times of proton spins, respectively. Generally speaking, the shorter the voxel's T1, the more signal it produces and it appears brighter on the scan. On the other hand, the longer the T2, the longer the signal is acquired, making the signal-producing tissue brighter. Water in bulk phase (e.g., CSF) has long T1 and T2 relaxation times; therefore, it appears dark on T1-weighted but bright on T2-weighted acquisitions. Gadolinium-based contrast agents, which lower T1 relaxation times, are often utilized to enhance brain tumors. Because several tumors compromise the brain–blood barrier, they permit entrance of contrast agents which lower the T1 time, making the tumor brighter on T1-weighted images. Vasogenic edema associated with brain tumors appears bright on T2-weighted images. Often, extremely high spatial resolution is needed (e.g., for visualization of cranial nerves), in which case the constructive interference steady state (CISS, also called Fast Imaging Employing Steady-state Acquisition [FIESTA]) sequence is utilized. The MRI technique of FLAIR can be utilized to dampen the signal from the CSF, which allows better visualization of infiltrative, non-enhancing tumor and is particularly useful for low-grade gliomas which typically do not enhance. Magnetic resonance spectroscopy (MRS) measures the levels of various metabolites in body tissues. It can be tuned to recognize specific tumor cellular metabolites. The level of these metabolites can be spatially overlaid with MRI images, putatively allowing better differentiation of tumor from normal tissue. However, to date, this approach has not found widespread clinical applicability.

Diffusion tensor imaging enables visualization of neural fiber directions and provides tractographic information. Conceptually, this could be used to potentially avoid hot spots and high doses within critical fiber tracts, but in practice, this approach is not routinely used. Functional MRI measures signal changes in the brain that are due to changing neural activity. The measurement is done through a mechanism referred to as the blood-oxygen-level-dependent (BOLD) effect, which is based on the fact that increased neural activity requires enhanced oxygen levels. Deoxygenated hemoglobin attenuates the MRI signal, while in the oxygenated state it enhances the signal, leading to a T2 signal increase related to increased neural activity.

The desired MRI sequences are co-registered with CT images in the treatment-planning software with the help of specially designed mutual information-seeking algorithms and edited with human input. This co-registration allows delineation of the most pertinent regions of interest in the framework of the treatment-planning CT.

After an acceptable treatment plan has been created, the patient is positioned using appropriate external immobilization and three-point alignment, following which setup verification of the relevant anatomy and/or fiducials is performed. The simplest modality for this is the radiographic film. Port films are compared to digitally reconstructed radiographs from the treatment-planning system and setup corrections are applied as necessary. Electronic devices such as the electronic portal imaging device (EPID) have substituted radiographic film with an electronic screen. Conventionally, the megavoltage photon beam is used to obtain the verification image. The Compton interaction responsible for image creation results in very low tissue contrast, making it difficult to interpret the images in the absence of fiducials or dense bone. Recent technologic advances have introduced in-room imaging with kilovoltage photon beams, in which the portion of photoelectric interactions significantly increase, resulting in a very substantial increase in tissue contrast and therefore image quality. X-ray sources and imaging panels are mounted on modern linear accelerators, allowing them to acquire partial-volume CT type image sets, referred to as cone beam CT. This allows volumetric information at the time of the patient setup to be compared with the 3D image sets on which the treatment plans were generated. Necessary shifts can be applied to best match the treatment-planning conditions.

Volume Definition

Treatment-planning volumes are based on reports 50 and 62 of the International Commission on Radiation Units and Measurements (ICRU).[58,59] Gross tumor volume (GTV) represents grossly identifiable disease.[58,59] For glioblastoma, this includes the T1-enhancing abnormality on MRI. For non-enhancing low-grade glioma, this is usually the FLAIR abnormality on MRI. The clinical target volume (CTV) includes the subclinical microscopic tumor extent as well as the resection cavity. For glioblastoma, two CTVs are delineated: (1) T2-hyperintense abnormality plus resection cavity and 2-cm margin treated to 46 Gy and (2) T1-enhancing abnormality plus resection cavity and 2-cm margin treated to 60 Gy cumulative dose. Uniform expansion may result in an excessively large volume with unnecessary dose to normal surrounding tissues. The CTV is therefore reduced around natural barriers to tumor growth, such as the skull, ventricles, and the falx. In addition, the CTV margin may be limited in areas near critical organs.

The planning target volume (PTV) is also referred to as the "dosimetric margin," which has two components.[50] The internal margin accounts for variations in size, shape, and position of the CTV in relation to anatomic reference points. In the CNS, this is usually not a major component and is mainly due to physiologic variations, such as the possible changes in the mass effect from cerebral edema that may increase or decrease over the course of treatment. Setup margin is added to take into account uncertainties in patient-to-beam positioning, although this may be reduced by utilizing appropriate immobilization devices. Dosimetric margins as low as 3 to 5 mm are acceptable with optimal immobilization devices and daily volumetric image guidance. For treatment plans emphasizing homogeneous dose delivery, the maximum dose to PTV should be generally less than 110% of the prescription dose, and 95% of the target should receive at least the prescription dose.

Organs at Risk

OARs are critical normal structures whose relative radiation sensitivity and proximity to the CTV may significantly modify the prescribed dose and the treatment-planning strategy. It is especially important to limit the

TABLE 5.3	Normal Tissue Tolerance of Intracranial Organs at Risk	
	QUANTEC Recommended Dose Constraint	
Organ	**Conventional Fractionation**	**Hypofractionation**
Brain	Maximum dose to 72 Gy	5–10 mL to 12 Gy
Brain stem	Entire brain stem to ≤54 Gy Maximum dose to 1–10 mL to 59 Gy	1 fraction: Maximum dose to 12.5 Gy
Cochlea	Mean dose to ≤45 Gy (more conservatively ≤35 Gy)	1 fraction: Prescription dose ≤14 Gy
Optic nerves/chiasm	Maximum dose < 55 Gy	1 fraction: Maximum dose < 8 Gy
Spinal cord	Maximum dose to 50 Gy	1 fraction: maximum dose to 13 Gy 3 fractions: maximum dose to 20 Gy

From Lawrence YR, Li XA, Naqa I, et al. Radiation dose-volume effects in the brain. *Int J Radiat Oncol Biol Phys.* 2010;76(3 Suppl):S20–S27.

risk of late toxicities by respecting the dose tolerances of normal structures, especially when long-term survival is expected. The relationship between the planning organ-at-risk volume (PRV) and the OAR is analogous to that of the PTV and the CTV.[50] For each OAR, when part of the organ or the whole organ is irradiated above the accepted tolerance level, the maximum dose should be reported[50] and evaluated using the corresponding dose–volume histogram (DVH).

Recent publications of Quantitative Analyses of Normal Tissue Effects in the Clinic based on a review of published series have established recommended dose constraints for the brain, brain stem, optic nerves/chiasm, cochlea, and spinal cord (Table 5.3). It must be remembered that these are extrapolated estimates, and when two plans both yield OAR doses below a defined dose threshold, the plan with the lower OAR dose would often (but not always) be dosimetrically, and possibly clinically, superior.

The spinal cord, visual apparatus, and brain stem are among the most critical normal structures to be considered in the CNS, given the devastating consequences that can arise from damage to these structures. Damage to the spinal cord can result in pain, paresthesias, sensory deficits, paralysis, Brown-Sequard syndrome, and bowel/bladder incontinence, and even complete paralysis and death.[51] With conventional fractionation of 2 Gy per day for the full cord cross section, the alpha–beta ratio has been estimated to be as low as 0.87 Gy, suggesting a strong dose-per-fraction response relationship (i.e., exquisite sensitivity to damage as the dose per fraction increases). In addition, doses of 50, 60, and 69 Gy have been estimated to be associated with 0.2%, 6.0%, and 50% rates of myelopathy, respectively. In the case of re-irradiation, a 25% increase in spinal cord tolerance (presumably from completed repair of prior DNA-damaging events) 6 months after the initial course of conventionally fractionated radiotherapy has been proposed.[52]

Although damage to the brain stem can result in symptoms similar to those seen in the spinal cord, the brain stem is also critical in providing motor and sensory

innervation to the head and neck via the cranial nerves, as well as the regulation of respiratory and cardiac function. A maximal dose constraint of 54 Gy is generally considered to have a minimal risk of causing severe neurological effects, and small volumes (1–10 cc) may be irradiated to as much as 59 Gy with a continued small risk of side effects.[53] Furthermore, series on dose-escalated proton radiotherapy for skull base tumors have demonstrated that the ventral surface of the brain stem may be somewhat radioresistant, with surface doses as high as 64 CGE and 53 CGE to the brain stem center resulting in high rates of toxicity-free survival.[54]

Radiation-induced optic neuropathy (RION) can result in profound and irreversible visual loss approximately 10 to 20 months after treatment, with a median onset of 18 months after treatment.[55] The alpha–beta ratio is estimated to be quite small, suggesting a very strong dose-per-fraction effect. With conventional fractionation, a dose of 50 Gy is associated with a near-zero incidence of RION. This risk increases to between 3% and 7% at doses of 55 to 60 Gy and becomes more substantial with rates of 7% to 20% reported for doses of >60 Gy at traditional fraction sizes.[56] The retina is another radiosensitive structure, where radiation-induced retinopathy can mimic the symptoms of diabetic retinopathy. The threshold dose for radiation retinopathy is estimated to be at 30 to 35 Gy, with lower doses associated with a near-zero risk of retinopathy and >50 Gy associated with approximately a 5% chance of retinopathy. Consequentially, most protocols set 45 Gy as the maximum dose constraint for the retina.[57]

The pathogenesis of radiotherapy-induced cognitive decline may at least partially involve a neural stem cell compartment located in the subgranular zone of the hippocampal dentate gyrus. Preclinical and clinical studies have demonstrated not just the importance of this neural stem cell compartment on memory function but also its exquisite radiosensitivity.[58] In Radiation Therapy Oncology Group (RTOG) 0933, a prospective clinical trial of whole-brain radiotherapy for brain metastases, conformal avoidance of the hippocampal dentate gyrus using intensity-modulated radiotherapy reduced the rate of memory decline, as compared to historical controls.[59] These findings were subsequently confirmed in the randomized phase III trial, NRG CC001, and provided the first direct clinical evidence that the application of advanced radiotherapy techniques to minimize hippocampal dose may prevent radiotherapy-induced cognitive decline.[60] However, the precise radiobiologic dose tolerance of the hippocampal dentate gyrus remains unclear. Exploratory analysis of patients enrolled on RTOG 0933 demonstrated that a dose to 100% of the hippocampal dentate gyrus correlated with severity of memory decline, suggesting that better memory preservation might be attainable with lower hippocampal dose.[59] In a prospective study of benign and low-grade tumor treated with photon radiotherapy without hippocampal avoidance, >7.3 Gy in 2-Gy fractions to 40% of the hippocampal dentate gyrus was associated with long-term impairment in list-learning recall.[61]

Temporal lobe injury (TLI) can be associated with symptoms such as dizziness, memory impairment, disorientation, and personality changes or with more specific symptoms such as temporal lobe epilepsy.[62] Data from studies on nasopharyngeal cancer patients have established 70 Gy as a threshold for an increased incidence of TLI.[63] Some authors treating skull base tumors have proposed a D2cc of 74 Gy as an absolute threshold dose.[64]

Intensity-Modulated Radiation Therapy

Intensity-modulated radiation therapy (IMRT) is an advanced form of 3D conformal radiation therapy (CRT). While CRT delivers an irregularly shaped beam of uniform intensity, IMRT modulates the intensity of the photon beam across the treated area by delivering multiple subfields (segments), each of irregular shape and of different photon intensities. There are four major advantages of utilizing IMRT for CNS tumors: (1) shape dose around concave PTVs (such as with some meningiomas); (2) improve the homogeneity of the delivered dose to complex-shaped PTVs; (3) permit simultaneous integrated dose delivery using two or more PTV dose levels (such as for glioblastoma); and (4) improve dose homogeneity to the target in regions where large variations of external contours exist (such as in the case of posterior fossa lesions or spinal cord meningiomas).

These advantages of IMRT techniques are achieved through "inverse planning," during which dosimetric objectives are set for tumor coverage and for OAR avoidance. An optimization algorithm is then employed to find the optimal photon fluence that meets the predetermined dosimetric objectives. After the optimal photon fluence has been found, another optimization algorithm is employed to determine the optimal way (i.e., the shape, the number, and the intensity of segments) to deliver the calculated fluence. In order to fully utilize the power of IMRT, the irradiated tissue should be as static as possible during delivery, the dosimetric objectives for planning

should not be unrealistic, and great care should be given to contour targets and OARs, which include lenses, eye globes, optic nerves, chiasm, brain stem, temporal lobes, pituitary gland, inner ears, general brain parenchyma, and spinal cord.

Immobilization can help reduce the uncertainty/setup margins when creating PTVs. Margins should be set based on a realistic assessment of setup uncertainties and the quality of immobilization. During IMRT planning, unrealistic desired objectives could lead to suboptimal plans. For instance, if aiming to cover the PTV with a homogeneous dose of 60 Gy, while constraining the maximum dose to the adjacent chiasm to 40 Gy, the planning algorithm will substantially increase the needed monitor units and generate a large number of very tiny area segments, which might not be deliverable due to machine limitations. Good IMRT plans can achieve better than 5%/mm dose gradient while still preserving good target dose uniformity.

Proton Therapy

Proton therapy, a form of particle therapy, is becoming increasingly more accessible and available. Its dosimetric advantages of reduced entrance dose and finite distal range permit greater sparing of OARs in close proximity to the tumor target, especially distal to the beam. This becomes particularly important in the treatment of radioresistant tumors in eloquent locations, such as skull base chordoma and chondrosarcoma, where a dose escalation to 70 Gy or higher in close proximity to the brain stem, optic nerves, temporal lobes, and cochlea is required for optimal local control. In addition, reduced integral dose, due to the finite range of proton therapy and fewer proton beams needed to optimally treat the tumor target, may have important implications in terms of secondary malignancy risk reduction and adverse cognitive and other functional effects.[65] In the setting of craniospinal irradiation, proton therapy has been observed to have significant clinical benefits in terms of acute toxicities and is postulated to minimize the risk of multiple long-term toxicities. Several trials testing the potential benefits of proton therapy for novel CNS tumor indications are ongoing.

SIMULATION PROCEDURES
Positioning

When simulating CNS tumor patients, positioning becomes very important, and appropriate devices should be used to aid in immobilization, reproducibility, and setup. If marks or tattoos are used for localization or setup purposes, these setup marks should be in easily locatable and reproducible positions. Marks on steeply sloping surfaces, ears, nose, lips, and chin, should be avoided whenever possible. In some settings, there is benefit from positioning the head on a pituitary head-board for posteriorly located tumors (e.g., occipital lobes or posterior fossa). For patients requiring craniospinal irradiation, it is often useful to have the patient supine with the chin slightly extended such that the exit beam of the posteroanterior (PA) spine field does not pass through the patient's oral cavity. CT simulation, 3D treatment planning, and IMRT allow for different head and neck positions in most situations as non-coplanar beams can be used to avoid entry and exit dose to OARs.

Immobilization

There exist a variety of commercially available head immobilization devices, most of which use thermoplastic or other materials, such as expandable foam or plastic beads in a vacuum bag. They are adaptable for flexion or extension when the patient is in the supine position. Variability of setup should not be >2 or 3 mm with a thermoplastic mask. To obtain more accurate and/or rigid head positioning and immobilization, a modified stereotactic aquaplast mask with reinforcement strips may be used to help ensure reproducibility and setup.

Once the patient is placed in the appropriate positioning device, they are scanned, typically using between 1 and 3 mm slice thickness. The clinician may need to decide at the time of simulation where the isocenter should be placed. After completion of treatment planning in virtual reality (see subsequent text), verification films should be obtained before treatment; these may include orthogonal radiographs to verify the isocenter and films of any custom-shaped portal fields. Isocenter films (with or without portal images) are usually obtained throughout the course of treatment to verify the accuracy of the treatment setup. Volumetric imaging capabilities now offer more detailed imaging verification of the patient setup. The frequency of image guidance is dictated by patient-specific criteria, and in some cases, daily guidance is required. Newer technologies incorporate volumetric image guidance with each delivered fraction. The most modern technologies also provide for monitoring and sometimes even correcting for intra-fraction motion.

Generally, special custom immobilization devices are used for patients with spinal cord tumors to ensure setup reproducibility and are especially crucial for patients undergoing craniospinal irradiation, where surface matching to skin marks represents the first estimate, which must be validated and verified with an anatomic imaging correlate. The immobilization devices must fit the physical dimensions of the CT scan or MRI scanner and should be constructed of materials compatible with the imaging modality.

Simulation

In this chapter, the reader may assume that patients are simulated in the supine position using volumetric CT-based setup, unless otherwise stated. The primary body planes are transverse, sagittal, and coronal, with body axes anterior, posterior, right, left, superior, and inferior. Isocentric treatment machines rotate 360 degrees around a transverse plane of the patient's body, and treating in a coronal or sagittal plane requires the treatment couch to be rotated.

For CT simulation involving the brain, the patient is placed in the positioning device and scanned and the isocenter or reference markers are selected and marked on the thermoplastic mask. For intracranial disease, a single-field or opposed-beam two-field arrangements are usually not considered acceptable, as they deliver excessive dose to normal tissues in the beam paths. The exception is a short course of palliative radiation therapy to the whole brain or cervical spinal cord using an opposed lateral beam arrangement. An optimum beam arrangement typically consists of multiple non-coplanar beams or intensity- modulated techniques that are typically helically or volumetrically modulated. Modern randomized trials have categorically demonstrated the cognitive, endocrine, and intelligence quotient sparing benefits of more conformal brain treatment techniques. When applicable, the contralateral uninvolved hemisphere of the brain should be spared as much as possible. Beam exit through the thyroid gland, eyes, lacrimal gland, and oral cavity should also be avoided as much as possible.

Most lesions can be treated well with 6 to 10 MV photon beams. For more lateralized tumors, it is ideal to not include contralateral beams if possible. Typically, a homogeneous dose distribution within the target volume is desirable, with not more than 5% to 10% inhomogeneity in the irradiated volume. When IMRT is used, a practical time-saving approach uses the beam arrangement of an optimized non-coplanar 3D plan as a starting point. This can significantly shorten the treatment-planning effort and allows for greater freedom of optimization than a coplanar (i.e., two-dimensional) plan.

Specific Examples of Treatment Techniques

Whole-Brain Radiation Therapy

Whole-brain radiation therapy evolved in the early days of radiation therapy when precise anatomic definition of tumor was limited to plain radiography. With the advent of CT and MRI, more focal radiation techniques for brain tumors became the standard. Still, there are important clinical settings in which the brain and/or meninges are the target for which whole-brain radiation therapy is an essential component of therapy. These clinical situations with examples are reviewed in the following.

Acute Leukemia

The CNS is a known sanctuary site. After post-chemotherapy failures in the CNS and eyes were noted,

CNS- penetrating therapy such as intrathecal drugs and radiation therapy became important components of treatment of leukemia.[66] While the doses of radiotherapy are low, in the 12- to 18-Gy range, the target remains the entire brain, cranial meninges down to the level of C2, and the posterior retina and optic nerves. An example of a C2-whole-brain field for cranial prophylaxis is shown in Figure 5.1A. Opposed lateral fields in an aquaplast mask with a 2 to 3 degree posterior cant on the fields can help spare exit through the contralateral lens. The anterior border is set at the fleshy canthus of the eye, which corresponds to the anatomic equator of the eye. Radio-opaque markers placed on the fleshy canthus are very helpful for conventional simulation. For a CT simulation, the anterior border is placed at the posterior border of the lens, and the gantry angle is adjusted to make the beam nondivergent across the posterior aspect of both lenses. Placement of the block such that the entire posterior globe is included in the fields is important. At least a 1-cm margin should be included on the middle cranial and base of skull meninges. An appropriate amount of flash (~1 cm) should be provided over the convexity, and the soft tissue of the posterior neck should be shielded with a minimum 1-cm margin on the intracranial contents (Fig. 5.1A).

Brain Metastases

The RTOG conducted a number of trials in the early 1980s, evaluating whole-brain radiotherapy for brain metastases.[67] These trials established a palliative benefit for whole-brain radiation therapy. In subsequent studies, whole-brain radiotherapy with a stereotactic boost showed a survival and neurological function preservation benefit in selected patients with brain metastases.[68] Randomized trials of stereotactic radiosurgery (SRS) and whole-brain radiation versus SRS alone for 1 to 4 brain metastases showed equivalent survival with better cognitive preservation but suggested a local control benefit to whole-brain radiotherapy.[69,70]

Using 2-D techniques, an open flashing rectangular field with the inferior border collimated to a line connecting the superior orbital rim with the mastoid tip was used. Increasingly, CT simulation with multi-leaf collimator (MLC) blocking techniques has become common, allowing easier target definition and blocking. The target in whole-brain radiation is the brain parenchyma. Figure 5.1B illustrates a whole-brain field that includes the brain parenchyma with a 1-cm block margin. This typically blocks the lenses of the eyes, but occasionally adjustment of the leaves over the lenses is necessary. The advantage of including a "scalp block" is to avoid the tangent effect of the beam over the vertex scalp that often leads to a characteristic "reverse mohawk" bald patch among surviving patients. Inhomogeneities across the superior thinned parts of the head can also be reduced with simple field-within-a-field techniques.

Whole-brain radiation can cause mild to moderate memory deficits as early as 4 months after treatment.[71,72] RTOG 0614 demonstrated a modest improvement in cognition with the use of prophylactic memantine during whole-brain radiation.[73] In addition, NRG CC001 demonstrated that the use of intensity-modulated radiotherapy during whole-brain radiotherapy to conformally avoid the hippocampal dentate gyrus, where neural stem cells whose neurogenic differentiation subserves memory function are believed to reside, also improved cognition and patient-reported quality of life.[67,68] Based on the results of the NRG Oncology CC001 randomized trial, both prophylactic memantine and

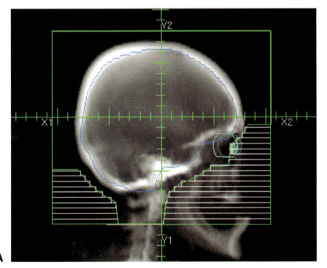
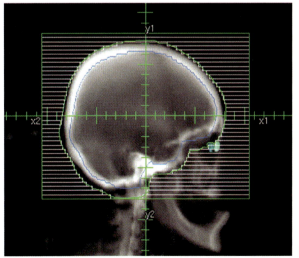

FIGURE 5.1. Sample whole-brain radiotherapy fields illustrating blocking for C2-whole-brain fields (**A**) that would be appropriate for leukemic prophylaxis and whole-brain fields with a scalp block (**B**) that would be appropriate for whole-brain radiotherapy of metastatic disease.

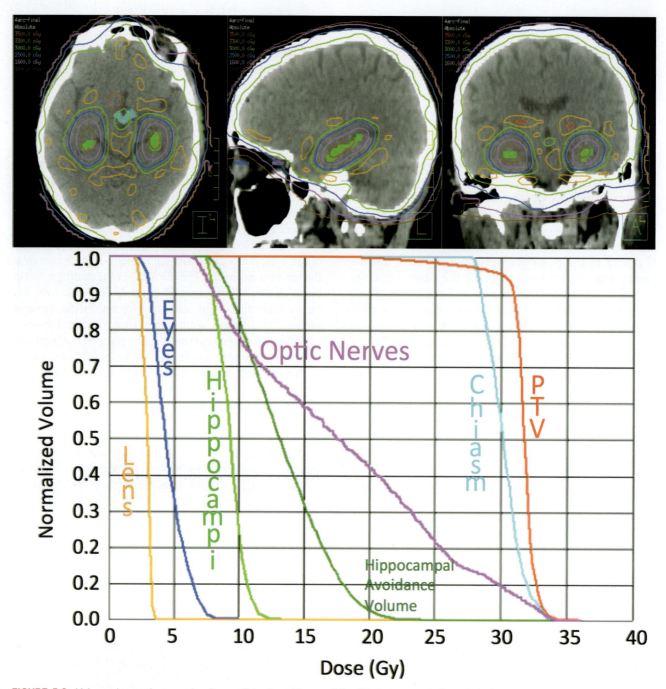

FIGURE 5.2. Volumetric arc therapy plan for conformal avoidance of the hippocampus during whole-brain radiotherapy. This IMRT plan was generated using the partial-field dual-arc planning technique. The following isodose lines are shown: 35 Gy (red), 33 Gy (orange), 30 Gy (green), 25 Gy (blue), 16 Gy (purple), and 10 Gy (brown). This technique significantly spares the hippocampus with 100% of the hippocampus receiving a dose of 8 Gy and a maximum hippocampal dose of less than 16 Gy.

hippocampal avoidance are now considered standard-of-care neuroprotective interventions during whole-brain radiotherapy (Fig. 5.2).

Craniospinal Irradiation

Certain neoplasms require treatment to the entire craniospinal axis. This may include medulloblastomas and PNETs, high-grade ependymomas, some germ cell tumors, pineoblastomas, disseminated CNS lymphoma, and leptomeningeal carcinomatosis or gliomatosis. Several positioning variations are used in clinical practice often in an immobilization cast to ensure daily positional reproducibility.[74] Patients are ideally treated in the supine position with the neck extended to avoid beams exiting the oral cavity. Conventional methods utilize field "feathering" to reduce hot or cold spots caused by imperfect fields matching between cranial and spine fields. This method feathered each junction on a weekly basis with the cranial fields' inferior border decreasing between 5 and 10 mm. The intracranial contents and upper one or two segments of the cervical cord are treated through opposed lateral fields, usually positioned so that the isocenter is at midline with the beam axes passing through the lateral canthi to minimize divergence into the contralateral eye. The collimator and couch are rotated to create a straight line through the inferior portion of the brain fields that removes the possibility of overlap with the posterior spine field. This can be visualized with the treatment-planning systems simulation software (see subsequent text). Customized blocks protect the normal head and neck tissues from the primary radiation beam; as mentioned previously, care must be taken not to underdose the cribriform plate. Figure 5.3A represents a typical cranial field with blocks for the lenses and collimator angled to match the divergence of the PA spine field. The inferior border of the initial "short" field is placed around C2 to C3, leaving adequate room for subsequent shifts in the match with the upper spine field, a technique commonly referred to as "feathering the gap."

Depending on length, the spine is treated through one or two posterior fields. It is customary practice to maximize the field length of the upper spinal field (40 cm at 100 cm source–skin distance [SSD]) and minimize the length of the lower spinal field, therefore simplifying planning for junction shifts (see in subsequent text). If 40 cm or less of length covers the spine inclusive of the end of the thecal sac (typically near the level of S3, this should be confirmed by MRI), a lower spine field is not necessary. All fields' central axes remain fixed; it is only the fields' lengths that are changed. Therefore, the caudal border of the lower PA spine field should be set inferior to S3 by a length equal to the two-field shifts and then blocked back to S3 using asymmetric collimators.

Matching the upper border of the spine field to the lower border of the cranial field requires strict attention to accuracy, as overlap (i.e., overdosing) in the upper cervical cord may have catastrophic outcomes for the patient. In one method, the collimator for the lateral cranial fields is angled to match the divergence of the upper border of the adjacent spinal field, and the treatment couch is angled so that the inferior border of the cranial field is perpendicular to the superior edge of the spinal field ("exact-match" technique). Both the rotation of the collimator and degree of couch rotation are calculated and typically range from 9 to 11 degrees. The drawback to this technique is that the couch rotation displaces the contralateral eye cephalad, so that it cannot be blocked without blocking the frontal brain tissue. This technique may also result in underdosing of the temporal lobes and the cribriform plate.

One method for craniospinal irradiation involves a 3D CT simulation of a patient in the supine position in a wooden box that encompasses the entire spinal canal. The patient's cranium extends outside the end of the box to allow for positioning, utilizing an aquaplast mask. This method, referred to as "simulated dynamic feathering," feathers the gap daily as opposed to the conventional methods where the fields are feathered after five fractions. The process is discussed in the following sections.

Simulation

The patient is placed in the vac bag, which provides comfort. An aquaplast mask is used to immobilize the cranium. The patient is aligned with the spine as straight as possible and no rotation of the cranium before scanning. A scout is usually needed to confirm that the patient is aligned and no adjustments are needed. An isocenter is placed in the CT room for the cranium fields only and the mask is marked. The isocenter is usually placed midline and will serve as a reference point for the spine field. Ideally, the spine isocenter is placed such that the couch is moved as little as possible between the brain and the spine fields. Generally, after the cranium fields are treated, the couch is shifted in two directions: toward the gantry and raised to accommodate the extended SSD of the PA spine field.

Treatment Planning

The cranial fields as well as the spine field are designed for the initial beams. Collimator and couch are rotated to prevent the overlap between the brain and spine fields using the treatment-planning system. The planning system allows visualization of beam divergence for all beams in the axial, sagittal, and coronal views. Once the initial fields have been designed, they are copied and labeled accordingly (Shift 1, 2, etc.). The cranial field's inferior border is increased by 5 mm, and the spine fields' superior border is decreased to match the inferior border of the brain fields. A total of 1.5 cm shift is used for this technique, which requires 3 shifts of 5 mm each shift. It is important to note that the spine field will not necessarily be 5 mm due to beam divergence as these fields are generally treated at extended SSDs (between 125 and 135 cm). The following shifts are created using the same process. The number of beams can be as many as 12 treated on a daily basis using the dynamic method; therefore, patient comfort is important as it contributes greatly to reproducibility. The number of shifts or junctions is physician dependent.

Plan optimization usually involves a forward planned field in field technique for the brain fields as well as for the spine field. However, it is possible to optimize the spine fields using inverse planning to cool off hot spots. The rationale for inverse planning the spine field is merely related to time. The control points needed for the spine field are generally higher than those of the brain

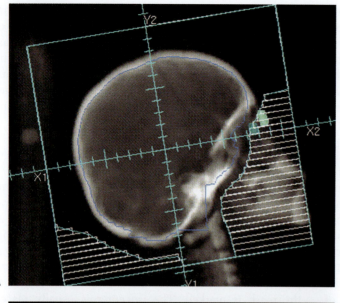

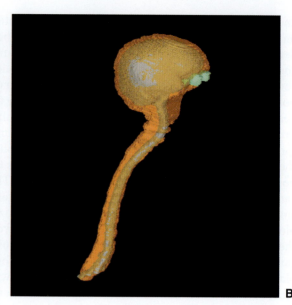

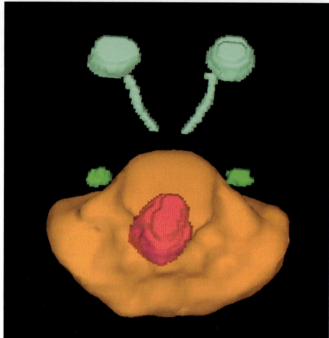

FIGURE 5.3. Sample whole-brain field with angled collimator for craniospinal radiotherapy of medulloblastoma (**A**). **B** represents the prescription dose cloud for craniospinal radiation of medulloblastoma. Note no loss of dose at the junction between the brain and the spine fields on account of a daily 3-feathered junction using the independent jaw. **C** illustrates the isodose cloud for an IMRT medulloblastoma posterior fossa boost specifically avoiding the cochlea (shown in green). The optic pathway is shown in aqua and the primary tumor is shown in pink.

fields. Figure 5.3B shows the dose cloud for such a craniospinal plan. Figure 5.3C shows the dose cloud for an IMRT-planned posterior fossa boost, sparing cochlea. Documenting junction match requires placing wires on the inferior border of brain fields before imaging the spine field for each junction shift.

Partial Brain Radiation

The era of 3D CRT in the 1990s allowed substantial reduction of unnecessary radiation to normal brain.

The anatomic location of the brain atop the head also maximized the benefits of non-coplanar beams, because vertex beam arrangements were available with a simple rotation of the treatment couch. While the wedge requirements of non-coplanar beam to produce homogeneous plans are more complicated, they are solvable.[75] In spite of this, the compensation requirements of such non-coplanar arrangements are more easily handled with IMRT inverse planning. In addition, intensity modulation can produce concave dose distributions around critical adjacent structures such as the optic chiasm, brain stem, and cochlea and thus provide more adequate dose sparing. IMRT also allows differential prescription of doses and simultaneously integrated boost plans that have made IMRT routine for contemporary partial brain irradiation. These techniques have been tested in a randomized trial, showing superior clinical benefits from reducing the volume of normal brain irradiated.[76]

Low-Grade Glioma

Low-grade gliomas, a heterogeneous group of tumors, include the most favorable pilocytic astrocytomas and the less favorable fibrillary astrocytomas with greater propensity to progress to a higher grade histology. Doses of 45 to 54 Gy in standard fraction sizes of 1.8 to 2 Gy per fraction with a typical 1 to 2 cm clinical margin on the radiographically defined GTV are used. Higher radiation doses have been studied but only resulted in increased toxicity with no survival benefit.

A helpful quantitative tool to evaluate brain plans is the conformity index. Originally utilized in radiosurgical planning, various conformity indices have now been described for external beam planning techniques. For an ideal plan, conformity indices approach 1. From a practical point of view, the indices have value in discriminating between generally acceptable treatment plans, since poorly conformal plans and plans that do not cover the target are usually quite apparent to the keen observer. The simplest conformity index can be defined as

Conformity Index = Treatment Volume/Target Volume

When the entire body is contoured in the planning system, the treatment volume is easily obtained from the DVH as the volume of the body receiving the prescription dose. A conformity index <1.2 indicates a highly conformal plan and should be an important and achievable planning goal. Proton therapy is being investigated for these tumors given the inherently lower integral dose in these long-term survivors.

High-Grade Glioma

Most high-grade gliomas are glioblastomas. Although temozolomide with radiation prolongs median survival by about 2 months with a small number of 5-year survivors, most patients invariably recur, requiring salvage therapy. While hypofractionated treatments and smaller treatment volumes are under investigation, the radiation standard remains 45 to 50 Gy to a clinical target including all surrounding postoperative FLAIR signals plus a 2-cm margin along continuous white matter tracks within the brain with a boost to a clinical target including the enhancing tumor or postoperative cavity plus a 1 to 2 cm margin. It is important to adjust clinical targets

along known anatomic white matter tracks to avoid unnecessary irradiation of the posterior fossa or contralateral brain, as both the tentorium and the falx are effective barriers to the spread of glial tumors. The standard dose remains 60 Gy. While radiotherapy dose escalation has demonstrated no survival benefit, these trials were conducted prior to the widespread adoption of concurrent and adjuvant temozolomide. The potential survival benefit of dose escalation with concomitant and adjuvant temozolomide remains the subject of an ongoing NRG oncology study.

Ependymoma

Ependymomas are uncommon primary glial CNS tumors that typically arise in the posterior fossa and cauda equina. Ependymomas in the cauda equina are most often low-grade myxopapillary type and carry a relatively favorable prognosis. Radiation therapy is reserved for incompletely resected or recurrent tumors. Ependymomas account for 5% to 10% of childhood intracranial tumors but occur in adults as well. Standard management involves complete surgical removal. Most authors agree that posterior fossa ependymomas should receive postoperative radiotherapy, as recurrence rates remain high even after complete surgical removal in this location. The addition of radiotherapy for supratentorial ependymomas after complete surgical resection is controversial, as this appears to be a more favorable subsite.

Meningiomas

Meningiomas are common CNS tumors, for which radiation therapy is a safe and effective treatment approach. Radiotherapy for meningiomas can be challenging because they often have irregular shapes and are located near critical structures. With the advent of IMRT, fractionated stereotactic radiotherapy (FSRT), SRS, and proton therapy, radiotherapeutic options in the management of meningiomas are now diverse. However, regardless of the modality, careful treatment planning is critical, since meningiomas are mostly benign tumors, and therefore the risk of serious late toxicities needs to be minimized.

Fusion of a contrast-enhanced MRI with the planning CT scan provides the optimal definition of the meningioma and adjacent OARs. In Europe, PET imaging (Ga-68 DOTATE) for radiotherapeutic planning is now available and approved. For well-demarcated lesions, the GTV and CTV are identical. Stereotactic positioning may be useful to reduce the margin for PTV, which takes into account the error in tumor volume delineation, errors inherent to image fusion, and for the variation in the day-to-day setup. With invasive tumors, such as those involving the sphenoid or cavernous sinuses, there is greater uncertainty, which must be considered in determining the CTV, and often a detailed evaluation of CT bone windows is a requirement.

The optimal beam arrangement is dictated by both the shape and the location of the lesion. With a large convexity lesion, for example, a potential arrangement may be three coplanar beams angled at 120 degrees from one another ("Mercedes Star") or a cruciform arrangement of four coplanar beams. The couch and gantry are then rotated so that each beam is shifted 10 degrees inferiorly with respect to the patient (Fig. 5.2). These arrangements minimize the cross-sectional area of the lesion within the beam's eye view. Other suggestions for beam arrangements are presented in the subsequent text, based on the region of the brain. The use of IMRT may be useful for concave-shaped lesions, and, in fact, now it is the most commonly used approach for meningiomas. With superficially located lesions, 6-MV photons are typically utilized owing to the short buildup depth; for more deeply situated tumors, such as cavernous sinus lesions, higher energy beams may be considered. Proton therapy, especially IMPT, is finding broader applicability in the treatment of meningiomas, based primarily on dosimetric considerations.

Pituitary Tumors

Fusion of a contrast-enhanced MRI with a contrasted planning CT scan provides the optimum definition of the suprasellar optic apparatus and the extensiveness of the tumor. The GTV is the pituitary adenoma, including any of its extension into adjacent anatomic regions. Generally, the entire content of the sella and, if appropriate, extension into the sphenoid or cavernous sinuses are included in the CTV. With appropriate immobilization devices and stereotactic positioning, PTV expansion of 0.3 to 0.5 cm gives excellent dose distribution with minimal dose to surrounding tissues. OARs to be contoured include the optic globes, lenses, optic nerves, optic chiasm, brain stem, residual pituitary gland, and temporal lobes.

The traditional three-field approach using wedged opposed laterals and an anterior or vertex beam superior to the eyes leads to unacceptably high doses to the temporal lobes. IMRT may be useful to further improve dose distribution, especially for irregularly shaped lesions. Beam energies of at least 6 MV should be used to spare surrounding structures, most notably the temporal lobes. Ten-megavolt photons provide a good balance between the depth dose and penumbra width, although for stereotactic plans with small margins, 6-MV photons may be more advantageous. IMRT and IMPT approaches are becoming more widespread in the treatment of several

pituitary adenomas. Non-randomized data also suggest that radiosurgical approaches lead to faster declines in hormone hypersecretion, and especially for growth-hormone secreting adenomas, this could be the preferred approach for several patients.

Spinal Tumors

The most favorable field arrangement will be determined by the location and adjacent OARs, and it may be a single PA field, opposed-lateral fields, a PA field with opposed laterals, opposed anterior–posterior (AP/PA) fields, or oblique wedge-pair fields. In some circumstances, IMRT may be useful to spare esophagus, heart, lung, kidney, and bowel, especially when higher doses need to be delivered. IMPT may also have these advantages in specific cases. When very long lengths of the spine need to be treated, proton therapy might be especially valuable to decrease the dose to multiple OARs in the exit beam. Some metastatic lesions may be suitable for treatment in a single fraction with spinal radiosurgery using appropriate immobilization and image guidance tools. In the cervical region, an opposed-lateral beam approach minimizes the dose to the anterior neck. When palliating a tumor in the cervicothoracic region, a split beam approach facilitates the match with another treatment field. In this case, the central axis is placed just above the shoulders and opposed-lateral beams are used to treat the upper spine, and a PA field is used for the area of the spine below the central axis. Tumors in the thoracic region can be treated with opposed lateral beams, a three-field approach using a PA field and opposed lateral beams, a two-field approach using AP/PA beams, or a posterior beam prescribed to an appropriate depth. When treating with a single posterior beam, the depth prescription should take into account the dose to the spinal cord to prevent accidental overdosing. In the lumbar region, AP/PA or PA fields reduce the exposure to the kidneys. In the sacral region, opposed lateral beams with or without a posterior beam or a four-field approach using AP/PA and opposed lateral beams may be useful. Comparison of various treatment setups by means of DVHs is recommended.

ACKNOWLEDGMENTS

The author would like to acknowledge the contributions of Lucien A Nedzi, Kevin S. Choe, Arnold Pompos, Ezequiel Ramirez, Volker W. Stieber, Kevin P. McMullen, Allan DeGuzman, and Edward G. Shaw to the writing of this chapter in the previous editions of this book.

KEY POINTS

- Multimodality therapy for CNS tumors may consist of medical therapy, surgical resection, radiation therapy, or some combination of the above.

- The therapeutic ratio of radiation therapy for CNS tumors has improved due to the introduction of new irradiation technologies, such as 3DCRT, IMRT, and proton therapy, and the development and availability of advanced imaging techniques such as MRI that help to better delineate targets and regions of avoidance.

- Modern radiation therapy for CNS tumors requires various novel imaging techniques that help to better understand the dosimetrically relevant composition of the tissue in the path of the radiation and verify the location of the target during dose delivery.

- Brain metastases can be treated with advanced radiotherapy techniques such as radiosurgery and/or hippocampal-avoidant whole-brain radiotherapy using IMRT to achieve optimal intracranial control and cognitive outcomes.

- Given their infiltrative nature, radiotherapy targeting of lower-grade and higher-grade gliomas typically involves a 1- to 2-cm margin around the resection and MR-visible residual tumor, neuroanatomically confined by structural barriers (e.g., tentorium or falx).

REVIEW QUESTIONS

1. (T/F) In patients diagnosed with a brain tumor, prophylactic use of anticonvulsants should be initiated irrespective of seizure history.

2. For radiotherapy planning of a resected high-grade glioma, the following MRI sequence(s) should be obtained:
   A. Preoperative T1-weighted sequence with contrast only
   B. Postoperative T1-weighted sequence with contrast only
   C. Preoperative T1-weighted sequence with contrast and preoperative T2/FLAIR sequence only
   D. Postoperative T2/FLAIR sequence only
   E. Pre- and postoperative T1-weighted sequences with contrast and pre- and postoperative T2/FLAIR sequences only

3. The following statements regarding radiobiologic tolerance of the brain stem and spinal cord are true except:
   A. A maximal dose constraint of 54 Gy is generally considered to have a minimal risk of causing severe neurological effects.
   B. 50 Gy at 2-Gy per fraction has been estimated to be associated with a 0.2% rate of myelopathy.
   C. Damage to the spinal cord can result in pain, paresthesias, sensory deficits, paralysis, Brown-Sequard syndrome, and bowel/bladder incontinence.
   D. Series on dose-escalated radiotherapy for skull base tumors have demonstrated that the dorsal surface of the brain stem may be relatively radioresistant.

4. (T/F) A radiosensitive neural stem cell compartment located in the subgranular zone of the hippocampal dentate gyrus may be central to radiotherapy-related memory toxicity.

5. All of the following statements are true regarding craniospinal irradiation except:
   A. The field length of the lower spine field should be maximized, whereas the field length of the upper spine field should be minimized.
   B. Medulloblastoma is an example of a neoplasm requiring craniospinal irradiation.
   C. When treating craniospinal irradiation in the supine position, the neck should be extended to avoid beams exiting the oral cavity.
   D. In the "exact-match" technique for matching the cranial fields to the upper spinal field, the collimator for the lateral cranial fields is angled to match the divergence of the upper border of the adjacent spinal field, and the treatment couch is angled so that the inferior border of the cranial field is perpendicular to the superior edge of the spinal field.

6. With conventional fractionation of 2 Gy per day for the full spinal cord cross section, the alpha–beta ratio has been estimated to be as low as:
   A. 10.0 Gy
   B. 5.0 Gy
   C. 2.0 Gy
   D. 0.87 Gy

ANSWERS

1. (F) In brain tumor patients who have no known seizure history, there is no evidence that prophylactic use of anticonvulsants prevents seizure risk.

2. E Both T2/FLAIR and contrast-enhanced T1-weighted sequences are critical to assessing regions of non-enhancing and enhancing tumor. Preoperative imaging provides an assessment of the preoperative extent of the tumor, while postoperative imaging provides visualization of the residual tumor to be targeted.

3. D Radiotherapy dose escalation for clival chordomas and clival/paraclival chondrosarcomas routinely increases radiotherapy exposure to the ventral surface of the brain stem (location of the corticospinal tracts) and has been shown to be associated with acceptable risk of brain stem toxicity.

4. (T) Preclinical and clinical studies have demonstrated that the radiosensitive and memory-specific neural stem cell compartment in the hippocampal dentate gyrus should be considered an organ at risk in radiotherapy planning.

5. A During craniospinal irradiation, it is customary practice to maximize the field length of the upper spinal field (40 cm at 100 cm source–skin distance [SSD]) and minimize the length of the lower spinal field, in order to simplify the planning for junction shifts.

6. D This estimate suggests a strong dose-per-fraction response relationship (i.e., exquisite sensitivity to damage as the dose per fraction increases), which is important given the devastating consequences that can arise from the damage to the spinal cord, including pain, paresthesias, sensory deficits, paralysis, Brown-Sequard syndrome, bowel/bladder incontinence, and even complete paralysis and death.[51]

REFERENCES

1. American CS. Cancer facts and figures. American Cancer Society; 2010.
2. CBTRUS. CBTRUS Statistical Report: Primary Brain and Central Nervous System Tumors Diagnosed in the United States in 2007–2011. Hinsdale, IL: Central Brain Tumor Registry of the United States; 2014.
3. Connolly E. Spinal cord tumors in adults. In: Youmans Y, ed. *Neurological Surgery*. vol 5. Philadelphia: WB Saunders; 1982:3196.
4. Sasanelli F. Primary intraspinal neoplasms in Rochester, Minnesota, 1935–1981. *Neuroepidemiology*. 1983;2:156–163.
5. IARC. WHO Classification of tumours of the central nervous system. IARC; 2007.
6. Preston-Martin S. Descriptive epidemiology of primary tumors of the spinal cord and spinal meninges in Los Angeles County, 1972–1985. *Neuroepidemiology*. 1990;9:106–111.
7. Cagney DN, Martin AM, Catalano PJ, et al. Incidence and prognosis of patients with brain metastases at diagnosis of systemic malignancy: a population-based study. *Neuro Oncol*. 2017;19(11):1511–1521.
8. Barnholtz-Sloan JS, Sloan AE, Davis FG, et al. Incidence proportions of brain metastases in patients diagnosed (1973 to 2001) in the Metropolitan Detroit Cancer Surveillance System. *J Clin Oncol*. 2004;22:2865–2872.
9. Byrne TN. Spinal cord compression from epidural metastases. *N Engl J Med*. 1992;327:614–619.
10. Gerszten P. Current surgical management of metastatic spinal disease. *Oncology*. 2000;14:1013–1024.
11. Loblaw DA, Laperriere NJ, Mackillop WJ. A population-based study of malignant spinal cord compression in Ontario. *Clin Oncol (R Coll Radiol)*. 2003;15:211–217.
12. Schaberg J, Gainor BJ. A profile of metastatic carcinoma of the spine. *Spine (Phila Pa 1976)*. 1985;10:19–20.
13. Bilsky MH, Lis E, Raizer J, et al. The diagnosis and treatment of metastatic spinal tumor. *Oncologist*. 1999;4:459–469.
14. Healey JH, Brown HK. Complications of bone metastases: surgical management. *Cancer*. 2000;88:2940–2951.
15. Wong DA, Fornasier VL, MacNab I. Spinal metastases: the obvious, the occult, and the impostors. *Spine (Phila Pa 1976)*. 1990;15:1–4.
16. Gilbert RW, Kim JH, Posner JB. Epidural spinal cord compression from metastatic tumor: diagnosis and treatment. *Ann Neurol*. 1978;3:40–51.
17. Patchell RA. A randomized trial of direct decompressive surgical resection in the treatment of spinal cord compression caused by metastasis. *J Clin Oncol*. 2003;21(1):67–86.
18. Pigott KH, Baddeley H, Maher EJ. Pattern of disease in spinal cord compression on MRI scan and implications for treatment. *Clin Oncol (R Coll Radiol)*. 1994;6:7–10.
19. O'Rourke T, George CB, Redmond J 3rd, et al. Spinal computed tomography and computed tomographic metrizamide myelography in the early diagnosis of metastatic disease. *J Clin Oncol*. 1986;4:576–583.
20. Ruff RL, Lanska DJ. Epidural metastases in prospectively evaluated veterans with cancer and back pain. *Cancer*. 1989;63:2234–2241.
21. Schiff D, Batchelor T, Wen PY. Neurologic emergencies in cancer patients. *Neurol Clin*. 1998;16:449–483.
22. Kaufmann TJ, Smits M, Boxerman J, et al. Consensus recommendations for a standardized brain tumor imaging protocol for clinical trials in brain metastases. *Neuro-Oncol*. 2020;22(6):757–772.
23. Ellingson BM, Wen PY, Cloughesy TJ. Modified criteria for radiographic response assessment in glioblastoma clinical trials. *Neurotherapeutics*. 2017;14(2):307–320.
24. Munley M. Bioanatomic IMRT treatment planning with dose function histograms. *Int J Rad Oncol Biol Phys*. 2002;54:126.
25. Nuutinen J, Sonninen P, Lehikoinen P, et al. Radiotherapy treatment planning and long-term follow-up with [(11)C]methionine PET in patients with low-grade astrocytoma. *Int J Radiat Oncol Biol Phys*. 2000;48:43–52.
26. Pirzkall A, McKnight TR, Graves EE, et al. MR-spectroscopy guided target delineation for high-grade gliomas. *Int J Radiat Oncol Biol Phys*. 2001;50:915–928.

27. Husband DJ, Grant KA, Romaniuk CS. MRI in the diagnosis and treatment of suspected malignant spinal cord compression. *Br J Radiol*. 2001;74:15–23.

28. Sarin R, Murthy V. Medical decompressive therapy for primary and metastatic intracranial tumours. *Lancet Neurol*. 2003;2:357–365.

29. French LA. The use of steroids in the treatment of cerebral edema. *Bull N Y Acad Med*. 1966;42:301–311.

30. Long DM, Hartmann JF, French LA. The response of human cerebral edema to glucosteroid administration: an electron microscopic study. *Neurology*. 1966;16:521–528.

31. Vecht CJ, Hovestadt A, Verbiest HB, et al. Dose-effect relationship of dexamethasone on Karnofsky performance in metastatic brain tumors: a randomized study of doses of 4, 8, and 16 mg per day. *Neurology*. 1994;44:675–680.

32. Wolfson AH, Snodgrass SM, Schwade JG, et al. The role of steroids in the management of metastatic carcinoma to the brain: a pilot prospective trial. *Am J Clin Oncol*. 1994;17:234–238.

33. Kalkanis SN, Eskandar EN, Carter BS, et al. Microvascular decompression surgery in the United States, 1996 to 2000: mortality rates, morbidity rates, and the effects of hospital and surgeon volumes. *Neurosurgery*. 2003;52:1251–1261; discussion 1261–1262.

34. Sorensen S, Helweg-Larsen S, Mouridsen H, et al. Effect of high-dose dexamethasone in carcinomatous metastatic spinal cord compression treated with radiotherapy: a randomised trial. *Eur J Cancer*. 1994;30A:22–27.

35. Bilsky MH. *Intensive and Postoperative Care of Intracranial Tumors*, 3rd ed. Raven Press; 1993:309–329.

36. Heimdal K, Hirschberg H, Slettebo H, et al. High incidence of serious side effects of high-dose dexamethasone treatment in patients with epidural spinal cord compression. *J Neurooncol*. 1992;12:141–144.

37. Weissman DE, Janjan NA, Erickson B, et al. Twice-daily tapering dexamethasone treatment during cranial radiation for newly diagnosed brain metastases. *J Neurooncol*. 1991;11:235–239.

38. Maranzano E, Latini P, Beneventi S, et al. Radiotherapy without steroids in selected metastatic spinal cord compression patients: a phase II trial. *Am J Clin Oncol*. 1996;19:179–183.

39. Bell BA, Smith MA, Kean DM, et al. Brain water measured by magnetic resonance imaging. Correlation with direct estimation and changes after mannitol and dexamethasone. *Lancet*. 1987;1:66–69.

40. Quinn JA, DeAngelis LM. Neurologic emergencies in the cancer patient. *Semin Oncol*. 2000;27:311–321.

41. Working Group on Status Epilepticus. Treatment of convulsive status epilepticus. Recommendations of the Epilepsy Foundation of America's Working Group on Status Epilepticus. *JAMA*. 1993;270:854–859.

42. Forsyth PA, Weaver S, Fulton D, et al. Prophylactic anticonvulsants in patients with brain tumour. *Can J Neurol Sci*. 2003;30:106–112.

43. Glantz MJ, Cole BF, Friedberg MH, et al. A randomized, blinded, placebo-controlled trial of divalproex sodium prophylaxis in adults with newly diagnosed brain tumors. *Neurology*. 1996;46:985–991.

44. Patchell RA, Tibbs PA, Walsh JW, et al. A randomized trial of surgery in the treatment of single metastases to the brain. *N Engl J Med*. 1990;322:494–500.

45. Vecht CJ, Haaxma-Reiche H, Noordijk EM, et al. Treatment of single brain metastasis: radiotherapy alone or combined with neurosurgery? *Ann Neurol*. 1993;33:583–590.

46. Mintz AH, Kestle J, Rathbone MP, et al. A randomized trial to assess the efficacy of surgery in addition to radiotherapy in patients with a single cerebral metastasis. *Cancer*. 1996;78:1470–1476.

47. Loblaw DA, Laperriere NJ. Emergency treatment of malignant extradural spinal cord compression: an evidence-based guideline. *J Clin Oncol*. 1998;16:1613–1624.

48. Young RF, Post EM, King GA. Treatment of spinal epidural metastases: randomized prospective comparison of laminectomy and radiotherapy. *J Neurosurg*. 1980;53:741–748.

49. Patchell RA, Tibbs PA, Regine WF, et al. Direct decompressive surgical resection in the treatment of spinal cord compression caused by metastatic cancer: a randomised trial. *Lancet*. 2005;366:643–648.

50. ICRU report 62. Prescribing, recording, and reporting photon beam therapy (Supplement to ICRU Report 50). International Commission on Radiation Units and Measurements; 1999.

51. Schultheiss TE, Kun LE, Ang KK, Stephens LC. Radiation response of the central nervous system. *Int J Radiat Oncol Biol Phys*. 1995;31:1093–1112.

52. Kirkpatrick JP, van der Kogel AJ, Schultheiss TE. The radiation dose-response of the human spinal cord. *Int J Radiat Oncol Biol Phys*. 2010;76:S42–S49.

53. Mayo C, Yorke E, Merchant TE. Radiation associated brainstem injury. *Int J Radiat Oncol Biol Phys*. 2010;76:S36–S41.

54. Debus J, Hug EB, Liebsch NJ, et al. Brainstem tolerance to conformal radiotherapy of skull base tumors. *Int J Radiat Oncol Biol Phys*. 1997;39:967–975.

55. Danesh-Meyer HV. Radiation-induced optic neuropathy. *J Clin Neurosci*. 2008;15:95–100.

56. Mayo C, Martel MK, Marks LB, Flickinger J, Nam J, Kirkpatrick J. Radiation dose-volume effects of optic nerves and chiasm. *Int J Radiat Oncol Biol Phys*. 2010;76:S28–S35.

57. Jeganathan VS, Wirth A, MacManus MP. Ocular risks from orbital and periorbital radiation therapy: a critical review. *Int J Radiat Oncol Biol Phys*. 2011;79:650–659.

58. Gondi V, Tome WA, Mehta MP. Why avoid the hippocampus? A comprehensive review. *Radiot Oncol*. 2010;97:370–376.

59. Gondi V, Pugh, SL, Tome, WA, et al. Preservation of memory with conformal avoidance of the hippocampal neural stem-cell compartment during whole-brain radiotherapy for brain metastases (RTOG 0933): a phase II multi-institutional trial. *J Clin Oncol*. 2014;32:3810–3816.

60. Brown PD, Gondi V, Pugh S, et al. Hippocampal avoidance during whole-brain radiotherapy plus memantine for patients with brain metastases: phase III trial NRG Oncology CC001. *J Clin Oncol*. 2020;38(10);1019–1029.

61. Gondi V, Hermann B, Mehta MP, et al. Hippocampal dosimetry predicts neurocognitive function impairment after fractionated stereotactic radiotherapy for benign or low-grade adult brain tumors. *Int J Radiat Oncol Biol Phys*. 2013;85:348–354.

62. Lee AW, Ng SH, Ho JH, et al. Clinical diagnosis of late temporal lobe necrosis following radiation therapy for nasopharyngeal carcinoma. *Cancer*. 1988;61:1535–1542.

63. Lee AW, Ng WT, Hung WM, et al. Major late toxicities after conformal radiotherapy for nasopharyngeal carcinoma-patient- and treatment-related risk factors. *Int J Radiat Oncol Biol Phys*. 2009;73:1121–1128.

64. Pehlivan B, Ares C, Lomax AJ, et al. Temporal lobe toxicity analysis after proton radiation therapy for skull base tumors. *Int J Radiat Oncol Biol Phys*. 2012;83:1432–1440.

65. Gross JP, Powell S, Zelko F, et al. Improved neuropsychological outcomes following proton therapy relative to X-ray therapy for pediatric brain tumor patients. *Neuro Oncol*. 2019;21(7);934–943.

66. Aur RJ, Simone JV, Hustu HO, et al. A comparative study of central nervous system irradiation and intensive chemotherapy early in remission of childhood acute lymphocytic leukemia. *Cancer*. 1972;29:381–391.

67. Borgelt B, Gelber R, Kramer S, et al. The palliation of brain metastases: final results of the first two studies by the Radiation Therapy Oncology Group. *Int J Radiat Oncol Biol Phys*. 1980;6:1–9.

68. Andrews DW, Scott CB, Sperduto PW, et al. Whole brain radiation therapy with or without stereotactic radiosurgery boost for patients with one to three brain metastases: phase III results of the RTOG 9508 randomised trial. *Lancet*. 2004;363:1665–1672.

69. Aoyama H, Shirato H, Tago M, et al. Stereotactic radiosurgery plus whole-brain radiation therapy vs stereotactic radiosurgery alone for treatment of brain metastases: a randomized controlled trial. *JAMA*. 2006;295:2483–2491.

70. Kocher M, Soffietti R, Abacioglu U, et al. Adjuvant whole-brain radiotherapy versus observation after radiosurgery or surgical resection of one to three cerebral metastases: results of the EORTC 22952-26001 study. *J Clin Oncol*. 2011;29:134–41.

71. Chang EL, Wefel JS, Hess KR, et al. Neurocognitive function of patients with brain metastasis who received either whole brain radiotherapy plus stereotactic radiosurgery or radiosurgery alone. *Lancet Oncol.* 2009;10:1037–1044.

72. Brown PD, Jaeckle K, Ballman KV, et al. Effect of radiosurgery alone vs radiosurgery with whole brain radiation therapy on cognitive function in patients with 1 to 3 brain metastases: a randomized clinical trial. *JAMA.* 2016;316(4);401–409.

73. Brown PD, Pugh S, Laack NN, et al. Memantine for the prevention of cognitive dysfunction in patients receiving whole-brain radiotherapy: a randomized, double-blind, placebo-controlled trial. *Neuro Oncol.* 2013;15(10);1429–1437.

74. Shiu AS, Chang EL, Ye JS, et al. Near simultaneous computed tomography image-guided stereotactic spinal radiotherapy: an emerging paradigm for achieving true stereotaxy. *Int J Radiat Oncol Biol Phys.* 2003;57:605–613.

75. Sherouse GW. A mathematical basis for selection of wedge angle and orientation. *Med Phys.* 1993;20:1211–1218.

76. Kumar N, Kumar R, Sharma S, et al. Impact of volume of irradiation on survival and quality of life in glioblastoma: a prospective phase II randomized comparison of RTOG and MDACC protocols. *Neurooncol Pract.* 2020;7(1):86–93.

6 Cancers of the Head and Neck

Yolanda I. Garces, Charles Mayo, Christopher Beltran, and Robert L. Foote

INTRODUCTION

Head and neck (H&N) cancer is a complex disease site to master because there are many factors that one has to consider. First, this group of malignancies encompasses more than just one disease site. H&N cancers include a wide variety of primary sites from the orbit, ear, and scalp cranially to the thyroid gland caudally. Further, H&N cancer physicians need to be proficient in the treatment of a wide variety of histologic subtypes, from the common squamous cell carcinomas to the rare sarcomas. This chapter focuses on the more common adult squamous cell carcinomas of the H&N as well as thyroid cancers given their increasing incidence; it will not include rare diseases. In addition, a solid understanding of H&N anatomy as well as the patterns of cancer spread, both local and nodal, is critical to the development of optimal treatment plans and strong decision-making. Finally, a well-integrated multidisciplinary team is also critical for treatment success.

INCIDENCE AND EPIDEMIOLOGY

An estimated 65,000 US citizens were afflicted with H&N cancer in 2019. Another 53,000 were diagnosed with thyroid cancer. The incidence of cancer overall is declining, which is predominantly due to increased cancer screening and smoking cessation in recent decades. However, the incidence is increasing for human papilloma virus (HPV)–related oropharyngeal cancer and thyroid cancer.[1] Alarmingly, the 5-year relative survival rates for larynx cancer have declined from 66% to 63% when comparing the 1975–1977 to the 2004–2010 cohorts, making larynx cancer one of the two cancers where there has been a statistically significant decline in the 5-year survival, the other being cancer of the uterine corpus.[2] However, a more recent National Cancer Data Base study is showing that non-T4, low nodal burden patients have similar outcomes with surgery or radiation.[3] In addition, an interesting retrospective study has shown that clinicians can use an age-adjusted comorbidity index to predict non–cancer-related deaths; older patients with more

comorbidities do poorly. The authors suggest that the Charlson comorbidity index score should be utilized to stratify patients on future clinical trials.[4] Further, a retrospective review performed at the Mayo Clinic showed that patients treated with definitive chemoradiotherapy were more likely to experience a non–cancer-related death when compared to patients treated with total laryngectomy and postoperative radiotherapy. The deaths were likely due to aspiration pneumonia, emphasizing the need for swallowing evaluations and therapy for patients who chose to undergo larynx preservation chemoradiotherapy.[5]

The main risk factor for H&N cancer remains current or past tobacco use. Concurrent alcohol use significantly augments the risk.[6] H&N cancer patients have often reduced or already quit smoking by the time they are seen by their health-care team.[7] However, relapse back to smoking remains high. Strong recommendations for quitting and remaining quit are essential to help improve treatment outcomes, and most health-care providers are good at asking and providing this advice. However, beyond asking and advising,[8] it is essential that cancer centers develop mechanisms to assist with behavioral counseling, providing appropriate cessation medications as well as tobacco cessation follow-up with patients to optimize outcomes.[9] It is well known that smoking cessation can reduce the risk of second primary cancers.[10] The epidemic of HPV-related oropharynx cancers among younger, relatively healthy individuals who never smoked is changing the perception of H&N cancer patients and survivors.

The causal relationship between HPV and oropharynx cancers was first described in 2000.[11] The incidence of HPV-related cancers is increasing in the United States and worldwide. HPV-related oropharynx cancers are occurring predominantly in never smoking younger men who are less than 60 years old.[12] These cancers are predominantly located in the tonsil, tongue base, or pharyngeal wall. It is felt that changes in sex behaviors in developed countries have led to this increase. Men also have higher rates of HPV prevalence than do women.[13] Interestingly, patients who have HPV-related tumors and are either never smokers or smoked less than 10 pack-years in their lifetime have a better prognosis.[14] Clinical trials are being conducted to exploit this benefit and to reduce the morbidity of treatment.

GENERAL TREATMENT RECOMMENDATIONS

General Principles

The treatment of H&N cancer with radiotherapy is typically complex, and intensity-modulated radiation therapy (IMRT) is utilized for the majority of patients. IMRT is typically delivered with volumetric-modulated arc therapy (VMAT) as discussed in the treatment section. The only general exception is for patients with early-stage larynx cancer, where we generally still utilize 3D-conformal fields, in which the outcomes are excellent and the risk of long-term complications is low due to the small field size (see Fig. 6.1A).[15] The field arrangement for an early-stage larynx patient typically is opposed laterals that enter "above" or "cranial to" the shoulders. One centimeter of bolus material is placed over the skin overlying the anterior commissure region for patients who have anterior commissure involvement and a "thin" neck with less than 1 cm of subcutaneous tissue between the skin and the anterior thyroid cartilage. Wedges with the heels placed anteriorly are utilized to keep the dose uniform throughout the target volume (see Fig. 6.1B).

However, it is fairly common for centers to utilize field-in-field techniques or dynamic wedges rather than physical wedges. The dose of radiation for invasive cancers typically ranges from 225 to 200 cGy per day to a total dose of 6,300 to 7,000 cGy, respectively. For some T2 larynx cancers, utilizing a BID fractionation of 120 cGy with at least a 6-hour interval between fractions to a total dose of 7,920 cGy provides increased local control.[16] There are dosimetric studies as well as early retrospective clinical data and trials that are evaluating carotid artery sparing techniques and hypofractionated stereotactic body radiation techniques (ClinicalTrial.gov Identifier NCT03548285 and NCT01984502) to minimize the possible long-term complications from definitive treatments including carotid stenosis and stroke.[17-16]

The vast majority of H&N patients have been treated with IMRT in the past decade with comparative effectiveness research showing that the primary reason for this being an improvement in xerostomia in patients who received IMRT and are able to undergo parotid sparing techniques.[20] These patients require a multidisciplinary team to best identify the most appropriate treatment options. Therefore, this section will focus on general treatment principles for optimal H&N treatment and then review the unique issues as they relate to H&N cancers including the following: target volumes and normal organ contouring, planning challenges for dosimetrists and physicists, image-guided and adaptive radiation therapy, and finally novel radiation therapy techniques like intensity-modulated particle therapy.

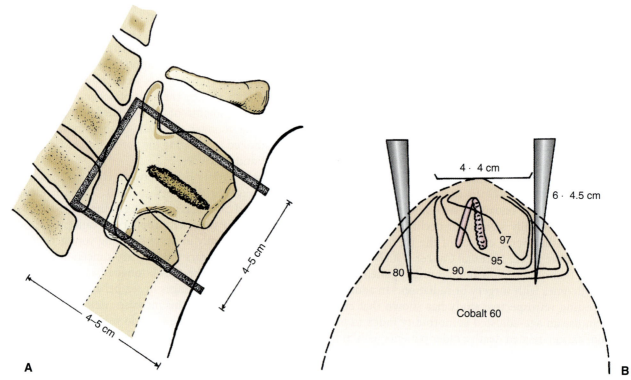

FIGURE 6.1. A: Early larynx (cT1N0) cancer treatment field. **B:** Early larynx (cT1N0) cancer isodoses.

General Treatment Recommendations

It is beyond the scope of this chapter to discuss which primary treatment option (surgery vs. radiation therapy) is best for patients, and it will focus primarily on definitive treatments for the majority of patients and discuss postoperative challenges for H&N cancer (squamous cell carcinomas and well-differentiated thyroid carcinoma) patients as well. Treatment volumes for both the primary and nodes[21-26,] are summarized by the disease site for the uninvolved neck to the N3 neck in Tables 6.1 and 6.2. The primary and nodal tumor volumes (gross tumor volume: GTVp, GTVn) are determined by radiologic imaging, which could include CT simulation with or without IV

TABLE 6.1	Primary Tumor Site and Gross Tumor Volume Delineations		
Tumor Site	**Subsites**		
Oropharynx:	**Tonsil**	**Base of Tongue**	**Soft Palate**
Primary	GTVp	GTVp	GTVp
CTV expansion	CTV includes 1–1.5 cm expansion and includes the adjacent structures, soft palate, base of tongue, and pharyngeal wall.	CTV includes ≥2 cm expansion on the GTVp and includes the vallecula and suprahyoid epiglottis, if the vallecula is involved.	CTV includes 1–1.5 cm expansion and includes the soft palate, tonsillar pillars, and pterygopalatine fossa.
Advanced disease	Include the nasopharynx, pterygoid musculature, or parapharyngeal space.	Oral tongue if involved.	Consider skull base if pterygopalatine fossa is involved.
Oral Cavity	**Buccal**	**Retromolar Trigone (RMT)**	**Anterior or Lateral Gingiva**
Primary	GTVp	GTVp	GTVp
CTV expansion	CTV includes the entire buccal space from buccal–gingival sulcus superior to inferior, infratemporal fossa, and lip commissure to the RMT.	CTV includes 1–1.5 cm expansion and includes the adjacent sites if the buccal mucosa, anterior tonsillar pillar, palate, or lingual nerve is involved.	CTV includes 1–1.5 cm expansion and includes the mandible/maxilla.
Advanced disease	As above.	Include the nasopharynx, pterygoid musculature, or parapharyngeal space.	As above.
Oral Cavity (continued):	**Oral Tongue**	**Floor of Mouth (FOM)**	**Hard Palate**
Primary	GTVp	GTVp	GTVp
CTV expansion	CTV includes 1.5–2 cm expansion and includes the tongue base if involved, as well as the intrinsic/extrinsic muscle of the tongue, FOM, glossotonsillar sulcus, and anterior tonsillar pillar (as necessary).	CTV includes 1–1.5 cm expansion and includes the geniohyoid and genioglossus muscles bilaterally and ipsilateral sublingual and submandibular glands.	CTV includes 1–1.5 cm expansion and includes the maxilla.
Advanced disease	As above.	Bilateral sublingual/submandibular glands if midline involvement.	As above.
Larynx:	**Subglottic**	**Glottic**	**Supraglottic**
Primary	GTVp	GTVp	GTVp
CTV expansion	CTV includes 1.0–1.5 cm expansion and includes the entire cricoid cartilage.	CTV includes 1.0–1.5 cm expansion and includes the entire thyroid and cricoid cartilages.	CTV includes 1.0–1.5 cm expansion and includes the entire supraglottic/glottic larynx and pre-epiglottic space.
Advanced disease	If tracheostomy was performed, include the tracheostomy site.	If tracheostomy was performed, include the tracheostomy site. If vallecular involvement, include the vallecular and pre-epiglottic space.	If tracheostomy was performed, include the tracheostomy site.

(continued)

TABLE 6.1   Primary Tumor Site and Gross Tumor Volume Delineations (*Continued*)

Tumor Site	Subsites		
Hypopharynx:	**Pyriform Sinus**	**Post-cricoid**	**Posterior Pharyngeal Wall**
Primary	GTVp	GTVp	GTVp
CTV expansion	CTV includes 1.5–2.0 cm expansion, includes the ipsilateral hemilarynx, and 2 cm below the cricoid cartilage.	CTV includes a 1.5–2.0 cm expansion and includes the entire larynx down to 2 cm below the cricoid cartilage.	CTV includes 1.5–2.0 cm expansion on the GTV and includes the entire posterior pharyngeal wall from the nasopharynx through the hypopharynx as a lower risk CTV.
Advanced disease	If lateral wall involvement, consider including the ipsilateral thyroid lobe.	As above.	As above.
Nasopharynx:			
Primary	GTVp		
CTV expansion	CTVp1 = GTVp + 5 mm +/– whole NPX, down to 1 mm if close to critical OARs	CTVp2 = GTVp + 10 mm + whole NPX, add 5 mm of posterior nasal cavity and posterior wall of maxillary sinus; include vomer (posterior ethmoid sinus); pterygoid fossa and parapharyngeal spaces	Additional notes for CTVp2: For T1/T2, include inferior half of sphenoid sinus and for T3/T4, include the entire sphenoid sinus; include 1/3 of clivus in no invasion and include entire clivus if involved. Mininum margin on GTV is 2 mm for these critical OARs
Advanced disease	For T3/T4 disease, include ipsilateral foramina ovale, rotundum, lacerum, and petrous tip.		
Thyroid:			
Primary	GTVp		
CTV expansion	CTV includes 1.0–1.5 cm expansion.		
Advanced disease	CTV expansion could include the hemilarynx or hemiesophagus if larynx or tracheoesophageal groove involvement is involved.		

TABLE 6.2   Target Volumes by Dose and Disease Site for the N0 through N3 Neck

Tumor Site	N Classification	CTV70 Gy	CTV63 Gy	CTV56 Gy	Notes	Additional Notes
Oropharynx (p16 negative)						
	N0 or N1 (in level II, III, or IV)	GTVp +/– GTVn	For N1 neck: IN +/– CN (II–IVa)[1] +/– VIIa[2]	For N0 neck: IN +/– CN (II–IVa) +/– VIIa[2]		Include ipsilateral Ib if the primary tumor extends to the oral cavity (retromolar trigone, oral tongue, inferior gingiva, oral side of anterior tonsillar pillar) or anterior involvement of level II.
	N2a–N2b	GTVp + GTVn	IN (Ib–IVa, Va,b, VIIa)[1,3]	CN (II–IVa) +/– VIIa[2]		

TABLE 6.2   Primary Tumor Site and Gross Tumor Volume Delineations (*Continued*)

Tumor Site	N Classification	CTV70 Gy	CTV63 Gy	CTV56 Gy	Notes	Additional Notes
	N2c	GTVp + GTVn	According to N classification on each side of the neck	According to N classification on each side of the neck		
	N3	GTVp + GTVn	IN (Ib–IVa, Va, b, VIIa)[3]	CN (II–IVa) +/– VIIa[2]		

HPV-mediated or p16-positive tumors have a different staging classification to reflect a better prognosis. However, similar principles apply while reviewing what nodal levels to include and should not be different than p16-negative tumors.

IN only for tonsil fossa tumors not infiltrating the BOT or soft palate for N0–N2a; MD discretion for N2b.

[1]If IVa is involved, then include IVb.

[2]Include VIIa for posterior pharyngeal wall tumors.

[3]Level VIIb should be included if bulky involvement of upper level II.

Oral Cavity

Tumor Site	N Classification	CTV70 Gy	CTV63 Gy	CTV56 Gy	Notes	Additional Notes
Buccal, alveolar ridge, floor of mouth, and oral tongue	N0-1 (in levels I, II or III)	GTVp +/– GTVn	For N1 neck: IN +/– CN (I–IVa)[4–6]	For N0 neck: IN +/– CN (I–IVa)[4,5]		
	N2a–N2b	GTVp + GTVn	IN (I–IVa)[1,3,6], Va,b Level V can be omitted if only levels I to II are involved.	CN (I–IVa)[4,5]		
	N2c	GTVp + GTVn	According to N classification on each side of the neck	According to N classification on each side of the neck		
	N3	GTVp + GTVn	IN (I–IVa)[1,3,6], Va, b	CN (I–IVa)[4]		

Unilateral treatment for N0–N2a if well lateralized and involve alveolar ridges, lateral floor of mouth, or buccal; at discretion of MD for N2b.

For lateral border of oral tongue that is N0–N1, one could also consider ipsilateral treatment if more than 1 cm from midline.

[1]If IVa is involved, then include IVb.

[3]Level VIIb should be included if bulky involvement of upper level II.

[4]Include level IVa if the primary extends to involve the oropharynx (anterior tonsillar pillar, tonsillar fossa, base of tongue) or if N1 node involved is at Level III.

[5]Level IIb could be omitted if no cervical nodes on the same side.

[6]Include ipsilateral level IX for buccal.

Tumor Site	N Classification	CTV70 Gy	CTV63 Gy	CTV56 Gy	Notes	Additional Notes
Larynx (excluding T1N0 glottic)	N0-N1 (in level II, III, or IV)	GTVp	For N1 neck: IN (II–IVa)[1,5,7,8]	For N0 neck: IN (II–IVa)[1,5,7,8] For N0 or N1 neck: CN (II–IVa)[5,8]		
	N2a–N2b	GTVp + GTVn	IN (II–IVa, Va,b)[1,3,7,8]	CN (II–IVa)[5,8]		

(*continued*)

TABLE 6.2   Primary Tumor Site and Gross Tumor Volume Delineations (*Continued*)

Tumor Site	N Classification	CTV70 Gy	CTV63 Gy	CTV56 Gy	Notes	Additional Notes
	N2c	GTVp + GTVn	According to N classification on each side of the neck	According to N classification on each side of the neck		
	N3	GTVp + GTVn	IN (Ib–IVa, Va,b, VI)[1,3]	CN (II–IVa)[5,8]		

[1]Include level IVb nodes if level IVa involved.

[3]Level VIIb should be included if bulky involvement of upper level II.

[5]Level IIb could be omitted if no cervical lymph nodes on the same side.

[7]Include level Ib nodes if anterior level II is involved.

[8]Include level VI nodes if subglottic or transglottic extension.

Tumor Site	N Classification	CTV70 Gy	CTV63 Gy	CTV56 Gy	Notes	Additional Notes
Hypopharynx	N0	GTVP		IN (II–IVa) + CN (II–IVa)[5]	Include VI if apex of piriform sinus, postcricoid and/or esophageal extension.	Include VIIa for posterior pharyngeal wall tumor.
	N1, N2a-b	GTVp + GTVn	IN (Ib–IVa, Va,b, VIIa)[1,3]	CN (II–IVa)[5]	Include VI if apex of piriform sinus, postcricoid and/or esophageal extension and/or N2b.	Include VIIa for posterior pharyngeal wall tumor.
	N2c	GTVp + GTVn	According to N classification on each side of the neck	According to N classification on each side of the neck		
	N3	GTVp + GTVn	IN (Ib–IVa, Va,b, VIIa, VI)[1,3]	CN (II–IVa)[5] Include Level VI for esophageal extension. Include VIIa for posterior pharyngeal wall primary tumors.		

Could consider unilateral treatment for a small well-lateralized tumor of piriform sinus.

[1]Include level IVb nodes if level IVa is involved.

[3]Level VIIb should be included if bulky involvement of upper level II.

[5]Level IIb could be omitted if no cervical lymph nodes on the same side.

Tumor Site	N Classification	CTV70 Gy	CTV63 Gy	CTV56 Gy	Notes	Additional Notes
Nasopharynx	N0	GTVp		IN and CN (II–V, VIIa, VIIb)	Level IV and Vb could be omitted for patients with no ipsilateral cervical involvement on the same side.	

TABLE 6.2 Primary Tumor Site and Gross Tumor Volume Delineations (*Continued*)

Tumor Site	N Classification	CTV70 Gy	CTV63 Gy	CTV56 Gy	Notes	Additional Notes
	N1 or N2	GTVp + GTVn	For N2 neck: IN +/− CN (II–V, VIIa, VIIb)	For N1 neck: CN (II-V, VIIa, VIIb)	Level IV and Vb could be omitted for patients with no ipsilateral cervical involvement on the same side. If III or IVa is involved, then include IVb.	Include Ib if submandibular gland involvement, and/or structures that drain to Ib, and/or level II (LN>2 cm and/or ENE). If Va,b is involved, then include Vc.
	N3	GTVp + GTVn	Bilateral neck involvement: IN +/− CN (Ib–IVb, Va,b,c, VIIa, VIIb)	Unilateral neck involvement: CN (Ib-IVb, Va,b,c, VIIa, VIIb)		
Thyroid		Treat all node levels including the upper mediastinum. Omit VIIa/b, Level Ia/b (unless level II involved), preauriculars.				
Post-Op Patients		For post-op patients, CTV60 Gy is for the primary tumor site post-op tumor bed and involved dissected neck. CTV54 Gy is for the clinically negative undissected neck. One could consider a simultaneous integrated boost for patients with positive margins (CTV66 Gy) all in 30 fractions.				

Always include next echelon lymph node level adjacent to involved nodes, for example, if level II nodes are involved, include level Ib; include level Ia if level Ib is involved, include V if IV is involved, include level VII if level VI is involved, etc.

These recommendations are for squamous cell carcinoma only of the primary tumor sites mentioned here.

Modified with permission from Gregoire V, Evans M, Le Q, et al. Delineation of the primary tumor Clinical Target Volumes (CTV-P) in laryngeal, hypopharyngeal, oropharyngeal and oral cavity squamous cell carcinoma: AIRO, CAC, DAHANCA, EORTC, GEORCC, GORTEC, HKNPCSG, HNCIG, IAG-KHT, LPRHHT, NCIC CTG, NCRI, NRG Oncology, PHNS, SBRT, SOMERA, SRO, SSHNO, TROG consensus guidelines. *Radiother Oncol.* 2018;126:3–24; Gregoire V, Ang K, Budach W, et al. Delineation of the neck node levels for head and neck tumors: a 2013 update. DAHANCA, EORTC, HKNPCSG, NCIC CTG, NCRI, RTOG, TROG consensus guidelines. *Radiother Oncol.* 2014;110(1):172–181; Biau J, Lapeyre M, Troussier I, et al. Selection of lymph node target volumes for definitive head and neck radiation therapy: a 2019 Update. *Radiother Oncol.* 2019;134:1–9. BOT, Base of tongue; CN, Contralateral neck; FOM, Floor of mouth; GTVn, GTV of involved node(s); GTVp, GTV of primary tumor; IN, Ipsilateral neck; OT, Oral tongue; RMT, Retromolar trigone.

Nasal and Paranasal Sinuses						
Maxillary Sinus	N0	GTVp		IN (Ib-III, VIIa, IX) and CN (Ib-III, VIIa)		Prophylactic neck RT for T3/4 squamous cell carcinoma or sinonasal undifferentiated carcinomas (SNUC).
	N1-3	GTVp	IN (Ib-V, VIIa, IX) [1,3]	CN (Ib-V, VIIa) [1,3]		
Ethmoid sinus	N0	GTVp		IN and CN, Levels II-III, VIIa for Kadish Stage > C and/or Hyams grade III/IV esthesioneuroblastoma		
	N1-N3	GTVp	IN (Ib-V, VIIa) [1,3]	CN (Ib-V, VIIa) [1,3]		

(continued)

Nasal and Paranasal Sinuses						
Nasal Cavity	N0	GTVp		IN (Ib-III, VIIa) and CN (Ib-III, VIIa)	Ipsilateral IX for anterior third nasal cavity involvement.	Prophylactic neck RT for T3/4 squamous cell carcinoma or SNUC.
	N1-N3	GTVp	IN (Ib-V, VIIa)[1,3]	CN (Ib-V, VIIa)[1,3]	Ipsilateral IX for anterior third nasal cavity involvement.	

Unilateral RT for maxillary sinus and nasal cavity tumors not crossing mid-line and without nodal contralateral neck involvement.

If contralateral neck nodes are involved, they should receive intermediate CTV dose level and not low CTV dose level.

[1]Include level IVb nodes if level Iva is involved.

[3]Level VIIb should be included if bulky involvement of upper level II.

contrast, contrast-enhanced CT, PET/CT, or MRI as well as a good clinical examination including nasopharyngolaryngoscopy. It is also beyond the scope of this chapter to discuss the various dose options for each disease site and/or the clinical scenario. The typical doses of 7,000, 6,300, and 5,600 cGy in 35 fractions for high-, intermediate-, and low-risk target volumes, respectively, for definitive cases are presented in Table 6.2. Similarly, postoperative radiation doses are 6,000 and 5,400 cGy in 30 fractions for the high- and low-risk target volumes, respectively. Consensus guidelines on clinical target volume (CTV) expansions are now allowing for a 5-mm expansion from the GTVp for high tumor burden and an additional 5 mm for lower tumor burden with these volumes called CTV-P1 (high-dose CTV) and CTV-P2 (intermediate-dose CTV).[23] These expansions are removed from air, bone, or other anatomic barriers to tumor spread (if those structures are not directly involved). These expansions do not apply for patients who have received induction chemotherapy and have recurrent disease and/or for use with adaptive radiation therapy techniques.

For postoperative patients, chemotherapy is added to radiation therapy primarily for fit patients with high-risk features of extracapsular extension and/or positive margins.[27] Chemotherapy is typically cisplatin-based, but there are ongoing clinical trials investigating various chemotherapy regimens for high-risk patients including docetaxel, cetuximab, and atezolizumab (Radiation Therapy Oncology Group (RTOG) 1216, NCT01810913). Of note, this trial includes patients with high-risk non-HPV-related oropharynx cancers. The phase II portion of the study closed in March of 2020; the study is now in the phase III portion of the trial, which includes the atezolizumab arm. There is an intermediate-risk group of patients for whom a recently closed clinical trial is looking

at the addition of cetuximab to adjuvant radiotherapy (RTOG 0920, NCT00956007). The patients eligible for this clinical trial have the following risk factors: perineural or lymphovascular invasion, a single lymph node greater than 3 cm or ≥ 2 lymph nodes (all less than 6 cm) with no extracapsular extension, close margins (within 5 mm), a T3 or T4 primary tumor of the oral cavity, oropharynx, or larynx, or a T2 oral cavity cancer with >5-mm depth of invasion. It is essential that all patients are seen promptly after surgery as the complexity of treatment planning and the social factors associated with H&N cancer patients can make a long and possibly toxic treatment challenging for patients. Ideally, the entire "package" of treatment from surgery to the completion of radiation therapy is delivered within 11 weeks from the date of surgery.[28]

Treatment volumes in the postoperative setting do differ slightly from definitive cases as one needs to consider the surgery performed and invasion of the tumor into adjacent sites for the primary and nodal disease CTV. Typically, no GTV is identified on the planning study since the primary tumor and involved nodes have been completely resected with negative margins. A pre-op GTV can be added as a guide, but this volume is not used for CTV or planning target volume (PTV) expansions. The nodal levels and volumes tend to be as described by the International Multi-Cooperative Group Consensus 2013 Neck Node Guidelines.[25] A simultaneous integrated boost (SIB) to 66 Gy in 30 fractions to the site of a positive margin is included in the treatment plan and is designed with the aid of surgical clips and/or a thorough review of the operative note, pathology report, preoperative imaging, and communication with the surgeon.

No data exist to support different treatment volumes or expansions for patients with HPV-related disease with or without extracapsular extension; however, there is great interest in decreasing the volume and dose or intensity of the radiation treatments for patients with favorable prognosis who have undergone resection. There are several studies looking at dose de-escalation and RT volume reductions in the setting or primary radiation therapy including the following Clinical-Trials.gov Identifiers: NCT03416153, NCT04012502, NCT03822897, NCT03107182, NCT02072148, NCT02281955, NCT02254278, NCT01706939, NCT01088802, NCT01302834, NCT02258659, NCT01663259, NCT01932697, and NCT02159703. Two of the de-escalation studies in the postoperative setting are highlighted as follows: First, the Eastern Cooperative Oncology Group (ECOG) is conducting a randomized phase II trial of transoral surgery followed by low-dose or standard-dose radiation therapy in HPV-related stage III to IVA patients who are at intermediate risk (ECOG E3311 trial, NCT01898494). Second, Mayo Clinic is conducting a single institution randomized trial that is offering patients twice-daily adjuvant hyperfractionated radiation therapy to 3,600 or 3,000 cGy in 150 cGy fractions over 2 weeks in combination with docetaxel for patients with or without extracapsular nodal extension, respectively, versus standard of care 6000 cGy with or without weekly cisplatin (DART-HPV, NCT02908477). There are studies with RT volume reductions that will be valuable to follow. These include two mucosal sparing studies (UPENN, AVOID and Mayo Clinic's mucosal sparing intensity-modulated proton therapy [IMPT] trials, NCT02159703 and NCT02736786, respectively).[29] Another important study to watch for longer-term results is Washington University's study of not radiating a pathologically uninvolved (pN0) neck after TORS (NCT00593840).[30] All these trials will likely inform future treatment options for this growing and favorable subgroup of patients.

Thyroid cancer patients can also be treated in the adjuvant setting. However, the role of adjuvant radiation therapy remains somewhat controversial for the differentiated thyroid cancers, given the lack of randomized trials. There are several retrospective series that support its use.[31–34] Because of this lack of evidence, the national guidelines, including those of the American Thyroid Association and the National Comprehensive Cancer Network, recommend that radiation therapy be discussed in those who have gross residual disease that is unresectable, is not radioiodine avid, and is threatening vital structures among those patients with papillary, follicular, and Hurthle cell cancers.[35,36] They also recommend adjuvant radiation for those patients with medullary cancers who have gross extrathyroidal extension and a positive margin or have medium- to high-volume extranodal extension.[37] Radiation therapy can help decrease the risk of local recurrence and may improve survival; studies support the use of IMRT.[38] Because of the associated acute side effects, many providers are reluctant to refer their patients for radiation therapy and few centers have expertise in this setting.

Anaplastic thyroid cancer (ATC) represents a rare form of thyroid cancer that does require intensive treatments if found when still locally and regionally confined. Success with aggressive surgery, radiation therapy, and chemotherapy[39–41] has led to a recently completed RTOG trial evaluating paclitaxel and pazopanib with radiation therapy (RTOG 0912, NCT01236547). Early results were reported in abstract form at ESMO 2020 and demonstrated a 1-year overall survival rate of 37.1% (95% CI: 21.1% to 53.2%) in the pazopanib arm. We await the final report of this trial.[42] The American Thyroid Association published the guidelines for the management of ATC in 2012 and advocates for an aggressive approach for patients with stage IVA or IVB resectable and select stage IVB unresectable patients.[37] Again, IMRT is an important component of treatment for these patients and clinical experience is valuable. See Figure 6.2 for a case example.

Organs-at-Risk Contouring and Dose Constraints

Contouring the organs at risk (OARs) for H&N cancer patients can be very complicated and time consuming. Oftentimes, contouring as many as 41 or more OARs as well as 3 to 9 target volumes (GTV, CTV, and/or PTVs) is required. These GTVs and CTVs can be in close proximity to radiosensitive structures (e.g., spinal cord, brachial plexus, optic structures, and salivary glands), so great care must be taken in contouring and planning as these structures are likely adjacent to steep dose gradients. In some cases, a specified expansion is placed on these OARs to develop a planning organ-at-risk volume (PRV). CTV expansions do not include bone, air, or adjacent organs unless they are involved. Further, PTV expansions of 3 mm are utilized for patients undergoing cone beam CT (CBCT) scan for patient setup based on studies of our immobilization system[43] and 2 to 3 mm for Brainlab ExacTrac. There are excellent atlases as well as anatomy books that can help with contouring of the OARs[44–48] as well as targets.[21,25] However, there is now an international consensus guideline that hopes to help improve interobserver differences in OAR contouring for clinical practice and trials.[49] The current dose constraints that are utilized for H&N cancer planning at Mayo Clinic are outlined in Table 6.3.

Consistently contouring OARs, receiving non-negligible doses, that are involved in toxicities of primary concern in the treatment of H&N cancer (e.g., xerostomia, dysphagia, mucositis, esophagitis, dysgeusia, osteoradionecrosis, laryngeal edema, esophageal stenosis, brachial plexopathy, myelopathy, brain, and brain stem necrosis) is important for enabling systematic learning from historic data to refine toxicity models and improve care. These structures include parotid glands, submandibular glands, oral cavity, lips, pharyngeal constrictors, cricopharyngeal inlet, larynx, esophagus, brachial plexi, spinal cord,

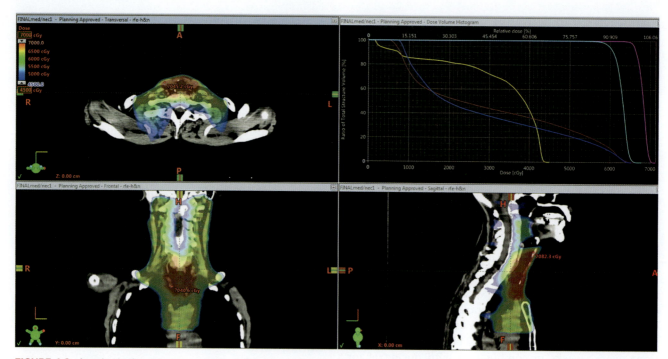

FIGURE 6.2. Anaplastic thyroid case example. A 60-year-old female presented with localized stage IVA (pT4 a N1 a M0) anaplastic thyroid carcinoma in 2012. At the time of her total thyroidectomy and central compartment node dissection, she was found to have anaplastic thyroid carcinoma arising from an encapsulated follicular variant of papillary thyroid carcinoma within the right lobe of her thyroid gland (3.4 × 2.8 × 2.5 cm mass). She had extrathyroidal extension as well as a focally positive margin. She had one out of two lymph nodes in the central compartment involved with anaplastic thyroid carcinoma. She had four right central neck compartment lymph nodes and one Delphian lymph node that were negative for carcinoma. She had no evidence of distant disease. She was then treated on RTOG 0912 with definitive radiation (6,600 and 5,940 cGy in 33 fractions delivered to her high- and low-risk regions, respectively). See the color wash figures in the axial, coronal, and sagittal planes. The DVH curves shown in the upper-right panel show the spinal cord (*yellow curve*) and right and left parotid glands (*blue and brown curves*, respectively). The patient has done well with no evidence of local-regional disease recurrence, but did develop biopsy-proven metastatic disease in her lungs and left lower extremity (adductor muscles, lymph nodes, and skin) in May 2014 which has been treated with stereotactic body radiation therapy, cryoablation, and surgery. Unfortunately, she later developed additional metastatic disease in the lungs, bone, and soft tissues and passed away in late 2016 but was NED in the head and neck region.

TABLE 6.3   Mayo Clinic Head and Neck Cancer Normal Tissue Dose Constraints for Standard Fractionation Adjuvant or Definitive Radiation Therapy

Structure	DVH End Point	Constraint Value	Planning Priority
Brain	Max [Gy]	<56 Gy	2
	V60 Gy [cc]	<1 cc	2
Brain stem	Max [Gy]	≤50 Gy	2
	V30 Gy [%]	<33%	2
Brain stem PRV	V54 Gy[cc]	<0.1 cc	2
Spinal cord	Max [Gy]	≤45 Gy	2
Cochlea	Mean [Gy]	≤35 Gy	2
External auditory canal	Mean [Gy]	<30 Gy	3
	V55 Gy [cc]	<0.03 cc	3
Mastoid	Mean [Gy]	<30 Gy	3
	V60 Gy [cc]	<0.1 cc	3
Semicircular canal	Mean [Gy]	<30 Gy	3
	V60 Gy [cc]	<0.1 cc	3
Eye	Mean [Gy]	≤20 Gy	2
	V50 Gy [cc]	<0.1 cc	2
	V40 Gy [%]	≤50%	2

TABLE 6.3 Mayo Clinic Head and Neck Cancer Normal Tissue Dose Constraints for Standard Fractionation Adjuvant or Definitive Radiation Therapy (*Continued*)

Structure	DVH End Point	Constraint Value	Planning Priority
Optic nerve	Max [Gy]	<50 Gy	2
	V54 Gy [cc]	<0.1 cc	1
Optic nerve PRV	Max [Gy]	<55 Gy	2
	V50 Gy [cc]	<0.1 cc	1
Optic chiasm	Max [Gy]	<50 Gy	2
	V54 Gy [cc]	<0.1 cc	1
Optic chiasm PRV	Max [Gy]	<55 Gy	2
	V55 Gy [cc]	<0.1 cc	1
Lacrimal gland	Max [Gy]	≤30 Gy	2
	Mean [Gy]	≤10 Gy	2
Lens	Max [Gy]	≤4 Gy	Report
Parotid gland	Mean [Gy]	<26 Gy	3
	V30 Gy [%]	≤50%	3
	V40 Gy [%]	<33%	3
Total parotid glands	Mean [Gy]	<39 Gy	3
Submandibular gland	Mean [Gy]	<39 Gy	3
Oral cavity	Mean [Gy]	≤40 Gy	3
	V30 Gy [%]	≤65%	3
	V35 Gy [%]	≤35%	3
Nasal cavity	Mean [Gy]	≤40 Gy	3
	V30 Gy [%]	≤65%	3
	V35 Gy [%]	≤35%	3
Lips	Max [Gy]	≤50 Gy	3
	Mean [Gy]	≤20 Gy	3
Mandible	Max [Gy]	<70 Gy	2
	V75 Gy [cc]	<1 cc	3
Pharyngeal constrictors and cricopharyngeal inlet	Mean [Gy]	≤50 Gy	2
	V55 Gy [%]	≤80%	2
	V65 Gy [%]	≤30%	2
Larynx (including supraglottis)	Max [Gy]	<60 Gy	2
	Mean [Gy]	≤35 Gy	2
	V50 Gy [%]	≤27%	2
Esophagus and cervical esophagus	Mean [Gy]	≤34 Gy	2
	V35 Gy [%]	≤50%	2
	V55 Gy [%]	≤40%	2
	V70 Gy [%]	≤20%	2
Brachial plexus	Max [Gy]	<63 Gy	2
Pituitary	Mean [Gy]		Report
Hypothalamus	Mean [Gy]		Report
Thyroid	Mean [Gy]		Report

PRV, planning organ-at-risk volume.

optic nerves and chiasm, brain, brain stem, retina, lacrimal glands, carotid arteries, cochlea, semicircular canals, lungs, mandible, lenses, pituitary gland, thyroid gland, external auditory canals, mastoid air cells, nasal cavity, and paranasal sinuses. For bilateral, parallel function structures (e.g., parotids, submandibular glands), both left and right structures should be contoured.

Dosimetric Considerations

Clearly defined nomenclature is critical to understanding dose constraints and goals of treatment planning. Dosimetrists understand that good plans are often a trade-off between target coverage and protection of normal structures. Figure 6.3 illustrates the nomenclature used in Tables 6.3 and 6.4 for defining the dose volume histogram (DVH) metrics. Planning priorities are requested where the physician requests a priority of 1, 2, 3, or "report" after careful contouring and discussion with the patient in terms of goals of therapy and the risks from the treatment. These priorities are designed to balance the doses to the targets and to the critical normal structures. Finally, a treatment plan is a combination of evaluation of the isodose curves and DVH metrics while taking into account target coverage and what was achievable for OARs. One can also "report" doses to structures that might not have strict or well-understood dose constraints like the thyroid gland, mastoids, or the semicircular canals. Finally, the entire plan should be reviewed to identify the location of "hot spots" and areas of target under coverage. For intensity-modulated proton plans, the commercial

physical dose calculation should be verified by a Monte Carlo physical dose calculation and discrepancies of ≥5% should be further evaluated. In addition, Monte Carlo linear energy transfer (LET) and radiobiologic equivalent (RBE) dose calculations are useful to identify the locations of high LET/RBE. Robust optimization should be utilized to account for daily translational setup variations of 3 to 5 mm and 3% range uncertainty. The normal tissue constraints utilized come from a combination of clinical experience, the Quantitative Analyses of Normal Tissue Effect in the Clinic (QUANTEC) supplement, and prior and ongoing RTOG studies.[50] See Table 6.3.

Table 6.4 describes the end point dictionary utilized for this clear nomenclature. Both absolute and relative values for dose and volume are used according to the issue addressed by the constraint. The nomenclature defines both input and output units. Output units are enclosed in square brackets. Limits on high doses are typically given a higher priority for the minimum dose to the hottest 0.03 cc subvolume of structure (D0.03 cc[Gy]) than for the maximum dose to any single pixel in the structure (Max[Gy]). Similarly, keeping a subvolume of a structure less than 0.1 cc receiving 54 Gy or more, for example in the optic nerve (V54 Gy <0.1 cc), is also more valuable than the Max[Gy] dose. In addition to monitoring volumes receiving a specified dose or more (e.g., PTV:V95%[%], percentage of PTV receiving 95% of the prescribed dose or more), we track the volume of target that is underdosed. For example, CTV:CV95%[cc] is the absolute volume of CTV that received 95% of the prescribed dose or less.

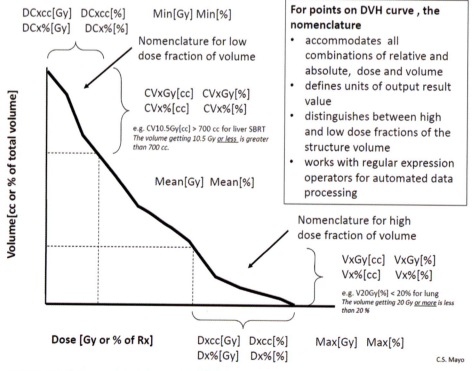

FIGURE 6.3. Dose versus volume nomenclature.

TABLE 6.4	End Point Dictionary
End Point Type	**Description**
Max [Gy]	Maximum dose in Gy.
Max [%]	Maximum dose as a percentage of the prescribed dose.
Min [Gy]	Minimum dose in Gy.
Min [%]	Minimum dose as a percentage of the prescribed dose.
Mean [Gy]	Mean dose in Gy.
Mean [%]	Mean dose as a percentage of the prescribed dose.
D{x1}cc[Gy]	{x1} cc of the volume received this dose or more. Dose expressed in Gy.
D{x1}cc[%]	{x1} cc of the volume received this dose or more. Dose expressed as a percentage of the prescribed dose.
D{x1}%[Gy]	{x1}% of the structure volume received this dose or more. Dose expressed in Gy.
D{x1}%[%]	{x1}% of the structure volume received this dose or more. Dose expressed as a percentage of the prescribed dose.
DC{x1}cc[Gy]	{x1} cc of the volume received this dose or less. Dose expressed in Gy.
DC{x1}cc[%]	{x1} cc of the volume received this dose or less. Dose expressed as a percentage of the prescribed dose.
DC{x1}%[%]	{x1}% of the structure volume received this dose or less. Dose expressed as a percentage of the prescribed dose.
DC{x1}%[Gy]	{x1}% of the structure volume received this dose or less. Dose expressed in Gy.
V{x1}Gy [cc]	The volume receiving {x1} Gy or more. Volume expressed in cc.
V{x1}Gy [%]	The volume receiving {x1} Gy or more. Volume expressed as a percentage of structure volume.
V{x1}%[cc]	The volume receiving {x1}% of the prescribed dose or more. Volume expressed in cc.
V{x1}% [%]	The volume receiving {x1}% of the prescribed dose or more. Volume expressed as a percentage of structure volume.
Volume [cc]	Volume of a structure in cc.
CV {x1}%[%]	The volume receiving {x1}% of the prescribed dose or less. Volume expressed as a percentage of the structure volume.
CV {x1}Gy[cc]	The volume receiving {x1} Gy or less. Volume expressed in cc.
CV {x1}%[cc]	The volume receiving {x1}% of the prescribed dose or less. Volume expressed in cc.
CV {x1}Gy[%]	The volume receiving {x1} Gy or less. Volume expressed as a percentage of the structure volume.
DHI [%]	Relative to the mean, the dose range encompassing 95% of the structure. 100*(D2.5%[Gy]–D97.5[Gy]/Mean[Gy]).

DHI, dose heterogeneity index.

Physics Challenges

Treatment planning is a negotiation with what is possible. It is typically not possible to meet all constraints for target coverage and for normal tissue sparing, since these structures are often adjacent or overlapping. Planning optimization can be made more efficient, quickly achieving treatment plans that reflect overall planning objectives, through the use of dose-sculpting structures in addition to constraints on normal and target tissues alone.

For targets, a planning volume or "IMRT_PTV" is created for each PTV dose level (e.g., IMRT_PTV5400, IMRT_PTV6300, IMRT_PTV7000) to reflect physician preferences for dose compromises to coverage of the PTV to spare OARs. Each volume is cropped away from the body surface by 3 mm to reduce skin dose. High-dose volumes are subtracted out of lower-dose volumes with a 1-mm margin.

A dose-limiting annulus (DLA) is created for each IMRT_PTV to use in the optimizer to drive the prescribed isodoses to conform to the PTV. Figure 6.4 illustrates the creation of DLAs, as 1- to 2-cm-thick shells around their respective IMRT_PTV with 1-mm gap. If an IMRT_PTV structure overlaps normal structures that are to be spared with a higher priority than the target (e.g., brain stem, optic nerve, or brachial plexus), then it should be subdivided into two parts that do and do not overlap the high priority OAR. A 1- to 3-mm margin is used to crop the non-overlapping portion of the IMRT_PTV out of the OAR. The overlapping portion is constructed as a Boolean subtraction of the non-overlapping portion from the IMRT_PTV. During optimization, this provides the spatial specificity needed to enable differentially driving doses to reflect physician objectives for the overlapping versus non-overlapping portions of the target volume.

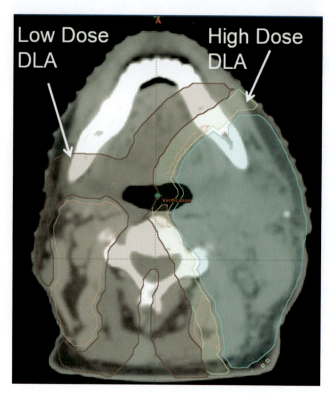

FIGURE 6.4. High- and low-dose limiting annulus (DLA).

of the disease region while remaining within the 22 cm constraint. For the first two arcs, the multi-leaf collimator leaves travel along the X-axis in the transverse planes. In the third arc, they travel in the superior/inferior direction. This third arc is valuable, providing a nearly orthogonal set of multi-leaf collimator leaf trajectories, compared to the ±30-degree pair, for the optimizer to use in dose delivery. Gantry rotation direction, that is, clockwise versus counter clockwise, should be alternated between the arcs to make most efficient use of delivery time.

For complex cases where there is substantial extension into the supraclavicular region, multiple prescribed dose levels, and high-dose gradients, it may be advantageous to add a 4th arc, also at 85 degrees, to fully span the superior–inferior extension of the disease. In this case, jaws should be set so that coverage in the superior/inferior direction should be split between the 3rd and 4th arcs with a 2-cm overlap enabling the optimizer to feather dose between the 3rd and 4th arcs.

Some treatment planning systems allow specification of the curve characterizing the fall off of the dose as you move away from the PTVs (e.g., a normal tissue objective). Setting unrealistically high priorities for these types of constraints or specifying unrealistically steep fall off can produce unintended consequences such as overly "soft" shoulders on PTV DVHs compromising coverage, dose bulging out in unexpected regions. When troubleshooting is hard to explain problems in dose distributions, check that overly aggressive parametrization of these types of constraints is not contributing.

Undesirable "hot" spots can be created in PTVs when the constraints on abutting OAR volumes are overly aggressive. Dose is like a balloon; when it is squeezed in one place, it tends to bulge out in another. When troubleshooting hot spots, be mindful of constraints on nearby OARs.

Buffer structures are created around critical normal structures to control dose gradients. Figure 6.5 illustrates a buffer around the spinal cord and brain stem. The beam arrangement includes three VMAT arc beams. Collimator angles are ±30 degrees for the first two arcs and 85 degrees with X jaws ≤22 cm. Jaws for the 85-degree collimator angle arc should be set to extend from the most inferior portion of the supraclavicular toward the superior extent

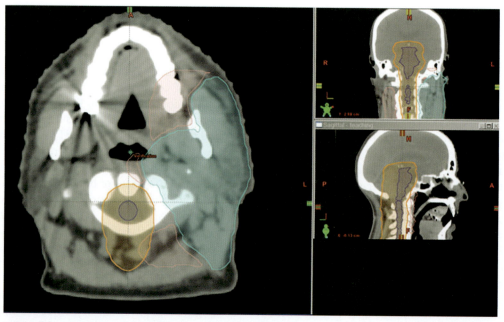

FIGURE 6.5. Cord/brain stem buffer.

During optimization, the following points need to be borne in mind:

- Maximum and minimum doses are set on IMRT PTVs; PTVs are used for plan evaluation only.
- Maximum doses are set on DLAs corresponding to IMRT_PTV minimum doses, to drive conformality.
- Use the OAR subdivided IMRT_PTV structures, with differential optimization constraints, to shape spatial compromises in coverage needed to spare high-priority OARs. Set maximum dose to cord ~4,000 cGy as needed. During optimization, push down volume at a matching dose (e.g., V40 Gy[%] in buffer to soften the dose gradient near the cord and push the 4,000 cGy line away from the cord/brain stem).
- Push low- and intermediate-dose levels to reduce mean parotid doses.
- Push low- and intermediate-dose levels to reduce mean submandibular gland doses.
- Push high- and intermediate-dose levels in brain down.
- Push low- and intermediate-dose levels on larynx to reduce the mean dose.
- Push high- and intermediate-dose levels in esophagus and superior and inferior constrictors down.
- Monitor DVH prescription constraints and add other constraints as needed.
- Be mindful of the potential of overly aggressive constraints (i.e., pushing for physically unrealistic dose distributions) to create dose heterogeneity or coverage issues.
- Where control of dose in specific spatial regions is an objective (e.g., controlling high doses in the nape of the neck), creating dose-sculpting structures that can be constrained in the optimizer is the most direct approach.

Figure 6.6 illustrates a dose distribution resulting from the use of this approach. The dose distribution shows the 7,000 cGy (yellow isodose line) covering the PTV_7000 while the 5,940 cGy (blue isodose line) covers the PTV_5940.

Treatment plans are typically produced within 1 to 2 hours by skilled planners. With the advent of writable scripting in treatment-planning systems, viable clinical treatment plans can be created with automation in minutes.[51–53] This approach is promising in the future for standardizing the baseline plan quality. It also has promise as a means to expand the number of individuals available to participate in initial planning, with efforts of highly skilled planners used to advantage on refinements.

Prior to treatment, the plans are delivered to a phantom (or other devices) to ensure the accurate delivery of the plan to a patient.

IMRT quality assurance (QA) measurements are carried out for each plan prior to treatment, to demonstrate that the system produces the expected absolute dose and dose distribution within acceptable limits. There are a broad range of devices used in clinical practice to carry out

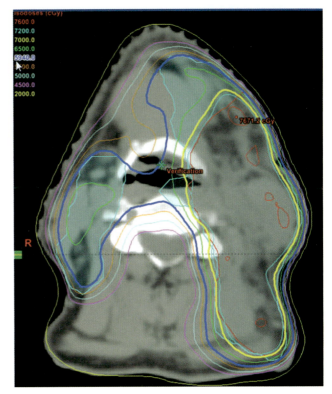

FIGURE 6.6. Dose distribution.

IMRT QA. Typically, the dose distribution is measured in one or more flat planes or in a curved plane embedded in a phantom. Typically, measurements are carried out with the beams irradiating the array at the treatment angles or a single angle. Measured doses are compared to doses predicted by the treatment-planning system for the measurement plane, examining dose profiles, the fraction of measurement points passing a gamma test, or both. Measurement devices typically use diode or ionization chamber arrays and radiochromic or radiographic films. Some devices additionally use a single-point ionization chamber for assessment of absolute dose. For planar devices, the user may select a measurement plane that specifically checks dose gradients near to critical structures, for example, a sagittal plane to check regions near the cord, brain stem, and larynx.

IMRT and VMAT utilize dynamic modification of several parameters (multileaf collimator, collimator, dose rate, gantry angle, etc.) during irradiation. Disagreement of measured and predicted doses may result from improper behavior of these components. In addition, other factors contribute to disagreement. Positioning errors (1–2 mm) are common. In addition, steep dose gradients perpendicular to the measurement planes can result in substantial differences in measured dose as a result of small (≤1 mm) errors in positioning of the device with respect to the gradient.

Response of measurement devices may vary with angle of irradiation. If the couch is not included in the verification plan, then attenuation may result in systematic errors. Calibration of the devices may vary over time. Random, spatially varying errors in the dose response of the detector range from 0.5% to 5%, depending on the type of detector used.

Treatment Delivery Including IGRT and ART

The delivery of radiation therapy is a key component to successful treatment. A plan has to do more than "look good on paper"; it must be deliverable. If a patient is unable to lay still due to a difficult setup or an uncomfortable immobilization device, the treatment might not be successful. Great care is taken in simulation for this reason. Our institutional practice for H&N cancer is to perform two simulations. At the first simulation, the 3- or 5-point thermoplastic mask (ORFIT Industries, Jericho, NY) with a bite block (Precise Bite, CIVCO Medical Solutions, Coralville, IA), mandibular fluoride carrier, or maxillary and mandibular fluoride carriers, oral sponges, adjustable oral stent with or without tongue depressor (TruGuard, Bionix), and/or customized oral stents, as appropriate, is fabricated. The oral stents are mandatory for nasal cavity, paranasal sinus, and oral cavity cancers to lower the dose to a large volume of the oral cavity. The oral stents are also helpful in patients with tongue base cancer to separate the soft palate from the tongue base. A standard H&N rest is customized using a Klarity mold (Klarity Medical Products, Newark, OH) with shims under the Klarity mold to allow for shrinking of the thermoplastic mask. The arms are at the patient sides with the hands holding a ring over the abdomen or holding indexable hand grips on the sides of the treatment table. The patient then returns after a minimum of 2 hours of mask cooling and drying for the CT simulation, which may be done with IV contrast. This allows the mask to cure and more closely replicates setting the patient up for treatment each day. The shims are removed from under the Klarity mold for the CT imaging. This has minimized our need for re-simulation due to patient factors like the mask feeling too tight or the interfraction flexion of the head, neck, and shoulders changing from simulation to treatment. To avoid dose errors and enhanced skin dose resulting from scatter, immobilization devices should be minimally attenuating, and not introduce significant dose errors if the immobilization system is mistakenly omitted from the treatment plan. The delivery of radiation therapy is image guided, as discussed in the following. We do not routinely utilize ART but do consider it on a case-by-case basis, as discussed in the following.

Image guided radiation therapy (IGRT) is an evolving area due to improved computing capabilities and advances in technology. For example, CBCTs can be obtained in treatment position on the linear accelerator and matched to the simulation CT using a 6-degrees-of-freedom (6-DOF) robotic treatment couch in just 1 to 2 minutes. Our institutional experience has shown this to be more accurate than 3-DOF and has been rapidly adopted as our standard.[43] We continue to use Brainlab ExacTrac (BrainLab, Feldkirchen, Germany) for small-field skull base cases. On-board daily imaging (OBI) is also a quite reasonable approach for aligning the bony anatomy; but very little soft tissue anatomy can be visualized and/or utilized. For large fields, we perform OBI to align the patient prior to CBCTs. Surface mapping is also helpful for initial positioning and detecting movement during treatment. If tumor size or shape changes or other systematic changes occur (weight loss or change in size, shape, and/or location of OARs), then no IGRT technique can adjust for this and one might need to adapt or change the original treatment plan. We counsel patients not to swallow during the simulation CT scan and while the beam is on during treatment.

Adaptative radiation therapy (ART) is evolving into its own field as well. If the patient has had significant tumor shrinkage or weight loss, the original plan may no longer be covering the intended treatment volume.[54] Alternatively, the OARs might be receiving more dose than intended. For example, it has been described that the parotid can shift medially into the high-dose volumes and receive more dose than intended, which would abolish the primary reason for IMRT.[55] Knowing when and how to replan a patient is still an area of active research and no standard has been developed for IMRT or IMPT.[56] How to accumulate the doses across the targets and OARs is a challenge. We often do not know when the volume change occurred. We do not precisely know how much dose the target or OARs have received. We do not know if it will make a clinically meaningful difference in outcomes to replan.[57,58] How this time- and labor-intensive replanning can be incorporated into a safe, efficient, and cost-effective workflow is yet to be determined. Adaptations made in the first weeks of treatment are likely to be more beneficial than adaptations made during the final weeks of treatment. Many questions remain to be answered. The radiation oncology community is poised to answer these questions to improve the outcomes of radiation therapy.

NOVEL RADIATION THERAPY AND THE FUTURE OF H&N CANCER TREATMENTS

Over the past two decades, charged particle radiation therapy has become an accepted and, some would argue, preferred treatment for appropriately selected H&N cancers. This has been made possible by the advent of intensity-modulated pencil beam spot scanning proton and carbon ion radiation therapy, and thereby intensity-modulated charged particle therapy (IMCPT). IMPT, in particular multi-field optimized (MFO) IMPT, allows the sculpting of the radiation dose around critical

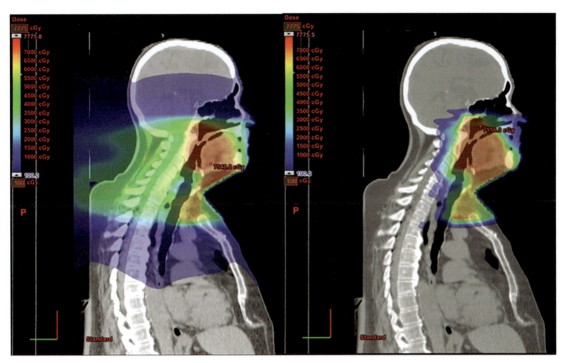

FIGURE 6.7. Comparison of IMRT (**left**) and IMPT (**right**) 7,000 cGy (RBE) plan for a definitive bilateral H&N cancer patient. Note the distinct difference in the doses below 5,000 cGy (RBE).

structures near the target area and good conformality to the target.[59] Figure 6.7 compares an IMRT plan to an MFO-IMPT plan for a H&N cancer treated primarily with radiation therapy including bilateral cervical lymph nodes. The conformality of the 7,000 cGy(RBE) dose level to the target is very similar, but there is a distinct difference in the doses below 5,000 cGy(RBE), with a clear advantage to the proton plan.

The advantage of proton therapy, and in particular MFO-IMPT, does not come without a cost. There are five key points that are of particular importance in H&N IMPT. First is the robustness of the plan to positional and range errors. In conventional IMRT planning, a PTV structure is created by adding an appropriate margin to the CTV. The dose to the PTV is, in general, an adequate surrogate of the CTV when positional uncertainties are considered. In proton therapy, the PTV concept no longer holds and this is especially true for H&N cancer treatments due to the large anatomical heterogeneities, that is, many bone–air-tissue interfaces. Some institutions have therefore dropped the PTV nomenclature and instead use optimization target volumes (OTVs) and *directly* evaluate the CTV (and critical structures) under positional (3–5 mm) errors and range uncertainty (3%). It is possible that two IMPT plans give very similar dose distributions, but under robustness conditions, one plan is severely degraded while the other only has minor perturbations. When evaluating robustness, it is important that the CTV does not encompass an air cavity as it is difficult to robustly cover air. For image guidance, we use a combination of surface mapping, in-room CT on

rails, and 6 DoF kV:kV matching matched to 2–3 mm in the head and cervical spine and 5 mm in the shoulders and clavicles.

They second key point is anatomical changes during the course of therapy. It is important for treating H&N cancer patients with IMPT to obtain a weekly CT scan in the treatment position and recast the plan on the new CT. We use an in-room CT on rails to obtain diagnostic quality images for treatment planning with the patient on the treatment table in the treatment position.[56] Not only would target coverage be compromised if the volumes change, but a critical structure that was previously being spared may now be receiving very high doses. These changes may have been insignificant in a more robust IMRT plan but have the potential to be devastating in the proton setting. Third is the quality of the dose calculation. Monte Carlo calculations are important in H&N treatments as there are many air–bone and air–tissue interfaces that are not well handled by analytical calculations.[60,61] A fourth consideration is the potential of an increased RBE at the end of range for the protons. This enhanced RBE may lead to unwanted hot spots and potential adverse effects.[62,63] The last key point is to understand the limitations of the treatment table and immobilization system that are being used and properly work around those limitations. For example, how does the neck flexion and neck skin folds change on a daily basis, are the shoulders in a reproducible position, or does the chin/mandible position change throughout the course of treatment. How will the treatment table and immobilization system perturb the proton beam or limit the available beam angle options? Minimizing these issues is the first step, but field arrangements can also be chosen that would reduce the impact of these uncertainties.

Finally, in this era of targeted agents and immunotherapies, the future of H&N cancer treatments is bright. Cetuximab added to radiation therapy was an initial success.[64] We await the results of RTOG 1216, which is adding docetaxel to cetuximab as one of the treatment arms. HPV-related malignancies likely have a better prognosis in never smokers and the different molecular mechanisms that underlie this difference could be further exploited. Similarly, the non-HPV-related malignancies might also have different molecular signatures that could be targeted.[65,66] Various immunotherapies are being explored for H&N cancers, including the following: monoclonal antibody therapies, cytokine therapies, cancer vaccines, adoptive T-cell immunotherapies, and immunologic targeting of stem cells.[46] Continued understanding and exploration of these molecular mechanisms and immune responses will play a crucial role in the future of H&N cancer radiation therapy.

ACKNOWLEDGMENTS

We would like to acknowledge Marlene Huston for assistance with manuscript preparation.

KEY POINTS

- H&N cancer represents a diverse collection of tumor sites and histologies. In addition to a highly functional multidisciplinary team, mastery of anatomy, patterns of spread, and tumor recurrence are needed to optimize patient outcomes.

- The main risk factor for H&N cancer remains current or past tobacco use; however, the incidence of HPV-related oropharynx cancer is increasing.

- Several studies have demonstrated markedly higher control rates for HPV-related oropharynx H&N cancers compared to HPV negative.

- The majority of patients with H&N cancer are treated with IMRT with VMAT technologies. IMPT is emerging as another means of further reducing long-term complications from radiotherapy.

- Radiation treatment volume delineation including the primary site and the appropriate nodal volumes varies per the primary site and the risk of nodal involvement.

- Postoperative chemotherapy is generally added to adjuvant radiation therapy for patients who have undergone surgery and have positive margins and/or extracapsular extension. Ideally, the entire package of treatment from surgery to completion of radiation therapy is delivered within 11 weeks.

- Radiation therapy can help decrease the risk of local recurrence and may improve survival in select thyroid cancer patients with gross residual disease and/or high nodal burden.

- Contouring the many H&N organs at risk (OARs) can be very time consuming and international consensus guidelines can help guide this effort.

- Clear nomenclature and definitions of dosimetric dose constraints are essential when negotiating what is possible for an individual treatment plan. Physicians, physicists, and dosimetrists work together to accomplish the best treatment plan possible for a patient.

- A variety of dose-limiting annuli and buffer structures are created to optimize IMRT plans.

- Daily IGRT is an essential component of successful therapy and begins with an optimal and individualized simulation with appropriate intra-oral devices, thermoplastic masks, and neck rests for comfortable immobilization. Tools for daily imaging include the following: surface mapping, kV CBCTs, in-room CT on rails, 6DoF kV-kV, orthogonal kV-kV, and/or ExacTrac.

- Adaptive radiotherapy is a rapidly evolving area that will help individualize treatments for patients who have changes in external contours and/or changes in size and shape of the gross disease and position of OARs due to rapid tumor shrinkage, weight loss, and/or positional changes.

- Proton therapy, in particular IMPT, is a complex endeavor and requires ongoing and intensive physician, physics, and dosimetric resources and support.

- Understanding and exploring molecular mechanisms and immune responses will play a crucial role in the future of H&N cancer radiation therapy.

REVIEW QUESTIONS

1. According to SEER (The Surveillance, Epidemiology, and Ends Results) data, the incidence of which type of H&N cancer is increasing when comparing a 1970 cohort to a 2000 cohort of patients?
   A. Larynx cancer
   B. HPV-related oropharyngeal cancer
   C. Oral cavity cancer
   D. Hypopharynx cancer

2. Which of the following is the most appropriate adjustment of CTV expansion in a 46-year-old never-smoking male with an HPV-related base of tongue cancer, given the favorable prognosis?
   A. Decrease
   B. None
   C. Increase

3. A patient presents with a large HPV-negative T3 N2a M0 tonsil squamous cell. The treating physician elects to utilize the consensus 5 + 5 mm expansions of the primary tumor for the high-dose and intermediate-dose CTVs, respectively. This is most appropriate for which of the following additional clinical scenarios (pick one)?
   A. The patient has had induction chemotherapy and the primary tumor has decreased by greater than 50% in volume.
   B. The patient will be embarking on definitive concurrent chemotherapy with radiation therapy.
   C. The patient has had prior cancer and this is actually a large recurrence.

4. Which of the following volumes is not used in proton beam therapy treatment planning?
   A. GTV
   B. CTV
   C. PTV
   D. OTV

5. What is the best time to perform a verification simulation on a patient receiving IMPT and chemotherapy for a cT4 N2c M0 HPV-mediated squamous cell carcinoma of the tonsil?
   A. Prior to the first treatment
   B. The day of the first treatment
   C. Between the first and third weeks of treatment
   D. Only if the patient loses weight or when significant changes in tumor volume are noted

ANSWERS

1. B   The incidence of HPV-related oropharyngeal cancers is increasing. This is particularly true in younger males. Studies have also shown that never smokers or light smokers have a better prognosis. Studies are being conducted to try to minimize treatment intensity and/or treatment volumes. The hope is that this will lead to fewer long-term complications while maintaining excellent tumor-related outcomes in this subgroup of patients.[1,29]

2. B   There are ongoing studies looking at various aspects of dose de-escalation to reduce toxicity but none are decreasing the margins.

3. B   5 + 5 mm high- and intermediate-dose CTVs are not utilized for patients who have had induction chemotherapy or have recurrent tumors. One might consider larger intermediate- and/or high-dose CTV expansions and might consider treating the pre-induction chemotherapy volumes to an intermediate dose and treating the remaining tumor to a higher dose. This remains controversial and is under investigation. In patients who have had prior treatment (surgery or radiation) and have recurrent disease, the areas of subclinical spread might not be the same as in a de-novo case. Again, caution when outlining tumor volumes by the treating physician is necessary.

4. C   PTV is not used in proton beam therapy treatment planning due to range uncertainties and beam path tissue inhomogeneity.[68]

5. C   The best time to perform verification CT simulations to check for changes in dose to the primary or the OARs changes is early in the course of a treatment. A modified plan can then be implemented. At Mayo Clinic, we perform weekly verification CT simulations. MD Anderson investigators have found the third week of treatment to be a crucial time for replanning cases. Waiting for weight loss or tumor shrinkage might be too late. Performing verifications prior to starting IMPT is also rare unless the patient reports a significant change (e.g., loss of postoperative edema, change in weight, or tumor progression) in a week or two from simulation to treatment.[56,59]

REFERENCES

1. Siegel RL, Miller KD, Jemal A. Cancer statistics, 2020. *CA Cancer J Clin.* 2020;70(1):7–30.
2. Siegel RL, Miller KD, Jemal A. Cancer statistics, 2015. *CA Cancer J Clin.* 2015;65(1):5–29.
3. Patel AS, Qureshi MM, Dyer MA, et al. Comparing surgical and nonsurgical larynx-preserving treatments with total laryngectomy for locally advanced laryngeal cancer. *Cancer.* 2019; 125:3367–3377.
4. Multidisciplinary Larynx Cancer Working Group, Mulcahy CF, Mohamed AS, Kanwar A, et al. Age-adjusted comorbidity and survival in locally advanced laryngeal cancer. *Head Neck.* 2018;40(9):2060–2069.
5. Kobic A, Lester SC, Kreofsky CR, et al. The impact of total laryngectomy on non-oncologic causes of death in patients treated with radiation therapy for larynx and hypopharynx cancer. *Int J Radiat Oncol Biol Phys.* 2017;99(2S):S121.
6. Scoccianti C, Cecchini M, Anderson AS, et al. European Code against Cancer 4th Edition: alcohol drinking and cancer. *Cancer Epidemiol.* 2015;39:S67–S74.
7. Garces Y, Offord KP, Croghan IT, et al. Tobacco use among radiation oncology outpatients (Abstract 1027). Paper presented at: American Society of Clinical Oncology 2004 July 15. *J Clin Oncol.* 2004;22:14S.
8. Prokhorov AV, Hudmon KS, Marani S, et al. Engaging physicians and pharmacists in providing smoking cessation counseling. *Arch Intern Med.* 2010;170(18):1640–1646.
9. Fiore MC, Jaen CR, Baker TB, et al. Treating Tobacco Use and Dependence: 2008 Update. Clinical Practice Guideline. Rockville, MD: U.S. Department of Health and Human Services Public Health Service May 2008; 2008.
10. Khuri FR, Lee JJ, Lippman SM, et al. Randomized phase III trial of low-dose isotretinoin for prevention of second primary tumors in stage I and II head and neck cancer patients. *J Natl Cancer Inst.* 2006;98(7):441–450.
11. Gillison ML, Koch WM, Capone RB, et al. Evidence for a causal association between human papillomavirus and a subset of head and neck cancers. *J Natl Cancer Inst.* 2000;92(9):709–720.
12. Chaturvedi AK, Anderson WF, Lortet-Tieulent J, et al. Worldwide trends in incidence rates for oral cavity and oropharyngeal cancers. *J Clin Oncol.* 2013;31(36):4550–4559.
13. Gillison ML, Broutian T, Pickard RK, et al. Prevalence of oral HPV infection in the United States, 2009–2010. *JAMA.* 2012; 307(7):693–703.
14. Ang KK, Harris J, Wheeler R, et al. Human papillomavirus and survival of patients with oropharyngeal cancer. *N Engl J Med.* 2010;363(1):24–35.
15. Chera BS, Amdur RJ, Morris CG, et al. T1N0 to T2N0 squamous cell carcinoma of the glottic larynx treated with definitive radiotherapy. *Int J Radiat Oncol Biol Phys.* 2010;78(2):461–466.
16. Trotti A, 3rd, Zhang Q, Bentzen SM, et al. Randomized trial of hyperfractionation versus conventional fractionation in T2 squamous cell carcinoma of the vocal cord (RTOG 9512). *Int J Radiat Oncol Biol Phys.* 2014;89(5):958–963.
17. Gomez D, Cahlon O, Mechalakos J, et al. An investigation of intensity-modulated radiation therapy versus conventional two-dimensional and 3D-conformal radiation therapy for early stage larynx cancer. *Radiat Oncol.* 2010;5:74.
18. Zumsteg ZS, Riaz N, Jaffery S, et al. Carotid sparing intensity-modulated radiation therapy achieves comparable locoregional control to conventional radiotherapy in T1–2N0 laryngeal carcinoma. *Oral Oncol.* 2015;51(7):716–723.
19. Schwartz DL, Sosa A, Chun S, et al. SBRT for early-stage glottis larynx cancer: initial clinical outcomes from a phase I clinical trial. *PLoS ONE.* 2017;12(3):1–10.
20. Ratko TA, Douglas GW, de Souza JA, et al. Radiotherapy treatments for head and neck cancer update. Comparative Effectiveness Review No. 144. (Prepared by Blue Cross and Blue Shield Association Evidence-based Practice Center under Contract No. 290–2007–10058.) AHRQ Publication No. 15-EHC001-EF. Rockville, MD: Agency for Healthcare Research and Quality; 2014. http://www.effectivehealthcare.ahrq.gov/reports/final.cfm. Accessed July, 2015.
21. Eisbruch A, Foote RL, O'Sullivan B, et al. Intensity-modulated radiation therapy for head and neck cancer: emphasis on the selection and delineation of the targets. *Semin Radiat Oncol.* 2002;12(3):238–249.
22. Clifford Chao KS, Tony W, Tim M. *Practical Essentials of Intensity Modulated Radiation Therapy.* 3rd ed. Philadelphia, PA: Lippincott Williams & Wilkins; 2013.
23. Gregoire V, Evans M, Le Q, et al. Delineation of the primary tumor clinical target volumes (CTV-P) in laryngeal, hypopharyngeal, oropharyngeal and oral cavity squamous cell carcinoma: AIRO, CAC, DAHANCA, EORTC, GEORCC, GORTEC, HKNPCSG, HNCIG, IAG-KHT, LPRHHT, NCIC CTG, NCRI, NRG Oncology, PHNS, SBRT, SOMERA, SRO, SSHNO, TROG consensus guidelines. *Radiother Oncol.* 2018;126:3–24.
24. Lee AW, Ng WT, Pan JJ, et al. International guideline for the delineation of the clinical target volumes (CTV) for nasopharyngeal carcinoma. *Radiother Oncol.* 2018;126(1):25–36.
25. Gregoire V, Ang K, Budach W, et al. Delineation of the neck node levels for head and neck tumors: a 2013 update. DAHANCA, EORTC, HKNPCSG, NCIC CTG, NCRI, RTOG, TROG consensus guidelines. *Radiother Oncol.* 2014;110(1):172–181.
26. Biau J, Lapeyre M, Troussier I, et al. Selection of lymph node target volumes for definitive head and neck radiation therapy: a 2019 Update. *Radiother Oncol.* 2019;134:1–9.
27. Bernier J, Cooper JS, Pajak TF, et al. Defining risk levels in locally advanced head and neck cancers: a comparative analysis of concurrent postoperative radiation plus chemotherapy trials of the EORTC (#22931) and RTOG (# 9501). *Head Neck.* 2005;27(10):843–850.
28. Swisher-McClure S, Lukens JN, Aggarwal C, et al. A phase 2 trial of Alternative Volumes of Oropharyngeal Irradiation for De-intensification (AVOID): omission of the resected primary tumor bed after transoral robotic surgery for human papilloma virus-related squamous cell carcinoma of the oropharynx. *Int J Radiat Oncol Biol Phys.* 2020;106(4):725–732.
29. Ang KK, Trotti A, Brown BW, et al. Randomized trial addressing risk features and time factors of surgery plus radiotherapy in advanced head-and-neck cancer. *Int J Radiat Oncol Biol Phys.* 2001;51(3):571–578.
30. Contrares JA, Spencer C, DeWees T, et al. Eliminating postoperative radiation to the pathologically node-negative neck: long-term results of a prospective phase II study. *J Clin Oncol.* 2019;37:2548–2555.
31. Meadows KM, Amdur RJ, Morris CG, et al. External beam radiotherapy for differentiated thyroid cancer. *Am J Otolaryngol.* 2006;27(1):24–28.
32. Schwartz DL, Lobo MJ, Ang KK, et al. Postoperative external beam radiotherapy for differentiated thyroid cancer: outcomes and morbidity with conformal treatment. *Int J Radiat Oncol Biol Phys.* 2009;74(4):1083–1091.
33. Beckham TH, Romesser PB, Groen AH, et al. Intensity-modulated radiation therapy with or without concurrent chemotherapy in nonanaplastic thyroid cancer with unresectable or gross residual disease. *Thyroid.* 2018;28(9):1180–1189.
34. Terezakis SA, Lee KS, Ghossein RA, et al. Role of external beam radiotherapy in patients with advanced or recurrent nonanaplastic thyroid cancer: Memorial Sloan-kettering Cancer Center experience. *Int J Radiat Oncol Biol Phys.* 2009;73(3):795–801.
35. Smallridge RC, Ain KB, Asa SL, et al. American Thyroid Association guidelines for management of patients with anaplastic thyroid cancer. *Thyroid.* 2012;22(11):1104–1139.
36. NCCN. Clinical Practice Guidelines in Oncology: Thyroid Carcinoma, Version 1.2015. http://www.nccn.org/professionals/physician_gls/pdf/thyroid.pdf. 2015.
37. Wells SA Jr, Asa SL, Dralle H, et al. Revised American Thyroid Association guidelines for the management of medullary thyroid carcinoma. *Thyroid.* 2015;25(6):567–610.
38. Urbano TG, Clark CH, Hansen VN, et al. Intensity modulated radiotherapy (IMRT) in locally advanced thyroid cancer: acute toxicity results of a phase I study. *Radiother Oncol.* 2007;85(1): 58–63.

39. Foote RL, Molina JR, Kasperbauer JL, et al. Enhanced survival in locoregionally confined anaplastic thyroid carcinoma: a single-institution experience using aggressive multimodal therapy. *Thyroid.* 2011;21(1):25–30.

40. Chen J, Tward JD, Shrieve DC, et al. Surgery and radiotherapy improves survival in patients with anaplastic thyroid carcinoma: analysis of the surveillance, epidemiology, and end results 1983–2002. *Am J Clin Oncol.* 2008;31(5):460–464.

41. Isham CR, Bossou AR, Negron V, et al. Pazopanib enhances paclitaxel-induced mitotic catastrophe in anaplastic thyroid cancer. *Sci Transl Med.* 2013;5(166):166ra163.

42. Sherman EJ, Harris J, Bible KC, et al. Randomized phase II study of radiation therapy and paclitaxel with pazopanib or placebo: NRG-RTOG 0912. *Ann Oncol.* 2020;31(4):S1085.

43. Courneyea L, Mullins J, Howard M, et al. Positioning reproducibility with and without rotational corrections for 2 head and neck immobilization systems. *Pract Radiat Oncol.* 2015;5(6):e575–e581.

44. Christianen ME, Langendijk JA, Westerlaan HE, et al. Delineation of organs at risk involved in swallowing for radiotherapy treatment planning. *Radiother Oncol.* 2011;101(3):394–402.

45. Hall WH, Guiou M, Lee NY, et al. Development and validation of a standardized method for contouring the brachial plexus: preliminary dosimetric analysis among patients treated with IMRT for head-and-neck cancer. *Int J Radiat Oncol Biol Phys.* 2008;72(5):1362–1367.

46. Yi SK, Hall WH, Mathai M, et al. Validating the RTOG-endorsed brachial plexus contouring atlas: an evaluation of reproducibility among patients treated by intensity-modulated radiotherapy for head-and-neck cancer. *Int J Radiat Oncol Biol Phys.* 2012;82(3):1060–1064.

47. van de Water TA, Bijl HP, Westerlaan HE, et al. Delineation guidelines for organs at risk involved in radiation-induced salivary dysfunction and xerostomia. *Radiother Oncol.* 2009;93(3):545–552.

48. Macdonald ME. *Diagnostic and Surgical Imaging Anatomy, Brain, Head and Neck, and Spine.* 2nd ed. Salt Lake City, UT: Amirsys; 2009.

49. Brouwer CL, Steenbakkers RJ, Bourhis J, et al. CT-based delineation of organs at risk in head and neck region: DAHANCA, EORTC, GORTEC, HKNPCSG, NCIC CTG, NCRI, NRG Oncology and TROG consensus guidelines. *Radiother Oncol.* 2015;117:83–90.

50. Marks LB, Yorke ED, Jackson A, et al. The use of normal tissue complication probability (NTCP) models in the clinic. *Int J Radiat Oncol Biol Phys.* 2010;76(30):S10–S19.

51. Huang Y, Yue H, Wang M, et al. Fully automated search for the optimal VMAT jaw settings based on Eclipse Scripting Application Programming Interface (ESAPI) and RapidPlan knowledge based planning. *J Appl Clin Med Phys.* 2018;19(3):177–182.

52. Hernandez Morales D, Shan J, Liu W, et al. Automation of routine elements for spot-scanning proton patient-specific quality assurance. *Med Phys.* 2019;46(1):5–14.

53. Amaloo C, Hayles L, Manning M, et al. Can automated treatment plans gain traction in the clinic? *J Appl Clin Med Phys.* 2019;20(8):29–35.

54. Schwartz DL, Dong L. Adaptive radiation therapy for head and neck cancer: can an old goal evolve into a new standard? *J Oncol.* 2011;pii:690595.

55. Jensen AD, Nill S, Huber PE, et al. A clinical concept for interfractional adaptive radiation therapy in the treatment of head and neck cancer. *Int J Radiat Oncol Biol Phys.* 2012;82(2):590–596.

56. Evans JD, Harper RH, Petersen M, et al. The importance of verification CT-QA scans in patients treated with IMRT for head and neck cancers. *Int J Part Ther.* 2020;7(1):41–53.

57. Chen AM, Daly ME, Cui J, et al. Clinical outcomes among patients with head and neck cancer treated by intensity-modulated radiotherapy with and without adaptive replanning. *Head Neck.* 2014;36(11):1541–1546.

58. Capelle L, Mackenzie M, Field C, et al. Adaptive radiotherapy using helical tomotherapy for head and neck cancer in definitive and postoperative settings: initial results. *Clin Oncol (R Coll Radiol).* 2012;24(3):208–215.

59. Frank SJ, Cox JD, Gillin M, et al. Multifield optimization intensity modulated proton therapy for head and neck tumors: a translation to practice. *Int J Radiat Oncol Biol Phys.* 2014;89(4):846–853.

60. Wan Chan Tseung H, Ma J, Beltran C. A fast GPU-based Monte Carlo simulation of proton transport with detailed modeling of nonelastic interactions. *Med Phys.* 2015;42(6):2967–2978.

61. Beltran C, Wan Chan Tseung H, Augustine KE, et al. Clinical implementation of a proton dose verification system utilizing a GPU accelerated Monte Carlo engine. *Int J Part Ther.* 2016;3(2):312–319.

62. Fossum CC, Beltran CJ, Whitaker TJ, et al. Biological model for predicting toxicity in head and neck cancer patients receiving proton therapy. *Int J Part Ther.* 2017;4(2):18–25.

63. Wan Chan Tseung HS, Ma J, Kreofsky CR, et al. Clinically applicable Monte Carlo-base biological dose optimization for the treatment of head and neck cancers with spot-scanning proton therapy. *Int J Radiat Oncol Biol Phys.* 2016;95(5):1535–1543.

64. Bonner JA, Harari PM, Giralt J, et al. Radiotherapy plus cetuximab for locoregionally advanced head and neck cancer: 5-year survival data from a phase 3 randomized trial, and relation between cetuximab-induced rash and survival. *Lancet Oncol.* 2010;11(1):21–28.

65. Sepiashvili L, Bruce JP, Huang SH, et al. Novel insights into head and neck cancer using next-generation "omic" technologies. *Cancer Res.* 2015;75(3):480–486.

66. Du Y, Peyser ND, Grandis JR. Integration of molecular targeted therapy with radiation in head and neck cancer. *Pharmacol Ther.* 2014;142(1):88–98.

67. Li Q, Prince ME, Moyer JS. Immunotherapy for head and neck squamous cell carcinoma. *Oral Oncol.* 2015;51(4):299–304.

68. Lee NY, et al. *Target Volume Delineation and Treatment Planning for Particle Therapy: A Practical Guide.* Springer; 2018. https://doi.org/10.1007/978-3-319-42478-1

7 Cancers of the Thorax/Lung

Gregory M.M. Videtic, Rupesh Kotecha, Neil M. Woody, and Kevin L. Stephans

INTRODUCTION

The chest is home to a range of pathologic processes because of the number and variety of structures it harbors. The present chapter reviews the principles and practice of radiation therapy (RT) for primary malignancies of the chest. In that regard, it will focus on the diagnoses of lung cancer, mesothelioma, and thymoma since the anatomic structures associated with these malignancies (e.g., lung parenchyma, pleura, mediastinum) account for both tumor and organs at risk (OARs) that need to be considered when delivering safe and effective radiation. A discussion of RT for other diseases of the thorax such as gastro-intestinal cancers (e.g., esophageal cancer), lymphomas, and sarcomas is dealt with elsewhere in this textbook.

Radiation plays a fundamental role in the management of thoracic tumors and encompasses all facets of oncologic care, from cure to palliation. In considering the procedures and processes required for RT planning and delivery, we will focus on relevant issues to the chest, including special approaches to simulation, target definition, dose and fractionation, dosimetric planning, and tolerance of normal structures, as well as selected tumor- and site-specific treatment techniques, for example, postoperative RT to the pleural cavity after an extra-pleural pneumonectomy (EPP) for malignant pleural mesothelioma (MPM). Specialty topics in RT including the use of stereotactic body RT (SBRT) and proton therapy (PT) will be addressed.

ANATOMY

Many of the normal structures in the thorax are very sensitive to irradiation and therefore it is incumbent on the specialists in radiation medicine to be expert in understanding the normal anatomy of the chest and the relationship of its various structures one to another in order to anticipate and predict the acute and late manifestations of RT on these organs and tissues. The thorax contains the heart, lungs, and other vital structures within a skeletal framework that also protects some of the abdominal organs.[1] The mediastinum occupies the central space of the thorax and is defined as the interval between the two pleural sacs. It is commonly divided into a superior mediastinum, above the level of the pericardium, and three lower divisions: anterior, middle, and posterior. The anterior mediastinum lies between the sternum and pericardium and most importantly contains the thymus. The middle mediastinum contains the pericardium, heart, and the main bronchi and other structures of the roots of the lungs. The posterior mediastinum, behind the pericardium, contains the esophagus and thoracic aorta. The superior mediastinum contains portions of the thymus, great vessels related to the heart, the trachea, the esophagus, and occasionally aberrant thyroid tissue. The two lungs and their pleural sacs are situated in the thoracic cavity. The pleura is a thin serous membrane adherent to various structures. When it lines up the thoracic wall and diaphragm, it is known as the parietal pleura and when it is reflected onto the lung, it is called the visceral pleura. The latter covers the whole surface of the lung parenchyma and tracks deeply into its fissures. The bronchi and pulmonary vessels, which extend from the trachea and heart, respectively, collectively form the root of the lung. The part of the medial surface where these structures enter the lung is known as the hilus. The trachea extends from the inferior end of the larynx to its point of bifurcation between the T5 and T7 vertebral levels dividing into right and left main bronchi. The esophagus extends from the lower end of the pharynx to the cardiac opening of the stomach. The heart is situated in the middle mediastinum and is enclosed in a fibroserous sac termed the "pericardium."

DIAGNOSTIC WORK-UP AND STAGING

A patient presenting with a suspected chest malignancy requires a thorough history and physical examination as well as selected diagnostic tests in order to confirm malignancy, identify the histologic tumor type, and determine the disease stage, all in order to direct treatment and management decisions. There are no cancer-specific laboratory studies to gauge the presence of the majority of thoracic tumors but certain tests including complete blood count, serum electrolytes, and liver function tests may point to paraneoplastic syndromes, the presence of metastatic disease, or cancer-associated phenomena such as malnutrition. Routine radiologic examinations include chest x-rays and computed tomography (CT). CT studies are valuable at identifying tumor location and size and at staging disease but have limitations with respect to recognizing mediastinal nodal disease or metastatic disease. 2-deoxy-2[^{18}F]fluoro-D-glucose positron emission tomography (FDG-PET) scanning is considered standard in the staging work-up of thoracic tumors. It can help distinguish inflammatory from neoplastic disease, it is more sensitive than CT at recognizing metastatic disease in regional lymph nodes (LNs), and it is more accurate in determining the clinical stage of the patient: for example, in lung cancer, up to 25% of patients judged potentially curable were found on PET to have incurable advanced disease.[2,3] Brain imaging is frequently utilized for staging, especially for certain diagnoses, for example, small cell lung cancer (SCLC), when there is a large burden of intra-thoracic disease or in patients who present with neurologic symptoms. Magnetic resonance imaging (MRI) is considered more sensitive than CT at detecting frank and occult metastatic disease. Pulmonary function tests (such as spirometry and diffusing capacity of the lung for carbon monoxide [DLCO]) are not staging tools but are used to predict a patient's tolerance to different treatment modalities such as surgery or RT.

- A range of diagnostic procedures may be employed in order to characterize a thoracic tumor.[4] These include sputum cytology, percutaneous fine needle aspiration (FNA), bronchoscopy, mediastinosocopy, thoracentesis, endobronchial ultrasound-guided (EBUS) FNA or core biopsy, thoracoscopy, and rarely, exploratory thoracotomy. The goal in choosing any of these procedures is to effectively and safely obtain tissues for histologic characterization, accurately map out the extent of disease in the chest (e.g., mediastinoscopy or EBUS sampling of mediastinal LNs), and to appropriately complete the staging. Research over the past decades has led to identifying specific molecular and genetic profiles of lung cancers that has revolutionized their clinical management with respect to the choice of effective systemic therapies.[5] To date, there is no routine role for such markers in making RT choices although this is an active area of investigation. The extent, or more formally the "stage," of cancer at the time of diagnosis is the key factor that defines prognosis and is a critical element in determining appropriate treatment based on patients

with a similar stage. The most widely accepted and clinically validated staging system is the tumor node metastasis (TNM) system maintained collaboratively by the American Joint Committee on Cancer (AJCC) and the International Union for Cancer Control.[6] The TNM system classifies cancers by the size and extent of the primary tumor (T), the degree of involvement of regional LN (N), and the presence or absence of distant metastases (M), and more recently, has been supplemented by carefully selected non-anatomic prognostic factors for certain cancers (e.g., tumor grade, and histology). Detailed LN maps have been published in order to facilitate consistent and appropriate labeling of regional thoracic LN levels. The International Association for the Study of Lung Cancer LN map is the recommended means of describing regional LN involvement for lung cancers.[7] The eighth edition of the TNM system is currently the accepted standard for staging patients diagnosed on or after January 1, 2017.[8] Given the limitations of standard radiographic staging tools, a current area of research is the role of blood-based biomarkers, such as circulating tumor cells, in the detection and staging of lung cancers.[9]

RT PRINCIPLES FOR THORACIC MALIGNANCIES

Introduction

There are general principles for planning thoracic RT that are valid across a range of malignancies since it is the normal anatomy of the thorax which imposes the most important constraints on the safe delivery of RT. These common principles when considering planning chest RT include the approaches to simulation, target delineation, motion control, definition of normal tissues and OARs, dose constraints, dose-limiting structures, and beam geometry. Specific thoracic RT dose prescriptions are determined by the tumor types being treated and by the particular indications for treatment which include preoperative, postoperative, definitive (both conventional and stereotactic), prophylactic, and palliative therapies.

The primary rationale for preoperative (also known as induction or neo-adjuvant) therapy is to facilitate complete surgical resection of disease, and yield a margin-negative (R0) resection, usually in the setting of locally advanced disease. Preoperative RT is typically administered in conjunction with chemotherapy. Doses delivered initiate tumor killing, both macroscopically and microscopically, without the expectation of total tumor eradication. Additionally, preoperative RT may "downsize" a tumor to alter the form of surgical resection required, for example, to change the operation from a pneumonectomy to lobectomy. It may also alter patterns of loco-regional failure by sterilizing micro-metastatic disease in regional LN chains and potentially affect overall survival. Pre-operative RT is typically well tolerated by most patients since their performance and medical status remain usually intact.

Postoperative (or adjuvant) RT is administered to patients showing high-risk features for loco-regional recurrence after surgical resection, that is, positive margins at the resection line (R1), gross residual disease (R2), or regional LN involvement. Doses employed reflect the need to eradicate microscopic disease primarily (except in the R2 setting). Given that patient status is often compromised after surgery, completing a planned course of postoperative RT is often challenging due to patient intolerance of expected side effects.

The rationale for definitive RT is to provide optimal intra-thoracic control of disease by ablating visible tumor and eradicating micro-metastatic disease. Because of the constraints imposed by normal thoracic structures on RT delivery, the potential doses for optimal gross tumor control by conventional RT may often not be achievable in the chest. This has led to pursuing other means of dose optimization for thoracic RT such as stereotactic delivery, integrating RT with chemotherapy (CHT), use of altered RT dose schedules (e.g., hyperfractionation), and exploration of different radiotherapy delivery technologies such as PT and use of radio-protectants.

As noted above, the most common indication for thoracic RT is for palliation of local symptoms attributable to advanced or metastatic disease. Since the primary goal of palliation is symptom relief, thoracic RT schedules in this setting tend to be short, and favor large doses per fraction with modest total doses, since late effects are not a critical consideration in patients with a limited life expectancy.

The role for prophylactic therapy in the management of thoracic tumors addresses the propensity of some thoracic malignancies for occult dissemination to the brain. For example, SCLC may find sanctuary in the brain despite its eradication extra-cranially. That is why prophylactic cranial irradiation (PCI) is routinely used with that diagnosis. PCI typically involves lower total RT doses and short treatment schedules.

Technical Factors

Simulation

RT simulation for thoracic malignancies is performed using a CT scan for delineation of the target volumes and the OARs. In general, patients are set up in the supine position with their arms above their head. In special scenarios, such as for patients with superior sulcus or Pancoast tumors, simulation can be performed in the akimbo position. For mesothelioma patients receiving adjuvant RT after EPP, the incision and drainage sites should be marked with radiopaque material and application of tissue-equivalent bolus over these sites and the chest wall should be considered at the time of simulation.

Localization

A volumetric CT scan should be acquired with a 3 mm slice thickness from the second or third cervical vertebrae to the third or fourth lumbar vertebrae to ensure adequate margin around the lungs for generation of digitally reconstructed radiographs, dosimetry calculations, and planning using non-coplanar fields.[10] The liver should be included in the simulation CT scan. Oral contrast can assist with delineation of the esophagus. Intravenous contrast (IV) contrast can be administered to assist with identification of the major blood vessels, which is especially important for patients with centrally located tumors and mediastinal LN involvement.[11,12] Alternatively, if a patient had previously undergone a diagnostic CT scan of the chest with IV contrast, this can be co-registered to a non-contrast simulation CT scan. Patients undergoing simulation for PT should have all contrast scans (oral or IV) performed after the treatment planning scans are done to ensure correct dose calculations with accurate proton stopping power values. Patients undergoing simulation for MR-guided RT (MRgRT) undergo an MR simulation with a defined breath-hold 3D MR scan for treatment planning. For patients with early-stage lung cancer undergoing SBRT, the isocenter should be placed in the center of the primary tumor volume. For patients undergoing treatment to a primary tumor and regional LNs, the isocenter should be placed in the center of the mediastinum near the carina. After placement of the isocenter and acquisition of a verification scan, external marks are placed on the patient or immobilization device to ensure accurate setup for treatment delivery.

Immobilization

Numerous immobilization devices are commercially available, including a simple thorax board, alpha cradle, vacuum-lock bag, and thermoplastic mold. Patients should be positioned in a reproducible manner that is comfortable enough to reduce intrafraction movement but reproducible enough to minimize interfraction setup errors. Patients undergoing SBRT can also be immobilized using a stereotactic frame. Patients simulated for MRgRT also have vendor-specific surface receiver coils placed above and below the patient during 3D MR scanning.

Motion Management

For patients undergoing treatment to thoracic sites, the effect of respiratory motion on target movement must be accounted for in simulation, treatment planning, and treatment delivery.[13,14] At the time of simulation, the motion of the primary tumor should be characterized and quantified. For the initial simulation scan, patients should be instructed to breathe at a normal pace. Motion management strategies are recommended for patients in whom the target motion exceeds 5 mm and include use of four-dimensional CT (4DCT) scan, physical restriction of motion, breath-hold techniques, and respiratory gating. A 4DCT scan can generate volumetric datasets representing the various phases of the respiratory cycle.[15] During acquisition of the 4DCT, imaging data are stored relative to a respiratory phase or amplitude either by use of an external motion detector, infrared-based respiratory position monitor device, or a belt wrapped around the patient's waist.[16] The 4DCT scan can reconstruct either 10 individual-phase CT scans or a reduced number of scans representing specific phases of respiration (e.g., 25%, 50%, 75%, and 100%) which can be viewed in a motion display.[17] The 4DCT image data set can also reconstruct a maximum intensity projection (MIP) to provide a rapid and reliable estimate of the maximum motion of the tumor through the respiratory cycle.[18] For accurate dosimetry analysis and dose calculation, an average intensity (AIP) data set should be generated from the 4DCT.[19] This AIP also represents the most accurate representation of the tumor center of mass and should be used for comparison with cone-beam CT images at the time of delivery to avoid potential systematic errors.[20] Physical restriction of tumor motion is most commonly performed with application of an abdominal belt or hoop.[21] Breath-hold is performed with an active breathing control (ABC) device to monitor the patient's inspiratory and expiratory breathing patterns.[22] A respiratory gating technique uses external patient signals (such as the movement of the chest wall), continuous tracking of the target volume itself, or surrogate fiducials to determine the RT beam-on time relative to tumor position. During the course of treatment, the patient breathes at a normal pace, but the treatment machine delivers the radiation treatment only during a specific interval based on the position of these signals.[16] Newer MRgRT technologies involve identification of a target for anatomical tracking (region of interest to be treated or avoided), creation of a boundary to identify the tracking region, visualization of the tracking algorithm as deformation of the volume occurs during cine imaging, and treatment delivery only when the target is within the boundary region.

Target Definition and Normal Structures

Target Volumes

The International Commission on Radiation Units (ICRU) Report No. 50 outlines the definitions for treatment volumes in RT planning.[23] For patients with thoracic malignancies, the gross tumor volume (GTV) includes the primary tumor volume and the involved regional LNs. Regional LNs are included in the GTV if they are metabolically active on PET-CT (standardized uptake values (SUV) = 1.5 × mean intensity of 1 cc

of the aorta volume or SUV > 3), ≥1 cm in short axis on CT scan, or found to be pathologically involved on bronchoscopy or mediastinoscopy. Regional hilar or mediastinal LNs should also be included if there is serial growth documented on diagnostic CT scans, if two or more nodes are visualized in a high-risk nodal station, or if nodes are visualized at the first echelon drainage or within 1 cm of the primary tumor. The primary tumor volume should be contoured on the lung window settings.[24] For tumors abutting the chest wall or mediastinum, the edge of the primary tumor can be modified using mediastinal window settings. Involved hilar and mediastinal LNs should be contoured using the mediastinal window setting. The primary tumor volume can be disjointed from the regional LNs, and LN contours can be noncontiguous.

For patients with thoracic malignancies, internal margins (IMs) and target volumes have to be considered and are defined in the ICRU Report No. 62.[25] The IM accounts for variations in size, shape, and position of the targets relative to the movements of respiration and is used to generate an internal target volume (ITV). When using a 4DCT scan, there are numerous approaches to reconstructing the image data for determining the ITV. Ezhil and colleagues evaluated the generation of the ITV using four different methods: (1) combining the GTV contours from each of the 10 respiratory phases, (2) combining the GTV contours from two extreme respiratory phases (0% and 50%), (3) defining the GTV contour using the MIP, and (4) defining the GTV contour using the MIP with modification based on visual verification of contours on individual respiratory phases.[26] Based on this comparison, methods (2) and (3) underestimated the ITV, and the use of MIP with modification based on visual verification was recommended. There are alternative methods of generating an ITV without use of 4DCT. For example, the targets can be contoured on the end of tidal volume inhale and exhale scans to create a composite structure to capture any possible tumor motion.[27,28] Alternatively, "slow" CT techniques (slice thickness 4 mm, index 3 mm, revolution time 4 seconds/slice) can be used to better capture potential tumor movement.[29] For patients being simulated with an ABC device, at least two confirmatory scans should be acquired to verify the position of the target during subsequent breath holds and these scans are used to generate the ITV.

The clinical target volume (CTV) includes the GTV and adds a margin for coverage of areas at risk for subclinical microscopic disease. For patients undergoing SBRT, the CTV representation is equivalent to the GTV. For patients undergoing RT for locally advanced non-small cell lung cancer, the CTV is created from a 0.5 to 1 cm expansion around the GTV or ITV. Data to support these RT expansions arise from a study by Giraud and colleagues who examined pathological specimens from 70 patients with NSCLC.[30] They determined that the mean microscopic extension was 2.69 and 1.48 mm for adenocarcinoma and squamous cell carcinoma cases, respectively. Moreover, to account for 95% of microscopic disease extension, a margin of 8 mm for adenocarcinoma and 6 mm for squamous cell carcinoma histologies was required. Similarly, pathological studies have also shown that the extent of microscopic nodal extracapsular extension is 0.7 mm and ≤3 mm in 95% of nodes.[31] For patients with SCLC, the CTV may also include the ipsilateral hilar LNs (station 10), if not already included in the GTV.

The planning target volume (PTV) includes the CTV and provides a margin for motion of the target and setup reproducibility between fraction delivery. With regard to internal motion, there should be at least a 1 cm expansion in the superior–inferior dimension and a 0.5 cm expansion in the axial dimension. In the free-breathing (non-ITV) setting, an additional setup margin of at least 0.5 cm should be added to create the final PTV.

Organs at Risk

As important as it is to accurately identify and contour the tumor volume, defining the OARs is equally important in creating an RT treatment plan. OARs should be outlined on all CT slices in which the structures exist and are in the field of irradiation.[32] The lungs should be individually contoured as right and left lung structures and then combined into a composite structure for dosimetry evaluation. The lung contours should represent the inflated lung volume and exclude the proximal bronchial tree, areas of atelectasis, scarring, pleural fluid, or large vessels. Considerable variability exists regarding the subtraction of the GTV, CTV, ITV, or PTV from the composite lung volume with no prospective evidence to support one particular method over another. SBRT protocols have used the proximal bronchial tree to differentiate central lung tumors (within 2 cm) from peripheral tumors. The proximal bronchial tree is composed of the distal 2 cm of the trachea, carina, right and left mainstem bronchi, right and left upper lobe bronchi, right middle lobe bronchus, left lingular bronchus, and the right and left lower lobe bronchi. These structures should be contoured using mediastinal window settings with inclusion of the outer wall of the airway.

The heart contour should include the pericardial sac extending from the superior aspect, defined as either the ascending arch of the aorta or the inferior aspect of the pulmonary artery passing midline, to the apex of the heart using mediastinal window settings. The esophagus should be contoured with inclusion of the outer edge of the muscular wall and adventitia from the inferior edge of the cricoid cartilage to the gastro-esophageal junction on mediastinal window settings. Of note, although oral contrast can be used for easier identification of the esophagus, this may distort the true dimensions of the structure. The spinal cord should be outlined on each slice as either the true spinal cord or the extent of the bony canal from the same cranial level as the esophagus contour (cricoid cartilage) to the bottom of the second lumbar vertebra. For patients with superior sulcus tumors, apical tumors,

or supraclavicular nodal metastases, the brachial plexus should be contoured. The brachial plexus is located posterior to the subclavian vessels between the anterior and middle scalene muscles from the interspace between the fourth and fifth cervical vertebra to the interspace between the first and second thoracic vertebra. For patients with tumors abutting the chest wall, the ribs and chest wall can be contoured by applying a 2 cm expansion in the lateral, anterior, and posterior dimension from the lung contours within 3 cm of the PTV. This should include the intercostal muscles but exclude other muscles, vertebral bodies, sternum, or the skin. For patients with lower lobe tumors, consideration should be given to contouring the stomach, liver, and kidneys, each individually and then combined into a composite whole kidney structure. For patients with implanted devices in the thorax, such as pacemakers and defibrillators, the devices should be contoured separately. For non-isocentric treatment techniques or non-coplanar beam entries, clinicians need to be aware of avoiding beam entrance through non-immobilized structures such as the chin or arms.

Dose-volume histograms (DVHs) are created to evaluate the radiation exposure to the OARs.[33] In general, the tolerance of each of the normal organs depends on the dose per fraction received and the total dose prescribed to the target, but the dose received to normal structures should be minimized. Examples of suggested constraints for conventionally fractionated RT treatments for thoracic malignancies are outlined in Table 7.1.

Integration of PET-CT into Treatment Planning

FDG-PET has not only enhanced the accuracy of staging patients with lung cancer, but is also useful in delineation of the primary tumor target, distinction between atelectasis and tumor, evaluation of mediastinum, and detection of distant metastatic disease.[34] PET remains investigational for delineation of tumor volumes in patients who previously received CHT, RT dose escalation, or other forms of response-adapted therapy.

PET-CT is useful in delineating the primary tumor extent, as the size and dimensions of the primary tumor measured on PET-CT correlate well with pathological examination.[35] There are numerous methods of utilizing PET in contouring, including use of the absolute SUV (typically 2.5),[36] a percentage of the maximum SUV, a fixed percent intensity level of the maximum activity in the primary tumor (typically 40%–55%),[37] or an SUV intensity threshold as referenced above the background level. The use of PET-CT for delineation of the primary tumor volume also reduces variability in target contouring between providers.[38] Compared to CT scans, however, FDG-PET tumor volumes can be larger than CT volumes since the slower acquisition time of the PET scan captures the integral movement of the primary tumor through respiration.[39] Therefore, the PET volume may correlate more closely with the ITV volume than the CT-derived GTV.[40]

TABLE 7.1	Suggested Normal Tissue Dose Constraints for Conventionally Fractionated External Beam Radiotherapy[33]			
Critical Structure	**DVH Parameters**	**Limits**	**Toxicity Rate**	**Toxicity Endpoint**
Spinal cord	Max. dose	50 Gy	0.2%	Myelopathy
Spinal cord	Max. dose	60 Gy	6%	Myelopathy
Spinal cord	Max. dose	69 Gy	50%	Myelopathy
Lung	V20[a]	≤30%	<20%	Symptomatic pneumonitis
Lung	Mean dose	7 Gy	5%	Symptomatic pneumonitis
Lung	Mean dose	13 Gy	10%	Symptomatic pneumonitis
Lung	Mean dose	20 Gy	20%	Symptomatic pneumonitis
Lung	Mean dose	24 Gy	30%	Symptomatic pneumonitis
Lung	Mean dose	27 Gy	40%	Symptomatic pneumonitis
Esophagus	Mean dose	<34 Gy	5%–20%	Grade 3+ esophagitis
Esophagus	V35[a]	<50%	<30%	Grade 2+ esophagitis
Esophagus	V50[a]	<40%	<30%	Grade 2+ esophagitis
Esophagus	V70[a]	<20%	<30%	Grade 2+ esophagitis
Heart (pericardium)	Mean dose	<26 Gy	<15%	Pericarditis
Heart (pericardium)	V30[a]	<46%	<15%	Pericarditis
Heart	V25[a]	<10%	<1%	Long-term cardiac mortality

[a] Vx = volume receiving ≥x Gy; DVH, dose-volume histogram.

It is important to note that FDG-PET may increase the GTV contour in cases where the adjacent tissue appears morphologically normal but has metabolic activity concerning for disease extension. At the same time, FDG-PET may be used to reduce the CT-derived tumor volume when the tumor is directly adjacent to a structure and no clear plane of separation is visualized. This is useful in cases of atelectasis or for tumors abutting the chest wall (see Figure 7.1).[41]

PET-CT is especially useful in evaluation of the mediastinum, where it has a higher sensitivity (84%) and specificity (89%) than CT scans (57% and 82%, respectively) or endoscopic ultrasound (78% and 71%, respectively).[42] In fact, when integrating FDG-PET findings into RT treatment planning, significant changes to target volume contours have been reported in 21% to 100% of cases, primarily due to the addition of mediastinal LN targets.[43] At the same time, given the high negative predictive value of FDG-PET, nodal regions without significant SUV uptake can be omitted from RT volumes.

A PET-CT scan is typically obtained during staging. This scan can be used in planning if it can be co-registered to the simulation CT scan. Differences in patient setup for acquisition of each scan and these differences must be accounted for when co-registering diagnostic to treatment planning studies. Alternatively, PET-CT scans may be obtained in the treatment position on a firm flat-top couch with the same immobilization device used for RT planning to minimize co-registration errors.[44] In either setting, consistent FDG-PET window and color settings should be utilized.

There are certain caveats to be aware of when interpreting FDG-PET images. False-positive findings can be seen in patients with inflammatory conditions, whereas false-negative readings may be obtained either when LNs are below the size threshold for detection (typically <1 cm) or when LNs are too close to the primary tumor volume.[45] Moreover, in patients who recently received CHT, the residual malignant cells may decrease their glucose uptake, resulting in false-negative findings.[43]

Elective Nodal Irradiation

Prior to the introduction of the CT scan into RT planning, lung cancer volumes were based on anatomic landmarks and encompassed the definable lung tumor on chest X-ray (CXR), any clinically involved LNs, and the regional nodes considered at risk. This approach of covering all the mediastinal LNs, independent of confirmed metastatic involvement, was termed "elective nodal irradiation" (ENI). Given improvements in pathological evaluation of the mediastinum (e.g., EBUS), wide spread integration of PET-CT, and multiple cohort studies and randomized controlled trials demonstrating lack of elective nodal failure, use of ENI has substantially diminished

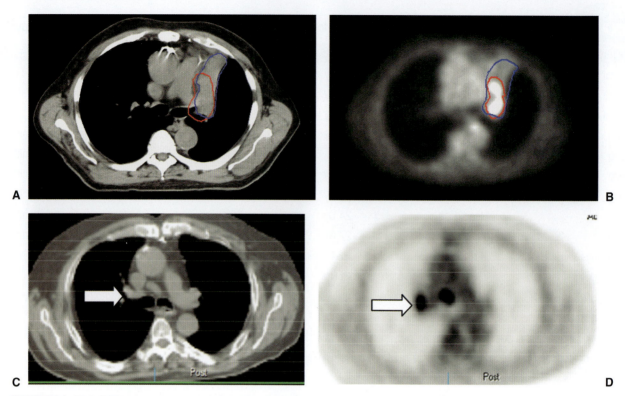

FIGURE 7.1. FDG-PET improves staging accuracy for nonsmall cell lung cancer. FDG-PET differentiates tumor from collapsed lung (**A** and **B**) and detects CT undetected node (*arrow* in **C** and **D**). *Blue*, CT lesion; *red*, PET hypermetabolic lesion.

in clinical practice.[46] Currently involved LN irradiation only is performed on modern cooperative group clinical trials and supported by consensus guidelines.

Treatment Planning

Dose

A range of dose/fractionation schedules is employed routinely in thoracic RT. Guidelines have been developed for selection of dose and fractionation in SCLC,[47] definitive management of NSCLC,[48–50] postoperative RT,[51] and palliation/poor performance status.[52,53] This section includes general dose and fractionation information for thoracic RT. Guidelines for specific disease sites and specific techniques (e.g., SBRT) are located in their respective sections.

Standard Fractionation

Standard fractionation using doses of 1.8 to 2 Gy per fraction has an established role in preoperative, definitive, and postoperative RT in the chest. Doses of 45 to 60 Gy in the preoperative setting may be used.[54–56] In the definitive setting, dose of 60 Gy is the standard of care.[57] In the postoperative setting, dose of 50 to 60 Gy in 1.8 to 2 Gy fractions is employed.[51,58,59] The postoperative dose range reflects that the resected tumor bed is treated to a dose of 50 Gy; a focal boost to a dose of 60 Gy is considered for areas of extracapsular extension or

resected bulky nodes. For areas of gross residual disease total doses of 66 to 70 Gy may be considered if normal tissue constraints can be met and these doses are contextualized within the usage of, and sequencing with, coordinated chemotherapy.

Hyperfractionation and Hypofractionation

Hyperfractionation is utilized in definitive thoracic RT. Hyperfractionation to a total dose of 69.6 Gy in 1.2 Gy fractions given BID (twice daily) with an interfraction interval of >6 hours has been employed in NSCLC and may be superior to standard fractionation when concurrent CHT is not used.[60,61] Accelerated hyperfractionation to total dose of 45 to 54 Gy given BID is routine in SCLC.[62,63] In NSCLC, continuous hyperfractionated accelerated RT to a dose of 54 Gy in 36 fractions given at 1.5 Gy TID (thrice daily) has been shown to be superior compared to standard once-daily fractionation in the absence of CHT.[64–66]

Accelerated hypofractionation may also provide advantages; for example, 40 to 45 Gy in 15 fractions are associated with comparable responses to standard fractionation.[67–69] A phase I dose-escalation study up to 60 Gy in 15 fractions has demonstrated feasibility and safety,[70] with long-term safety, efficacy, and comparisons to conventionally fractionated radiotherapy pending. Other hypofractionated regimens including split course regimens are also feasible and efficacious.[71] A meta-analysis of clinical trials has suggested a 2.5%

overall survival benefit at 5 years for the use of altered fractionation schedules.[72]

Palliation

The primary role of thoracic RT in metastatic lung cancer is the palliation of symptoms prior to the initiation of systemic CHT or in patients who are unable to receive systemic therapy at all. In the United States, 30 Gy in 10 fractions is commonly utilized. However, multiple prospective randomized trials of different dose/fractionation schedules have shown that thoracic symptoms can be treated safely and effectively with 1- or 2-fraction (e.g., 17 Gy at 8.5 Gy per fraction 1 week apart) schedules with no overall benefit to higher RT doses for symptom relief. Selected patients with good performance status may see modest survival benefits from higher-dose palliative regimens (30 Gy/10 fraction equivalent or higher) but at the expense of moderately higher esophageal toxicity.[53] Although these randomized clinical trials of palliative RT for lung cancer have been conducted in patients with NSCLC, the treatment approaches and results from such studies are readily applicable to the patient with symptoms related to SCLC.[73]

Technical Factors

Beam Energy

Appropriate beam energy is critical in the treatment planning of thoracic RT. For photon therapy, a 6 MV beam energy is generally the preferred choice to provide optimal PTV coverage particularly near lung tissue density interfaces. With higher-energy beams, high-energy secondary electrons travel resulting in dose loss in the boundary region.[74–76] This effect may not always be well represented in computerized treatment planning with heterogeneity calculation.[77] In addition, higher-energy beam neutron contamination is also introduced. Despite these limitations, higher-energy beams no higher than 10 MV may be occasionally helpful to provide improved dose homogeneity particularly in AP/PA arrangements where tissue density is more consistent. For delivery of SBRT, which often utilizes more hetereogeneous dose distributions for targets located within parallel tissue and may place a premium on speed of delivery given small margins and large dose per fraction, flattening filter free beams are often employed. Such beams exhibit a lower average energy profile than their filtered counterparts as they contain a broader mix of lower-energy photons that would otherwise have been removed by the flattening filter.

Heterogeneity

The chest is unique relative to other body sites as the lungs have significantly less electron density and thus significantly less attenuation of a RT beam occurs than in other surrounding tissues. These differences have the effect of changing the dose distribution substantially if the heterogeneity of tissue densities is not considered. Traditional thoracic RT was performed without heterogeneity correction but as these corrections are now routinely available in modern computer treatment planning systems, they are considered routine practice. Several algorithms for heterogeneity correction are presently available although convolution/superposition algorithms are most common. Corrections with pencil beam algorithms which were historically used have been shown to have reduced accuracy relative to other options.[78] Caution should be used when switching between homogeneous planning and accounting for heterogeneity (see Figure 7.2). Conversion factors have been suggested to adjust RT prescription dose but these conversions may be different between algorithms within a type and between types.[78,79] Monte Carlo algorithms which are increasingly becoming available in commercial planning systems may be particularly distinct from prior algorithms.[80] It is notable that when heterogeneity corrections are applied PTV surface dose decreases due to increased range of secondary electrons. This effect can be particularly pronounced with high-energy beams.[81]

Intensity-Modulated RT

Since its initial development in the 1980s, 3D conformal RT (3D-CRT) has long been a standard technique for dose delivery in lung cancer. This technique, while powerful, may not provide optimal sparing of nearby normal tissues. Several dosimetric studies have suggested that intensity-modulated RT (IMRT) can result in statistically significant improvements in dose distributions.[82–83] Retrospective data by Li et al. comparing 3D-CRT to IMRT did show reduction in loco-regional failure and improvement in overall survival with IMRT without improvement in the distant metastatic rate. Unfortunately prospective comparisons have not been performed and are unlikely to be forthcoming to validate the results of this retrospective comparison. Based on available data, some clinicians still question the routine use of IMRT for lung cancer.[84,85] First, some postulate that the mediastinal coverage to high dose with 3D-CRT may be aiding in controlling microscopic mediastinal spread. The higher conformality with IMRT could potentially reduce this incidental coverage. Second, IMRT is associated with a lower V20 and mean lung dose but is also associated with a higher low dose (V5) and the effect of this low dose cloud on lung toxicity has not been well elucidated.[83,85] Finally, there is a concern of motion interplay effect where tumor motion and MLC leaf motion could interact to perturb the expected dose distribution. However, studies have suggested this effect is likely to be small.[86,87] Despite these concerns, sufficient experience exists to suggest that IMRT may be safely and effectively employed in thoracic malignancies and may be particularly appropriate when normal tissue constraints cannot be met with 3D-CRT. It is important to note that a secondary analysis of the Radiation Therapy Oncology Group (RTOG 0617) demonstrated that IMRT use was associated with lower rates of high-grade pneumonitis as well as cardiac doses, while on the other hand

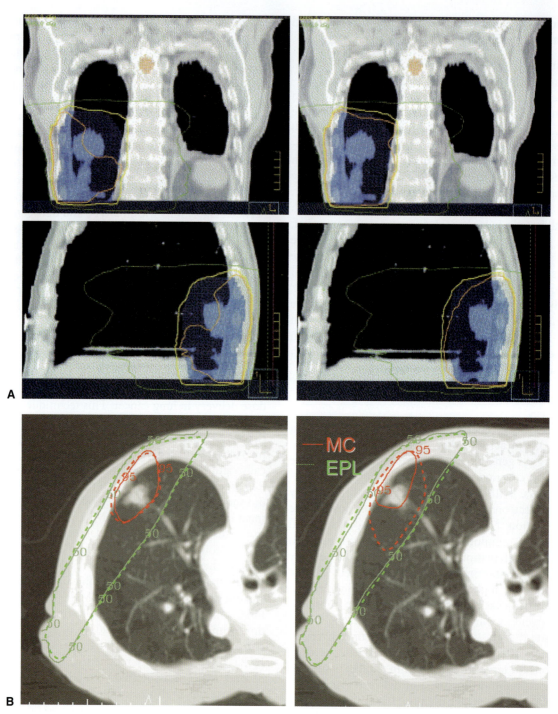

FIGURE 7.2. Tissue heterogeneity correction in lung cancer planning. **A:** Impact of heterogeneity correction on planning target volume (PTV) coverage in a patient with a tumor in the right lower lobe. This figure shows a remarkable under dosage of PTV in a plan generated by the traditional homogeneous prescription method with heterogeneity corrections (*right panel*) and the current heterogeneity-corrected prescription method (*left panel*) in the (a) sagittal and (b) coronal planes. Isodose lines are color coded as follows: *red*, 76 Gy; *orange*, 66 Gy (prescribed dose); *yellow*, 60 Gy; *green*, 20 Gy. **B:** Impact of calculation algorithm on isodose distribution in a lung treatment plan (two fields, 15-MV photons show isodose lines calculated with Monte Carlo [MC, *solid line*] and an equivalent path-length-based algorithm (EPL, *dashed line*). Figure 7.2A (left panel) shows that MC and EPL have almost same isodose distribution when heterogeneity correction is not turned on (i.e., the lung tissue is treated homogeneously), while Figure 7.2B (right panel) depicts remarkable overestimation of 95% isodose surface of the EPL-based dose computation comparing to that of MC calculation. (Courtesy of Indrin Chetty, Henry Ford Hospital, Detroit, Michigan)

not improving overall survival compared to 3D conformal treatments.[88] While a clear role for IMRT in all patients has not been observed, IMRT may be beneficial to achieve dose escalation although the optimal strategy for such dose escalation has not been determined.[58]

SPECIAL TOPICS IN RT DELIVERY

Stereotactic Body Radiation

SBRT is a radiation technique that allows for the precise delivery of large fractions of RT by multiple beams guided by a set of coordinates relating to the direct position of the tumor rather than external marks or anatomical structures. Given the high hypofractionated radiation doses and small treatment margins involved, SBRT requires both careful definition of target and non-target structures, and precise management of target motion and treatment setup.[89]

Indications

While medically inoperable stage I NSCLC remains its primary indication, SBRT is also utilized in the treatment of lung oligometasasis,[90] thoracic re-irradiation,[91–98] poor-risk stage I SCLC[99,100] and is under investigation for operable stage I NSCLC[101,102] as well as potentially as a boost to conventionally fractionated radiation in locally advanced NSCLC.[103,104]

Treatment Planning

SBRT requires careful immobilization of the patient followed by management of target motion so that it is limited to <5 to 10 mm. This may be accomplished by abdominal compression, respiratory gating using either controlled breath-hold or external surrogates, or tumor tracking/respiratory modeling. Tumor motion should be assessed by either fluoroscopy, 4DCT imaging at simulation, or cine-MR imaging, depending on the treatment technology, and verified by appropriate corresponding image-guided radiotherapy (IGRT) methodology during treatment.

In lung SBRT, a PTV can be created from a fixed expansion (1 cm superior–inferior, 5 mm axially) off the contoured GTV.[105] Alternatively it may be derived from the union of multiphasic CT GTVs (free-breathing, inhale, exhale) or 4DCT images into an ITV, which is then expanded uniformly by 5 mm yielding the PTV.[89] Expansion of the 4DCT ITV typically results in a smaller PTV and likely more consistently represents the actual tumor motion as well as center of mass.[106] Delivery technologies allowing for continuous tracking of the target volume allow for direct GTV to PTV expansions without use of an ITV.

Beam arrangements may consist of six or more non-coplanar open beams, IMRT beams, non-coplanar volumetric arcs (typically at least three arcs each offset by 30°–40°), non-isocentric beamlets, intensity-modulated arc therapy, or alternatively particle-based therapy.

Planning should utilize collapsed cone convolution, ray tracing, or Monte Carlo algorithms, as there is a suggestion that pencil beam algorithms may compromise tumor control due to potential for more variable underdosing.[107] Planning should focus on maximizing conformality and rapid dose falloff. Heterogeneity is acceptable and may be desirable for purposes of faster falloff provided critical serial structures are not overexposed. Per its protocol design, RTOG 0236 utilized homogeneous treatment planning prescribing 60 Gy in 3 fractions (see Figure 7.3). This has been estimated to correlate with a heterogeneity-corrected prescription of 54 Gy in 3 fractions;[79] however, care should be taken in interpreting this as the correction is based on estimates of attaining 95% coverage of the PTV periphery whereas other parameters such as mean dose to the GTV, ITV, and PTV may vary considerably; furthermore this correction is also sensitive to tumor size and location.[108]

Dose

SBRT prescriptions can range from 30 to 60 Gy in 1 to 8 fractions. Early series established a correlation with delivery of biologically equivalent dose of at least 100 to 105 Gy_{10} to improved LC[109,110] and reported excellent safety and tumor control regardless of tumor location. In the United States, clinical practice favors the results of the Indiana University phase I dose-escalation studies which ultimately formed the basis for RTOG 0236.[111] In the phase II setting, these researchers did find this dose was associated with a grade 3 or higher toxicity rate exceeding 50% in patients whose tumor fell within 2 cm of the proximal bronchial tree, termed "central" tumors by them[112] and this has led to the routine practice of dose selection as a function of tumor location. While this has caused concern regarding the safety of treating "central" tumors it is noted that Japanese series utilizing a lower-dose per fraction (10–12 Gy) did not report variability of toxicity by location.[109,113,114] Two recent randomized phase II trials comparing single fraction lung SBRT to fractionated schedules showed equivalency with respect to toxicity, local control (LC), and overall survival, and their results are encouraging adoption of these regimens for the routine treatment of peripheral lung cancers.[115,116]

Subsequent publications from the Netherlands validated 60 Gy in 8 fractions even for very large central tumors,[116] and several U.S. retrospective series similarly demonstrated the safety of SBRT for central lung lesions with fraction sizes of up to 10 Gy/fraction.[117,118] For "ultra-central" tumors, broadly categorized as tumors abutting the trachea, mainstem bronchus, or esophagus, a variety of risk-adapted hypofractionated schedules have been used including 60 Gy in 12 fractions,[119] 70 Gy in 10 fractions,[120] or 60 Gy in 15 fractions.[121] RTOG 0813, a dose escalation for SBRT of central lung tumors escalating dose from 50 Gy up to 60 Gy in 5 fractions was completed reaching the highest-dose level without interruption.[122] It showed no

Dose Distribution

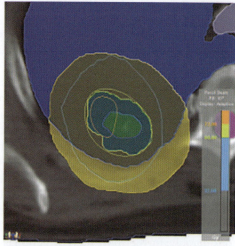

Overview Axial: PTV (Free + 5 mm axial, 1 cm SI)

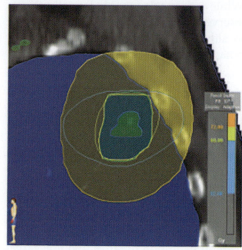

Overview Sagittal: PTV (Free + 5 mm axial, 1 cm SI)

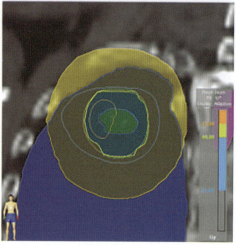

Overview Coronal: PTV (Free + 5 mm axial, 1 cm SI)

FIGURE 7.3. Representative dose distribution for a lung SBRT plan. The patient is a 75-year-old male with medically inoperable adenocarcinoma of the right upper lobe, T1aN0M0, stage IA, treated with 60 Gy in 3 fractions (per RTOG 0236) delivered by dynamic arcs. Motion management was by abdominal compression. Image guidance was by an infrared-based X-ray positioning system. Overall treatment time was 8 days. PTV = GTV + 1 cm superior–inferior and 0.5-cm radial expansion. *Green color fill* is the GTV, *yellow color* filled–ring represents a 2-cm planning structure to limit dose spillage, *light blue line* is 30 Gy, and *yellow line* is 60 Gy.

significant difference in toxicity rates with escalation but did not demonstrate improved LC.

Normal tissue constraints are still evolving with increased SBRT experience. Early experiences used few normal tissue constraints focusing purely on conformality. More recently, constraints have emerged from early experience,[123,124] though they still need to be validated in larger settings. Normal tissue constraints should be based on appropriate protocols for the target being treated such as RTOG trials # 0236, 0813, 0915, or large institutional experiences (see Table 7.2).

Treatment Delivery

IGRT, or image guidance during treatment, initially consisted of bony registration followed by port films, though modern approaches typically rely on CBCT and most recently MRI guidance. Free-breathing CT may not represent the true tumor center-of-mass due to respiratory motion, and a pitfall can be created by matching

free breathing CT to CBCT tumor at time of treatment, potentially introducing systematic error that occasionally exceeds the PTV expansion.[106] One should either use the average CT as the reference for matching or otherwise localize only to bony anatomy if using a free-breathing image while verifying that the CBCT tumor falls within the ITV. In the setting of MRgRT, a new breath-hold 3D MR scan is acquired at the time of treatment delivery, and rigid registration of the target volumes and deformable registration of the OARs, with physician editing as necessary, are performed.[125] In certain cases, such as single fraction treatment or with central lung SBRT, on table adaptive replanting can be expeditiously performed with full reoptimization of the dose fluences based on the current anatomy.[126,127] A tracking algorithm allows for continuous visualization and tracking of the target volume during treatment delivery cine-imaging. An in-room monitor can also be used to project the GTV and gating window for the patient.

TABLE 7.2 Suggested Normal Tissue Dose Constraints for Lung SBRT Based on a Range of Dose/Fractionation Schedules[115,122]

Critical Structure	Volume (cc)	Maximum Dose for Defined Volume (Fraction/Total) (in Gy) for a Given Lung SBRT Fractionation			Toxicity End Point
		1 Fraction	3 Fractions	5 Fractions	
Spinal cord	Point	14/14	7.3/21.9	6/30	Myelopathy
	<0.35	10/10	6/18	4.6/23	
	<1.2	7/7	4.1/12.3	2.9/14.5	
Lung	<1,500	7/7	3.5/10.5	2.5/12.5	Basic lung function
Lung	<1,000	7.4/7.4	3.8/11.4	2.7/13.5	Pneumonitis
Esophagus	Point	15.4/15.4	8.4/25.2	7/35	Stenosis/fistula
	<5	11.9/11.9	5.9/17.7	3.9/19.5	
Heart/pericardium	Point	22/22	10/30	7.6/38	Pericarditis
	<15	16/16	8/24	6.4/32	
Brachial plexus	Point	17.5/17.5	8/24	6.1/30.5	Neuropathy
	<3	14/14	6.8/20.4	5.4/27	
Rib[a]	Point	30/30	12.3/36.9	8.6/43	Pain or fracture
	<1	22/22	9.6/28.8	7/35	
	<30		10/30		
Skin	Point	26/26	11/33	7.9/39.5	Ulceration
	<10	23/23	10/30	7.3/36.5	
Great vessel	Point	37/37	15/45	10.6/53	Aneurysm
	<10	31/31	13/39	9.4/47	
Trachea and large bronchus	Point	20.2/20.2	10/30	8/40	Stenosis/fistula
	<4	10.5/10.5	5/15	3.3/16.5	

[a] The rib/chest wall as a critical structure: Factors associated with increasing chest wall toxicity are currently active areas of investigation. Tumor location, especially peripheral lesions, will increase the potential for any such risk. Therefore, since the goal of any plan is to optimize target treatment parameters, assessment of rib dosing must be ALARA (as low as reasonably achievable) and in no way adjusted to compromise target coverage or restrict potential delivery parameters for the sake of rib dosing. Rib "limits" provided in the table may in that respect be exceeded for an otherwise excellent plan.

SBRT, stereotactic body radiation therapy.

Outcomes

LC of the index lesion after lung SBRT is typically defined as the absence of tumor progression within 1 cm of the primary tumor site[105] and has historically ranged from 90% to 98%,[102,105,109,113,114,119,128,129] consistent with prospective surgical series showing a loco-regional failure rate of 5% to 7% for lobectomy and 8% to 17% for sub-lobar resection.[130,131] A pooled meta-analysis of 40 SBRT studies totaling 4,850 patients and 23 surgical studies (lobar or sub-lobar resection, 7,071 patients in total) likewise suggest no significant differences in LC.[129] SBRT is remarkably well tolerated in the medically inoperable population. Pulmonary function is well conserved with generally <3% risk of radiation pneumonitis, and even in patients with extremely compromised pulmonary function exhibiting overall survival (OS) outcomes at or above the mean,[132–134] suggesting there is no lower limit to pulmonary function for SBRT provided patients are medically stable. Neuropathic pain and rib fractures may occur with 10% to 15% of treatments of targets abutting the chest wall, though symptoms are generally modest

and potentially less common than in surgical series.[135,136] Skin ulcers,[137] brachial plexopathy,[138] and bronchial[139] or esophageal fistulas[140] have been reported, though they are extremely uncommon and risk is modifiable during the planning process when identified.

Endobronchial Brachytherapy

Endobronchial brachytherapy is a useful method of achieving palliation after previous radiation for recurrent centrally located obstructive lesions. In most reports, rates of relief from hemoptysis and obstructive symptoms are high, while cough is less frequently improved.[52,141–143] A range of dose regimens have been used with most using weekly dosing such as 7 Gy × 3. Potential complications include pneumothorax from the endobronchial catheter, as well as 5% to 10% risk of high-grade hemoptysis due to the combination of cumulative treatment dose and recurrence of resistant central disease. Mesh-based brachytherapy sewn to the surgical staple line has also been investigated in conjunction is sub-lobar resection of early-stage NSCLC but is associated with increased risk of complications without improving recurrence rates.[131]

Proton Therapy

Although modern photon therapy advancements, such as IMRT, IGRT, and MRgRT, have improved treatment planning and delivery of RT, the doses needed to control or eradicate disease for most thoracic malignancies typically exceed the safety tolerance of many of the key thoracic OARs. Consequently, the physical properties of PT, where the majority of the proton dose is deposited across a very narrow range with little to no "exit" dose in the remainder of the thoracic structures, known as the Bragg peak, have supported the continuous development of this technology for patients with thoracic malignancies. The two treatment planning and delivery techniques used in PT, passively scattered PT and active scanning PT (also referred to as "pencil beam scanning [PBS] PT"), utilize a high-energy proton beam to cover the target volume.[144] PBS is the newer form of PT delivery and, unlike passively scattered PT, is able to conform the dose of the proximal edge of the target volume, in addition to the distal edge, and has led to the development of intensity-modulated PT (IMPT).[145] Similar to IMRT, IMPT delivers RT using multiple individual heterogeneous fields, with the summation of all of the fields yielding a homogeneous isodose distribution across the target volume. Given the superior dosimetry of PT to photon therapy but with lack of certainty on how this impacts patient outcomes, PT is being evaluated in a number of clinical studies in patients with thoracic malignancies.

For patients with medically inoperable early-stage NSCLC, dosimetric studies comparing PT and photon therapy have demonstrated a potential for reduction of dose to key OARs.[146] For example, a meta-analysis of 72 photon SBRT series and 9 PT studies in patients with early-stage NSCLC demonstrated a higher 5-year overall survival in patients treated with PT (60% vs. 41.3%, $p = 0.005$), attributed to a reduced risk of high-grade pneumonitis (grade 3+ 0.9% vs. 3.4%, $p = 0.001$) or any pneumonitis (4.8% vs. 6.9%, $p = 0.05$).[147]

Limitations in dose-escalation with photon therapy for patients with locally advanced NSCLC have also led to exploring the role of PT in this setting. In the absence of phase III data comparing modalities, results from a National Cancer Database (NCDB) study comparing the outcomes of patients with NSCLC treated with photon therapy and PT are suggestive in that they demonstrated a higher overall survival after propensity-matching analysis (22% vs. 16%, $p = 0.025$) in PT-treated patients, especially those with stage II–III disease.[148] That said, a Bayesian adaptive randomized controlled trial of passively scattered PT and IMRT recently reported no difference in grade 3 radiation pneumonitis or local failure between the two treatment arms.[149] Results from RTOG 1308, a phase III trial that intends to randomize over 300 medically

inoperable patients with locally advanced NSCLC to PT or photon therapy (70 Gy in 35 fractions) along with concurrent chemotherapy will be critical since its primary endpoint is overall survival.[150]

PT has also been utilized for patients with limited-stage SCLC, recurrent locally advanced NSCLC, and patients with intact-lung MPM.[151] Finally, given the peri-cardiac location of thymic malignancies and their generally decades-long natural history allowing for development of potential late effects,[152,153] the use of PT for this patient population has been supported by the National Comprehensive Cancer Network guidelines.

There are important caveats to the use of PT in the chest. These involve differences compared to photon approaches including principles of motion management, incorporation of cross-sectional image guidance at time of treatment delivery, robust treatment planning accounting for interplay effects, and careful evaluation for need for adaptive replanning. As with other evolving RT technologies, increasing experience with PT appears to predict for better treatment profiles.[149]

LUNG CANCER
Introduction

In 2019, an estimated 228,150 new cases of lung cancer were diagnosed in the United States, with an estimate of 155,400 lung cancer–related deaths.[154] NSCLC represents about 75% to 85% of lung cancer diagnosis,[154] while SCLC makes up approximately 10% to 15%.[155] Although the use of the TNM staging system is standard for NSCLC, SCLC has traditionally been classified as either limited (LSCLC) or extensive stage (ESCLC), with disease confined to a hemithorax considered limited and all other presentations considered extensive. The AJCC eighth edition cancer staging handbook now recommends that TNM staging be normative for SCLC.[6] The primary risk factor for lung cancer is a history of smoking. Risk may increase by contributions from exposure asbestos and other industrial irritants. Successful promotion of smoking cessation is largely credited with recent decreases in the incidence and mortality rates of lung cancer, particularly in men.[156]

NSCLC
Stage I

Stage I NSCLC comprises only 10% to 15% of all lung cancer diagnoses. The standard of care for stage I disease is lobectomy, which results in excellent LC (95%) and overall survival, ranging from 60% to 80%.[130] Given the risk factors associated with NSCLC, however, many patients cannot tolerate surgical resection. These patients historically fare poorly with observation[157] and are treated with either 3D-CRT or doses ranging from 60 to 74 Gy in conventional fractionation, though as high as 100 Gy has been investigated.[158–160] SBRT is achieving LC rates in the medically inoperable population approaching those of surgical resection,[105,109,129] along with excellent LC and overall survival in limited use in the operable population.[101,102] The reader is referred to the section on SBRT for further details. More hypofractionated courses in conventional RT such as 60 Gy in 15 fractions have been recently described as both safe and effective.[121,161]

Stage II

Stage II NSCLC is even less common than stage I,[154] and almost universally treated surgically as the need for nodal coverage typically prevents radiation doses from reaching levels which would attain equivalent LC.[55,159,162] Patients unable to tolerate surgical resection can be treated with concurrent or sequential chemoradiotherapy, or RT alone if unable to tolerate the additional of CHT.[70] Similar dose and targeting strategies as those discussed for stage III disease apply here as well.

Stage III

Operable and Surgically Resectable

Stage III is the most challenging NSCLC presentation due to its tumor and nodal heterogeneity. A decision point in the management of many stage III patients is the role, if any, of surgery in addition to CHT and RT (known collectively as trimodality therapy). Much like stage II disease, the LC achieved with definitive chemoradiotherapy does not reach the levels attained by the addition of surgical resection due to limitations of normal tissue toxicity on radiation dose for fields including significant portions of the mediastinum.[159,162] However, the predominant cause of mortality in lung cancer is distant metastatic failure, hence bringing into question the role of any local therapy. Two randomized trials in this patient population have compared definitive chemoradiotherapy to induction chemoradiotherapy followed by surgical resection. The Intergroup 0139 study randomized 396 patients with technically resectable surgically staged IIIA (N2) NSCLC to either (1) definitive RT to 61 Gy concurrent with 2 cycles of CHT or (2) the same CHT concurrent with RT to 45 Gy followed by resection. There was no benefit to overall survival afforded by the surgery despite progression-free survival being improved.[55] A second randomized study, European Organisation for Research and Treatment of Cancer (EORTC) 08941, showed no difference in either of these survival endpoints for trimodality therapy compared to chemoradiotherapy.[163] Patient selection is critical in this patient group, and the risks of surgery based on a particular patient's cardio-pulmonary status must be balanced with respect to the LC benefit of surgical resection.

For those who receive trimodality therapy, the most common induction regimen is 45 Gy in 25 fractions with concurrent CHT.[164] Phase II trials have explored the safety, efficacy, and outcomes for dose-escalated RT (60 Gy/30 fractions) in this setting,[165,166] but to date no phase III data show superiority of this approach.

Definitive RT

The standard of care for nonoperative treatment of stage III NSCLC is concurrent CHT and RT given as 60 Gy in 30 fractions (see Figure 7.4) based on the most current phase III randomized study showing no advantage, and potentially some detriment, to dose escalation beyond 60 Gy in 30 fractions.[57] RTOG 0617 randomly assigned 544 patients to receive either 60 Gy in 30 fractions or 74 Gy in 37 fractions, with or without the addition of cetuximab to standard CHT. There was an unexpected overall survival detriment to high-dose radiation and notably also a decrease in LC. The addition of cetuximab likewise increased toxicity without benefit to overall survival. Finally, altered fractionation

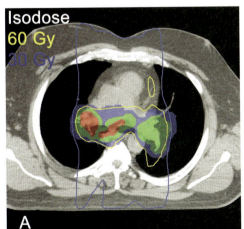
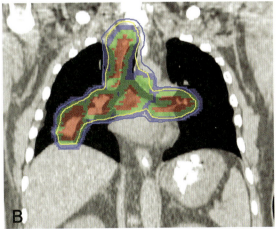

FIGURE 7.4. Sixty-year-old male with stage IIIB T1N3 (biopsy-proven contralateral hilar lymph nodes) M0 adenocarcinoma of the RLL lung, treated with definitive chemoradiotherapy consisting of weekly carboplatin/paclitaxel and concurrent RT followed by consolidation carboplatin/paclitaxel; RT given as 60 Gy/30 fx delivered with 6 MV photons via 7-field IMRT prescribed per plan to the 98.5% IDL. Representative axial **(A)** and coronal **(B)** CT planning images.

does not appear to have significant benefit in the setting of concurrent CHT.[60] For patients who cannot tolerate concurrent CHT with RT, sequential therapy is recommended. When delivering sequential therapy or RT alone, there may be a benefit to dose escalation.[167–169] A significant development in NSCLC over the past 5 years has been the introduction of immune checkpoint inhibitors into comprehensive therapy. The recent PACIFIC trial demonstrated a substantial improvement in overall survival with the use of anti-PD-L1 inhibitors as consolidative therapy for patients who do not progress after completion of definitive chemoradiation in stage III NSCLC[170] compared to standard consolidative chemotherapy.

In the definitive setting, ENI is not recommended.[171,172] While local failure inside the high-dose volume is a significant contributor to treatment failure, recurrence in omitted potential elective nodal regions was low in a prospective series.[173]

Early randomized trials examined the role of PCI in both NSCLC and SCLC and did find that rates of brain metastasis were reduced in both diseases; however, unlike in SCLC where PCI improved survival,[174] a modern randomized study in NSCLC showed no benefit despite some reduction in the frequency of future brain metastasis.[175]

Postoperative Radiation

While four randomized trials have confirmed a survival advantage for the addition of adjuvant CHT for resected stage II–III NSCLC,[176–180] adjuvant radiation has a more limited range of indications. In N2+ disease the Lung Cancer Study Group (included in postoperative radiation [PORT] meta-analysis) demonstrated improved LC for PORT without a survival detriment.[181,182] A subset analysis of a randomized adjuvant CHT study[183] and reviews of the surveillance, epidemiology, and end results, and NCDB also suggest the potential for a survival advantage when modern techniques and smaller fields are utilized in the setting of resected stage III NSCLC.[184]

PORT is typically delivered sequentially after completion of CHT; however, in the setting of positive margins, concurrent delivery is an alternative.[59] The target volume for PORT is the bronchial stump and hilum, as well as known clinically and pathologically involved mediastinal nodal stations. Intervening nodal stations may be covered as well. Recommended dose is 50 Gy in 25 fractions for patients with negative margins. Dose should be increased to 54 to 60 Gy in 27 to 30 fractions for close or positive margins.

Stage IV

The primary role of radiation in metastatic NSCLC is the palliation of symptoms prior to the initiation of systemic CHT or in patients who are unable to receive systemic therapy at all. The reader is referred to the section on Dose given earlier.

SMALL CELL LUNG CANCER

Limited Disease

Thoracic RT
Dose/Fractionation

The standard of care in the treatment of LSCLC is 45 Gy given as BID fractions of 1.5 Gy for a total of 30 fractions over 3 weeks. Initially demonstrated to be superior to a once-daily fractionation schedule in the landmark phase III Intergroup 0096 study,[62] this dose/fractionation schedule was reconfirmed as the standard of care by the results of the CONVERT (Concurrent ONce daily VErsus twice daily RT) phase III trial in which patients were randomized to either 45 Gy/1.5 Gy BID in 30 fractions or 66 Gy in 33 once-daily fractions, both starting with the second cycle of CHT.[185] Another phase III trial is also being carried out investigating dose escalation. Final results from CALGB 30610/RTOG 0538, a trial in which patients were to be randomized to either 70 Gy/2 Gy once-daily over 7 weeks or 45 Gy/1.5 Gy BID, remain pending.

Timing/Sequencing/Duration

In fit patients, thoracic RT should be administered early, rather than late, in the course of administering CHT cycles since early initiation is associated with improved survival as shown in a range of randomized trials and three major meta-analyses.[186–188] Within this concept of RT timing, overall treatment duration may in fact be the most important factor associated with LC and overall survival in LS-SCLC.[186] De Ruysscher and colleagues have promoted the concept of SER, an acronym for the "Start of any treatment until the End of RT," in the treatment of LS-SCLC. Their analysis suggests the SER is the most important predictor with respect to outcomes. The biological rationale for this observation is that shortening the overall time of RT delivery (i.e., acceleration) reduces the potential for triggering accelerated repopulation in SCLC stem cells, which could lead to resistant cells.

Treatment Volume

In 1987, the Southwest Oncology Group (SWOG) investigated the question of treatment volume in SCLC in a phase III trial.[189] Patients were randomized to treatment with either a pre-CHT or a post-CHT target designed at the time of RT planning. The study showed that the RT target can be restricted to the residual visible tumor (post-CHT target) without increasing the risk of local failure. Almost 35 years after SWOG 7924 was completed, Hu et al. published in 2020 results of the only other randomized that has addressed the same question of pre- versus post-CHT target delineation in treated LSCLC, however with the trial now conducted in the era of modern RT planning, including access to PET staging and 3D conformal radiotherapy.[190] The study confirmed that it is appropriate to use the post-CHT target for treatment planning because it is not associated with increased rates of failure or changes in overall survival.

Designing SCLC targets without ENI had once been controversial[191] but is now considered accepted practice in most clinical centers, as long as PET imaging is used as a planning tool.[192] This was first supported by the prospective study from van Loon and colleagues[193] that involved PET-based planning when designing the thoracic target. It showed that omission of ENI only resulted in a 3% rate of out-of-target nodal failures. More recently, the randomized CONVERT trial, which specifically omitted ENI and showed better than expected overall survival compared to historic controls as well as lower toxicity rates than expected, provides further evidence that a non-ENI strategy can be considered safe and effective.[185]

Extensive Disease

Thoracic RT

In incurable ESCLC, thoracic RT is conventionally used for relief and palliation of local symptoms. In 1999, a novel role for thoracic RT in advanced-stage SCLC patients was published by Jeremic and colleagues.[63] In this phase III study, ESCLC patients who had received induction CHT and had shown response were randomized to either accelerated hyperfractionated thoracic RT (50.4 Gy/36 BID fractions over 18 days) and concurrent low-dose daily CHT or to CHT alone. The 5-year OS rate for those receiving thoracic RT compared to those not receiving it was 9.1% vs. 3.7%, respectively, and was statistically significant. These results however did not prompt widespread introduction of thoracic RT in the care of ESCLC patients. Slotman et al.[194] reported the results of a phase III trial looking at the impact on overall survival of adding thoracic RT after PCI compared to PCI alone for ESCLC patients who showed any response after 4 to 6 cycles of CHT. The thoracic RT consisted of 30 Gy in 10 fractions. The primary endpoint of this study was improvement in overall survival at 1 year by the addition of RT and was not met. Secondary endpoints of LC as well as 2-year overall survival were improved however which has prompted some clinicians to use it in selected patients. RTOG 0937 was a randomized phase II study comparing PCI alone to PCI and consolidative RT to the chest and to a limited number of partially responding distant metastases. Its results did not show any improvement in overall survival in the experimental arm.[195] In light of the recent addition of immunotherapy to the standard systemic management of ESCLC, the role of thoracic RT remains even more indeterminate. Thus, the addition of thoracic RT cannot be considered to be a standard of care at this time.

PCI in LSCLC and ESCLC

Indications

PCI is considered standard of care for LSCLC patients. In 1999, Auperin and colleagues published a meta-analysis of completed randomized trials of PCI in SCLC[174] and reported that it yields a 25.3% decreased incidence of brain metastases at 3 years with overall and disease-free survivals in the PCI group by 5.4% and 8.8%, respectively, at 3 years, compared to patients not receiving PCI.

In 2007, the EORTC reported the results of a phase III trial in which ESCLC patients were randomized to PCI or observation after CHT.[196] At 1 year, the PCI patients were found to have a significantly lower rate of symptomatic brain metastases but more strikingly, improved 1-year (27% vs. 13%) survivals compared to the patients in the no-PCI arm. In response to these findings, Takahashi and colleagues subsequently conducted a phase III trial in which patients with ESCLC were randomized following chemotherapy and in the absence of progression to PCI versus brain MRI monitoring. The study did not show any difference in terms of OS between the two arms.[197] The role of PCI in this patient population remains controversial.

Dose and Toxicity in PCI

The total dose used in PCI is modest: 25 Gy in 10 fractions delivered by opposed lateral fields remains the standard of care in LSCLC based on phase III data showing no benefits to dose escalation.[198] Doses in ESCLC can be more variable given the advanced disease stage. Currently, concerns about neurotoxicity in long-term survivors have become a major issue with use of PCI. PCI-related neurocognitive toxicities appear dose dependent.[199] In a meta-analysis of two RTOG studies evaluating PCI, it was observed that the addition of PCI relative to observation led to a decline in objective and self-reported cognitive functioning at 6 and 12 months after treatment.[200] In efforts to potentially reduce this toxicity, an ongoing cooperative group study, NRG CC003, is currently being conducted to define the role of IMRT-based hippocampal-avoidance whole brain RT (HA-WBRT) in SCLC patients undergoing PCI since the hippocampus is part of the brain that is important for memory.[201] This phase II/III study includes patients with limited or extensive-stage disease who are then randomized to receive PCI with or without HA-WBRT.

MESOTHELIOMA

Introduction

MPM is an uncommon tumor strongly associated with asbestos exposure. MPM is staged according to the AJCC staging system.[202] Medically fit, potentially resectable patients are treated surgically with EPP or with pleurectomy and decortication (P/D). Controversy exists regarding the optimal surgical approach, but combined modality treatment can have good outcomes in favorable patients.[203–207] Studies suggest that any surgical resection is preferable to RT alone from a LC standpoint.[208] Patients who are unresectable are treated palliatively with CHT and RT as needed.[209]

Indications

Historically there have been two conventional indications for RT for MPM: (1) as adjuvant therapy following definitive surgical resection with EPP and (2) for palliation of symptoms. With recent surgical evolution shifting away from EPP and to more limited P/D second to toxicity in this group of patients with a limited prognosis[210] there has been increasing use of IMRT-based consolidative treatment of the residual involved pleura.[208,211-213] This treatment is complex and challenging with a target volume consisting of the residual ipsilateral pleural margin excluding the fissures and attempting to spare as much of the central portion of the lung as possible. Reported XRT doses range from 45 to 50 Gy to the pleura with intermittent use of a boost to 54 to 60 Gy to gross residual disease with the final dose limited by normal tissue tolerance.[211,214] The large size of the treatment field, complex contouring of the target to include pleural reflections, and presence of many adjacent normal tissue structures make such plans quite complex. While early reports suggest the possibility of substantial increase in overall survival after P/D with hemi-thoracic IMRT compared to focal palliative radiation (2y OS 58% vs. 28%, $p = 0.003$), toxicity can be substantial, and additional multicenter randomized trials are actively accruing.

RT prophylaxis to drain or biopsy sites is a controversial indication due to conflicting results from a small number of randomized trials, with the most current suggesting rates of surgical track recurrences are not improved by its addition.[215,216]

Simulation

For mesothelioma it is crucial to encompass the entire extent of the pleural surface within the CT simulation scan. Particular attention to the lower boarder of the scan is critical as the diaphragm can extend as low as L3 and this recess is a common site of failure.[217] All scars and drain sites should be identified with radiopaque wire. Clinicians should consider application of bolus to drain sites or areas of chest wall invasion. After P/D, the standard principles of thoracic RT should be followed. For patients who can tolerate, we have found deep-inspiration breath-hold gating to be useful in the setting of post-P/D hemi-thoracic IMRT, by both reducing/eliminating ITV expansion along the diaphragm and more critically increasing the total lung volume, allowing better sparing of the expanded central lung when treating the full pleural rim.

Target Volume

After EPP, the CTV for adjuvant RT is defined as the entire resected pleural surfaces (chest wall, pericardium, diaphragmatic crural insertions, any reconstructed diaphragm, ipsilateral hilum, and mediastinal boundary). Surgical clips can aid in the delineation of the medial aspect of the diaphragm, inferior diaphragmatic insertion, and sterno-pericardial recess in particular. IMRT studies have suggested this sterno-pericardial recess is a particular site of recurrence.[208] A boost to the ipsilateral mediastinum can be applied in the setting of resected N2 disease, positive margins, or residual disease. CTV-PTV expansion is typically 5 to 10 mm.[212]

Dose/Fractionation

In the adjuvant setting, 54 Gy at 2 Gy per fraction is standard following R0 resection for EPP. An example of the resulting treated PTV is shown in Figure 7.5. In cases of positive margin or pathologically involved mediastinal nodes, a boost to a total dose of 60 Gy in 2 Gy fractions is recommended.[217,218] Following P/D or as definitive RT, doses of 45 to 50.4 Gy with a boost to 54 to 60 Gy for residual disease have been employed with acceptable toxicity and control.[212] For palliative treatment, minimal doses of 40 Gy and at least 4 Gy per fraction appear to be associated with improved symptom control, compared to conventional palliative schedules, for example, 30 Gy in 10 fractions.[219-221]

Treatment Planning

Adjuvant RT following EPP was historically performed with AP/PA fields and electrons to supplement dose in key areas.[217] IMRT is now recommended in this setting as it allows for better sparing of normal tissues, and outcomes do not appear to be inferior to conventional field arrangements.[222] Rates of severe pulmonary toxicity with IMRT however may be higher than expected due to the delivery approach selected.[218,223,224] To minimize the risk of pulmonary toxicity, dosimetrists need to avoid beam entry through the remaining lung and to restrict the mean lung dose to the contralateral lung to 8.5 Gy or less. Following P/D, only an IMRT approach is indicated. A substantial difference in planning technique for the post-EPP, cavity versus with an intact lung is that post-EPP, the center of the resection cavity (which is a fluid-filled space) can serve as a repository for hot spots without restriction of dose; however with an intact lung, in addition to constraints on the contralateral lung, sparing the center of the residual intact lung takes on more critical importance with additional planning constraints.

THYMOMA

Indications

Thymomas represent the most common tumor in the anterior mediastinum.[225,226] Most patients present with localized disease and surgical resection provides histologic conformation of the diagnosis and is often curative as a single modality. In addition to the completeness of surgical resection, the Masaoka stage and specific histologic classification of the tumor are important prognostic factors.[225-229] Adjuvant therapy is the most common RT indication and is generally recommended for patients who present with stages III–IV but is controversial for stage II. Definitive RT is offered to the rare patients who is medically inoperable or who as a tumor which is also surgically unresectable. Patients with Masaoka stage I thymomas (macroscopically and microscopically encapsulated) are managed with surgical resection

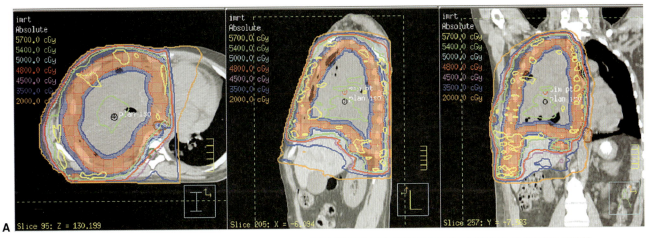

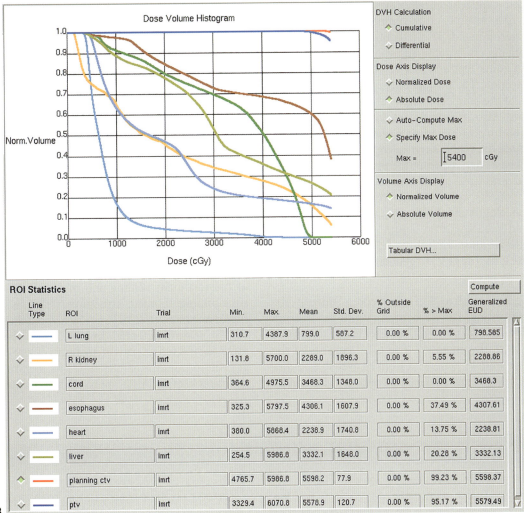

FIGURE 7.5. (A) Representative axial, coronal, and sagittal images from the treatment plan and **(B)** the DVH for a 40-year-old male with right thoracic epithelioid mesothelioma treated with 3 cycles induction chemotherapy, then a right extrapleural pneumonectomy followed by adjuvant right pleural space IMRT-based radiotherapy (54 Gy in 27 fractions). The mean lung dose is 7.99 Gy.

alone. Local recurrences are rare (<5%) and patients may be salvaged with repeat excision.[230] For Masaoka stage II disease (microscopic transcapsular invasion or macroscopic invasion into surrounding fatty tissue with or without adherence to the mediastinal pleura or pericardium), modern retrospective studies had failed to demonstrate a LC benefit to adjuvant RT[230] but a recent meta-analysis suggests a possible survival and control benefit to postoperative RT.[231] Adjuvant RT is generally recommended for patients with stage III thymomas (macroscopic invasion into nearby organs such as the pericardium, great vessels, or lung) since only 50%

of patients undergo complete surgical resection and the local recurrence remains considerable even in this setting.[232–235]

Thymic carcinomas are considerably rarer than thymomas, and patients often present with locally advanced disease.[227] Patients often undergo multimodality treatment including upfront surgical resection with adjuvant CHT and RT.[236,237] Adjuvant RT may provide a locoregional control and possible survival benefit in patients with resected thymic carcinomas, although data from different retrospective reviews are conflicting.[230,235–238]

Postoperative RT

A dose of 45 to 50 Gy is recommended for adjuvant RT in the setting of a negative or close-margin resection. For patients with a microscopically involved resection margin, a dose of 54 to 60 Gy is recommended. A dose of 60 to 70 Gy is recommended for patients with gross residual disease. Patients undergoing adjuvant RT for a resected thymic carcinoma typically receive 60 Gy after complete surgical resection. The postoperative CTV should be referenced off of pre-surgical imaging and reflect the operative findings. Also it should contain any gross residual disease visible on postoperative imaging studies. The CTV should include the visible surgical clips in the tumor bed, the tumor bed as derived from the preoperative extent of disease, and other areas at risk for subclinical microscopic disease. In patients with a positive resection margin, the radiation oncologist should discuss the findings with the surgeon and pathologist to ensure adequate coverage of the at-risk regions. Typically, a 0.5 to 1 cm margin is added to the CTV (or ITV) to generate the PTV.

Preoperative RT

Typically, a dose of 45 to 50 Gy is recommended in the preoperative setting, delivered in conventional fraction sizes of 1.8 to 2.0 Gy per fraction. ENI is not warranted in patients with thymomas.[239] The GTV consists of the visible tumor volume, generated from all available studies including CT scans and FDG-PET scans. A CTV can be

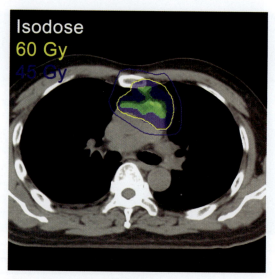

FIGURE 7.6. 66-year-old male with resected thymic carcinoma and positive margins. Representative axial CT image from postoperative TRT plan of 60 Gy in 30 fx at 2 Gy/fx delivered with 6 MV photons via two VMAT arc fields prescribed to the 96.9% isodose line (IDL).

generated with a 0.5 to 1 cm margin to account for extension of microscopic disease. If a 4DCT scan is acquired at the time of simulation, an ITV can then be generated. Typically, a 0.5 to 1 cm margin is added to the CTV (or ITV) to generate the PTV.

Treatment Planning

Patients treated with either 3D-CRT or IMRT need planning techniques designed to maximize the conformality of the treatment volume and minimize the dose to the surrounding thoracic structures.[234] PT is currently of increasing interest. IMRT may be favored due to perceived cardiac sparing potential. In 3D-CRT, the beam arrangement should reflect patient anatomy, extent of the RT target volume, and proximity to OARs. Figure 7.6 provides an example of an IMRT approach in the adjuvant setting.

KEY POINTS

- The treatment of thoracic malignancies with RT is challenging because of the limitations in dose delivery imposed by a range of highly sensitive normal structures in the thorax.

- Lung cancer is the most common thoracic malignancy and also kills more cancer patients than any other because one half of newly diagnosed patients are essentially incurable at presentation. Palliative therapy is therefore the most common RT indication.

- Technological and planning improvements in RT delivery, such as IMRT, adoption of motion management,

integration of 4DCT into planning, and consistent use of DVHs, have enhanced our understanding of the benefits and side effect potential of treatment to the chest.

- SBRT has created a new paradigm of RT care by offering medically inoperable lung cancer patients with early-stage disease the possibility of safe and effective cure.

- Ongoing refinements in RT delivery, such as particle therapies, are geared toward minimizing toxicity in potentially curable patients.

REFERENCES

1. O'Rahilly R, Müller F, Carpenter S, et al. *Basic Human Anatomy: A Regional Study of Human Structure.* Hanover, NA: Dartmouth Medical School; 2004.

2. Vansteenkiste JF, Stroobants SG. The role of positron emission tomography with 18F-fluoro-2-deoxy-D-glucose in respiratory oncology. *Eur Respir J.* 2001;17:802–820.

3. Pieterman RM, van Putten JW, Meuzelaar JJ, et al. Preoperative staging of non-small-cell lung cancer with positron-emission tomography. *N Engl J Med.* 2000;343:254–261.

4. Rengan R, Chetty IJ, Decker R, et al. Lung cancer. In: Perez CA, Halperin EC, Brady LW, Wazer DE, eds. *Perez & Brady's Principles and Practice of Radiation Oncology.* 6th ed. Wolters Kluwer, Lippincott, Wilkins and Williams; 2013.

5. Suster DI, Mino-Kenudson M. Molecular pathology of primary non-small cell lung cancer. *Arch Med Res.* 2020;51:784–798.

6. Part VII Thorax. In: Amin MB, Edge S, Greene F, et al., eds. *AJCC Cancer Staging Handbook.* 8th ed. Chicago, IL: Springer; 2018: 423–470.

7. Rusch VW, Asamura H, Watanabe H, et al. The IASLC lung cancer staging project: a proposal for a new international lymph node map in the forthcoming seventh edition of the TNM classification for lung cancer. *J Thorac Oncol.* 2009;4:568–577.

8. Kay FU, Kandathil A, Batra K, et al. Revisions to the tumor, node, metastasis staging of lung cancer (8th edition): rationale, radiologic findings and clinical implications. *World J Radiol.* 2017;9:269–279.

9. Maharjan N, Thapa N, Tu J. Blood-based biomarkers for early diagnosis of lung cancer: areview article. *JNMA J Nepal Med Assoc.* 2020;58:519–524.

10. Senan S, De Ruysscher D, Giraud P, et al. Literature-based recommendations for treatment planning and execution in high-dose radiotherapy for lung cancer. *Radiother Oncol.* 2004;71:139–146.

11. Cascade PN, Gross BH, Kazerooni EA, et al. Variability in the detection of enlarged mediastinal lymph nodes in staging lung cancer: a comparison of contrast-enhanced and unenhanced CT. *AJR Am J Roentgenol.* 1998;170:927–931.

12. Patz EFJr, Erasmus JJ, McAdams HP, et al. Lung cancer staging and management: comparison of contrast-enhanced and non-enhanced helical CT of the thorax. *Radiology.* 1999;212:56–60.

13. Seppenwoolde Y, Shirato H, Kitamura K, et al. Precise and real-time measurement of 3D tumor motion in lung due to breathing and heartbeat, measured during radiotherapy. *Int J Radiat Oncol Biol Phys.* 2002;53:822–834.

14. Mageras GS, Pevsner A, Yorke ED, et al. Measurement of lung tumor motion using respiration-correlated CT. *Int J Radiat Oncol Biol Phys.* 2004;60:933–941.

15. Underberg RWM, Lagerwaard FJ, Cuijpers JP, et al. Four-dimensional CT scans for treatment planning in stereotactic radiotherapy for stage I lung cancer. *Int J Radiat Oncol Biol Phys.* 2004;60: 1283–1290.

16. Keall PJ, Mageras GS, Balter JM, et al. The management of respiratory motion in radiation oncology report of AAPM task group 76. *Med Phys.* 2006;33:3874–3900.

17. Rosu M, Balter JM, Chetty IJ, et al. How extensive of a 4D dataset is needed to estimate cumulative dose distribution plan evaluation metrics in conformal lung therapy? *Med Phys.* 2007;34:233–245.

18. Underberg RW, Lagerwaard FJ, Slotman BJ, et al. Use of maximum intensity projections (MIP) for target volume generation in 4DCT scans for lung cancer. *Int J Radiat Oncol Biol Phys.* 2005;63: 253–260.

19. Glide-Hurst CK, Hugo GD, Liang J, et al. A simplified method of four-dimensional dose accumulation using the mean patient density representation. *Med Phys.* 2008;35:5269–5277.

20. Woody NM, Stephans KL, Videtic GMM, et al. Systematic errors in lung stereotactic body radiation therapy (SBRT): a caution on mixing and matching target delineation methods and planning CTs. *J Radiat Oncol.* 2015;4:185–191

21. Negoro Y, Nagata Y, Aoki T, et al. The effectiveness of an immobilization device in conformal radiotherapy for lung tumor: reduction of respiratory tumor movement and evaluation of the daily setup accuracy. *Int J Radiat Oncol Biol Phys.* 2001;50:889–898.

22. Wong JW, Sharpe MB, Jaffray DA, et al. The use of active breathing control (ABC) to reduce margin for breathing motion. *Int J Radiat Oncol Biol Phys.* 1999;44:911–919.

23. International Commission on Radiation Units and Measurements. ICRU report 50. prescribing, recording, and reporting photon beam therapy. 1993.

24. Harris KM, Adams H, Lloyd DC, et al. The effect on apparent size of simulated pulmonary nodules of using three standard CT window settings. *Clin Radiol.* 1993;47:241–244.

25. International Commission on Radiation Units and Measurements. ICRU report 62. prescribing, recording and reporting photon beam therapy (supplement to ICRU report 50). 1999.

26. Ezhil M, Vedam S, Balter P, et al. Determination of patient-specific internal gross tumor volumes for lung cancer using four-dimensional computed tomography. *Radiat Oncol.* 2009;4:4–18.

27. Balter JM, Ten Haken RK, Lawrence TS, et al. Uncertainties in CT-based radiation therapy treatment planning associated with patient breathing. *Int J Radiat Oncol Biol Phys.* 1996;36:167–174.

28. Shih HA, Jiang SB, Aljarrah KM, et al. Internal target volume determined with expansion margins beyond composite gross tumor volume in three-dimensional conformal radiotherapy for lung cancer. *Int J Radiat Oncol Biol Phys.* 2004;60:613–622.

29. Lagerwaard FJ, Van Sornsen dK, Nijssen-Visser MR, et al. Multiple "slow" CT scans for incorporating lung tumor mobility in radiotherapy planning. *Int J Radiat Oncol Biol Phys.* 2001;51:932–937.

30. Giraud P, Antoine M, Larrouy A, et al. Evaluation of microscopic tumor extension in non-small-cell lung cancer for three-dimensional conformal radiotherapy planning. *Int J Radiat Oncol Biol Phys.* 2000;48:1015–1024.

31. Yuan S, Meng X, Yu J, et al. Determining optimal clinical target volume margins on the basis of microscopic extracapsular extension of metastatic nodes in patients with non-small-cell lung cancer. *Int J Radiat Oncol Biol Phys.* 2007;67:727–734.

32. Kong FS, Ritter T, Quint DJ, et al. Consideration of dose limits for organs at risk of thoracic radiotherapy: atlas for lung, proximal bronchial tree, esophagus, spinal cord, ribs, and brachial plexus. *Int J Radiat Oncol Biol Phys.* 2011;81:1442–1457.

33. Marks LB, Yorke ED, Jackson A, et al. Use of normal tissue complication probability models in the clinic. *Int J Radiat Oncol Biol Phys.* 2010;76(3 Suppl):S10–S19.

34. MacManus M, Nestle U, Rosenzweig KE, et al. Use of PET and PET/CT for radiation therapy planning: IAEA expert report 2006–2007. *Radiother Oncol.* 2009;91:85–94.

35. Yu HM, Liu YF, Hou M, et al. Evaluation of gross tumor size using CT, 18F-FDG PET, integrated 18F-FDG PET/CT and pathological analysis in non-small cell lung cancer. *Eur J Radiol.* 2009;72:104–113.

36. Hong R, Halama J, Bova D, et al. Correlation of PET standard uptake value and CT window-level thresholds for target delineation in CT-based radiation treatment planning. *Int J Radiat Oncol Biol Phys.* 2007;67:720–726.

37. Yaremko B, Riauka T, Robinson D, et al. Thresholding in PET images of static and moving targets. *Phys Med Biol.* 2005;50: 5969–5982.

38. Caldwell CB, Mah K, Ung YC, et al. Observer variation in contouring gross tumor volume in patients with poorly defined non-small-cell lung tumors on CT: the impact of 18FDG-hybrid PET fusion. *Int J Radiat Oncol Biol Phys.* 2001;51:923–931.

39. Nestle U, Kremp S, Schaefer-Schuler A, et al. Comparison of different methods for delineation of 18F-FDG PET-positive tissue for target volume definition in radiotherapy of patients with non-small cell lung cancer. *J Nucl Med.* 2005;46:1342–1348.

40. De Ruysscher D, Wanders S, Minken A, et al. Effects of radiotherapy planning with a dedicated combined PET-CT-simulator of patients with non-small cell lung cancer on dose limiting normal tissues and radiation dose-escalation: a planning study. *Radiother Oncol.* 2005;77:5–10.

41. Lavrenkov K, Partridge M, Cook G, et al. Positron emission tomography for target volume definition in the treatment of non-small cell lung cancer. *Radiother Oncol.* 2005;77:1–4.

42. Toloza EM, Harpole L, McCrory DC. Noninvasive staging of non-small cell lung cancer: a review of the current evidence. *Chest.* 2003;123:137S–146S.

43. Nestle U, Kremp S, Grosu AL. Practical integration of [18F]-FDG-PET and PET-CT in the planning of radiotherapy for non-small cell lung cancer (NSCLC): the technical basis, ICRU-target volumes, problems, perspectives. *Radiother Oncol.* 2006;81:209–225.

44. Grgic A, Nestle U, Schaefer-Schuler A, et al. FDG-PET-based radiotherapy planning in lung cancer: optimum breathing protocol and patient positioning—an intraindividual comparison. *Int J Radiat Oncol Biol Phys.* 2009;73:103–111.

45. Rodriguez Fernandez A, Gomez Rio M, Llamas Elvira JM, et al. Diagnosis efficacy of structural (CT) and functional (FDG-PET) imaging methods in the thoracic and extrathoracic staging of non-small cell lung cancer. *Clin Transl Oncol.* 2007; 9:32–39.

46. Li R, Yu L, Lin S, et al. Involved field radiotherapy (IFRT) versus elective nodal irradiation (ENI) for locally advanced non-small cell lung cancer: a meta-analysis of incidence of elective nodal failure (ENF). *Radiat Oncol.* 2016;11:124–131.

47. Kong FM, Lally BE, Chang JY, et al. ACR appropriateness criteria(R) radiation therapy for small-cell lung cancer. *Am J Clin Oncol.* 2013;36:206–213.

48. Chang JY, Kestin LL, Barriger RB, et al. ACR appropriateness criteria(R) nonsurgical treatment for locally advanced non-small-cell lung cancer: good performance status/definitive intent. *Oncology (Williston Park)* 2014;28:706,10, 712, 714 passim.

49. De Ruysscher D, Faivre-Finn C, Nestle U, et al. European organisation for research and treatment of cancer recommendations for planning and delivery of high-dose, high-precision radiotherapy for lung cancer. *J Clin Oncol.* 2010;28:5301–5310.

50. Gewanter RM, Rosenzweig KE, Chang JY, et al. ACR appropriateness criteria: nonsurgical treatment for non-small-cell lung cancer: good performance status/definitive intent. *Curr Probl Cancer.* 2010;34:228–249.

51. Decker RH, Langer CJ, Rosenzweig KE, et al. ACR appropriateness criteria: postoperative adjuvant therapy in non-small cell lung cancer. *Am J Clin Oncol.* 2011;34:537–544.

52. Rosenzweig KE, Chang JY, Chetty IJ, et al. ACR appropriateness criteria: nonsurgical treatment for non-small-cell lung cancer: poor performance status or palliative intent. *J Am Coll Radiol.* 2013;10:654–664.

53. Rodrigues G, Videtic GMM, Sur R, et al. Palliative thoracic radiotherapy in lung cancer: an American Society for Radiation Oncology evidence-based clinical practice guideline. *Pract Radiat Oncol.* 2011;1:60–671.

54. Rusch VW, Giroux DJ, Kraut MJ, et al. Induction chemoradiation and surgical resection for superior sulcus non-small-cell lung carcinomas: long-term results of southwest oncology group trial 9416 (intergroup trial 0160). *J Clin Oncol.* 2007;25:313–318.

55. Albain KS, Swann RS, Rusch VW, et al. Radiotherapy plus chemotherapy with or without surgical resection for stage III non-small-cell lung cancer: a phase III randomised controlled trial. *Lancet.* 2009;374:379–386.

56. Vyfhuis MAL, Burrows WM, Bhooshan N, et al. Implications of pathologic complete response beyond mediastinal nodal clearance with high-dose neoadjuvant chemoradiation therapy in locally advanced, non-small cell lung cancer. *Int J Radiat Oncol Biol Phys.* 2018 Jun 1;101:445–452.

57. Bradley JD, Paulus R, Komaki R, et al. Standard-dose versus high-dose conformal radiotherapy with concurrent and consolidation carboplatin plus paclitaxel with or without cetuximab for patients with stage IIIA or IIIB non-small-cell lung cancer (RTOG 0617): a randomised, two-by-two factorial phase 3 study. *Lancet Oncol.* 2015;16:187–199.

58. Bradley JD, Paulus R, Graham MV, et al. Phase II trial of postoperative adjuvant paclitaxel/carboplatin and thoracic radiotherapy in resected stage II and IIIA non-small-cell lung cancer: promising long-term results of the radiation therapy oncology group--RTOG 9705. *J Clin Oncol.* 2005;23:3480–3487.

59. Keller SM, Adak S, Wagner H, et al. A randomized trial of postoperative adjuvant therapy in patients with completely resected stage II or IIIA non-small-cell lung cancer. eastern cooperative oncology group. *N Engl J Med.* 2000;343:1217–1222.

60. Curran WJJr, Paulus R, Langer CJ, et al. Sequential vs. concurrent chemoradiation for stage III non-small cell lung cancer: randomized phase III trial RTOG 9410. *J Natl Cancer Inst.* 2011;103:1452–1460.

61. Cox JD, Azarnia N, Byhardt RW, et al. A randomized phase I/II trial of hyperfractionated radiation therapy with total doses of 60.0 Gy to 79.2 Gy: possible survival benefit with greater than or equal to 69.6 Gy in favorable patients with radiation therapy oncology group stage III non-small-cell lung carcinoma: report of radiation therapy oncology group 83–11. *J Clin Oncol.* 1990;8:1543–1555.

62. Turrisi AT, Kim K, Blum R, et al. Twice-daily compared with once-daily thoracic radiotherapy in limited small-cell lung cancer treated concurrently with cisplatin and etoposide. *N Engl J Med.* 1999;340:265–271.

63. Jeremic B, Shibamoto Y, Nikolic N, et al. Role of radiation therapy in the combined-modality treatment of patients with extensive disease small-cell lung cancer: a randomized study. *J Clin Oncol.* 1999;17:2092–2099.

64. Saunders M, Dische S, Barrett A, et al. Continuous, hyperfractionated, accelerated radiotherapy (CHART) versus conventional radiotherapy in non-small cell lung cancer: mature data from the randomised multicentre trial. CHART steering committee. *Radiother Oncol.* 1999;52:137–148.

65. Belani CP, Choy H, Bonomi P, et al. Combined chemoradiotherapy regimens of paclitaxel and carboplatin for locally advanced non-small-cell lung cancer: a randomized phase II locally advanced multi-modality protocol. *J Clin Oncol.* 2005;23:5883–5891.

66. Saunders M, Dische S, Barrett A, et al. Continuous hyperfractionated accelerated radiotherapy (CHART) versus conventional radiotherapy in non-small-cell lung cancer: a randomised multicentre trial. CHART steering committee. *Lancet.* 1997;350:161–165.

67. Amini A, Lin SH, Wei C, et al. Accelerated hypofractionated radiation therapy compared to conventionally fractionated radiation therapy for the treatment of inoperable non-small cell lung cancer. *Radiat Oncol.* 2012;7:33–40.

68. Murray N, Coy P, Pater JL, et al. Importance of timing for thoracic irradiation in the combined modality treatment of limited-stage small-cell lung cancer. the national cancer institute of Canada clinical trials group. *J Clin Oncol.* 1993;11:336–344.

69. Gore E, Bae K, Langer C, et al. Phase I/II trial of a COX-2 inhibitor with limited field radiation for intermediate prognosis patients who have locally advanced non-small-cell lung cancer: radiation therapy oncology group 0213. *Clin Lung Cancer.* 2011;12:125–130.

70. Westover KD, Loo BW Jr, Gerber DE, et al. Precision hypofractionated radiation therapy in poor performing patients with non-small cell lung cancer: phase 1 dose escalation trial. *Int J Radiat Oncol Biol Phys.* 2015;93:72–81.

71. Slotman BJ, Njo KH, de Jonge A, et al. Hypofractionated radiation therapy in unresectable stage III non-small cell lung cancer. *Cancer.* 1993;72:1885–1893.

72. Mauguen A, Le Pechoux C, Saunders MI, et al. Hyperfractionated or accelerated radiotherapy in lung cancer: an individual patient data meta-analysis. *J Clin Oncol.* 2012;30:2788–2797.

73. Videtic GM. The role of radiation therapy in small cell lung cancer. *Curr Oncol Rep.* 2013;15:405–410.

74. Ekstrand KE, Barnes WH. Pitfalls in the use of high energy X rays to treat tumors in the lung. *Int J Radiat Oncol Biol Phys.* 1990;18:249–252.

75. Yorke E, Harisiadis L, Wessels B, et al. Dosimetric considerations in radiation therapy of coin lesions of the lung. *Int J Radiat Oncol Biol Phys.* 1996;34:481–487.

76. Miller RC, Bonner JA, Kline RW. Impact of beam energy and field margin on penumbra at lung tumor-lung parenchyma interfaces. *Int J Radiat Oncol Biol Phys.* 1998;41:707–713.

77. Wang L, Yorke E, Desobry G, et al. Dosimetric advantage of using 6 MV over 15 MV photons in conformal therapy of lung cancer: Monte Carlo studies in patient geometries. *J Appl Clin Med Phys.* 2002;3:51–59.

78. Vanderstraeten B, Reynaert N, Paelinck L, et al. Accuracy of patient dose calculation for lung IMRT: a comparison of Monte Carlo, convolution/superposition, and pencil beam computations. *Med Phys.* 2006;33:3149–3158.

79. Knoos T, Wieslander E, Cozzi L, et al. Comparison of dose calculation algorithms for treatment planning in external photon beam therapy for clinical situations. *Phys Med Biol.* 2006;51:5785–5807.

80. Li J, Galvin J, Harrison A, et al. Dosimetric verification using Monte Carlo calculations for tissue heterogeneity-corrected conformal treatment plans following RTOG 0813 dosimetric criteria for lung cancer stereotactic body radiotherapy. *Int J Radiat Oncol Biol Phys.* 2012;84:508–513.

81. Klein EE, Morrison A, Purdy JA, et al. A volumetric study of measurements and calculations of lung density corrections for 6 and 18 MV photons. *Int J Radiat Oncol Biol Phys.* 1997;37:1163–1170.

82. Grills IS, Yan D, Martinez AA, et al. Potential for reduced toxicity and dose escalation in the treatment of inoperable non-small-cell lung cancer: a comparison of intensity-modulated radiation therapy (IMRT), 3D conformal radiation, and elective nodal irradiation. *Int J Radiat Oncol Biol Phys.* 2003;57:875–890.

83. Liu HH, Wang X, Dong L, et al. Feasibility of sparing lung and other thoracic structures with intensity-modulated radiotherapy for non-small-cell lung cancer. *Int J Radiat Oncol Biol Phys.* 2004;58:1268–1279.

84. Bezjak A, Rumble RB, Rodrigues G, et al. Intensity-modulated radiotherapy in the treatment of lung cancer. *Clin Oncol (R Coll Radiol).* 2012;24:508–520.

85. Chan C, Lang S, Rowbottom C, et al. Intensity-modulated radiotherapy for lung cancer: current status and future developments. *J Thorac Oncol.* 2014;9:1598–1608.

86. Li HS, Chetty IJ, Solberg TD. Quantifying the interplay effect in prostate IMRT delivery using a convolution-based method. *Med Phys.* 2008;35:1703–1710.

87. Chui C, Yorke E, Hong L. The effects of intra-fraction organ motion on the delivery of intensity-modulated field with a multileaf collimator. *Med Phys.* 2003;30:1736–1746.

88. Chun SG, Hu C, Choy H, et al. Impact of intensity-modulated radiation therapy technique for locally advanced non-small-cell lung cancer: asecondary analysis of the NRG Oncology RTOG 0617 randomized clinical trial. *J Clin Oncol.* 2017; 35:56–62.

89. Yang M, Timmerman R. Stereotactic ablative radiotherapy uncertainties: delineation, setup and motion. *Semin Radiat Oncol.* 2018;28:207–217.

90. Tree AC, Khoo VS, Eeles RA, et al. Stereotactic body radiotherapy for oligometastases. *Lancet Oncol.* 2013;14:e28–e37.

91. Peulen H, Karlsson K, Lindberg K, et al. Toxicity after reirradiation of pulmonary tumours with stereotactic body radiotherapy. *Radiother Oncol.* 2011;101:260–266.

92. Trakul N, Harris JP, Le QT, et al. Stereotactic ablative radiotherapy for reirradiation of locally recurrent lung tumors. *J Thorac Oncol.* 2012;7:1462–1465.

93. Liu H, Zhang X, Vinogradskiy YY, et al. Predicting radiation pneumonitis after stereotactic ablative radiation therapy in patients previously treated with conventional thoracic radiation therapy. *Int J Radiat Oncol Biol Phys.* 2012;84:1017–1023.

94. Reyngold M, Wu AJ, McLane A, et al. Toxicity and outcomes of thoracic re-irradiation using stereotactic body radiation therapy (SBRT). *Radiation Oncology.* 2013;8:99.

95. Valakh V, Miyamoto C, Micaily B, et al. Repeat stereotactic body radiation therapy for patients with pulmonary malignancies who had previously received SBRT to the same or an adjacent tumor site. *J Cancer Res Ther.* 2013;9:680–685.

96. Trovo M, Minatel E, Durofil E, et al. Stereotactic body radiation therapy for re-irradiation of persistent or recurrent non-small cell lung cancer. *Int J Radiat Oncol Biol Phys.* 2014;88:1114–1119.

97. Hearn JW, Videtic GM, Djemil T, et al. Salvage stereotactic body radiation therapy (SBRT) for local failure after primary lung SBRT. *Int J Radiat Oncol Biol Phys.* 2014.

98. Parks J, Kloecker G, Woo S, et al. Stereotactic body radiation therapy as salvage for intrathoracic recurrence in patients with previously irradiated locally advanced non-small cell lung cancer. *Am J Clin Oncol.* 2014;39:147–153.

99. Videtic GM, Stephans KL, Woody NM, et al. Stereotactic body radiation therapy-based treatment model for stage I medically inoperable small cell lung cancer. *Pract Radiat Oncol.* 2013;3:301–306.

100. Shioyama Y, Nakamura K, Sasaki T, et al. Clinical results of stereotactic body radiotherapy for stage I small-cell lung cancer: a single institutional experience. *J Radiat Res.* 2013;54:108–112.

101. Onishi H, Shirato H, Nagata Y, et al. Stereotactic body radiotherapy (SBRT) for operable stage I non-small-cell lung cancer: can SBRT be comparable to surgery? *Int J Radiat Oncol Biol Phys.* 2011;81:1352–1358.

102. Lagerwaard FJ, Verstegen NE, Haasbeek CJ, et al. Outcomes of stereotactic ablative radiotherapy in patients with potentially operable stage I non-small cell lung cancer. *Int J Radiat Oncol Biol Phys.* 2012;83:348–353.

103. Feddock J, Arnold SM, Shelton BJ, et al. Stereotactic body radiation therapy can be used safely to boost residual disease in locally advanced non-small cell lung cancer: a prospective study. *Int J Radiat Oncol Biol Phys.* 2013;85:1325–1331.

104. Karam SD, Horne ZD, Hong RL, et al. Dose escalation with stereotactic body radiation therapy boost for locally advanced non small cell lung cancer. *Radiat Oncol.* 2013;8:179.

105. Timmerman R, Paulus R, Galvin J, et al. Stereotactic body radiation therapy for inoperable early stage lung cancer. *JAMA.* 2010;303:1070–1076.

106. Wang L, Hayes S, Paskalev K, et al. Dosimetric comparison of stereotactic body radiotherapy using 4D CT and multiphase CT images for treatment planning of lung cancer: evaluation of the impact on daily dose coverage. *Radiother Oncol.* 2009;91:314–324.

107. Latifi K, Oliver J, Baker R, et al. Study of 201 non-small cell lung cancer patients given stereotactic ablative radiation therapy shows local control dependence on dose calculation algorithm. *Int J Radiat Oncol Biol Phys.* 2014;88:1108–1113.

108. Zhuang T, Djemil T, Qi P, et al. Dose calculation differences between Monte Carlo and pencil beam depend on the tumor locations and volumes for lung stereotactic body radiation therapy. *J Appl Clin Med Phys.* 2013;14:4011.

109. Onishi H, Shirato H, Nagata Y, et al. Hypofractionated stereotactic radiotherapy (HypoFXSRT) for stage I non-small cell lung cancer: updated results of 257 patients in a Japanese multi-institutional study. *J Thorac Oncol.* 2007;2:S94–S100.

110. Kestin L, Grills I, Guckenberger M, et al. Dose-response relationship with clinical outcome for lung stereotactic body radiotherapy (SBRT) delivered via online image guidance. *Radiother Oncol.* 2014;110:499–504.

111. Timmerman R, Papiez L, McGarry R, et al. Extracranial stereotactic radioablation: results of a phase I study in medically inoperable stage I non-small cell lung cancer. *Chest.* 2003;124:1946–1955.

112. Timmerman R, McGarry R, Yiannoutsos C, et al. Excessive toxicity when treating central tumors in a phase II study of stereotactic body radiation therapy for medically inoperable early-stage lung cancer. *J Clin Oncol.* 2006;24:4833–4839.

113. Uematsu M, Shioda A, Suda A, et al. Computed tomography-guided frameless stereotactic radiotherapy for stage I non-small cell lung cancer: a 5-year experience. *Int J Radiat Oncol Biol Phys.* 2001;51:666–670.

114. Haasbeek CJ, Lagerwaard FJ, Slotman BJ, et al. Outcomes of stereotactic ablative radiotherapy for centrally located early-stage lung cancer. *J Thoracic Oncol.* 2011;6:2036–2043.

115. Videtic GM, Paulus R, Singh AK, et al. Long term follow-up on NRG Oncology RTOG 0915 (NCCTG N0927): a randomized phase II study comparing 2 stereotactic body radiation therapy schedules for medically inoperable patients with stage I peripheral non-small cell lung cancer. *Int J Radiat Oncol Biol Phys.* 2019;103:1077–1084.

116. Singh AK, Gomez-Suescun JA, Stephans KL, et al. One versus three fractions of stereotactic body radiation therapy for peripheral stage I-II non-small cell lung cancer: a randomized, multi-institution, phase 2 trial. *Int J Radiat Oncol Biol Phys.* 2019;105:752–759.

117. Senthi S, Haasbeek CJ, Slotman BJ, et al. Outcomes of stereotactic ablative radiotherapy for central lung tumours: a systematic review. *Radiother Oncol.* 2013;106:276–282.

118. Chang JY, Li QQ, Xu QY, et al. Stereotactic ablative radiation therapy for centrally located early stage or isolated parenchymal recurrences of non-small cell lung cancer: how to fly in a "no fly zone". *Int J Radiat Oncol Biol Phys.* 2014;88: 1120–1128.

119. Tekatli H, Haasbeek N, Dahele M, et al. Outcomes of hypofractionated high-dose radiotherapy in poor-risk patients with "Ultracentral"non-small cell lung cancer. *J Thorac Oncol.* 2016;11:1081–1089.

120. Li Q, Swanick CW, Allen PK, Gomez DR, et al. Stereotactic ablative radiotherapy (SABR) using 70 Gy in 10 fractions for non-small cell lung cancer: exploration of clinical indications. *Radiother Oncol.* 2014;112:256–261.

121. Cheung P, Faria S, Ahmed S, et al. Phase II study of accelerated hypofractionated three-dimensional conformal radiotherapy for stage T1-3 N0 M0 non-small cell lung cancer: NCIC CTG BR.25. *J Natl Cancer Inst.* 2014;106:dju164 1-8.

122. Bezjak A, Paulus R, Gaspar LE, et al. Safety and efficacy of a five-fraction stereotactic body radiotherapy schedule for centrally located non-small-cell lung cancer: NRG oncology/RTOG 0813 trial. *J Clin Oncol.* 2019;37:1316–1325.

123. Timmerman R, Bastasch M, Saha D, et al. Optimizing dose and fractionation for stereotactic body radiation therapy. normal tissue and tumor control effects with large dose per fraction. *Front Radiat Ther Oncol.* 2007;40:352–365.

124. Lagerwaard FJ, Haasbeek CJ, Smit EF, et al. Outcomes of risk-adapted fractionated stereotactic radiotherapy for stage I non-small-cell lung cancer. *Int J Radiat Oncol Biol Phys.* 2008;70:685–692.

125. Finazzi T, Haasbeek CJA, Spoelstra FOB, et al. Clinical outcomes of stereotactic MR-guided adaptive radiation therapy for high-risk lung tumors. *Int J Radiat Oncol Biol Phys.* 2020;107:270–278.

126. Finazzi T, Palacios MA, Spoelstra FOB, et al. Role of on-table plan adaptation in MR-guided ablative radiation therapy for central lung tumors. *Int J Radiat Oncol Biol Phys.* 2019;104:933–941.

127. Henke LE, Olsen JR, Contreras JA, et al. Stereotactic MR-guided online adaptive radiation therapy (SMART) for ultracentral thorax malignancies: results of a phase 1 trial. *Adv Radiat Oncol.* 2018;4:201–209.

128. Fakiris AJ, McGarry RC, Yiannoutsos CT, et al. Stereotactic body radiation therapy for early-stage non-small-cell lung carcinoma: four-year results of a prospective phase II study. *Int J Radiat Oncol Biol Phys.* 2009;75:677–682.

129. Zheng X, Schipper M, Kidwell K, et al. Survival outcome after stereotactic body radiation therapy and surgery for stage I non-small cell lung cancer: a meta-analysis. *Int J Radiat Oncol Biol Phys.* 2014;90:603–611.

130. Ginsberg RJ, Rubinstein LV. Randomized trial of lobectomy versus limited resection for T1 N0 non-small cell lung cancer. lung cancer study group. *Ann Thorac Surg.* 1995;60:615–622; discussion 622–623.

131. Fernando HC, Landreneau RJ, Mandrekar SJ, et al. Impact of brachytherapy on local recurrence rates after sublobar resection: results from ACOSOG Z4032 (alliance), a phase III randomized trial for high-risk operable non-small-cell lung cancer. *J Clin Oncol.* 2014;32:2456–2462.

132. Stephans KL, Djemil T, Reddy CA, et al. Comprehensive analysis of pulmonary function test (PFT) changes after stereotactic body radiotherapy (SBRT) for stage I lung cancer in medically inoperable patients. *J Thorac Oncol.* 2009;4:838–844.

133. 133 Henderson M, McGarry R, Yiannoutsos C, et al. Baseline pulmonary function as a predictor for survival and decline in pulmonary function over time in patients undergoing stereotactic body radiotherapy for the treatment of stage I non-small-cell lung cancer. *Int J Radiat Oncol Biol Phys.* 2008;72:404–409.

134. Stanic S, Paulus R, Timmerman RD, et al. No clinically significant changes in pulmonary function following stereotactic body radiation therapy for early- stage peripheral non-small cell lung cancer: an analysis of RTOG 0236. *Int J Radiat Oncol Biol Phys.* 2014;88:1092–1099.

135. Voroney JP, Hope A, Dahele MR, et al. Chest wall pain and rib fracture after stereotactic radiotherapy for peripheral non-small cell lung cancer. *J Thorac Oncol.* 2009;4:1035–1037.

136. Stephans KL, Djemil T, Tendulkar RD, et al. Prediction of chest wall toxicity from lung stereotactic body radiotherapy (SBRT). *Int J Radiat Oncol Biol Phys.* 2012;82:974–980.

137. Hoppe BS, Laser B, Kowalski AV, et al. Acute skin toxicity following stereotactic body radiation therapy for stage I non-small-cell lung cancer: who's at risk? *Int J Radiat Oncol Biol Phys.* 2008;72:1283–1286.

138. Forquer JA, Fakiris AJ, Timmerman RD, et al. Brachial plexopathy from stereotactic body radiotherapy in early-stage NSCLC: dose-limiting toxicity in apical tumor sites. *Radiother Oncol.* 2009;93:408–413.

139. Corradetti MN, Haas AR, Rengan R. Central-airway necrosis after stereotactic body-radiation therapy. *N Engl J Med.* 2012; 366:2327–2329.

140. Stephans KL, Djemil T, Diaconu C, et al. Esophageal dose tolerance to hypofractionated stereotactic body radiation therapy: risk factors for late toxicity. *Int J Radiat Oncol Biol Phys.* 2014.

141. Gejerman G, Mullokandov EA, Bagiella E, et al. Endobronchial brachytherapy and external-beam radiotherapy in patients with endobronchial obstruction and extrabronchial extension. *Brachytherapy.* 2002;1:204–210.

142. Ung YC, Yu E, Falkson C, et al. The role of high-dose-rate brachytherapy in the palliation of symptoms in patients with non-small-cell lung cancer: a systematic review. *Brachytherapy.* 2006;5: 189–202.

143. de Aquino Gorayeb MM, Gregorio MG, de Oliveira EQ, et al. High-dose-rate brachytherapy in symptom palliation due to malignant endobronchial obstruction: a quantitative assessment. *Brachytherapy.* 2013;12:471–478.

144. Liu H, Chang JY. Proton therapy in clinical practice. *Chin J Cancer.* 2011;30:315–326.

145. Chang JY, Jabbour SK, De Ruysscher D, et al. Consensus statement on proton therapy in early-stage and locally advanced non-small-cell lung cancer. *Int J Radiat Oncol Biol Phys.* 2016;95: 505–516.

146. Macdonald OK, Kruse JJ, Miller JM, et al. Proton beam radiotherapy versus three-dimensional conformal stereotactic body radiotherapy in primary peripheral, early-stage non-small-cell lung carcinoma: a comparative dosimetric analysis. *Int J Radiat Oncol Biol Phys.* 2009;75:950–958.

147. Chi A, Chen H, Wen S, et al. Comparison of particle beam therapy and stereotactic body radiotherapy for early stage non-small cell lung cancer: a systematic review and hypothesis-generating meta-analysis. *Radiother Oncol.* 2017;123:346–354.

148. Higgins KA, O'Connell K, Liu Y, et al. National cancer database analysis of proton versus photon radiation therapy in non-small cell lung cancer. *Int J Radiat Oncol Biol Phys.* 2017;97:128–137.

149. Liao Z, Lee JJ, Komaki R, et al. Bayesian adaptive randomization trial of passive scattering proton therapy and intensity-modulated photon radiotherapy for locally advanced non-small-cell lung cancer. *J Clin Oncol.* 2018;36:1813–1822.

150. Comparing photon therapy to proton therapy to treat patients with lung cancer. https://clinicaltrials.gov/ct2/show/NCT01993810, accessed 9/30/20.

151. Pan HY, Jiang S, Sutton J, et al. Early experience with intensity modulated proton therapy for lung-intact mesothelioma: a case series. *Pract Radiat Oncol.* 2015;5:e345–e353.

152. Parikh RR, Rhome R, Hug E, et al. Adjuvant proton beam therapy in the management of thymoma: adosimetric comparison and acute toxicities. *Clin Lung Cancer.* 2016;17:362–366.

153. Vogel J, Berman AT, Lin L, et al. Prospective study of proton beam radiation therapy for adjuvant and definitive treatment of thymoma and thymic carcinoma: early response and toxicity assessment. *Radiother Oncol.* 2016; 118:504–509.

154. Miller KD, Nogueira L, Mariotto AB, et al. Cancer treatment and survivorship statistics, 2019. *CA Cancer J Clin.* 2019; 69:363–385.

155. Govindan R, Page N, Morgensztern D, et al. Changing epidemiology of small-cell lung cancer in the United States over the last 30 years: analysis of the surveillance, epidemiologic, and end results database. *J Clin Oncol.* 2006;24:4539–4544.

156. Edwards BK, Noone AM, Mariotto AB, et al. Annual report to the nation on the status of cancer, 1975–2010, featuring prevalence of comorbidity and impact on survival among persons with lung, colorectal, breast, or prostate cancer. *Cancer.* 2014;120: 1290–1314.

157. McGarry RC, Song G, des Rosiers P, et al. Observation-only management of early stage, medically inoperable lung cancer: poor outcome. *Chest.* 2002;121:1155–1158.

158. Noordijk EM, vd Poest Clement E, Hermans J, et al. Radiotherapy as an alternative to surgery in elderly patients with resectable lung cancer. *Radiother Oncol.* 1988;13:83–89.

159. Sibley GS, Mundt AJ, Shapiro C, et al. The treatment of stage III non small cell lung cancer using high dose conformal radiotherapy. *Int J Radiat Oncol Biol Phys.* 1995;33:1001–1007.

160. Manon RR, Jaradat H, Patel R, et al. Potential for radiation therapy technology innovations to permit dose escalation for non-small-cell lung cancer. *Clin Lung Cancer.* 2005;7:107–113.

161. Soliman H, Cheung P, Yeung L, et al. Accelerated hypofractionated radiotherapy for early-stage non-small-cell lung cancer: long-term results. *Int J Radiat Oncol Biol Phys.* 2011;79:459–465.

162. Machtay M, Paulus R, Moughan J, et al. Defining local-regional control and its importance in locally advanced non-small cell lung carcinoma. *J Thorac Oncol.* 2012;7:716–722.

163. van Meerbeeck JP, Kramer GW, Van Schil PE, et al. Randomized controlled trial of resection versus radiotherapy after induction chemotherapy in stage IIIA-N2 non-small-cell lung cancer. *J Natl Cancer Inst.* 2007;99:442–450.

164. Albain KS, Rusch VW, Crowley JJ, et al. Concurrent cisplatin/etoposide plus chest radiotherapy followed by surgery for stages IIIA (N2) and IIIB non-small-cell lung cancer: mature results of southwest oncology group phase II study 8805. *J Clin Oncol.* 1995;13:1880–1892.

165. Edelman MJ, Suntharalingam M, Burrows W, et al. Phase I/II trial of hyperfractionated radiation and chemotherapy followed by surgery in stage III lung cancer. *Ann Thorac Surg.* 2008;86:903–910.

166. Suntharalingam M, Paulus R, Edelman MJ, et al. Radiation therapy oncology group protocol 02-29: a phase II trial of neoadjuvant therapy with concurrent chemotherapy and full-dose radiation therapy followed by surgical resection and consolidative therapy for locally advanced non-small cell carcinoma of the lung. *Int J Radiat Oncol Biol Phys.* 2012;84:456–463.

167. Rosenzweig KE, Fox JL, Yorke E, et al. Results of a phase I dose-escalation study using three-dimensional conformal radiotherapy in the treatment of inoperable non small cell lung carcinoma. *Cancer.* 2005;103:2118–2127.

168. Narayan S, Henning GT, Ten Haken RK, et al. Results following treatment to doses of 92.4 or 102.9 Gy on a phase I dose escalation study for non-small cell lung cancer. *Lung Cancer.* 2004;44:79–88.

169. Bradley JD, Moughan J, Graham MV, et al. A phase I/II radiation dose escalation study with concurrent chemotherapy for patients with inoperable stages I to III non-small-cell lung cancer: phase I results of RTOG 0117. *Int J Radiat Oncol Biol Phys.* 2010; 77:367–372.

170. Antonia SJ, Villegas A, Daniel D, et al. Durvalumab after chemoradiotherapy in stage III non-small-cell lung cancer. *N Engl J Med.* 2017;377:1919–1929.

171. Rosenzweig KE, Sura S, Jackson A, et al. Involved-field radiation therapy for inoperable non small cell lung cancer. *J Clin Oncol.* 2007;25:5557–5561.

172. Belderbos JS, Kepka L, Spring Kong FM, et al. Report from the international atomic energy agency (IAEA) consultants' meeting on elective nodal irradiation in lung cancer: non-small-cell lung cancer (NSCLC). *Int J Radiat Oncol Biol Phys.* 2008;72:335–342.

173. Yuan S, Sun X, Li M, et al. A randomized study of involved-field irradiation versus elective nodal irradiation in combination with concurrent chemotherapy for inoperable stage III non small cell lung cancer. *Am J Clin Oncol.* 2007;30:239–244.

174. Auperin A, Arriagada R, Pignon JP, et al. Prophylactic cranial irradiation for patients with small-cell lung cancer in complete remission. prophylactic cranial irradiation overview collaborative group. *N Engl J Med.* 1999;341:476–484.

175. Gore EM, Bae K, Wong SJ, et al. Phase III comparison of prophylactic cranial irradiation versus observation in patients with locally advanced non-small-cell lung cancer: primary analysis of radiation therapy oncology group study RTOG 0214. *J Clin Oncol.* 2011;29:272–278.

176. Winton T, Livingston R, Johnson D, et al. Vinorelbine plus cisplatin vs. observation in resected non-small-cell lung cancer. *N Engl J Med.* 2005;352:2589–2597.

177. Douillard JY, Rosell R, De Lena M, et al. Adjuvant vinorelbine plus cisplatin versus observation in patients with completely resected stage IB-IIIA non-small-cell lung cancer (adjuvant navelbine international trialist association [ANITA]): a randomised controlled trial. *Lancet Oncol.* 2006;7:719–727.

178. Pignon JP, Tribodet H, Scagliotti GV, et al. Lung adjuvant cisplatin evaluation: a pooled analysis by the LACE collaborative group. *J Clin Oncol.* 2008;26:3552–3559.

179. Strauss GM, Herndon 2ndJE, Maddaus MA, et al. Adjuvant paclitaxel plus carboplatin compared with observation in stage IB non-small-cell lung cancer: CALGB 9633 with the cancer and leukemia group B, radiation therapy oncology group, and north central cancer treatment group study groups. *J Clin Oncol.* 2008;26:5043–5051.

180. Arriagada R, Dunant A, Pignon JP, et al. Long-term results of the international adjuvant lung cancer trial evaluating adjuvant cisplatin-based chemotherapy in resected lung cancer. *J Clin Oncol.* 2010;28:35–42.

181. Weisenberger. Effects of postoperative mediastinal radiation on completely resected stage II and stage III epidermoid cancer of the lung. the lung cancer study group. *N Engl J Med.* 1986;315:1377–1381.

182. PORT Meta-Analysis Trialists Group. Postoperative radiotherapy for non-small cell lung cancer. *Cochrane Database Syst Rev.* 2003;(1):CD002142.

183. Douillard J, Rosell R, De Lena M, et al. Impact of postoperative radiation therapy on survival in patients with complete resection and stage I, II, or IIIA non-small-cell lung cancer treated with adjuvant chemotherapy: the adjuvant navelbine international trialist association (ANITA) randomized trial. *Int J Radiat Oncol Biol Phys.* 2008;72:695–701.

184. Lally BE, Zelterman D, Colasanto JM, et al. Postoperative radiotherapy for stage II or III non-small-cell lung cancer using the surveillance, epidemiology, and end results database. *J Clin Oncol.* 2006;24:2998–3006.

185. Faivre-Finn C, Snee M, Ashcroft L, et al. Concurrent once-daily versus twice-daily chemoradiotherapy in patients with limited-stage small-cell lung cancer (CONVERT): an open-label, phase 3, randomised, superiority trial. *Lancet Oncol.* 2017;18:1116–1125.

186. De Ruysscher D, Pijls-Johannesma M, Bentzen SM, et al. Time between the first day of chemotherapy and the last day of chest radiation is the most important predictor of survival in limited-disease small-cell lung cancer. *J Clin Oncol.* 2006;24:1057–1063.

187. Pijls-Johannesma MC, De Ruysscher D, Lambin P, et al. Early versus late chest radiotherapy for limited stage small cell lung cancer. *Cochrane Database Syst Rev.* 2005;(1):CD004700.

188. Fried DB, Morris DE, Poole C, et al. Systematic review evaluating the timing of thoracic radiation therapy in combined modality therapy for limited-stage small-cell lung cancer. *J Clin Oncol.* 2004;22:4837–4845.

189. Kies MS, Mira JG, Crowley JJ, et al. Multimodal therapy for limited small-cell lung cancer: a randomized study of induction combination chemotherapy with or without thoracic radiation in complete responders; and with wide-field versus reduced-field radiation in partial responders: a southwest oncology group study. *J Clin Oncol.* 1987;5:592–600.

190. Hu X, Bao Y, Xu YJ, et al. Final report of a prospective randomized study on thoracic radiotherapy target volume for limited-stage small cell lung cancer with radiation dosimetric analyses. *Cancer.* 2020;126:840–849.

191. Videtic GM, Belderbos JS, Spring Kong FM, et al. Report from the international atomic energy agency (IAEA) consultants' meeting on elective nodal irradiation in lung cancer: small-cell lung cancer (SCLC). *Int J Radiat Oncol Biol Phys.* 2008;72:327–334.

192. Farrell MJ, Yahya JB, Degnin et al. Elective nodal irradiation for limited-stage small-cell lung cancer: survey of US radiation oncologists on practice patterns. *Clin Lung Cancer.* 2020;21:443–449.

193. van Loon J, De Ruysscher D, Wanders R, et al. Selective nodal irradiation on basis of (18)FDG-PET scans in limited-disease small-cell lung cancer: a prospective study. *Int J Radiat Oncol Biol Phys.* 2010;77:329–336.

194. Slotman BJ, van Tinteren H, Praag JO, et al. Use of thoracic radiotherapy for extensive stage small-cell lung cancer: a phase 3 randomised controlled trial. *Lancet.* 2015;385:36–42.

195. Gore EM, Hu C, Sun AY, et al. Randomized phase II study comparing prophylactic cranial irradiation alone to prophylactic cranial irradiation and consolidative extracranial irradiation for extensive-disease small cell lung cancer (ED SCLC): NRG oncology RTOG 0937. *J Thorac Oncol.* 2017;12:1561–1570.

196. Slotman B, Faivre-Finn C, Kramer G, et al. Prophylactic cranial irradiation in extensive small-cell lung cancer. *N Engl J Med.* 2007;357:664–672.

197. Takahashi T, Yamanaka T, Seto T, et al. Prophylactic cranial irradiation versus observation in patients with extensive-disease small-cell lung cancer: a multicentre, randomised, open-label, phase 3 trial. *Lancet Oncol.* 2017;18:663–671.

198. Le Pechoux C, Dunant A, Senan S, et al. Standard-dose versus higher-dose prophylactic cranial irradiation (PCI) in patients with limited-stage small-cell lung cancer in complete remission after chemotherapy and thoracic radiotherapy (PCI 99-01, EORTC 22003-08004, RTOG 0212, and IFCT 99-01): a randomised clinical trial. *Lancet Oncol.* 2009;10:467–474.

199. Wolfson AH, Bae K, Komaki R, et al. Primary analysis of a phase II randomized trial radiation therapy oncology group (RTOG) 0212: impact of different total doses and schedules of prophylactic cranial irradiation on chronic neurotoxicity and quality of life for patients with limited-disease small-cell lung cancer. *Int J Radiat Oncol Biol Phys.* 2011;81:77–84.

200. Gondi V, Paulus R, Bruner DW, et al. Decline in tested and self-reported cognitive functioning after prophylactic cranial irradiation for lung cancer: pooled secondary analysis of radiation therapy oncology group randomized trials 0212 and 0214. *Int J Radiat Oncol Biol Phys.* 2013;86:656–664.

201. Whole-brain radiation therapy with or without hippocampal avoidance in treating patients with limited stage or extensive stage small cell lung cancer. https://clinicaltrials.gov/ct2/show/NCT02635009, accessed October 10, 2020.

202. Pleural mesothelioma. In: Part VII Thorax. In: Amin MB, Edge S, Greene F, et al., eds. *AJCC Cancer Staging Handbook.* 8th ed. Chicago, IL: Springer; 2018:457–470.

203. Sugarbaker DJ, Flores RM, Jaklitsch MT, et al. Resection margins, extrapleural nodal status, and cell type determine postoperative long-term survival in trimodality therapy of malignant pleural mesothelioma: results in 183 patients. *J Thorac Cardiovasc Surg.* 1999;117:54,63; discussion 63–65.

204. Flores RM, Pass HI, Seshan VE, et al. Extrapleural pneumonectomy versus pleurectomy/decortication in the surgical management of malignant pleural mesothelioma: results in 663 patients. *J Thorac Cardiovasc Surg.* 2008;135:620,6, 626.e1–3.

205. Lang-Lazdunski L, Bille A, Lal R, et al. Pleurectomy/decortication is superior to extrapleural pneumonectomy in the multimodality management of patients with malignant pleural mesothelioma. *J Thorac Oncol.* 2012;7:737–743.

206. Treasure T, Lang-Lazdunski L, Waller D, et al. Extra-pleural pneumonectomy versus no extra-pleural pneumonectomy for patients with malignant pleural mesothelioma: clinical outcomes of the mesothelioma and radical surgery (MARS) randomised feasibility study. *Lancet Oncol.* 2011;12:763–772.

207. Kostron A, Friess M, Inci I, et al. Propensity matched comparison of extrapleural pneumonectomy and pleurectomy/decortication for mesothelioma patients. *Interact Cardiovasc Thorac Surg.* 2017;24:740–746.

208. Rimner A, Spratt DE, Zauderer MG, et al. Failure patterns after hemithoracic pleural intensity modulated radiation therapy for malignant pleural mesothelioma. *Int J Radiat Oncol Biol Phys.* 2014;90:394–401.

209. Vogelzang NJ, Rusthoven JJ, Symanowski J, et al. Phase III study of pemetrexed in combination with cisplatin versus cisplatin alone in patients with malignant pleural mesothelioma. *J Clin Oncol.* 2003;21:2636–2644.

210. Chance WW, Rice DC, Allen PK, et al. Hemithoracic intensity modulated radiation therapy after pleurectomy/decortication for malignant pleural mesothelioma: toxicity, patterns of failure, and a matched survival analysis. *Int J Radiat Oncol Biol Phys.* 2015;91:149–156.

211. Baldini EH. Radiation therapy options for malignant pleural mesothelioma. *Semin Thorac Cardiovasc Surg.* 2009;21:159–163.

212. Rosenzweig KE, Zauderer MG, Laser B, et al. Pleural intensity-modulated radiotherapy for malignant pleural mesothelioma. *Int J Radiat Oncol Biol Phys.* 2012;83:1278–1283.

213. Gupta V, Mychalczak B, Krug L, et al. Hemithoracic radiation therapy after pleurectomy/decortication for malignant pleural mesothelioma. *Int J Radiat Oncol Biol Phys.* 2005;63:1045–1052.

214. Minatel E, Trovo M, Bearz A, et al. Radical radiation therapy after lung-sparing surgery for malignant pleural mesothelioma: survival, pattern of failure, and prognostic factors. *Int J Radiat Oncol Biol Phys.* 2015;93:606–613.

215. O'Rourke N, Garcia JC, Paul J, et al. A randomised controlled trial of intervention site radiotherapy in malignant pleural mesothelioma. *Radiother Oncol.* 2007;84:18–22.

216. Boutin C, Rey F, Viallat JR. Prevention of malignant seeding after invasive diagnostic procedures in patients with pleural mesothelioma:a randomized trial of local radiotherapy. *Chest.* 1995;108:754–758.

217. Rusch VW, Rosenzweig K, Venkatraman E, et al. A phase II trial of surgical resection and adjuvant high-dose hemithoracic radiation for malignant pleural mesothelioma. *J Thorac Cardiovasc Surg.* 2001;122:788–795.

218. Allen AM, Czerminska M, Janne PA, et al. Fatal pneumonitis associated with intensity-modulated radiation therapy for mesothelioma. *Int J Radiat Oncol Biol Phys.* 2006;65:640–645.

219. Ball DL, Cruickshank DG. The treatment of malignant mesothelioma of the pleura: review of a 5-year experience, with special reference to radiotherapy. *Am J Clin Oncol.* 1990;13:4–9.

220. de Graaf-Strukowska L, van der Zee J, van Putten W, et al. Factors influencing the outcome of radiotherapy in malignant mesothelioma of the pleura--a single-institution experience with 189 patients. *Int J Radiat Oncol Biol Phys.* 1999;43:511–516.

221. Gordon WJr, Antman KH, Greenberger JS, et al. Radiation therapy in the management of patients with mesothelioma. *Int J Radiat Oncol Biol Phys.* 1982;8:19–25.

222. Gomez DR, Hong DS, Allen PK, et al. Patterns of failure, toxicity, and survival after extrapleural pneumonectomy and hemithoracic intensity-modulated radiation therapy for malignant pleural mesothelioma. *J Thorac Oncol.* 2013;8:238–245.

223. Miles EF, Larrier NA, Kelsey CR, et al. Intensity-modulated radiotherapy for resected mesothelioma: the Duke experience. *Int J Radiat Oncol Biol Phys.* 2008;71:1143–1150.

224. Rice DC, Stevens CW, Correa AM, et al. Outcomes after extrapleural pneumonectomy and intensity-modulated radiation therapy for malignant pleural mesothelioma. *Ann Thorac Surg.* 2007;84:1685,92; discussion 1692–1693.

225. Azarow KS, Pearl RH, Zurcher R, et al. Primary mediastinal masses:a comparison of adult and pediatric populations. *J Thorac Cardiovasc Surg.* 1993;106:67–72.

226. Cowen D, Hannoun-Levi JM, Resbeut M, et al. Natural history and treatment of malignant thymoma. *Oncology (Williston Park).* 1998;12:1001,5; discussion 1006.

227. Zhu G, He S, Fu X, et al. Radiotherapy and prognostic factors for thymoma: a retrospective study of 175 patients. *Int J Radiat Oncol Biol Phys.* 2004;60:1113–1119.

228. Regnard JF, Magdeleinat P, Dromer C, et al. Prognostic factors and long-term results after thymoma resection: a series of 307 patients. *J Thorac Cardiovasc Surg.* 1996;112:376–384.

229. Masaoka A, Monden Y, Nakahara K, et al. Follow-up study of thymomas with special reference to their clinical stages. *Cancer.* 1981;48:2485–2492.

230. Kondo K, Monden Y. Therapy for thymic epithelial tumors: a clinical study of 1,320 patients from japan. *Ann Thorac Surg.* 2003;76:878,84; discussion 884–885.

231. Rimner A, Yao X, Huang J, et al. Postoperative radiation therapy is associated with longer overall survival in completely resected stage II and III thymoma: an analysis of the international thymic malignancies interest group retrospective database. *J Thorac Oncol.* 2016;11:1785–1792.

232. Myojin M, Choi NC, Wright CD, et al. Stage III thymoma: pattern of failure after surgery and postoperative radiotherapy and its implication for future study. *Int J Radiat Oncol Biol Phys.* 2000;46:927–933.

233. Strobel P, Bauer A, Puppe B, et al. Tumor recurrence and survival in patients treated for thymomas and thymic squamous cell carcinomas: a retrospective analysis. *J Clin Oncol.* 2004;22:1501–1509.

234. Fan C, Feng Q, Chen Y, et al. Postoperative radiotherapy for completely resected Masaoka stage III thymoma: a retrospective study of 65 cases from a single institution. *Radiat Oncol.* 2013;8:199,717X-8-199.

235. Chang JH, Kim HJ, Wu HG, et al. Postoperative radiotherapy for completely resected stage II or III thymoma. *J Thorac Oncol.* 2011;6:1282–1286.

236. Hsu HC, Huang EY, Wang CJ, et al. Postoperative radiotherapy in thymic carcinoma: treatment results and prognostic factors. *Int J Radiat Oncol Biol Phys.* 2002;52:801–805.

237. Ruffini E, Van Raemdonck D, Detterbeck F, et al. Management of thymic tumors: a survey of current practice among members of the European society of thoracic surgeons. *J Thorac Oncol.* 2011;6:614–623.

238. Ruffini E, Detterbeck F, Van Raemdonck D, et al. Thymic carcinoma: a cohort study of patients from the European society of thoracic surgeons database. *J Thorac Oncol.* 2014;9:541–548.

239. Ruffini E, Mancuso M, Oliaro A, et al. Recurrence of thymoma: analysis of clinicopathologic features, treatment, and outcome. *J Thorac Cardiovasc Surg.* 1997;113:55–63.

8 Breast Cancer

Susan G.R. McDuff, Colin E. Champ, Sua Yoo, and Rachel C. Blitzblau

INTRODUCTION

Radiotherapy plays an essential role in the definitive management of in situ and invasive breast carcinoma. This chapter reviews factors relevant to breast radiation treatment planning, including breast and regional nodal anatomy, breast cancer biology, and indications for adjuvant radiotherapy after breast conserving surgery and mastectomy. Patient positioning, treatment techniques, target volumes, and dose fractionation are discussed for different clinical scenarios.

Anatomy

The breast is positioned within the superficial fascia on the anterior chest wall (Fig. 8.1). It extends from the second rib superiorly to the inframammary fold, typically at the sixth rib. Horizontally, the breast spans from the lateral sternal edge to the midaxillary line. Breast tissue extending into the axilla is referred to as the axillary tail of Spence. The pectoral fascia, serratus anterior, external oblique muscles, and upper rectus sheath form the posterior border of the breast. The retromammary bursa consists of loose areolar tissue located between the glandular breast elements and deep fascia of the pectoralis major. This space allows for breast mobility along the chest wall. Anteriorly, the breast is attached to the skin by fibrous connective tissue septa called suspensory or Cooper's ligaments. These ligaments insert perpendicularly to the superficial fascia below the dermis and attach posteriorly to the deep fascia, providing structural support without impairing mobility. Infiltration of these ligaments by malignancy leads to skin retraction and dimpled appearance of the breast.

The breast consists of 15 to 20 lobes arranged radially around the nipple. Each lobe contains 20 to 40 terminal ductal lobular units (TDLU), which represent the functional unit of the breast. A TDLU contains clusters of tubuloalevolar glands or lobules that drain into a terminal duct. Terminal ducts coalesce to form interlobular ducts, and ducts from each lobe join to empty into a larger lactiferous duct. Typically, 5 to 10 main lactiferous ducts converge to open at the nipple. The glandular breast tissue with its branching duct system is embedded in subcutaneous adipose tissue and surrounded by supportive connective tissues, blood vessels, nerves, and lymphatics. The upper outer quadrant contains the most glandular tissue and is the most common site of breast carcinoma.

Blood Vessels

The internal mammary (IM) and lateral thoracic arteries provide the majority of the breast blood supply (Fig. 8.2). The IM artery (internal thoracic artery) is a branch of the subclavian artery and delivers blood to greater than 50% of the breast. It descends vertically across intercostal spaces lateral to the sternum and branches into perforating arteries that supply the medial and central breast. The lateral thoracic artery is a branch of the axillary artery and primarily supplies the upper outer quadrant. The pectoral branch of the thoracoacromial artery runs between the pectoralis major and minor to supply the posterior breast. The subscapular artery and lateral branches of the third to fifth posterior intercostal arteries provide minor contributions to the arterial blood supply. Venous drainage is primarily through tributaries of the axillary vein and perforating branches of the internal thoracic and posterior intercostal veins.

Lymphatic Drainage

A dense network of lymphatic vessels exists within the breast, and approximately 35% of patients with breast cancer have positive lymph nodes at presentation.[1] The axilla is most commonly involved, followed by the IM and supraclavicular regions, respectively. The probability of drainage to the infraclavicular or interpectoral regions is <2%.[2] Lymphatic drainage patterns vary based on breast "quadrant" (upper outer, upper inner, lower outer, lower inner, and central).[2-4] The dominant drainage site is the axilla regardless of location; however, IM drainage is much more frequent for medial or central breast lesions.[5]

Axillary nodes are categorized into three levels based on their position relative to the pectoralis minor muscle (Fig. 8.3). Level I contains axillary nodes situated lateral to the pectoralis minor. Level II nodes lie posterior to the pectoralis minor and include the interpectoral (Rotter) nodes situated between the pectoralis minor and major.

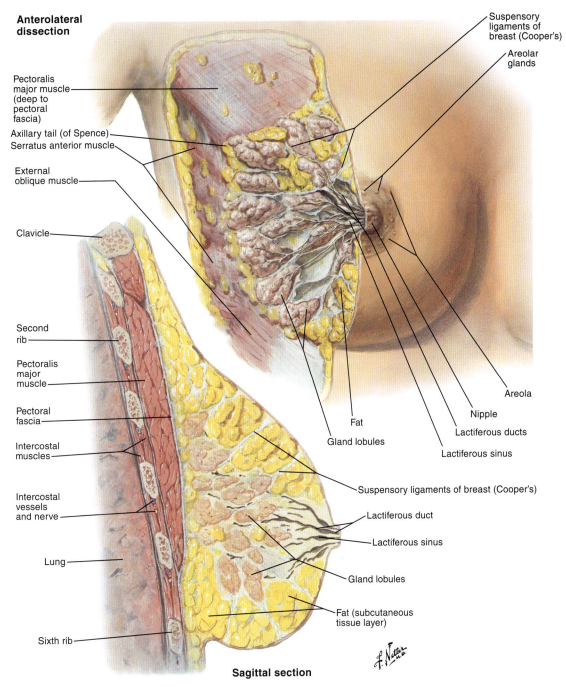

Anterolateral dissection

Pectoralis major muscle (deep to pectoral fascia)

Axillary tail (of Spence)

Serratus anterior muscle

External oblique muscle

Clavicle

Second rib

Pectoralis major muscle

Pectoral fascia

Intercostal muscles

Intercostal vessels and nerve

Lung

Sixth rib

Sagittal section

Suspensory ligaments of breast (Cooper's)

Areolar glands

Areola

Nipple

Lactiferous ducts

Lactiferous sinus

Fat

Gland lobules

Suspensory ligaments of breast (Cooper's)

Lactiferous duct

Lactiferous sinus

Gland lobules

Fat (subcutaneous tissue layer)

FIGURE 8.1. Mammary gland (coronal and sagittal sections). Reprinted with permission from Netter FH. *Atlas of Human Anatomy*, 5th edition. Philadelphia, PA: Saunders-Elsevier.

Level III (infraclavicular) nodes are located medial to the medial border of the pectoralis minor and inferior to the clavicle. Supraclavicular lymph nodes lie within the supraclavicular fossa, between the anterior scalene and sternocleidomastoid muscles. Adjacent nodes above the cricoid cartilage are considered lower cervical nodes and categorized as metastatic disease. Nodal involvement typically exhibits progressive, orderly spread from level I to adjacent axillary levels then the supraclavicular region.[6] Reported rates of "skip metastases" range from 1.5% to 19.2%.[7]

A complete axillary lymph node dissection is usually limited to surgical levels I and II, which differ from radiologically defined axillary levels. A level I and II axillary dissection removes all nodes below the axillary vein, extending medially behind the pectoralis minor and laterally to the point where the axillary vein crosses the latissimus dorsi tendon. In an effort to reduce surgical morbidity, surgeons typically do not skeletonize the axillary vessels. In contrast, the NRG Oncology breast contouring atlas defines axillary level II as beginning where the axillary vessels cross the pectoralis muscle laterally

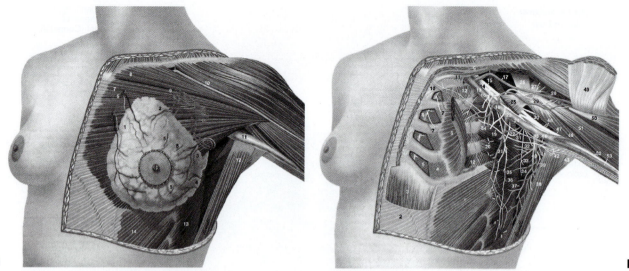

A　**B**

FIGURE 8.2. Normal anatomy of the breast, chest wall muscles, and vasculature. **(A)** 1. Perforating branches from internal mammary artery and vein; 2. Pectoral branches from thoracoacromial artery and vein; 3. External mammary branch from lateral thoracic artery and vein; 4. Branches from subscapular and thoracodorsal arteries and veins; 5. Lateral branches of third, fourth, and fifth intercostal arteries and veins; 6. Internal mammary artery and veins; 7. Sternocostal head of pectoralis major muscle; 8. Clavicular head of pectoralis major muscle; 9. Axillary artery and vein; 10. Cephalic vein; 11. Axillary sheath; 12. Latissimus dorsi muscle; 13. Serratus anterior muscle; 14. External abdominal oblique muscle. **(B)** 1. External abdominal oblique muscle; 2. Rectus sheath; 3. Rectus abdominis muscle; 4. Internal intercostal muscle; 5. Transverse thoracic muscle; 6. Pectoralis minor muscle; 7. Perforating branches from internal mammary artery and vein; 8. Internal mammary artery and vein; 9. Cut edge of pectoralis major muscle; 10. Sternoclavicular branch of thoracoacromial artery and vein; 11. Subclavius muscle and Halsted ligament; 12. External intercostal muscle; 13. Axillary vein; 14. Axillary artery; 15. Lateral cord of brachial plexus; 16. Lateral pectoral nerve (from the lateral cord); 17. Cephalic vein; 18. Thoracoacromial vein; 19. Intercostobrachial nerve; 20. Lateral cutaneous nerves; 21. Lateral thoracic artery and vein; 22. Scapular branches of lateral thoracic artery and vein; 23. Medial pectoral nerve (from medial cord); 24. Ulnar nerve; 25. Pectoralis minor muscle; 26. Coracoclavicular ligament; 27. Coracoacromial ligament; 28. Cut edge of deltoid muscle; 29. Acromial and humeral branches of thoracoacromial artery and vein; 30. Musculocutaneous nerve; 31. Medial cutaneous nerve of arm; 32. Subscapularis muscle; 33. Lower subscapular nerve; 34. Teres majormuscle; 35. Long thoracic nerve; 36. Serratus anterior muscle; 37. Latissimus dorsi muscle; 38. Latissimus dorsi muscle; 39. Thoracodorsal nerve; 40. Thoracodorsal artery and vein; 41. Scapular circumflex artery and vein; 42. Branching of intercostobrachial nerve; 43. Teres majormuscle; 44. Medial cutaneous nerve of forearm; 45. Subscapular artery and vein; 46. Posterior humeral circumflex artery and vein; 47. Median nerve; 48. Coracobrachialis muscle; 49. Pectoralis major muscle; 50. Biceps brachii muscle, long head; 51. Biceps brachii muscle, short head; 52. Brachial artery; 53. Basilic vein; 54. Pectoral branch of thoracoacromial artery and vein. Reprinted with permission from Osborne MP, Boolbol SK. Breast anatomy and development. In: Harris JR, Lippmann ME, Morrow M, Osborne CK, eds. *Diseases of the Breast,* 4th edition. Philadelphia, PA: Lippincott Williams & Wilkins, 2010.

and extending until the vessels cross the medial border of the muscle. This volume is typically superior to standard surgical fields.

IM nodes are situated in intercostal spaces within 3 cm of the sternal edge. Most of these lymph nodes are located medial to the IM vessels within the first and second intercostal spaces and lateral to the IM vessels within the third intercostal space.[8] Lymphatic drainage infrequently occurs to IM nodes only (<2%), but drainage from ~20% of patients with early breast cancer flows to both axillary and IM nodes.[4] In the absence of grossly abnormal IM nodes, this nodal region is not typically dissected.

EPIDEMIOLOGY

Breast cancer is the most common noncutaneous malignancy among women, with an estimated cumulative lifetime risk of approximately 12% in the United States (US). The American Cancer Society estimates that 268,600 new cases of invasive breast cancer and 48,100 new cases of carcinoma in situ will be diagnosed among US women in 2019. An additional 2,670 new cases are anticipated among US men. Breast cancer is the second leading cause of cancer death among women. Female and male breast cancer deaths in the US are expected to be approximately 41,760 and 500, respectively, in 2019.[9] While breast cancer incidence has been relatively stable for the past decade, death rates have decreased by approximately 1.9% per year between 2002 and 2011, and slowed to 1.3% per year between 2011 and 2017.[9,10]

Greater than 90% of breast cancer cases are sporadic; however, several risk factors are associated with breast cancer development. Increasing age is a major risk factor, with incidence rising sharply above age 40 and peaking at ages 75 to 79. This pattern is reflected in recommendations to initiate screening mammography at age 40 or 50 for women at normal risk for breast cancer.[11–13] Longer duration of endogenous estrogen exposure also appears to play a role. This hormonal effect likely accounts for the

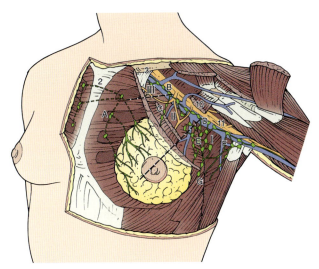

FIGURE 8.3. Lymphatic drainage of the breast showing lymph node groups and levels. 2. Substernal cross-drainage to contralateral internal mammary lymphatic chain; 3. Subclavius muscle and Halsted ligament; 10. Pectoralis minor muscle; 11, Axillary artery and vein. Internal mammary lymph nodes (A); apical lymph nodes (B); interpectoral (Rotter) lymph nodes (C); axillary vein lymph nodes (D); central lymph nodes (E); scapular lymph nodes (F); external mammary lymph nodes (G). Level I lymph nodes: lateral to lateral border of pectoralis minor muscle; level II lymph nodes: behind pectoralis minor muscle; level III lymph nodes: medial to medial border of pectoralis minor muscle. Reprinted with permission from Burstein HJ, Harris JR, Morrow M. Malignant tumors of the breast. In: DeVita VT, Lawrence, TS, Rosenberg SA, eds. *DeVita, Hellman, and Rosenberg's Cancer: Principles & Practice of Oncology*, 9th edition. Philadelphia, PA: Lippincott Williams & Wilkins, 2011.

association between breast cancer and nulliparity, early menarche, older age at first pregnancy, and delayed menopause.[14–16] Exogenous hormone exposure from postmenopausal hormone replacement therapy has also been associated with increased breast cancer risk.[17,18] A small increase in relative risk has been demonstrated among women currently or recently using oral contraceptives.[19]

Ionizing radiation is a well-established environmental risk factor for breast cancer development. A dose-dependent relationship exists between radiation exposure and breast cancer, with greater risk with exposure at a younger age.[20,21] Cumulative breast cancer incidence ranges from 13% to 20% by age 40 to 45 among women who received chest radiotherapy during childhood, adolescence, or young adulthood.[22] Increased breast cancer risk is noted as early as 8 years after therapeutic chest irradiation, and the risk does not plateau with longer follow-up. Consequently, National Comprehensive Cancer Network (NCCN) guidelines recommend early initiation of breast cancer screening for women who have undergone thoracic irradiation between the ages of 10 and 30. For women <25 years old, annual clinical encounters are recommended starting 8 years after radiation. For women with age 25, annual screening mammogram should begin 8 years after thoracic radiotherapy but not

prior to age 30, and annual breast MRI is recommended starting 8 years after RT but not prior to age 25.[13]

Approximately 5% to 10% of breast cancers are hereditary.[23] Most cases have been linked to mutations in BRCA1 or BRCA2, which are tumor suppressor genes involved in maintaining chromosomal stability. Lifetime breast cancer risk is 28% to 84% among BRCA mutation carriers, with diagnosis often occurring at a younger age compared to sporadic cases.[24] BRCA mutation carriers also have an increased risk of bilateral breast cancer and ovarian cancer, which can influence further workup and treatment decisions.[25] Genetic testing should be considered for patients with breast cancer meeting any of the following criteria: diagnosis at age ≤45, triple-negative breast cancer diagnosed ≤60, *less than* three breast cancer primaries, male breast cancer at any age, personal history of ovarian cancer, known BRCA mutation within the family, or significant family history of breast and/or ovarian cancer.[26]

CLINICAL PRESENTATION AND HISTOLOGIC SUBTYPES

Breast cancer typically presents as an abnormality on screening mammogram or a palpable breast mass. Less common presentations include bloody nipple discharge, axillary adenopathy, and breast skin changes such as erythema, thickening, or peau d'orange. The upper outer quadrant is the region most commonly involved site by both in situ and invasive carcinoma. Primary tumor location is not correlated with prognosis.[27] Axillary lymph node status is the most important predictor of disease-free and overall survival in non-metastatic breast cancer.[28] Approximately 5% of patients in the US have distant disease upon presentation.[29,30]

Noninvasive breast cancer, or carcinoma in situ (Tis), represents a proliferation of abnormal cells that do not extend beyond ducts or lobules into surrounding stroma. Rates of ductal in situ carcinoma (DCIS) diagnosis have increased dramatically with rising use of screening mammography, and DCIS now represents approximately 20% of breast cancers diagnosed by screening.[31] DCIS most often presents as microcalcifications on mammogram, and it is estimated that approximately 15% to 60% of DCIS cases progress to invasive ductal carcinoma (IDC) without treatment.[32] By contrast, lobular carcinoma in situ (LCIS) is typically an incidental pathologic finding. LCIS is associated with increased breast cancer risk in the ipsilateral and contralateral breast, however, there is controversy regarding whether it represents a precursor lesion for breast cancer.[33] In 2018, LCIS was removed from AJCC staging system as it is treated as a benign entity.[34]

IDC is the most common invasive histologic subtype, followed by invasive lobular carcinoma. Invasive carcinomas extend through the basement membrane to directly infiltrate surrounding breast tissue, often resulting in a stellate or spiculated appearance. This infiltration provides access to lymphatic and blood vessels, facilitating spread to adjacent lymph nodes and distant hematogenous sites. Compared to IDC, lobular carcinomas are more likely to be multifocal and diffusely infiltrative, resulting in poorly defined margins on exam and imaging.[35] Rarer histologic subtypes include tubular, mucinous, papillary, and micropapillary. Hormone receptor and HER2 status have been increasingly recognized as prognostic factors in breast cancer regardless of histologic subtype. Four major subgroups of breast cancer have been defined as a function of gene expression patterns (related to proliferation, hormone receptor expression, HER2 expression, and expression of basal epithelial markers) and include luminal A, luminal B, HER2-enriched, and basal like.[36]

Inflammatory breast cancer (IBC) is an aggressive breast cancer subtype with a higher propensity for lymphatic and distant spread compared to other invasive carcinomas. IBC typically presents with rapid development of breast tenderness, warmth, erythema, skin thickening, and/or peau d'orange appearance. Skin changes are secondary to tumor emboli within dermal lymphatics. Due to this dermal lymphatic involvement, most women with IBC have positive nodes and approximately one-third have metastatic disease upon presentation. Neglected primary tumors may have a similar appearance to IBC, however, there is a longer interval between initial symptoms and development of skin changes.

PATIENT SELECTION

Breast Conservation

Large randomized trials have established that breast conservation, consisting of partial mastectomy followed by adjuvant radiotherapy, provides equivalent outcomes to mastectomy in the treatment of early stage invasive and in situ breast carcinoma.[37,38] The whole breast with or without regional lymph nodes is irradiated to eradicate microscopic residual disease and minimize the risk of local recurrence. A large meta-analysis has demonstrated improved breast cancer survival with adjuvant radiotherapy after breast conserving surgery.[39]

Breast conservation candidates must be motivated to preserve their breasts and should not have any contraindication to adjuvant radiotherapy. Contraindications to breast conservation include widespread disease that cannot be incorporated in a local excision, extensive suspicious microcalcifications, persistently positive margins, and pregnancy at the time of radiotherapy. Collagen vascular disease,[40] prior ipsilateral breast irradiation, tumor size relative to breast size or location resulting in suboptimal cosmetic results, and genetic predisposition to breast cancer may be relative contraindications as well. Young patient age, in and of itself, is not a contraindication to breast conservation, as excellent outcomes have been

reported for these patients with breast conservation as well.[41] Large pendulous breasts are not a contraindication to breast conservation, but may affect patient positioning considerations during radiation therapy.

Postmastectomy

Locoregional postmastectomy radiotherapy is associated with significantly improved outcomes for women with node-positive breast cancer. A recent meta-analysis of randomized controlled trials by the Early Breast Cancer Trialists' Collaborative Group (EBCTCG) showed relative risk reductions of 32% for locoregional recurrence and 20% for breast cancer mortality among all node-positive women receiving radiotherapy after mastectomy and axillary dissection.[42] These results are driven largely by the large British Columbia and Danish Breast Cancer Cooperative Group trials, which showed improved overall survival with postmastectomy locoregional radiotherapy for node-positive women.[43-45] While guidelines universally endorse postmastectomy radiotherapy for patients with four or more positive axillary nodes, recommendations have been mixed for patients with one to three positive axillary nodes.[46-50]

The EBCTCG meta-analysis did not show any improvement in locoregional control or breast cancer mortality with postmastectomy radiotherapy for node-negative women.[42] However, several guidelines recommend at least consideration of postmastectomy radiotherapy for patients with T3 and T4 tumors or positive margins.[46,48,49] Additional factors such as lymphovascular invasion, high-grade histology, multicentric disease, skin or nipple involvement, and young age or premenopausal status have also been associated with postmastectomy recurrence and therefore may influence decisions regarding adjuvant radiotherapy.[51,52]

Treatment Following Neoadjuvant Chemotherapy

Neoadjuvant chemotherapy is increasingly administered in the modern era, particularly for patients with locally advanced, triple negative, or HER2-positive disease. Historically, the advantage of neoadjuvant chemotherapy largely related to facilitating surgical resection. In more recent years, trials such as CREATE-X and KATHERINE have established neoadjuvant chemotherapy as a powerful method for risk stratification and for selection of patients who may benefit from escalation of adjuvant therapy (i.e., those who do not have a robust response to neoadjuvant therapy).[53,54] Currently, NCCN guidelines recommend use of the highest pre or posttreatment stage to make decisions regarding PMRT in the setting of neoadjuvant chemotherapy. However, patients who achieve a pathologic complete response (pCR) in the axilla have very low rates of locoregional recurrence and optimal adjuvant radiation in this setting remains an area of question.[55] To this end, the NSABP B51/RTOG 1304 trial is an ongoing randomized study of patients with clinical T1–T3, N1 breast cancer who achieve a nodal pCR following neoadjuvant chemotherapy. Patients who receive breast conserving surgery are randomized to whole breast radiation with or without regional radiation and patients who receive a mastectomy are randomized to PMRT or no radiotherapy.[56] Results of this trial are eagerly anticipated in order to help inform adjuvant radiotherapy decision-making for patients who achieve a pCR after neoadjuvant chemotherapy.

Omission of Radiotherapy

Consideration of omission of radiotherapy after breast conserving surgery may be appropriate for a highly selected patient group. One such population is women over the age of 70 with small (<2 cm), estrogen receptor positive, node-negative tumors. Ten-year results of the CALGB 9343 trial showed that patients who received tamoxifen alone, without adjuvant radiotherapy, had slightly higher rates of local recurrence (9% vs. 2%), but with no difference in overall survival.[57] PRIME II was a similar trial that randomized patients over 65 with estrogen-receptor positive tumors up to 3 cm taking endocrine therapy to receive adjuvant radiation or no radiation.[58] At 5 years, patients who did not receive radiation had higher rates of local recurrence (4% vs. 1%) but no difference in OS.[58] Breast conserving surgery without adjuvant radiotherapy may also be appropriate for women with completely resected, small DCIS that is low or intermediate grade.[59] Similarly, the randomized RTOG 9804 trial shows a statistically significant reduction in local recurrence risk for small completely resected DCIS, but with very low recurrence rates in both arms.[60] However, newer studies reveal that abbreviated courses of radiation therapy, especially in women with low-risk disease, can be delivered in as few as 5 total fractions with low rates of side effects.[61] Thus, a thorough discussion of the risks and benefits of radiation therapy versus observation should be discussed with patients.

SIMULATION

Historically, simulation for breast radiation was performed on a conventional simulator with asymmetric collimators and a breast tilt board.[62] Currently, most treatment centers in the US utilize computed tomography (CT)-based treatment planning.

Supine Intact Breast

The patient is placed in the supine position with arms up on abreast board, vac-lock, or other immobilization device. A tilt should be applied to the immobilization device in order to isolate breast tissue below the clavicle. The head is turned slightly to the contralateral side if regional nodal irradiation is planned. The clinical

boundaries of breast are marked with radio-opaque fiducial wire. The medial border is placed at midline over the sternum, and the lateral border is placed at the mid-axillary line. The superior border is placed at the inferior aspect of the clavicular head, and the inferior border is placed approximately 2 cm below the inframammary fold. For an intact breast, adjustment of wires may be required to allow approximately 2 cm margin around palpable breast tissue, particularly for large-breasted women. A fiducial wire is also placed over the lumpectomy scar and any drain sites. A fiducial wire can also be placed circumferentially around clinical breast tissue to assist in target delineation. If nodal volumes are to be included, a catheter can be placed 3 cm lateral to the midline sternal catheter toward the contralateral side to facilitate field design encompassing the IM nodes. Although these catheters are placed as guides, target delineation is largely based on CT volumes as discussed below.

A scout CT scan is obtained to verify patient positioning and setup. Axial 3-mm CT slices are then acquired. The superior border of the CT scan should be at least 4 cm above the superior border for breast-only treatment or above the angle of the mandible if treating supraclavicular nodes. The inferior border should be at least 4 cm below the inferior catheter. For breath-hold technique (further discussion below), the inferior border is lowered to encompass the tracking device on the patient's abdomen. Axial CT images are reviewed at the time of simulation to identify any needed positioning changes.

A stable reference point is set at the middle of the breast in the longitudinal direction, at the center of the patient in the lateral direction and at the mid-chest level in the vertical direction. This reference point is projected on the skin with the room lasers and alignment marks are made on the patient with marker and protected with clear stickers. These can be subsequently used during positioning on the treatment table as a stable point from which to shift to treatment isocenter. At some institutions, tattoos are used to delineate alignment marks. An isocenter may also be selected at the time of simulation.

Prone

Prone positioning for whole breast radiation can be considered largely for patients who will not receive nodal irradiation[63]; although some institutions have published experiences for prone regional nodal radiation.[64,65] Improved dose homogeneity and decreased lung dose have been observed with this technique.[66,67] Effect on cardiac dose varies depending on patient anatomy.[67,68] Prone setup may be particularly beneficial for women with large breasts by facilitating reduced separation.[69]

The patient is initially placed in the supine position with arms up, and catheters are placed to demarcate the clinical limits of breast tissue as described for supine simulation. The patient is then positioned in prone position on a prone breast board with the ipsilateral breast suspended in the open area of the breast board with both arms up. The contralateral breast is pulled away beneath the patient with the support of the contralateral breast board plate. The head can be turned toward the treated side, away from the treated side, or in a neutral position depending on prone breast board style and patient comfort.

A scout CT scan is obtained to verify patient positioning and setup. Axial 3-mm CT images are then obtained with similar superior and inferior borders as discussed for supine positioning. Breath-hold technique is not utilized in the prone position. A stable reference point is set at the middle of the breast in the longitudinal direction, at the center of the board in the lateral direction and at the level of the contralateral breast board plate. This reference point is marked on the patient skin. Indexing and leveling marks are also made on the patient, primarily on the back and arms, to maximize reproducibility on the treatment table. This is particularly important for prone position due to greater inter-fraction setup variability compared to supine position.[70]

Repeat simulation in supine position is typically performed for tumor bed boost planning. For certain tumor locations and/or large breasts, a lateral decubitus position is preferable to supine position for en face treatment. In other cases, boost may be best performed in the prone position, most commonly with mini-tangent fields. If needed, repeat simulation should be performed near the end of whole breast irradiation (WBI) to allow for any changes in tumor bed or seroma.

Postmastectomy

The patient is immobilized in the supine position with both arms above the head. The mastectomy scar, drain sites, and clinical boundaries of breast tissue are marked with a radio-opaque wire as described for intact breast simulation. If intact, the contralateral breast can be used to determine the appropriate location of the inferior, lateral,

and superior borders. The CT scan is then performed as described for breast conservation. A stable reference point is set on the patient, and alignment marks are made as discussed above.

Deep Inspiration Breath Hold

The patient is simulated in supine position as discussed above. Respiratory gating or active breathing control can be used to monitor respiration. Respiratory gating utilizes a reflective marker placed on the patient during simulation and treatment. Marker motion with respiration is tracked by an infrared camera, and the respiratory pattern is displayed as a waveform. The patient practices deep inspiration and breath hold a few times. Gating thresholds are set at the amplitude level where the patient is able to perform stable deep inspiration breath hold over 15 to 20 seconds. Axial CT images are obtained during breath hold within this optimal breath-hold threshold, as well as during free breathing.

Active breathing control is an alternative technique in which the patient breathes through a mouthpiece that is connected to a breathing control device. This apparatus has respiratory flow monitors and valves to control inspiration and expiration. The valves are closed to immobilize breathing motion temporarily when the patient reaches the optimal inspiratory phase of the respiratory cycle. A nose clip prevents air leakage and facilitates accurate inspiratory volume measurement. Axial CT images are obtained during this preselected respiratory phase, as well as during free breathing.

Deep inspiration breath-hold facilitates reduced cardiac dose compared to free breathing during treatment of left-sided breast cancer for many patients.[71,72] Breath hold can also be considered for treatment of right-sided breast cancer for select patients for cardiac, liver, or pulmonary protection.[73] Breath hold and free breathing images are compared at the time of simulation to determine which position provides better cardiac sparing (Fig. 8.4).

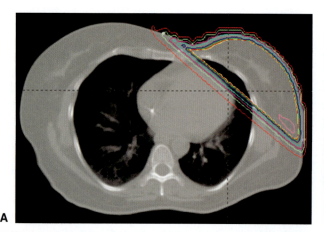
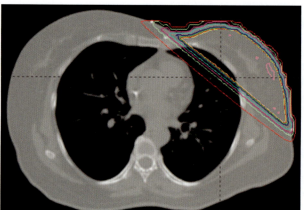

FIGURE 8.4. Cardiac sparing with (A) free breathing versus (B) breath hold for treatment of left-sided breast cancer. Isodose curves are shown at the same level within the breast for a patient simulated in **(A)** free breathing and **(B)** deep inspiratory breath hold.

TREATMENT PLANNING: TARGET DELINEATION

Breast cancer was historically treated using clinical body landmarks. In the current era of CT-based three-dimensional treatment planning, targets can be more precisely delineated. CT images from simulation are exported from the CT acquisition software and imported to the treatment planning software. Normal structures, including lungs, heart, and potentially other structures such as the spinal cord, brachial plexus, and contralateral breast, are contoured on the acquired CT images. Target structures, including the breast or chest wall are contoured. Regional lymph nodes consisting of axillary levels I, II, and III, supraclavicular, and IM nodes are also contoured in the setting of nodal treatment. In the intact breast setting, the lumpectomy cavity is contoured including seroma, architectural distortion of the tissue, and any surgical clips present in the breast.

Contouring is generally performed manually by the treating physician and planning dosimetrist. However, automated contouring is increasingly utilized with newer treatment planning software.[74] Studies show that even amongst experts, there is significant inter-observer variability in contouring of breast, chest wall, and regional nodal targets.[75] Published guidelines are available from NRG Oncology (RTOG) and ESTRO regarding delineation of the breast, chest wall, and regional draining nodal basins.[76,77] While individual patient anatomy may not strictly conform to the example images in these atlases, these guidelines provide a starting point for practitioners, and continue to be utilized in current cooperative group protocols. Recent guideline comparisons indicate that ESTRO guidelines may be preferred for treating early-stage breast cancer, whereas RTOG guidelines may be preferred for treating locally advanced disease.[78,79] However, some areas at risk for recurrence seen in modern patterns of failure analyses are not included in either atlas (e.g., cranial to the cricoid cartilage, posterolateral neck, junction of IMN and SCV volumes, fourth and fifth intercostal spaces, etc.) and one may consider inclusion of these regions for select patients.[80,81]

Breast Conservation

The desired target in the breast conservation setting is the entire ipsilateral breast. Care must be taken to ensure adequate coverage of the tumor bed, particularly if this is located to one edge of the breast tissue. Treatment of regional nodes may be appropriate after breast conservation as well. Nodal irradiation has been universally considered to be indicated in the setting of four or more involved axillary lymph nodes. Comprehensive nodal irradiation is more controversial in the setting of one to three positive lymph nodes. However, data recently reported from the MA20 and EORTC 22922 trials, in which patients with one to three positive nodes were randomized to whole breast or chest wall irradiation with or without radiotherapy to lymph node targets, indicate at least a trend toward survival benefit with the addition of nodal irradiation.[82,83]

Additionally, after publication of the ACOSOG Z0011 study showing non-inferior outcomes for patients who do not receive axillary dissection in the setting of one or two positive sentinel lymph nodes, an increasing number of patients are not undergoing axillary dissection after identification of a positive sentinel node.[84,85] An analysis of the radiotherapy treatment patterns on the ACOSOG Z0011 study showed that approximately 15% of patients did receive a third field to the supraclavicular region. Approximately 50% of patients received coverage of the lower axilla interpreted as high tangents, regardless of treatment arm.[86]

The EORTC 10981-22023 AMAROS trial showed equivalence of radiotherapy to axillary dissection in controlling the axilla in the setting of positive sentinel lymph node biopsy after breast conservation[83] with a significantly lower rate of lymphedema. Therefore, it may be increasingly common to consider regional nodal radiotherapy rather than axillary dissection in the setting of a small number of positive sentinel nodes. In this context, it may be particularly important for the radiation oncologist to consider inclusion of at least lower axillary levels in high tangent fields versus full nodal irradiation with a third field depending on individual patient risk. Of note, if axillary nodes were not dissected, the full axilla and supraclavicular nodes (rather than a supraclavicular field alone without attention to the lower axilla) should be covered if nodal treatment is desired.

Postmastectomy

The desired target volumes in the setting of postmastectomy radiotherapy include the chest wall, axillary and supraclavicular nodal regions, and often, the IM lymph nodes. Though IM nodes were included in the large randomized trials evaluating postmastectomy radiotherapy, inclusion of IM nodes in the setting of PMRT remains controversial. Ten-year results from trials comparing outcomes for patients with stages I and II breast cancer treated with mastectomy and postoperative radiotherapy with or without treatment of the IM nodes demonstrated no difference in overall survival.[87] The recently reported MA20 and EORTC22922 trials evaluating inclusion of nodal treatment or not, also included IM coverage in addition to axillary and supraclavicular treatment. The recently reported DBCG-IMN study was a population-based cohort study that enrolled 3,089 patients with unilateral early-stage, node-positive breast cancer. Patients with right-sided disease received treatment with inclusion of IMN and patients with left-sided disease received regional treatment without IMN coverage. At 8 years, inclusion of IMN radiation was associated with a 3.7% increase in overall survival and a 2.5% decrease in breast cancer mortality.[88] For many practitioners the decision regarding inclusion of IM nodes may be performed on an individual patient basis to achieve a balance between local recurrence risk and morbidity of treatment. In particular, consideration may be given to exclusion of IM nodes when treating left-sided breast cancer, given concern for cardiotoxicity.

TREATMENT PLANNING: FIELD DESIGN

Tangent Fields for Intact Breast

Tangential fields are designed to encompass the entire breast as defined by the treating physician (Fig. 8.5A–D). It is important to allow adequate clearance of breast tissue. The entire contoured tumor bed should be included within the tangential fields with adequate margin. A margin of at least 2 cm around the tumor bed within the tangential field is frequently used to allow for variation in setup. The isocenter is generally set along the chest wall, midway between the superior and inferior aspects of the field. If treatment of only lower axillary levels is desired, without inclusion of upper axillary or supraclavicular nodes, high tangents can be considered. In this situation the upper level of the tangents is raised to ensure coverage of the desired axillary levels, generally at least level I, possibly also level II depending on individual patient risk. It is important to note that inclusion of levels I and II may be best achieved by contouring these axillary levels to ensure appropriate coverage within tangents.

Tangent Fields for Chest Wall

The entire ipsilateral chest wall target, as defined by the treating clinician, should be included within the tangential fields (Fig. 8.5E–G). Fields may require modification to ensure inclusion of the entire mastectomy scar and drain sites. When drain sites fall significantly outside the tangents, an abutting electron field can be utilized to supplement superficial dose in these areas if clinically appropriate.

Inclusion of Nodal Targets

Breast/chest wall and regional nodal treatment traditionally entails matching the superior boarder of opposed tangent fields to the inferior boarder of an anterior oblique supraclavicular field that is half-beam blocked inferiorly (Fig. 8.5E–G). This can be accomplished with single isocenter or dual isocenter methods. Couch rotation and collimator angulation can be used to match diverging field edges and minimize normal tissue toxicity from overlap.[48–51] The use of half-blocked or over-rotated tangents minimizes tangent beam divergence into the lung.

Three-Field Single Isocenter

In this technique the single isocenter is set along the match line at the bottom of the clavicular head (Fig. 8.5E). For the tangential fields, the superior jaw is set to zero at the level of the isocenter and the inferior jaw is opened to the inferior marking wire to encompass the entire chest wall target. Couch rotation and collimator angulation are set to zero so that no diverging field occurs at the junction with half-blocked fields. The supraclavicular field is designed with an inferior jaw set to zero at the level of the isocenter and the superior jaw is set to the level of the bottom of the cricoid cartilage. The supraclavicular field is obliqued slightly to avoid the spinal cord. The medial jaw edge is set to the lateral vertebral bodies, and custom MLCs can be used to shape this field medially and laterally. The lateral field edge is set to cover desired axillary levels and supraclavicular nodes, depending on the clinical situation and desired axillary targets. While this technique has the advantage of simpler setup and imaging on the treatment machine, one drawback is that the tangent field length is limited to 20 cm, and tools for modulating dose are often restricted further. The superior border of the tangent, that is, match line, can be adjusted up or down to compensate for this. However, lowering the matched line can result in inadequate dose coverage for the superior breast tissue area and increases in the ipsilateral lung dose.

Three-Field Dual Isocenter

With this technique, the supraclavicular field isocenter and borders are placed as described for the single isocenter method. However, for tangential field design, an isocenter is set along the chest wall approximately equal depth from medial and lateral tangential fields and midway between the superior and inferior borders of the field (Fig. 8.5F). In order to create a non-overlapping matching plane between the superior border of the tangents and the inferior border of the half-beam blocked supraclavicular field, couch rotation and collimator angulation are utilized for the medial and lateral tangential fields. Modern treatment planning software can often perform this automatically and it can then be visually double-checked within the computer planning software. While this technique requires more complicated setup and imaging on the treatment machine, it allows the tangential fields to be greater than 20 cm. This may be required for patients with larger habitus or breast size.

IM Nodal Coverage

If the IM nodes are to be treated, multiple methods have been described to ensure coverage. These include partially wide tangent fields (Fig. 8.5E–F), extended tangent fields, and matching electron/photon fields (Fig. 8.5G). Dosimetric comparison studies have determined that the partially wide tangent technique provides the optimal

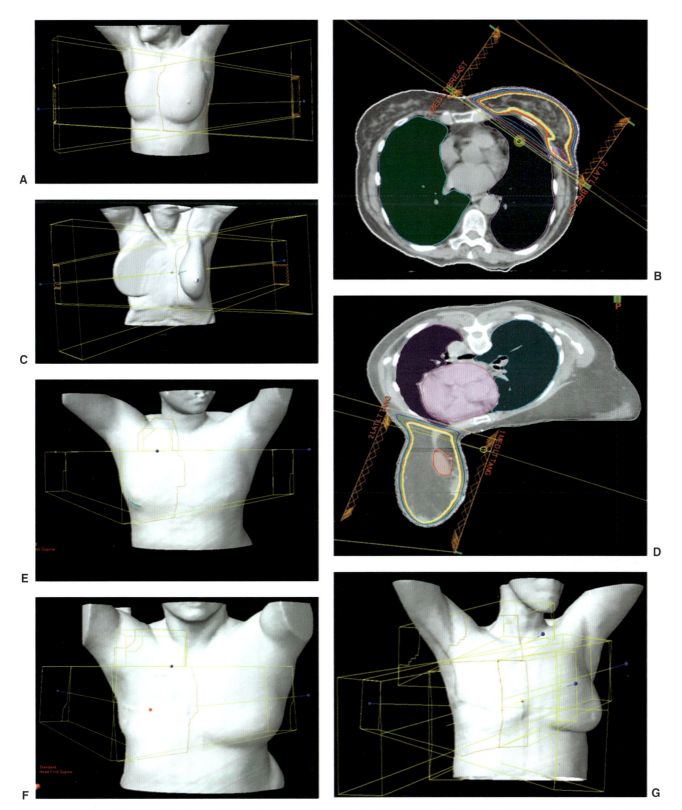

FIGURE 8.5. Tangent, supraclavicular, and internal mammary field design. **(A)** Medial and lateral tangent fields with field entry shapes displayed on skin rendering with patient in supine position. **(B)** Isodose curves for the same supine patient. The isocenter (*yellow circle*) is located within the patient at a point that is approximately midway along the central axis. **(C)** Medial and lateral tangent fields are shown with field entry shapes displayed on skin rendering with patient in prone position. **(D)** Isodose curves for the same prone patient. The isocenter (*yellow circle*) is located medial to the breast, outside the body. The tumor bed is in red. **(E)** Single isocenter three-field beam arrangement. The shared isocenter is marked by a blue sphere. The internal mammary nodes are included within partially wide tangents. **(F)** Dual isocenter three-field beam arrangement. The oblique nodal field isocenter is marked by a blue sphere. The isocenter for the tangents is within the patient at the location of the red dot. The internal mammary nodes are included within partially wide tangents. **(G)** Matched electron beam arrangement. An electron field is matched medially to opposed tangents and superiorly to the anterior oblique field to encompass the internal mammary nodes and lower inner chest wall.

blend of target coverage and normal tissue sparing.[89–91] For patients requiring a matched electron field, split electron fields using a lower energy below the third intercostal space can help to lower cardiac dose.[92]

Supraclavicular/Axillary Field

The supraclavicular and desired axillary nodal levels are generally included in a single anterior oblique photon field angled off the spinal cord. The starting angle is often 15°, but this can be adjusted as needed based on patient anatomy. Historically dose was prescribed to a depth of 3 cm. However, dose should be prescribed to adequately encompass the contoured nodal volumes within the full prescription dose using modern CT-based treatment planning (Fig. 8.6A–B). Field borders are set based on contoured nodal volumes and custom MLCs can be utilized to avoid spinal cord medially and the shoulder joint as appropriate laterally. Avoidance of skin flash superiorly in the supraclavicular region can decrease acute skin reaction and may preserve a strip of lymphatics within the skin to help minimize risk of upper extremity lymphedema.

Posterior Axillary Field

If deeper axillary nodal volumes cannot be adequately encompassed within a minimum dose of 4500 cGy through a single anterior oblique supraclavicular/axillary field without excessive hot spots, the dose to deeper axillary structures can be supplemented with a posterior axillary field. This field is designed to oppose the supraclavicular/axillary field. Conventional field borders are the clavicle superiorly and the tangential match line inferiorly. The lateral and medial borders are based on patient anatomy and contoured axillary nodal targets (Fig. 8.6C–E). The dose contribution from this field is low, typically in the range of 25 to 50 cGy per day to supplement the dose from the anterior oblique supraclavicular field.

Alternatively, a full posterior oblique opposed field can be used to provide supplemental coverage of the entire supraclavicular/axillary field (Fig. 8.6F–H). This field is designed with a non-divergent medial border to avoid spinal cord dose. In this setting, the dose is generally prescribed to a midpoint, and the anterior–posterior field weighting can be adjusted as desired based on patient anatomy, target coverage, and placement of dose hotspots. In the setting of either posterior field utilization, mixed beam energy, forward planned electronic compensation, or field-in-field techniques may also be utilized to improve dose homogeneity.

Dose Modulation

The large variability in tissue thickness within the breast poses a challenge in achieving a homogeneous dose distribution. Lack of scatter from lung tissue contributes to insufficient coverage near the central chest wall region, leading to higher dose elsewhere when a plan is normalized to provide adequate coverage near the chest wall. Hotspots are typically greater in women with large breasts due to greater separation. Traditionally, wedges have been utilized to improve dose homogeneity.[93–96] Physical wedges (typically 15°, 30°, 45°, or 60°) are placed along the desired plane with the heel compensating for the thinnest area of breast tissue. Field size is limited within the wedge plane, with maximum dimension depending on wedge angle. Alternatively, dynamic wedges use collimator jaw movement while the beam is on to modulate dose. This allows additional wedge angles, avoids manual wedge placement by the therapists, and permits larger field size. Patient-customized physical compensators can also be used, although construction of these devices is impractical due to the required labor and time involved.[97,98] Mixed beam energies represent another simple method of improving dose homogeneity with standard tangential fields.[99,100]

Several studies have shown reduced short-term toxicity and improved cosmesis with intensity modulated radiation therapy (IMRT) compared to wedge-based tangential whole breast radiotherapy.[101–106] Improved cardiac dose sparing has been proposed as an additional benefit.[107–113] Breast IMRT studies have utilized various techniques including "field-in-field" or multi-segmented 3D conformal radiotherapy, inverse and forward planned techniques, and dynamic or segmental multileaf collimator modes. Helical tomotherapy and volume modulated arc therapy (VMAT) have been introduced as additional methods of dose modulation.

The American Society for Radiation Oncology (ASTRO) recently recommended against routine usage of IMRT to deliver whole breast radiotherapy. This was one of the five recommendations released in 2013 for the Choosing Wisely® campaign, identifying treatment options that should be carefully considered to avoid overuse.[114] Inverse planned IMRT should be limited to specific breast cancer cases such as patients with unusual anatomy, where this technique will more likely provide significant clinical benefit.[115–118]

Electronic tissue compensation (ECOMP) represents an alternative method of modulating dose to achieve homogeneous dose distribution. ECOMP involves forward planning to modify the fluence distribution manually within each tangential field to improve dose homogeneity. Treatment planning software subsequently converts the fluence maps to dynamic multileaf collimation sequences for treatment delivery. ECOMP does not require optimization process, but skilled manual fluence modification is required. It provides similar target coverage and normal tissue sparing compatible to inverse planning IMRT.[119,120]

Normal Tissue Dose Constraints

The primary organs at risk during breast and chest wall irradiation are the lungs and heart. Dose to the

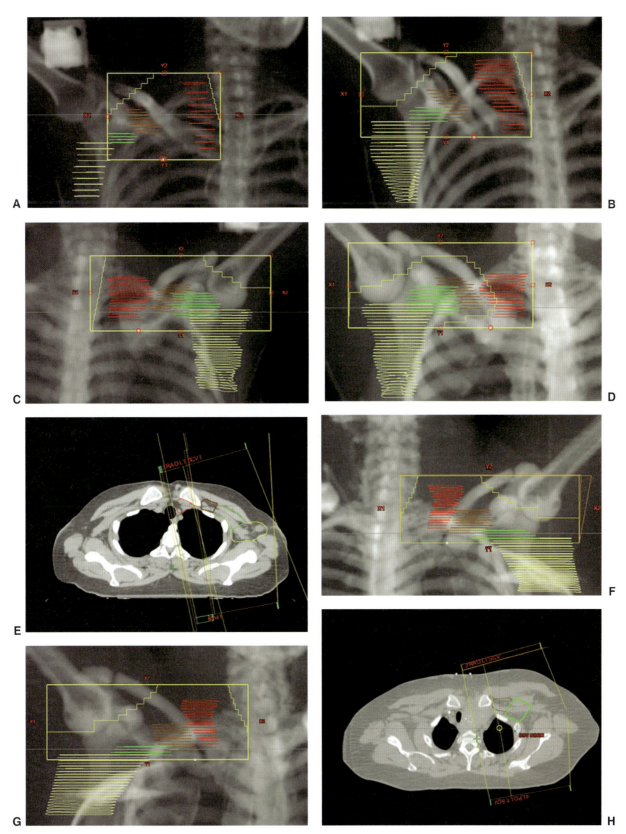

FIGURE 8.6. Supraclavicular and axillary nodal fields. **(A)** Digital reconstructed radiograph (DRR) of a nodal field for a patient has undergone a complete axillary dissection. The anterior oblique field has been shaped to include only the undissected axilla and supraclavicular region. **(B)** DRR of a nodal field for a patient who has not undergone an axillary dissection or for whom full axillary coverage is indicated. The field extends farther laterally than is seen in panel A to encompass the entire axilla and supraclavicular region. **(C–E)** DRRs for a right anterior oblique field **(C)** and partial posterior axillary boost beam **(D)** with an axial image **(E)** showing both fields. **(F–H)** DRRs for a right anterior oblique field **(F)** and full opposed left posterior oblique field **(G)** with an axial image **(H)** showing both fields. Axillary level I is *yellow*, II is *green*, III is *brown*, and supraclavicular nodal region is *red*.

opposite breast should also be minimized to reduce risk of radiation-induced contralateral breast cancer. Lung dose is strongly correlated with radiation pneumonitis, and V_{20Gy} ≤20% has been associated with significantly lower incidence of radiation pneumonitis.[121] However, achieving an ipsilateral lung V_{20Gy} ≤20% can be difficult when IM nodes are targeted. Symptomatic radiation pneumonitis is rare with ipsilateral lung V_{20Gy} <30%.[122,123] Ipsilateral lung dose-volume constraints of V_{20Gy} ≤20% and V_{20Gy} ≤30% are commonly accepted in breast treatment planning.[124]

Breast radiotherapy has been associated with cardiac mortality in numerous trials predating the era of CT-based radiation treatment planning.[125–127] More recent studies indicate that radiotherapy-associated cardiac toxicity has decreased with the advent of modern treatment planning techniques.[128–130] Normal Tissue Complication Probability models in the Quantitative Analyses of Normal Tissue Effects in the Clinic guidelines estimate a <1% risk of cardiac mortality at 15 years with a cardiac V_{25Gy} <10%.[131] A large population-based case–control study of patients with prior radiotherapy for breast cancer showed a linear increase in major coronary events of 7.4% per Gray mean radiation dose to the heart with no apparent threshold.[132] Shielding blocks or multi-leaf collimators should be used to minimize radiation dose to the heart. Prone positioning, deep inspiratory breath hold, and dose modulation techniques discussed above may also facilitate lower cardiac doses.

Treatment Imaging

The CT dataset is used to create digitally reconstructed radiographs for orthogonal setup films (AP and lateral) and beam's eye view for each tangential treatment field. Port films and kV on-board imaging are performed before delivering the first treatment to confirm isocenter location, patient positioning and field shape in relation to patient anatomy target area. Imaging frequency during the treatment course depends on numerous factors, including daily setup variability, patient positioning, and utilization of respiratory gating. Free-breathing treatment in supine position typically requires less frequent imaging than breath-hold or prone breast treatment. Supine treatment with respiratory gating requires port images for the first few days to confirm patient breath-hold level. Prone position typically requires daily orthogonal setup imaging since the treatment area is difficult to visualize.

DOSE AND FRACTIONATION

Breast Conservation

WBI has historically delivered 45 to 50 Gy in 25 to 28 fractions at 1.8 to 2 Gy per fraction. However, 10-year data from multiple large randomized trials have demonstrated the non-inferiority of hypofractionated whole breast radiotherapy (42.5 Gy in 16 fractions[133] or 40.05 Gy in 15 fractions[134,135]) for patients with invasive breast cancer. The Canadian trial included only node-negative patients and placed restrictions on breast size and treatment hot spots.[133] The UK START trials had broader inclusion criteria, including approximately 25% node-positive patients.[134] The recently reported DBCG HYPO trial is the first randomized trial to include a subset of patients with DCIS (13% of the cohort), with no difference in locoregional recurrence in this subset between standard and hypofractionation arms.[135]

Hypofractionated WBI should be strongly considered, given the high-quality evidence supporting its safety and efficacy. This was highlighted in one of the ASTRO 2013 Choosing Wiselyre® commendations, stating not to initiate radiotherapy in women aged 50 years or older with early-stage invasive breast cancer without considering a hypofractionated treatment schedule.[114] In 2018, ASTRO updated guidelines on dose and fractionation schedules for patients receiving whole breast radiation with or without inclusion of the lower axilla, and determined that the preferred dose-fractionation scheme is hypofractionated whole breast radiotherapy to a dose of 4000 cGy in 15 fractions or 4250 cGy in 16 fractions.[136,137] These updated guidelines do not limit hypofractionation use as a function of age, stage (provided the intent is to treat the whole breast without an additional field to cover regional lymph nodes), chemotherapy receipt, or several other patient-specific variables. Prone positioning and advanced dose modulation strategies may help to improve dose homogeneity and increase the number of patients appropriate for hypofractionation. Data supporting more hypofractionated regimens have recently been reported in the UK FAST and FAST FORWARD trials.[138] In the UK FAST trial, patients aged 50 years or older with node-negative early breast cancer were randomized to receive 50 Gy in 25 fractions versus 28.5 or 30 Gy in 5 once-weekly fractions to the whole breast.[139] Although not powered for local control, at 10 years, 28.5 Gy in 5 fractions was determined to be comparable to 50 Gy in 25 fractions in terms of cosmesis (but normal tissue effects were higher following 30 Gy in 5 once-weekly fractions). In the UK FAST FORWARD trial, patients were randomized to 40 Gy in 15 fractions versus 26 or 27 Gy in 5 fractions over a period of 1 week. At 5 years, 26 Gy in 5 daily fractions was non-inferior to 40 Gy/15 fractions for local control and cosmesis/toxicity (while 27 Gy in 5 fractions was associated with higher normal tissue effect risk).[61]

If nodal targets are included in the treatment of the intact breast setting, treatment planning and dose coverage are similar to those described in the postmastectomy setting. Hypofractionated radiotherapy in the treatment of lymph nodes is more commonly used in other countries than it currently is in the US.[140,141] Patients with N1 disease were included on the UK START trials, and a subset of patients received hypofractionated nodal irradiation. Additionally, the original British Columbia postmastectomy radiotherapy trial utilized a hypofractionated course (37.5 Gy in 16 fractions). This regimen was well-tolerated; however, no fractionation randomization was included in this trial.[45] More recently, a Chinese randomized, non-inferiority trial was conducted investigating hypofractionated postmastectomy radiation for patients with locally advanced disease. In this trial, patients were randomized to receive 50 Gy in 25 fractions versus 43.5 Gy in 15 fractions, and hypofractionated PMRT was determined to be non-inferior to standard fractionated radiotherapy in terms of local control and toxicity.[142] A notable limitation is that IM nodes were not included in this trial.

Postmastectomy

Standard prescribed dose to the chest wall and IM nodes is 45 to 50.4 Gy in 25 to 28 fractions. In most cases, chest wall bolus is utilized to ensure adequate dose to the skin and superficial subcutaneous tissue. Significant heterogeneity exists in the accepted bolus thickness and schedule.[124] Bolus use may be modified based on the clinical situation and estimated patient risk. More frequent bolus schedules, including possibly daily bolus, may be considered for the patients at highest risk, particularly those with IBC.

Tumor Bed Boost

Randomized controlled trials have demonstrated improved local tumor control with additional radiotherapy to the tumor bed for patients with invasive breast cancer in the setting of breast conservation.[143–145] A greater absolute benefit was observed for younger patients. There are no level one data evaluating boost for DCIS, but practitioners often extrapolate from the invasive data and utilize a boost in these patients. This is particularly true in the setting of close or positive margins and for young patients, supported by one series that showed a benefit for boost in women younger than 40 years of age.[146] A recent multi-institutional retrospective study pooled data for over 4,000 patients with DCIS and tumor bed boost was associated with reduced in breast tumor recurrence.[147] BIG 3-07/TROG 07.01 is an ongoing randomized trial of tumor bed boost for women with non-low-risk DCIS. Local recurrence analysis has not yet been reported, however, initial toxicity assessment indicates that tumor bed boost is associated with worse cosmesis.[148] A tumor bed boost usually consists of 10 Gy to 16 Gy at 2 to 2.5 Gy per fraction delivered to the lumpectomy cavity, typically with 1.5 to 2.5 cm additional margin. Boosting to a total tumor bed dose greater than 60 Gy should be considered in patients with positive margins.

Tumor bed boost is typically administered by en face electrons, with beam energy chosen based on tumor depth. A normalization point can be set at D-max for the chosen electron energy and dose prescribed to the desired isodose level. Alternatively, dose can be prescribed to a specific depth. Photons may be necessary to provide adequate coverage for deep tumors depending on patient anatomy. In this case, generally a four to five beam bouquet is used, often in a non-coplanar arrangement to minimize exit dose into the lungs, heart, or contralateral breast, or mini-tangents can be used with similar angles and beam arrangement as the tangential breast fields, with the treatment field reduced to include the lumpectomy cavity and expansions. Brachytherapy can also be utilized to deliver the boost dose, although this is rarely performed.[144] Historically, the boost has been administered sequentially after WBI; however, studies are ongoing to investigate simultaneous integrated photon boost.[149]

Mastectomy Scar Boost

A radiotherapy boost is commonly administered to the mastectomy scar in the postmastectomy setting based on extrapolation of tumor bed boost data; however, practice patterns vary widely.[150] While most local recurrences after mastectomy occur at or near the scar,[151] no randomized controlled trials have examined whether additional radiotherapy provides any benefit. One retrospective review has shown reduced local recurrence and improved survival in patients with stage II–III breast cancer receiving a chest wall boost above 50.4 Gy.[152,153] Another retrospective analysis indicated that chest wall boost did not significantly improve local control, and did increase the risk of reconstruction complications.[154] Mastectomy scar boost typically consists of 10 Gy at 2 to 2.5 Gy per fraction delivered by en face electrons to a margin of 2 to 3 cm around the scar. Additional dose above 60 Gy may be considered in particularly high-risk settings such as IBC or other skin involvement.

PARTIAL BREAST IRRADIATION

Accelerated partial breast irradiation (APBI) is an alternative to WBI for a subset of patients with low-risk breast cancer. APBI targets the lumpectomy cavity with a small margin of normal surrounding tissue. This limited treatment volume is based on studies showing that most local recurrences occur in or near the tumor bed after breast-conserving therapy.[155–159] Irradiation of a smaller normal tissue volume allows delivery of a higher dose per fraction and shorter total treatment course. This may offer improved patient convenience and treatment accessibility, as well as decreased healthcare system costs.

Patient Selection

Appropriate patient selection for use of partial breast irradiation is essential, and several groups have released selection guidelines, highlighting a favorable-risk patient population with small tumors, negative margins, and no lymph node involvement.[160] APBI is typically not recommended for younger women or patients with invasive lobular histology. Recently, long-term follow-up from two large randomized studies have rendered additional support for the safety of a partial breast approach for select patients.[161,162] In the NSABP-B39/RTOG 0413 trial, 4,216 women with unifocal DCIS or invasive tumors up to 3 cm and negative margins were randomized to receive whole breast RT (50 Gy in 25 fractions) versus APBI delivered either via twice daily external beam radiation (38.5 Gy in 5 days, 73% of cohort) or 34 Gy brachytherapy.[162] At 10 years, the incidence of in-breast tumor recurrence was higher with APBI (4.6% vs. 3.9%), however, absolute difference between arms was small and treatment-related toxicity was similar. In the RAPID trial, 2,135 women with unifocal DCIS or invasive tumors up to 3 cm were randomized to receive whole breast radiation (either 50 Gy in 25 fractions or 42.56 Gy in 16 fractions) versus APBI as 38.5 Gy twice daily external beam radiation.[161] In contrast to NSABP-B39, APBI was found to be non-inferior in preventing in breast tumor recurrence, however, adverse cosmesis was more common with APBI as measured by nurses and patients.[162] Less toxicity has been generally been observed with once-daily partial breast approaches. For example, the IMPORT-LOW trial randomized patients with low-risk early stage breast cancer to receive 40 Gy in 15 fractions to either the whole or partial breast, and partial breast radiotherapy was determined to be non-inferior in terms of local relapse and had less toxicity.[163]

Treatment Planning

Several techniques can be utilized to deliver APBI, including brachytherapy, intraoperative radiotherapy (IORT), and external beam radiotherapy (EBRT). The longest follow-up is available for brachytherapy, but the optimal APBI method has not been determined.[164] The above NSABP B-39/RTOG 0413 trial randomizing patients to APBI or WBI allowed use of multicatheter brachytherapy, MammoSite balloon catheter, or three-dimensional conformal radiation therapy (3D-CRT) in the APBI treatment arm.

Simulation for treatment planning entails CT in prone or supine position as described previously for WBI. The lumpectomy cavity, including surgical clips and postoperative changes, is outlined. Typical postoperative clinical target volume (CTV) for EBRT-based APBI consists of the lumpectomy cavity expanded by 1 to 1.5 cm.[165–172] An additional 0.5 to 1 cm is generally added to generate the planning target volume (PTV), accounting for setup variability and patient motion. The seroma cavity with 1 to 2 cm margin is the recommended PTV for brachytherapy-based APBI.[173]

Promising cosmetic and local control outcomes have been demonstrated with brachytherapy-based APBI. The Budapest randomized controlled trial demonstrated excellent local control and superior cosmesis with interstitial APBI compared to WBI at 10 years.[174] Similar results have been shown in small single-institution series and the RTOG 95-17 phase II trial using multicatheter interstitial brachytherapy.[175–177] Implantation for interstitial brachytherapy is typically performed under general anesthesia. The tumor bed is localized by CT or an Integrated Brachytherapy Unit to visualize surgical clips, and catheters are inserted into the tumor bed and surrounding tissue. Repeat CT or orthogonal x-ray imaging is performed to reconstruct catheter placement for dosimetric planning. The most common interstitial catheter dose regimens are 45 to 50 Gy over 4 days, 32 to 34 Gy in twice daily 4 Gy fractions over 4 to 5 days, and 36.4 Gy in twice daily 5.2 Gy fractions over 4 days (HDR).[174–176]

Intracavitary and hybrid brachytherapy techniques have recently gained favor due to increased reproducibility and easier use compared to interstitial catheter placement. Available devices, including MammoSite, Contura, SAVI, Axxent, and ClearPath, are typically placed into the lumpectomy cavity at the time of surgery or postoperatively under image guidance. A CT scan is performed to evaluate the quality of the implant, including assessment of conformity to the cavity and distance to skin (ideally 7 mm). Several dosimetric optimization methods have been described.[178] Data from the American Society of Breast Surgeons MammoSite registry show excellent cosmesis and local control comparable to WBI in a highly selected patient population receiving 34 Gy in 3.4 Gy fractions twice daily over 5 days.[179]

IORT involves delivery of a single dose to the lumpectomy bed at the time of resection. Two randomized controlled trials have shown slightly higher local recurrence rates with IORT compared to external beam WBI, though low in both arms.[180,181] The TARGIT technique delivers approximately 20 Gy to the tumor bed surface from a point source of 50 kV x-rays within a spherical applicator (1.5–5 cm diameter, selected to fit tumor bed dimensions).[180] Electron Intra-Operative Radiation Therapy uses a linear accelerator to deliver 21 Gy to the tumor bed intraoperatively with 3 to 12 MeV electrons.[181]

Numerous EBRT techniques have been utilized to deliver APBI without requiring specialized equipment or training. 3D-CRT entails using three to five noncoplanar conformal fields with different wedge angles, while IMRT utilizes four to five coplanar or noncoplanar fields with dynamic MLC movement. Beam orientations should be selected to minimize dose to the critical normal structures. VMAT utilizes one or two partial arcs with varying speed of gantry rotation, MLC movement and dose rate. Prescription dose is typically 3.85

Gy twice daily to 38.5 Gy administered within 1 week. Notably, several studies utilizing these widely available external beam techniques have demonstrated suboptimal cosmetic outcomes.[165,170,172] Increased rates of subcutaneous fibrosis and fair to poor cosmesis have been associated with large volumes of breast tissue receiving relatively high dose.[170,172] An analysis of patients treated with 3D-CRT APBI showed high rates of excellent to good cosmesis when the ipsilateral breast volume receiving more than 50% of the prescribed dose remained below 40%.[182]

KEY POINTS

- Nodal involvement is common in breast cancer, with axillary nodes most frequently involved regardless of tumor location within the breast.

- Adjuvant WBI is standard after breast conserving surgery to reduce locoregional recurrence risk and improve survival. Postmastectomy radiotherapy is typically recommended for patients with nodal involvement, particularly greater than three positive lymph nodes.

- Prone positioning may facilitate improved dose homogeneity and reduced normal tissue dose for certain patients, particularly in the setting of large, pendulous breasts.

- Contouring target volumes, including tumor bed and nodal regions (if indicated), facilitates field design with CT-based three-dimensional treatment planning.

- Medial and lateral tangential fields are designed to encompass the entire breast or chest wall with adequate margin to allow for setup variation.

- An anterior oblique field is utilized to cover the supraclavicular nodes and undissected axilla. This field is matched inferiorly with opposed tangents using a single or dual isocenter technique. IM nodal coverage may be achieved with partially wide tangents, extended tangents, or matched electron fields.

- Wedges may be used to improve dose homogeneity within the breast. Newer dose modulation methods include electronic compensation and "field-in-field" techniques.

- Cardiac dose should be minimized using multi-leaf collimators. Deep inspiratory breath hold or prone position may also facilitate reduced cardiac dose.

- Conventional whole breast radiotherapy fractionation is 45 to 50 Gy in 25 to 28 fractions. Hypofractionated whole breast radiotherapy is also appropriate for many patients. Commonly used dose regimens are 40.05 in 15 fractions or 42.5 Gy in 16 fractions.

- Tumor bed boost is generally performed with en face electrons to treat the lumpectomy cavity plus 1.5 to 2.5 cm margin.

- APBI is typically limited to older patients with small tumors and no nodal involvement. Treatment modalities include brachytherapy, IORT, and EBRT.

REVIEW QUESTIONS

1. Which of the following is *not* a risk factor for development of breast cancer?
   A. BRCA1 mutation
   B. Young age
   C. Radiation exposure
   D. Early menarche

2. Which of the following is a potential benefit from treatment in breath hold?
   A. Decreased radiation dose to heart
   B. Decreased radiation dose to ipsilateral lung

   C. Easier patient setup and shorter treatment time
   D. Better axillary nodal coverage

3. Which of the following is a disadvantage of three-field single isocenter versus three-field dual isocenter technique?
   A. Increased contralateral lung dose
   B. Supraclavicular nodal coverage omitted
   C. More complicated setup
   D. Tangent field size limited to 20 × 20 cm

4. All of the following are techniques used to cover IM nodes *except*
A. Partially wide tangents
B. Three-field dual isocenter
C. Extended tangents
D. Matching photon and electron fields

5. Which of the following is a typical expansion on the lumpectomy cavity to generate a CTV for tumor bed boost?
A. 0.5 cm
B. 1 cm
C. 2 cm
D. 3 cm

ANSWERS

1. B Breast cancer incidence rises with increasing age. Therefore, older age rather than young age is a risk factor for developing breast cancer. Additional risk factors include BRCA1 and BRCA2 mutations, radiation exposure, early menarche, nulliparity, and late menopause.

2. A Deep inspiration breath hold often facilitates decreased cardiac dose when treating left-sided breast cancer. Longer treatment time and more difficult patient setup are required for respiratory gating with the breath-hold technique. Ipsilateral lung dose and nodal coverage are not significantly affected by breath hold.

3. D Tangent field size is limited to 20 × 20 cm for three-field single isocenter technique. Patient setup and imaging is simpler with a single isocenter compared to dual isocenter. Both techniques include an anterior oblique field for supraclavicular nodal coverage. Contralateral lung dose does not differ between techniques.

4. B Three-field dual isocenter technique is utilized to cover supraclavicular nodes and the undissected axilla. Partially wide tangents, extended tangents, and matching photon/electron fields can be used to cover IM nodes

5. C The tumor bed boost CTV typically includes the lumpectomy cavity with a 1.5 to 2.5 cm margin.

REFERENCES

1. Jatoi I, Chen BE, Anderson WF, et al. Breast cancer mortality trends in the United States according to estrogen receptor status and age at diagnosis. *J Clin Oncol.* 2007;25(13):1683–1690.
2. Blumgart EI, Uren RF, Nielsen PM, et al. Predicting lymphatic drainage patterns and primary tumour location in patients with breast cancer. *Breast Cancer Res Treat.* 2011;130(2):699–705.
3. Estourgie SH, Nieweg OE, Olmos RA, et al. Lymphatic drainage patterns from the breast. *Ann Surg.* 2004;239(2):232–237.
4. Kawase K, Gayed IW, Hunt KK, et al. Use of lymphoscintigraphy defines lymphatic drainage patterns before sentinel lymph node biopsy for breast cancer. *J Am Coll Surg.* 2006;203(1):64–72.
5. Handley RS, Thackray AC. Invasion of the internal mammary lymph glands in carcinoma of the breast. *Br J Cancer.* 1947;1(1):15–20.
6. Danforth DN, Jr, Findlay PA, McDonald HD, et al. Complete axillary lymph node dissection for stage I-II carcinoma of the breast. *J Clin Oncol.* 1986;4(5):655–662.
7. Wang H, Mao XY, Zhao TT, et al. Study on the skip metastasis of axillary lymph nodes in breast cancer and their relation with Gli1 expression. *Tumour Biol.* 2012;33(6):1943–1950.
8. Stibbe EP. The internal mammary lymphatic glands. *J Anat.* 1918;52(Pt 3):257–264.
9. American Cancer Society. Breast Cancer Facts & Figures 2019–2020. 2019, American Cancer Society: Atlanta.
10. Howlader N, Krapcho M, Garshell J, et al. SEER Cancer Statistics Review, 1975–2011. 2014, National Cancer Institute: Bethesda, MD.
11. U.S. Preventive Services Task Force. Screening for Breast Cancer: U.S. Preventive Services Task Force Recommendation Statement. *Ann Intern Med.* 2009;151(10):716–726.
12. Smith RA, Manassaram-Baptiste D, Brooks D, et al. Cancer screening in the United States, 2015: a review of current American Cancer Society guidelines and current issues in cancer screening. *CA Cancer J Clin.* 2015;65(1):30–54.
13. National Comprehensive Cancer Network. Breast Cancer Screening and Diagnosis (version 1.2020). https://www.nccn.org/professionals/physician_gls/pdf/breast-screening.pdf. Accessed September 28, 2020.
14. Collaborative Group on Hormonal Factors in Breast Cancer. Menarche, menopause, and breast cancer risk: individual participant meta-analysis, including 118 964 women with breast cancer from 117 epidemiological studies. *Lancet Oncol.* 2012;13(11):1141–1151.
15. Reeves GK, Pirie K, Green J, et al. Reproductive factors and specific histological types of breast cancer: prospective study and meta-analysis. *Br J Cancer.* 2009;100(3):538–544.
16. Kelsey JL, Gammon MD, John EM. Reproductive factors and breast cancer. *Epidemiol Rev.* 1993;15(1):36–47.
17. Beral V. Breast cancer and hormone-replacement therapy in the Million Women Study. *Lancet.* 2003;362(9382):419–427.
18. Manson JE, Chlebowski RT, Stefanick ML, et al. Menopausal hormone therapy and health outcomes during the intervention and extended poststopping phases of the Women's Health Initiative randomized trials. *Jama.* 2013;310(13):1353–1368.
19. Collaborative Group on Hormonal Factors in Breast Cancer. Breast cancer and hormonal contraceptives: collaborative reanalysis of individual data on 53 297 women with breast cancer and 100 239 women without breast cancer from 54 epidemiological studies. *Lancet.* 1996;347(9017):1713–1727.
20. Drooger JC, Hooning MJ, Seynaeve CM, et al. Diagnostic and therapeutic ionizing radiation and the risk of a first and second primary breast cancer, with special attention for BRCA1 and BRCA2 mutation carriers: a critical review of the literature. *Cancer Treat Rev.* 2015;41(2):187–196.
21. Preston DL, Mattsson A, Holmberg E, et al. Radiation effects on breast cancer risk: a pooled analysis of eight cohorts. *Radiat Res.* 2002;158(2):220–235.
22. Henderson TO, Amsterdam A, Bhatia S, et al. Systematic review: surveillance for breast cancer in women treated with chest radiation for childhood, adolescent, or young adult cancer. *Ann Intern Med.* 2010;152(7):444–455; w144–154.

23. Collaborative Group on Hormonal Factors in Breast Cancer. Familial breast cancer: collaborative reanalysis of individual data from 52 epidemiological studies including 58,209 women with breast cancer and 101,986 women without the disease. *Lancet.* 2001;358(9291):1389–1399.

24. Nicoletto MO, Donach M, De Nicolo A, et al. BRCA-1 and BRCA-2 mutations as prognostic factors in clinical practice and genetic counselling. *Cancer Treat Rev.* 2001;27(5):295–304.

25. Carter RF. BRCA1, BRCA2 and breast cancer: a concise clinical review. *Clin Invest Med.* 2001;24(3):147–157.

26. National Comprehensive Cancer Network. Genetic/Familial High-Risk Assessment: Breast, Ovarian, and Pancreatic (version 1. 2021). https://www.nccn.org/professionals/physician_gls/pdf/genetics_bop.pdf Accessed September 28, 2020.

27. Fisher B, Slack NH, Ausman RK et al. Location of breast carcinoma and prognosis. *Surg Gynecol Obstet.* 1969;129(4):705–716.

28. Fitzgibbons PL, Page DL, Weaver D, et al. Prognostic factors in breast cancer. College of American Pathologists Consensus Statement 1999. *Arch Pathol Lab Med.* 2000;124(7):966–978.

29. Jemal A, Ward E, Thun MJ. Recent trends in breast cancer incidence rates by age and tumor characteristics among U.S. women. *Breast Cancer Res.* 2007;9(3):R28.

30. Sariego J. Patterns of breast cancer presentation in the United States: does geography matter? *Am Surg.* 2009;75(7):545–549; discussion 549–550.

31. Kerlikowske K. Epidemiology of ductal carcinoma in situ. *J Natl Cancer Inst Monogr.* 2010;2010(41):139–141.

32. Burstein HJ, Polyak K, Wong JS, et al. Ductal carcinoma in situ of the breast. *N Engl J Med.* 2004;350(14):1430–1441.

33. Jorns J, Sabel MS, Pang JC. Lobular neoplasia: morphology and management. *Arch Pathol Lab Med.* 2014;138(10):1344–1349.

34. Hortobagyi GN, Connolly JL, D'Orsi CJ, Yang WT. Breast. In: Amin MB, Edge S, Greene F, et al., eds. American Joint Committee on Cancer. AJCC cancer staging manual, 8th ed. Springer, 2017:589–636.

35. Pestalozzi BC, Zahrieh D, Mallon E, et al. Distinct clinical and prognostic features of infiltrating lobular carcinoma of the breast: combined results of 15 International Breast Cancer Study Group Clinical Trials. *J Clin Oncol.* 2008;26(18):3006–3014.

36. Horton JK, Jagsi R, Woodward WA, et al. Breast cancer biology: clinical implications for breast radiation therapy. *IJROBP.* 2018;100:23–37.

37. Fisher B, Anderson S, Bryant J, et al. Twenty-year follow-up of a randomized trial comparing total mastectomy, lumpectomy, and lumpectomy plus irradiation for the treatment of invasive breast cancer. *N Engl J Med.* 2002;347(16):1233–1241.

38. Fisher B, Land S, Mamounas E, et al. Prevention of invasive breast cancer in women with ductal carcinoma in situ: an update of the National Surgical Adjuvant Breast and Bowel Project experience. *Semin Oncol.* 2001;28(4):400–418.

39. Darby S, McGale P, et al. Effect of radiotherapy after breast-conserving surgery on 10-year recurrence and 15-year breast cancer death: meta-analysis of individual patient data for 10,801 women in 17 randomised trials. *Lancet.* 2011;378(9804):1707–1716.

40. Fleck R, McNeese MD, Ellerbroek NA, et al. Consequences of breast irradiation in patients with pre-existing collagen vascular diseases. *Int J Radiat Oncol Biol Phys.* 1989;17(4):829–833.

41. Cao JQ, Truong PT, Olivotto IA, et al. Should women younger than 40 years of age with invasive breast cancer have a mastectomy? 15-year outcomes in a population-based cohort. *Int J Radiat Oncol Biol Phys.* 2014;90(3):509–517.

42. McGale P, Taylor C, et al. Effect of radiotherapy after mastectomy and axillary surgery on 10-year recurrence and 20-year breast cancer mortality: meta-analysis of individual patient data for 8135 women in 22 randomised trials. *Lancet.* 2014;383(9935):2127–2135.

43. Overgaard M, Jensen MB, Overgaard J, et al. Postoperative radiotherapy in high-risk postmenopausal breast-cancer patients given adjuvant tamoxifen: Danish Breast Cancer Cooperative Group DBCG 82c randomised trial. *Lancet.* 1999;353(9165):1641–1648.

44. Overgaard M, Hansen PS, Overgaard J, et al. Postoperative radiotherapy in high-risk premenopausal women with breast cancer who receive adjuvant chemotherapy. Danish Breast Cancer Cooperative Group 82b Trial. *N Engl J Med.* 1997;337(14):949–955.

45. Ragaz J, Olivotto IA, Spinelli JJ, et al. Locoregional radiation therapy in patients with high-risk breast cancer receiving adjuvant chemotherapy: 20-year results of the British Columbia randomized trial. *J Natl Cancer Inst.* 2005;97(2):116–126.

46. NCCN Guidelines version 1.2015. Breast Cancer. (2015); Available from: http://www.nccn.org/professionals/physician_gls/pdf/breast.pdf.

47. Goldhirsch A, Winer EP, Coates AS, et al. Personalizing the treatment of women with early breast cancer: highlights of the St Gallen International Expert Consensus on the Primary Therapy of Early Breast Cancer 2013. *Ann Oncol.* 2013;24(9):2206–2223.

48. Belkacemi Y, Fourquet A, Cutuli B, et al. Radiotherapy for invasive breast cancer: guidelines for clinical practice from the French expert review board of Nice/Saint-Paul de Vence. *Crit Rev Oncol Hematol.* 2011;79(2):91–102.

49. Wenz F, Sperk E, Budach W, et al. DEGRO practical guidelines for radiotherapy of breast cancer IV: radiotherapy following mastectomy for invasive breast cancer. *Strahlenther Onkol.* 2014;190(8):705–714.

50. Souchon R, Sautter-Bihl ML, Sedlmayer F, et al. Radiation oncologists' view on the zurich consensus. *Breast Care (Basel).* 2013;8(6):448–452.

51. Rowell NP. Radiotherapy to the chest wall following mastectomy for node-negative breast cancer: a systematic review. *Radiother Oncol.* 2009;91(1):23–32.

52. Katz A, Strom EA, Buchholz TA, et al. The influence of pathologic tumor characteristics on locoregional recurrence rates following mastectomy. *Int J Radiat Oncol Biol Phys.* 2001;50(3):735–742.

53. von Minckwitz G, Huang CS, Mano MS, et al. Trastuzumab Emtansine for Residual Invasive HER2-Positive Breast Cancer. *NEJM.* 2019;380:617–628.

54. Masuda N, Lee SJ, Ohtani S, et al. Adjuvant capecitabine for breast cancer after preoperative chemotherapy, *N Engl J Med.* 2017;376:2147–2159.

55. Mamounas EP, Anderson SJ, Dignam JJ, et al. Predictors of locoregional recurrence following neoadjuvant chemotherapy: results from combined analysis of NSABP B-18 and B-27. *J Clin Oncol.* 2012;30(32):3960–3966.

56. Standard or Comprehensive Radiation Therapy in Treating Patients With Early-Stage Breast Cancer Previously Treated With Chemotherapy and Surgery. http://clinicaltrials.gov/ct2/show/NCT01872975?term=nsabp+b51&draw=2&rank=1

57. Hughes KS, Schnaper LA, Bellon JR, et al. Lumpectomy plus tamoxifen with or without irradiation in women age 70 years or older with early breast cancer: long-term follow-up of CALGB 9343. *J Clin Oncol.* 2013;31(19):2382–2387.

58. Kunkler IH, Williams LJ, Jack WJL, et al. Breast-conserving surgery with or without irradiation in women aged 65 years or older with early breast cancer (PRIME II): a randomised controlled trial. *Lancet Oncol.* 2015;16:266–273.

59. Hughes LL, Wang M, Page DL, et al. Local excision alone without irradiation for ductal carcinoma in situ of the breast: a trial of the Eastern Cooperative Oncology Group. *J Clin Oncol.* 2009;27(32):5319–5324.

60. McCormick B, Winter K, Hudis C, et al. RTOG 9804: a prospective randomized trial for good-risk ductal carcinoma in situ comparing radiotherapy with observation. *J Clin Oncol.* 2015;33:709–715.

61. Brunt AM, Haviland JS, Wheatley DA, et al. Hypofractionated breast radiotherapy for 1 week versus 3 weeks (FAST-Forward): 5-year efficacy and late normal tissue effects results from a ulticentre, non-inferiority, randomised, phase 3 trial. *Lancet.* 2020;23:395:1613–1626.

62. Hartsell WF, Kelly CA, Schneider L, et al. A single isocenter three-field breast irradiation technique using an empiric simulation and asymmetric collimator. *Med Dosim.* 1994;19(3):169–173.

63. Alonso-Basanta M, Ko J, Babcock M, et al. Coverage of axillary lymph nodes in supine vs. prone breast radiotherapy. *Int J Radiat Oncol Biol Phys.* 2009;73(3):745–751.

64. Shin SM, No HS, Vega RM, et al. Breast, chest wall, and nodal irradiation with prone set-up: results of a hypofractionated trial with a median follow-up of 35 months. *Pract Radiat Oncol.* 2016;6:e81–e88.

65. Deseyne P, Speleers B, De Neve W, et al. Whole breast and regional nodal irradiation in prone versus supine position in left sided breast cancer. *Radiat Oncol.* 2017;12:89.

66. Griem KL, Fetherston P, Kuznetsova M, et al. Three-dimensional photon dosimetry: a comparison of treatment of the intact breast in the supine and prone position. *Int J Radiat Oncol Biol Phys.* 2003;57(3):891–899.

67. Lymberis SC, deWyngaert JK, Parhar P, et al. Prospective assessment of optimal individual position (prone versus supine) for breast radiotherapy: volumetric and dosimetric correlations in 100 patients. *Int J Radiat Oncol Biol Phys.* 2012;84(4):902–909.

68. Kirby AM, Evans PM, Donovan EM, et al. Prone versus supine positioning for whole and partial-breast radiotherapy: a comparison of non-target tissue dosimetry. *Radiother Oncol.* 2010;96(2):178–184.

69. Krengli M, Masini L, Caltavuturo T, et al. Prone versus supine position for adjuvant breast radiotherapy: a prospective study in patients with pendulous breasts. *Radiat Oncol.* 2013;8:232.

70. Mitchell J, Formenti SC, DeWyngaert JK. Interfraction and intrafraction setup variability for prone breast radiation therapy. *Int J Radiat Oncol Biol Phys.* 2010;76(5):1571–1577.

71. Hayden AJ, Rains M, Tiver K. Deep inspiration breath hold technique reduces heart dose from radiotherapy for left-sided breast cancer. *J Med Imaging Radiat Oncol.* 2012;56(4):464–472.

72. Swanson T, Grills I, Ye H, et al. Six-year experience routinely using moderate deep inspiration breath-hold for the reduction of cardiac dose in left-sided breast irradiation for patients with early-stage or locally advanced breast cancer. *Am J Clin Oncol.* 2013;36(1):24–30.

73. Bergom C, Currey A, Desai N, et al. Deep inspiration breath hold: techniques and advantages for cardiac sparing during breast cancer irradiation. *Front Oncol.* 2018;8:87.

74. Velker VM, Rodrigues GB, Dinniwell R, et al. Creation of RTOG compliant patient CT-atlases for automated atlas based contouring of local regional breast and high-risk prostate cancers. *Radiat Oncol.* 2013;8:188.

75. Li XA, Tai A, Arthur DW, et al. Variability of target and normal structure delineation for breast cancer radiotherapy: an RTOG Multi-Institutional and Multiobserver Study. *Int J Radiat Oncol Biol Phys.* 2009;73(3):944–951.

76. White J, Tai D, Arthur T, et al. *Breast Cancer Atlas for Radiation Treatment Planning: Consensus Definitions*, R.T.O.G. (RTOG), Editor.

77. Offersen BV, Boersma LJ, Kirkove C, et al. ESTRO consensus guideline on target volume delineation for elective radiation therapy of early stage breast cancer. *Radiother Oncol.* 2015;114:3–10.

78. Loganadane GK, Truong PT, Taghian AG, et al. Comparison of nodal target volumes definition in breast cancer radiotherapy according to RTOG versus ESTRO atlases. A practical review from the TransAtlantic Radiation Oncology Network (TRONE). *IJROBP.* 2020;107(3):437–448.

79. Gee HE, Moses L, Stuart K, et al. Contouring consensus guidelines in breast cancer radiotherapy: comparison and systematic review of patterns of failure. *J Med Imaging Radiat Oncol.* 2018;63:102–115.

80. DeSelm C, Yang TJ, Cahlon O, et al. A 3-Dimensional Mapping Analysis of Regional Nodal Recurrences in Breast Cancer. *IJROBP.* 2019;103(3):583–591.

81. Kowalski ES, Feigenberg SJ, Cohen J, et al. Optimal target delineation and treatment techniques in the era of conformal photon and proton breast and regional nodal irradiation. *Pract Radiat Oncol.* 2020;10(3):174–182.

82. Whelan TJ, Olivotto I, Ackerman I, et al. NCIC-CTG MA.[20]: an intergroup trial of regional nodal irradiation in early breast cancer. *J Clin Oncol.* 2011;29(18_suppl):LBA1003.

83. Donker M, van Tienhoven G, Straver ME, et al. Radiotherapy or surgery of the axilla after a positive sentinel node in breast cancer (EORTC 10981-22023 AMAROS): a randomised, multicentre, open-label, phase 3 non-inferiority trial. *Lancet Oncol.* 2014;15(12):1303–1310.

84. Giuliano AE, Hunt KK, Ballman KV, et al. Axillary dissection vs no axillary dissection in women with invasive breast cancer and sentinel node metastasis: a randomized clinical trial. *JAMA.* 2011;305(6):569–575.

85. Robinson KA, Pockaj BA, Wasif N, et al. Have the American College of Surgeons Oncology Group Z0011 trial results influenced the number of lymph nodes removed during sentinel lymph node dissection? *Am J Surg.* 2014;208(6):1060–1064; discussion 1063–1064.

86. Jagsi R, Chadha M, Moni J, et al. Radiation field design in the ACOSOG Z0011 (Alliance) Trial. *J Clin Oncol.* 2014;32(32):3600–3606.

87. Hennequin C, Bossard N, Servagi-Vernat S, et al. Ten-year survival results of a randomized trial of irradiation of internal mammary nodes after mastectomy. *Int J Radiat Oncol Biol Phys.* 2013;86(5):860–866.

88. Thorsen LB, Offersen BV, Danø H, et al. DBCG-IMN: a population-based cohort study on the effect of internal mammary node irradiation in early node positive breast cancer. *JCO.* 2016;34(4):314–320.

89. Arthur DW, Arnfield MR, Warwicke LA, et al. Internal mammary node coverage: an investigation of presently accepted techniques. *Int J Radiat Oncol Biol Phys.* 2000;48(1):139–146.

90. Pierce LJ, Butler JB, Martel MK, et al. Postmastectomy radiotherapy of the chest wall: dosimetric comparison of common techniques. *Int J Radiat Oncol Biol Phys.* 2002;52(5):1220–1230.

91. Sonnik D, Selvaraj RN, Faul C, et al. Treatment techniques for 3D conformal radiation to breast and chest wall including the internal mammary chain. *Med Dosim.* 2007;32(1):7–12.

92. Oh JL, Buchholz TA. Internal mammary node radiation: a proposed technique to spare cardiac toxicity. *J Clin Oncol.* 2009;27(31):e172–e173.

93. Kutcher GJ, et al. Treatment planning for primary breast cancer: a patterns of care study. *Int J Radiat Oncol Biol Phys.* 1996;36(3):731–737.

94. Solin LJ, Chu JC, Sontag MR, et al. Three-dimensional photon treatment planning of the intact breast. *Int J Radiat Oncol Biol Phys.* 1991;21(1):193–203.

95. Garavaglia G, Porepp C, Jozefowsky M. Improved dose distribution homogeneity in conservative breast cancer irradiation. *Radiother Oncol.* 1991;22(4):245–247.

96. Beavis AW. Treatment planning challenges in breast irradiation: the ideal and the practical. *Clin Oncol.* 2006;18(3):200–209.

97. Mageras GS, Mohan R, Burman C, et al. Compensators for three-dimensional treatment planning. *Med Phys.* 1991;18(2):133–140.

98. Hansen VN, Evans PM, Shentall GS, et al. Dosimetric evaluation of compensation in radiotherapy of the breast: MLC intensity modulation and physical compensators. *Radiother Oncol.* 1997;42(3):249–256.

99. Lief EP, Hunt MA, Hong LX, et al. Radiation therapy of large intact breasts using a beam spoiler or photons with mixed energies. *Med Dosim.* 2007;32(4):246–253.

100. Ramsey CR, Chase D, Scaperoth D, et al. Improved dose homogeneity to the intact breast using three-dimensional treatment planning: technical considerations. *Med Dosim.* 2000;25(1):1–6.

101. Donovan E, Bleakley N, Denholm E, et al. Randomised trial of standard 2D radiotherapy (RT) versus intensity modulated radiotherapy (IMRT) in patients prescribed breast radiotherapy. *Radiother Oncol.* 2007;82(3):254–264.

102. Barnett GC, Wilkinson JS, Moody AM, et al. Randomized controlled trial of forward-planned intensity modulated radiotherapy for early breast cancer: interim results at 2 years. *Int J Radiat Oncol Biol Phys.* 2012;82(2):715–723.

103. Mukesh MB, Barnett GC, Wilkinson JS, et al. Randomized controlled trial of intensity-modulated radiotherapy for early breast cancer: 5-year results confirm superior overall cosmesis. *J Clin Oncol.* 2013;31:4488–4495.

104. Pignol JP, Olivotto I, Rakovitch E, et al. A multicenter randomized trial of breast intensity-modulated radiation therapy to reduce acute radiation dermatitis. *J Clin Oncol.* 2008;26(13):2085–2092.

105. Harsolia A, Kestin L, Grills I, et al. Intensity-modulated radiotherapy results in significant decrease in clinical toxicities compared with conventional wedge-based breast radiotherapy. *Int J Radiat Oncol Biol Phys.* 2007;68(5):1375–1380.

106. McDonald MW, Godette KD, Butker EK, et al. Long-term outcomes of IMRT for breast cancer: a single-institution cohort analysis. *Int J Radiat Oncol Biol Phys.* 2008;72(4):1031–1040.

107. Lohr F, El-Haddad M, Dobler B, et al. Potential effect of robust and simple IMRT approach for left-sided breast cancer on cardiac mortality. *Int J Radiat Oncol Biol Phys.* 2009;74(1):73–80.

108. Beckham WA, Popescu CC, Patenaude VV, et al. Is multibeam IMRT better than standard treatment for patients with left-sided breast cancer? *Int J Radiat Oncol Biol Phys.* 2007;69(3):918–924.

109. Hong L, Hunt M, Chui C, et al. Intensity-modulated tangential beam irradiation of the intact breast. *Int J Radiat Oncol Biol Phys.* 1999;44(5):1155–1164.
110. Bhatnagar A, Brandner E, Sonnik D, et al. Intensity modulated radiation therapy (IMRT) reduces the dose to the contralateral breast when compared to conventional tangential fields for primary breast irradiation. *Breast Cancer Res Treat.* 2006;96(1):41–46.
111. Freedman GM, Anderson PR, Li J, et al. Intensity modulated radiation therapy (IMRT) decreases acute skin toxicity for women receiving radiation for breast cancer. *Am J Clin Oncol.* 2006;29(1):66–70.
112. Mast ME, van Kempen-Harteveld L, Heijenbrok MW, et al. Left-sided breast cancer radiotherapy with and without breath-hold: does IMRT reduce the cardiac dose even further? *Radiother Oncol.* 2013;108(2):248–253.
113. Coon AB, Dickler A, Kirk MC, et al. Tomotherapy and multifield intensity-modulated radiotherapy planning reduce cardiac doses in left-sided breast cancer patients with unfavorable cardiac anatomy. *Int J Radiat Oncol Biol Phys.* 2010;78(1):104–110.
114. Hahn C, Kavanagh B, Bhatnagar A et al. Choosing wisely: the American Society for Radiation Oncology's top 5 list. *Pract Radiat Oncol.* 2014;4(6):349–355.
115. ASTRO releases list of five radiation oncology treatments to question as part of national Choosing Wisely® campaign. 2013 [cited (2015) 2/19/(2015)]; Available from: http://www.choosingwisely.org/astro-releases-list-of-five-radiation-oncology-treatments-to-question-as-part-of-national-choosing-wisely-campaign/.
116. McCormick B, Hunt M. Intensity-modulated radiation therapy for breast: is it for everyone? *Semin Radiat Oncol.* 2011;21(1):51–54.
117. Teh BS, Lu HH, Sobremonte S, et al. The potential use of intensity modulated radiotherapy (IMRT) in women with pectus excavatum desiring breast-conserving therapy. *Breast J.* 2001;7(4):233–239.
118. Cendales R, Vasquez J, Arbelaez JC, et al. Intensity modulated radiotherapy (IMRT) with simultaneous integrated boost (SIB) in a patient with left breast cancer and pectus excavatum. *Clin Transl Oncol.* 2012;14(10):747–754.
119. Caudell JJ, De Los Santos JF, Keene KS, et al. A dosimetric comparison of electronic compensation, conventional intensity modulated radiotherapy, and tomotherapy in patients with early-stage carcinoma of the left breast. *Int J Radiat Oncol Biol Phys.* 2007;68(5):1505–1511.
120. Al-Rahbi ZS, Ravichandran R, Binukumar JP, et al. A dosimetric comparison of radiotherapy techniques in the treatment of carcinoma of breast. *J Cancer Ther.* 2013;4(11a):10–17.
121. Gokula K, Earnest A, Wong LC. Meta-analysis of incidence of early lung toxicity in 3-dimensional conformal irradiation of breast carcinomas. *Radiat Oncol.* 2013;8:268.
122. Blom Goldman U, Wennberg B, Svane G, et al. Reduction of radiation pneumonitis by V20-constraints in breast cancer. *Radiat Oncol.* 2010;5:99.
123. Lind PA, Wennberg B, Gagliardi G, et al. Pulmonary complications following different radiotherapy techniques for breast cancer, and the association to irradiated lung volume and dose. *Breast Cancer Res Treat.* 2001;68(3):199–210.
124. Blitzblau RC, Horton JK. Treatment planning technique in patients receiving postmastectomy radiation therapy. *Pract Radiat Oncol.* 2013;3(4):241–248.
125. Cuzick J, Stewart H, Rutqvist L, et al. Cause-specific mortality in long-term survivors of breast cancer who participated in trials of radiotherapy. *J Clin Oncol.* 1994;12(3):447–453.
126. Gyenes G, Rutqvist LE, Liedberg A, et al. Long-term cardiac morbidity and mortality in a randomized trial of pre- and postoperative radiation therapy versus surgery alone in primary breast cancer. *Radiother Oncol.* 1998;48(2):185–190.
127. Favourable and unfavourable effects on long-term survival of radiotherapy for early breast cancer: an overview of the randomised trials. Early Breast Cancer Trialists' Collaborative Group. *Lancet.* 2000;355(9217):1757–1770.
128. Giordano SH, Kuo YF, Freeman JL, et al. Risk of cardiac death after adjuvant radiotherapy for breast cancer. *J Natl Cancer Inst.* 2005;97(6):419–424.
129. Rutter CE, Chagpar AB, Evans SB. Breast cancer laterality does not influence survival in a large modern cohort: implications for radiation-related cardiac mortality. *Int J Radiat Oncol Biol Phys.* 2014;90(2):329–334.
130. Darby SC, McGale P, Taylor CW, et al. Long-term mortality from heart disease and lung cancer after radiotherapy for early breast cancer: prospective cohort study of about 300,000 women in US SEER cancer registries. *Lancet Oncol.* 2005;6(8):557–565.
131. Gagliardi G, Constine LS, Moiseenko V, et al. Radiation dose-volume effects in the heart. *Int J Radiat Oncol Biol Phys.* 2010;76(3 Suppl):S77–S85.
132. Darby SC, Ewertz M, McGale P, et al. Risk of ischemic heart disease in women after radiotherapy for breast cancer. *N Engl J Med.* 2013;368(11):987–998.
133. Whelan TJ, Pignol JP, Levine MN, et al. Long-term results of hypofractionated radiation therapy for breast cancer. *New Engl J Med.* 2010;362(6):513–520.
134. Haviland JS, Owen JR, Dewar JA, et al. The UK Standardisation of Breast Radiotherapy (START) trials of radiotherapy hypofractionation for treatment of early breast cancer: 10-year follow-up results of two randomised controlled trials. *Lancet Oncol.* 2013;14(11):1086–1094.
135. Offersen BV, Alsner J, Nielsen HM, et al. Hypofractionated versus standard fractionated radiotherapy in patients with early breast cancer or ductal carcinoma in situ in a randomized phase III trial: the DBCG HYPO trial. *J Clin Oncol.* published online September 10, 2020.
136. Smith BD, Bentzen SM, Correa CR, et al. Fractionation for whole breast irradiation: an American Society for Radiation Oncology (ASTRO) evidence-based guideline. *Int J Radiat Oncol Biol Phys.* 2011;81(1):59–68.
137. Smith BD, Bellon JR, Blitzblau R, et al. Radiation therapy for the whole breast: executive summary of an American Society for Radiation Oncology (ASTRO) evidence-based guideline. *Pract Radiat Oncol.* 2018;8:145–152.
138. Agrawal RK, Alhasso A, et al. First results of the randomised UK FAST Trial of radiotherapy hypofractionation for treatment of early breast cancer (CRUKE/04/015). *Radiother Oncol.* 2011;100(1):93–100.
139. Brunt AM, Haviland JS, Sydenham M, et al. Ten-year results of FAST: a randomized controlled trial of 5-fraction whole-breast radiotherapy for early breast cancer. *J Clin Oncol.* 2020;38(28):3261–3272.
140. Koukourakis MI, Panteliadou M, Abatzoglou IM, et al. Postmastectomy hypofractionated and accelerated radiation therapy with (and without) subcutaneous amifostine cytoprotection. *Int J Radiat Oncol Biol Phys.* 2013;85(1):e7–e13.
141. Holloway CL, Panet-Raymond V, Olivotto I. Hypofractionation should be the new 'standard' for radiation therapy after breast conserving surgery. *Breast.* 2010;19(3):163–167.
142. Wang SL, Fang H, Song YW, et al. Hypofractionated versus conventional fractionated postmastectomy radiotherapy for patients with high-risk breast cancer: a randomised, non-inferiority, open-label, phase 3 trial. *Lancet Oncol.* 2019;20(31):352–360.
143. Romestaing P, Lehingue Y, Carrie C, et al. Role of a 10-Gy boost in the conservative treatment of early breast cancer: results of a randomized clinical trial in Lyon, France. *J Clin Oncol.* 1997;15(3):963–968.
144. Polgar C, Fodor J, Orosz Z, et al. Electron and high-dose-rate brachytherapy boost in the conservative treatment of stage I-II breast cancer first results of the randomized Budapest boost trial. *Strahlenther Onkol,* 2002;178(11):615–623.
145. Bartelink H, Horiot JC, Poortmans PM, et al. Impact of a higher radiation dose on local control and survival in breast-conserving therapy of early breast cancer: 10-year results of the randomized boost versus no boost EORTC 22881-10882 trial. *J Clin Oncol.* 2007;25(22):3259–3265.
146. Omlin A, Amichetti M, Azria D, et al. Boost radiotherapy in young women with ductal carcinoma in situ: a multicentre, retrospective study of the Rare Cancer Network. *Lancet Oncol.* 2006;7(8):652–656.
147. Moran MS, Zhao Y, Ma S, et al. Association of radiotherapy boost for ductal carcinoma in situ with local control after whole-breast radiotherapy. *JAMA Oncol.* 2017;3(8):1060–1068.

148. King MT, Link EK, Whelan TJ, et al. Quality of life after breast-conserving therapy and adjuvant radiotherapy for non-low-risk ductal carcinoma in situ (BIG 3-07/TROG 07.01): 2-year results of a randomised, controlled, phase 3 trial. *Lancet Oncol.* 2020;21:685–698.

149. Freedman GM, White JR, Arthur DW, et al. Accelerated fractionation with a concurrent boost for early stage breast cancer. *Radiother Oncol.* 2013;106(1):15–20.

150. Mayadev J, Einck J, Elson S, et al. Practice patterns in the delivery of radiation therapy after mastectomy among the University of California Athena Breast Health Network. *Clin Breast Cancer,* 2015;15(1):43–47.

151. Gilliland MD, Barton RM, Copeland EM. 3rd. The implications of local recurrence of breast cancer as the first site of therapeutic failure. *Ann Surg.* 1983;197(3):284–287.

152. Taghian A, Jeong JH, Mamounas E, et al. Patterns of locoregional failure in patients with operable breast cancer treated by mastectomy and adjuvant chemotherapy with or without tamoxifen and without radiotherapy: results from five national surgical adjuvant breast and bowel project randomized clinical trials. *J Clin Oncol.* 2004;22(21):4247–4254.

153. Panoff JE, Takita C, Hurley J, et al. Higher chest wall dose results in improved locoregional outcome in patients receiving postmastectomy radiation. *Int J Radiat Oncol Biol Phys.* 2012;82(3):1192–1199.

154. Naoum GE, Salama L, Ho A, et al. The impact of chest wall boost on reconstruction complications and local control in patients treated for breast cancer. *Int J Radiat Oncol Biol Phys,* 2019;105(1):155–164.

155. Fowble B, Solin LJ, Schultz DJ, et al. Breast recurrence following conservative surgery and radiation: patterns of failure, prognosis, and pathologic findings from mastectomy specimens with implications for treatment. *Int J Radiat Oncol Biol Phys.* 1990;19(4):833–842.

156. Veronesi U, Marubini E, Mariani L, et al. Radiotherapy after breast-conserving surgery in small breast carcinoma: long-term results of a randomized trial. *Ann Oncol.* 2001;12(7):997–1003.

157. Liljegren G, Holmberg L, Bergh J, et al. 10-Year results after sector resection with or without postoperative radiotherapy for stage I breast cancer: a randomized trial. *J Clin Oncol.* 1999;17(8):2326–2333.

158. Fisher ER, Anderson S, Redmond C, et al. Ipsilateral breast tumor recurrence and survival following lumpectomy and irradiation: pathological findings from NSABP protocol B-06. *Semin Surg Oncol.* 1992;8(3):161–166.

159. Clark RM, McCulloch PB, Levine MN, et al. Randomized clinical trial to assess the effectiveness of breast irradiation following lumpectomy and axillary dissection for node-negative breast cancer. *J Natl Cancer Inst.* 1992;84(9):683–689.

160. Correa C, Harris EE, Leonardi MC, et al. Accelerated partial breast irradiation: executive summary for the update of an ASTRO evidence based consensensus statement. *Pract Radiat Oncol.* 2019;7(2):73–79.

161. Whelan TJ, Julian JA, Berrang TS, et al. External beam accelerated partial breast irradiation versus whole breast irradiation after breast conserving surgery in women with ductal carcinoma in situ and node-negative breast cancer (RAPID): a randomised controlled trial. *Lancet.* 2019;394:2165–2172.

162. Vicini FA, Cecchini RS, White JR, et al. B39: long-term primary results of accelerated partial breast irradiation after breast-conserving surgery for early-stage breast cancer: a randomised, phase 3, equivalence trial. *Lancet.* 2019;394:2155–2164.

163. Coles CE, Griffin CL, Kirby AM, et al. Partial-breast radiotherapy after breast conservation surgery for patients with early breast cancer (UK IMPORT LOW trial): 5-year results from a multicentre, randomised, controlled, phase 3, non-inferiority trial. *Lancet.* 2017;390(10099):1048–1060.

164. Smith BD, Arthur DW, Buchholz TA, et al. Accelerated partial breast irradiation consensus statement from the American Society for Radiation Oncology (ASTRO). *Int J Radiat Oncol Biol Phys.* 2009;74(4):987–1001.

165. Olivotto IA, Whelan TJ, Parpia S, et al. Interim cosmetic and toxicity results from RAPID: a randomized trial of accelerated partial breast irradiation using three-dimensional conformal external beam radiation therapy. *J Clin Oncol.* 2013;31(32):4038–4045.

166. Shah C, Wilkinson JB, Lanni T, et al. Five-year outcomes and toxicities using 3-dimensional conformal external beam radiation therapy to deliver accelerated partial breast irradiation. *Clin Breast Cancer.* 2013;13(3):206–211.

167. Berrang TS, Olivotto I, Kim DH, et al. Three-year outcomes of a Canadian multicenter study of accelerated partial breast irradiation using conformal radiation therapy. *Int J Radiat Oncol Biol Phys.* 2011;81(5):1220–1227.

168. Kim Y, Parda DS, Trombetta MG, et al. Dosimetric comparison of partial and whole breast external beam irradiation in the treatment of early stage breast cancer. *Med Phys.* 2007;34(12):4640–4648.

169. Livi L, Meattini I, Marrazzo L, et al. Accelerated partial breast irradiation using intensity-modulated radiotherapy versus whole breast irradiation: 5-year survival analysis of a phase 3 randomised controlled trial. *Eur J Cancer.* 2015;51:451–463.

170. Liss AL, Ben-David MA, Jagsi R, et al. Decline of cosmetic outcomes following accelerated partial breast irradiation using intensity modulated radiation therapy: results of a single-institution prospective clinical trial. *Int J Radiat Oncol Biol Phys.* 2014;89(1):96–102.

171. Chafe S, Moughan J, McCormick B, et al. Late toxicity and patient self-assessment of breast appearance/satisfaction on RTOG 0319: a phase 2 trial of 3-dimensional conformal radiation therapy-accelerated partial breast irradiation following lumpectomy for stages I and II breast cancer. *Int J Radiat Oncol Biol Phys.* 2013;86(5):854–859.

172. Leonard KL, Hepel JT, Hiatt JR, et al. The effect of dose-volume parameters and interfraction interval on cosmetic outcome and toxicity after 3-dimensional conformal accelerated partial breast irradiation. *Int J Radiat Oncol Biol Phys.* 2013;85(3):623–629.

173. Shah C, Vicini F, Wazer DE, et al. The American Brachytherapy Society consensus statement for accelerated partial breast irradiation. *Brachytherapy.* 2013;12(4):267–277.

174. Polgar C, Fodor J, Major T, et al. Breast-conserving therapy with partial or whole breast irradiation: ten-year results of the Budapest randomized trial. *Radiother Oncol.* 2013;108(2):197–202.

175. Vicini FA, Antonucci JV, Wallace M, et al. Long-term efficacy and patterns of failure after accelerated partial breast irradiation: a molecular assay-based clonality evaluation. *Int J Radiat Oncol Biol Phys.* 2007;68(2):341–346.

176. King TA, Bolton JS, Kuske RR, et al. Long-term results of wide-field brachytherapy as the sole method of radiation therapy after segmental mastectomy for T(is,1,2) breast cancer. *Am J Surg.* 2000;180(4):299–304.

177. Rabinovitch R, Winter K, Kuske R, et al. RTOG 95-17, a Phase II trial to evaluate brachytherapy as the sole method of radiation therapy for Stage I and II breast carcinoma–year-5 toxicity and cosmesis. *Brachytherapy.* 2014;13(1):17–22.

178. Dickler A, Kirk MC, Chu J, et al. The MammoSite™ breast brachytherapy applicator: a review of technique and outcomes. *Brachytherapy.* 2005;4(2):130–136.

179. Shah C, Badiyan S, Ben Wilkinson J, et al. Treatment efficacy with accelerated partial breast irradiation (APBI): final analysis of the American Society of Breast Surgeons MammoSite((R)) breast brachytherapy registry trial. *Ann Surg Oncol.* 2013;20(10):3279–3285.

180. Vaidya JS, Wenz F, Bulsara M, et al. Risk-adapted targeted intraoperative radiotherapy versus whole-breast radiotherapy for breast cancer: 5-year results for local control and overall survival from the TARGIT-A randomised trial. *Lancet.* 2014;383(9917):603–613.

181. Veronesi U, Orecchia R, Maisonneuve P, et al. Intraoperative radiotherapy versus external radiotherapy for early breast cancer (ELIOT): a randomised controlled equivalence trial. *Lancet Oncol.* 2013;14(13):1269–1277.

182. Mellon EA, Sreeraman R, Gebhardt BJ, et al. Impact of radiation treatment parameters and adjuvant systemic therapy on cosmetic outcomes after accelerated partial breast irradiation using 3-dimensional conformal radiation therapy technique. *Pract Radiat Oncol.* 2014;4(3):e159–e166.

9 Cancers of the Gastrointestinal Tract

David Carpenter, Jordan Torok, Christopher G. Willett, Fang-Fang Yin, and Brian G. Czito

INTRODUCTION

Radiotherapy, in combination with chemotherapy, has a significant role in the treatment of cancers of the esophagus, stomach, liver, pancreas, rectum, and anus. The role of combined-modality therapy in the treatment of these diseases has been defined by numerous prospective clinical trials conducted over the past 20 years. This chapter highlights the technical aspects of treatment of gastrointestinal cancer, with particular emphasis on anatomic target definitions and modern treatment planning techniques.

ESOPHAGEAL CANCER

In 2020, there will be an estimated 18,440 new cases of esophageal cancer in the United States and 16,170 related deaths.[1] While esophageal and gastric cancers are often described together, they are distinct malignancies—anatomically, etiologically, and therapeutically. Squamous cell carcinoma and adenocarcinoma are the predominant histologies in esophageal cancer, attributable to specific risk factors for each.[2] The incidence of adenocarcinoma in the United States rose dramatically from the 1970s through the mid-2000s, with more contemporary reports demonstrating a plateau over the past 10 to 15 years.[3,4] Internationally, there is significant geographic variation in the incidence of esophageal cancer,[5] where the predominant histology in endemic regions is squamous cell carcinoma.[6,7] Radiation therapy (RT) plays an important role in the management of esophageal cancer, particularly in the neoadjuvant setting for locally advanced disease.

DIAGNOSTIC EVALUATION

A complete diagnostic workup is crucial in defining the maximal extent of locoregional disease prior to treatment. Due to the limitations of each of the diagnostic modalities in staging this disease, no single study should be solely relied upon to define the extent of tumor during treatment planning.

Description of the mucosal extent of disease is best defined visually by upper endoscopy, often delineating tumor beyond what is appreciated by imaging modalities. Review of endoscopy reports and/or discussion with the gastroenterologist is imperative. Tumor extent is characterized by endoscopic distance from the incisors and location of the tumor in reference to the gastroesophageal junction (GEJ). These measurements may be inconsistent and imprecise between exams; however, they should be noted and compared to radiologic findings to ensure general consistency between modalities. The cervical esophagus begins approximately 15 cm from the incisors at the level of the cricopharyngeus muscle, transitioning to the upper thoracic esophagus at the level of the sternal notch (~20 cm), the middle thoracic esophagus at the lower border of the azygos vein (~25 cm), the lower thoracic esophagus at the lower border of the pulmonary vein (~30 cm), and concluding at the GEJ located ~40 cm from the incisors.[8] Adenocarcinoma of the GEJ is further characterized by Siewert classification. Siewert types I (tumor center is located 1–5 cm above the gastric cardia) and II (1 cm above to 2 cm below the gastric cardia) are generally managed as esophageal cancers, while type III (2–5 cm below) lesions are characterized as gastric cancers.[9]

Endoscopic ultrasound (EUS) is an established modality for local staging in experienced hands. The accuracy of EUS for T stage is generally reported to be between 80% and 90% for esophageal cancer, with higher accuracy for tumors that penetrate the muscularis propria (T3).[10] Regional staging by EUS, which characterizes both nodal size and architecture, has been reported to have ~75% accuracy. Fine-needle aspiration may augment the accuracy of the procedure for determining lymph node involvement.

Axial imaging of the chest and abdomen with computed tomography (CT) or magnetic resonance imaging (MRI) can detect lymphadenopathy beyond the range of EUS and distant metastases. Positron emission tomography (PET) is more accurate than CT or EUS in detecting distant metastases and may increase diagnostic specificity for regional and distant lymphadenopathy.[11,12] Integrated PET/CT takes advantage of the improved spatial resolution of CT, making this a complementary study to the local staging provided by EUS.

Among patients with concerning respiratory symptoms at presentation, or for any patient with a cervical or upper esophageal tumor, bronchoscopy should be considered to evaluate for fistula within the tracheobronchial tree prior to treatment planning. Although presence of a fistula is a poor prognostic factor and traditionally considered a contraindication to radiotherapy, there exist multiple reports of irradiating these patients with potential closure of the fistula and improved survival compared to chemotherapy or supportive care alone.[13–15] Consideration should be given to endoscopically stenting these patients.[14]

TREATMENT OPTIONS

The optimal coordination of surgery, chemotherapy, and radiotherapy continues to be studied by large multi-institutional studies in patients with esophageal and GEJ cancers. Surgical resection has long been the foundation of curative strategies for locoregionally confined esophageal and GEJ cancers, with multimodality therapy indicated for most cases.[16]

Definitive resection is generally indicated for early stage (T1N0) esophageal cancers.[17] Patients with locally advanced disease (at least T2 and/or N+) are generally managed with neoadjuvant chemoradiotherapy (CRT), largely based on results from the CROSS trial. In this trial, patients with T1N1 or T2-3N0-1 esophageal or GEJ cancer were randomized to preoperative CRT or surgery alone. Trimodality therapy was associated with improved complete resection rates, a pathological complete response rate of ~30%, and an overall survival benefit (median survival 49.4 vs. 24 months).[18,19] Perioperative chemotherapy may also be considered for locally advanced GEJ tumors based on results of the FLOT4 trial, which showed improved overall survival (50 vs. 35 months) and comparable toxicity with perioperative FLOT4 chemotherapy as compared to perioperative ECF/ECX (MAGIC regimen) in patients with locally advanced gastric (44%) or GEJ cancers (24% Siewert type I; 32% II/III).[20]

Adjuvant treatment of GEJ tumors in the United States has largely been informed by Intergroup 0116, which demonstrated an overall survival benefit of CRT, compared to surgery alone.[21] All patients had adenocarcinomas, the majority of which were gastric cancers, with GEJ tumors making up about 20% of the population. Phase II data support CRT in the adjuvant setting, particularly in patients with pT3+ and/or node-positive disease.[22] Adjuvant RT alone is of uncertain benefit. Dated trials using antiquated techniques and/or unusual fractionation schemes showed either no improvement or even a possible detrimental effect to RT alone.[23,24]

Surgical resection may not benefit all patients with potentially resectable disease after CRT. Randomized trials of the addition of surgical resection to initial chemoradiotherapy for locally advanced squamous cell carcinomas of the esophagus have shown improved locoregional control but no significant improvement in patient survival.[25–27] In patients with unresectable disease, CRT represents the standard of care.[28]

TREATMENT PLANNING

Simulation

Patients are generally simulated in the supine position, with arms extended over the head using a wing-board or similar device, to ensure reproducibility and to allow treatment with oblique or lateral fields. Although prone positioning may be less reproducible, it may be advantageous for some patients with middle or lower esophageal lesions. Prone positioning is reported to move the esophageal lumen anteriorly, an average of 1.7 cm from the spinal cord, compared to supine positioning.[29] It should be noted that despite such maneuvers, periesophageal tissue posterior to the esophagus still remains fixed to the vertebral column. If treatment fields will encompass any portion of the stomach, the patient, the patient is often simulated and treated with an empty stomach (minimum 3 h NPO) to reduce gastric distension and improve target reproducibility. Oral contrast may aid in localizing the mucosal extent of esophageal cancers. In addition, respiratory movement of the left hemidiaphragm can be noted and incorporated into parameters of the planning target volume (PTV) for GEJ tumors. Studies of four-dimensional CT-simulation (4DCT) of esophageal cancers have demonstrated significant primary tumor, as well as nodal (celiac), movement with respiration in all directions.[30,31] Using 4DCT, optimal PTV coverage for proximal and middle esophageal cancer involves asymmetrical margins, while conventional margins (i.e., uniform 1.0 cm expansion from CTV) provide ideal conformity for distal tumors.[32] At all sites, interfractional esophageal motion is significantly larger than intrafractional motion.[33] Given wide patient variation in such target motion, individual assessment of target motion is preferred to standardized internal target margins for all patients.

Radiotherapy Target

For patients treated neoadjuvantly or definitively with radiotherapy, the gross tumor volume (GTV) includes the maximal extent of gross disease as defined by the combination of all staging modalities. CT is used to define the radial and regional extent of gross disease, while longitudinal tumor boundaries may not be as distinct. Small tumors (T1 or T2) may not be discernable on CT. Oral contrast may assist in defining extent of mucosal irregularity.

Upper endoscopy may provide the most accurate assessment of longitudinal mucosal tumor boundaries, but it may be difficult to precisely correlate these measurements with a planning CT. EUS is probably the best modality for defining both longitudinal and radial extent of the primary tumor. By coordinating with the endoscopist, the superior and inferior tumor boundaries can be referenced to an intrathoracic structure such as the top of the aortic arch or GE junction rather than just the incisors.[34]

PET imaging is also useful in defining the GTV. With clinical judgment, the GTV may be expanded to include fluorodeoxyglucose (FDG)-avid tissue not appreciated as tumor with other imaging. Other areas of tumor extension may be less appreciated on PET, particularly in the longitudinal dimension.[35] Given the risks of false-negative imaging, target contours should not be reduced to include only abnormal volumes defined by PET.[36] While PET may improve target delineation, its contribution to improving treatment efficacy seems limited.[37]

The clinical target volume (CTV) includes areas of microscopic risk of disease from either primary tumor extension or nodal metastases not detected by clinical staging. The lymphatic drainage of the esophagus is primarily longitudinal with channels that may extend several centimeters before perforating the muscularis propria to communicate with adventitial lymphatics.[38] Autopsy studies in patients dying of esophageal cancer have found lymphangitic carcinomatosis of the esophageal wall in up to one-third of patients, with *in situ* or invasive skip lesions at a distance of 2 to 10 cm in 13% of patients.[39] Thus, in the preoperative or definitive setting, radiotherapy ports for esophageal cancer have traditionally included a generous longitudinal margin of mucosa. Although initial fields in RTOG 85–01 treated the entire esophagus for 30 Gy,[40] subsequent trials have limited the longitudinal margin to 5 cm.[41] With 3D target definition, this 5 cm margin is comparable to a 3 to 4 cm CTV of longitudinal margin of esophagus from the GTV (assuming 1 cm PTV and 0.5 to 1 cm to block edge for dosimetric buildup). For tumors of the lower esophagus and GEJ, a 3 to 4 cm inferior extension of the CTV often includes proximal stomach. Pathologic study of resected squamous cell carcinoma and adenocarcinoma has shown the general risk of microscopic extension to be limited to 3 and 5 cm, respectively.[42]

CTV radial expansion should include 1 to 2 cm of adjacent soft tissue, which is generally well within the CTV boundary required for regional nodal coverage. In the CROSS trial, GTV to PTV expansion included a 1.5 cm radial margin and a 4 cm longitudinal margin, with the distal margin shortened to 3 cm when tumor extended to the stomach.[18] It is important to note that these expansions did not include a CTV. Recurrences at the border of the treatment fields were rare (~2%), suggesting these margins are adequate at least when followed by esophagectomy.[43]

The regional lymphatics included within the CTV depend on the anatomic location of the primary tumor. Huang et al. examined the pattern of lymph node metastases based on location in patients undergoing esophagectomy and lymphadenectomy.[44] To summarize, upper thoracic tumors more commonly involved cervical, upper, and middle mediastinal lymph nodes, while lower thoracic tumors more commonly involved middle to lower mediastinal and abdominal nodes. For primary tumors of the esophagus, the CTV should be extended radially to include periesophageal lymph nodes around the GTV, with the longitudinal extent of the normal esophagus included within the CTV. The periesophageal lymph nodes lie in the posterior mediastinum in the soft tissue immediately surrounding the esophagus. Although conventional radiotherapy fields have accommodated these nodes by a 2- to 2.5-cm margin on the esophagus, such guidelines do not account for the often asymmetric and variable distribution of this tissue surrounding the esophagus. Thus, the CTV should be contoured based on individual patient anatomy. Given a >40% rate of subclinical metastases to the supraclavicular lymph nodes for upper esophageal cancers as defined by surgical dissections,[45] extension of the CTV to this region is usually indicated for tumors in this location. Similarly, if the upper esophagus is within the CTV, adjacent paratracheal lymphatics should be included in addition to periesophageal tissue. When CTV includes the mid-esophagus, the subcarinal lymph-node region should be included at the same axial levels. Treatment of the thoracic hilar or anterior mediastinal lymph nodes is not usually indicated unless they are grossly involved on pretreatment imaging.

Distal esophageal tumors that extend to or involve the GEJ pose a threat to upper abdominal lymph nodes. Pericardial lymph nodes (medial and lateral borders of gastric cardia) and celiac lymph nodes are, therefore, included in the CTV. While splenic hilar lymph nodes may be at risk for T3 or T4 GEJ tumors,[46] failure rates were low in the CROSS study, where ~25% had GEJ tumors and these lymph nodes were not electively treated.[43] With extension of tumor inferiorly/laterally into the gastric cardia, lymph nodes of the entire celiac axis and splenic hilar nodes are at risk as described in the gastric cancer section.

Target identification is inherently more challenging in the postoperative setting. Using preoperative staging studies and operative findings, the original extent of the primary cancer (and gross nodal disease) should be reconstructed on the planning CT and included within the CTV. In addition, gastroesophageal anastomosis should be identified and included. Although there may be temptation to exclude the anastomosis among patients where it lies high in the thorax or even lower neck, such an omission has been associated in one series with a 29% anastomotic recurrence rate (compared to 0% with treatment).[47]

Normal Tissue Tolerances

The percentage of total lung receiving >20 Gy should be kept to <30%, and preferably <20%, if achievable.[48,49] Among patients treated neoadjuvantly, postoperative pulmonary complications have been inversely associated with the absolute volume of lung spared 5 Gy.[50,51] The mean dose to the whole heart should not exceed 30 Gy. Heart V40 should be kept to <30% and the V25 to <50%, minimizing high doses to the left ventricle in particular.[52] The spinal cord should not receive >45 Gy.

Radiotherapy Dose

RTOG 94–05[41] evaluated the radiotherapy dose for definitive treatment of esophageal cancer in conjunction with concurrent chemotherapy. No differences in locoregional control or overall survival were detected between the 50.4 and 64.8 Gy arms of the trial, with a trend toward inferior outcome with high-dose CRT. Similarly, the more recent ARTDECO trial examined dose escalation from 50.4 Gy to 61.6 Gy, given with concurrent chemotherapy for patients with T2-4N0-3M0 esophageal cancer. Despite higher toxicity, augmented radiotherapy dose was not associated with significantly improved local control or overall survival.[53] Thus, 50.4 Gy at 1.8 Gy/fraction is the recommended dose for patients with esophageal cancer treated definitively with radiation. In the neoadjuvant setting, the CROSS trial utilized a lower total dose of 41.4 Gy at 1.8 Gy/fraction to a single volume.[18] It is important to note that this was in a well-selected patient population fit for surgery, with 94% of patients subsequently undergoing esophagectomy. In practice, many patients may not ultimately go to surgery where a total dose of 41.4 Gy may be inadequate. An alternative approach is to deliver 45 Gy at 1.8 Gy/fraction to the initial CTV, with consideration of a 5.4 Gy boost to gross disease. In this manner, a definitive dose is administered even if the patient ultimately does not undergo surgery. Whether this additional dose results in increased perioperative complications compared to that used in the CROSS regimen is unknown.

In the postoperative setting, 45 Gy at 1.8 Gy/fraction is considered standard based on Intergroup 0116.[54] Boost treatment beyond 45 Gy for such indications as close or involved surgical margins may be cautiously considered in the setting of normal tissue and patient tolerances.

RADIOTHERAPY FIELDS AND TECHNIQUES

Traditional field borders for esophageal cancers have generally been defined with 2 cm lateral (radial) margins beyond the esophagus and a 5 cm longitudinal margin from tumor (superior–inferior).[41] To account for setup uncertainty, the PTV should be expanded by a minimum of 5 to 10 mm, depending on the frequency of image guidance. Without the aid of more sophisticated technologies such as 4D imaging, fluoroscopy with upper gastrointestinal contrast may assist in defining field size as such internal movement may not simply be limited to the superior and inferior dimensions. At present, 4D CT is the preferred technology to assess target motion, with the understanding that organ motion is related not only to respiration but also to irregular physiological motion.

Given the complex geometric targets associated with esophageal cancers and the proximity of normal organs, the increased conformity of intensity-modulated radiotherapy (IMRT) may provide dosimetric advantages compared to standard radiotherapy techniques (see Fig. 9.1). Use of this technology should account for the challenges of respiratory and cardiac motion, the potential intolerance of large volumes of the lung to even modest doses of radiation, and the undesirability of dose inhomogeneity within the PTV. Its careful implementation has been associated in pooled retrospective analysis with improved overall survival, presumably secondary to decreased exposure of the lungs and heart compared to traditional techniques.[55–59] A propensity score-based comparison of 676 patients with stage Ib-IVa esophageal cancer demonstrated significantly improved long-term overall survival, locoregional control, and non–cancer-related death following IMRT as compared to 3D-CRT.[60]

A growing body of data suggests that, in comparison to 3DCRT and IMRT, proton beam therapy (PBT) may offer significant improvements in cardiopulmonary sparing[61,62] and decreased postoperative complications.[63,64] Intensity-modulated proton therapy (IMPT), also referred to as pencil beam scanning, may offer additional organ sparing over IMRT[64] or conventional PBT.[65] A recently published phase IIB trial of PBT (80% passive scattering) versus IMRT for esophageal cancer demonstrated reduced risk and severity of adverse events in patients treated with PBT, with similar rates of progression-free survival across arms (51% vs. 51% at 3 years).[66]

Chemotherapy

Based on Intergroup 0116, 5-FU-based CRT is typical for adjuvant CRT.[54] Patients initially received 5-FU (425 mg/m^2), with leucovorin (20 mg/m^2) for 5 days. Chemoradiotherapy began 28 days later with reduced doses of 5-FU (400 mg/m^2) and leucovorin on the first 4 days and last 3 days of radiotherapy. Two more monthly cycles of chemotherapy were given a month after completion of radiotherapy. Grade 3 or higher hematologic and gastrointestinal toxicity associated with this regimen was seen in 54% and 33% of patients, respectively.

For patients treated with definitive chemoradiotherapy of the esophagus, the optimal agent(s), dose, and schedule of systemic therapy are currently unknown. RTOG 85–01 established the clear superiority of chemoradiotherapy over radiotherapy alone for patients with squamous cell

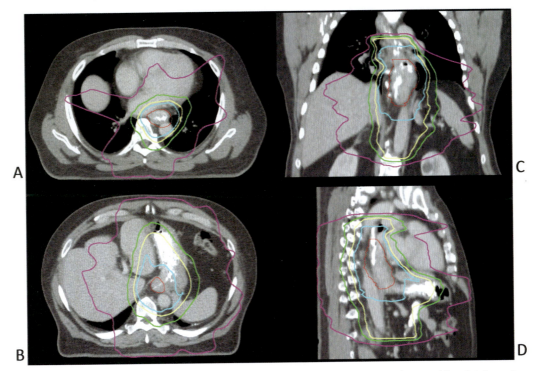

FIGURE 9.1. 60-year-old male patient with uT3N0 borderline resectable adenocarcinoma of the distal esophagus treated with neoadjuvant chemoradiotherapy utilizing a three-arc VMAT technique. Axial (**A, B**), coronal (**C**), and sagittal (**D**) views showing GTV (red) and 48.6 Gy (cyan), 41.4 Gy (yellow), 30 Gy (light green), and 15 Gy (magenta) isodose lines.

carcinoma of the esophagus.[40] Cisplatin (75 mg/m^2) was administered on the first and fifth week of radiotherapy with 5-FU (1,000 mg/m^2) for 4 days. Two additional cycles of cisplatin and 5-FU were administered after completion of radiotherapy. Rates of grade 3 or higher hematologic and gastrointestinal toxicity were comparable to those seen in the Intergroup trial. Initial randomized trials of neoadjuvant chemoradiotherapy have similarly included various schedules of concurrent cisplatin, generally with 5-FU as well.[67–70] The CROSS regimen included carboplatin at an area under the curve of 2 mg/mL/min and paclitaxel 50 mg/m^2, both given weekly[18] with radiotherapy in resectable esophageal cancer patients. Acute toxicity was considerably less than observed in earlier trials containing 5-FU, with grade 3+ hematologic, and all other nonhematologic toxicity reported in 7% and 13% of patients, respectively.

For resectable adenocarcinomas of the GEJ treated with perioperative chemotherapy, FLOT4 represents the current standard of care based on the results of the German FLOT4 trial.[20] In patients with locally advanced gastric (44%) or GEJ (56%) tumors, the FLOT4 regimen (four preoperative and four postoperative 2-week cycles of 50 mg/m^2 docetaxel, 85 mg/m^2 oxaliplatin, 200 mg/m^2 leucovorin, and 2600 mg/m^2 fluorouracil as a 24-hour infusion on day 1) demonstrated superior overall survival (median 50 months versus 35 months) and a comparable toxicity profile to a control arm of three preoperative and three postoperative cycles of ECF/ECX ("MAGIC" regimen).[71] This trial is discussed further in the gastric cancer chapter. Caution should be taken when extrapolating these data to adenocarcinoma of the lower or mid-thoracic esophagus. Prospective trials of perioperative chemotherapy with and without neoadjuvant chemoradiation for esophageal and GEJ tumors are ongoing.

PROGNOSIS

For locally advanced, unresectable esophageal cancers, the 5-year overall survival after definitive chemoradiotherapy was 26% in RTOG 85–01.[28] Five-year overall survival among patients undergoing trimodality therapy and perioperative chemotherapy have been reported as high as 47%[18] and 50%,[20] respectively. Surgical or endoscopic treatment of T1 esophageal cancer results in a 5-year survival of ~80%.[72]

GASTRIC CANCER

In 2020, there will be an estimated 27,600 new cases of gastric cancer in the United States, with 11,010 deaths attributed to the disease.[1] As with esophageal cancer, there is marked variation in the incidence of gastric cancer based on geographic region.[5] Gastric cancer is predominantly of adenocarcinoma histology, with diffuse and intestinal subtypes. Distal gastric cancers have been decreasing in incidence, while more proximal/cardia lesions have become more common.[73] The use of radiation in the management of gastric cancer has declined alongside improvements in systemic therapy.

DIAGNOSTIC EVALUATION

Upper endoscopy is critical in delineating the location and extent of mucosal disease involvement. The location of the tumor "epicenter" and its extension to the GEJ/distal esophagus should be determined based on endoscopy reports and/or discussion with the gastroenterologist. The Siewert classification can be useful in differentiating true gastric cancers from GEJ cancers.[9] As with esophageal cancer, EUS may play an important role in the local and regional staging of gastric cancer. EUS accuracy in determining both correct T- and N-stage is ~80%.[74-76]

Contrast-enhanced CT of the chest, abdomen and pelvis is performed to evaluate for regional lymph nodes and distant metastases but is limited in the detection of peritoneal implants.[77] The addition of PET to CT increases specificity for diagnosing lymph node metastases[78] and distant metastases.[79] However, PET has limited diagnostic sensitivity for peritoneal metastases[80] and for diffuse-type/signet-ring gastric cancers.[81-83] Thus, its role in gastric cancer staging remains somewhat poorly defined. Staging laparoscopy with cytology of peritoneal washings may be obtained for patients with ≥T1b disease undergoing curative-intent therapy,[84-86] with positive peritoneal cytology indicating M1 disease even in the absence of a radiographic correlate.

TREATMENT OPTIONS

The optimal treatment paradigm for gastric cancer remains an active area of investigation. Upfront surgical resection is indicated for early stage gastric cancers (T1N0). For more advanced cases, local recurrence and/or regional failure occurs in a significant number of patients following curative resection.[87] Intergroup 0116 investigated the use of adjuvant CRT in a heterogeneous patient population including T1N+, T2-4N0-2 gastric cancers as well as a smaller proportion of GEJ cancers.[54] The addition of adjuvant CRT to surgical resection resulted in a significant reduction in local regional failure and an improvement in survival (median survival 35 vs. 27 months).[21] As a result, adjuvant CRT became the standard treatment for patients with gastric cancer in North America. Critics have suggested the clinical benefit of radiotherapy may be limited following standard of care surgery, as opposed to D0 resection performed for the majority of patients in the Intergroup 0116 trial.[88] The Korean ARTIST trial addressed this criticism by comparing the use of adjuvant chemotherapy to CRT in patients undergoing a D2 resection, demonstrating a significant reduction in locoregional relapse with CRT but no difference in overall survival.[89] Subset analysis from the ARTIST trial suggested that patients with node-positive disease were more likely to benefit from CRT, prompting a subsequent trial (ARTIST II) comparing adjuvant chemotherapy to adjuvant CRT in this population. The ARTIST II trial was terminated upon interim analysis showing no difference in 3-year fluorodeoxyglucose (FDG)-avid between chemotherapy with (73%) or without (78%) radiation.[90]

Perioperative chemotherapy has become an increasingly utilized treatment paradigm for advanced gastric cancer.[91] The UK MAGIC trial compared this approach (utilizing an ECF regimen) to surgical resection alone in a heterogeneous patient population of mostly gastric (~75%) but also GEJ and distal esophageal cancers. The perioperative chemotherapy regimen was associated with tumor downstaging and a significant improvement in overall survival (5-year 36% vs. 23%).[71] More recently, the German FLOT4 trial demonstrated a further overall survival benefit to perioperative FLOT chemotherapy compared to the ECF/ECX regimen used in the MAGIC trial for cT2 and/or cN+ resectable gastric cancer (median OS 50 m vs. 35 m).[20]

Recent trials have explored the addition of CRT to perioperative chemotherapy regimens. The Dutch CRITICS trial compared perioperative chemotherapy (ECX) to preoperative chemotherapy (ECX), followed by adjuvant CRT with concurrent capecitabine and cisplatin for patients with stage IB-IVA resectable gastric or GEJ adenocarcinoma undergoing at least D1 node dissection.[92] No survival difference was observed between arms. Given poor rates of postoperative treatment compliance in both arms and known correlation of tumor downstaging and resectability to overall survival, subsequent studies have focused on the potential benefit of CRT in the neoadjuvant setting. RTOG 9904, a single-arm phase II study, demonstrated the feasibility of neoadjuvant CRT, with pathologic complete response rates >20%.[93] The role of neoadjuvant radiotherapy in the context of modern perioperative chemotherapy regimens is being addressed in the ongoing TOPGEAR[94] and CRITICS-II[95] trials.

For unresectable disease, some patients can be downstaged with neoadjuvant therapy, but the optimal approach is unknown. Therapy for the majority of these patients is typically palliative. The role of RT in this setting is largely based on historical trials. The addition of chemotherapy to RT improved survival,[96] while the comparison of CRT to chemotherapy alone appeared to result in more long-term survivors.[97] Most contemporary trials have focused on improving combination chemotherapy efficacy for these patients.

TREATMENT PLANNING
Simulation

Patients are generally simulated in the supine position with arms extended over the head using a wing-board or similar device. An empty stomach (minimum 3 h NPO) may be useful to reduce gastric distension and improve target reproducibility. Oral contrast is typically given, which in the preoperative or definitive setting can help identify mucosal extent of disease. In the postoperative setting, oral contrast helps identify anatomical structures, including the gastric remnant and anastomosis. IV contrast is routinely given to assist in the detection of lymphadenopathy. 4D CT is useful for defining organ and target motion related to respiration, which can be incorporated into parameters of the PTV.[98] Other strategies for estimating the extent of organ motion include fluoroscopic imaging with contrast and the use of fiducial markers.[99]

Radiotherapy Target

In the neoadjuvant and definitive settings, the GTV includes the maximal extent of gross disease as defined by upper endoscopy and imaging modalities, primarily CT and EUS. The CTV includes areas at risk for microscopic disease from either primary tumor extension or nodal metastases not detected by clinical staging. Areas at risk for local and regional recurrence have been identified, most notably from a seminal re-operation series.[87] The CTV includes all the perigastric lymph nodes along the lesser and greater curvatures of the stomach. Adequate longitudinal normal mucosal margin within the CTV should be generated (~5 cm). For proximal gastric tumors, cranial extension of CTV may include distal esophagus with associated periesophageal lymphatics. For very distal gastric cancers, caudal extension including a portion of the duodenum is appropriate. Tumors of the gastric cardia or fundus (especially if T3) often include the medial left hemidiaphragm.

In addition to the perigastric lymph nodes, the following nodal stations should generally be included in the CTV for gastric tumors: the celiac, porta hepatis (including gastrohepatic and hepatoduodenal), suprapancreatic (along the splenic artery), splenic hilar, supra- and infrapyloric (above and below the pylorus), pancreaticoduodenal (tissue around and posterior to the pancreatic head), and local para-aortic/retroperitoneal lymph nodes (along the cranial-caudal extent of the stomach). These can vary somewhat depending on extent and location of the primary tumor.

Similar principles for target identification exist in the postoperative setting. Using preoperative staging studies and operative findings, the original extent of the primary cancer (and gross nodal disease) should be reconstructed on the planning CT and included within the CTV. An available contouring atlas is helpful for identification of regional nodes on CT in patients with both intact and postoperative anatomy.[100] Among gastric tumors that involve only the upper one-third of the stomach with minimal lymphatic tumor involvement pathologically, cautious consideration can be given for exclusion of the infrapyloric and pancreaticoduodenal lymph nodes.[101]

Similarly, lesions of the lower one-third of the stomach may have a lower propensity for involvement of the splenic hilar lymph nodes.[101]

Normal Tissue Tolerances

The amount of small bowel receiving over 45 Gy should be minimized without compromising target coverage. Any small bowel within a possible boost volume should generally be kept <50 Gy. At least 75% of one kidney or the composite of one whole kidney should be kept <18 to 20 Gy. If the large majority of one kidney receives doses >20 Gy, consideration should be given to a quantitative renal scan prior to treatment to ensure sufficient function of the other kidney. Sixty (and preferably much less) percent of the liver should be kept <30 Gy and the whole liver should not receive a mean dose >25 Gy. Heart and spinal cord constraints are similar to those described for esophageal cancer.

RADIOTHERAPY DOSE

In the neoadjuvant setting, 45 Gy at 1.8 Gy/fraction was utilized in RTOG 9904 and is the dose being used in the ongoing TOPGEAR and CRITICS-II trials.[94,95] In the postoperative setting, 45 Gy at 1.8 Gy/fraction is the standard dose based on Intergroup 0116.[54] Boost treatment beyond 45 Gy may be considered cautiously in select cases with close or involved surgical margins, with regard given to normal tissue and patient tolerances.

Radiotherapy Fields and Techniques

The PTV should integrate organ motion assessment based on 4DCT. For 3D planning, a minimum of an additional 5 mm margin is necessary for dosimetric coverage of the PTV. Postoperative field design continues to be influenced by the Intergroup 0116 trial. Smalley et al.[101] describe the traditional borders as follows: the superior field border includes the left hemidiaphragm, though it may be significantly higher for proximal gastric tumors whose anastomoses are in the thorax. In order to include the infrapyloric and pancreaticoduodenal nodes, the inferior field border is generally placed at L3. The left lateral border extends sufficiently to include the lateral border of the perigastric lymph nodes of the greater curvature and the splenic hilum. The medial border is placed to include the porta hepatis and the medial extent of the preoperative tumor volume. Using this technique, the addition of lateral or oblique fields to AP–PA ports may have some benefit. The gastric fundus and adjacent perigastric lymph nodes often necessitate posterior extension such that straight lateral fields are unable to spare the entire spinal cord or a significant amount of kidney. In addition, the contribution of lateral fields should be limited to <20 Gy when involving the liver. The anterior borders of lateral and oblique fields must cover the preoperative extent of the ventral gastric wall.

Modern 3D conformal treatment planning should incorporate CT-defined volumes while accounting for volumes included in traditional ports to avoid undertreatment. Customized field techniques may be advantageous for some patients depending on the anatomic extent of target. Oblique fields optimized to avoid spinal cord or kidney while covering the PTV may often prove superior to straight lateral fields. 3D treatment planning with five or more fields has demonstrated superior sparing of normal structures in comparison to the AP–PA technique used in Intergroup 0116,[102] with clinically significant reductions in treatment-related toxicity.[103] The dosimetric benefit achieved was largely from reduction in kidney and spinal cord doses, at the expense of small increases in dose to the liver.

Dosimetric studies of IMRT in the postoperative treatment of gastric cancer have reported a possible improvement in target coverage and sparing of critical structures,[104] most notably in reducing kidney exposure,[105–107] compared to conventional techniques. However, clinically apparent renal dysfunction has not been described as a common problem after treatment with more conventional techniques, such as among patients treated in Intergroup 0116.[54] While some reports have demonstrated similar rates of acute toxicity between patients treated with 3D CRT and IMRT,[108,109] other modern retrospective series have shown IMRT to significantly reduce grade 3+ toxicity with similar survival outcomes to 3D-CRT.[110]

Chemotherapy

Intergroup 0116 employed an adjuvant/concurrent regimen of 5-FU as described in the esophageal section. This has subsequently served as the backbone for most CRT regimens. The RTOG investigated combination and alternate regimens in both the preoperative and postoperative settings. RTOG 9904 utilized an induction regimen of 5-FU (200 mg/m^2) by continuous infusion on days 1 to 21 and cisplatin (20 mg/m^2) on days 1 to 5 for 2 cycles, followed by concurrent 5-FU (300 mg/m^2) 5 days a week and paclitaxel (45 mg/m^2) weekly during radiotherapy.[93] RTOG 0114 conducted a randomized phase II study comparing an intensified regimen of paclitaxel, cisplatin, and 5-FU (PCF) induction, followed by a PF-based-CRT regimen to a non-5-FU containing regimen of PC induction followed by PC CRT.[111] The PCF arm closed early due to excess toxicity, while the PC arm did not improve outcomes compared to INT 0116. Intergroup trial CALGB 80101 compared the INT 0116 5-FU regimen used before and after CRT to a regimen similar to that used in the MAGIC trial containing epirubicin (50 mg/m^2 d1), cisplatin (60 mg/m^2 d1), and 5-FU (200 mg/m^2/d1-21, ECF).[112] The CRT component was the same in both arms with 5-FU given via continuous infusion at a dose of 200 mg/m^2/d. No significant difference in survival was observed

between the arms. A possible alternative to intravenous 5-FU is daily oral capecitabine (825 mg/m^2 BID) as used in the ARTIST trial,[89] although there is no prospective evidence comparing the two in gastric cancer. Additional agents used in the adjuvant setting include S-1 and oxaliplatin. While fluoropyrimidine-based CRT has been a consistent theme across trials, the optimal neoadjuvant regimen remains an area of active investigation.

For patients receiving perioperative chemotherapy without radiotherapy, FLOT4 represents the current standard of care. The German FLOT4 trial demonstrated superior overall survival of the FLOT4 regimen of four preoperative and four postoperative 2-week cycles of 50 mg/m^2 docetaxel, 85 mg/m^2 oxaliplatin, 200 mg/m^2 leucovorin, and 2600 mg/m^2 fluorouracil as a 24-hour infusion on day as compared to the MAGIC trial regimen of three cycles of preoperative and postoperative epirubicin, cisplatin, and 5-FU or gemcitabine (ECF/ECX).[20] Rates of adverse events were comparable between arms. Therefore, ECF/ECX should not be routinely recommended for locally advanced gastric cancer.

Prognosis

The outcome of patients with gastric cancer varies depending on the geographic region of the patient. The 5-year overall survival from the ARTIST trial based in South Korea was ~75%,[89] compared to a 5-year survival of 45% in the experimental arm from the FLOT4 trial and ~40% in the combined-modality arm from INT 0116.[21] The 5-year survival rate was <30% in the surgery alone arms from the INT 0116 and MAGIC trials,[71] compared to 60% to 70% in the surgery alone arms from recent Japanese and Korean studies.[113,114] This may partially be explained by more advanced patients included in the North American and European trials but may also reflect differences in the biology of the disease, surgical experience, and screening practices resulting in stage migration between the countries.

HEPATOCELLULAR CARCINOMA

Liver cancer is the third-leading cause of global cancer death. In the United States, the incidence of liver and intrahepatic biliary cancers is increasing,[115] with an estimated 42,810 new cases in 2020.[1] Outcomes for hepatocellular carcinoma (HCC) are closely correlated to underlying etiology and hepatic function. Recent technological advancements in radiotherapy have expanded its role in multidisciplinary management of HCC.

DIAGNOSTIC EVALUATION

HCC requires multidisciplinary evaluation across hepatologists, transplant surgeons, diagnostic and interventional radiologists, and medical, surgical, and radiation oncologists. Patients at high risk for developing HCC, including those with cirrhosis or chronic hepatitis B (HBV) infection, are typically screened biannually with abdominal ultrasound with or without alpha-fetoprotein (AFP).[116] Hepatic lesions ≥1 cm on ultrasound should be further characterized by contrast-enhanced MRI or CT that include arterial, portal, and delayed phases. Biopsy is not typically necessary, as application of the Liver Imaging Reporting Data System (LI-RADS) in high-risk patients yields a diagnostic sensitivity and specificity of 60% to 85% and 87% to 96%, respectively.[117] Imaging characteristics consistent with HCC include larger lesion size, enhancing capsule appearance on portal and post-contrast phases, nonperipheral lesion washout in portal and venous phases, and ≥50% lesion growth within a 6-month timeframe.[118]

Initial work up for HCC includes assessment of co-morbidities, liver reserve, and staging. Clinical examination should address signs and symptoms of decompensated liver disease. General labwork includes a complete metabolic profile (transaminases, bilirubin, alkaline phosphatase, albumin, creatinine, and BUN), complete blood count (platelets), coagulation studies (PT/INR), and tumor markers (AFP, CA 19-9 and CEA as indicated). Childs–Pugh classification is commonly used to estimate hepatic functional reserve.[119] Model for End-Stage Liver Disease (MELD) score is a measure of 3-month mortality that is particularly useful for transplantation cases,[120] while Albumin-Bilirubin (ALBI) grading offers a more objective alternative to Childs–Pugh classification (i.e., clinical evaluation of ascites and encephalopathy are not considered) with comparable prognostic performance.[121]

Imaging should include contrasted CT or MRI of the abdomen and pelvis as well as CT chest to assess for distant disease. Bone scan may be obtained when osseous metastases are suspected based on history and examination. PET imaging is not generally obtained for HCC, having a low sensitivity and high specificity.[122] A variety of staging systems exist for HCC, including the Barcelona Clinic Liver Cancer (BCLC) system, American Joint Committee on Cancer (AJCC), Okuda, and Cancer of the Liver Italian Program (CLIP) systems.

TREATMENT OPTIONS

Transplantation and surgical resection should be considered as first-line therapy for HCC, with 5-year overall survival rates of 45% to 80% and 10% to 50%, respectively.[123,124] However, less than 30% of patients with newly diagnosed HCC are candidates for transplantation or surgical resection. For nonoperative candidates with disease localized to the liver, therapeutic options include radiofrequency and microwave ablation (RFA/MWA), cryotherapy, percutaneous injection with ethanol or acetic acid, intra-arterial therapies including intra-arterial

chemotherapy, trans-arterial chemoembolization (TACE), bland embolization, radioembolization, and radiotherapy using a variety of techniques including brachytherapy, IMRT, stereotactic body radiotherapy (SBRT), proton therapy, and heavy ion therapy.

Percutaneous ablation became the most common modality for treating unresectable HCC confined to the liver following a series of trials demonstrating the superiority of ablation to percutaneous ethanol and acetic acid injection.[125,126] RFA and MWA are thermal modalities involving high-frequency current, with limited comparative data suggesting similar rates of local control and toxicity.[127,128] Potential advantages of MWA over RFA include the ability to treat multiple lesions simultaneously, less procedural time, and less "heat sink" effect due to a greater degree of direct heating versus thermal conductance at higher frequencies.[129] Thermal ablation complication rates range from 0% to 30%, and include abscess formation, hemorrhage, biliary leakage, and stricture. Lesion size >3 cm is a relative contraindication to ablative therapy due to lower rates of local control.[130] RFA and MWA are also generally avoided for tumors located, either along the liver edge due to difficulty with access, or, particularly for RFA, near blood vessels due to "heat sink" effect. Prospective comparisons of ablation to SBRT, including the PROVE-HCC trial, are currently ongoing.[131]

No consensus exists for optimal embolization technique; however, a growing number of recent trials have examined TACE in comparison and in combination with other local modalities. Unlike ablation and radiotherapy approaches, TACE is considered a palliative rather than curative treatment modality. TACE is often used alone or alongside RFA or SBRT for patients with lesions too large or numerous for other local therapies.[132] Relative contraindications to TACE include >50% liver involvement, limited hepatic reserve, prior transjugular intrahepatic portosystemic shunting, and vascular invasion (aside from first or second branch portal vein invasion treated with additional radiotherapy).[133] Radiotherapy and TACE in combination have shown superior outcomes to TACE alone.[134,135] Radioembolization with Y-90 is a preferred embolization approach for patients with macrovascular invasion.[136]

The use of radiotherapy for HCC was historically limited due to high toxicity and low efficacy with conventional techniques. Tumor dose was limited by associated hepatotoxicity to 30 to 40 Gy, with local control rates <30%.[137] Recent technical advances in cross-sectional imaging and conformal radiotherapy techniques have enabled the delivery of curative doses with favorable toxicity rates.[138] Multiple phase I and II trials of SBRT for HCC have demonstrated both excellent local control (85%–100%) and low rates of grade 3 toxicity[139–141] despite including patients with lesions >3 cm, adverse tumor locations (inferior border, hepatic dome), vascular involvement, limited hepatic function, and multiple prior local therapies. Similar clinical outcomes and toxicity profiles have been observed with proton therapy.[142] Common indications for radiotherapy include large lesion size, obstructive jaundice, portal vein thrombosis, and failure of other local treatment modalities. Relative contraindications to SBRT include large burden extrahepatic disease, Child–Pugh C disease (B8-9 disease is controversial), tumor proximity to luminal gastrointestinal (GI) structures (although more protracted RT courses may be appropriate in this situation), and <700 cc liver sparing.[143] Ongoing phase III trials compare SBRT to ablation as first-line therapy for localized unresectable HCC and in combination with sorafenib for metastatic disease.[131,144]

TREATMENT PLANNING

Simulation

Patients undergoing radiotherapy for HCC are generally simulated in the supine position with arms elevated in a customized immobilization device. Imaging should be used to account for organ motion,[145] with tri-phasic contrast administration for arterial, portal, and delayed venous series preferred. Emerging 4D MRI imaging has the potential to provide better lesion delineation.[146] Additional strategies for reducing hepatic motion include breath holding, active breathing control, and abdominal compression. Abdominal compression may push bowel closer to target volumes, notably for left-sided tumors. One to two glasses of water 30 minutes prior to simulation and treatment may reduce bowel gas and corresponding artifact.

Radiotherapy Target

For SBRT to HCC localized to the liver, arterial, portal, and delayed series are useful for accurately delineating GTV. Where tumor extent is not apparent on simulation images, contrasted MRI or CT images should be fused using deformable registration.[147] Portal thrombus should be included in GTV, including cases with benign radiographic characteristics on contrasted imaging.[148] These varying phase volumes are combined into an internal target volume (ITV). Depending on tumor size, location, motion extent, immobilization, and on-treatment imaging capabilities, ITV to PTV expansion should generally be 5 to 10 mm.

Normal Tissue Tolerances

HCC is generally a radiosensitive tumor, with SBRT dose largely dependent on normal tissue toxicity. Radiation-induced liver disease, characterized by anicteric hepatomegaly, ascites, and disproportionally elevated alkaline phosphatase, is rarely seen in the setting of modern conformal radiotherapy.[149] The probability of liver toxicity during radiotherapy can be estimated with the prospectively validated Lyman–Kutcher–Burman model.[150,151] Evaluation of hepatic reserve in patients undergoing resection includes sparing, at an absolute minimum, uninvolved liver at the following rates: 40% in the context of cirrhosis, 30% in the context of prior chemotherapy, and 20% in other instances. Less than 700 cc of remaining functional liver is a relative contraindication to radiotherapy, with 500 cc as an absolute cutoff.[152] QUANTEC recommendations for median uninvolved liver dose include <13 Gy for 3-fraction plans, <18 Gy for 5-fraction plans, and <6 Gy in the context of Child–Pugh B disease.[152] Efforts to spare uninvolved liver beyond these near-absolute cut-offs are warranted.

In the context of 3-fraction plans, GI luminal structures should be kept to 3 cc <21 Gy, the heart to 1 cc <30 Gy, the chest wall to 30 cc < 30 Gy, bilateral kidneys to V15 <35%, and spinal cord to 1 cc <18 Gy.[153] Similar to the "no fly zone" of the central bronchi for lung SBRT, irradiation of central hepatic lesions should account for biliary stricture risk associated with a central biliary tree. A 1.5 cm extension beyond the portal vein (extending from the spleno-portal confluence to the main portal bifurcation into right and left portal veins) should generally be limited in 5-fraction plans to a V40 <21 cc and a V37 <24 cc (BED_{10} of 72 Gy and 66 Gy, respectively).[154]

Radiotherapy Dose

A variety of fractionation schemes are widely used for SBRT. Common dose prescriptions include 48 to 54 Gy over 3 fractions for small, peripheral lesions, 50 Gy over 5 fractions, 40 Gy over 5 fractions for patients with Childs–Pugh B disease, 50 Gy over 10 fractions for tumors near hollow viscera, and 30 Gy over 5 fractions for larger tumors, while always prioritizing normal tissue constraints. More protracted RT courses delivering higher BED courses may be similarly effective. For palliative cases, whole liver irradiation can be delivered with a single 8 Gy fraction or to 21 Gy over 7 fractions.[155]

Radiotherapy Fields and Techniques

Conformal radiotherapy techniques are essential when delivering curative doses while minimizing dose-limiting toxicities of the liver parenchyma, central biliary tree, and GI luminal structures (see Fig. 9.2). SBRT may be delivered as IMRT, particularly when prioritizing conformality of nonelliptical target volumes and reduction of normal tissue volumes receiving low radiation doses. However, volumetric modulated arc therapy (VMAT) offers quicker treatment times and less heterogeneity within target volumes.[156] PBT may allow for further dose escalation with improved normal tissue (including liver) sparing.[157]

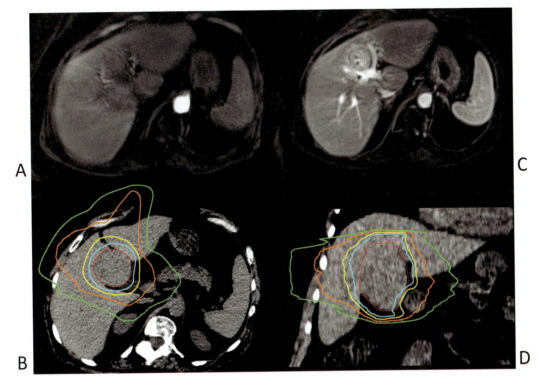

FIGURE 9.2. 63-year-old woman with a cT1bN0 hepatocellular carcinoma of the right hepatic lobe adjacent to the gallbladder fossa in the setting of Childs–Pugh A6 cirrhosis, treated with a 5-fraction SBRT plan utilizing a 2-arc VMAT technique. Diagnostic MRI axial T1 arterial (**A**) and portal venous (**B**) images, as well as axial (**C**) and coronal (**D**) views showing tri-phasic ITV (red) and 50 Gy (cyan), 40 Gy (yellow), 25 Gy (orange), and 15 Gy (green) isodose lines.

Chemotherapy

Systemic chemotherapy for HCC is generally reserved for patients with extrahepatic disease or for those who have progressed following locoregional therapies. Acceptable first-line therapies include sorafenib,[158] lenvatinib,[159] atezolizumab and bevacizumab,[160] and FOLFOX.[161] The optimal sequencing of systemic therapies is currently unknown.

Prognosis

Mortality of HCC correlates closely to underlying etiology, with death most commonly due to intrahepatic recurrence. Rates of 5-year overall survival for HCC following transplantation and surgical resection range from 45% to 80% and 10% to 50%, respectively.[123,124] For unresectable cases, 2-year local control is similarly 80% to 85% for RFA (for smaller lesions) and SBRT.[162] Survival rates for patients with metastatic disease are generally <1 year.[158,160]

PANCREATIC CANCER

In the year 2020, the American Cancer Society estimated 57,600 new pancreatic cancers in the United States.[1] They also predicted 47,050 deaths from this disease,

highlighting the unfavorable prognosis of this cancer at any stage and the need for more effective therapies.

DIAGNOSTIC EVALUATION

The pretreatment diagnostic evaluation is crucial for identification of patients who are candidates for surgical resection, those with borderline/unresectable disease, and patients with distant metastases. Abdominal CT and MRI remain the most useful modalities for defining local disease extent and for detecting metastases within the abdomen. Resectability criteria are based on tumor involvement of adjacent arteries and veins, which can be assessed with these imaging modalities. Refinements in abdominal CT imaging, such as acquisition of thin sections, dual-phase contrast imaging, 3D reconstruction, and use of multi-detector CT, have greatly improved the accuracy in defining local tumor extension. With these techniques, accurate prediction of resectability has been reported in up to 87% of patients.[163] In addition to CT or MRI, EUS in experienced hands may add further information regarding tumor extent, vascular involvement, and regional adenopathy. EUS is also useful for obtaining a cytological diagnosis. Endoscopic retrograde cholangiopancreatography (ERCP) is a useful technique as it can be utilized as both a diagnostic tool to collect brushings, which can confirm malignancy within the biliary and/or pancreatic ducts, and as a therapeutic tool for biliary stent placement, which can relieve extrinsic compression from the pancreatic tumor. Imaging from ERCP can also be reviewed to assist in defining tumor boundaries based on abnormalities of the biliary and/or pancreatic ducts.

The roles of PET imaging and staging laparoscopy for detecting metastatic disease not seen on pancreatic protocol CT or MRI remain controversial. Select institutions utilize one or both approaches for patients deemed high risk for metastatic disease based on clinical characteristics such as borderline resectability/unresectability, primary tumor size, nodal burden, CA19-9 levels, and/or clinical symptoms.[164,165] Where diagnostic laparotomy is employed, positive cytology establishes a pathologic M1 diagnosis.[166]

TREATMENT OPTIONS

Where feasible, surgery is the backbone of curative therapy for pancreatic cancer.[167] Given the high rates of both local failure and distant metastases following resection alone,[168,169] multimodality treatment has improved clinical outcomes across all stages of disease. The optimal combination and sequencing of multimodality therapies remain an active area of investigation across all stages of pancreatic cancer.

For resectable disease, two historical treatment paradigms have evolved in parallel. In the United States, the Gastrointestinal Tumor Study Group (GITSG) trial established adjuvant chemoradiation as standard of care, showing improved overall survival compared to surgery alone.[170] More contemporary retrospective data demonstrate improved overall survival of adjuvant chemoradiation over surgery alone regardless of age, tumor size, margin status, or node status.[171,172] Adjuvant chemotherapy is now standard of care in Europe for resected disease, having demonstrated improved survival compared to resection alone.[173,174] Randomized comparisons between adjuvant chemotherapy and chemoradiation demonstrate conflicting results and are difficult to interpret due to limitations in trial design and the use of outdated therapies.[175–178]

For borderline resectable disease, multimodality therapy is typically given in the neoadjuvant setting. Some of the theoretic advantages of this strategy include local tumor downstaging to facilitate an R0 resection, better oxygenation of the target tissues during chemoradiation, reduced risk of intraoperative seeding, and improved treatment tolerance compared to adjuvant therapy. Neoadjuvant therapy may also allow for identification of patients with rapidly progressive disease who are not likely to benefit from curative-intent surgical resection, which carries a high degree of associated morbidity.[179] A recent Korean phase II/III trial demonstrated improved 2-year overall survival with neoadjuvant chemoradiation as compared to upfront surgery and adjuvant chemoradiation.[180] The PREOPANC trial showed significantly improved disease-free survival, locoregional failure-free survival, and R0 resection rates for patients with resectable or borderline resectable pancreatic cancer treated with neoadjuvant chemoradiation and adjuvant chemotherapy compared to immediate surgery and adjuvant chemotherapy. Overall survival was not significantly different between treatment arms.[181] The addition and sequencing of chemoradiotherapy to neoadjuvant chemotherapy remain an actively evolving paradigm.

Patients with unresectable cancers who have a favorable functional status can be considered for noncurative approaches, including chemoradiotherapy or chemotherapy alone. Two randomized studies have not shown any survival benefit with the addition of RT to initial chemotherapy among patients with unresectable disease.[182,183] Additional reports have demonstrated improved survival with combined-modality therapy compared to radiotherapy alone,[184] chemotherapy alone,[185,186] or supportive care.[187] In light of these conflicting data, one approach for patients without local symptoms is to offer initial systemic therapy, followed by combined-modality therapy or SBRT in patients without disease progression. Among symptomatic patients, local therapy with radiation is likely to be an effective palliative tool and, therefore, should be considered alongside chemotherapy in the upfront setting.

Patients who present with metastatic disease are typically best managed with systemic chemotherapy, although short palliative courses of radiotherapy for symptoms, such as pain, may be beneficial in some instances.

TREATMENT PLANNING
Simulation

Patients should be simulated in the supine position with arms over the head using a wing-board or similar device to ensure reproducibility and to allow treatment with multiple field orientations. Use of oral contrast is helpful to identify the duodenal C-loop as an important reference for field design. Intravenous contrast during CT planning aids in detection of vascular landmarks and target definition, and, similar to HCC, a tri-phasic protocol optimized for pancreas imaging (acquisition during arterial, portal-venous, and delayed phases of contrast) may be useful. Diagnostic films should be reviewed in conjunction with planning CT images. Respiratory motion can be significant within the radiation target areas, as is generally accounted for by use of 4D CT and/or fiducial placement. These approaches allow for quantification of duodenal C-loop motion and ensure appropriate coverage of the target regions. Motion management may be appropriate in instances of significant motion.

Radiotherapy Target

Accurate target definition is especially important, given the proximity of dose-limiting organs at risk to target volumes. For unresectable tumors or those treated neoadjuvantly, the GTV includes the primary tumor (including vessels involved by tumor) and any radiographically enlarged lymph nodes. The CTV includes a 1 to 2 cm margin of soft tissue around the primary tumor, involved nodes, and further margin for microscopic extension involving at-risk abdominal lymph node basins. Given the proximity of the pancreatic head to duodenum, the adjacent medial wall is included. For cases with gross duodenal invasion, the entire circumference of duodenum should be included. In the postoperative setting, surgical and pathological information should be carefully reviewed at the time of treatment planning to assist with target delineation. The postoperative CTV includes the postoperative bed, anastomoses, and the abdominal lymph nodes at risk. Often a postoperative boost volume (CTV2) is delineated, which attempts to reconstruct the preoperative tumor volume. The RTOG has published a contouring atlas to assist with postoperative target delineation, which is also useful for identifying nodal areas at risk when radiation is delivered neoadjuvantly.[188]

Brunner et al.[189] have provided an excellent analysis of nodal regions at risk based on pathologic specimens from 175 cancers of the pancreatic head. Peripancreatic nodal regions at >5% risk of nodal metastasis include the following (in order of decreasing frequency): posterior pancreaticoduodenal area, superior–inferior border of the pancreatic head, anterior pancreaticoduodenal area, hepatoduodenal ligament (porta hepatis), superior margin of pancreatic body, and along the superior mesenteric artery. Thus, a CTV that includes a small rim of peripancreatic soft tissue in all directions of the pancreatic head and neck will include all but the nodes along the porta hepatis, superior mesenteric artery (SMA), aorta, and celiac artery, which should also be included within the CTV. Although the locations of the celiac artery and SMA have traditionally been described in relationship to T12 and L1, respectively, data from angiography[190] suggest enough individual variability to warrant CT-imaging rather than relying solely on bony landmarks. Although the paraaortic lymph nodes are considered a distant site of disease for staging purposes, given the >20% risk of subclinical metastases,[189] they should be included in the CTV. Retroperitoneal metastases primarily arise anterior to the aorta and inferior vena cava, between the vessels, or lateral to the aorta. The risk of subclinical metastases lateral to the cava or retroaortic/retrocaval is <5%; therefore, these regions can generally be omitted from the CTV.[191] In the craniocaudal dimension, the majority of paraaortic nodal involvement is between the celiac artery superiorly and the level of the renal veins inferiorly (except for tumors >3 cm, where the CTV volume should extend inferiorly to level of inferior mesenteric artery).[192] For tumors involving the pancreatic tail, inclusion of the suprapancreatic lymph nodes (along splenic vessels) and splenic hilum is recommended. Additionally, elective treatment of inferior pancreaticoduodenal lymph nodes may be excluded in these patients, allowing for relative sparing of the right kidney.

SBRT and/or hypofractionation for pancreatic cancer was recently added to the NCCN guidelines for select cases of locally advanced disease.[193] Given the predominance of tumor recurrence within radiotherapy ports even when small local fields are used,[194] initial reports of SBRT for unresectable pancreatic cancer described treating the primary tumor only.[195–197] Whether to electively treat regional lymphatics, based on pathologic nodal involvement reported in up to 76% of patients undergoing surgical resection,[189,192] remains an area of investigation. Inclusion of involved peripancreatic lymph nodes has demonstrated favorable rates of local control and toxicity across a range of SBRT and hypofractionated schemes.[198,199] However, the absolute benefit of elective nodal coverage for SBRT remains unknown.[200]

Normal Tissue Tolerances

The amount of small bowel receiving 45 Gy should be minimized without compromising target coverage. Any small bowel within the boost volume of treatment should be limited and not receive >50 Gy, though up to 55 Gy may be cautiously delivered to small portions of the duodenum wall if clinically indicated. At least 75% of one kidney or the composite of one whole kidney should be kept <18 to 20 Gy. If the large majority of one kidney will receive doses >20 Gy, consideration should be given to a quantitative renal scan prior to treatment to ensure sufficient function of the other kidney. Sixty percent of the liver should be kept <30 Gy (and preferably much less). The spinal cord should not receive >45 Gy. With careful planning, these constraints should be achievable.

For 5-fraction SBRT plans, published constraints for the combined small bowel and stomach include 1 cc below 33 Gy, 3cc below 20 Gy, and 9 cc below 15 Gy. At least 50% of the liver should not exceed 12 Gy. At least 75% of the bilateral kidneys should be kept <12 Gy. Point doses to the spinal cord should not exceed 8 Gy.[196]

Radiotherapy Dose

The only randomized data in pancreatic cancer regarding conventionally fractionated radiotherapy dose is the GITSG trial for unresectable tumors. No difference in patient outcome was detected between 40 and 60 Gy (split course schedule with concurrent 5-FU).[184] The radiotherapy and imaging techniques of this trial are outdated by current standards. Meanwhile, more recent data demonstrate persistently high rates of local failure at higher doses.[183,201] Thus, current radiotherapy dose guidelines are primarily based on normal organ tolerance to upper abdominal radiation. Elective nodal stations (CTV) are treated to 45 Gy at 1.8 Gy/fraction. A subsequent boost of 5.4 Gy is delivered to the GTV or CTV2 (postoperatively). Higher boost doses may be considered for unresectable patients or those with positive margins when dose can be delivered within the constraints of normal organs (especially small bowel). A range of hypofractionated and SBRT fractionation schemes have been reported, with ASTRO guidelines recommending doses of 33 to 40 Gy over 5 fractions for locally advanced pancreatic cancer and 30 to 36 Gy over 5 fractions for borderline resectable pancreatic cancer.[202]

Radiotherapy Fields and Techniques

Utilizing 3-D techniques, the pancreas may be treated with a four-field approach with disproportionate weighting of the anterior and posterior fields to reduce dose to the liver from the lateral fields. To account for setup error and target movement, a PTV margin of 1 cm beyond the CTV is advised. If respiratory motion and image-guided setup techniques are utilized, PTV margins as small as 5 mm can be considered. Given the movement of upper abdominal organs due to respiration, greater margin in the superior to inferior dimension may be prudent.[203] Field edges are devised at an additional 5 to 10 mm beyond the PTV to provide dosimetric coverage. The use of highly conformal radiotherapy techniques should account for substantial *inter-* and *intrafraction* variations in the pancreas position. Study of pancreas movement by cine MRI demonstrate larger and more variable changes in pancreas position than often appreciated, especially in the craniocaudal dimension, which do not necessarily correlate well with diaphragm location.[204] Similarly, image guidance based on bony landmarks has been found to correlate with accurate pancreas target setup in only 20% of treatments when compared to tumor fiducial markers, even when using respiratory gating.[205]

3D treatment planning with four to six noncoplanar beams has been objectively compared to traditional four-field techniques and may provide some dosimetric advantages, particularly in sparing the kidneys.[206] Deviation from traditional field orientations may be considered among patients with dosimetric challenges due to atypical target volumes or normal organs (e.g., one kidney). The use of IMRT for pancreatic cancers may also provide some dosimetric advantages by sparing kidneys, bowel, and liver,[201,207,208] as well as enabling possible dose escalation to the GTV.[209] A few institutions have reported

patient outcomes after treatment with IMRT with favorable tolerance and expected survival.[207,210] Robust evidence that IMRT is superior to less advanced techniques, however, is lacking. When utilized, IMRT should account for target motion and avoid dosimetric hot spots.

A growing body of single and multi-institutional experiences describes SBRT and hypofractionated techniques for treatment of pancreatic cancer.[195–199] Due to variability in target volume delineation and more limited experience with SBRT for pancreatic cancer, prescription doses using SBRT have varied widely. SBRT planning typically consists of 4D-CT simulation and utilization of advanced respiratory motion management techniques such as deep inspiratory breath hold or abdominal compression to minimize the size of target volume while accounting for organ motion. Fiducial markers can be placed and utilized as part of image-guided radiation therapy (IGRT) to assist with treatment setup. Treatment delivery with linear accelerator-based RT typically utilizes VMAT or IMRT with multiple noncoplanar beams to maximize dose gradient and minimize high dose to nontarget normal tissues in close proximity to the target (see Fig. 9.3). Recent development of real-time adaptive RT using a MRI-Linac showed promise in minimizing the dose to critical organs and improving the localization accuracy.[146]

Chemotherapy

Given the high rates of distant metastatic disease, systemic treatment with chemotherapy is a critical component to the management of pancreatic cancer across all stages. The CONKO 001 trial established the role of adjuvant chemotherapy for resectable disease, showing superior overall and disease-free survival with single-agent gemcitabine versus observation.[173] Subsequent phase III trials of patients with resectable disease and good performance status have demonstrated superior survival outcomes with newer, multidrug regimens including oxaliplatin, irinotecan, fluorouracil, and leucovorin (FOLFIRINOX)[174] and gemcitabine plus capecitabine.[211] For borderline resectable disease, chemotherapy has increasingly shifted from the adjuvant to neoadjuvant setting.[181] Potential advantages of neoadjuvant chemotherapy include improved rates of R0 resection and identification of patients with early distant progression prior to surgery. First-line neoadjuvant systemic therapies include FOLFIRINOX, gemcitabine, and albumin-bound paclitaxel, and, for patients with BRCA1/2 mutations, gemcitabine and cisplatin.[193] These regimens may be used before or after concurrent chemoradiation or SBRT in the neoadjuvant setting. For metastatic disease, first-line regimens include FOLFIRINOX,[212] gemcitabine, and albumin-bound paclitaxel,[213] or gemcitabine alone as dictated by functional status.

Chemotherapy has a long history of utilization as a radiosensitizer for patients with pancreatic cancer. Among unresectable patients, a randomized trial conducted by

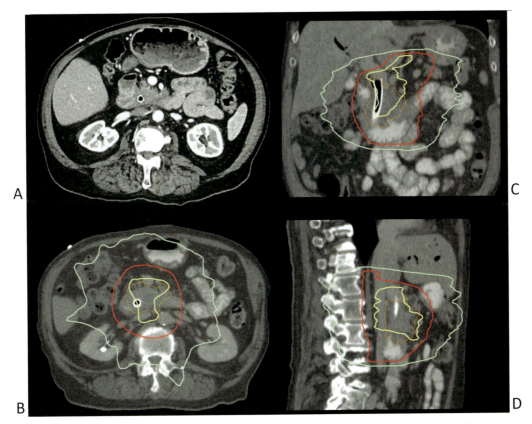

FIGURE 9.3. 66-year-old male patient with a uT2N0 borderline resectable adenocarcinoma of the pancreas head, with <180° abutment of the celiac axis, superior mesenteric artery, and portal vein, treated with eight cycles of FOLFIRINOX, followed by a 5-fraction SBRT plan utilizing a three-arc VMAT technique. Diagnostic arterial-phase axial images (**A**) and axial (**B**), coronal (**C**), and sagittal (**D**) views showing tri-phasic ITV (orange) as well as 33 Gy (yellow), 25 Gy (red), and 12 Gy (green) isodose lines.

the GITSG established the superiority of bolus 5-FU concurrent with radiotherapy over radiotherapy alone.[185] In current practice, continuous venous infusion 5-FU or oral capecitabine are now more commonly utilized with RT, although the data to support their use are extrapolated from larger randomized studies of patients treated with combined-modality therapy for rectal cancer.[214,215] Gemcitabine has been repeatedly studied concurrently with radiation both among unresectable patients and in the postoperative setting, with conflicting data from small randomized studies regarding its efficacy compared to 5-FU based regimens.[216,217] Toxicity with combined-modality therapy using gemcitabine is dependent on the inverse relationship between gemcitabine schedule and dose related to radiation field size and dose.[218] Without standardized parameters or large trials showing benefit over 5-FU based therapy and radiation, gemcitabine delivered concurrently with radiation should be approached with caution.

Prognosis

The prognosis for all patients with pancreatic cancer is poor across all stages of disease. The median survival for patients presenting with metastatic disease treated with modern chemotherapy techniques remains less than 1 year.[212,213] Among locally advanced patients who receive chemotherapy alone or combined-modality therapy, median survival is about 16 months.[183] For patients with resectable pancreatic cancer, the median survival is 35 to 54 months, with a 5-year overall survival rate of approximately 20% to 40%.[174,181] Innovative approaches are necessary to change the natural progression of this disease before significant improvements in outcomes can be made.

COLORECTAL CANCER

In 2020, an estimated 104,610 cancers of the colon and 43,340 cancers of the rectum will be diagnosed in the United States.[1] Radiotherapy plays an important role in the management of rectal cancers, particularly in the neoadjuvant setting, and is uncommonly indicated in the treatment of colon cancer.

DIAGNOSTIC EVALUATION

Careful diagnostic evaluation is essential for accurate staging and selection of patients for neoadjuvant strategies, as well as for determining appropriate target definition during treatment planning. During the patient history, careful attention should be given to bowel-related symptoms and indicators of local tumor extension into other pelvic structures (bladder/prostate or pelvic wall). The radiation oncologist's digital rectal examination should assess the distance of the tumor from the anal verge, size, and location; degree of circumferential involvement; and palpable morphology. The mobility of palpable lesions is described as mobile, tethered, or fixed; the latter implies initial unresectability. Proximal rectal cancers that are not palpable are referenced to the anal verge by endoscopy. Measurements from flexible endoscopies should be relied upon with caution as they are notoriously imprecise and inconsistent between exams. Measurements from rigid proctoscopy tend to be more reliable.

EUS and MRI have been reported as superior to CT in both determination of tumor depth of penetration (T stage) and detection of perirectal adenopathy.[219] High-resolution MRI may be of particular benefit in predicting involvement of circumferential resection margin.[220,221] Pelvic CT or MRI is indicated for the evaluation of pelvic lymphatic stations beyond perirectal lymph nodes. Among patients with locally advanced disease, PET may detect liver metastases in up to 8% of patients in whom distant disease was not identified by other modalities.[222] PET generally does not have sufficient spatial resolution to determine depth of tumor penetration nor consistently distinguish perirectal adenopathy from adjacent primary tumor.

TREATMENT OPTIONS

The use of adjuvant or neoadjuvant RT for rectal cancer is generally reserved for patients whose tumors penetrate the bowel wall ($\geq$T3) and/or are node positive as determined by EUS or MRI. Among such patients, randomized trials demonstrate superior local control and overall survival with the use of adjuvant combined-modality therapy compared to surgery alone.[223–225] Two paradigms have emerged in the neoadjuvant treatment of locally advanced rectal cancer: a short course of hypofractionated RT and a long course of chemoradiation (CRT). The German Rectal Cancer Study Group found a significant downstaging effect and higher rate of sphincter-preservation with long-course preoperative CRT, as compared to adjuvant CRT.[226] Preoperative CRT also demonstrated significantly increased local control in long-term follow-up (10-year local relapse rate of 7% vs. 10%, $p = 0.048$).[227] Concurrently, Dutch investigators found that a short course of preoperative hypofractionated RT improved local control compared to patients undergoing total mesorectal excision (TME) alone (10-year LR 5% vs. 11%, $p<0.0001$).[228] Two phase III trials showed no differences in clinical outcomes between neoadjuvant short-course radiotherapy and

long-course CRT, using bolus 5FU[229] and a more contemporary continuous infusion,[230] respectively. A more recent phase III trial compared short-course RT, followed by chemotherapy to long-course CRT, showing similar R0 resection rates, similar long-term overall survival, and decreased acute toxicity with short course RT.[231,232] No consensus exists for optimal neoadjuvant therapy in locally advanced rectal cancer.

Total neoadjuvant therapy (TNT) is an actively evolving treatment paradigm for patients with locally advanced rectal cancer, including those at high risk for margin-positive resection (i.e., T4 disease, mesorectal fascial involvement, or node-positive low-lying tumors). While distant failure has become the leading cause of death for locally advanced rectal cancer,[233] phase III trials have shown no benefit to adjuvant chemotherapy following chemoradiation and surgery.[234,235] Poor compliance with adjuvant therapy in these trials (~40%–60%) prompted investigation of oxaliplatin-based neoadjuvant chemotherapy before or after chemoradiation in the neoadjuvant setting (i.e., TNT). In addition to improved treatment compliance (85%–100%), advantages of TNT include higher rates of resectability and pathologic complete response (pCR; <20% vs. 30%–50%).[236–239] Potential drawbacks to TNT include potential for disease progression in poor responders and increased surgical complications; however, local progression during TNT is exceedingly rare, with similarly low rates of distant progression at time of surgery.[238] Moreover, no differences in surgical complications or surgeon-reported difficulty are reported following TNT compared to neoadjuvant CRT alone.[238] The use of TNT toward identifying patients for whom surgery may be omitted (i.e., "watch and wait") should generally be limited to centers with experienced multidisciplinary teams.[240] For the 20% to 25% of patients that achieve a complete clinical response,[241] 5-year local recurrence-free survival with close surveillance is 70% at 5 years.[242]

Adjuvant radiotherapy for patients with colon cancer is not routinely indicated. Although retrospective series have shown favorable local control outcomes with the use of adjuvant radiotherapy among patients with T4 tumors or selected T3 tumors with positive lymph nodes,[243–245] this has not been corroborated in clinical trials.[246] Preoperative treatment may be considered in patients whose tumors are considered unresectable at presentation.

TREATMENT PLANNING FOR RECTAL CANCERS

Simulation

Proper patient positioning can significantly reduce the amount of small bowel within the pelvis and limit toxicity from treatment. In addition to decreasing the volume of bowel receiving maximal organ tolerance (45–50 Gy), reduction of bowel receiving doses as low as 5 Gy has been associated with improved patient tolerance to pelvic radiation.[247–249] Maximal small bowel displacement out of the pelvis is achieved with prone positioning and bladder distension.[250] Multiple studies have documented significant reduction in pelvic small-bowel volume with use of a belly-board device[251–253] or lower abdominal wall compression.[254] Without the use of a belly-board or lower abdominal wall compression, ~25% of patients will have more small bowel in the pelvis with prone positioning compared to supine on fluoroscopy (more commonly in obese patients).[254] Although these efforts displace bowel from the pelvis, they may also be less reproducible and be associated with variation in patient setup, which is undesirable when employing highly conformal radiation techniques.

The anal verge should be marked with a radiopaque marker, while rectal contrast may be utilized to assist with radiographic identification of the primary lesion. Taping the buttocks laterally may reduce their self-bolusing effect on the perianal skin during treatment. Patients who have undergone abdominoperineal resection should have the perineal scar marked and included in the initial pelvic fields with appropriate posterior bolus as necessary, given that perineal recurrence has been described in 8% to 30% of patients in the absence of adjuvant RT,[255–257] and as low as 2% when the scar is adequately treated.[258]

Radiotherapy Target

Myerson et al.[259] and Roels et al.[260] provide a review of CT-based treatment planning for rectal cancer. For patients treated preoperatively, the GTV includes the primary tumor and any radiographically enlarged lymph nodes. All clinical, endoscopic, and imaging information should be used to define the maximal extent of the rectal tumor. Relying solely on one modality risks underestimation of the tumor extent and inaccurate field design (especially within boost portals). Although not mandatory in treatment planning, the addition of PET to CT in GTV contouring has been shown to increase the target size by an average of 25%[261] and leads to change in treatment fields in 17% of patients.[262] Soft-tissue extension or suspected infiltration of rectal tumors into adjacent mesorectal fat, particularly posteriorly, should be included within the GTV. Patients who initially present with a limited number of liver and/or lung metastases and respond favorably to upfront systemic therapy may undergo metastasectomy with subsequent curative-intent local treatment. In such cases, radiotherapy target delineation and dose should correspond to T- and N-staging from MRI/EUS performed at time of initial diagnostic workup.

The CTV encompasses all the perirectal tissue/mesorectum, presacral space, and lymphatics of the internal iliac chain (which are not commonly dissected at the time of surgery). A report of 269 cases of rectal cancer that recurred in the pelvis after surgery alone emphasized the predilection for rectal cancer recurrence in the posterior pelvis, specifically the presacral space. Among patients undergoing anterior resection, 93% recurred at or posterior to the colorectal anastomosis.[263] Other studies of rectal cancer failure patterns have shown infrequent recurrence above the S1–S2 interspace, lateral pelvic nodes, or in the anal sphincter.[264,265] In the upper pelvis, the CTV should extend cephalad to include the sacral promontory, posteriorly to include the anterior wall of the sacrum, and laterally to encompass vasculature and presacral soft tissue to the border of the iliopsoas muscles. In the mid-pelvis, the CTV includes similar tissues with care taken to include perirectal fat anterior to the rectum. In addition, 1 to 2 cm of posterior bladder or uterus may be included if at risk of subclinical extension of disease for patients who have adjacent, locally advanced lesions. In the lower pelvis, the CTV includes all the perirectal fat inferiorly and laterally extending to the levator ani muscles. It should extend to the posterior wall of the prostate or vagina. A larger margin of anterior pelvic organs may be indicated for tumors with documented invasion (T4). The inclusion of the external iliac lymph nodes is generally reserved for patients with T4 tumors, which extend into anterior organs of the pelvis (prostate, bladder, vagina, and cervix/uterus) for whom these nodes are at risk. This modification is supported by failure patterns[263] from patients treated with surgery alone. However, in a series of patients with T4 rectal cancers where external iliac lymph nodes were not routinely included within RT portals, regional recurrence of disease still occurred almost exclusively within the radiotherapy field.[266] Tumors of the lower rectum, which extend to the dentate line of the anal canal, have a theoretical risk of failure in the inguinal lymph nodes. A report of 184 patients with such lesions revealed only six groin failures (5-year actuarial rate of 4%) without elective radiotherapy to the inguinal lymph nodes.[267] Thus, for patients with low-lying rectal cancers, the added toxicity of treatment to the inguinal nodes should be weighed against clinical benefit if deemed clinically negative during initial staging.

The CTV should also include a minimum of 2 cm of normal rectum cephalad and caudad to the primary tumor. With a subsequent PTV expansion of at least 1 cm (without IGRT) around the CTV, this will provide a minimum 4 cm longitudinal margin from GTV to block edge (assuming an additional 0.5 to 1 cm margin beyond PTV to block edge for dosimetric buildup). With use of daily image-guidance, smaller CTV to PTV margins may be utilized. Given the distensibility of the rectum, more PTV margin may be indicated anteriorly, especially for anterior wall tumors of the mid- and upper rectum. Bladder, small bowel, and femoral heads should also be contoured for evaluation of normal tissue tolerance.

In the postoperative setting, treatment volumes are similar except that with the removal of the primary lesion, the entire preoperative tumor bed should be reconstructed and included within the CTV (often identified separately as a boost volume—CTV2). Review of preoperative imaging, operative reports, and surgical clip placement is imperative. As mentioned earlier, the perineal scar should be included in the initial fields for patients who have undergone abdominoperineal resection.

To account for internal target motion and patient setup variability, a PTV is delineated beyond the CTV. In the absence of IGRT, PTV margin of at least 1 cm is appropriate. However, retrospective study of interfraction variability has shown that patient setup without IGRT can easily approach these margins, especially among patients with large body mass index treated in the prone position.[268] Intrafraction movement of the mesorectum averages <4 mm in various dimensions, but significant individual variability is observed.[269]

Normal Tissue Tolerances

The amount of small bowel receiving 45 Gy should be minimized without compromising target coverage. Any small bowel within the boost volume of treatment should generally not exceed 50 Gy. In addition to maximum dose, acute intestinal side effects from pelvic radiotherapy have been found to correlate with volume of bowel receiving doses as low as 5 Gy.[248,249] Thus, bowel exposure at any dose should be minimized. The femoral heads and necks should receive <45 to 50 Gy,[270] and preferably <40 Gy. Blocking in the lateral fields excludes the anterior genitalia in addition to small bowel and bladder.

Radiotherapy Dose

A paucity of data addresses the optimal radiotherapy dose in the treatment of rectal cancer. One retrospective study supporting current dosing guidelines showed superior local control with adjuvant radiotherapy doses ≥45 Gy compared to patients who received lower doses.[271] With CRT, 45 Gy given in 1.8 Gy fractions is the currently accepted dose and fractionation for initial pelvic fields in the adjuvant setting based on its repeated use in clinical trial designs.[225,272] After the initial 45 Gy, a boost of 5.4 to 9 Gy is generally given to the tumor bed and adjacent lymphatics (CTV2). In the neoadjuvant setting, the radiotherapy dose depends on the use of short- or long-course RT. In the former approach, five daily 5 Gy fractions are administered to a single volume for a total cumulative dose of 25 Gy.[273] Long-course CRT doses are similar to those used in the adjuvant setting, typically 45 Gy with a 5.4 Gy boost to the GTV[230,274] or treatment of the entire volume to 50.4 Gy.[226] In any case, careful attention should be made to minimize small bowel within the field. Treating beyond a cumulative dose of 50 Gy should generally only be considered when small bowel can be completely excluded from the high-dose region of treatment.

Radiotherapy Fields and Techniques

Patients are commonly treated with a three-field technique consisting of a PA and laterals (see Fig. 9.4). When inclusion of the anterior pelvis is indicated (e.g., treatment of the external iliac lymph nodes, more anterior-lying rectosigmoid lesions, or larger habitus patients), an additional AP field may be advantageous to improve dose homogeneity. High-energy photons and appropriate beam wedging and weighting are mandatory to ensure a homogeneous dose distribution within the pelvis.

Traditional field design has been based on bony landmarks as well as the location of contrast-enhanced bowel, rectum, and the anal verge. The superior border of the PA (and AP) fields generally covers the sacral promontory, while the inferior border is placed at least 3 to 4 cm distal to the primary lesion. For upper rectal cancers, the distal border need not include the entire anal canal but should extend to approximately the level of the dentate line (about 2 to 3 cm from the anal verge) to encompass the entire mesorectum. The lateral borders of the PA field should include 1.5 to 2 cm margin beyond the pelvic brim, with appropriate blocking of almost all of the femoral head. Lateral fields should cover the anterior bony margin of sacrum with 1.5 to 2 cm margin posteriorly to allow for setup variation and dosimetric coverage. Anteriorly, the field includes the internal iliac lymph nodes by placing its border at approximately the posterior edge of pubic symphysis, while ensuring adequate anterior coverage of the primary tumor/mesorectum. In the superior–anterior portion of the field, it is usually possible to block a portion of small bowel. Similarly, the anterior genitalia in most patients should be blocked in the lateral fields. Custom boost fields are devised that include the GTV (or tumor bed) with an approximate 2 to 3 cm margin. A three-field technique or laterals alone will often suffice.

CT-based planning is necessary to account for the variability inherent in individual patient anatomy. The caudal extent of the CTV should be a minimum of 2 cm caudal to gross disease, including the entire mesorectum to the pelvic floor. The lateral CTV should include the mesorectum and only a few millimeters of the levator muscles unless radiographically involved. Involvement of adjacent organs and/or pelvic sidewall requires a more generous margin (1–2 cm). In the mid-pelvis, the CTV extends to the pelvic sidewall and musculature posterolaterally. Anteriorly, the posterior 1 cm of the bladder is included to account for variation in bladder position.[276] The superior extent of the rectal CTV is a minimum of 2 cm cephalad to gross disease, including the rectosigmoid junction. A minimum of 7 to 8 mm margin around the internal iliac vessels is included up to the common iliac bifurcation, including at least 1 cm anterior to the sacrum. CTV to PTV expansion depends on treatment technique and the use of IGRT. The PTV margin should be 7 to 10 mm when using IMRT with IGRT. Conventional field borders

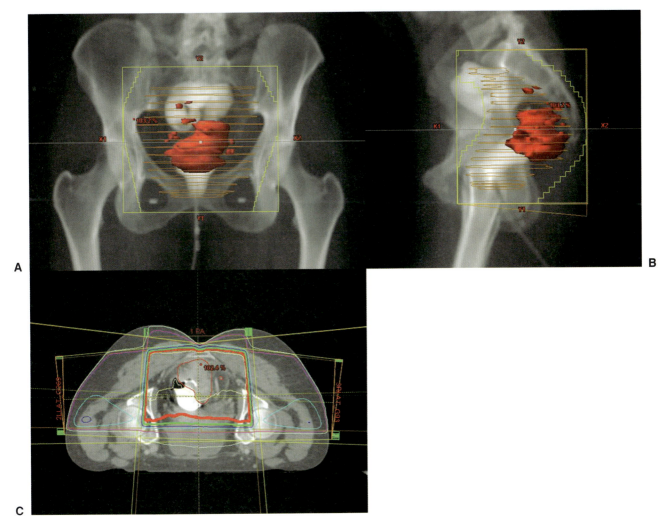

FIGURE 9.4. 41-year-old woman with a cT3N+ adenocarcinoma of the distal rectum treated with a 3-field technique. Beam's eye view of PA (**A**) and lateral (**B**) fields. Note the GTV (red) and CTV (orange) including mesorectum and rectal contrast. Axial view (**C**) showing field arrangement and dosimetry (red and light green lines denote the 98% and 95% isodose lines, respectively). Prescription dose was 4,500 cGy in daily 180 cGy fractions.

are generally expanded another 5 to 10 mm in order to achieve sufficient dosimetric target coverage.

Dosimetric studies comparing IMRT to traditional techniques in rectal cancer have shown clinically significant reductions in dose to bowel, bladder, pelvic bones, and femoral heads while achieving superior target coverage, homogeneity, and conformality.[277–280] The successful implementation of IMRT in the management of rectal cancer has been reported from multiple institutions, generally with dose escalation to the GTV with favorable outcomes.[281–283] A retrospective review of 92 patients treated at the Mayo Clinic in Arizona demonstrated a 32% incidence of grade ≥2 gastrointestinal toxicity among patients treated with IMRT compared to 62% ($p = 0.006$) among patients treated with conventional fields during the same era.[284] However, prospective data from the RTOG 0822 trial failed to demonstrate a significant difference in grade ≥2 toxicity between IMRT-based preoperative CRT and

historical 3D-CRT controls from RTOG 0247.[285] Challenges of IMRT planning include accounting for internal movement, distensibility of pelvic organs (rectum, bowel, and bladder) and dose inhomogeneity produced by some treatment planning systems.

Chemotherapy

Adjuvant and neoadjuvant radiotherapy have traditionally been delivered with concurrent 5-FU. In the postoperative setting, protracted venous infusion (PVI) of 5-FU (225 mg/m²/day) throughout the course of pelvic radiotherapy has been shown to decrease tumor recurrence and improve overall survival compared to the administration of bolus 5-FU,[272] although not confirmed in a subsequent trial.[286] Despite this, continuous infusion 5-FU became the standard in subsequent neoadjuvant trials.[226] More contemporary studies have found the use of capecitabine, an orally administered 5-FU premetabolite, is at least equivalent if not superior to PVI 5-FU in conjunction with pelvic radiation for rectal cancer.[214,287] Multiple studies have attempted to integrate additional chemotherapeutics, namely oxaliplatin, into the neoadjuvant and adjuvant fluoropyrimidine backbone with concurrent radiation. The majority of these studies found no improvement in clinical outcome at the expense of added toxicity.[287–289] For locally advanced disease, modern chemotherapy regimens administered in the neoadjuvant setting in sequence with chemoradiation or short-course radiotherapy include capecitabine and oxaliplatin (CAPEOX) and 5-fluorouracil (5-FU), leucovorin, and oxaliplatin (FOLFOX).

Treatment Planning for Colon Cancer

Management of colon cancer involves the same chemotherapeutic and radiation principles as rectal cancer. Decubitus positioning at simulation and during treatment may reduce the amount of small bowel in the treatment field. The initial CTV generally includes the tumor bed and adjacent lymphatics, with a subsequent boost to the tumor bed (or tumor preoperatively). Review of preoperative imaging, operative reports, and identification of surgical clips demarcating the tumor bed are essential in order to define targets and design fields that may improve local control and the prognosis of this disease.

Prognosis

The incidence and mortality of colorectal cancer in the United States has been declining in recent years, most likely as a result of screening practices.[1] Based on the Dutch TME results, 10-year overall survival for TNM stage I, II, and III patients are ~70%, 55%, and 40%, respectively.[228] The inclusion criteria for the German rectal trial more closely approximate those patients eligible for neoadjuvant CRT (cT3-4 and/or N+; TNM stages II-III), where 10-year overall survival was ~60%.[227] Long-term data from the International Watch and Wait Database demonstrate an 85% 5-year overall survival rate for patients who achieve a complete response to TNT.[242]

ANAL CANCER

In 2020, there were an estimated 8,590 new cases and approximately 1,350 deaths from anal cancer in the United States.[1] Historically, abdominoperineal resection (APR) was the standard of care in the management of anal cancer.[290,291] Although this procedure resulted in cure for many patients, there were significant drawbacks, including permanent colostomy and high rates of morbidity and mortality. In 1974, Nigro et al. introduced chemotherapy and radiation as a novel treatment approach in the management of anal cancer.[292] Since Nigro's publications, phase

III randomized trials have examined different strategies of chemotherapy and radiation administration.[293–298] Given the favorable results of definitive chemoradiation, this sphincter-preserving approach is the standard of care for this disease.

DIAGNOSTIC EVALUATION

Potential candidates for chemoradiation should undergo a complete history and physical examination. Risk factors for HIV infection should be reviewed, with a low threshold for obtaining corresponding laboratory testing. Careful review of gastrointestinal and genitourinary symptoms may indicate extension of tumor beyond what is otherwise clinically or radiographically detected. It is necessary to perform thorough clinical evaluation of inguinal lymph nodes, digital rectal examination, and proctoscopy to determine tumor extent. Thorough examination of the perianal skin is imperative for accurate treatment planning as this often reveals disease beyond what is visible on imaging studies. When patients have severe anal discomfort that inhibits adequate examination, proctoscopy should be scheduled under anesthesia. In females, pelvic examination is indicated to rule out vaginal extension and to screen for synchronous gynecological cancers (HPV-related).

Axial CT imaging of the chest, abdomen, and pelvis is critical for appropriate staging. Anal cancer most commonly spreads by local and lymphatic invasion, with approximately 13% of cases involving distant metastases at initial presentation.[299] Distant metastases are most commonly seen in the liver and lungs.[300,301] As an alternative to CT or MRI, PET/CT can be useful for assessing disease extent and often assists in treatment planning. Multiple reports have shown that PET/CT alters staging in about 20% of patients compared to conventional imaging due to improved sensitivity in detection of primary tumor, involved regional lymph nodes and distant metastases.[302–306] Winton et al. reported that initial diagnostic PET/CT altered design of radiation treatment fields in 8 of 61 (13%) patients with anal cancer.[302] Similarly, a series of 50 patients from Australia reported 19% of cases underwent treatment planning revision based on pelvic or nodal inguinal involvement on PET/CT.[305] All patients should have a biopsy to confirm invasive malignancy at the primary site. In patients with suspicious inguinal adenopathy, biopsy may be performed to clarify the diagnosis and to determine radiation treatment volumes and doses.

TREATMENT OPTIONS

Patients with anal carcinoma *in situ* (anal intraepithelial neoplasia or AIN) and select cases of tumors involving the perianal skin (which do not extend past the anal verge) should initially be considered for local excision. When these lesions cannot be adequately excised without significantly compromising anal function, definitive RT alone or chemoradiation should be considered. Patients with invasive carcinoma of the anal canal should generally be treated with definitive chemoradiotherapy. The addition of mitomycin-C and 5-FU to radiotherapy has been shown to improve local control, colostomy-free survival, and disease-free survival.[293–295] Multiple subsequent phase III randomized trials have failed to identify a superior chemotherapeutic regimen to mitomycin-C and 5-FU.[296–298]

APR is usually reserved as salvage treatment for patients with persistent or recurrent disease after radiotherapy. When considering salvage APR, it should be noted that randomized data have shown delayed tumor regression up to 26 weeks after completion of therapy.[297] Therefore, in the absence of progression, a decision to proceed with APR for persistent disease should typically be delayed until at least 6 months and perhaps up to 1 year after completion of therapy in select circumstances.

TREATMENT PLANNING

Simulation

After clinical and radiographic staging, CT-based simulation is performed for radiation treatment planning. If available, PET/CT at the time of simulation may be helpful to define local and regional target structures. Patients can be simulated in the supine or prone position, as there are benefits to each approach in the appropriate clinical setting. Prone setup with a false tabletop allows for improved small bowel avoidance and may be useful in individuals with a large pannus and pelvic node involvement. Supine positioning is usually more reproducible, potentially allowing for reduced PTV margins and smaller treatment fields. Typically, if IMRT treatment planning is used, patients should be simulated in the supine position with legs slightly abducted (frog-legged) with semi-rigid immobilization using a vacuum-locked bag or alpha-cradle. Patients are instructed to maintain a full bladder for simulation and treatment to decrease the amount of small bowel within the pelvis. In males, the external genitalia are typically positioned midline and inferiorly such that setup is reproducible, while being cognizant of proximity to the anal verge. In females, a vaginal dilator can be placed to help delineate the genitalia and displace the vulva, vagina, and urethra away from the primary tumor. A radiopaque marker should be placed at the anal verge. The clinical extent of any visible or palpable perianal tumor should be demarcated with radio-opaque catheters, as this may not be apparent on simulation imaging. It may be helpful to place a catheter with rectal contrast in the anal canal at the time of simulation for tumor delineation. In patients with adequate renal function, IV contrast facilitates identification of the pelvic and groin vasculature (which approximates at-risk nodal regions). Oral contrast identifies small bowel as an avoidance structure during treatment planning. For tumors involving the perianal skin or superficial inguinal nodes, bolus should be placed as necessary for adequate dosing of gross disease. Routine use of bolus may not be necessary as the tangential effect of IMRT may minimize skin sparing. In situations where adequate dosing of superficial targets is uncertain, *in vivo* diode dosimetry with the first treatment fraction can ensure appropriate dose at the skin surface.

Radiotherapy Target

Target volume definition is generally performed per ICRU 50 recommendations.[307] GTV should include all primary tumor and involved lymph nodes, utilizing information from physical examination, endoscopic findings, diagnostic imaging, and simulation planning study for delineation. CTV should include the GTV plus areas at risk for microscopic spread from the primary tumor and at-risk nodal areas. If the primary tumor cannot be determined with available information (such as after local excision), the anal canal may be used as a surrogate target. At-risk nodal regions include the mesorectum, presacral, internal iliac, external iliac, and inguinal nodes.[308] Ortholan et al.[309] published a study of 181 patients with anal cancer without inguinal nodal involvement at diagnosis, demonstrating 5-year inguinal recurrence rates of 2% and 16% in patients with and without inguinal irradiation, respectively. Pelvic and inguinal nodes should therefore be routinely treated in most patients. The presacral nodal volume is typically defined as an approximately 1 cm strip over the anterior sacral prominence. To contour the internal and external iliac nodes, an approximate 0.7 cm margin beyond iliac arteries and veins (1–1.5 cm anteriorly on external iliac vessels) is generally sufficient. In order to include the obturator lymph nodes, external and internal iliac volume contours should be joined parallel to the pelvic sidewall. The inguinal node volume extends beyond the external iliac contour along the femoral artery from approximately the upper edge of the superior pubic rami to approximately 2 cm caudal to saphenous/femoral artery junction. The medial and lateral borders may be defined by adductor longus and sartorius muscles, respectively. Several published atlases are helpful to review when defining elective nodal CTVs.[275,310,311] The above descriptions are generalizations, and target volume should be individualized based on the anatomy of each patient and tumor distribution.

When using IMRT, a separate CTV volume for each planned treatment dose tier is contoured. A common approach includes three clinical volumes: a gross disease volume, a high-risk elective nodal volume (including gross disease), and a low-risk elective nodal volume (including gross disease and high risk elective nodal volume).[312,313] Alternatively, a gross disease volume with a single elective nodal volume can be used to deliver the prescribed course.[314–321]

In defining the gross disease CTV around the primary tumor, an approximate 2.5 cm margin around GTV should be used with manual editing to avoid muscle or bone at low risk for tumor infiltration. To define the gross disease CTV around involved nodes, a 1 cm expansion should be made beyond the contoured involved lymph node with manual editing to exclude areas at low risk for tumor infiltration. The entire mesorectum is generally included within the volume defined as gross disease CTV for the purposes of treatment planning.

The high-risk elective nodal volume typically includes the gross disease CTV including the entire mesorectum, presacral nodes, and bilateral internal and external iliac lymph nodes inferior to the sacroiliac joint as per conventional field definitions utilized in RTOG 98-11.[296] In patients with gross inguinal nodal involvement, the bilateral or unilateral inguinal nodes may be included in the high-risk elective nodal volume. The low-risk elective nodal volume should include the gross disease CTV and high-risk elective nodal CTV as well as presacral, bilateral internal, and external iliac nodes above the inferior border of the sacroiliac joint to the bifurcation of the internal and external iliac vessels located approximately at the L5/S1 vertebral body junction. If there is no obvious involvement of the bilateral inguinal nodes, these are only included in the low-risk elective nodal volume.

The PTV should account for effects of organ and patient movement and inaccuracies in beam and patient setup. PTV expansions should typically be 0.5 to 1.0 cm from CTV, depending on use of image guidance and physician practice with treatment setup for each defined CTV. To account for differences in bladder and rectal filling, a more generous CTV to PTV margin is applied in these regions. Future development of real-time adaptive RT will potentially reduce this margin. When using IMRT, especially with small PTV margins, use of daily image guidance with kV orthogonal imaging of the bony anatomy is recommended. Additionally, cone beam CT should be performed prior to the first treatment and periodically to ensure target soft tissue volumes remain within the appropriate PTV and ensure bladder filling is relatively stable. These volumes may be manually edited to limit the borders to the skin surface for treatment planning purposes.

Normal Tissue Tolerances

With IMRT, dose to small bowel, bladder, pelvic/femoral bones, and external genitalia can be sculpted and minimized despite close proximity of these organs to target volumes. When contouring these structures, it is typically best to demarcate normal tissues on axial CT at least 2 cm above and below the PTV. Contouring atlases offer excellent guidance on defining organs at risks (OARs).[310,311] Once the OARs have been identified, the chief aim of IMRT planning is to limit the dose to these structures without compromising PTV coverage. The extent to which OARs can be avoided largely depends on the location and extent of tumor involvement at presentation as

well as the extent to which the bowel extends into the lower pelvis and a given individual's anatomy.

The amount of small bowel treated to >45 Gy should be minimized. Although this is generally achievable due to the inferior location of the boost target volume, acute intestinal side effects from pelvic radiotherapy have been found to correlate with volume of bowel receiving dose levels as low as 5 Gy.[248,249] Devisetty et al. published a multi-institution, dosimetric analysis which found that limiting the volume of bowel receiving 30 Gy (V30 Gy) to less than 450 cc significantly reduced acute GI toxicity (8% vs. 33%).[322] Defoe et al. showed lower rates of acute GI toxicity, with V30 Gy less than 310 cc and V40 Gy less than 70 cc.[323] Emami et al. estimate a dose of 50 Gy to 1/3 of the small bowel is associated with 5% likelihood of obstruction or perforation at 5 years.[324] To minimize late small bowel toxicity, the Quantitative Analysis of Normal Tissue Effects in the Clinic (QUANTEC) analysis reviewed available clinical data for small bowel dose and recommends minimizing volume receiving greater than 45 Gy to less than 195 cc when contouring the entire potential peritoneal space.[325]

There are limited clinical data correlating bladder dose–volume relationships to increased GU toxicity in anal cancer. Extrapolating from other cancer treatment sites, normal tissue complication probability models suggest that risk of serious GU complications with bladder doses <65 Gy is low.[326] The risk of clinical complications appears to increase with larger volumes of bladder receiving high dose. Marks et al. estimate that limiting 50% of the bladder to less than 40 to 50 Gy will limit complications to less than 5% to 10% (based on cervical cancer clinical literature).[327]

Retrospective data demonstrate a cumulative 5-year pelvic fracture rate of 14.0% among women receiving radiation treatment for anal cancer versus 7.5% among women who did not receive RT.[328] There are limited empirical data on dose–response relationships for femoral neck complications. Emami et al. reported a tolerance dose of 52 Gy to the entire femoral neck to limit the risk of complication to less than 5%.[324] Bedford et al. have recommended limiting the volume of femoral neck receiving 52 Gy to less than 10%.[329] The femoral heads and necks should receive <45 to 50 Gy,[270] and preferably <40 Gy.

Sexual dysfunction is a late effect of RT for anal cancer with significant impact on quality of life.[330,331] Pelvic radiotherapy has been associated with high rates of impotence and sterility in young men, as well as dyspareunia, vaginal bleeding, and vaginal dryness in women. Limited data on dose–response relationships between late sexual toxicity and genitalia dose are available. As with other pelvic OARs where data are limited, it is advisable to minimize genitalia dose without compromising PTV coverage.

Dosimetric hot spots within the perianal skin should generally be avoided to minimize treatment breaks for skin toxicity and resultant detriments in local control.[332,333] In the absence of infection, treatment breaks for skin toxicity should be avoided by instituting early, aggressive supportive measures.

Given patient variation with respect to OAR position and areas of tumor involvement, practical dose constraint guidelines are challenging. In tumors without gross nodal involvement, it is often possible to limit OAR doses even further. In tumors with gross nodal involvement within the pelvis, compromise of PTV coverage may be necessary to limit doses to the small bowel. Normal tissue dose constraints from RTOG 05-29 are a reasonable guide to assist with IMRT treatment planning.[315]

Radiotherapy Dose

The appropriate dose for elective nodal sites has not been well defined. In RTOG 87-04, 30.6 Gy in 1.8 Gy fractions was delivered to initial pelvic fields with the superior border placed at the L4–L5 interspace.[295] Subsequently, the superior field borders were reduced to the bottom of the sacroiliac joints, and the pelvis and inguinal nodes continued treatment to 36 Gy. Finally, 10×10 cm fields that included the primary tumor and lowermost pelvis were treated to cumulative doses of 45 to 50.4 Gy. In RTOG 98–11, the initial pelvic fields were treated to 30.6 Gy, with the superior border placed at L5–S1.[296] Reducing the superior border to the bottom of the sacroiliac joints, the lower pelvis was treated to 45 Gy. The inguinal lymph nodes electively received 36 Gy. In the ACT II study, all patients received a dose of 30.6 Gy in 1.8 Gy fractions to the pelvis and inguinal nodes, with the superior border placed at least 3 cm above the SI joints.[297] A second volume including the gross primary tumor plus 3 cm margin was prescribed an additional 19.8 Gy for a total dose of 50.4 Gy. Among patients with macroscopic nodal involvement on CT, all gross disease plus margin was prescribed 50.4 Gy.

RTOG 05-29 was the first phase II prospective study utilizing IMRT for the treatment of anal cancer.[315] The prescription parameters designated a single elective nodal volume inclusive of mesorectum, presacrum, bilateral internal and external iliac, and bilateral inguinal regions as outlined in the RTOG atlas.[275] A simultaneous integrated boost (SIB) plan was utilized to treat the elective nodal volume plus areas of gross tumor and nodal involvement with slightly different dose prescriptions, depending on tumor stage and nodal volume. T2N0 tumors received 42 Gy elective nodal and 50.4 Gy to the anal tumor in 28 fractions. T3-4N0-3 tumors received 45 Gy elective nodal and 50.4 Gy for involved nodes <3 cm, 54 Gy for involved nodes >3 cm and 54 Gy to the anal tumor in 30 fractions.

Although successive pelvic field reductions probably address the gradient of risk for micrometastatic disease within lymph nodes, retrospective series suggest that doses as low as 30 Gy with concurrent chemotherapy may be sufficient to achieve control of subclinical disease

within nodes or at the primary site after excisional biopsy of small lesions.[334–336] The SIB approach offers the convenience of developing a single treatment plan with reduced planning complexity, albeit with a lower biological dose delivered to the elective nodal areas. Utilization of SIB dose painting implements 1.5 Gy per fraction to the elective nodal region, and such doses are not well studied. When concurrently treating multiple targets at different doses per fraction (i.e., IMRT), higher total doses may be indicated for regions receiving <1.8 Gy/day.[315] Only small primary tumors that have completely responded to radiation should be treated to 45 to 50.4 Gy. Larger tumors (T3/T4) and incompletely responding tumors should receive at least 50.4 to 54 Gy. Multiple retrospective series have reported superior local control rates in this dose range compared to lower doses.[334,337,338]

Radiotherapy Fields and Techniques

The treatment of patients with anal cancer can be technically challenging, given the complex geometric distribution of targets, particularly the inguinal nodes, in relationship to normal pelvic structures. By reducing radiation to normal structures, IMRT minimizes toxicities and treatment interruptions. Institutional experiences.[312,313,316–321,339] and a single phase II, multi-institutional prospective study[315] have shown the feasibility of IMRT with improvements in acute toxicity, compared to historical studies. Although no direct comparison of IMRT to conventional radiotherapy planning has been performed, utilization of IMRT is recommended to minimize treatment toxicity and associated treatment breaks. Due to the high precision of IMRT, planning and delivery of RT requires a thorough understanding of the local and regional progression patterns to define PTV and surrounding normal organs. A knowledgeable treatment planning team is required to optimally utilize IMRT planning algorithms ensuring homogeneous dose to target areas while reducing dose to normal tissues (see Fig. 9.5).

If IMRT planning is not available, alternative approaches utilizing treatment field design based on bony anatomy may be feasible. A wide AP photon field, which includes the inguinal lymph nodes, is simulated with a narrow PA field that excludes the femoral neck (may include a small portion of the medial femoral head for margin on the obturator nodes). Due to divergence, it is sometimes possible to match the lateral exit of the narrow PA beam with the surface entrance of the wide AP photon beam and provide sufficient dosimetric coverage of the groins.[340] More commonly, however, supplemental anterior electrons are indicated. The lateral exit of the narrow PA field is marked anteriorly on the patient's groins (done at time of fluoroscopic simulation). This serves as the medial border for each electron supplement. The lateral border of each electron supplement is placed at or 1 cm lateral (due to beam constriction) to the surface entrance

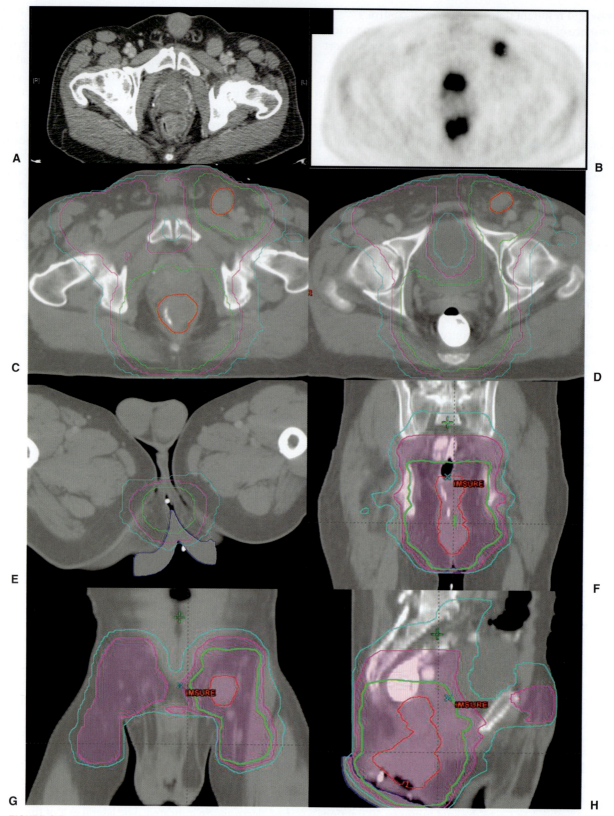

FIGURE 9.5. 60-year-old male patient with T2N2 squamous cell carcinoma of the anal canal. Diagnostic CT (**A**) and with PET (**B**) indicate abnormal FDG avidity in left inguinal lymph node and anal canal. Sequential 9-field IMRT treatment plans were delivered. Axial (**C, D, E**), coronal (**F, G**) and sagittal (**H**) dosimetry, with GTV (red) and 54 Gy (Green), 45 Gy (magenta), 30.6 Gy (cyan) isodose lines.

of the wide anterior photon beam. During treatment, particular attention must be given to any shifts made with the PA field to ensure similar movement in the anterior electron field junctions. Radiopaque wire placed on these junctions may assist with proper setup when porting the PA field. To reduce the complexities associated with electron groin setups, photons have also been used to supplement the lateral inguinal lymph nodes using the same AP photon field and setup. This can be achieved with multileaf collimation.[341,342]

For patients treated with conventional radiotherapy techniques, gross tumor should be boosted with reduced fields encompassing primary tumor and involved nodes with a 2 to 3 cm margin to the field edge. When possible, a composite representation of dose between the initial and boost treatments should be created to ensure normal organ tolerance is not exceeded during the boost phase of treatment. A variety of beam arrangements may be used. Separate boost fields for involved inguinal lymph nodes are usually necessary, but care should be taken not to concurrently overlap any tissues irradiated by the boost treatment to the anus.

Chemotherapy

Careful coordination of the timing of concurrent chemotherapy with the delivery of radiation is important for successful treatment of anal cancer. The addition of mitomycin-C (10 mg/m^2 on days 1 and 29 of radiotherapy) to 5-FU (1 g/m^2/day for 96 hours on days 1–4 and 29–32 of radiotherapy) was established as a standard of care by the results of RTOG 87-04,[295] which compared both drugs to concurrent 5-FU alone. With this approach, treatment should generally begin on a Monday or Tuesday so that radiotherapy may be given on each day of chemotherapy delivery (4 days of 5-FU). As an alternative to mitomycin-C, multiple institutions have reported excellent results with cisplatin and 5-FU concurrent with radiation.[343,344] However, the ACT II trial failed to demonstrate superior outcomes with cisplatin + 5-FU versus mitomycin-C + 5-FU with concurrent radiotherapy.[297] In RTOG 98-11, cisplatin and 5-FU, given as induction therapy and concurrent

with RT, demonstrated inferior long-term survival to RT concurrent with mitomycin-C and 5-FU.[345]

Prognosis

The ACT II trial reported 5-year progression-free, colostomy-free, and overall survival rates of 69%, 68%, and 79%, respectively among patients receiving combined-modality therapy with RT, mitomycin-C, and 5-FU.[297] Among patients who experience local failure, approximately 50% have been salvaged with surgical resection.[295]

KEY POINTS

- Esophageal cancers are most commonly treated with neoadjuvant chemoradiation and carboplatin/paclitaxel, followed by surgical resection. The role of surgical resection in squamous cell carcinoma is less clear, with no associated improvement in overall survival.

- Gastric cancers are most commonly treated with perioperative chemotherapy, with current trials exploring the addition of neoadjuvant chemoradiation to this paradigm.

- Pancreatic cancers are practically classified as resectable, borderline resectable, unresectable, and metastatic. Within multimodality management, neoadjuvant chemoradiation is commonly given for borderline resectable disease, while chemoradiation or SBRT may be considered for unresectable disease.

- Rectal malignancies are treated with neoadjuvant 5-FU based chemoradiation, hypofractionated short-course radiation alone, or sequential hypofractionated short-course radiation and chemotherapy prior to surgical resection

- For anal cancers, sphincter sparing is achieved with radiotherapy combined with 5-FU and mitomycin.

REVIEW QUESTIONS

1. Which of the following nodal areas would not be routinely included in a cT3N1 rectal adenocarcinoma?
   A. presacral
   B. internal iliac
   C. external iliac
   D. mesorectum

2. For a T2N1 gastric cardia cancer, which of the following regions may be excluded from the RT treatment fields?
   A. gastric remnant
   B. splenic hilum nodes
   C. celiac axis
   D. porta
   E. pancreaticoduodenal nodes

3. The following nodal areas are routinely encompassed in both anal cancer and rectal cancer treatment volumes with the exception of which of the following:
A. inguinal nodes
B. mesorectum
C. external iliac
D. presacral

4. Which of the following are appropriate adjuvant therapies for resected pancreatic cancer:
A. Adjuvant chemotherapy
B. Adjuvant chemoradiation
C. Clinical trial
D. All of the above

5. The appropriate concurrent chemoradiation regimen for resectable esophageal cancer is which of the following:
A. CDDP and RT
B. Carboplatin/paclitaxel and RT
C. CDDP/mitomycin and RT
D. Capecitabine and RT

ANSWERS

1. C	4. D
2. E	5. B
3. A	

REFERENCES

1. Siegel RL, Miller KD, Jemal A. Cancer statistics, 2020. *CA Cancer J. Clin.* 2020;70:7–30.
2. Engel LS, et al. Population attributable risks of esophageal and gastric cancers. *J Natl Cancer Inst.* 2003;95:1404–1413.
3. Pohl H, Sirovich B, Welch HG. Esophageal adenocarcinoma incidence: are we reaching the peak? *Cancer Epidemiol Biomarkers Prev.* 2010;19:1468–1470.
4. Njei B, McCarty TR, Birk JW. Trends in esophageal cancer survival in United States adults from 1973 to 2009: a SEER database analysis. *J Gastroenterol Hepatol.* 2016;31:1141–1146.
5. Torre LA, et al. Global cancer statistics, 2012. *CA Cancer J Clin.* 2015;65:87–108.
6. Tran GD, et al. Prospective study of risk factors for esophageal and gastric cancers in the Linxian general population trial cohort in China. *Int J Cancer.* 2005;113:456–463.
7. Gholipour C, Shalchi RA, Abbasi M. A histopathological study of esophageal cancer on the western side of the Caspian littoral from 1994 to 2003. *DisEsophagus.* 2008;21:322–327.
8. Rice TW, Ishwaran H, Ferguson MK, et al. Cancer of the esophagus and the esophagogastric junction: an eighth edition staging primer. *J Thorac Oncol.* 2017;12:36–42.
9. Siewert JR, Stein HJ. Classification of adenocarcinoma of the oesophagogastric junction. *Br J Surg.* 1998;85:1457–1459.
10. Lightdale CJ, Kulkarni KG. Role of endoscopic ultrasonography in the staging and follow-up of esophageal cancer. *J Clin Oncol.* 2005;23:4483–4489.
11. Flamen P, et al. Utility of positron emission tomography for the staging of patients with potentially operable esophageal carcinoma. *J Clin Oncol.* 2000;18:3202–3210.
12. van Vliet EPM, Heijenbrok-Kal MH, Hunink MGM, et al. Staging investigations for oesophageal cancer: a meta-analysis. *Br J Cancer.* 2008;98:547–557.
13. Gschossmann JM, et al. Malignant tracheoesophageal fistula in patients with esophageal cancer. *Cancer.* 1993;72:1513–1521.
14. Yamada S, Takai Y, Ogawa Y, et al. Radiotherapy for malignant fistula to other tract. *Cancer.* 1989;64:1026–1028.
15. Burt M, et al. Malignant esophagorespiratory fistula: management options and survival. *Ann Thorac Surg.* 1991;52:1222–1228; discussion 1228–1229.
16. Rice TW, et al. Worldwide esophageal cancer collaboration. *Dis Esophagus.* 2009;22:1–8.
17. Mariette C, et al. Surgery alone versus chemoradiotherapy followed by surgery for stage I and II esophageal cancer: final analysis of randomized controlled phase III trial FFCD 9901. *J Clin Oncol.* 2014;32:2416–2422.
18. van Hagen P, et al. Preoperative chemoradiotherapy for esophageal or junctional cancer. *N Engl J Med.* 2012;366:2074–2084.
19. Shapiro J, et al. Neoadjuvant chemoradiotherapy plus surgery versus surgery alone for oesophageal or junctional cancer (CROSS): long-term results of a randomised controlled trial. *Lancet Oncol.* 2015;16:1090–1098.
20. Al-Batran S-E, et al. Perioperative chemotherapy with fluorouracil plus leucovorin, oxaliplatin, and docetaxel versus fluorouracil or capecitabine plus cisplatin and epirubicin for locally advanced, resectable gastric or gastro-oesophageal junction adenocarcinoma (FLOT4): a randomised, phase 2/3 trial. *Lancet.* 2019;393:1948–1957.
21. Smalley SR, et al. Updated analysis of SWOG-directed intergroup study 0116: a phase III trial of adjuvant radiochemotherapy versus observation after curative gastric cancer resection. *J Clin Oncol.* 2012;30:2327–2333.
22. Adelstein DJ, et al. Mature results from a phase II trial of postoperative concurrent chemoradiotherapy for poor prognosis cancer of the esophagus and gastroesophageal junction. *J Thorac Oncol.* 2009;4:1264–1269.
23. Fok M, Sham JS, Choy D, et al. Postoperative radiotherapy for carcinoma of the esophagus: a prospective, randomized controlled study. *Surgery.* 1993;113:138–147.
24. Teniere P, Hay JM, Fingerhut A, et al. Postoperative radiation therapy does not increase survival after curative resection for squamous cell carcinoma of the middle and lower esophagus as shown by a multicenter controlled trial. French University Association for Surgical Research. *Surg Gynecol Obstet.* 1991;173:123–130.
25. Stahl M, et al. Chemoradiation with and without surgery in patients with locally advanced squamous cell carcinoma of the esophagus. *J Clin Oncol.* 2005;23:2310–2317.
26. Bedenne L, et al. Chemoradiation followed by surgery compared with chemoradiation alone in squamous cancer of the esophagus: FFCD 9102. *J Clin Oncol.* 2007;25:1160–1168.
27. Vellayappan BA, et al. Chemoradiotherapy versus chemoradiotherapy plus surgery for esophageal cancer. *Cochrane Database Syst Rev.* 2017;8:CD010511.
28. Cooper JS, et al. Chemoradiotherapy of locally advanced esophageal cancer: long-term follow-up of a prospective randomized trial (RTOG 85-01). *JAMA.* 1999;281:1623–1627.
29. Corn BW, et al. Significance of prone positioning in planning treatment for esophageal cancer. Int J Radiat Oncol Biol Phys. 1991;21:1303–1309.
30. Patel AA, et al. Implications of respiratory motion as measured by four-dimensional computed tomography for radiation treatment planning of esophageal cancer. Int J Radiat. Oncol Biol Phys. 2009;74:290–296.
31. Dieleman EMT, et al. Four-dimensional computed tomographic analysis of esophageal mobility during normal respiration. *Int J Radiat Oncol Biol Phys.* 2007;67:775–780.

32. Wang W, et al. Comparison of planning target volumes based on three-dimensional and four-dimensional CT imaging of thoracic esophageal cancer. *Onco Targets Ther*. 2016;9:4785–4791.

33. Gao H, et al. Impact of esophageal motion on dosimetry and toxicity with thoracic radiation therapy. *Technol Cancer Res Treat*. 2019;18:1533033819849073.

34. Thomas E, Crellin A, Harris K, et al. The role of endoscopic ultrasound (EUS) in planning radiotherapy target volumes for oesophageal cancer. *Radiother Oncol*. 2004;73:149–151.

35. Konski A, et al. The integration of 18-fluoro-deoxy-glucose positron emission tomography and endoscopic ultrasound in the treatment-planning process for esophageal carcinoma. *Int J Radiat Oncol Biol Phys*. 2005;61:1123–1128.

36. Vrieze O, et al. Is there a role for FGD-PET in radiotherapy planning in esophageal carcinoma? *Radiother Oncol*. 2004;73:269–275.

37. Muijs CT, et al. Clinical validation of FDG-PET/CT in the radiation treatment planning for patients with oesophageal cancer. *Radiother Oncol*. 2014;113:188–192.

38. Sannohe Y, Hiratsuka R, Doki K. Lymph node metastases in cancer of the thoracic esophagus. *Am J Surg*. 1981;141:216–218.

39. Mandard AM, et al. Autopsy findings in 111 cases of esophageal cancer. *Cancer*. 1981;48:329–335.

40. Herskovic A, et al. Combined chemotherapy and radiotherapy compared with radiotherapy alone in patients with cancer of the esophagus. *N Engl J Med*. 1992;326:1593–1598.

41. Minsky BD, et al. INT 0123 (Radiation Therapy Oncology Group 94-05) phase III trial of combined-modality therapy for esophageal cancer: high-dose versus standard-dose radiation therapy. *J Clin Oncol*. 2002;20:1167–1174.

42. Gao X-S, et al. Pathological analysis of clinical target volume margin for radiotherapy in patients with esophageal and gastroesophageal junction carcinoma. *Int J Radiat Oncol Biol Phys*. 2007;67:389–396.

43. Oppedijk V, et al. Patterns of recurrence after surgery alone versus preoperative chemoradiotherapy and surgery in the CROSS trials. *J Clin Oncol*. 2014;32:385–391.

44. Huang W, et al. Pattern of lymph node metastases and its implication in radiotherapeutic clinical target volume in patients with thoracic esophageal squamous cell carcinoma: a report of 1077 cases. *Radiother Oncol*. 2010;95:229–233.

45. Akiyama H, Tsurumaru M, Udagawa H, et al. Radical lymph node dissection for cancer of the thoracic esophagus. *Ann Surg*. 1994;220:364–372; discussion 372–373.

46. Meier I, et al. Adenocarcinoma of the esophagogastric junction: the pattern of metastatic lymph node dissemination as a rationale for elective lymphatic target volume definition. *Int J Radiat Oncol Biol Phys*. 2008;70:1408–1417.

47. Yu E, et al. Is extended volume external beam radiation therapy covering the anastomotic site beneficial in post-esophagectomy high risk patients? *Radiother Oncol*. 2004;73:141–148.

48. Marks LB, et al. Use of normal tissue complication probability models in the clinic. *Int J. Radiat Oncol Biol Phys*. 2010;76:S10–S19.

49. Kong F-M, et al. Final toxicity results of a radiation-dose escalation study in patients with non–small-cell lung cancer (NSCLC): predictors for radiation pneumonitis and fibrosis. *Int J Radiat Oncol Biol Phys*. 2006;65:1075–1086.

50. Tucker SL, et al. Dose–volume modeling of the risk of postoperative pulmonary complications among esophageal cancer patients treated with concurrent chemoradiotherapy followed by surgery. *Int J Radiat Oncol Biol Phys*. 2006;66:754–761.

51. Wang S-L, et al. Investigation of clinical and dosimetric factors associated with postoperative pulmonary complications in esophageal cancer patients treated with concurrent chemoradiotherapy followed by surgery. *Int J Radiat Oncol Biol Phys*. 2006;64:692–699.

52. Gagliardi G, et al. Radiation dose–volume effects in the heart. *Int J Radiat Oncol Biol Phys*. 2010;76:S77–S85.

53. Hulshof MCCM, et al. A randomized controlled phase III multicenter study on dose escalation in definitive chemoradiation for patients with locally advanced esophageal cancer: ARTDECO study. *J Clin Oncol*. 2020;38:281–281.

54. Macdonald JS, et al. Chemoradiotherapy after surgery compared with surgery alone for adenocarcinoma of the stomach or gastroesophageal junction. *N Engl J Med*. 2001;345:725–730.

55. Chandra A, et al. Feasibility of using intensity-modulated radiotherapy to improve lung sparing in treatment planning for distal esophageal cancer. *Radiother Oncol*. 2005;77:247–253.

56. Mayo CS, et al. Hybrid IMRT for treatment of cancers of the lung and esophagus. *Int J Radiat Oncol Biol Phys*. 2008;71:1408–1418.

57. Chen Y-J, et al. Helical tomotherapy for radiotherapy in esophageal cancer: a preferred plan with better conformal target coverage and more homogeneous dose distribution. *Med Dosim*. 2007;32:166–171.

58. Hsu F-M, et al. Association of clinical and dosimetric factors with postoperative pulmonary complications in esophageal cancer patients receiving intensity-modulated radiation therapy and concurrent chemotherapy followed by thoracic esophagectomy. *Ann Surg Oncol*. 2009;16:1669–1677.

59. Xu D, Li G, Li H, et al. Comparison of IMRT versus 3D-CRT in the treatment of esophagus cancer: a systematic review and meta-analysis. *Medicine*. 2017;96:e7685.

60. Lin SH, et al. Propensity score-based comparison of long-term outcomes with 3-dimensional conformal radiotherapy vs intensity-modulated radiotherapy for esophageal cancer. *Int J Radiat Oncol Biol Phys*. 2012;84:1078–1085.

61. Lin SH, et al. Proton beam therapy and concurrent chemotherapy for esophageal cancer. *Int J Radiat Oncol Biol Phys*. 2012;83:e345–e351.

62. Warren S, et al. An analysis of plan robustness for esophageal tumors: comparing volumetric modulated arc therapy plans and spot scanning proton planning. *Int J Radiat Oncol Biol Phys*. 2016;95:199–207.

63. Wang J, et al. Predictors of postoperative complications after trimodality therapy for esophageal cancer. *Int J Radiat Oncol Biol Phys*. 2013;86:885–891.

64. Chuong MD, et al. Improving outcomes for esophageal cancer using proton beam therapy. *Int J Radiat Oncol Biol Phys*. 2016;95:488–497.

65. Yu J, et al. Motion-robust intensity-modulated proton therapy for distal esophageal cancer. *Med Phys*. 2016;43:1111–1118.

66. Lin SH, et al. Randomized phase IIB trial of proton beam therapy versus intensity-modulated radiation therapy for locally advanced esophageal cancer. *J Clin Oncol*. 2020;38:1569–1579.

67. Burmeister BH, et al. Surgery alone versus chemoradiotherapy followed by surgery for resectable cancer of the oesophagus: a randomised controlled phase III trial. *Lancet Oncol*. 2005;6:659–668.

68. Bosset JF, et al. Chemoradiotherapy followed by surgery compared with surgery alone in squamous-cell cancer of the esophagus. *N Engl J Med*. 1997;337:161–167.

69. Tepper J, et al. Phase III trial of trimodality therapy with cisplatin, fluorouracil, radiotherapy, and surgery compared with surgery alone for esophageal cancer: CALGB 9781. *J Clin Oncol*. 2008;26:1086–1092.

70. Walsh TN, et al. A comparison of multimodal therapy and surgery for esophageal adenocarcinoma. *N Engl J Med*. 1996;335:462–467.

71. Cunningham D, et al. Perioperative chemotherapy versus surgery alone for resectable gastroesophageal cancer. *N Engl J Med*. 2006;355:11–20.

72. Merkow RP, et al. Treatment trends, risk of lymph node metastasis, and outcomes for localized esophageal cancer. *J Natl Cancer Inst*. 2014;106.

73. Powell J, McConkey CC. Increasing incidence of adenocarcinoma of the gastric cardia and adjacent sites. *Br J Cancer*. 1990;62:440–443.

74. Yoshida S, et al. Diagnostic ability of high-frequency ultrasound probe sonography in staging early gastric cancer, especially for submucosal invasion. *Abdom Imaging*. 2005;30:518–523.

75. Saito N, Takeshita K, Habu H, et al. The use of endoscopic ultrasound in determining the depth of cancer invasion in patients with gastric cancer. *Surg Endosc*. 1991;5:14–19.

76. Ganpathi IS, So JB-Y, Ho K-Y. Endoscopic ultrasonography for gastric cancer. *Surg Endosc*. 2006;20:559–562.

77. Kim SJ, et al. Peritoneal metastasis: detection with 16--or 64--detector row CT in patients undergoing surgery for gastric cancer. *Radiology*. 2009;253:407–415.

78. Chen J, et al. Improvement in preoperative staging of gastric adenocarcinoma with positron emission tomography. *Cancer*. 2005;103:2383–2390.

79. Smyth E, et al. A prospective evaluation of the utility of 2-deoxy-2-[18F] fluoro-D-glucose positron emission tomography and computed tomography in staging locally advanced gastric cancer. *Cancer*. 2012;118:5481–5488.

80. Yoshioka T, et al. Evaluation of 18F-FDG PET in patients with advanced, metastatic, or recurrent gastric cancer. *J Nucl Med*. 2003;44:690–699.

81. Mukai K, et al. Usefulness of preoperative FDG-PET for detection of gastric cancer. *Gastric Cancer*. 2006;9:192–196.

82. Kim S-K, et al. Assessment of lymph node metastases using 18F-FDG PET in patients with advanced gastric cancer. *Eur J Nucl Med Mol Imaging*. 2006;33:148–155.

83. Stahl A, et al. FDG PET imaging of locally advanced gastric carcinomas: correlation with endoscopic and histopathological findings. *Eur J Nucl Med Mol Imaging*. 2003;30:288–295.

84. Leake P-A, et al. A systematic review of the accuracy and indications for diagnostic laparoscopy prior to curative-intent resection of gastric cancer. *Gastric Cancer*. 2012;15 Suppl 1:S38–S47.

85. Sarela AI, Lefkowitz R, Brennan MF, et al. Selection of patients with gastric adenocarcinoma for laparoscopic staging. *Am J Surg*. 2006;191:134–138.

86. Bentrem D, Wilton A, Mazumdar M, et al. The value of peritoneal cytology as a preoperative predictor in patients with gastric carcinoma undergoing a curative resection. *Ann Surg Oncol*. 2005;12:347–353.

87. Gunderson LL, Sosin H. Adenocarcinoma of the stomach: areas of failure in a re-operation series (second or symptomatic look) clinicopathologic correlation and implications for adjuvant therapy. *Int J Radiat Oncol Biol Phys*. 1982;8:1–11.

88. Hundahl SA, Macdonald JS, Benedetti J, et al. Surgical treatment variation in a prospective, randomized trial of chemoradiotherapy in gastric cancer: the effect of undertreatment. *Ann Surg Oncol*. 2002;9:278–286.

89. Park SH, et al. Phase III trial to compare adjuvant chemotherapy with capecitabine and cisplatin versus concurrent chemoradiotherapy in gastric cancer: final report of the adjuvant chemoradiotherapy in stomach tumors trial, including survival and subset analyses. *J Clin Oncol*. 2015;33:3130–3136.

90. Park SH, et al. ARTIST 2: Interim results of a phase III trial involving adjuvant chemotherapy and/or chemoradiotherapy after D2-gastrectomy in stage II/III gastric cancer (GC). *J Clin Oncol*. 2019;37:4001–4001.

91. Sada YH, et al. National trends in multimodality therapy for locally advanced gastric cancer. *J Surg Res*. 2019;237:41–49.

92. Cats A, et al. Chemotherapy versus chemoradiotherapy after surgery and preoperative chemotherapy for resectable gastric cancer (CRITICS): an international, open-label, randomised phase 3 trial. *Lancet Oncol*. 2018;19:616–628.

93. Ajani JA, et al. Phase II trial of preoperative chemoradiation in patients with localized gastric adenocarcinoma (RTOG 9904): quality of combined modality therapy and pathologic response. *J Clin Oncol*. 2006;24:3953–3958.

94. Leong T, et al. TOPGEAR: a randomized, phase III trial of perioperative ECF chemotherapy with or without preoperative chemoradiation for resectable gastric cancer: interim results from an international, intergroup trial of the AGITG, TROG, EORTC and CCTG. *Ann Surg Oncol*. 2017;24:2252–2258.

95. Slagter AE, et al. CRITICS-II: a multicentre randomised phase II trial of neo-adjuvant chemotherapy followed by surgery versus neo-adjuvant chemotherapy and subsequent chemoradiotherapy followed by surgery versus neo-adjuvant chemoradiotherapy followed by surgery in resectable gastric cancer. *BMC Cancer*. 2018;18:877.

96. Moertel C, Reitemeier R, Childs D, et al. COMBINED 5-FLUOROURACIL AND SUPERVOLTAGE RADIATION THERAPY OF LOCALLY UNRESECTABLE GASTROINTESTINAL CANCER. *Lancet*. 1969;294:865–867.

97. Schein PS, Group GTS. A comparison of combination chemotherapy and combined modality therapy for locally advanced gastric carcinoma. *Cancer*. 1982;49:1771–1777.

98. Yamashita H, et al. Four-dimensional measurement of the displacement of metal clips or postoperative surgical staples during 320-multislice computed tomography scanning of gastric cancer. *Radiat Oncol*. 2012;7:137.

99. Wang J, et al. Quantifying the interfractional displacement of the gastroesophageal junction during radiation therapy for esophageal cancer. *Int J Radiat Oncol Biol Phys*. 2012;83:e273–e280.

100. Wo JY, et al. Gastric lymph node contouring atlas: A tool to aid in clinical target volume definition in 3-dimensional treatment planning for gastric cancer. *Pract Radiat Oncol*. 2013;3:e11–e19.

101. Smalley SR, et al. Gastric surgical adjuvant radiotherapy consensus report: rationale and treatment implementation. *Int J Radiat Oncol Biol Phys*. 2002;52:283–293.

102. Leong T, et al. 3D Conformal radiotherapy for gastric cancer—results of a comparative planning study. *Radiother Oncol*. 2005;74:301–306.

103. Ringash J, et al. Post-operative radiochemotherapy for gastric cancer: adoption and adaptation. *Clin Oncol*. 2005;17:91–95.

104. Ringash J, et al. IMRT for adjuvant radiation in gastric cancer: a preferred plan? *Int J Radiat Oncol Biol Phys*. 2005;63:732–738.

105. Dahele M, et al. Adjuvant radiotherapy for gastric cancer: a dosimetric comparison of 3-dimensional conformal radiotherapy, tomotherapy® and conventional intensity modulated radiotherapy treatment plans. *Med Dosim*. 2010;35:115–121.

106. Wieland P, et al. IMRT for postoperative treatment of gastric cancer: covering large target volumes in the upper abdomen: a comparison of a step-and-shoot and an arc therapy approach. *Int J Radiat Oncol Biol Phys*. 2004;59:1236–1244.

107. Trip AK, et al. IMRT limits nephrotoxicity after chemoradiotherapy for gastric cancer. *Radiother Oncol*. 2014;112:289–294.

108. Chakravarty T, et al. Intensity-modulated radiation therapy with concurrent chemotherapy as preoperative treatment for localized gastric adenocarcinoma. *Int J Radiat Oncol Biol Phys*. 2012;83:581–586.

109. Ren F, et al. Efficacy and safety of intensity-modulated radiation therapy versus three-dimensional conformal radiation treatment for patients with gastric cancer: a systematic review and meta-analysis. *Radiat Oncol*. 2019;14:84.

110. Moningi S, et al. IMRT reduces acute toxicity in patients treated with preoperative chemoradiation for gastric cancer. *Adv Radiat Oncol*. 2020;5:369–376.

111. Schwartz GK, et al. Randomized phase II trial evaluating two paclitaxel and cisplatin-containing chemoradiation regimens as adjuvant therapy in resected gastric cancer (RTOG-0114). *J Clin Oncol*. 2009;27:1956–1962.

112. Fuchs CS, et al. Adjuvant chemoradiotherapy with epirubicin, cisplatin, and fluorouracil compared with adjuvant chemoradiotherapy with fluorouracil and leucovorin after curative resection of gastric cancer: results from CALGB 80101 (Alliance). *J Clin Oncol*. 2017;35:3671.

113. Sasako M, et al. Five-year outcomes of a randomized phase III trial comparing adjuvant chemotherapy with S-1 versus surgery alone in stage II or III gastric cancer. *J Clin Oncol*. 2011;29:4387–4393.

114. Noh SH, et al. Adjuvant capecitabine plus oxaliplatin for gastric cancer after D2 gastrectomy (CLASSIC): 5-year follow-up of an open-label, randomised phase 3 trial. *Lancet Oncol*. 2014;15:1389–1396.

115. Akinyemiju T, et al. The burden of primary liver cancer and underlying etiologies from 1990 to 2015 at the global, regional, and national level: results from the global burden of disease study 2015. *JAMA Oncol*. 2017;3:1683–1691.

116. Marrero JA, et al. Diagnosis, staging, and management of hepatocellular carcinoma: 2018 practice guidance by the American Association for the Study of Liver Diseases. *Hepatology*. 2018;68:723–750.

117. Cerny M, et al. LI-RADS for MR imaging diagnosis of hepatocellular carcinoma: performance of major and ancillary features. *Radiology.* 2018;288:118–128.
118. Mitchell DG, Bruix J, Sherman M, et al. LI-RADS (Liver Imaging Reporting and Data System): summary, discussion, and consensus of the LI-RADS Management Working Group and future directions. *Hepatology.* 2015;61:1056–1065.
119. Albers I, Hartmann H, Bircher J, et al. Superiority of the Child-Pugh classification to quantitative liver function tests for assessing prognosis of liver cirrhosis. *Scand J Gastroenterol.* 1989;24:269–276.
120. Durand F, Valla D. Assessment of the prognosis of cirrhosis: Child--Pugh versus MELD. *J Hepatol.* 2005;42:S100–S107.
121. Johnson PJ, et al. Assessment of liver function in patients with hepatocellular carcinoma: a new evidence-based approach—the ALBI grade. *J Clin Oncol.* 2015;33:550.
122. Lin C-Y, et al. 18F-FDG PET or PET/CT for detecting extrahepatic metastases or recurrent hepatocellular carcinoma: a systematic review and meta-analysis. *Eur J Radiol.* 2012;81:2417–2422.
123. Pang TCY, Lam VWT. Surgical management of hepatocellular carcinoma. *World J Hepatol.* 2015;7:245.
124. Hwang S, Moon D-B, Lee S-G. Liver transplantation and conventional surgery for advanced hepatocellular carcinoma. *Transpl Int.* 2010;23:723–727.
125. Lin S-M, Lin C-J, Lin C-C, et al. Randomised controlled trial comparing percutaneous radiofrequency thermal ablation, percutaneous ethanol injection, and percutaneous acetic acid injection to treat hepatocellular carcinoma of 3 cm or less. *Gut.* 2005;54:1151–1156.
126. Lencioni RA, et al. Small hepatocellular carcinoma in cirrhosis: randomized comparison of radio-frequency thermal ablation versus percutaneous ethanol injection. *Radiology.* 2003;228:235–240.
127. Majumdar A, et al. Management of people with early-or very early-stage hepatocellular carcinoma. *Cochrane Database Syst Rev.* 2017;3:CD011650.
128. Xu Y, et al. Microwave ablation is as effective as radiofrequency ablation for very-early-stage hepatocellular carcinoma. *Chin J Cancer.* 2017;36:14.
129. Kim C. Understanding the nuances of microwave ablation for more accurate post-treatment assessment. *Future Oncol.* 2018;14:1755–1764.
130. Shiina S, et al. Radiofrequency ablation for hepatocellular carcinoma: 10-year outcome and prognostic factors. *Am J Gastroenterol.* 2012;107:569.
131. Identifier NCT0340260, Trial comparing PLA to HIGRT therapy (PROVE-HCC); 2018 Jan 18. Clinicaltrials.gov [Internet]. Bethesda (MD): National Library of Medicine (US). Available at https://clinicaltrials.gov/ct2/show/NCT0340260. Accessed July 14, 2020.
132. Veltri A, et al. Radiofrequency thermal ablation (RFA) after transarterial chemoembolization (TACE) as a combined therapy for unresectable non-early hepatocellular carcinoma (HCC). *Eur Radiol.* 2006;16:661–669.
133. Tsurusaki M, Murakami T. Surgical and locoregional therapy of HCC: TACE. *Liver Cancer.* 2015;4:165–175.
134. Yasuda S, et al. Radiotherapy for large hepatocellular carcinoma combined with transcatheter arterial embolization and percutaneous ethanol injection therapy. *Int J Oncol.* 1999;15:467–473.
135. Wu D-H, Liu L, Chen L-H. Therapeutic effects and prognostic factors in three-dimensional conformal radiotherapy combined with transcatheter arterial chemoembolization for hepatocellular carcinoma. *World J Gastroenterol.* 2004;10:2184.
136. Tsai AL, et al. Use of yttrium-90 microspheres in patients with advanced hepatocellular carcinoma and portal vein thrombosis. *J Vasc Interv Radiol.* 2010;21:1377–1384.
137. Stillwagon GB, et al. 194 hepatocellular cancers treated by radiation and chemotherapy combinations: toxicity and response: a Radiation Therapy Oncology Group Study. *Int J Radiat Oncol Biol Phys.* 1989;17:1223–1229.
138. Murray LJ, Dawson LA. Advances in stereotactic body radiation therapy for hepatocellular carcinoma. *Semin Radiat Oncol.* 2017;27:247–255.
139. Sapir E, et al. Stereotactic body radiation therapy as an alternative to transarterial chemoembolization for hepatocellular carcinoma. *Int J Radiat Oncol Biol Phys.* 2018;100:122–130.
140. Bujold A, et al. Sequential phase I and II trials of stereotactic body radiotherapy for locally advanced hepatocellular carcinoma. *J Clin Oncol.* 2013;31:1631–1639.
141. Lasley FD, et al. Final results of a phase II trial of stereotactic body radiotherapy (SBRT) in patients with hepatocellular carcinoma (HCC) with Child-Pugh class A (CPC-A). *J Clin Oncol.* 2014;32:4103–4103.
142. Fukuda K, et al. Long-term outcomes of proton beam therapy in patients with previously untreated hepatocellular carcinoma. *Cancer Sci.* 2017;108:497–503.
143. Dawson LA. Overview: where does radiation therapy fit in the spectrum of liver cancer local-regional therapies? *Semin Radiat Oncol.* 2011;21:241–246.
144. Radiation Therapy Oncology Group. RTOG 1112: Randomized phase III study of sorafenib versus stereotactic body radiotherapy followed by sorafenib in hepatocellular carcinoma. Available at: https://www.rtog.org/ClinicalTrials/. Accessed July 21, 2020.
145. Deshpande S. To study tumor motion and planning target volume margins using four dimensional computed tomography for cancer of the thorax and abdomen regions. *J Med Phys.* 2011;36:35–39.
146. Stemkens B, Paulson ES, Tijssen RHN. Nuts and bolts of 4D-MRI for radiotherapy. *Phys Med Biol.* 2018;63:21TR01.
147. Yu JI, et al. Evaluation of anatomical landmark position differences between respiration-gated MRI and four-dimensional CT for radiation therapy in patients with hepatocellular carcinoma. *Br J Radiol.* 2013;86:20120221–20120221.
148. Hong TS, et al. Interobserver variability in target definition for hepatocellular carcinoma with and without portal vein thrombus: radiation therapy oncology group consensus guidelines. *Int J Radiat Oncol Biol Phys.* 2014;89:804–813.
149. Ingold JA, Reed GB, Kaplan HS, et al. Radiation hepatitis. *Am J Roentgenol Radium Ther Nucl Med.* 1965;93:200–208.
150. Dawson LA, et al. Analysis of radiation-induced liver disease using the Lyman NTCP model. *Int J Radiat Oncol Biol Phys.* 2002;53:810–821.
151. Ben-Josef E, et al. Phase II trial of high-dose conformal radiation therapy with concurrent hepatic artery floxuridine for unresectable intrahepatic malignancies. *J Clin Oncol.* 2005;23:8739–8747.
152. Pan CC, et al. Radiation-associated liver injury. *Int J Radiat Oncol Biol Phys.* 2010;76:S94–S100.
153. Scorsetti M, Clerici E, Comito T. Stereotactic body radiation therapy for liver metastases. *J Gastrointest Oncol.* 2014;5:190.
154. Osmundson EC, et al. Predictors of toxicity associated with stereotactic body radiation therapy to the central hepatobiliary tract. *Int J Radiat Oncol Biol Phys.* 2015;91:986–994.
155. Soliman H, et al. Phase II trial of palliative radiotherapy for hepatocellular carcinoma and liver metastases. *J Clin Oncol.* 2013;31:3980–3986.
156. Bae SH, Jang WI, Park HC. Intensity-modulated radiotherapy for hepatocellular carcinoma: dosimetric and clinical results. *Oncotarget.* 2017;8:59965–59976.
157. Kim JY, et al. Normal liver sparing by proton beam therapy for hepatocellular carcinoma: comparison with helical intensity modulated radiotherapy and volumetric modulated arc therapy. *Acta Oncol.* 2015;54:1827–1832.
158. Llovet JM, et al. Sorafenib in advanced hepatocellular carcinoma. *N Engl J Med.* 2008;359:378–390.
159. Ikeda K, et al. Phase 2 study of lenvatinib in patients with advanced hepatocellular carcinoma. *J Gastroenterol.* 2017;52:512–519.
160. Finn RS, et al. Atezolizumab plus bevacizumab in unresectable hepatocellular carcinoma. *N Engl J Med.* 2020;382:1894–1905.
161. Qin S, et al. Randomized, multicenter, open-label study of oxaliplatin plus fluorouracil/leucovorin versus doxorubicin as palliative chemotherapy in patients with advanced hepatocellular carcinoma from Asia. *J Clin Oncol.* 2013;31:3501–3508.
162. Lee J, Shin I-S, Yoon WS, et al. Comparisons between radiofrequency ablation and stereotactic body radiotherapy for liver malignancies: meta-analyses and a systematic review. *Radiother Oncol.* 2020;145:63–70.
163. Vargas R, Nino-Murcia M, Trueblood W, et al. MDCT in Pancreatic adenocarcinoma: prediction of vascular invasion and resectability using a multiphasic technique with curved planar reformations. *AJR Am J Roentgenol.* 2004;182:419–425.

164. Kauhanen SP, et al. A prospective diagnostic accuracy study of 18F-fluorodeoxyglucose positron emission tomography/computed tomography, multidetector row computed tomography, and magnetic resonance imaging in primary diagnosis and staging of pancreatic cancer. *Ann Surg.* 2009;250:957–963.

165. White R, et al. Current utility of staging laparoscopy for pancreatic and peripancreatic neoplasms. *J Am Coll Surg.* 2008;206:445–450.

166. Ferrone CR, et al. The influence of positive peritoneal cytology on survival in patients with pancreatic adenocarcinoma. *J Gastrointest Surg.* 2006;10:1347–1353.

167. Doi R, et al. Surgery versus radiochemotherapy for resectable locally invasive pancreatic cancer: final results of a randomized multi-institutional trial. *Surg Today.* 2008;38:1021–1028.

168. Griffin JF, et al. Patterns of failure after curative resection of pancreatic carcinoma. *Cancer.* 1990;66:56–61.

169. Tepper J, Nardi G, Suit H. Carcinoma of the pancreas: review of MGH experience from 1963 to 1973—analysis of surgical failure and implications for radiation therapy. *Cancer.* 1976;37:1519–1524.

170. Kaiser MH, Ellenberg SS. Pancreatic cancer: adjuvant combined radiation and chemotherapy following curative resection. *Arch Surg.* 1985;120:899–903.

171. Hsu CC, et al. Adjuvant chemoradiation for pancreatic adenocarcinoma: the Johns Hopkins Hospital—Mayo Clinic collaborative study. *Ann Surg Oncol.* 2010;17:981–990.

172. Corsini MM, et al. Adjuvant radiotherapy and chemotherapy for pancreatic carcinoma: the Mayo Clinic experience (1975–2005). *J Clin Oncol.* 2008;26:3511–3516.

173. Oettle H, et al. Adjuvant chemotherapy with gemcitabine vs observation in patients undergoing curative-intent resection of pancreatic cancer: a randomized controlled trial. *JAMA.* 2007;297:267–277.

174. Conroy T, et al. FOLFIRINOX or gemcitabine as adjuvant therapy for pancreatic cancer. *N Engl J Med.* 2018;379:2395–2406.

175. Regine WF, et al. Fluorouracil-based chemoradiation with either gemcitabine or fluorouracil chemotherapy after resection of pancreatic adenocarcinoma: 5-year analysis of the U.S. Intergroup/RTOG 9704 phase III trial. *Ann Surg Oncol.* 2011;18:1319–1326.

176. Smeenk HG, et al. Long-term survival and metastatic pattern of pancreatic and periampullary cancer after adjuvant chemoradiation or observation: long-term results of EORTC trial 40891. *Ann Surg.* 2007;246:734.

177. Neoptolemos JP, et al. A randomized trial of chemoradiotherapy and chemotherapy after resection of pancreatic cancer. *N Engl J Med.* 2004;350:1200–1210.

178. Liao W-C, et al. Adjuvant treatments for resected pancreatic adenocarcinoma: a systematic review and network meta-analysis. *Lancet Oncol.* 2013;14:1095–1103.

179. Ujiki MB, Talamonti MS. Guidelines for the surgical management of pancreatic adenocarcinoma. *Semin Oncol.* 2007;34:311–320.

180. Jang J-Y, et al. Oncological benefits of neoadjuvant chemoradiation with gemcitabine versus upfront surgery in patients with borderline resectable pancreatic cancer: a prospective, randomized, open-label, multicenter phase 2/3 trial. *Ann Surg.* 2018;268:215–222.

181. Versteijne E, et al. Preoperative chemoradiotherapy versus immediate surgery for resectable and borderline resectable pancreatic cancer: Results of the dutch randomized phase III PREOPANC trial. *J Clin Oncol.* 2020;38:1763–1773.

182. Klaassen DJ, MacIntyre JM, Catton GE, et al. Treatment of locally unresectable cancer of the stomach and pancreas: a randomized comparison of 5-fluorouracil alone with radiation plus concurrent and maintenance 5-fluorouracil--an Eastern Cooperative Oncology Group study. *J Clin Oncol.* 1985;3:373–378.

183. Hammel P, et al. Effect of chemoradiotherapy vs chemotherapy on survival in patients with locally advanced pancreatic cancer controlled after 4 months of gemcitabine with or without erlotinib: the LAP07 randomized clinical trial. *JAMA.* 2016;315:1844–1853.

184. Moertel CG, et al. Therapy of locally unresectable pancreatic carcinoma: a randomized comparison of high dose (6000 rads) radiation alone, moderate dose radiation (4000 rads+ 5-fluorouracil), and high dose radiation+ 5-fluorouracil. The gastrointestinal tumor study group. *Cancer.* 1981;48:1705–1710.

185. Group GTS. Treatment of locally unresectable carcinoma of the pancreas: comparison of combined-modality therapy (chemotheraphy plus radiotherapy) to chemotheraphy alone1. *J Natl Cancer Inst.* 1988;80:751–755.

186. Loehrer Sr PJ, et al. A randomized phase III study of gemcitabine in combination with radiation therapy versus gemcitabine alone in patients with localized, unresectable pancreatic cancer: E4201. *J Clin Oncol.* 2008;26:4506–4506.

187. Shinchi H, et al. Length and quality of survival after external-beam radiotherapy with concurrent continuous 5-fluorouracil infusion for locally unresectable pancreatic cancer. *Int J Radiat Oncol Biol Phys.* 2002;53:146–150.

188. Goodman KA, et al. Radiation Therapy Oncology Group consensus panel guidelines for the delineation of the clinical target volume in the postoperative treatment of pancreatic head cancer. *Int J Radiat Oncol Biol Phys.* 2012;83:901–908.

189. Brunner TB, et al. Definition of elective lymphatic target volume in ductal carcinoma of the pancreatic head based on histopathologic analysis. *Int J Radiat Oncol Biol Phys.* 2005;62:1021–1029.

190. Kao GD, Whittington R, Coia L. Anatomy of the celiac axis and superior mesenteric artery and its significance in radiation therapy. *Int J Radiat Oncol Biol Phys.* 1993;25:131–134.

191. Nagakawa T, et al. Clinical study of lymphatic flow to the paraaortic lymph nodes in carcinoma of the head of the pancreas. *Cancer.* 1994;73:1155–1162.

192. Kayahara M, et al. Analysis of paraaortic lymph node involvement in pancreatic carcinoma: a significant indication for surgery? *Cancer.* 1999;85:583–590.

193. Tempero MA. NCCN guidelines updates: pancreatic cancer. *J Natl Compr Canc Netw.* 2019;17:603–605.

194. Tokuuye K, et al. Small-field radiotherapy in combination with concomitant chemotherapy for locally advanced pancreatic carcinoma. *Radiother Oncol.* 2003;67:327–330.

195. Chang DT, et al. Stereotactic radiotherapy for unresectable adenocarcinoma of the pancreas. *Cancer.* 2009;115:665–672.

196. Dholakia AS, et al. A phase 2 multicenter study to evaluate gemcitabine and fractionated stereotactic body radiation therapy for locally advanced pancreatic adenocarcinoma. *Int J Radiat Oncol Biol Phys.* 2013;87:S28.

197. Chuong MD, et al. Stereotactic body radiation therapy for locally advanced and borderline resectable pancreatic cancer is effective and well tolerated. *Int J Radiat Oncol Biol Phys.* 2013;86:516–522.

198. Moningi S, et al. The role of stereotactic body radiation therapy for pancreatic cancer: a single-institution experience. *Ann Surg Oncol.* 2015;22:2352–2358.

199. Crane CH. Hypofractionated ablative radiotherapy for locally advanced pancreatic cancer. *J Radiat Res.* 2016;57 Suppl 1: i53–i57.

200. Bernard V, Herman JM. Pancreas SBRT: who, what, when, where, and how.… *Pract Radiat Oncol.* 2020;10:183–185.

201. Milano MT, et al. Intensity-modulated radiotherapy in treatment of pancreatic and bile duct malignancies: toxicity and clinical outcome. *Int J Radiat Oncol Biol Phys.* 2004;59:445–453.

202. Palta M, et al. Radiation therapy for pancreatic cancer: executive summary of an ASTRO clinical practice guideline. *Pract Radiat Oncol.* 2019;9:322–332.

203. Bussels B, et al. Respiration-induced movement of the upper abdominal organs: a pitfall for the three-dimensional conformal radiation treatment of pancreatic cancer. *Radiother Oncol.* 2003;68:69–74.

204. Feng M, et al. Characterization of pancreatic tumor motion using cine MRI: surrogates for tumor position should be used with caution. *Int J Radiat Oncol Biol Phys.* 2009;74:884–891.

205. Jayachandran P, et al. Interfractional uncertainty in the treatment of pancreatic cancer with radiation. *Int J Radiat Oncol Biol Phys.* 2010;76:603–607.

206. Higgins PD, Sohn JW, Fine RM, et al. Three-dimensional conformal pancreas treatment: comparison of four- to six-field techniques. *Int J Radiat Oncol Biol Phys.* 1995;31:605–609.

207. Ben-Josef E, et al. Intensity-modulated radiotherapy (IMRT) and concurrent capecitabine for pancreatic cancer. *Int J Radiat Oncol Biol Phys.* 2004;59:454–459.

208. van der Geld YG, et al. Evaluation of four-dimensional computed tomography-based intensity-modulated and respiratory-gated radiotherapy techniques for pancreatic carcinoma. *Int J Radiat Oncol Biol Phys.* 2008;72:1215–1220.

209. Brown MW, et al. A dosimetric analysis of dose escalation using two intensity-modulated radiation therapy techniques in locally advanced pancreatic carcinoma. *Int J Radiat Oncol Biol Phys.* 2006;65:274–283.

210. Fuss M, et al. Image-guided intensity-modulated radiotherapy for pancreatic carcinoma. *Gastrointest Cancer Res.* 2007;1:2–11.

211. Neoptolemos JP, et al. Comparison of adjuvant gemcitabine and capecitabine with gemcitabine monotherapy in patients with resected pancreatic cancer (ESPAC-4): a multicentre, open-label, randomised, phase 3 trial. *Lancet.* 2017;389:1011–1024.

212. Conroy T, et al. FOLFIRINOX versus gemcitabine for metastatic pancreatic cancer. *N Engl J Med.* 2011;364:1817–1825.

213. Von Hoff DD, et al. Increased survival in pancreatic cancer with nab-paclitaxel plus gemcitabine. *N Engl J Med.* 2013;369:1691–1703.

214. Hofheinz R-D, et al. Chemoradiotherapy with capecitabine versus fluorouracil for locally advanced rectal cancer: a randomised, multicentre, non-inferiority, phase 3 trial. *Lancet Oncol.* 2012;13:579–588.

215. Meta-analysis Group In Cancer et al. Efficacy of intravenous continuous infusion of fluorouracil compared with bolus administration in advanced colorectal cancer. *J Clin Oncol.* 1998;16:301–308.

216. Li C-P, et al. Concurrent chemoradiotherapy treatment of locally advanced pancreatic cancer: gemcitabine versus 5-fluorouracil, a randomized controlled study. *Int J Radiat Oncol Biol Phys.* 2003;57:98–104.

217. Mukherjee S, et al. Gemcitabine-based or capecitabine-based chemoradiotherapy for locally advanced pancreatic cancer (SCALOP): a multicentre, randomised, phase 2 trial. *Lancet Oncol.* 2013;14:317–326.

218. Crane CH, et al. Combining gemcitabine with radiation in pancreatic cancer: understanding important variables influencing the therapeutic index. *Semin Oncol.* 2001;28:25–33.

219. Kim NK, Kim MJ, Yun SH, et al. Comparative study of transrectal ultrasonography, pelvic computerized tomography, and magnetic resonance imaging in preoperative staging of rectal cancer. *Dis Colon Rectum.* 1999;42:770–775.

220. Group MS, MERCURY Study Group. Diagnostic accuracy of preoperative magnetic resonance imaging in predicting curative resection of rectal cancer: prospective observational study. *BMJ.* 2006;333:779.

221. MERCURY Study Group. Extramural depth of tumor invasion at thin-section MR in patients with rectal cancer: results of the MERCURY study. *Radiology.* 2007;243:132–139.

222. Calvo FA, et al. 18F-FDG positron emission tomography staging and restaging in rectal cancer treated with preoperative chemoradiation. *Int J Radiat Oncol Biol Phys.* 2004;58:528–535.

223. Tumor Study Group, G. Prolongation of the disease-free interval in surgically treated rectal carcinoma. *N Engl J Med.* 1985;312:1465–1472.

224. Douglass HO Jr, et al. Survival after postoperative combination treatment of rectal cancer. *N Engl J Med.* 1986;315:1294–1295.

225. Krook JE, et al. Effective surgical adjuvant therapy for high-risk rectal carcinoma. *N Engl J Med.* 1991;324:709–715.

226. Sauer R, et al. Preoperative versus postoperative chemoradiotherapy for rectal cancer. *N Engl J Med.* 2004;351:1731–1740.

227. Sauer R, Liersch T, Merkel S, et al. Preoperative versus postoperative chemoradiotherapy for locally advanced rectal cancer: results of the German CAO/ARO/AIO-94 randomized phase III trial. *J Clin.* 2012;30:1926–1933.

228. van Gijn W, et al. Preoperative radiotherapy combined with total mesorectal excision for resectable rectal cancer: 12-year follow-up of the multicentre, randomised controlled TME trial. *Lancet Oncol.* 2011;12:575–582.

229. Bujko K, et al. Long-term results of a randomized trial comparing preoperative short-course radiotherapy with preoperative conventionally fractionated chemoradiation for rectal cancer. *Br J Surg.* 2006;93:1215–1223.

230. Ngan SY, et al. Randomized trial of short-course radiotherapy versus long-course chemoradiation comparing rates of local recurrence in patients with T3 rectal cancer: Trans-Tasman Radiation Oncology Group trial 01.04. *J Clin Oncol.* 2012;30:3827–3833.

231. Bujko K, et al. Long-course oxaliplatin-based preoperative chemoradiation versus 5× 5 Gy and consolidation chemotherapy for cT4 or fixed cT3 rectal cancer: results of a randomized phase III study. *Ann Oncol.* 2016;27:834–842.

232. Cisel B, et al. Long-course preoperative chemoradiation versus 5× 5 Gy and consolidation chemotherapy for clinical T4 and fixed clinical T3 rectal cancer: long-term results of the randomized Polish II study. *Ann Oncol.* 2019;30:1298–1303.

233. Peeters KCMJ, et al. The TME trial after a median follow-up of 6 years: increased local control but no survival benefit in irradiated patients with resectable rectal carcinoma. *Ann Surg.* 2007;246:693–701.

234. Bosset J-F, et al. Fluorouracil-based adjuvant chemotherapy after preoperative chemoradiotherapy in rectal cancer: long-term results of the EORTC 22921 randomised study. *Lancet Oncol.* 2014;15:184–190.

235. Sainato A, et al. No benefit of adjuvant fluorouracil leucovorin chemotherapy after neoadjuvant chemoradiotherapy in locally advanced cancer of the rectum (LARC): long term results of a randomized trial (I-CNR-RT). *Radiother Oncol.* 2014;113:223–229.

236. Fernandez-Martos C, et al. Chemoradiation, surgery and adjuvant chemotherapy versus induction chemotherapy followed by chemoradiation and surgery: long-term results of the Spanish GCR-3 phase II randomized trial. *Ann Oncol.* 2015;26:1722–1728.

237. Sclafani F, et al. PAN-EX: a pooled analysis of two trials of neoadjuvant chemotherapy followed by chemoradiotherapy in MRI-defined, locally advanced rectal cancer. *Ann Oncol.* 2016;27:1557–1565.

238. Garcia-Aguilar J, et al. Effect of adding mFOLFOX6 after neoadjuvant chemoradiation in locally advanced rectal cancer: a multicentre, phase 2 trial. *Lancet Oncol.* 2015;16:957–966.

239. Habr-Gama A, et al. Local recurrence after complete clinical response and watch and wait in rectal cancer after neoadjuvant chemoradiation: impact of salvage therapy on local disease control. *Int J Radiat Oncol Biol Phys.* 2014;88:822–828.

240. Benson AB, et al. NCCN guidelines insights: rectal cancer, Version 6.2020: featured updates to the NCCN guidelines. *J Natl Compr Canc Netw.* 2020;18:806–815.

241. Al-Sukhni E, Attwood K, Mattson DM, et al. Predictors of pathologic complete response following neoadjuvant chemoradiotherapy for rectal cancer. *Ann Surg Oncol.* 2016;23:1177–1186.

242. van der Valk MJM, et al. Long-term outcomes of clinical complete responders after neoadjuvant treatment for rectal cancer in the International Watch & Wait Database (IWWD): an international multicentre registry study. *Lancet.* 2018;391:2537–2545.

243. Willett CG, et al. Adjuvant postoperative radiation therapy for colonic carcinoma. *Ann Surg.* 1987;206:694–698.

244. Willett CG, et al. Does postoperative irradiation play a role in the adjuvant therapy of stage T4 colon cancer? *Cancer J Sci Am.* 1999;5:242–247.

245. Ludmir EB, Palta M, Willett CG, et al. Total neoadjuvant therapy for rectal cancer: an emerging option. *Cancer.* 2017;123:1497–1506.

246. Martenson JA Jr, et al. Phase III study of adjuvant chemotherapy and radiation therapy compared with chemotherapy alone in the surgical adjuvant treatment of colon cancer: results of intergroup protocol 0130. *J Clin Oncol.* 2004;22:3277–3283.

247. Baglan KL, et al. The dose-volume realationship of acute small bowel toxicity from concurrent 5-FU-based chemotherapy and radiation therapy for rectal cancer. *Int J Radiat Oncol Biol Phys.* 2002;52:176–183.

248. Robertson JM, Lockman D, Yan D, et al. The dose–volume relationship of small bowel irradiation and acute grade 3 diarrhea during chemoradiotherapy for rectal cancer. *Int J Radiat Oncol Biol Phys.* 2008;70:413–418.

249. Tho LM, et al. Acute small bowel toxicity and preoperative chemoradiotherapy for rectal cancer: investigating dose–volume relationships and role for inverse planning. *Int J Radiat Oncol Biol Phys.* 2006;66:505–513.

250. Kim TH, et al. Comparison of the belly board device method and the distended bladder method for reducing irradiated small bowel volumes in preoperative radiotherapy of rectal cancer patients. *Int J Radiat Oncol Biol Phys.* 2005;62:769–775.

251. Martin J, et al. Treatment with a belly-board device significantly reduces the volume of small bowel irradiated and results in low acute toxicity in adjuvant radiotherapy for gynecologic cancer: results of a prospective study. *Radiother Oncol.* 2005;74:267–274.

252. Olofsen-van Acht M, et al. Reduction of irradiated small bowel volume and accurate patient positioning by use of a bellyboard device in pelvic radiotherapy of gynecological cancer patients. *Radiother Oncol.* 2001;59:87–93.

253. Pinkawa M, et al. Dose-volume histogram evaluation of prone and supine patient position in external beam radiotherapy for cervical and endometrial cancer. *Radiother Oncol.* 2003;69:99–105.

254. Gallagher MJ, et al. A prospective study of treatment techniques to minimize the volume of pelvic small bowel with reduction of acute and late effects associated with pelvic irradiation. *Int J Radiat Oncol Biol Phys.* 1986;12:1565–1573.

255. Moossa AR, et al. Factors influencing local recurrence after abdominoperineal resection for cancer of the rectum and rectosigmoid. *Br J Surg.* 1975;62:727–730.

256. Roberson SH, Heron HC, Kerman HD, et al. Is anterior resection of the rectosigmoid safe after preoperative radiation? *Dis Colon Rectum.* 1985;28:254–259.

257. Ciatto S, Pacini P. Radiation therapy of recurrences of carcinoma of the rectum and sigmoid after surgery. *Acta Radiol Oncol.* 1982;21:105–109.

258. Schild SE, et al. Postoperative adjuvant therapy of rectal cancer: an analysis of disease control, survival, and prognostic factors. *Int J Radiat Oncol Biol Phys.* 1989;17:55–62.

259. Myerson R, Drzymala, R. Technical aspects of image-based treatment planning of rectal carcinoma. *Semin Radiat Oncol.* 2003;13:433–440.

260. Roels S, et al. Definition and delineation of the clinical target volume for rectal cancer. *Int J Radiat Oncol Biol Phys.* 2006;65:1129–1142.

261. Bassi MC, et al. FDG-PET/CT imaging for staging and target volume delineation in preoperative conformal radiotherapy of rectal cancer. *Int J Radiat Oncol Biol Phys.* 2008;70:1423–1426.

262. Anderson C, et al. PET-CT fusion in radiation management of patients with anorectal tumors. *Int J Radiat Oncol Biol Phys.* 2007;69:155–162.

263. Hruby G, et al. Sites of local recurrence after surgery, with or without chemotherapy, for rectal cancer: implications for radiotherapy field design. *Int J Radiat Oncol Biol Phys.* 2003;55:138–143.

264. Syk E, Torkzad MR, Blomqvist L, et al. Local recurrence in rectal cancer: anatomic localization and effect on radiation target. *Int J Radiat Oncol Biol Phys.* 2008;72:658–664.

265. Yu T-K, et al. Patterns of locoregional recurrence after surgery and radiotherapy or chemoradiation for rectal cancer. *Int J Radiat Oncol Biol Phys.* 2008;71:1175–1180.

266. Sanfilippo NJ, et al. T4 rectal cancer treated with preoperative chemoradiation to the posterior pelvis followed by multivisceral resection: patterns of failure and limitations of treatment. *Int J Radiat Oncol Biol Phys.* 2001;51:176–183.

267. Taylor N, et al. Elective groin irradiation is not indicated for patients with adenocarcinoma of the rectum extending to the anal canal. *Int J Radiat Oncol Biol Phys.* 2001;51:741–747.

268. Robertson JM, Campbell JP, Yan D. Generic planning target margin for rectal cancer treatment setup variation. *Int J Radiat Oncol Biol Phys.* 2009;74:1470–1475.

269. Tournel K, et al. Assessment of intrafractional movement and internal motion in radiotherapy of rectal cancer using megavoltage computed tomography. *Int J Radiat Oncol Biol Phys.* 2008;71:934–939.

270. Grigsby PW, Roberts HL, Perez CA. Femoral neck fracture following groin irradiation. *Int J Radiat Oncol Biol Phys.* 1995;32:63–67.

271. Brizel HE, Tepperman BS. Postoperative adjuvant irradiation for adenocarcinoma of the rectum and sigmoid. *Am J Clin Oncol.* 1984;7:679–685.

272. O'Connell MJ, et al. Improving adjuvant therapy for rectal cancer by combining protracted-infusion fluorouracil with radiation therapy after curative surgery. *N Engl J Med.* 1994;331:502–507.

273. Kapiteijn E, et al. Preoperative radiotherapy combined with total mesorectal excision for resectable rectal cancer. *N Engl J Med.* 2001;345:638–646.

274. Roh MS, et al. Preoperative multimodality therapy improves disease-free survival in patients with carcinoma of the rectum: NSABP R-03. *J Clin Oncol.* 2009;27:5124–5130.

275. Myerson RJ, et al. Elective clinical target volumes for conformal therapy in anorectal cancer: a radiation therapy oncology group consensus panel contouring atlas. *Int J Radiat Oncol Biol Phys.* 2009;74:824–830.

276. Nuyttens JJ, Robertson JM, Yan D, et al. The variability of the clinical target volume for rectal cancer due to internal organ motion during adjuvant treatment. *Int J Radiat Oncol Biol Phys.* 2002;53:497–503.

277. Engels B, et al. Preoperative helical tomotherapy and megavoltage computed tomography for rectal cancer: impact on the irradiated volume of small bowel. *Int J Radiat Oncol Biol Phys.* 2009;74:1476–1480.

278. Urbano MTG, et al. Intensity-modulated radiotherapy in patients with locally advanced rectal cancer reduces volume of bowel treated to high dose levels. *Int J Radiat Oncol Biol Phys.* 2006;65:907–916.

279. Duthoy W, et al. Clinical implementation of intensity-modulated arc therapy (IMAT) for rectal cancer. *Int J Radiat Oncol Biol Phys.* 2004;60:794–806.

280. Mok H, et al. Intensity modulated radiation therapy (IMRT): differences in target volumes and improvement in clinically relevant doses to small bowel in rectal carcinoma. *Radiat. Oncol.* 2011;6:63.

281. De Ridder M, et al. Phase II study of preoperative helical tomotherapy for rectal cancer. *Int J Radiat Oncol Biol Phys.* 2008;70:728–734.

282. Freedman GM, et al. Phase I trial of preoperative hypofractionated intensity-modulated radiotherapy with incorporated boost and oral capecitabine in locally advanced rectal cancer. *Int J Radiat Oncol Biol Phys.* 2007;67:1389–1393.

283. Aristu JJ, et al. Phase I-II trial of concurrent capecitabine and oxaliplatin with preoperative intensity-modulated radiotherapy in patients with locally advanced rectal cancer. *Int J Radiat Oncol Biol Phys.* 2008;71:748–755.

284. Samuelian JM, et al. Reduced acute bowel toxicity in patients treated with intensity-modulated radiotherapy for rectal cancer. *Int J Radiat Oncol Biol Phys.* 2012;82:1981–1987.

285. Garofalo M, et al. RTOG 0822: a phase II study of preoperative (PREOP) chemoradiotherapy (CRT) utilizing IMRT in combination with capecitabine (C) and oxaliplatin (O) for patients with locally advanced rectal cancer. *Int J Radiat Oncol Biol Phys.* 2011;81:S3–S4.

286. Smalley SR, et al. Phase III trial of fluorouracil-based chemotherapy regimens plus radiotherapy in postoperative adjuvant rectal cancer: GI INT 0144. *J Clin Oncol.* 2006;24:3542–3547.

287. O'Connell MJ, et al. Capecitabine and oxaliplatin in the preoperative multimodality treatment of rectal cancer: surgical end points from National Surgical Adjuvant Breast and Bowel Project trial R-04. *J Clin Oncol.* 2014;32:1927–1934.

288. Aschele C, et al. Primary tumor response to preoperative chemoradiation with or without oxaliplatin in locally advanced rectal cancer: pathologic results of the STAR-01 randomized phase III trial. *J Clin Oncol.* 2011;29:2773–2780.

289. Gérard J-P, et al. Clinical outcome of the ACCORD 12/0405 PRODIGE 2 randomized trial in rectal cancer. *J Clin Oncol.* 2012;30:4558–4565.

290. Klotz RG Jr, Pamukcoglu T, Souilliard DH. Transitional cloacogenic carcinoma of the anal canal. Clinicopathologic study of three hundred seventy-three cases. *Cancer.* 1967;20:1727–1745.

291. Frost DB, Richards PC, Montague ED, et al. Epidermoid cancer of the anorectum. *Cancer.* 1984;53:1285–1293.

292. Nigro ND, Vaitkevicius VK, Considine B, Jr. Combined therapy for cancer of the anal canal: a preliminary report. *Dis Colon Rectum.* 1974;17:354.

293. Anal Cancer Trial Working Party, U. Epidermoid anal cancer: results from the UKCCCR randomised trial of radiotherapy alone versus radiotherapy, 5-fluorouracil, and mitomycin. *Lancet.* 1996;348:1049–1054.

294. Bartelink H, et al. Concomitant radiotherapy and chemotherapy is superior to radiotherapy alone in the treatment of locally advanced anal cancer: results of a phase III randomized trial of the European Organization for Research and Treatment of Cancer Radiotherapy and Gastrointestinal Cooperative Groups. *J Clin Oncol.* 1997;15:2040–2049.

295. Flam M, et al. Role of mitomycin in combination with fluorouracil and radiotherapy, and of salvage chemoradiation in the definitive nonsurgical treatment of epidermoid carcinoma of the anal canal: results of a phase III randomized intergroup study. *J Clin Oncol.* 1996;14:2527–2539.

296. Ajani JA, et al. Fluorouracil, mitomycin, and radiotherapy vs fluorouracil, cisplatin, and radiotherapy for carcinoma of the anal canal: a randomized controlled trial. *JAMA.* 2008;299:1914–1921.

297. James RD, et al. Mitomycin or cisplatin chemoradiation with or without maintenance chemotherapy for treatment of squamous-cell carcinoma of the anus (ACT II): a randomised, phase 3, open-label, 2 × 2 factorial trial. *Lancet Oncol.* 2013;14:516–524.

298. Peiffert D, et al. Induction chemotherapy and dose intensification of the radiation boost in locally advanced anal canal carcinoma: final analysis of the randomized UNICANCER ACCORD 03 trial. *J Clin Oncol.* 2012;30:1941–1948.

299. Howlader N, et al. SEER cancer statistics review, 1975–2009 (vintage 2009 populations). (2012).

300. Boman BM, et al. Carcinoma of the anal canal. A clinical and pathologic study of 188 cases. *Cancer.* 1984;54:114–125.

301. Clark MA, Hartley A, Geh JI. Cancer of the anal canal. *Lancet Oncol.* 2004;5:149–157.

302. Winton E de, et al. The impact of 18-fluorodeoxyglucose positron emission tomography on the staging, management and outcome of anal cancer. *Br J Cancer.* 2009;100:693–700.

303. Cotter SE, et al. FDG-PET/CT in the evaluation of anal carcinoma. *Int J Radiat Oncol Biol Phys.* 2006;65:720–725.

304. Trautmann TG, Zuger JH. Positron Emission Tomography for pretreatment staging and posttreatment evaluation in cancer of the anal canal. *Mol Imaging Biol.* 2005;7:309–313.

305. Nguyen BT, et al. Assessing the impact of FDG-PET in the management of anal cancer. *Radiother Oncol.* 2008;87:376–382.

306. Krengli M, et al. FDG-PET/CT imaging for staging and target volume delineation in conformal radiotherapy of anal carcinoma. *Radiat Oncol.* 2010;5:10.

307. Jones D. ICRU report 50-prescribing, recording and reporting photon beam therapy. *Med Phys.* 1994;21:833–834.

308. Godlewski G, Prudhomme, M. Embryology and anatomy of the anorectum. Basis of surgery. *Surg Clin North Am.* 2000;80:319–343.

309. Ortholan C, et al. Anal canal cancer: management of inguinal nodes and benefit of prophylactic inguinal irradiation (CORS-03 Study). *Int J Radiat Oncol Biol Phys.* 2012;82:1988–1995.

310. Ng M, et al. Australasian Gastrointestinal Trials Group (AGITG) contouring atlas and planning guidelines for intensity-modulated radiotherapy in anal cancer. *Int J Radiat Oncol Biol Phys.* 2012;83:1455–1462.

311. Gay HA, et al. Pelvic normal tissue contouring guidelines for radiation therapy: a Radiation Therapy Oncology Group consensus panel atlas. *Int J Radiat Oncol Biol Phys.* 2012;83:e353–e362.

312. Pepek JM, et al. Intensity-modulated radiation therapy for anal malignancies: a preliminary toxicity and disease outcomes analysis. *Int J Radiat Oncol Biol Phys.* 2010;78:1413–1419.

313. Bazan JG, et al. Intensity-modulated radiation therapy versus conventional radiation therapy for squamous cell carcinoma of the anal canal. *Cancer.* 2011;117:3342–3351.

314. Brooks CJ, et al. Organ-sparing Intensity-modulated Radiotherapy for Anal Cancer using the ACTII Schedule: a comparison of conventional and intensity-modulated radiotherapy plans. *Clin Oncol.* 2013;25:155–161.

315. Kachnic LA, et al. RTOG 0529: a phase 2 evaluation of dose-painted intensity modulated radiation therapy in combination with 5-fluorouracil and mitomycin-C for the reduction of acute

316. Milano MT, et al. Intensity-modulated radiation therapy (IMRT) in the treatment of anal cancer: toxicity and clinical outcome. *Int J Radiat Oncol Biol Phys.* 2005;63:354–361.

317. Kachnic LA, et al. Dose-painted intensity-modulated radiation therapy for anal cancer: a multi-institutional report of acute toxicity and response to therapy. *Int J Radiat Oncol Biol Phys.* 2012;82:153–158.

318. DeFoe SG, et al. Concurrent chemotherapy and intensity-modulated radiation therapy for anal carcinoma—clinical outcomes in a large National Cancer Institute-designated integrated cancer centre network. *Clin Oncol.* 2012;24:424–431.

319. Vieillot S, et al. IMRT for locally advanced anal cancer: clinical experience of the Montpellier Cancer Center. *Radiat Oncol.* 2012;7:45.

320. Dasgupta T, et al. Intensity-modulated radiotherapy vs. conventional radiotherapy in the treatment of anal squamous cell carcinoma: a propensity score analysis. *Radiother Oncol.* 2013;107:189–194.

321. Mitchell MP, et al. Intensity-modulated radiation therapy with concurrent chemotherapy for anal cancer: outcomes and toxicity. *Am J Clin Oncol.* 2014;37:461–466.

322. Devisetty K, et al. A multi-institutional acute gastrointestinal toxicity analysis of anal cancer patients treated with concurrent intensity-modulated radiation therapy (IMRT) and chemotherapy. *Radiother Oncol.* 2009;93:298–301.

323. DeFoe SG, Kabolizadeh P, Heron DE, et al. Dosimetric parameters predictive of acute gastrointestinal toxicity in patients with anal carcinoma treated with concurrent chemotherapy and intensity-modulated radiation therapy. *Oncology.* 2013;85:1–7.

324. Emami B, et al. Tolerance of normal tissue to therapeutic irradiation. *Int J Radiat Oncol Biol Phys.* 1991;21:109–122.

325. Kavanagh BD, et al. Radiation dose–volume effects in the stomach and small bowel. *Int J Radiat Oncol Biol Phys.* 2010;76:S101–S107.

326. Viswanathan AN, Yorke ED, Marks LB, et al. Radiation dose–volume effects of the urinary bladder. *Int J Radiat Oncol Biol Phys.* 2010;76:S116–S122.

327. Marks LB, Carroll PR, Dugan TC, et al. The response of the urinary bladder, urethra, and ureter to radiation and chemotherapy. *Int J Radiat Oncol Biol Phys.* 1995;31:1257–1280.

328. Baxter NN, Habermann EB, Tepper JE, et al. Risk of pelvic fractures in older women following pelvic irradiation. *JAMA.* 2005;294:2587–2593.

329. Bedford JL, Khoo VS, Webb S, et al. Optimization of coplanar six-field techniques for conformal radiotherapy of the prostate. *Int J Radiat Oncol Biol Phys.* 2000;46:231–238.

330. Bentzen AG, et al. Impaired health-related quality of life after chemoradiotherapy for anal cancer: late effects in a national cohort of 128 survivors. *Acta Oncol.* 2013;52:736–744.

331. Das P, et al. Long-term quality of life after radiotherapy for the treatment of anal cancer. *Cancer.* 2010;116:822–829.

332. John M, et al. Dose escalation in chemoradiation for anal cancer: preliminary results of RTOG 92-08. *Cancer J Sci Am.* 1996;2:205–211.

333. Weber DC, Kurtz JM, Allal AS. The impact of gap duration on local control in anal canal carcinoma treated by split-course radiotherapy and concomitant chemotherapy. *Int J Radiat Oncol Biol Phys.* 2001;50:675–680.

334. Rich TA, Ajani JA, Morrison WH, et al. Chemoradiation therapy for anal cancer: radiation plus continuous infusion of 5-fluorouracil with or without cisplatin. *Radiother Oncol.* 1993;27:209–215.

335. Hu K, et al. 30 Gy may be an adequate dose in patients with anal cancer treated with excisional biopsy followed by combined-modality therapy. *J Surg Oncol.* 1999;70:71–77.

336. Hatfield P, Cooper R, Sebag-Montefiore D. Involved-field, low-dose chemoradiotherapy for early-stage anal carcinoma. *Int J Radiat Oncol Biol Phys.* 2008;70:419–424.

337. Ferrigno R, et al. Radiochemotherapy in the conservative treatment of anal canal carcinoma: retrospective analysis of results and radiation dose effectiveness. *Int J Radiat Oncol Biol Phys.* 2005;61:1136–1142.

morbidity in carcinoma of the anal canal. *Int J Radiat Oncol Biol Phys.* 2013;86:27–33.

338. Constantinou EC, et al. Time-dose considerations in the treatment of anal cancer. *Int J Radiat Oncol Biol Phys*. 1997;39:651–657.

339. Salama JK, et al. Concurrent chemotherapy and intensity-modulated radiation therapy for anal canal cancer patients: a multicenter experience. *J Clin Oncol*. 2007;25:4581–4586.

340. Brown PD, Kline RW, Petersen IA, et al. Irradiation of the inguinal lymph nodes in patients of differing body habitus: a comparison of techniques and resulting normal tissue complication probabilities. *Med Dosim*. 2004;29:217–222.

341. Watson BA, et al. Use of segmental boost fields in the irradiation of inguinal lymphatic nodes. *Med Dosim*. 1999;24:27–32.

342. Dittmer PH, Randall ME. A technique for inguinal node boost using photon fields defined by asymmetric collimator jaws. *Radiother Oncol*. 2001;59:61–64.

343. Hung A, et al. Cisplatin-based combined modality therapy for anal carcinoma: a wider therapeutic index. *Cancer*. 2003;97:1195–1202.

344. Gerard JP, et al. Treatment of anal canal carcinoma with high dose radiation therapy and concomitant fluorouracil-cisplatinum. Long-term results in 95 patients. *Radiother Oncol*. 1998;46:249–256.

345. Gunderson LL, et al. Long-term update of US GI intergroup RTOG 98-11 phase III trial for anal carcinoma: survival, relapse, and colostomy failure with concurrent chemoradiation involving fluorouracil/mitomycin versus fluorouracil/cisplatin. *J Clin Oncol*. 2012;30:4344–4351.

10 Cancer of the Genitourinary Tract: Prostate, Bladder, and Testicular Cancer

Stephanie M. Yoon, Andrew S. Lim, and Albert Chang

INTRODUCTION

Epidemiology

Prostate cancer is the most common solid malignancy in men in the United States, with 191,930 men expected new cases and 33,330 men were estimated to have died from prostate cancer in 2020.[1] Approximately 1 in 12 men will be diagnosed with prostate cancer in their lifetime, with the incidence of prostate cancer increasing with age.[1] Since implementation of prostate-specific antigen (PSA) screening in the 1990s, prostate cancer mortality rates had dropped dramatically, with one in seven men dying from their disease.[2,3] While screening has led to the earlier detection and treatment of prostate cancer, particularly low-risk disease, the incidence of advanced metastatic disease has been increasing from 2010 to 2015.[4]

Clinical Anatomy

The prostate consists of four anatomic zones: peripheral, central, transitional, and the anterior fibromuscular zone. The prostate gland lies posterior to the pubic symphysis, anterior to the rectum, inferior to the bladder neck, and superior to the urogenital diaphragm. The urethra courses through the gland as it descends from the bladder neck to the urogenital diaphragm. A normal prostate gland is 20 to 30 cc, with the peripheral zone representing two thirds of this volume. The majority of prostate cancer arises from the peripheral zone and is often multifocal. Neurovascular bundles reside along the lateral surfaces of the prostate and attach to the base at the superior pedicles and to the apex at the inferior pedicles.

Local Growth Patterns

The prostatic capsule has an inner layer of smooth muscle and an outer layer of connective tissue though the capsule is ill-defined at the apex. Tumor that extends beyond the capsule of the prostate may involve the bladder neck, seminal vesicles, periprostatic fat, and neurovascular bundles. Lower urinary tract symptoms are derived from coexisting benign prostatic hyperplasia; however, tumors that invade superiorly into the bladder neck or into the membranous urethra can cause similar obstructive urinary symptoms. Extracapsular extension occurs most commonly at the posterolateral aspect of the gland, where the superior pedicles course along the prostate base, which may lead to erectile dysfunction. Tumor invasion of seminal vesicles may manifest as hematospermia. While some patients present with symptoms of bulky tumors, many patients in the era of PSA screening are diagnosed with prostate cancer without ever developing symptoms.

Regional and Distant Metastasis

Prostate cancer metastasizes through the blood and lymphatic systems. The prostate gland is predominantly drained by the obturator and internal iliac nodes.[5] The external iliac, presacral, and pre-sciatic nodes are also involved with prostatic lymphatic drainage. Distant metastasis most commonly results in osteoblastic bone lesions to the axial skeleton.

PRINCIPLES OF RADIATION THERAPY IN PROSTATE CANCER

Treatment with radiotherapy for prostate cancer spans multiple indications including (1) definitive treatment of localized disease, (2) adjuvant treatment following radical prostatectomy (RP), (3) salvage therapy following disease recurrence, and (4) palliation of locally advanced and metastatic disease.

Modern radiation therapy (RT) techniques for prostate cancer include external beam photon and particle beam treatments, low-dose rate (LDR), and high-dose rate (HDR) brachytherapy radioisotope implantation. External beam radiation (EBRT) involves three-dimensional (3D) planning with CT and/or MRI, as well as conformal treatment planning and delivery with inverse planning and intensity-modulated radiotherapy (IMRT). Stereotactic body radiotherapy (SBRT) is a newer technique with improved setup accuracy that delivers high doses of radiation up to five fractions and is increasingly adopted for the treatment of localized prostate cancer. Brachytherapy, either performed alone or in combination with EBRT, is another method of delivering escalated doses of radiation to the prostate.

These advanced treatment techniques are possible when used in conjunction with image guidance, which utilizes fiducial markers, ultrasound, and/or cone-beam CT.[6] The prostate is a moving target surrounded by deformable normal structures. The unpredictable position and motion of the prostate gland put neighboring structures, most importantly the rectum and bladder, at risk for injury during radiation treatment. Delivering high-radiation doses necessary to adequately treat prostate cancer not only requires smaller treatment margins to minimize normal tissue toxicity but also accurate target localization and tracking. Inadequate targeting of the prostate can also lead to underdosing of the tumor, inferior therapeutic outcomes, and increased toxicity.[6-8] Therefore, target volume delineation, tumor localization, patient immobilization, and treatment delivery must be carefully considered.

Altogether, the advancement in treatment techniques has allowed for safe delivery of higher-radiation doses, which correlate with improved PSA control [9-11] and over-all survival[12] with only modest changes in toxicity and patient-reported quality of life.[13,14]

CLINICAL ASSESSMENT

Diagnosis

A nodule palpated on digital rectal examination (DRE) warrants further evaluation with a transrectal ultrasound (TRUS)-guided biopsy to rule out cancer. With routine PSA screening, it is often an elevated absolute PSA level or abnormal PSA kinetics that prompts a biopsy as a palpable nodule is often not present at the time of diagnosis. The sensitivity of DRE for the detection of prostate cancer is low at 51%, and specificity of 59%.[15] An extended sextant biopsy consisting of at least 12 biopsy cores is recommended.[16] A pathologist makes the definitive diagnosis and assigns a Gleason primary and secondary grade to the biopsy specimen as an indication of tumor aggressiveness. Unfortunately, TRUS-guided biopsies tend to underdiagnose and understage prostate cancers. The sensitivity of a single biopsy session is 70% to 80%, thus approximately one third of prostate cancers are not detected on first biopsy.[17] Moreover, roughly half of detected cancers are less than the final Gleason scores (GS) assigned on prostatectomy samples.[18] MRI-guided or MRI-ultrasound fusion biopsies have been suggested to improve the staging accuracy of biopsies, especially after negative TRUS-guided biopsies.[19,20] Among patients with prior negative TRUS-guided biopsies, MR-ultrasound fusion biopsies have improved cancer detection rates by 20% to 40%.[21,22] The extent of the primary tumor, PSA level, and Gleason grade are used to determine the patient's risk group, which ultimately guides decision-making regarding treatment (Tables 10.1 and 10.2).

Risk Stratification

As previously mentioned, the clinical tumor stage, Gleason grade, and pretreatment PSA level are the most important prognostic indicators that determine a patient's risk group.

TABLE 10.1	2018 American Joint Committee on Cancer (AJCC) Clinical Primary Tumor (T) Staging for Prostate Cancer (8th Edition)[40]
TX	Primary tumor cannot be assessed
T0	No evidence of primary tumor
T1	Clinically inapparent tumor that is not palpable
T1a	Tumor incidental histologic finding in 5% or less of tissue resected
T1b	Tumor incidental histologic finding in >5% of tissue resected
T1c	Tumor identified by needle biopsy found in one or both sides, but not palpable (e.g., because of elevated PSA)
T2	Tumor is palpable and confined within the prostate
T2a	Tumor involves one-half of one side or less
T2b	Tumor involves more than one-half of one side but not both sides
T2c	Tumor involves both sides
T3	Extraprostatic tumor that is not fixed or does not invade adjacent structures[a]
T3a	Extraprostatic extension (unilateral or bilateral)
T3b	Tumor invades the seminal vesicle(s)
T4	Tumor is fixed or invades adjacent structures other than seminal vesicles: external sphincter, rectum, bladder, levator muscles, and/or pelvic wall

[a] Invasion into prostatic apex or into (but not beyond) the prostatic capsule is not classified as T3, but as T2.

PSA, prostate-specific antigen.

From Amin MB GD, Vega LR, Edge SB, Greene FL, Byrd DR, Brookland RK, Washington MK, Compton CC. AJCC *Cancer Staging Manual*, 8th Edition. Chicago, IL: American College of Surgeons; 2018 reproduced with permission of SNCSC.

TABLE 10.2	International Society of Urological Pathology (ISUP) Gleason Grade Group Risk Stratification System
Group 1	Gleason score ≤ 6; only composed of discrete, well-formed glands
Group 2	Gleason score 3 + 7 = 7; predominantly well-formed glands with lesser component of poorly formed/fused/cribiform glands
Group 3	Gleason score 4 + 3 = 7; predominantly poorly formed/fused/cribiform glands with lesser component of well-formed glands
	• If > 95% consists of poorly formed/fused/cribiform glands or lack of glands on core or at radical prostatectomy, the <5% component of well-formed glands is not factored into grading system.
Group 4	Gleason score 4 + 4 = 8, 3 + 5 = 8, or 5 + 3 = 8
	• Only poorly formed/fused/cribiform glands
	• Predominantly well-formed glands and less component lacking glands (poorly formed/fused/cribiform glands can be a minor component)
	• Predominantly lacking glands and lesser component of well-formed glands (poorly formed/fused/cribiform glands a minor component)
Group 5	Gleason score 9–10; lacking gland formation (or with necrosis) with or without poorly formed/fused/cribiform glands
	• If > 95% consists of poorly formed/fused/cribiform glands or lack of glands on core or at radical prostatectomy, the <5% component of well-formed glands is not factored into grading system.

The National Comprehensive Cancer Network (NCCN) stratifies patients into five risk categories (Table 10.3): very low, low, intermediate, high, and very high. Similarly, the American Joint Commission on Cancer (AJCC) prognostic groups are based on tumor stage, GS, and pretreatment PSA. However, broad heterogeneity can exist within a particular risk group, and newer classification systems incorporating factors such as age, percentage of positive biopsy cores,[23] and multi-gene molecular testing[24,25] are increasingly used to further risk stratify patients.

The role of prognostic multi-gene molecular testing is playing an increasing role in aiding in treatment decisions in clinical situations where uncertainty about disease progression remains beyond what is provided by life expectancy and clinical nomograms. Four molecular tests are currently utilized, with several others in development. Decipher is one genomic test prognostic for cancer outcomes for patients with newly diagnosed localized prostate cancer at the time of biopsy and after RP with high-risk features on surgical pathology. It is a whole-transcriptome RNA expression oligonucleotide microarray for formalin-fixed paraffin-embedded (FFPE) tissue specimens. In the setting of localized prostate cancer at the time of biopsy, Decipher reports the likelihood for having non-organ confined (pT3) or grade group ≥3 disease at the time of RP, as well as the likelihood for lymph node metastasis, biochemical recurrence, and prostate-cancer–specific mortality. This test is generally reserved for very-low to intermediate-risk prostate cancer patients with at least 10 years of life expectancy and who are candidates for either active surveillance or definitive therapy.[26–28] Decipher has also been tested among patients who may benefit in having additional treatment after RP. These patients include those with adverse pathology or who had biochemical recurrence/PSA persistence after prostatectomy. Adverse features following prostatectomy include positive margins, any pT3 disease, or persistent/rising PSA above nadir. In this setting, this test reports the likelihood for distant metastasis, postoperative radiation sensitivity, and prostate-cancer–specific mortality. This test would help patients and clinicians in discussing additional treatment such as adjuvant versus salvage radiation and/or whether to initiate androgen deprivation therapy (ADT).[29–31]

Prolaris is a quantitative real-time PCR for 31 cell cycle–related genes and 15 control genes that, like Decipher, has also been studied in the localized prostate cancer and post-radical prostatectomy settings.[32–34] This test predicts the likelihood for biochemical recurrence in both settings. It has also reported the likelihood for metastasis, non-organ confined disease (pT3 or higher and/or Grade Group ≥3) during RP, and prostate-cancer–specific mortality. Oncotype DX-Prostate is a quantitative real-time PCR for 12 prostate-cancer–related genes and 5 control genes. This test has primarily been studied among men with low-to-intermediate risk-localized prostate cancer at the time of biopsy to aid in discussion to pursue active surveillance or definitive therapy, and has not yet been tested among men who have already undergone RP.[35,36] This test reports the probability for metastasis, adverse features during RP (pT3 or higher and/or Grade Group ≥3), and prostate-cancer–specific mortality. Finally, ProMark is an 8-biomarker proteomic assay that analyzes proteins specific to prostate cancer directly from intact tissue biopsies. This test has primarily been tested among men with very-low-or low-risk disease who are being managed conservatively with active surveillance and reports the likelihood for prostate-cancer–specific mortality.[37] This test would also aid in discussions regarding continuing active surveillance or initiating definitive treatment.

TABLE 10.3	Prostate Cancer Recurrence Risk Group by National Comprehensive Cancer Network Criteria (2020 Version)
Clinically localized	
Very Low	Has all of the following: • T1c • Grade Group 1 • PSA < 10 ng/mL • Fewer than 3 prostate biopsy fragments/cores positive, ≤50% cancer in each fragment/core • PSA density <0.15 ng/mL/g
Low Risk	Has all of the following: • T1-T2a • Grade Group 1 • PSA <10 ng/mL

Intermediate Risk	Has all of the following:
	 • No high-risk group features
	 • No very-high-risk group features
	 • Has one or more intermediate risk factors (IRF):
	   • T2b-T2c
	   • Grade Group 2 or 3
	   • PSA 10–20 ng/mL
	 Favorable intermediate:
	 • 1 IRF
	 • Grade Group 1 or 2
	 • <50% biopsy cores positive
	 Unfavorable intermediate:
	 • 2 or 3 IRFs
	 • Grade Group 3
	 • ≥50% biopsy cores positive

High Risk	Has no very-high-risk features and has at least one high-risk feature: • T3a *or* • Grade Group 4 or 5 or • PSA >20 ng/mL
Very High Risk (Locally advanced)	Has at least one of the following: • T3b–T4 • Primary Gleason pattern 5 • 2 or 3 high-risk features • >4 cores with Grade Group 4 or 5
Metastatic	
	Any T, N1 or Any T, Any N, M1

PSA, prostate-specific antigen.

A large prospective study of 3,966 newly diagnosed localized prostate cancer patients reported the clinical utility of three tissue-based gene expression classifiers test (Decipher, Prolaris, and Oncotype DX)[38]; 18.8% of patients underwent a gene expression classifier test, and these patients were more likely to have lower PSA level, lower GS, lower clinical tumor stage, and fewer positive biopsy cores ($P < 0.05$). Active surveillance rates were 46.2% for patients whose genomic classifier whose results were above the specified threshold, while 75.9% of patients underwent active surveillance if the classifier resulted in below the specified threshold, and 57.9% of patients who did not undergo genomic testing underwent active surveillance ($P < 0.001$). It was estimated that for every nine men with favorable risk disease who undergo genomic classifier, one additional patient may have their disease initially managed with active surveillance. In another clinical utility study utilizing two prospective registries of 3,455 patients who have undergone RP, molecular testing with Decipher changed management recommendations in 39% of patients, which resulted in needing to test three patients to change one treatment decision.[39] Moreover, implementing treatment recommendations for patients with genomic high-risk disease led to improvements in early biochemical control. Sixty-one percent of patients who had genomic high-risk tumors and received adjuvant RT led to 2-year PSA recurrence of 3% compared to 25% of genomic high-risk patients who did not undergo adjuvant radiation.

Staging

The clinical tumor stage represents the size and extent of detectable tumor. DRE has previously been the main tool in making this determination but with routine PSA screening, prostate cancers are predominantly diagnosed at earlier stages. Non-palpable (T1c) disease represents the most common clinical stage. As such, many imaging modalities are used adjunctively to provide more accurate staging information. The AJCC clinical staging system for primary tumor is shown in Table 10.1.[40]

Ultrasound

Tumor under TRUS appears as a hypoechoic lesion in the peripheral zone. TRUS is widely utilized as a tool to provide visual guidance for prostate biopsy or to measure the volume of the prostate gland itself, as well as for brachytherapy seed placement.[41] However, when used as a diagnostic tool alone without the addition of biopsy, ultrasound is unreliable and has limited value for evaluating the full extent of disease. A hypoechoic lesion under ultrasound has a sensitivity of 85.5% and specificity of 28.4%. Nearly one third of prostate cancers are not identifiable on TRUS.[42]

Computed Tomography

CT does not play a role in either prostate cancer detection or primary tumor staging, due to its inadequate soft-tissue contrast discrimination between the prostate and underlying levator ani musculature. It may only accurately predict local tumor extent up to 65% of the time.[43] The main role for CT is nodal and distant metastatic staging. Nodal metastases occur relatively late in prostate cancer disease progression. While neither CT nor standard MRI is able to detect microscopic nodal metastases, CT may detect lymph nodes larger than 1 cm in diameter (along the short axis), with a sensitivity of about 36%.[44] Metastatic bone lesions can be detected and monitored with CT as well. While there are other imaging modalities superior to CT in detecting osseous metastasis, CT scans can better discriminate malignant from benign etiologies. Pelvic CT is recommended for patients with intermediate- to very-high-risk disease, and when nomogram predicts greater than 10% probability for pelvic lymph node involvement.

Magnetic Resonance Imaging

MR imaging has played an increasingly important role for the assessment of prostate cancer. Multiparametric MR images (mpMRI) include high-resolution T2-weighted imaging and additional sequences, which could include diffusion-weighted imaging (DWI)–associated apparent diffusion coefficient (ADC) image, dynamic contrast-enhanced MRI (DCE-MRI), and MR spectroscopy (MRS). High-resolution T2-weighted imaging provides exquisite definition of the prostate zonal anatomy. Imaging for prostate cancer detection and staging often requires an endorectal and pelvic phased-array coil at 1.5T, although 3T MR scanners have superior signal-to-noise ratio (SNR) such that excellent image quality can be achieved even without endorectal coils.

Other MR sequences can increase the predictive power of T2-weighted images for diagnosis. DWI helps differentiate benign from malignant tissue by inferring cellular density by measuring Brownian motion of interstitial water molecules. Prostate cancer has a lower ADC than normal prostate, and this property can aid in detecting prostate cancer.[45] DWI sequences can also potentially be used to monitor treatment response and detect recurrent disease. DCE-MRI adds information about prostatic vascularization through a series of high-temporal-resolution T1-weighted images following the administration of contrast. Finally, proton MRS is a functional imaging technique that aids in localizing prostate cancer by detecting levels of choline and citrate, which accumulate in prostate cancer and benign prostate tissues, respectively.

mpMRI aids in detecting disease not only within the prostate but also for extracapsular extension and (ECE) and seminal vesical invasion (SVI). The sensitivity and specificity for ECE on multiparametric MRI have reported to range from 13% to 93% and 49% to 97%, respectively.[46–50] mpMRI is equivalent to CT for detecting nodal disease involvement.[51] The ranges in sensitivity and specificity reported for MR imaging have been in part due to interobserver variability. With increased reader experience and maturation of the technology, the accuracy of mpMRI for local tumor staging has improved over the recent years.

Bone Scan and Positron Emission Tomography

In patients with intermediate to high-risk disease, imaging evaluation is indicated to identify occult metastatic disease. A bone scan is recommended for patients at high risk for developing skeletal metastases, which include those with the following features: T2 and PSA >10 ng/mL, high-or very-high-risk disease, or symptomatic disease. In one large North American population-based study, the sensitivity of bone scans in detecting osseous metastasis was 90.8%, with specificity of 76.3%. While the positive predictive value was only 5.7%, the negative predictive value was 99.8%. This overall yielded an accuracy of 76.5% in detecting bone metastasis.[52]

When the results of a bone scan are equivocal, or when a patient has biochemical recurrence after primary treatment, newer imaging modalities are recommended to detect for metastatic disease. F-18 sodium fluoride PET/CT scans detect F-18 sodium fluoride absorbed within bone matrix undergoing bone remodeling. This scan can detect bone metastases better than conventional bone scans with a sensitivity of 87% to 100%, though with a lower specificity of 62% to 89%.[53,54] C-11 choline and F-18 fluciclovine (Axumin) PET/CT or PET/MRIs are used to detect small volume disease in either the bone or soft tissues. These tracers highlight the increased cell membrane and protein synthesis, respectively, in prostate cancer cells. F-18 fluciclovine scans have reported to have a sensitivity of 55% to 90% and specificity of 56% to 100%.[55,56]

Newer tracers include gallium-68 prostate-specific membrane antigen (PSMA) and C-11 acetate, and hold promise for improving the detection of occult metastases. However, neither is approved for use by the U.S. Food and Drug Administration at this time. Emerging results on PSMA PET have primarily been in the setting of recurrent disease after primary treatment. A systematic review and meta-analysis reported the sensitivity and specificity of PSMA PET on a per-patient basis to be 86%.[57] More recently, a large multi centered prospective single-arm trial of PSMA PET in men with biochemically recurrent prostate cancer after prostatectomy demonstrated a positive predictive value of 84% to 92% with an overall detection rate of 75% that improved significantly with rising levels of PSA.[58] Studies are beginning to show that PSMA PET is able to detect more cancerous lesions compared to conventional imaging in the biochemically recurrent setting, especially for recurrent disease located in pelvic lymph nodes and extra-pelvic sites.[59] A prospective trial acquired both F-18 fluciclovine and PSMA PET scans in 50 patients with biochemically recurrent prostate cancer after prostatectomy.[59] PSMA PET had significantly higher overall detection rates (56%) compared to F-18 fluciclovine (26%) with an odds ratio of 4.8 ($p = 0.0026$), and remained superior for both pelvic and extrapelvic regions. Novel tracers that also bind to prostate-specific transmembrane protein such as 18F-DCFPyL have shown to yield excellent sensitivity and specificity for prostate cancer at metastatic and pelvic nodal sites as well.[60] With improved detection rates, the impact of PSMA on treatment practice, such as salvage radiotherapy, is currently being investigated, and detailed further under "Treatment Planning for Definitive EBRT-Lymph Nodes". Trials evaluating the utility of PSMA PET for upfront staging for patients newly diagnosed with prostate cancer are still investigational.

Gleason Grade

The Gleason system is based on the morphologic architecture of prostate cancer and is the most common method for histologic grading.[61] The Gleason grade applies to adenocarcinomas, but not to squamous cell carcinomas, sarcomas, or transitional cell carcinomas of the prostate. The Gleason grading scale ranges from 1 (most differentiated) to 5 (least differentiated). The GS is the sum of the two most prevalent Gleason grades observed within a tissue sample. If only two grades are seen in a biopsy core, the first number is the most predominant grade and the second number is that of the secondary grade. The GS ranges from 2 to 10, with 10 being the most malignant. In contemporary clinical practice, GS is broken down into five grade groups (Table 10.2).[62] Gleason grade groupings are akin to the risk stratification of Gleason scoring; however, the primary advantage is that Gleason grade groups discriminate Gleason patterns 3+4, and 4+3, whereas the GS for both these patterns is 7.[62-64] A GS of <6 is rarely encountered on needle biopsy due to a prevailing change in Gleason grading by pathologists, which has led to a shift in GS over time with higher GS being more prevalent in the PSA era even as other clinical risk features have declined.[65]

Prostate-Specific Antigen

Several guidelines are available regarding PSA screening. The American Urologic Association guidelines recommend a shared decision to pursue PSA screening every 1 to 2 years for men aged 55 to 69 years old.[66] For men 40 to 54 years of age, individualized screening decisions are recommended based on personal risk factors and family history. Screening is not recommended for men younger than 40 or older than 70 years old with life expectancy of less than 10 years.

An elevated PSA may prompt a biopsy. However, in addition to prostate cancer, elevated PSAs may result from benign prostatic hypertrophy (BPH), prostatitis, trauma, TURP, prostate biopsy, or recent ejaculation, which may lead to false–positive results. Other supplementary tests and considerations are available to help decide if a biopsy is necessary, including free PSA levels, PSA velocity, PSA density, family history, and DRE. A PSA above 10 ng/mL correlates with a 50% to 75% chance of diagnosis. A moderately elevated PSA between 4 and 10 ng/mL correlates to only a 20% to 30% risk of prostate cancer and can be difficult to interpret, especially if BPH is also present. In this range, a PSA density (serum total PSA level divided by prostate volume) greater than 0.15, a free PSA below 10% of total serum PSA level, and a PSA velocity above 0.75 ng/mL/year should further heighten suspicion for prostate cancer and prompt TRUS-guided needle biopsies of the prostate to be performed by a urologist.[67-69]

Prostate cancer antigen 3 (PCA3) is increasingly utilized for screening in addition to PSA testing. PCA3 is a noncoding RNA biomarker that is overexpressed in prostate cancer.[70,71] PCA3 has a lower sensitivity but higher specificity, and a better positive and negative predictive values compared to PSA. PCA3 is measured in the urine after prostate massage and digital exam. PCA3 testing is suggested to be clinically useful to predict the presence of prostate cancer in patients with prior negative biopsies.

TREATMENT OPTIONS
Treatment Algorithms

Treatment recommendations are determined by the initial risk groupings shown in Table 10.4. This section will focus on the treatment paradigms for localized prostate cancer.

Watchful Waiting

Watchful waiting, or passive observation, is an appropriate strategy in asymptomatic patients who do not expect to derive a survival benefit from treatment either due to advanced age or competing co morbid illness. This approach defers upfront treatment with the expectation to deliver palliative therapy for symptomatic disease. One randomized trial compared RP with watchful waiting. The Scandinavian Prostate Cancer Group Study Number 4 (SPCG-4) is a trial that predated routine PSA screening but found a disease-specific and overall survival benefit for RP in patients younger than 65 years, but no survival benefit in patients 65 years or older.[72] The PIVOT trial randomizing patients to RP versus observation did not demonstrate a statistically significant improvement in all-cause mortality in the entire cohort of patients. However, on a subset analysis, RP was suggested to improve survival in patients with intermediate-risk disease but not in patients with low- or high-risk disease.[73] In some clinical contexts, monitoring should still include routine

TABLE 10.4	Treatment Planning Recommendations by Risk Stratification for Clinically Localized Prostate Cancer with 3D Conformal or Intensity-Modulated External Beam Radiation Therapy Utilized at the University of California Los Angeles
GROUP 1	Low risk
CTV =	Prostate
PTV expansion =	0.5 cm
Dose/Fraction =	78–80 Gy in 1.8–2.0 Gy/fx[a]
GROUP 2	Favorable Intermediate Risk
CTV =	Prostate + proximal 1 cm of seminal vesicle
PTV expansion =	0.5 cm
Dose/Fraction =	78–80 Gy in 1.8–2.0 Gy/fx[a]
GROUP 3	Unfavorable Intermediate Risk
RT dose and volumes the same as for GROUP 4	
Androgen Deprivation Therapy: 4–6 months of ADT starting 2 months before initiation of RT.	
GROUP 4	High Risk (PSA ≥20 or Gleason ≥8 or T stage ≥T3)
CTV1 =	Prostate + proximal 2 cm of seminal vesicles or entire seminal vesicles of grossly involved
CTV2 =	Pelvic lymph nodes
PTV1 expansion =	0.5 cm
PTV2 expansion =	0.5 cm
PTV 1 Dose/Fraction	45.0–50.4 Gy in 1.8–2.0 Gy/fx
PTV2 Dose/Fraction =	78.0–80 Gy in 1.8–2.0 Gy/fx[b]
Androgen Deprivation Therapy: 24–36 months starting 2 months before, 2 months during, and 20–32 months after RT	

[a] At the University of California Los Angeles (UCLA) most low-risk and intermediate-risk patients can also receive LDR or HDR brachytherapy or SBRT. The minimum prostate dose for all patients receiving definitive external beam radiation therapy alone is 78 Gy unless there is a medical contraindication.
[b] At UCLA most patients receive LDR or HDR brachytherapy boost following whole pelvic irradiation to 45 Gy.

CTV, clinical target volume; PTV, planning target volume.

DRE and PSA no more frequently than every 6 months as changes in examination or PSA level may prompt patients to start therapy in anticipation of new symptoms.

Active Surveillance

In contrast to watchful waiting, active surveillance involves serial DRE, PSA, and surveillance biopsies with the expectation to intervene with definitive treatment at the time of disease progression. Active surveillance is an alternative to definitive treatment for younger men and low-risk disease. A prospective cohort from the University of Toronto is one of the most mature and comprehensive data sets to date to demonstrate the safety and feasibility of active surveillance. In this series, predominantly low (GS≤ 6 or PSA≤ 10) and select favorable intermediate-risk (PSA≤15 or GS≤ 3+4 = 7) patients underwent active surveillance, and were offered definitive intervention if PSA doubling time was <3 years, Gleason upgrade (to 4+3 or greater), or had unequivocal clinical progression. The 15-year estimate of prostate-cancer–

specific death was 5.6%, and the risk of death due to other causes in this cohort was 9.2 times greater.[74] The recently published UK ProtecT trial also found no all-cause or prostate-cancer–specific survival benefit, with early intervention compared to active surveillance.[75] This trial randomized patients with localized prostate cancer to either active surveillance, RP, or RT with concurrent ADT. While no survival benefit was found with early intervention, patients undergoing either RP or radiation and ADT had significantly less clinical and metastatic disease progression, compared to those under active surveillance. Thus, immediate radical treatment is effective in preventing disease progression but has not yet led to all-cause or disease-specific survival.

Radical Prostatectomy

Approximately 40% to 50% of patients select to undergo an RP initially.[76] RP involves removal of the prostate, the surrounding capsule, seminal vesicles, and the ampullae of the vas deferens. There are a variety of approaches to the procedure: retropubic, perineal, and laparoscopic, which may be robot assisted. The advent of the nerve-sparing RP in the early 1980s, increasing chances for retaining sexual potency, as well as more recent refinements in surgical techniques, such as laparoscopic or robotic RP, have ensured that RP remains a popular treatment option.

Prostatectomy results in a risk of impotence and at least some degree of urinary incontinence.[77,78] Nerve-sparing techniques may decrease these rates although most patients still report significant sexual dysfunction even following nerve-sparing RP.[77,79] More recently, there has been an increased use of surgery for high-risk localized (T3 disease, high GS or PSA) or locally advanced disease, which may necessitate a higher rate of adjuvant radiation for residual disease after nerve-sparing surgery. In a multi-institutional retrospective cohort study among men with Gleason 9-10 disease, 8.7% and 34.1% of men who underwent RP ultimately received adjuvant and salvage radiotherapy, respectively.[80] Though no completed prospective randomized trials have compared RP to RT, it appears that cure rates are similar.

External Beam Radiation Therapy

EBRT is commonly utilized to treat men with clinically localized or locally advanced prostate cancer. EBRT alone may be applied to any clinical stage—T1 to T4—but is also often used with ADT for selected higher-risk patients. EBRT is also utilized as either adjuvant or salvage therapy in the post-prostatectomy setting for patients with clinical high-risk features or with a rising PSA following RP.

In the past, EBRT for prostate cancer consisted of a 4-field box or bilateral 120° arcs that were delineated using bony landmarks or a single CT slice to include the prostate, seminal vesicles, and pelvic lymph nodes. Using these non-conformal techniques, prescription doses to the prostate were limited to 64 to 70 Gy due to significant volumes of normal tissues that were included in the irradiation field, in particular the small bowel and rectum. Conformal RT simulation, planning, and treatment became increasingly available in the late 1980s, and one analysis estimated that a 10% increase in minimum tumor dose could be achieved without increasing acute or chronic toxicity.[81] IMRT was introduced in the mid-1990s and is now routinely used for prostate cancer treatment. 3D planning and IMRT allows for the safe planning and delivery of dose-escalated RT over 74 Gy, which has shown to improve biochemical free survival.[12]

Androgen Deprivation Therapy

For high-risk prostate cancer patients, RT with long-term ADT is the standard of care. The question of ADT added to RT was first evaluated in a series of randomized trials of patients with locally advanced (T3–T4) or high-grade prostate cancer (Gleason 8 to 10). These trials ultimately showed that the addition of ADT to conventional dose EBRT improved biochemical control and decreased the risk for metastasis, death from prostate cancer, and all-cause mortality for these patients.[82–84] Earlier trials delivered <70 Gy of RT. However, the benefits of ADT remain in the era of dose-escalated radiotherapy ($\geq$70 Gy). For patients with the high-risk disease, 18 to 36 months of ADT along with dose-escalated conventional EBRT appears better than either EBRT alone or EBRT delivered with shorter duration ADT (4–6 months).[85–89]

For intermediate-risk prostate cancer, short-term ADT and RT are recommended. The role of ADT in intermediate-risk disease has been addressed in two randomized trials which suggest a benefit to shorter course antiandrogen therapy (4–6 months) when treated with a conventional dose RT of <70 Gy.[84,90] The role of ADT for patients treated with higher-dose RT is an area of active evaluation at this time and is the subject of RTOG 0815, and final results are anticipated. There does not appear to be meaningful benefit in cancer-specific or overall survival with short-term ADT in men with clinical low-risk disease by NCCN risk criteria even when treated with RT dose <70 Gy.[90]

Emerging data have shown improvement in at least a biochemical recurrence-free survival (bRFS) benefit, with the addition of ADT to salvage radiotherapy. RTOG 9601 compared salvage radiation therapy (SRT) with SRT + ADT with high-dose bicalutamide.[91] The study randomized post-RP patients with pT3N0 or pT2N0 with positive margins who developed elevated PSA from 0.2 to 4.0 ng/mL to RT + placebo (64.8 Gy in 36 fractions of 1.8 Gy) versus RT + ADT (24 months of bicalutamide, 150 mg daily). Twelve-year biochemical failure was 44% in the RT + ADT group versus 67.9% in the RT + placebo group. Actuarial overall survival rates at 12 years were 76.3% and 71.3%, respectively (hazard ratio for death of 0.77 with a two-sided $p = 0.04$). Twelve-year incidence of metastatic disease progression was lower in the RT +ADT compared to RT + placebo group ($p = 0.005$). The GETUG-AFU 16 trial also demonstrated improved 5-year bRFS with the addition of ADT, compared to radiation alone.[92] In this trial, post-RP patients with postoperative PSA between 0.2 and 2.0 ng/mL were randomized to RT alone versus RT + ADT (6 months of goserelin), where 66 Gy in 33 fractions were delivered to both groups. Five-year bRFS rates were 62% versus 80%, respectively ($p < 0.0001$). However, no overall survival difference was found in this trial. While the optimal duration of ADT is unknown, many clinicians have used the results of GETUG-AFU 16 trial to justify a shorter course of ADT to 6 months.

A recent re-analysis of RTOG 9601 data was presented at the American Society for Radiation Oncology (ASTRO)'s 61st annual meeting in Chicago suggested that post-RP patients whose PSAs were $\leq$0.6 ng/mL may not derive a survival benefit with ADT.[93] At the time when RTOG 9601 was conducted, it was standard to allow PSAs to rise to high levels prior to initiating salvage radiation. Contemporary practice has changed, and clinicians are initiating salvage radiotherapy at lower PSA levels. This re-analysis found that patients with post-RP PSAs of ≤ 0.6 ng/mL were actually twice as likely to die from other causes when ADT was added (HR for death was 4.14 among patients with very low PSA levels of 0.2–0.3 ng/mL). Identifying patients who benefit from ADT based on tumor genetics will be analyzed in the BALANCE/NRG GU-006 trial.

Brachytherapy

Interstitial brachytherapy alone is an appropriate definitive treatment option for low-risk and select intermediate-risk patients with intact prostates. Brachytherapy as monotherapy has several advantages over EBRT, including the convenience of undergoing a 1-day outpatient procedure, rapid dose fall-off outside the prostate, and less issues presented by organ motion during treatment planning and delivery. Prostate brachytherapy is also commonly used in combination with EBRT to 45 to 50.4 Gy, particularly for patients with adverse risk features to improve bRFS as brachytherapy provides dose escalation to the prostate while minimizing toxicities. The ASCENDE-RT study showed the 9-year bRFS was estimated to be 83% in EBRT + brachytherapy boost group compared to 62% with dose-escalated EBRT (78 Gy) alone for both intermediate risk ($p = 0.003$) and high-risk patients ($p = 0.048$). Despite improvements in this primary outcome, this trial was underpowered to find significant differences in overall survival and prostate-cancer–specific survival with brachytherapy boost. Other similar randomized trials of combination EBRT + HDR brachytherapy boost, compared to EBRT alone, have also shown improved biochemical and clinical recurrence-free survival.[94–96] Long-term data from RTOG 0321 of combination EBRT + HDR brachytherapy boost reported favorable 5- and 10-year survival of 95% and 76%, respectively, with relatively low late grade 3 or higher toxicity rates.[96] As risk of disease extending beyond the prostate capsule increases, other modalities should be considered for definitive treatment.

LDR radioisotopic implants are performed using I-125, Pd-103, or more recently Cs-131 seeds, which are placed transperineally through a template. HDR brachytherapy involves needle placement of catheters that are used for afterloading of an Ir-192 source. Brachytherapy performs comparably to surgery or EBRT for low-risk patients.

Some disadvantages with brachytherapy include the requirement for anesthesia and risk of acute urinary retention. Relative contraindications to brachytherapy include large prostate size (>60 cc), a prominent median lobe, or significant preexisting obstructive urinary symptoms, as these may be associated with technical difficulty in performing an adequate implant or increased risks of complications. A mounting body of literature also supports the use of salvage brachytherapy for locally recurrent prostate cancer after prior definitive RT, although results at this time are limited to single-institution experiences.[97–101]

Other Treatments

Other focal therapies such as cryotherapy and high-intensity focused ultrasound (HIFU) are alternative treatment options for both primary and salvage treatment for prostate cancer. Long-term data and efficacy are limited; therefore, these therapies are not recommended as routine to treat localized prostate cancer. Cryotherapy is a minimally invasive procedure that freezes cancerous tissue. For low-risk localized prostate cancer, 5-year bRFS has reported to range from 65% to 92%.[102] Cryotherapy has shown to have inferior bRFS for locally advanced disease (cT2c-T3) in a randomized trial comparing cryotherapy to EBRT alone, as well as worse sexual dysfunction.[103,104] For patients who present with localized recurrent disease after primary radiotherapy, focal salvage therapy has reported to yield a 5-year bRFS ranging from 46% to 54%.[105,106] Cryotherapy may be an option for patients with biopsy-proven recurrence after previous RT.

Utilization of HIFU for primary treatment for localized prostate cancer has also been explored. One multi-institutional prospective study of 625 men with predominantly intermediate to high-risk localized prostate cancer found the rate of 5-year failure free, cancer-specific, and overall survival were 88%, 100%, and 99%, respectively.[107] Ninety-eight percent of patients reported urinary continence during short-term follow-up. Like cryotherapy, HIFU is a viable treatment option for radiorecurrent prostate cancer. In a prospective registry study of 81 men, median bRFS was 63 months, and 5-year overall survival was 88%. 3.7% of men experienced grade 3+ rectal fistula and severe urinary incontinence.[108]

TREATMENT PLANNING FOR DEFINITIVE EXTERNAL BEAM RADIATION

Target Volume Definition

Prostate

The International Commission on Radiation Units and Measurements (ICRU) has defined volumes for treatment planning that account for the extent of the known gross tumor, the areas of likely microscopic extension, and daily variations in patient setup and tumor position. Definitions of GTV, clinical target volume (CTV), and planning target volume (PTV) are shown in Table 10.5. The prostate is most commonly delineated on a treatment planning CT. Use of MRI is recommended to aid in delineating the prostate gland, especially at the apical region.[109] In addition, the penile bulb is well defined on MRI.

TABLE 10.5   International Commission on Radiation Units and Measurements Designated Tumor Volumes and Definitions

Tumor Volumes	
Gross tumor volume (GTV)	The palpable or visible extent of the tumor
Clinical target volume (CTV)	Gross tumor volume plus a margin for suspected subclinical disease
Planning target volume (PTV)	Clinical target volume plus a margin to account for variations in size, shape, and position relative to the treatment beam

The GTV is the extent of gross tumor identified on DRE and imaging. CTV is the entire prostate and the proximal seminal vesicles. Additional margin is added to account for variation in daily treatment setup and organ motion to define the PTV. The amount of margin added to the CTV to define the PTV has been the subject of extensive study and discussion. While it is important to make margins generous enough to consistently encompass gross and microscopic tumor by the prescribed dose, there is also a compelling reason to keep the margins as small as possible near organs of limited tolerance, such as the rectum posteriorly and the bladder superiorly. In general, a PTV margin of 0.5 to 0.7 cm is added around the prostate (and seminal vesicles) to account for coverage of extracapsular microscopic tumor extension, setup variability, and organ motion when using a daily kV cone beam CT for treatment alignment. As an example, treatment guidelines from RTOG 0924 suggest that the PTV be defined as the CTV plus a 0.5 to 1.0 cm margin depending on institutional policy. These volumes are then used for treatment planning using either 3D-CRT or IMRT techniques.

The prostate should be contoured between the genitourinary (GU) diaphragm to the bladder neck without the surrounding pelvic muscles. Gold seed fiducials or Calypso beacon transponders are often utilized to improve the accuracy of daily patient setup. Three gold markers may be placed in different planes within the prostate transrectally. Daily prostate position can then be confirmed and positional adjustments made based on 2D alignments between digitally reconstructed radiographs (DRRs) with electronic portal imaging or 3D alignments between CT and kV cone beam CT.

Daily imaging for prostate localization includes daily cone-beam CT, ultrasound, radiographic imaging of implanted radiopaque fiducial markers, or electromagnetic transponders (Fig. 10.1).[110–115] Adjustments can then be made on a daily basis, ensuring accurate localization and targeting of the PTV at the start of treatment. These techniques fall under the category of a collection of adaptive RT practices termed image-guided radiotherapy (IGRT).[116]

Prostate movement and the margin necessary to compensate for it have been studied in detail. Ten Haken et al. reported maximal superior, inferior, anterior, and posterior prostate movement of 1, 1.25, 2, and 0.75 cm, respectively.[117] The overall average movement was 0.5 cm, most often in the anterior and superior direction, while the average left-to-right movement was <0.05 cm. Nevertheless, residual errors in prostate position of over 7 mm after pretreatment localization and adjustment of prostate position clearly demonstrate the influence of intra-fraction movement. In a limited trial using fluoroscopy, Dawson et al. demonstrated breathing-related movement of the prostate, which increased with the amplitude of the breathing cycle (deep breathing vs. shallow). Movement of the prostate even varied within the same patients based on prone or supine positioning, with greater movement observed in the prone position.[118] Just as observed by others, the magnitude of movement

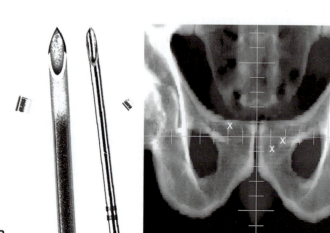
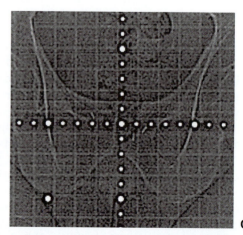

A, B   C

FIGURE 10.1. The position of the implanted markers, shown in a digitally reconstructed radiograph (DRR) can be used for daily localization of the prostate, shown with the proper alignment of a cone-beam CT scan.

was greatest in the anterior–posterior and cranial–caudal directions while minimal lateral movement was seen using non-IGRT techniques.[119,120] A recent clinical assessment of prostate displacement and its impact on PTV margins in setting of SBRT for definitive treatment reported similar values for both inter- and intra-fractional prostate motion.[6]

Seminal Vesicles

While the prostate gland is always in the CTV, a decision must be made as to whether the seminal vesicles and pelvic lymph nodes are included. The seminal vesicles are superior and posterior to the prostate gland, attaching at the base. The clinical risk factors of stage, GS, and PSA can be related to risk of seminal vesicle involvement, similar to lymph node risk.[121] Ninety percent of seminal vesicle involvement is limited to the proximal 2 cm, and therefore some argue that only the proximal portion of the seminal vesicles adjacent to the prostate needs to be included in the target volume.[122] Some advocate for the CTV to include the base of the seminal vesicles if the risk of seminal vesicle is less than 15% and for the CTV to include the entire seminal vesicles if risk of involvement is above 15%. To date, no study documents improved local control or survival if seminal vesicles are electively irradiated for the risk of clinically undetected microscopic disease; however, intuitively it seems important to include these structures in patients with unfavorable risk disease, so that likely potential sites of local disease in its entirety are treated. Including the seminal vesicles, lymph nodes, or both within the target volumes increases the field size and may potentially increase the acute side effects and long-term complications.[123] The RTOG 0924 clinical trial, which randomizes patients with unfavorable intermediate or favorable high-risk disease to high dose radiotherapy with or without whole pelvic radiation, required the entire seminal vesicles to be treated at least to 45 Gy in both arms and for the proximal 1.0 cm of the seminal vesicle tissue to be included in the boost target volumes.

Lymph Nodes

The benefit of pelvic lymph node irradiation has been a controversial topic over many years. Lymph node irradiation is not standard for low- or favorable intermediate-risk prostate cancer and is controversial for unfavorable intermediate- to high-risk disease.[124] Whole pelvis radiotherapy is generally recommended for T3-T4 tumors, GS 8-10, lymph node involvement, and seminal vesicle invasion. RTOG 9413 suggested that patients with a risk of lymph node involvement of at least 15% may benefit from pelvic lymph node irradiation. Patients were randomized to whole pelvic radiation versus prostate-only radiation, as well as to short-term neoadjuvant and concurrent ADT versus adjuvant ADT starting at the completion of RT. No statistically significant differences were found in progression-free or overall survival between the two study questions that patients were randomized

to: neoadjuvant ADT versus adjuvant ADT; and pelvic RT compared with prostate only RT. Nevertheless, a trend toward improved progression-free survival was found in favor of the pelvic and neoadjuvant ADT arm compared with the other three arms.[123] Additionally, when the size of the pelvic field was separately evaluated, it appeared that there was a direct benefit when using a whole pelvic field as compared to a mini-pelvic field or prostate-only treatment with 7-year progression-free survival of 40%, 35%, and 27%, respectively ($p = 0.02$).[125] The potential survival benefit of whole pelvic irradiation is the subject of RTOG 0924, which randomizes patients with unfavorable intermediate-risk disease and favorable high-risk disease to ADT with prostate-only irradiation or ADT with whole pelvis irradiation, and results are anticipated.

Current imaging technology, including CT, MRI, and lymphangiograms, has limited accuracy for detecting pelvic lymph node metastasis. Therefore, until improved methods for detecting pelvic lymph node metastases are developed, clinicians will be limited to using risk factor assessment and clinical judgment in deciding whether pelvic lymph nodes should be encompassed in the target volumes. The superior accuracy of PSMA PET scans in detecting pelvic nodal and distant metastasis over current standard-of-care imaging in both the biochemically recurrent and in the upfront setting holds potential to impact definitive treatment planning. One recent study used ^{68}Ga-PSMA PET/CT scans of 73 patients with intermediate-risk or higher localized prostate cancer to compare standard target volumes used during CT-based radiation planning with PSMA positive disease.[126] This study found that CT-based CTVs covered 94.5% of primary lesions but only 80% of pelvic lymph node lesions were detected on PSMA PET scans. Moreover, the median size of lymph node-positive lesions was 6 mm, which underscored that a proportion of lymph node metastases will be missed on the basis of size and morphologic criteria used on CT or MRI.

Accurate targeting is critically important if 3D conformal or IMRT-based treatment techniques are utilized to treat the pelvic lymph nodes, yet there is significant heterogeneity in how pelvic lymph nodes are contoured even amongst experienced GU radiation oncologists.[127] A consensus definition was established to make pelvic nodal volumes more uniform.[128] Based upon this consensus, the pelvic lymph node volumes to be irradiated include distal common iliac, presacral lymph nodes (S1–S3), external iliac lymph nodes, internal iliac lymph nodes, and obturator lymph nodes. Lymph node CTVs include the vessels (artery and vein) and a 0.7-cm radial margin without extending into bowel, bladder, bone, and muscle. Volumes begin at the L4/L5 interspace (recommended on RTOG 0924) and end at the superior aspect of the pubic bone. The treatment of presacral lymphatics is somewhat controversial as these nodes are infrequently problematic clinically and are rarely an isolated site of recurrence if left untreated. Therefore, they are not included in the standard pelvic lymph node dissection. Their inclusion in the radiation field necessitates that the posterior margin be expanded significantly, encompassing additional rectum and large bowel, and unless using 3D conformal or IMRT techniques may result in increased irradiation of the rectum with increased risk of acute and long-term side effects. The role of radiation in patients with known pelvic lymph node disease is less clear. However, as both RTOG 8531 and the European Organisation for Research and Treatment of Cancer (EORTC) studies of high-risk prostate cancer allowed positive pelvic lymph nodes at diagnosis, treatment of patients with positive lymph nodes with both irradiation and ADT is a reasonable course of action.[129,130]

Field Setup

Simulation, Immobilization, and Localization

Day-to-day setup variations can result in significant treatment errors.[131] Volumetric planning with CT simulation is recommended. CT images are obtained at 1- to 5-mm intervals through the levels to be encompassed within the treatment fields, though thin axial slices of 3 mm or finer are preferred.

Patients typically lie supine, with arms folded on the chest with a comfortably full bladder and an empty rectum. They are immobilized in the planned treatment position with a body mold with attention toward patient comfort and maximal daily reproducibility. Common options for immobilization include an Alpha Cradle, thermoplastic cast material similar to Aquaplast, and "vacuum lock" molds. Alternatively, for ease of position adjustment, some practitioners utilize supine position without an immobilization device if daily prostate localization techniques are employed. An advantage of the prone position is to shift the seminal vesicles forward, away from the rectum, potentially improving rectal sparing.[132] On the other hand, prone positioning may be associated with more internal organ motion, including respiratory motion particularly in men with any degree of obesity.[118]

Patients are asked to have a comfortably full bladder and empty rectum to minimize dose to critical structures. Intrarectal balloons may be expanded within the rectum to stabilize the prostate position, reducing the concerns over inter- and intra-fraction organ motion (Fig. 10.2). However, use of these devices may be inconvenient for daily treatment and somewhat uncomfortable for the patient. External marks are placed on the patient or immobilization device to designate a preliminary isocenter position. These locations may be delineated with radiopaque markers taped to the patient in the *x*, *y*, and *z* axes that can be referenced to the image set, facilitating the transposition of the isocenter from the treatment plan to the patient at the time of treatment.

Simulation involves a CT scan from the mid-abdomen to mid-femur. Superiorly, the scan should include L4-5 intervertebral disc level and the lesser trochanters interiorly. Contrast agents, such as IV contrast, a retrograde urethrogram, and oral contrast, are optional.

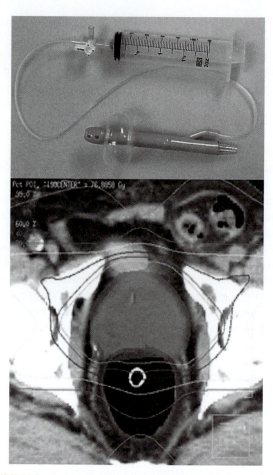

FIGURE 10.2. An intrarectal balloon device (*top panel*) can be used for stabilization of prostate position during external beam radiation therapy (*bottom panel*). Courtesy Dr. Mark Ritter.

MRI fusion with T2-weighted scans can also be done to provide better soft-tissue resolution of the apex, extraprostatic extension, seminal vesical invasion, and penile bulb. Target volumes and organs-at-risk (OARs) can then be delineated.

There are many options for image guidance, including cone beam CT, ultrasound localization system, or implanted fiducials. Selection of image guidance methods depends on patient factors and institutional experience. For instance, hip prosthesis may limit cone beam CT due to artifact. Many centers use daily imaging for prostate localization (Fig. 10.1). Adjustments can then be made on a daily basis, ensuring adequate localization and targeting of the PTV at the start of treatment.

Treatment Planning and Technique

Once the process of defining the patient positioning and localization have been determined, the process of treatment planning can commence. CT planning has now largely supplanted the setting of fields using 2D fluoroscopic techniques. Compared with the estimated general localization provided by bony landmarks in 2D planning, the size, shape, and location of the prostate and particularly the seminal vesicles can be visualized and defined

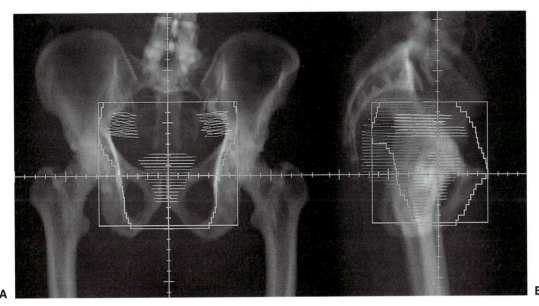

FIGURE 10.3. Digitally reconstructed radiograph (DRR) images are shown demonstrating typical anterior (**A**) and lateral (**B**) treatment fields encompassing the prostate, seminal vesicles, and regional pelvic nodes.

more precisely with CT planning. The seminal vesicles drape around the rectum in some patients, and standard blocking in 2D fields set using rectal contrast may not provide adequate coverage of these structures. Identification of the prostate apex on axial CT is sometimes difficult and may be facilitated with MRI or with sagittal and coronal reconstruction of CT data sets.

IMRT is currently the most common method of treatment planning for prostate cancer. For CT-based planning, CT images are entered into a treatment planning software package. The prostate, seminal vesicles, and lymph node regions are outlined by the physician, and can be expanded by adding appropriate margins to establish the CTVs and PTVs. Normal structures are outlined, including bladder, rectum, penile bulb, femoral heads, loops of small bowel, or any other structures to which the physician may wish to limit dose. RTOG 0924 recommends that the PTV margin be in the range of 0.5 to 1.5 cm, and depends on the institution's confidence in patient set-up and image guidance technique. The potential ability to use smaller PTV margins is a benefit with image guidance. If bladder fullness is inconsistent from treatment to treatment, superior and inferior margins may need to be more generous and accommodating. Examples of recommended OAR dose tolerances are provided in Table 10.6.[128]

Treatment planning software packages allow manipulation of virtual 3D reconstructions of these volumes, providing a variety of views for the planner, including bird's eye view perspectives (Fig. 10.3). These features are designed to allow the user to manipulate beam orientation (gantry, table, and collimator angles) and shaping (blocking or multi-leaf collimation) to encompass targets and avoid normal structures.

For forward-planned 3D CRT planning, high-energy beams from 6 to 10 MV are routinely used for pelvic lymph node and prostate irradiation. The software allows

rapid calculation of the dose that can be displayed on the overlying images in the form of isodose lines or surfaces (Figs. 10.4 and 10.5). Additional tools including dose–volume histograms (DVHs) help the clinician to compare treatment plans to determine the optimal plan for coverage of target volumes and avoidance of normal tissue structures (Figs. 10.6 and 10.7).

The application of IMRT technology to prostate cancer external beam planning has enabled further improvements in normal tissue DVHs, mainly due to the ability of this technology to achieve convex dose distributions, reducing rectal dose. The clinical significance of this advancement toward reducing rectal toxicity remains undetermined although some groups have suggested that with the combination of image guidance and IMRT, high-dose EBRT can be delivered without increases in toxicity compared to that observed in historical control groups treated to lower doses with less sophisticated techniques.[133] For instance, Zelefsky et al. noted an actuarial rate of grade 2 or greater rectal toxicity at 10 years of 13% in patients using 3D CRT and 5% using IMRT ($p < 0.0001$).[134] Of note, IMRT patients received higher doses of RT to target compared to 3D CRT patients, but IGRT was also used with much greater frequency in the IMRT group.

Inverse planning is a process that starts with the contouring of the target and normal tissue volumes on an axial CT image set—just as for 3D CRT planning. However, instead of inputting a candidate beam arrangement into the planning software and calculating a dose distribution for that plan, the IMRT software package uses an optimization algorithm to find a beam "solution" that minimizes a set of "cost functions." Typically, the process begins with a certain number of axial beam angles for the algorithm to utilize. Each beam is subdivided into square "beamlets" that represent the incremental movement of multi-leaf collimator leaves across the field in

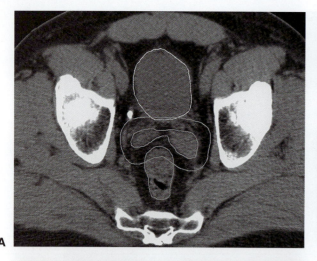

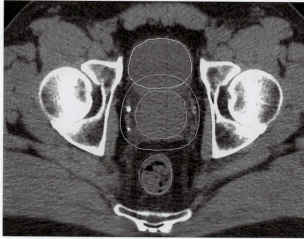

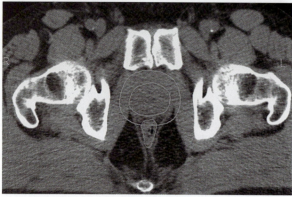

FIGURE 10.4. Three axial treatment planning computed tomography images are shown at the levels of the seminal vesicles (**A**), mid-prostate (**B**), and lower-prostate (**C**). The outlined clinical target volume (CTV) encompassing the seminal vesicles and the prostate is shown along with the planning target volume (PTV) expansion around the CTV. The normal bladder and rectum are also contoured.

1 cm or less increments. The algorithm "modulates" the fluence through each of these beamlets in an iterative process, evaluating and comparing each candidate plan to identify a better one. Each plan is evaluated for dose coverage of target volumes, as well as dose avoidance for normal tissue structures. Target coverage and normal tissue structure sparing are prioritized based on clinical judgment, and a cost for achieving or failing to achieve each objective is assigned. The algorithm will iterate until it identifies a plan that best achieves the stated objectives. Once the optimization algorithm produces a plan, a formal dose calculation is performed, and a quality assurance procedure is followed to ensure that the delivered dose will be within a desired level of accuracy. For the prostate, where the target shape and volume are relatively consistent from patient to patient, a template can be established to make the treatment planning process more efficient. Examples of typical dose constraints for rectum, bladder, femoral heads, and both large and small bowel are given in Table 10.6. The sparing of the penile bulb is controversial as different authors have come to differing conclusions about the utility of sparing the penile bulb in preserving sexual function.[135] However, it is clear that if a penile bulb dose constraint is observed that it should not be at the cost of decreasing dose to the PTV. Volumetric-modulated arc treatment plan (VMAT) is similar to IMRT in that radiation dose is modulated during treatment, but VMAT continuously delivers radiation while the treatment machine gantry rotates around the patient. An example of a volumetric-modulated arc treatment plan is shown in Figure 10.8.

In the past, the sharp dose gradients that was created using highly conformal techniques created a concern for missing the target due to inter- and intrafraction setup uncertainty and organ motion. However, careful delineation of treatment volumes, patient setup and immobilization, and implementation of IGRT ensure the accuracy of treatment delivery to minimize marginal misses due to setup error or changes in prostate position.

Dose Fractionation

Under conventional fractionation, prophylactic dose to the pelvic LN is 1.8 to 2.0 Gy/fx to 45–50.4 Gy, with a comedown boosts cover the prostate to at least 74 Gy (ideally 78–80 Gy). At UCLA, involved lymph nodes are typically treated to 60 Gy in 25 fractions, with consideration of normal organ dose tolerance. Dose escalation has shown to significantly improve biochemical cure rates. The rationale for IMRT versus 3D CRT is to improve conformality and to create steep gradients between the PTV and adjacent structures, namely the bladder and rectum. This is the motivation behind all forms of IMRT, such as step and shoot, sliding window, helical fan beam, and

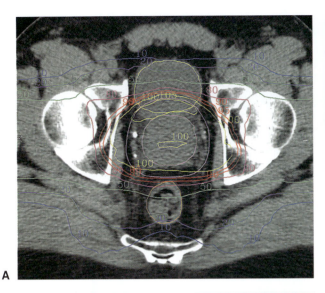

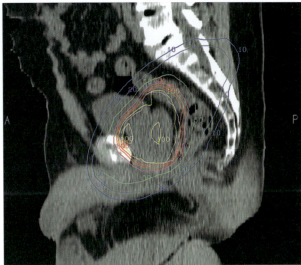

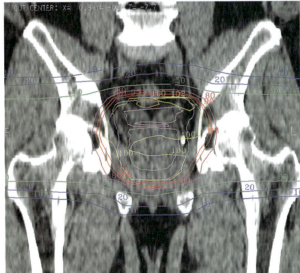

FIGURE 10.5. Axial (**A**), reconstructed sagittal (**B**), and coronal (**C**) computed tomography images are shown with contoured normal tissue structures (bladder and rectum) and target volumes (prostate and seminal vesicles). Isodose lines conforming to the planning target volume (PTV) are overlaid, depicting the dose distribution of a three-dimensional (3D) conformal radiation treatment plan.

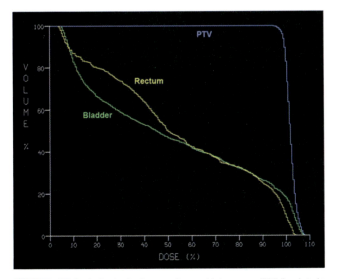

FIGURE 10.6. A typical dose–volume histogram (DVH) plot is shown for bladder, rectum, and planning target volume (PTV) from a three-dimensional (3D) conformal radiation treatment plan.

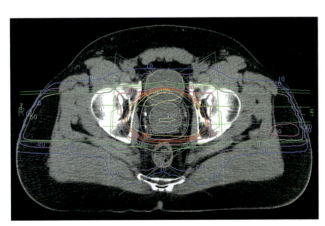

FIGURE 10.7. An axial computed tomography image with isodose lines is shown from a 3D-conformal radiation treatment plan utilizing a four-field technique with lateral and anterior inferior oblique beams.

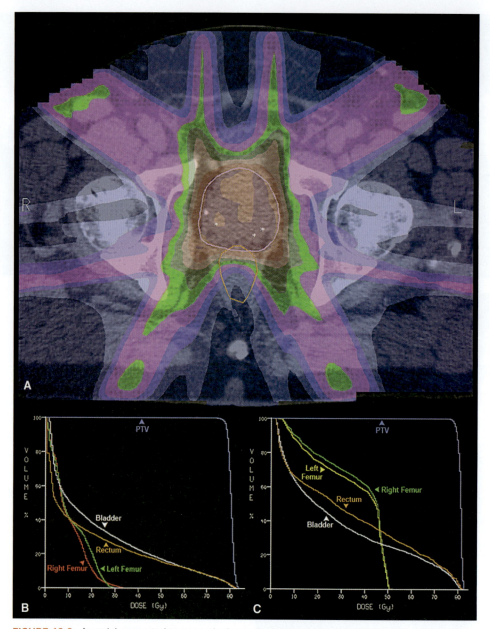

FIGURE 10.8. An axial computed tomography image is shown from a volumetric-modulated arc therapy (VMAT) plan. The dose distribution is demonstrated using a dose "color-wash" and depicts the concave dose distribution achieved for the rectum. This results in the improved normal tissue dose–volume histogram as compared with a four-field, 3D-conformal treatment.

VMAT. As advances in treatment techniques have allowed more conformal treatment of the target volumes with decreased dose to normal tissues, improved outcomes have been documented with increased doses of >74 Gy to the prostate. With the advent of 3D CRT, IMRT, and other highly conformal techniques, doses have been escalated without significant increases in acute side effects or late complications.[136]

Several randomized trials give strong evidence that dose escalation above 70 Gy may significantly improve prostate cancer biochemical cure rates. A landmark trial at MD Anderson Cancer Center compared 70 to 78 Gy using 3D CRT techniques treand found that patients receiving the higher dose had significantly improved bRFS, particularly

those patients with a pretreatment PSA above 10 ng/mL or with higher-risk clinical features.[137] Toxicity, however, was increased as a function of the volume of rectum treated to higher doses. Another significant randomized trial of dose escalation used a combination of external beam photon radiotherapy with a proton beam boost. Zeitman et al. reported that mostly low–intermediate-risk prostate cancer patients receiving 79.2 Gy had a 15% absolute reduction in the risk of biochemical recurrence at 10 years as compared to those receiving 70.2 Gy (32.4% vs. 16.7%).[9] Given the lack of biologic difference between protons and photons, there was no reason to presume that these results were unique to the use of a proton boost. Using this technique, although there was a slight increase in mild acute

TABLE 10.6	Dose Volume Histogram Constraints for Organs at Risk [a,128]	
Structure	**Dose**	**Volume**
Rectum	2 data points	
	50 Gy	≤50%
	70 Gy	≤20%
Bladder	2 data points	
	55 Gy	≤50%
	70 Gy	≤30%
Femoral Heads	50 Gy	<5%
Small Bowel	52 Gy	0% at or above
Large Bowel	Same as rectum	
Penile Bulb	No constraints	
Iliac Crests	No constraints	

[a] Dose constraints are based on conventional fractionation (1.8–2.0 Gy per day).

rectal toxicity, there was no significant difference in clinically substantial toxicity rates or patient-reported quality of life.[138] Most recently, results of NRG Oncology/RTOG 0126 with low-intermediate risk patients showed lower biochemical failure rates and distant metastasis rates at 8 years after receiving 79.2 Gy compared to 70.2 Gy.[139] At present, dose-escalated radiation has not resulted in clear differences in rates of prostate-cancer–specific death or overall survival. When dose-escalation is performed using conformal techniques, toxicity rates seem to be acceptable.[9,77,140]

The use of a smaller number of treatments delivered at a higher daily dose (hypofractionation) is being increasingly adopted. Hypofractionation has been suggested to improve prostate cancer control and decrease overall cost and treatment time, while still achieving acceptable long-term rates of toxicity. Recent reports have supported modest hypofractionation with daily fractions of 2.5 to 3.1 Gy as being efficacious without increased risks of toxicity.[141-145] Late toxicity data from moderate hypofractionation suggest favorable and similar rates of long-term urinary and bowel adverse events compared with conventional fractionated radiotherapy.[143-146] A summary of moderate hypofractionation trials is found in Table 10.7.

A number of reports have retrospectively analyzed biochemical control of prostate cancer using EBRT, LDR, or HDR brachytherapy, or the combination of these modalities.[147,148] Based on α/β corrections that take into account different radiation fraction sizes, it has been suggested that the α/β for prostate cancer is not actually in the range of 10 Gy (as commonly used for most tumor cells), but rather in the range of 1.2 to 3.0 Gy. Therefore, treating prostate cancer with larger fraction sizes, to an appropriate lower total dose yet equivalent biologic equivalent dose, would theoretically result in an increase in the therapeutic ratio. Thus, by using larger radiation fraction sizes, one might decrease overall treatment dose, time, and cost with a similar rate of late toxicity and an increase in expected biologic efficacy for prostate cancer.

Extreme hypofractionation with SBRT at doses in excess of 5 to 8 Gy delivered in four to five fractions has been reported from a number of single institutions' experiences.[149-152] In a recent pooled cohort study of 2,142 men

TABLE 10.7	Summary of Select Trials for Moderate Hypofractionation in the Treatment of Prostate Cancer				
Trial	**Patient eligibility**	**Hypofractionation**	**Conventional fractionation**	**Outcome**	**Toxicity**
Italian[144]	High risk	62 Gy at 3.1 Gy/fx	80 Gy at 2 Gy/fx	• 15% vs. 26% pts had biochemical failure after median f/u of 70 months • 5-year OS 92% vs. 82%	• 86% vs. 79% freedom from late ≥G2 GU toxicity ($p = 0.68$) • 86.5% vs. 84.6% freedom from late ≥G2 GI toxicity ($p = 0.57$)
Fox Chase[141]	Intermediate and high risk	70.2 Gy at 2.7 Gy/fx	76 Gy at 2 Gy/fx	• 5-year biochemical or clinical disease failure 23.3% vs. 21.4% ($p = 0.745$)	• No late GU or GI toxicity differences • If patients have IPSS>12, urinary function worse after hypofxn
RTOG 0415[142]	Low risk	70 Gy at 2.5 Gy/fx	73.8 Gy at 1.8 Gy/fx	• 5-year DFS 86.3% vs. 85.3% (HR 0.85, 95% CI 0.64–1.14) • 5-year BF 6.3% vs. 8.1% (HR 0.77, 95% CI 0.51–1.17)	• Late G2 and G3 GU and GI toxicities were significantly higher in hypofractionation arm

(continued)

TABLE 10.7	Summary of Select Trials for Moderate Hypofractionation in the Treatment of Prostate Cancer (*Continued*)				
Trial	**Patient eligibility**	**Hypofractionation**	**Conventional fractionation**	**Outcome**	**Toxicity**
CHHiP[143]	Intermediate and high risk	57 or 60 Gy at 3 Gy/fx	74 Gy at 2 Gy/fx	• 5-year bRFS 85.9% (57 Gy) vs. 90.6% (60 Gy) vs. 88.3% (74 Gy) • 60 Gy non-inferior to 74 Gy	• 5-year late ≥G2 GU events were 6.6% (57 Gy) 11.9% (60 Gy) vs. 9.1% (74 Gy) • 5-year late ≥G2 GI events were 11.3% (57 Gy) vs. 11.7% (60 Gy) vs. 13.7% (74 Gy)
PROFIT[145]	Intermediate risk	60 Gy at 3 Gy/fx	78 Gy at 2 Gy/fx	• 5-year bRFS was 85% (both arms) • 60 Gy non-inferior to 78 Gy	• Late ≥G3 GU toxicities were 3.0 vs. 2.1% • Late ≥G3 GI toxicities were 2.7% vs. 1.5%

bRFS, biochemical recurrence free survival; DFS, disease-free survival; Fx, fraction; G2/3, grade 2 or 3; GI, gastrointestinal; GU, genitourinary; HR, hazard ratio; hypofxn, hypofractionation IPSS, International Prostate Symptom Score; OS, overall survival; pt, patient.

across 10 single-institutional and 2 multi-institutional phase II trials of SBRT for low to intermediate-risk prostate cancer, 7-year cumulative rates of biochemical recurrence were 4.5%, 8.6%, and 14.9% for low, favorable intermediate, and unfavorable intermediate-risk patients, respectively. 7-year cumulative incidence of late grade 3 or higher GU and gastrointestinal (GI) toxicities were 2.4% and 0.4%, respectively.[11] As longer-term follow-up data for SBRT in prostate cancer ermerge, this technique is increasingly adopted for patients with low and intermediate-risk prostate cancers. At UCLA, we prescribe 40 Gy in 5 fractions to the prostate. A summary of select trials of SBRT for definitive treatment for prostate cancer is provided in Table 10.8.

TABLE 10.8	Summary of Select Trials for Extreme Hypofractionation or Stereotactic Body Radiotherapy (SBRT) in the Treatment of Prostate Cancer				
Trial	**Patient eligibility**	**Hypo-fractionation**	**EQD2 (α/β at 1.5)**	**Outcome**	**Toxicity**
SHARP trial, Madsen et al.[149]	Low risk	33.5 Gy at 6.7 Gy/fx	78.5 Gy	• Median time to PSA nadir 18 months • 2-year bRFS 90%	• No G3 toxicities • G1-2 Late GU toxicity 45% • G1-2 acute GI toxicity 37%
King et al.[150]	Low or favorable intermediate risk	36.25 Gy at 7.25 Gy/fx	90.6 Gy	• 4-year bRFS 94%	• After median f/u 2.7 years, 3% had G3 GU toxicity • None had G3 GI toxicity • Low-grade toxicities substantially less if tx given QOD vs. QD
Katz et al.[151]	Low to high risk	35.0–36.25 Gy at 7–7.25 Gy/fx	85–90.6 Gy	• 8-year DFS 93.6% (low risk) vs. 84.3% (intermediate) vs. 65.0% (high) • Unfavorable intermediate risk had similar outcomes as high-risk disease (7-year DFS 68.2% and 65%)	—
Meier et al.[152]	Low or intermediate risk	40 Gy at 8 Gy/fx	109 Gy	• 5-year DFS 97.3% (low risk) and 97.1% (intermediate) • Superior to historic controls ($p = 0.0008$)	• 1.2% (low) and 1.5% (intermediate) risk patients experienced G3 GU toxicity • No G4-5 toxicity

bRFS, biochemical recurrence-free survival; DFS, disease-free survival; EQD2, equivalent dose in 2 Gy per fraction; f/u, follow-up; fx, fraction; G1/2, grade 1 or 2; GI, gastrointestinal; GU, genitourinary; PSA, prostate-specific antigen; tx, treatment.

TREATMENT PLANNING FOR ADJUVANT OR SALVAGE EXTERNAL BEAM RADIATION

Adjuvant versus Salvage External Beam Radiation Following Radical Prostatectomy

Adjuvant radiation (ART) refers to immediate postoperative EBRT following prostatectomy due to the presence of high-risk pathologic features even with undetectable PSA. Three phase III randomized trials, The South West Oncology Group (SWOG) 8794, EORTC 22991, and ARO 96-02 support the use of ART.[153–155] These trials provide level I evidence supporting a decline in biochemical failure, metastasis, and prostate-cancer–specific death, with an improvement in overall survival with the use of ART.[153] SWOG 8794 randomized men (stage pT3N0M0 disease or positive surgical margins) to observation or ART arms where the radiation dose ranged from 60 to 64 Gy, with treatment portals included the prostatic fossa and para-prostatic tissues. With over 12 years of follow-up, the use of ART was associated with a 50% relative reduction in the risk of PSA recurrence in the ART group ($p < 0.001$). The use of ART yielded an absolute 10% improvement in metastasis-free survival at 10 years (71% vs. 61%, $p = 0.016$) and an 8% improvement in overall survival (66% vs. 74%, $p = 0.023$). Interestingly, the magnitude of benefit was similar for those with or without detectable PSA postoperatively although the utility of ART in context of ultra-sensitive PSA remains to be determined.[156] Two additional randomized trials support similar benefit in biochemical control of prostate cancer using ART although follow-up in these studies is insufficient to address more clinically meaningful endpoints.[154,155]

The role of salvage RT (SRT) for patients with a detectable and rising PSA after RP has not been evaluated in randomized trials (although certainly a significant portion of patients on both the SWOG and EORTC trials had detectable PSA at the time of irradiation and as such would be consistent with salvage therapy). In general, approximately 30% to 40% of patients given SRT will have long-term disease control. Preoperative, pathologic, and other clinical features have been utilized to construct a nomogram predicting the likelihood of PSA control, which was subsequently validated in a large multi-institutional data set.[157,158] A recent single-institution retrospective review of 1,106 patients receiving SRT from 1987–2003 demonstrated that early SRT significantly reduced the risk for 10-year biochemical failure, distant metastasis, and prostate cancer mortality.[159]

The balance between ART and early SRT remains to be determined. Early results from several randomized trials directly comparing ART with SRT have been recently emerging. The results of the RADICALS-RT (NCT 00541047) trial was presented at the European Society of Medical Oncology (ESMO) Congress 2019. This trial enrolled 1,396 patients after RP with postoperative PSA of <0.2 ng/mL with at least one of the following features: pT3/4 disease, GS 7-10, preoperative PSA ≥10 ng/mL, or positive surgical margins. Patients were then randomized to ART or early SRT, where 52.5 to 66 Gy in 20 to 33 fractions were delivered to the postoperative bed. After median follow-up of 5 years, progression-free survival 85% with ART vs. 88% with early SRT (HR 1.10, 95% CI 0.81-1.49, $p = 0.56$). Self-reported urinary incontinence and grade 3-4 urethral trictures at 1 year were worse in the ART arm. Overall rates were <5% for acute urinary toxicity and <1% for GI toxicity. The results of the RAVES trial were also reported around the same. This trial aimed to answer whether early SRT was non-inferior to ART with respect to biochemical failure.[160] Similar to RADICALS, patients were randomized to ART or early SRT, where 64 Gy in 32 fractions were delivered to the prostate bed. 8-year freedom from biochemical failure was 79% with ART and 76% with salvage RT (HR with respect to SRT was 1.03, 90% CI 0.65-1.63, $p = 0.91$). While both groups demonstrated freedom from biochemical failure, it did not meet protocol-defined levels of non-inferiority. Salvage radiotherapy did spare approximately half the men from pelvic radiotherapy, and was associated with lower levels of urinary toxicity. The GETUG-AFU 17 trial also aimed to compare ART to early SRT among men with pT3/4a disease or positive surgical margins after RP, but was closed early due to unexpectedly low event rates. While the study was under powered to find a significant difference in its primary endpoint, 5-year event-free survival rates were 92% and 90% in ART and SRT groups, respectively.[161] Fewer men in SRT experienced late grade 2 or worse GU toxicities and erectile dysfunction compared to those receiving ART. Therefore, SRT could spare men from over-treatment and untoward side effects from treatment. All three of these trials were included in the ARTISTIC meta-analysis, which used a prospective framework for adaptive analysis. This study analyzed 2,153 patients over median follow-up ranging from 60 to 78 months. Consistent with results from the aforementioned individual trials, event-free survival was high for both ART (89%) and SRT (88%) (HR 0.95, $p = 0.70$).[162] Early SRT remains to be the preferred treatment for men with biochemically recurrent prostate cancer after prostatectomy, as it gives men the opportunity to spare radiotherapy and treatment-related toxicities.

Target Volume Definition

Post-prostatectomy target volume delineation is subject to significant variation, especially in the posterior and superior aspects. Several target volume definition guidelines were created to improve interobserver variability. The randomized trials of ART in general utilized large fields and 2D treatment techniques; therefore, there was no need to precisely define target volume. Consensus guidelines have been published defining recommended anatomic boundaries of the CTV for RT delivered in the postoperative setting.[163–165] The definition of treatment volumes for ART or SRT for patients who have undergone previous RP is difficult as there is usually no palpable or visible disease on imaging to constitute a GTV. The vesicourethral anastomosis (VUA), periurethral, and perivesicular tissues should all be treated as these are the most common sites of recurrence following RP.[166,167] Some practitioners also encompass lymph node regions as described earlier, but pelvic nodal irradiation in the postoperative setting is controversial and will be addressed with RTOG 0534. Residual microscopic disease within the "prostate bed" is targeted by delineating the CTV at the preoperative location of the prostate and seminal vesicles. This can be accomplished using CT planning, and contouring an elongated "dumbbell-shaped" volume encompassing the plane between the posterior bladder and anterior rectum (Fig. 10.9).

Surgical clips remaining from prostatectomy, preoperative staging information, and postoperative pathology report information that are valuable in delineating the CTV.

The VUA can frequently be identified in relation to the urinary diaphragm on a CT scan sagittal reconstruction, ultrasound, or MRI. Given the prior location of the prostate at the level of the pubic symphysis, the region extending anteriorly to posteriorly from the pubic symphysis to the rectum should be included in the CTV. The most recent consensus guidelines only include the seminal vesicles if they were pathologically involved at the time of the surgical resection. If not including the seminal vesicles, the superior border should be either at or 0.5 cm above the cut of the vas deferens, or alternatively, at the level of the most superior surgical clip. In addition, ~1–2 cm of posterior bladder and bladder wall are also included to account for the shifting of the bladder into the space previously occupied by the prostate. The inferior border should be ~1 cm below the VUA; however, if there is concern that the initial prostate tumor may have been apical, then the inferior border of the CTV should end immediately superior to the penile bulb.[164] Lateral borders of the CTV should extend to the medial edge of the sacrorectogenitopubic fascia or the obturator internus bilaterally.

Advancements in imaging, such as F-18 fluciclovine and PSMA PET scans, have improved nodal or distant disease detection rates among men with biochemically recurrent disease after RP, and these imaging modalities are increasingly being utilized in this setting. With better ability to target disease detected on imaging, the paradigm in treating men with biochemically or clinically recurrent disease is evolving. For example, one study reported that PSMA PET directed therapy alone led to at least a 50% reduction in PSA for 80% of men with biochemical recurrence.[58] In a study from the University of California San Francisco, whose aim was to determine whether standard nodal radiation fields would cover areas of prostate cancer recurrence found on PSMA PET, the authors found that 30% of men would have nodal disease recurrence that would otherwise not be covered by standard pelvic nodal volumes.[168] A prospective survey conducted among physicians at UCLA revealed that the information gleaned from PSMA-PET scans altered treatment management decisions for over 50% of patients with biochemically recurrence.[169] Discovery of pelvic nodal or extrapelvic disease was significantly associated with changes in implemented treatment management. PSMAPET may soon impact the approach and treatment volume design for post-prostatectomy radiation in the near future.

Treatment Technique

Several IGRT methods have been developed to provide consistent localization of the prostate bed and reduce daily setup error, including Calypso beacon localization, daily portal imaging with implanted gold seed fiducials, ultrasound, and daily cone-beam imaging or kilovoltage imaging. The use of IGRT in the postoperative setting is not as clearly established as that in the definitive setting although the fundamental principles and rationale remain the same. These techniques are useful in detecting the location of the VUA, which, in turn, depends on variability in rectal and bladder distention. Similarly, use of IMRT in the postoperative setting has not been well studied at present. Given the somewhat poorly defined treatment volume that includes a large portion of bladder and rectum as well as the typically utilized RT doses of <70 Gy, the benefit of IMRT may be

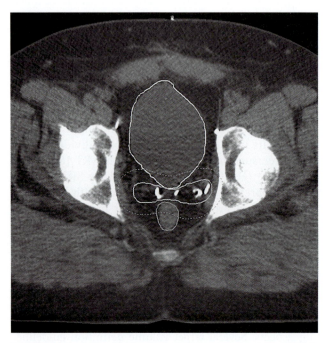

FIGURE 10.9. A "dumbbell"-shaped clinical target volume (CTV) is outlined to encompass the "prostate bed" between the bladder and rectum to facilitate treatment planning in the adjuvant or salvage situation after radical prostatectomy. Surgical clips are visible and also aid in defining the CTV.

limited. However, use of both IGRT and IMRT may allow dose escalation in the postoperative setting, which some have suggested will correlate with improvements in outcome just as it has in the definitive RT setting.[170]

Dose Fractionation

Doses of 64.8 to 70.2 in 1.8 to 2.0 Gy/fraction are used postoperatively. To date, there have been few studies investigating the role of dose escalation in the adjuvant or salvage setting. Ost et al. reported on the clinical outcome and safety of ART in 104 patients treated with IMRT and a median dose of 74 Gy.[171] The 3- and 5-year actuarial bRFS rates were 93%, a 20% gain as compared to the bRFS rate seen in the randomized trials with doses of 60 to 64 Gy. These results are limited by the study's retrospective nature, the short follow-up, and the impact of stage migration as compared to the randomized ART trials, which enrolled patients from the late 1980s to early 1990s. Despite the higher dose, acute and late toxicities were rare, with only 4% of patients experiencing late grade 3 toxicities (all GU). It is possible that the use of IMRT allowed dose distributions that partially spared the posterior and lateral rectal walls, thus minimizing late rectal toxicity. King et al. recently evaluated a series of retrospective reviews to assess the impact of RT dose on outcome in the adjuvant and salvage setting.[170] The authors found that the dose-response relationships were suggestive of a larger burden of disease for salvage patients with a detectable PSA and approximately one-tenth of this disease burden for adjuvant patients. They estimated an increase in the bRFS rate of ~3%/Gy over the range of 60 to 70 Gy. Of note, this is similar to the 2% to 3% improvement in biochemical event-free survival (bEFS) observed per 1 Gy increase in radiation in the four randomized trials of dose escalation for definitive radiation of the prostate. Most practitioners utilize RT doses ranging from 64.8 Gy to70.2 Gy in 1.8 to 2 Gy fractions.

Moderate hypofractionated RT has gained interest in the postoperative setting. A retrospective study comparing patients receiving a median dose of 65 Gy in 2.5 Gy per fraction vs. a median cumulative dose of 66 Gy with conventional fractionation did not demonstrate any differences in GU and GI toxicity with accounting for baseline function and similar biochemical progression-free survival with a median follow up of 38.6 months for all patients.[172] A phase 1-2 study of 124 patients receiving 62.5 Gy in 2.5 G per fraction to the prostate bed and 45 Gy in 25 fractions to the pelvic nodes demonstrated no acute Grade ≥3 GI toxicity and 0.8% grade 3 GU toxicity. Late grade ≥2 GI and GU toxicity were 1.1% and 7.3%, respectively. Five-year biochemical progression-free survival was 86.5%.[173] The phase III NRG-GU003 trial comparing hypofractionated versus conventional fractionation has completed accrual and is awaiting reporting of the primary endpoint evaluating patient-reported GI and GU symptoms.

TREATMENT PLANNING FOR BRACHYTHERAPY

Indications

Advances in brachytherapy techniques have made it a popular, effective, and safe treatment for localized prostate cancer. Compared to EBRT, brachytherapy implants follow the daily motion of the prostate, and dosimetry primarily depends on source arrangement within the prostate. Brachytherapy is categorized by dose rates defined in ICRU report 38. LDR brachytherapy ranges between 0.4 and 2.0 Gy/h, medium dose rate (MDR) between 2.0 and 12.0 Gy/h, and HDR above 12.0 Gy/h. Radioactive seed implant alone is effective in treating low-risk prostate cancer and indicated in select patients with intermediate-risk disease.[174,175] Men with larger, higher-grade tumors with higher PSA levels have a substantial risk of having disease outside the prostate. These patients may be best treated by a combination of EBRT and brachytherapy.[175] In a recent multi-institutional retrospective cohort study, dose escalation with combination EBRT and brachytherapy boost with ADT was associated with better cancer-specific mortality and time to distant metastases compared to RP or EBRT alone for men with Gleason 9-10 disease.[80]

While patient selection for brachytherapy is influenced by institutional practice and skills of the treating physician, caution is recommended for patients with a prostate size ≥60cc and bothersome urinary symptoms (IPSS ≥ 15), a TURP within recent 3 to 6 months, pubic arch interference, the presence of rectal fistulas, the inability to lie in lithotomy position, or the inability to undergo anesthesia.

Target Volume Definition

The clinical target volume is the prostate gland. Inclusion of the seminal vesicles and extracapsular areas depends on the patient's risk group, operator, and institution.

Localization and Treatment

The present era of low-energy permanent radioisotopic implantation for prostate cancer traces its origins to Scardino and Carlton at Baylor College of Medicine in the 1960s and Whitemore and Harris at Memorial Sloan Kettering Cancer Center in the 1970s, where an open, retropubic approach was used to perform implants using freehand placement of needles containing gold or iodine radioisotopes.[176] Unfortunately, this technique was associated with inhomogeneous dose distribution, inexact dosimetry, and disappointing local control and disease-free survival. By the mid-1980s, the retropubic technique was largely abandoned in favor of a transperineal approach.[177]

Soon thereafter, ultrasonography and a transperineal implant approach using a rigid template guidance system was developed.[178] Two ultrasound-based planning approaches are generally used, either a preplan designed with the prostate in treatment position or an intraoperative plan approach. With the preplanned technique, transverse TRUS images are recorded at 5-mm intervals from the base to the apex of the prostate gland using a stepping device attached to the ultrasound probe and the patient in the dorsal lithotomy position. The physician may evaluate the pubic arch during this procedure to determine any potential for bone interference with needle insertion. The ultrasound software projects the template grid over each successive prostate image. Typically, seven to nine images are displayed at 5-mm increments, and the prostate volume is contoured by the physician on each image. The prostate itself or the prostate with a margin of 2 to 5 mm around the prostate may be defined as the PTV. Various software packages can be used for planning a 3D implant volume, determining the number of needles, their placement according to template coordinates, and the number of seeds inserted per needle, prior to the actual implant.

With intraoperative planning, all these steps are performed in one setting in the operating suite, tailoring the plan to the individual. Without a preplan, there may be a risk of ordering too few or too many seeds; however, the intraoperative planning approach has the significant advantage in that the planning images are of the patient under anesthesia, minimizing discrepancies between the planning images and the actual anatomy and geometry. Furthermore, some treatment planning software packages now allow the users to register the location of sources as they are implanted and recalculate dosimetry in "real-time," allowing further adjustments and refinements to be made in the treatment plan to accommodate inaccuracies in needle placement and intraoperative prostate shift and swelling.

Seeds are usually spaced 0.5 to 1 cm apart in the transverse (right to left), anterior–posterior, and the superior–inferior planes. Computer-generated isodose curves predict the delivered dose, assuming the implant is completed as planned (Fig. 10.10). During the implant process each needle is guided to its predetermined position with the template placed against the perineum by the use of an on-screen template grid system and direct ultrasound visualization (Fig. 10.11).

The specified number of radioactive seeds is implanted from the base to the apex of the gland as each needle is withdrawn, using either individual seeds—seeds linked together with custom-assembled spacers—or fixed-space seeds embedded within a polymer strand cut to the desired length. After completion of the seed placement, cystoscopy or fluoroscopy may be utilized to assess for inadvertent seed localization within the bladder or urethra, and a Foley catheter may be placed. After anesthesia recovery and proper assessment of exposure rates outside the patient, most patients are safely released home and instructed to return for subsequent postimplant dosimetry studies.

A postimplant CT scan and dosimetry should be done on each patient to evaluate implant quality, thereby

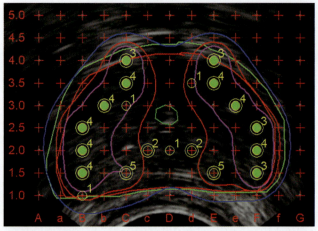

FIGURE 10.10. A typical preoperative or intraoperative prostate ultrasound is shown with the central urethra, prostate (clinical target volume), and prostate + 2 mm (planning target volume) contours. The loading positions and number of intended I-125 seeds to be implanted in each position are indicated at specific template coordinates, and the 290 Gy, 217.5 Gy, and 145 Gy isodose lines are shown. Courtesy of Dr. Vrinda Narayana.

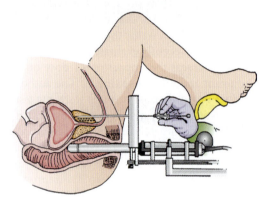

FIGURE 10.11. Transperineal prostate brachytherapy with transrectal ultrasound visualization and seed placement via needle insertion using template guidance.

detecting any consistent underdosing or inhomogeneities. The positions of all seeds are identified; the target and normal tissues are contoured (urethra and rectum at minimum, bladder neck, penile bulb, or neurovascular bundle). The CTV is the entire prostate for low-risk disease, with consideration of including proximal 1 cm of the seminal vesicles for intermediate risk or higher. A PTV margin could be considered to account for any uncertainties in the procedure (i.e., image registration). Dose distributions are calculated (Fig. 10.12). This allows calculation of various dose–volume metrics, such as the D_{90} and D_{100}, the doses that cover 90% and 100% of the prostate volume, respectively, as well as the V_{100}, the volume of the prostate receiving at least 100% of the prescribed dose. The reporting of these metrics is important in the medical literature to enable comparisons between treatment results and also for individual prostate seed brachytherapy programs to enable ongoing assessment of implant quality and correlation with disease and toxicity

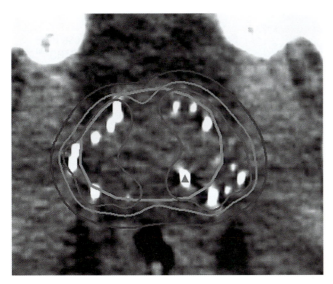

FIGURE 10.12. An axial computed tomography image is shown in a postimplant patient. Based upon the positions of the seeds and the contour of the prostate clinical and planning target volumes, one can assess the adequacy of the dose distribution, as shown by the overlaid 290, 217.5, and 145 Gy isodose lines. Courtesy of Dr. Vrinda Narayana.

Isotopes and Dose

Several isotopes have been used for prostate LDR—permanent interstitial prostate brachytherapy (Table 10.9). The most extensive experience with permanent interstitial, LDR implants has been with iodine-125 (I-125), which has been used for >40 years. Some radiobiologic evidence raised concerns that the dose-rate of ~8 cGy/h from I-125 was too low for prostate cancer doubling times, so palladium-103 (Pd-103), with a higher dose rate near 20 cGy/h, has been advocated.[179] Since the energy of Pd-103 is still low and similar to that of I-125, 21 versus 28 keV, this isotope retains the advantage of delivering a relatively low dose to surrounding organs and minimal exposure to the public. Clinical comparisons between the two isotopes have revealed no significant difference in biochemical control.[180] More recently, Cesium-131 has been FDA-approved for permanent prostate brachytherapy. Cs-131 has an energy (29 keV) similar to I-125, but a shorter half-life (9.7 days). Although early experience with this isotope has been positive, the follow-up is short, and there is no data to suggest superiority over I-125 or Pd-103.[181] Although given the shorter half-life of Pd-103 and Cs-131, these two isotopes may be associated with greater short-term urinary toxicity with the potential to also have earlier resolution of urinary irritative and obstructive symptoms.

The American Association of Physics and Medicine Task Group 43 (TG-43), published in 1995, altered the dose calculation algorithm used for I-125, and its recommendations have been broadly implemented.[182] As a result, prescription doses previously described as being 160 Gy have been lowered to 145 Gy as calculated under TG-43 with no change in implant activity, distribution, or geometry. This has consequently divided the prostate

outcomes. This enables any necessary adjustments to treatment techniques and procedures. Postimplant bleeding and edema can have significant effects on prostate volume. Given that this is a dynamic process, it can have significant implications for postimplant CT dosimetry. Practitioners may have varying preferences for the time interval between the implant procedure and when to perform postimplant dosimetry imaging, but it is important that implant programs remain consistent in their planning and dosimetry procedures to apply their dosimetry lessons toward quality improvement.

TABLE 10.9 Isotopes Used for Interstitial Prostate Implant

Isotope	Implant	$t\frac{1}{2}$ (days)	Time to 90% of Dose (days)	Energy (keV)	Prescription dose
Iodine-125	LDR	60.0	204	28	Monotherapy: 145–160 Gy Combination: 108–110
Cesium-131	LDR	9.7	33	30	Monotherapy: 100–115 Gy Combination: 70–80
Palladium-103	LDR	17.0	58	21	Monotherapy: 110–125 Gy Combination: 90–100
Iridium-192	HDR	74.0	—	380	See Table 10.10

Combination, combined therapy of external beam radiation to 40–50 Gy with brachytherapy.

HDR, high dose rate; LDR, low dose rate.

brachytherapy dosimetry literature into "pre-TG-43" and "TG-43" eras, an important consideration for clinicians' interpretation of older I-125 publications. Similarly, the dose for Pd-103 implant was 115 Gy before the National Institute of Standards and Technology 1999 Guidelines (NISTG-99) and 125 Gy afterward.[183]

Analysis of matched peripheral dose calculations within the Memorial Sloan-Kettering Cancer Center I-125 implant experience found that the 5-, 10-, and 15-year local relapse-free survival was 78%, 56%, and 30% among patients receiving doses of at least 140 Gy (126 Gy by TG-43), compared with 64%, 38%, and 21% among those receiving <140 Gy (126 Gy by TG-43).[177] Using modern transperineal prostate brachytherapy techniques with CT-based postimplant dosimetry, Stock et al. reported that patients receiving a D_{90} 140 Gy (using TG-43 criteria) had a 92% rate of 4-year biochemical control compared with only 68% for patients receiving a D_{90} < 140 Gy.[184]

Based on these experiences and others, the American Brachytherapy Society has published guidelines for transperineal permanent brachytherapy for prostate cancer, recommending prescription doses of 145 Gy (TG-43) for I-125 and 125 Gy for Pd-103 (after NISTG-99) as monotherapy.[185] For combination therapy, an EBRT dose of 40 to 50 Gy should be combined with 100 to 110 Gy (TG-43) I-125 or 90 to 100 Gy (NISTG-99) Pd-103 implantation. For Cs-131, an experienced group of users has developed consensus recommendations for prostate implantation, which includes a monotherapy prescription dose of 115 Gy and a boost prescription dose of 85 Gy, with special attention to urethral and rectal dosing.[181] Recommended dose prescriptions are summarized in Table 10.9.

Use of HDR iridium-192 (Ir-192) brachytherapy has become increasingly popular at many centers, either as monotherapy or as a boost in combination with EBRT. As with LDR brachytherapy, the HDR technique employs TRUS-guided transperineal placement of needles and catheters either via a template or by freehand, which is fixed to the perineum. Real-time, ultrasound-based dose planning software may be utilized. Planning may be accomplished using CT, ultrasound, or MRI images taken with the catheters in place. Targets and normal structures are contoured, and dwell times for source positions can be calculated to optimize delivery of the desired dose to the PTV while minimizing normal tissue dose. The hollow catheters can then be loaded by remote afterloading Ir-192 HDR unit either in single or in multiple insertions. Treatment is hypofractionated, generally using two or more large fractions delivered at dose rates of ~100 Gy/h. This is the main theoretical advantage of HDR brachytherapy and may result in a superior radiobiologic effect

TABLE 10.10	Summary of Published High-Dose Rate Dose Prescriptions from GEC/ESTRO[190]
HDR Monotherapy	**Combination EBRT and HDR Boost**
34–38 Gy in 4 fractions	*EBRT prescription*
31.5 Gy in 3 fractions	45 Gy in 25 fractions over 5 weeks
26 Gy in 2 fractions	46 Gy in 23 fractions over 4.5 weeks
	37.5 Gy in 15 fractions over 3 weeks
	35.7 Gy in 13 fractions over 2.5 weeks
	HDR Boost prescription
	15 Gy in 3 fractions
	11–22 Gy in 2 fractions
	12–15 Gy in 1 fraction

EBRT, External beam radiation; HDR, high dose rate.

compared with LDR brachytherapy, particularly for disease with adverse risk features.[80,186]

Although several centers and multi-institutional experience have been published on HDR brachytherapy, no randomized trials have compared outcomes of HDR monotherapy with modern dose-escalated EBRT.[187,188] A variety of dose and fractionation schedules have been reported.[189,190] A summary from Groupe Européen de Curiethérapie (GEC) and the European Society for Radiotherapy & Oncology (ESTRO) guidelines of published HDR dose fractionation schemas in both settings of monotherapy and combination with EBRT are shown in Table 10.10, as well as ideal dose constraints to OAR are shown in Table 10.11.

TABLE 10.11	Brachytherapy Planning Aims and Dose Constraints for Organs at Risk[190,279]	
	Low-dose rate implant	**High-dose rate implant**
Target aim	D90% > 90%–100% D100% > 100% V150% > 70% (<50% ideal)	D90% > 100% V100% > 95% (PTV)
Organ at risk		
Urethra	D5% > 150% D30% > 125%	D0.1 cc > 120 Gy (EQD2) D30% > 103 Gy (EQD2)
Rectum	V100% > 1.0–1.3 cc	D2cc > 75 Gy (EQD2)

PROGNOSIS

The likelihood of biochemical, local, and distant failure as well as disease-specific survival after RT for prostate cancer is related to tumor stage, grade, and pretreatment PSA level.[191–193] As discussed earlier, additional factors contribute to long-term prognosis, including radiation dose, the use of adjunctive androgen ablative therapy, PSA kinetics, and tumor volume. Posttreatment factors such as PSA nadir also have predictive value in estimating biochemical and distant failure.[194] Provider experience and treatment volume have also been demonstrated to influence the likelihood of recurrence and the need for salvage hormonal therapy for both brachytherapy and external beam radiation.[195]

At an RTOG symposium in Phoenix, numerous candidate definitions of biochemical failure were evaluated, and a definition was endorsed of the posttreatment nadir PSA plus 2 ng/mL as being the threshold for defining clinically meaningful biochemical failure after primary EBRT for prostate cancer.[195] The Phoenix definition was initially only defined for those receiving EBRT or brachytherapy with at most short-term androgen therapy.[196] However, others have suggested that it is applicable to those treated with EBRT along with long-term ADT.[197] Biochemical failure by the Phoenix definition has been demonstrated to correlate with patient survival although the risk of death from prostate cancer following biochemical failure is dependent upon both the clinical features of the cancer and patient's age, and as a result it is not a reasonable surrogate for patient survival in most patients.[197,198] Following biochemical failure patient risk group, the time to PSA failure and the PSA kinetics during failure may help further elucidate those patients at high risk of distant metastasis and prostate-cancer–specific mortality.[199–201]

Brachytherapy outcomes have also improved significantly with enhanced techniques, and multi-institutional and randomized trial data are now becoming available in the literature, which should provide more generalizable experiences as opposed to single-institutional case series, which are more prone to selection, individual practitioner experience/technique, and other biases. RTOG 9805 examined LDR monotherapy for patients with low-risk prostate cancer treated at 27 different institutions with I-125 LDR monotherapy to 145 Gy.[202] At 5 years, the biochemical failure-free survival rates exceeded 90%, which was comparable with other published brachytherapy series and with surgical or EBRT outcomes. Recently, a small Italian randomized trial comparing RP with LDR brachytherapy for low-risk patients showed no differences in 5-year bRFS rates between these two treatment modalities.[203] Brachytherapy patients were noted to have persistent increased GU irritative side effects, but superior urinary continence and erectile function compared with RP patients. ASCENDE-RT trial compared dose-escalated EBRT with EBRT with LDR brachytherapy boost for patients with high-risk disease.[204] EBRT was delivered to 78 Gy and minimum peripheral dose with I-125 was 115 Gy. Men randomized to the dose-escalated EBRT arm were twice as likely to experience biochemical failure compared to the combination EBRT and LDR brachytherapy arm. The estimated 9-year biochemical progression free survival was 62% for EBRT alone versus 83% in the combination therapy arm. While a biochemical failure difference was found, there was no evidence of improvement in overall survival with combination EBRT and LDR brachytherapy. RTOG study 0321 examined combined EBRT with HDR brachytherapy boost for patients with a slightly higher intermediate risk group of patients.[188] Treatment was delivered with EBRT to 45 Gy and two 9.5 Gy HDR boost fractions (total 19 Gy boost) within an overall treatment time of <8 weeks. At 29 months, the estimated rate of grade 3 through 5 GU and GI adverse events was 2.4%, demonstrating the feasibility of EBRT/HDR treatment in the multi-institutional setting and an acceptable level of adverse events. Finally, a prospective (but not randomized) study for intermediate to high-risk patients utilized ~9 months ADT with either 76 Gy EBRT as compared to 45 Gy EBRT with 18 Gy HDR boost given in two fractions and demonstrated a small but not statistically significant difference in 5-year bRFS between treatment arms. Lower rates of late grade 2 rectal toxicity in the HDR-treated patients were observed (13% vs. 3%, $p < 0.005$).[205]

CONCLUSION

Significant advances have been made in the treatment of prostate cancer with RT over the recent years that have resulted in improvements in disease control with decreased risks of toxicity and serious adverse impacts upon long-term patient quality of life. However, these advances have depended upon closer detail to the process of planning and delivery of RT to the prostate. The optimal selection of radiation modalities either alone or in combination and the timing and duration of ADT in this setting remain to be established. Nevertheless, RT is an attractive and viable treatment option for men with prostate cancer.

KEY POINTS

- Prostate cancer is the most common non-cutaneous malignancy in men in the United States and is the second-most common cause of cancer-related deaths in men.

- Clinical T stage, Gleason grade, and pretreatment PSA are the most important factors used for risk stratification.

- Definitive treatment involves treatment of the entire prostate gland.

- While the prostate gland is always in the target volume, a decision must be made as to whether the seminal vesicles and pelvic lymph nodes are included.

- There are many options for image guidance (IGRT), including CBCT, ultrasound localization system, or implanted fiducials.

- Post-prostatectomy target volume delineation is subject to significant variation, but the vesicourethral anastomosis (VUA), periurethral, and perivesicular tissues should all be treated as these are the most common sites of recurrence following RP.

- The prostate gland itself, with minimal margin, is the target for radioisotopic implant.

BLADDER CANCER

Introduction

Bladder cancers are fairly common cancers of the urinary tract, affecting 81,400 adults in the United States each year. It is the fourth most common tumor in men and the ninth most common cancer in women.[1] The majority of bladder cancers in the United States are transitional cell carcinomas (TCCs), while the majority in the rest of the world are squamous cell carcinomas. Curable bladder cancer can be conceptualized in several categories: (1) superficial and require superficial therapy (e.g., TURBT[transurethral resection of bladder tumor]), (2) muscle invasive—candidate for either radical cystectomy or bladder preservation (3) Muscle invasive—candidate for radical cystectomy but not bladder preservation (4) muscle invasive—ineligible for surgery. Radiotherapy plays a pivotal role in bladder preservation and can also be utilized in the postoperative setting. Radiotherapy is not used for superficial bladder cancers. This section will focus on patient selection and radiotherapy delivery for bladder preservation and postoperative radiotherapy.

CLINICAL ASSESSMENT

Risk Stratification

The most important assessment in the risk stratification of patients with bladder cancer is the depth of invasion of the primary tumor. Once bladder cancer reaches the muscularis propria, the risk of locoregional spread is much higher; thus, more aggressive definitive therapy is required. The risk of lymph node spread for superficial tumors is 5% or less compared to 20% for tumors that have reached the muscularis propria, and 20% to 40%

for tumors that have invaded beyond the muscularis propria.[206] Thankfully, the majority of bladder cancers are limited to the mucosal surface.

Muscle invasive TCC of the bladder can be curable, but unfortunately half of all patients with muscle-invasive disease will die of bladder cancer within 5 years regardless of therapy. Identifying optimal therapeutic options for these patients requires an understanding of the diagnostic studies that yield proper staging and risk stratification.

Diagnostic Studies and Staging

The classic presentation of bladder cancer is painless gross or microscopic hematuria, which occurs in up to 80% of cases. Urinary urgency, frequency, and dysuria without hematuria may occur in up to 30% of patients. Initial urologic evaluation must include urine cytology and cystoscopy with possible transurethral biopsy/TURBT during cystoscopy. If a suspicious lesion appears high-grade, solid, or muscle invasive on cystoscopy, further evaluation of the upper urinary tract, abdomen, and pelvis with a triphasic CT is recommended prior to TURBT for presence of more advanced disease, suspicious lymph nodes, or synchronous upper tract lesions. MRI of the pelvis could be considered for local staging. The purpose of TURBT is to identify the clinical stage and histologic grade of the disease, all while resecting all visible tumor. Specimens from TURBT should generally contain some muscles to properly evaluate for muscle invasion. If muscle invasion is discovered at the time of TURBT, the patient should have CT scan of chest and additional bloodwork.

The standard staging system utilized is the tumor, nodal, and metastasis (TNM) staging system (Table 10.12). The system is based on sub dividing patients into groups by the

TABLE 10.12   2018 American Joint Committee on Cancer (AJCC) Staging for Bladder Cancer (8th Edition)[40]

Primary Tumor (T)	
TX	Primary tumor cannot be assessed
T0	No evidence of primary tumor
Ta	Noninvasive papillary carcinoma
Tis	Carcinoma *in situ*: "flat tumor"
T1	Tumor invades lamina propria (subepithelial connective tissue)
T2	Tumor invades muscularis propria
T2a	Tumor invades superficial muscularis propria (inner half)
T2b	Tumor invades deep muscularis propria (outer half)
T3	Tumor invades perivesical tissue
T3a	Microscopically
T3b	Macroscopically (extravesical mass)
T4	Extravesical tumor directly invades any of the following: prostatic stroma, seminal vesicles, uterus, vagina, pelvic wall, or abdominal wall
T4a	Tumor invades prostatic stroma, uterus, vagina
T4b	Tumor invades pelvic wall, abdominal wall

Regional Lymph Nodes (N)

Nx	Regional lymph nodes cannot be assessed
N0	No regional lymph node metastasis
N1	Single regional lymph node metastasis in the true pelvis (perivesical, obturator, internal and external iliac, or presacral lymph node)
N2	Multiple regional lymph nodes metastases in the true pelvis
N3	Lymph node metastasis to the common iliac nodes

Distant Metastasis (M)

Mx	Distant metastasis cannot be assessed
M0	No distant metastasis
M1	Distant metastasis
M1a	Distant metastasis limited to lymph nodes beyond the common iliacs
M1b	Non–lymph node distant metastasis

Stage Grouping

Stage 0a	Ta	N0	M0
Stage 0is	Tis	N0	M0
Stage I	T1	N0	M0
Stage II	T2a–T2b	N0	M0
Stage IIIA	T3a–T4a	N0	M0
	T1–T4a	N1	M0
Stage IIIB	T1–T4a	N2, N3	M0
Stage IVA	T4b	Any N	M0
	Any T	Any N	M1a
Stage IVB	Any T	Any N	M1b

From Amin MB GD, Vega LR, Edge SB, Greene FL, Byrd DR, Brookland RK, Washington MK, Comptom CC. AJCC *Cancer Staging Manual*, 8th Edition. Chicago, IL: American College of Surgeons; 2018 reproduced with permission of SNCSC.

extent of local tumor invasion and the presence or absence of nodal or distant metastases. In this system, T-staging, based upon the depth of invasion of the primary tumor (T), conveys important prognostic information. The most useful assessment is whether the tumor is organ-confined (≤T2) or non–organ-confined (≥T3). The utility of available methods for determining the degree of muscle invasiveness preoperatively is modest with accuracy at most of 70% even with the combination of cystoscopic evaluation and TURBT when compared to pathologic examination following cystectomy. Determining the extent of muscle invasion at biopsy also requires adequate sampling of the bladder wall muscle. In addition to depth of invasion, other factors to be determined at the time of staging include the size and location of the lesion, the presence of carcinoma in situ (CIS), the histologic type, and the degree of differentiation. The majority (90%) of bladder cancers in the United States are transitional cell malignancies, and for these by consensus definition, the degree of differentiation is limited to low-grade and high-grade. With rare exception, muscle-invasive (T2 or greater) urothelial cancer is high-grade. Given the high incidence of multicentric disease, examination of specimens taken from clinically uninvolved areas of the bladder is also recommended.

TREATMENT OPTIONS

As mentioned earlier, bladder cancer is divided into superficial (Tis-T1), muscle invasive (T2), and more advanced disease (T3-4). Superficial cancers do not require surgery, systemic chemotherapy, or radiotherapy. They can be managed with TURBT, followed by superficial therapy with intravesicular mitomycin C or bacilli Calmette–Guerin (BCG). BCG is the preferred therapy for most superficial disease (Tis), papillary tumors (Ta), and tumors, confined to the mucosa (T1) of all grades (low and high). Mitomycin C can be used for low-grade, Ta tumors. Superficial tumors have a high recurrence rate of 50% or greater at 5 years. Many of these recurrences will progress to muscle invasion. Bladder conserving surgery using TURBT alone may be appropriate treatment for select early stage patients, particularly for patients who are poor candidates for aggressive interventions.[207]

TURBT is also a critical component of multimodality treatment strategies for more advanced disease, and the completeness of resection is an important predictor of local control and survival. Even for noninvasive disease, recurrence after TURBT alone is common, particularly for high-grade lesions.[208] Recurrence rates can be decreased by the use of weekly intravesical BCG for 6 weeks, resulting in 70% to 80% 5-year survival for T1 tumors.[209,210] However, many patients have difficulty completing the full course of BCG due to bothersome urinary frequency, cystitis, and dysuria.[211] With progression from T1 to muscle-invasive disease, radical cystectomy has been the standard recommendation; however, some would argue that at this point, organ-preserving therapy with radiation and chemotherapy may also be an option.[212,213]

Patients with muscle invasive cancer who are surgical candidates can be treated with either cystectomy with or without chemotherapy or with selective bladder preservation with TURBT followed by chemoradiation. No clinical trial has directly compared cystectomy to bladder preservation, but the data seems to indicate that overall survival rates are comparable.[206,214] Generally, the eligibility criteria for bladder preservation with TURBT and chemoradiotherapy are tumor size < 5 cm, unifocal, T2–T3, no CIS, complete TURBT, no hydronephrosis, good bladder function, and adherence close follow-up.

Non–Bladder Sparing Treatment Approaches for Muscle Invasive Disease

Five-year overall survival estimates in modern radical cystectomy series are approximately 50%. Radical cystectomy includes en bloc removal of the bladder, distal ureters, perivesicular fat, proximal urethra, prostate, seminal vesicles, and vas deferens in males. In females, the bladder, distal ureters, perivesicular fat, entire urethra, uterus, fallopian tubes, ovaries, cervix, and vaginal cuff are removed. Radical cystectomy may be followed by various reconstruction options, which is beyond the scope of this chapter.

Local control rates with radical cystectomy are high. However, the risk of pelvic relapse may approach 30% in patients who are found to have extravesicular extension (T3b) or positive lymph nodes, and may approach 70% in patients with positive margins.[215,216] These high locoregional recurrence rates generated interest in chemotherapy and radiotherapy in the adjuvant or neoadjuvant setting.

An approximately 5% overall survival benefit has been observed when neoadjuvant chemotherapy is utilized prior to radical cystectomy for patients with muscle-invasive bladder cancer.[217] Initially, dose-dense MVAC (methotrexate, vinblastine, doxorubicin, cisplatin) was the chemotherapy of choice in the neoadjuvant setting. However, gemcitabine and cisplatin have been shown to be equally effective and less toxic, and are alternatives for neoadjuvant chemotherapy.[218] It is worth noting that more than half of patients will have notable downstaging when neoadjuvant chemotherapy is utilized. More than one quarter may have a complete response. Responders to chemotherapy enjoy a higher overall survival, but they still require definitive therapy (chemoradiation or cystectomy). Adjuvant chemotherapy has also demonstrated disease-free and overall survival benefits in several studies, but neoadjuvant chemotherapy is favored because responders may be eligible for bladder-sparing approaches.[219]

A meta-analysis of five randomized trials did not show a benefit to preoperative radiotherapy compared to cystectomy alone.[220] Overall, preoperative radiotherapy is not commonly utilized because irradiated bowel is less suitable for ileal conduit reconstructions and the data behind neoadjuvant chemotherapy are stronger.

Interest in postoperative radiotherapy stems from the high rates of locoregional recurrence in the setting of pT3b-T4 or positive margins after cystectomy. The local recurrence rates in these situations are at least 30%.[215,221] Interest in postoperative radiotherapy is growing since adjuvant chemotherapy has not provided locoregional control benefit, nor are there any effective salvage treatment options. Recent trials have also suggested that improved locoregional control after adjuvant radiation and chemotherapy may also improve disease-free and overall survival benefits.[222,223] Approximately six trials are open or in development internationally to evaluate the benefit of postoperative radiotherapy. Additional trials determining the efficacy of postoperative radiation in combination with chemotherapy or immunotherapy may soon develop as well.[224] It is worth noting that postoperative radiotherapy to the pelvis after cystectomy would require a relatively large treatment field, which is likely to cause more bowel toxicity since pelvic organs are no longer displacing the small bowel from the true pelvis. In early adjuvant radiation studies from the 1970–1980s, close to 50%–60% of patients would experience significant long-term GI or stomal adverse effects due to a combination of using older radiation techniques and complications from cystectomy.[225–227] With more modern, conformal radiation techniques, significant late GI toxicities have lowered to 7%–36%.[223,228]

Bladder-Sparing Approaches for Muscle Invasive Disease

This section will focus on selective bladder-sparing techniques. There are two populations appropriate for this approach: (1) patients who are medically operable but would like to preserve their bladder rather than have radical en bloc removal of the bladder and surrounding GU/gynecological organs and (2) patients who are medically inoperable. For select patients in the first subgroup, selective bladder preservation with TURBT, followed by chemoradiation, is an appropriate treatment option. Definitive chemoradiation or radiation alone is recommended for the second subgroup of patients.

The history of bladder preservation strategies began as early as the 1980s, when investigators attempted to preserve the bladder. Definitive radiotherapy series demonstrated that half of the patients may be recurrence-free at 5 years, but overall survival was notably lower than cystectomy series, only 20% to 40%.[229–234] When investigators at the University of Paris noted a very high complete pathologic response rate

following combined maximal TURBT and neoadjuvant chemoradiotherapy (5FU/cisplatin), they attempted to elucidate what factors would allow patients to avoid cystectomy altogether.[235]

Investigators at the University of Paris, University of Erlangen (Germany), and Massachusetts General Hospital each developed bladder preservation strategies that involved TURBT, chemoradiation, and restaging cystoscopy at some point mid-way to two thirds of the way through chemoradiation to assess response. Non-responders were sent for cystectomy. Since then, there have been multiple RTOG trials published on selective bladder preservation (Table 10.14). The current treatment paradigm involves an initial maximal TURBT, concurrent cisplatin-based chemoradiotherapy to the entire pelvis up to 40 to 45 Gy with a cystoscopy 3 to 4 weeks later with biopsy. If the tumor has decreased to ≤T1, there are two options. The first of which is to boost the entire bladder with an additional 8 Gy, followed by boosting the tumor only with an additional 12 Gy. The second option is to boost the entire bladder with an additional 20 Gy. Target volumes and fields are described in a subsequent section.

Overall, contemporary series show equivalent 5-year overall survival when cystectomy is compared to selective bladder preservation (TURBT + chemoradiation) (Tables 10.13 and 10.14). In a pooled analysis of 5 RTOG bladder preservation trials, 5- and 10-year overall survival were 57% and 36%, respectively.[236] 5- and 10-year disease-specific survival were 71% and 65%, respectively, which is comparable to historic cystectomy series. Again, selective bladder preservation and radical cystectomy have never been directly compared in a randomized trial.

Functional outcomes after selective bladder preservation are excellent. In a recent analysis of late toxicity for 157 patients treated on 4 RTOG protocols revealed that there were no grade 4 toxicities or treatment-related deaths.[237] Further, only 7% of patients experienced late grade 3 or greater pelvic toxicity (6% GU and 2% GI), and the toxicities resolved in all but one patient. Overall quality of life after combined modality therapy is excellent for the majority of patients with only ~30% requiring a cystectomy. In

TABLE 10.13 Approximate 5-Year Relapse-Free and Overall Survival After Radical Cystectomy for Bladder Cancer by Stage[206]

Stage	RFS (%)	OS (%)
Ta–T1 N0	80–90	75–85
T2–T3a N0	75–90	65–75
T3b–T4 N0	50–60	40–50
Node+	30–40	20–30

RFS, Recurrence-free survival; OS, overall survival.

TABLE 10.14	Radiation Therapy Oncology Group (RTOG) Protocols for Muscle Invasive Bladder Cancer (1985–2009)[280,281]			
Protocol	**Induction Treatment**	**Number of Patients**	**Complete Response (%)**	**5-Year Survival (%)**
85–12	TURBT, XRT + Cis	42	66	52
88–02	TURBT, MCV, XRT + Cis	91	75	51
89–03	TURBT, +/- MCV, XRT + Cis	123	59	49
95–06	TURBT, 5-FU, XRT + Cis	34	67	NA
97–06	TURBT, XRT (BID) + Cis + adj MCV	52	74	NA
99–06	TURBT, Tax, XRT + Cis; adj Cis + Gem	84	81	56

addition, for those with a retained bladder, >75% are able to retain normal urinary function by urodynamic studies, and >85% with no bothersome urinary side effects.[238]

For patients who are not candidates for cystectomy or selective bladder preservation, chemoradiation or radiation alone is recommended. Locoregional recurrence is often high with radiation alone, and BC2001 trial demonstrated superior 2-year locoregional recurrence-free survival when patients with muscle-invasive bladder cancer were treated with concurrent chemoradiation with 5FU and mitomycin C compared to radiation alone (67% vs. 54%, respectively; $p = 0.03$). Of patients who developed local recurrence, significantly less proportion of patients developed invasive local recurrence after chemoradiation (11% vs. 19%, $p = 0.01$). However, this study was not powered to find improvement in overall survival. Interestingly, in an attempt to reduce treatment toxicity, subset of patients BC2001 was randomized to standard whole bladder radiation versus reduced high-dose volume radiation.[239] Rather than the entire bladder with 1.5 cm margin be irradiated to full prescription dose (64 Gy in 32 fractions or 55 Gy in 20 fractions), the reduced high-dose radiation group had this volume irradiated to 80% of prescription dose, and a smaller volume (GTV + 1.5cm) was treated to full dose. This trial did not demonstrate any improvement in 2-year local recurrence-free survival or late toxicity in the reduced high-dose radiation group. Overall, 2-year grade 3-4 late toxicities were low (5.4% vs. 2.4%), with minimal difference in bladder capacity.

The median age of patients diagnosed with muscle-invasive bladder cancer United States is 73 years. Concerns whether older patients would be able to tolerate potentially curative treatments (surgery, radiation, and/or chemotherapy) were raised, which led to undertreatment of older patients. In a propensity-matched retrospective review of patients (<75 years vs. ≥75 years old) with cT2-T4a disease treated with selective bladder preservation showed comparable disease-specific survival, emergency department visits during treatment, hospitalizations, and early discontinuation of treatment between younger and older patients.[240] Thus, clinicians should not deny patients from potentially curable therapies based on age alone. For older patients not suitable for cystectomy or daily radiation treatments, hypofractionated radiotherapy can be considered. In the recent HYBRID trial, treating the whole bladder to 36 Gy in 6 weekly fractions with image guidance yielded acceptable local control and toxicity.[241] Two-year cumulative incidence of local progression was 17%, and 1-year OS was 63% after. Rates of grade ≥3 late toxicity at 12 months was 4.3%.

Palliative Radiotherapy

Patients with advanced bladder tumors who are not eligible for cystectomy will often have metastatic disease. These patients may be managed with chemotherapy and reassessed for the appropriateness of concurrent chemoradiation. A randomized trial conducted in the United Kingdom randomized patients with advanced symptomatic bladder primaries to 35 Gy in 10 fractions or 21 Gy in 3 fractions. Sixty-eight percent of patients had symptomatic improvement and there was no difference between the two arms.[242]

TREATMENT PLANNING FOR BLADDER-SPARING APPROACHES

The traditional means of treating bladder cancer with external beam radiotherapy is a four-field box. There are several separate fields: (1) the whole pelvic field, (2) the bladder field, and (3) the final tumor boost. If selective bladder preservation is the goal, a treatment break for re-evaluation will take place after the whole pelvic treatment. If the patient is medically inoperable, the patient will not have a treatment break and continue to receive full course of chemoradiation.

Whole Pelvic Field

The whole pelvic field is typically treated with high-energy photons (6 to 15 MV) and a 3D conformal planning technique. The whole pelvic field in bladder cancer

AP and PA Fields   ## Lateral Fields

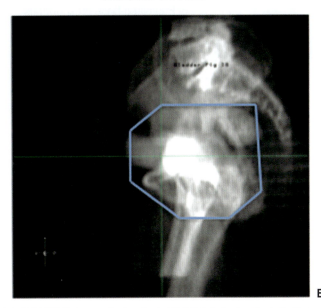

A   **B**

FIGURE 10.13. Whole pelvic fields for bladder cancer. Small/mini-pelvis field (45 Gy): superior border is S2/S3; inferior border is bottom of the obturator foramen. The border is 1/5 to 2.0 cm lateral to the medial aspect of the pelvic bone. Blocks can be used for the femoral heads. The lateral beams have the same superior and inferior borders as the AP/PA beams. The anterior field border is 1 cm anterior to the bladder or 1 cm anterior to the pubic symphysis, whichever is more anterior. The posterior border is 2.5 cm posterior to the bladder or any visible tumor. The whole bladder field (54 Gy) is the bladder with a 2-cm block margin. The tumor boost field (64 Gy) is a 2 cm expansion on the primary tumor (**A**). Bladder (**B**).

radiotherapy targets the external and internal iliac lymph nodes, the bladder, and the obturator lymph nodes, and provides a margin around the bladder and prostate. The common iliacs are not targeted because irradiation of bowel must be limited, and because the highest risk of nodal disease is in the external and internal iliac lymph node chains. Therefore, the superior border of all fields in the four-field box is at the mid-sacroiliac joint (approximately S2–S3 vertebral bodies). The inferior border of all four fields should adequately cover the prostate or in women the proximal 2 cm of urethra. In women, the inferior border should not be so low that the vulva is irradiated to a high dose. Therefore, the inferior border is at the bottom of the obturator foramen or 2 cm below the tumor, whichever is lower. The posterior border of the lateral fields is 2 cm posterior to the bladder and internal iliac lymph nodes. Up to half of the rectum should be blocked. The anterior border is 1 to 2 cm anterior to the external iliac lymph nodes and bladder. The lateral border of the anterior and posterior fields should extend 1.5 to 2 cm beyond the pelvic inlet. The whole pelvic field is treated to 39.6–50.4 Gy in 1.8 Gy per fraction. Per RTOG 0926, the whole pelvic field was treated to 41.6 Gy in 23 fractions. The femoral heads should be blocked to keep the total dose below 45 Gy. During the treatment of the pelvic field, patients can be treated with a full bladder to displace small bowel from the field. Point doses to the bowel should remain below

50 Gy. The volume of bowel receiving 45 Gy should be limited to less than 195 cc (Fig. 10.13).

IMRT with daily image guidance could be utilized. The GTV is the pre-TURBT tumor volume found on CT, MRI, or PET/CT (select cases). CTV would include the entire bladder, prostatic urethra, and prostate (men) or 2 cm proximal urethra (women), and regional lymphatics (obturator, internal iliac, and external iliac lymph nodes) up to the border of S1-2. PTV margin is 0.7 cm around the regional lymph nodes. PTV margins surrounding the bladder/prostate/urethra is anisotropically expanded by 0.5 cm, with exception of the superior aspect, which is expanded by 1.5 cm to account for daily variation in bladder size and position. This region is also be treated to 39.6–50.4 Gy.

Per NCCN guidelines, elective treatment to lymph nodes is optional for patient with no clinical lymph node involvement. From available evidence, there does not seem to be strong benefit in prophylactic nodal irradiation for clinically node-negative patients. In a randomized trial of whole pelvic versus bladder only irradiation, 5-year disease-free survival rates were comparable between the two groups (47.1% and 46.9%, respectively). Similar rates of bladder preservation and 5-year overall survival were also observed.[243] Furthermore, the rate of pelvic lymph node recurrences were low (5%) in the chemoradiation group in the BC2001 trial, which compared radiation alone versus chemoradiation for patients with T2-4N0 bladder cancer.

TABLE 10.15 Summary of Published Dose Prescriptions for Selective Bladder Preservation or Definitive Chemoradiation for Muscle-Invasive Bladder Cancer

Trial	Whole Pelvis	Bladder	Notes
RTOG*[281]	39.6–45 Gy	Boost to 60–65Gy	*See Table 10.14 for comprehensive list of trials. Dose prescription recommendation also includes RTOG 0926 (NCT00981656) RTOG 9706 and 9906 used hyperfractionated regimens. Others were conventionally fractionated
BC2001[282]	—	64 Gy in 32 fx 55 Gy in 20 fx	
HYBRID[241]	—	36 Gy in 6 weekly fx	Primarily reserved for older patients with poor performance status

Subsequent Boost Fields: Bladder Only or Bladder Followed by Tumor Only

Patients undergoing selective bladder preservation will have a treatment break after initial treatment to the pelvic fields. The patient can be simulated with an empty bladder during treatment of the bladder and/or tumor fields. Patients may have significant irritative voiding symptoms and urinary frequency after initial treatment to the pelvis, which may make treatment with a full bladder difficult. For the boost to the entire bladder or the tumor volume, an anisotropic expansion of 0.5 cm with exception to superior aspect (1.5 cm) around these structures would create the PTV$_{boost}$ volume. Coning down from the bladder to the tumor is advantageous because it may allow in minimizing radiation dose to normal bladder, which may impact subsequent bladder function. However, it should only be done if there is sufficient confidence that the original tumor will not be missed. Keep in mind that the dose of the final treatment is 60 to 66 Gy, which is the approximate tolerance for the whole bladder. A summary of common dose fractionation regimens is shown in Table 10.15.

TREATMENT PLANNING FOR ADJUVANT EXTERNAL BEAM RADIATION

Postoperative radiotherapy may be indicated for pathologic stage T3 or for positive margins. Consensus guidelines from RTOG were recently developed and validated for adjuvant radiotherapy.[244] Briefly if, there are positive surgical margins, the cystectomy bed, regional pelvic lymph nodes, and presacral lymph nodes should be treated to 45–50.4 Gy, with boost to 54–60 Gy to positive margins or extranodal disease. Alternatively,

if there are negative surgical margins but pT3 then one can forego radiating the cystectomy bed and just treat the regional pelvic lymph nodes, and presacral lymph nodes. Outlining the CTV for the cystectomy bed is described in Table 10.16.

FOLLOW-UP

Patients treated for muscle-invasive disease (stage T2 or greater) should be followed with urine cytology and cystoscopy every 3 to 6 months for 2 years, with imaging of the chest, upper tract, abdomen, and pelvis. If the patient has undergone cystectomy, urine cytology is still warranted to assess for abnormal cells from the upper tract or ureters.

PROGNOSIS

Survival from bladder cancer is largely determined by distant metastasis; therefore, ongoing prospective trials are focusing on incorporating novel combinations of cytotoxic chemotherapy, targeted agents, and immunotherapy. Radical cystectomy remains the standard treatment for muscle-invasive bladder cancer. It provides excellent rates of local control, and a 5-year survival that ranges from 30% to 90% depending on the extent of disease and risk for distant metastasis (Table 10.13). Multimodality treatment using TURBT, chemotherapy, and radiotherapy provides high rates of complete disease response, and survival that is comparable to radical cystectomy (Table 10.14). Furthermore, 60% to 70% of patients treated with multimodality, bladder-preserving treatment strategies are able to retain their native bladder, offering the potential of superior long-term bladder function and patient quality of life.

TABLE 10.16	**Radiation Therapy Oncology Group (RTOG) Consensus Anatomic Guidelines for Cystectomy Bed clinical target volume for Post-operative Radiotherapy[244]**
Superior	The contour extends 2 cm superior to the superior aspect of the pubic symphysis.
Anterior	The contour extends to the posterior aspect of the pubic rami/symphysis. Above and below the pubic symphysis, the contour stops anteriorly at the planes defined by extending lines superiorly and inferiorly from the posterior aspect of the symphysis.
Posterior	The contours abut the anterior one third of the external ano rectal circumference without extending into the ano rectum. Above the level of the rectum, the contour stops posteriorly at the plane defined by extending a line superior from the anterior border of the rectum.
Lateral	The contour extends to the medial border of the obturator internus muscles bilaterally. Inferior to the obturator internus muscles, the lateral border of the contour extends to the vaginal wall or the prostate bed.
Inferior	The contour stops 2–3 mm (1 axial CT slice) above the penile bulb for males and 1 cm below the lower pole of the obturator foramen for females.

KEY POINTS

- Bladder cancer is one of the most common cancers in adults in the United States: it is the fourth most common in men and the ninth most common in women.

- Most bladder cancers are superficial (Tis, Ta, T1) and require superficial therapy only with maximal TURBT and intravesicular therapy (mitomycin C or bacillus calmette guerin).

- One of the most important distinctions from a radiation oncologist's perspective is whether a patient has muscle-invasive ($\geq$T2) disease or not. Such patients should be treated with chemoradiation or cystectomy (unless metastatic).

- The factors that exclude medically operable patients from attempted bladder preservation include tumor size >5 cm, diffuse disease, inability to perform maximal TURBT, T4 disease, hydronephrosis, inability to tolerate chemotherapy, and metastatic disease.

- Selective bladder preservation refers to a strategy in which patients with a good or complete response noted

on cystoscopy after 40 to 50 Gy of chemoradiation to the whole pelvis continue radiotherapy for an additional 10 to 25 Gy to the bladder only. Non-responders are referred for radical cystectomy. Medically inoperable patients do not require a treatment break since there is no cystectomy salvage option.

- Complete response rates after TURBT and chemoradiation are 70% to 80%.

- There are no trials that directly compare cystectomy to chemoradiation. A 5-year overall survival for patients that are eligible for bladder preservation is approximately 50%, which is comparable to patients who undergo cystectomy.

- Eighty percent of the patients who survive 5 years will have an intact bladder. Most patients report satisfactory bladder function.

- Example dose constraints: Rectum V55 Gy <50%, bowel V45 <195 cc, femoral head D_{max} <50 Gy.

TESTICULAR CANCER

Introduction

Testicular cancer is the most common malignancy in men between the ages of 15 and 35 years.[1] Testicular cancer only accounts for approximately 1% of all malignancies in adults and <0.2% of all deaths. Between 1975 and 2004, the incidence of germ cell tumors increased by 71.9% in the United States for men 15–49 years of age. The incidence increased from 2.9 (1975) to 5.9 (2004) per 100,000 patients.

The most established risk factor for testicular cancer is a history of cryptorchidism, which increases the risk of testicular cancer five times.[245] Orchiopexy lowers the risk for developing testicular cancer. However, only 10% of patients with testicular cancer will have a history of cryptorchidism. Interestingly, cryptorchidism also increases the risk of cancer in the contralateral normally descended testis. Patients with a first-degree relative with testicular cancer are also at higher risk for developing this tumor. Testicular cancer is 5.4 times more common in white men compared to black men.

Germ cell tumors account for 95% of testicular cancers, of which they are divided into seminomatous and nonseminomatous germ cell tumors (NSGCT). The purpose of this chapter is to describe the treatment approach for stage I and stage II seminomas. NSGCT and later stage seminomas are treated with chemotherapy alone. NSGCT are once considered more dangerous than seminomas, and at one time were responsible for more than 10% of all cancer deaths in men aged 25 to 34 years. Today, NSGCTs are highly curable with platinum-based multiagent chemotherapy alone; therefore, radiotherapy plays a minor role for this subset of testicular tumors.[246] Radiotherapy is much more important in the treatment of seminoma. Some early stage seminomas have a prognosis so favorable that they may be treated with transinguinal orchiectomy alone. Patients who require treatment can enjoy a long life after treatment, increasing the focus on minimizing long-term sequelae of treatment.[247]

CLINICAL ASSESSMENT

The most common presentation of testicular cancer is a painless testicular nodule or mass.[245] Up to half of patients will actually have pain in the testicle at diagnosis. A detailed history and physical examination should be obtained, querying for history of cryptorchidism, and prior inguinal or scrotal surgery. A physical examination including testicular and abdominal examination should be undertaken. The normal pattern of nodal drainage leads directly from the testis to the para-aortic lymph nodes. In patients with a history of inguinal or scrotal surgery, the risk of aberrant drainage to the inguinal nodes may be increased, so this area should be examined. Transillumination of the testicle may distinguish between solid and cystic swelling of the scrotum. All patients should be referred for a testicular ultrasound. The characteristic appearance of a seminoma is a well-circumscribed hypoechoic mass.

Since more than half of all solid swellings of the testis are malignant, all patients with suspicious solid testicular masses should undergo radical inguinal orchiectomy to establish diagnoses. Patients with testicular cancer should undergo a CT scan of the abdomen to identify liver or infradiaphragmatic lymph node metastases. Chest imaging should be obtained to exclude pulmonary metastases.

Laboratory studies should include completed blood count, serum chemistry, and liver function studies. Serum lactate dehydrogenase (LDH), α-fetoprotein (AFP), and serum β-human chorionic gonadotropin (β-HCG) titers are prognostic and should be obtained. These serum markers also aid the clinician in distinguishing between pure seminoma and other germ cell tumors and are very useful in monitoring treatment response. AFP or β-HCG levels may be elevated in up to 90% of NSGCT. A modest elevation of β-HCG may be found in 15% to 20% of patients with pure seminoma, whereas an elevated AFP raises the suspicion of mixed tumor. The latter should be treated as nonseminomatous disease even if histologic evaluation does not support this finding. Elevation of these markers after treatment raises concern for residual or recurrent disease.

TREATMENT OPTIONS

During radical inguinal orchiectomy, there should be no violation of the scrotum, nor should the mass simply be biopsied. Patients can subsequently be managed based on their stage of disease. The AJCC staging system incorporates primary tumor, size of regional lymph nodes, presence or absence of distant metastases, and tiered levels of serum LDH, α-fetoprotein, and β-HCG (Table 10.17). Alternative staging systems exist, including the Royal Marsden Staging, which divides patients into stage I (confined to testis), IIA (<2-cm lymph nodes), IIB

TABLE 10.17	2018 American Joint Committee on Cancer (AJCC) Pathological Staging for Testicular Cancer (8th Edition)[40]
Primary Tumor (pT)	
pTX[a]	Primary tumor cannot be assessed
pT0	No evidence of primary tumor (e.g., histologic scar in testis)
pTis	Germ cell neoplasia *in situ*
pT1	Tumor limited to the testis (including rete testis invasion) without lymphovascular invasion
pT1a*	Tumor smaller than 3 cm in size
pT1b*	Tumor 3 cm or larger in size
pT2	Tumor limited to the testis (including rete testis invasion) without lymphovascular invasion *or* Tumor invading hilar soft tissue or epididymis or penetrating visceral mesothelial layer covering the external surface of the tunica albuginea with or without lymphovascular invasion
pT3	Tumor directly invades the spermatic cord soft tissue with or without lymphovascular invasion
pT4	Tumor invades scrotum with or without lymphovascular invasion

TABLE 10.17	2018 American Joint Committee on Cancer (AJCC) Pathological Staging for Testicular Cancer (8th Edition)[40] (*Continued*)

Primary Tumor (pT)

Regional Lymph Nodes (N)

NX	Regional lymph nodes cannot be assessed
N0	No regional lymph node metastasis
N1	Metastasis with a lymph node mass ≤2 cm in greatest dimension and ≤ 5 lymph nodes positive, none greater than 2 cm in greatest dimension
N2	Metastasis with a lymph node mass, >2 cm but not >5 cm in greatest dimension; or >5 lymph nodes positive, none >5 cm or evidence of extranodal extension of tumor
N3	Metastasis with a lymph node mass >5 cm in greatest dimension

Distant Metastasis (M)

M0	No distant metastasis
M1	Distant metastasis
M1a	Non-retroperitoneal nodal or pulmonary metastasis
M1b	Non-pulmonary visceral metastasis, microscopically confirmed

Serum Tumor Markers (S)

SX	Marker studies not available or not performed
S0	Marker study levels within normal limits
S1	LDH < 1.5 × upper limit of normal *and* hCG (mIU/mL) <5,000 *and* AFP (ng/mL) <1,000
S2	LDH 1.5–10 × upper limit of normal *or* hCG (mIU/mL) 5,000–50,000 *or* AFP (ng/mL) 1,000–10,000
S3	LDH > 10 × upper limit of normal *or* hCG (mIU/mL) >50,000 *or* AFP (ng/mL) >10,000

Stage Grouping

Stage 0	pTis	N0	M0	S0
Stage I	pT1–4	N0	M0	SX
Stage IA	pT1	N0	M0	S0
Stage IB	pT2–4	N0	M0	S0
Stage IS	Any pT/TX	N0	M0	S1–3 (measured post-orchiectomy)
Stage II	Any pT/TX	N1–3	M0	SX
Stage IIA	Any pT/TX	N1	M0	S0–1
Stage IIB	Any pT/TX	N2	M0	S0–1
Stage IIC	Any pT/TX	N3	M0	S0–1
Stage III	Any pT/TX	Any N	M1	SX
Stage IIIA	Any pT/TX	Any N	M1a	S0–1
Stage IIIB	Any pT/TX	N1–3	M0	S2
	Any pT/TX	Any N	M1a	S2
Stage IIIC	Any pT/TX	N1–3	M0	S3
	Any pT/TX	Any N	M1a	S3
	Any pT/TX	Any N	M1b	Any S

* Subclassification for pT1 applies only to pure seminoma.

[a] With exception for pTis and pT4, extent of primary tumor is classified by radical orchiectomy. TX may be used for other categories in the absence of radical orchiectomy.

LDH, lactate dehydrogenase; hCG, human chorionic gonadotropin; AFP, α-fetoprotein.

From Amin MB GD, Vega LR, Edge SB, Greene FL, Byrd DR, Brookland RK, Washington MK, Comptom CC. AJCC *Cancer Staging Manual*, 8th Edition. Chicago, IL: American College of Surgeons; 2018 reproduced with permission of SNCSC.

(2- to 5-cm lymph nodes), IIC (>5-cm lymph nodes), stage III (nodes above and below the diaphragm), and stage IV (extralymphatic metastases). There is also an International Germ Cell Cancer Collaborative Group (IGCCG) classification, which divides tumors into good prognosis (no non-pulmonary visceral metastases), intermediate prognosis (non-pulmonary visceral metastases), and poor prognosis.[247]

Stage I Seminoma

Patients with stage I seminoma enjoy a variety of options, including active surveillance, radiotherapy, and single-agent chemotherapy after radical inguinal orchiectomy.

Observation/Active Surveillance

Overall, several studies have shown that early stage patients who are observed after inguinal orchiectomy have a 15% to 25% risk of relapse at 5 years.[248,249] Withholding radiotherapy from these patients is advantageous because most of these patients would not relapse, and relapses are salvaged relatively easily. Observation protocols involve H&P and CT abdomen and pelvis scan at 3, 6, and 12 months during the first year, then 6 to 12 months for 2 and 3 year, then every 12 to 24 months for 4 to 5 years after diagnosis. CT chest is obtained only when clinically indicated, and serum tumor markers are optional during follow-ups. The decision to continue surveillance beyond five years is up to the discretion of the physician. The effect of multiple CT scans in this population has not been well studied, and the theoretical increase in the risk of secondary malignancy should be discussed.

A study published by Kaiser retrospectively evaluated 502 patients with stage I seminoma who were treated with active surveillance, chemotherapy, or radiotherapy after orchiectomy. Recurrence-free survival at 5 years was 97.2% to 98.3% in the radiotherapy and chemotherapy groups compared with 89.2% in the group of patients who were observed. The salvage treatment of relapsed seminoma is quite effective, resulting in no difference in overall survival or cause-specific survival between groups.[250] A study on a much larger group of 6,764 patients in the Surveillance, Epidemiology, and End Results database demonstrated that radiotherapy was associated with an improved cause-specific survival at 20 years with a hazard ratio of 0.37.[251] At 20 years, the difference in cause-specific survival was statistically significant, but quite small (cause-specific survival was 98.7% vs. 99.2%). The avoidance of medical expenses, time off from work, decreased sperm count, radiotherapy-associated fatigue, and increased risk of second malignancy is attractive to patients and oncologists. In fact, between 1998 and 2011, the rates of observation after orchiectomy increased from approximately 24% to 54%.[252] A subset of patients with stage I seminoma may be at higher risk of relapse, including those with larger tumors (>4 cm) and rete testis invasion.[253] A large group of researchers from Spain has published a nomogram that incorporates tumor size as a continuous variable and presence or absence of rete testis invasion.[254]

Radiotherapy

When patients are unsuitable for observation due to tumor factors (large tumors or tumors with rete testis invasion) or patient factors (patient choice, or inability to follow up with surveillance protocol), patients should be offered adjuvant treatment with chemotherapy or radiotherapy.

Chemotherapy

Single-agent chemotherapy with carboplatin is generally preferred over radiotherapy because it is associated with less long-term toxicity compared to radiation, and yields excellent prognosis. The rates of chemotherapy administration increased from 1.5% to 16%, while the utilization of adjuvant radiotherapy decreased from 71% to 29%.[252] The Medical Research Counsel TE19/EORTC 30982 trial, single-agent carboplatin (1 cycle, AUC 7) was compared to adjuvant RT in 1,447 patients for stage I seminomas treated with orchiectomy.[255] The majority of patients receiving radiotherapy had treatment to the para-aortic strip to 20–30 Gy in 2Gy per fraction. At 5 years, carboplatin was not inferior to adjuvant radiotherapy for stage I seminomas treated with orchiectomy, with recurrence-free survival rates ~95%. The number of contralateral germ cell tumors were also lower in the patients who received carboplatin compared to radiotherapy (0.3% vs. 1.7%). The most common sites of relapse after radiotherapy were outside of the radiation field (supradiaphragmatic or inguinal), whereas patients treated with carboplatin most commonly relapsed in the para-aortic nodes.

In summary, stage I seminoma has a very good prognosis. Some patients are at such low risk of relapse that observation is the optimal strategy. Relapses have good salvage rates, which makes observation an even more attractive option. For those patients who require adjuvant treatment to prevent relapse, either single-agent chemotherapy or adjuvant para-aortic radiotherapy are options. With radiotherapy, para-aortic lymph nodes are usually treated to 20 Gy in 10 fractions. With either treatment, relapse rates are approximately 5% at 5 years. Cause-specific survival for stage I seminoma remains >90% for all patients.

Of note, chemotherapy is preferred in patients with congenital horseshoe kidney. Horseshoe kidney is associated with aberrant lymphatic drainage, which makes traditional para-aortic and dog-leg fields possibly less efficacious. Furthermore, the presence of midline renal tissue would predispose the patient to high rates of radiation-induced nephritis.

Stage II Seminoma

Stage II seminoma is characterized by the presence of regional infradiaphragmatic lymph node involvement. Biopsy confirmation of lymph node involvement is generally not considered necessary. Seminoma is very sensitive to chemotherapy and radiation, so lymph node dissection is not part of the treatment for these patients. All patients with positive lymph nodes require inguinal orchiectomy, followed by adjuvant treatment with chemotherapy or radiotherapy.

Patients referred for radiotherapy usually have stage IIA and occasionally stage IIB disease. They should be treated with 20–25.5 Gy to the para-aortic and ipsilateral iliac lymph nodes (dog-leg field), followed by a boost to enlarged lymph nodes. Nodes less than 2 cm should be boosted to 30 Gy, and nodes of 2 to 5 cm should be boosted to 36 Gy or more.

Stage II with Bulky (>5 cm) Lymph Nodes

Patients with lymph nodes greater than 5 cm should not be managed with radiotherapy. Bulky lymph nodes portend a high risk of distant relapse; therefore, the standard of care for these patients is platinum-based, multiagent systemic chemotherapy.[256] Even in the presence of bulky lymph nodes, cure rates are nearly 90%.[257] The management of relapsed disease is similar to the management of bulky disease in that platinum-based multiagent chemotherapy is the preferred strategy. The efficacy of multiagent chemotherapy was demonstrated in the SWENOTECA study, where men with clinical stage IIB or higher disease were treated with four cycles of etoposide and cisplatin. No relapses were found in men with clinical stage IIB disease treated with chemotherapy, while 14.9% of patients who had clinical stage IIC experienced relapse.

Following chemotherapy for bulky node-positive disease, many patients will have residual disease detected on follow-up imaging.[258] Viable tumor cells were predominantly noted when residual mass was greater than 3 cm. Overall, approximately 50% of residual masses disappeared during surveillance, and patients are encouraged to have follow-up imaging until residual retroperitoneal mass resolves.[259] The data indicate that consolidative radiotherapy to residual masses does not decrease rates of relapse.[260,261] A surgical series from Memorial Sloan-Kettering Cancer Center indicates that in 55 patients with residual masses after chemotherapy who underwent retroperitoneal lymph node dissection, no patient with a residual mass less than 3 cm had viable tumor. Therefore, patients with residual masses less than 3 cm are typically observed.

TREATMENT PLANNING

Planning radiotherapy for seminoma requires knowledge of the typical patterns of disease spread. The right and left testes differ slightly in their lymphatic drainage.

The right testicular lymphatic trunks terminate in the sentinel nodes along the inferior vena cava and common iliac vein. The left testicular lymphatic trunks travel along the spermatic vein to drain into the lateral aortic nodes at the left renal vein pedicle. Right testicular lymphatics may cross over directly to the left PA nodes, but left testicular lymphatics generally cross to the right only after extensive involvement of the first station nodes. Tumor may spread in a retrograde fashion to nodes surrounding the vena cava and aorta. Further extension may occur via the thoracic duct to the left supraclavicular region or by the transdiaphragmatic lymphatics to the mediastinum. Although the primary drainage is to the retroperitoneal area, some lymphatic channels may also drain to the iliac lymph nodes. Normal lymphatic drainage may be altered if the patient has had an orchiopexy, herniorrhaphy, or other surgical procedures in the pelvis or inguinal region. Early tumor involvement of the epididymis increases the risk of external iliac nodal involvement.

Most published data on radiotherapy for testicular cancer utilizes opposed anteroposterior fields with megavoltage photons.

The most common site of lymph node metastasis is the para-aortic lymph nodes.[262,263] Therefore, traditional radiotherapy fields have encompassed the PA nodes and ipsilateral pelvic nodes.[264,265] Under usual circumstances, pelvic nodal involvement occurs in only 2% to 3% of patients. A British trial published a comparison of the para-aortic field to the traditional dog-leg field in 478 men with stage I seminoma.[266] The total dose was 30 Gy in 15 fractions. Acute toxicity was less common and less severe in the patients treated with para-aortic radiation only. Sperm counts were also significantly higher in men on the para-aortic radiotherapy arm. There was no difference in relapse rates between patients treated with para-aortic compared to combined para-aortic and dog-leg fields. As a result, patients with stage I seminoma who are treated with adjuvant radiotherapy are often treated with para-aortic fields only.

In stage II patients, the para-aortic and ipsilateral pelvic nodes should be treated, and if the para-aortic disease is bulky, consideration may be given to including the contralateral pelvic nodes. Although in the past inguinal nodes and the orchiectomy incision have been treated, more recent information indicates that this may be unnecessary, even if the inguinal area has been violated by surgery. Surveillance studies have shown an extremely low risk of relapse at these sites; therefore, adding the hemiscrotum and inguinal nodal region to the treatment portal is normally not required and should be avoided if possible because of the resulting significant dose to the remaining testicle.[267] Patients with a history of inguinal or pelvic surgery were also thought to be at risk for altered lymphatic drainage, and it has been recommended that the treatment fields be altered to include the pelvic nodes.[268] However, several authors challenge this practice since recurrence rates in surveillance studies are extremely low.[265,269]

The contralateral, remaining testis should be placed in a scrotal shield to minimize radiation and prevent azoospermia.

IMRT can be used to irradiate the at-risk areas, but the combination of multiple beams vastly increases the amount of tissue that receives low doses of radiation. The effect of such a large volume irradiated to a low dose is very important to consider in this group of young patients. Generally, anteroposterior opposed fields are the preferred means to irradiate the lymph nodes.

RADIATION TREATMENT FIELDS

Para-Aortic Fields for Stage I

In patients with no history of pelvic or scrotal surgery and stage I disease, the para-aortic lymph node region may be treated with equally weighted AP/PA fields. The fields should target the retroperitoneal lymph nodes but not necessarily the ipsilateral renal hilar nodes. Preferably, one should contour the aorta and inferior vena cava from the bottom of the T11 vertebrae to the bottom of L5.

The superior border should be placed at the bottom of the T11 vertebral body. The inferior border will be placed at the bottom of the L5 vertebral body. The lateral borders should encompass the tips of the transverse processes of the vertebrae, which is approximately 10 cm wide. For left-sided testicular cancer, ensure the left renal hilum is included in the field. The para-aortic field is depicted in the left panel of Figure 10.14.

In patients with stage II disease the treatment volume should be a para-aortic field with ipsilateral dog leg. The superior border of the para-aortic field should be placed at the bottom of the T11 vertebral body. The inferior border of the dog-leg field should be placed at the top of the acetabulum. The medial border of the dog-leg field extends from the contralateral transverse process of L5 to the medial border of the ipsilateral obturator foramen. The lateral border of the lower aspect of the dog-leg field is delineated by a line from the top of the ipsilateral transverse process of L5 to the superolateral border of the ipsilateral acetabulum. The dog-leg field is depicted in the right panel of Figure 10.14. For patients with a history of ipsilateral inguinal surgery, where the lymphatics may have been disrupted, the ipsilateral inguinal nodes and the inguinal scar should also be targeted.

Alternatively, fields can be delineated volumetrically. Wilder et al. suggests creating a para-aortic CTV by expanding the contoured vena cava by 1.2 cm and aorta 1.9 cm while excluding bone and bowel.[270] The dog-leg

AP Para-aortic Field

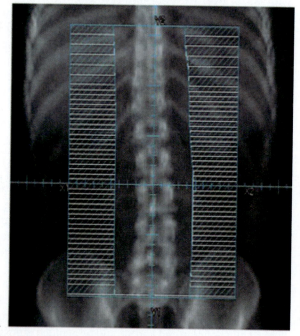

AP Dog-leg Field

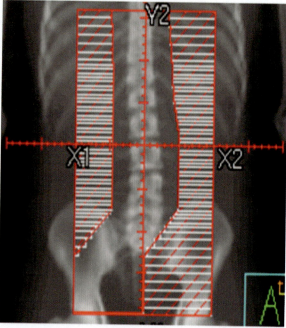

FIGURE 10.14. Example of filed arrangement based on bony landmarks. AP Para-aortic field. The superior border is T11; the inferior border is L5. The spinous processes of the vertebral bodies are covered **(A)**. AP dog-leg field used for stage II seminoma **(B)**. The common and external iliac vessels are treated down to the upper border of the acetabulum. If gross nodes are present, nodes should be identified on computed tomography-based planning and treated with a 0.8-cm GTV to CTV expansion.

CTV is created by expanding the contoured ipsilateral iliac vessels (common, internal, and external iliac vessels) by 1.2 cm also excluding bone, and bowel. The superior is the T11/T12 interspace, and inferior border is the top of the acetabulum. Again, for patients with a history of ipsilateral inguinal surgery, where the lymphatics may have been disrupted, the ipsilateral inguinal nodes and the inguinal scar should also be targeted. The CTV for involved lymph nodes is a 0.8-cm 3D expansion excluding bone, and bowel.

Dosage and Fractionation

Dosage for Stage I

In addition to field size reduction, randomized data supports reducing the dose of radiotherapy from 30 to 20 Gy. The MRC TE 18 non-inferiority trial randomized 625 patients to 20 Gy in 10 fractions or 30 Gy in 15 fractions to the para-aortic strip from T11 to L5.[271] At 2 years, the relapse rate in both arms was 3% to 4%. There was no difference in relapse rates at longer follow-up. There was only one death from seminoma in the study. There was significantly less acute fatigue in the 20 Gy arm, but this difference disappeared by the twelfth week. At Princess Margaret Hospital, 25 Gy in 1.25 Gy daily fractions has been used for more than two decades without an in-field recurrence.[272]

Dosage for Stage II

Stage II seminomas treated with radiotherapy should receive 20 to 25.5 Gy to the entire para-aortic and dog-leg field with a boost to 30 Gy for involved lymph nodes (stage IIA) or 36 Gy (stage IIB), which can be delivered concurrently or sequentially.

PROGNOSIS

Successful treatment of germ cell tumors offers the potential for many years of productive life following treatment. Treatment results vary significantly with tumor histology and disease stage (Table 10.18). Pure seminoma, even when metastatic to retroperitoneal nodes, can be cured in the majority of patients. Stage I seminoma is associated with a 15% to 20% risk of relapse when treated with orchiectomy alone; however, virtually all recurrences can be successfully salvaged, and disease-specific survival approaches 100%.[263,272] For stage I disease treated with inguinal orchiectomy and infra-diaphragmatic radiation approaches, relapse rates are approximately 3% to 4%.[255,265,269,271] Virtually all recurrences will be outside the irradiated area, and again, nearly all recurrences are successfully salvaged, most by systemic chemotherapy.

TABLE 10.18	Outcome Following Primary Radiation Therapy for Early Stage Seminoma and Chemotherapy for Bulky or Advanced Stage Seminoma[247,276]	
Stage	Post-orchiectomy Treatment	5-yr Progression-Free Survival (%)
I	Radiotherapy	95–100
IIA, IIB	Radiotherapy	85–95
IIC and III (M1a)	Chemotherapy	~80
III (M1b)	Chemotherapy	~70

Relapse rates for stage II patients depend on the bulk of disease and are higher than for stage I disease, yet are still only in the range of 5% to 15%. Nonetheless, due to excellent salvage options, post-orchiectomy radiotherapy results in disease-specific survival rates above 90%.[273–275] Patients with bulky disease treated with cisplatin-based chemotherapy still have excellent survival rates, with long-term survival possible even in advanced metastatic disease.[275,276]

Because of the success in treating testicular cancer, increased attention is paid to the long-term sequelae resulting from treatment, particularly impaired fertility, secondary malignancies, and cardiac disease. Men with seminoma commonly have impaired spermatogenesis at baseline; however, use of proper radiotherapy techniques is critical to minimize dose to the remaining testicle and preserve fertility. Second malignancies are increasingly recognized as a significant problem after radiotherapy and/or chemotherapy for testicular cancer, perhaps occurring in close to 20% of patients treated for testicular cancer.[277] Current trends toward increased use of surveillance in selected patients and avoidance of mediastinal irradiation should decrease the rates of these serious late effects. In addition, the adoption of smaller volumes and lower doses of RT is predicted to significantly reduce the risk of second malignancy following RT without compromising long-term survival.[278]

The relatively indolent course, predictable patterns of early progression, and marked sensitivity to both radiation and chemotherapy make seminoma one of the most curable malignancies. Testicular germ cell tumors have become a model for curable cancer, with cure being the goal of treatment while optimizing the risks of late effects even in advanced disease. Clinical outcome and survival for nonseminomatous disease are slightly less than that expected for seminoma, but with cisplatin-based treatment, it is still quite good.

KEY POINTS

- Testicular cancer is the most common cancer in males of age 15 to 35 years. It is more common in Caucasian males.

- Testicular cancer is divided into NSGCTs and seminomas. Seminomas almost never have a positive α-fetoprotein (α-FP or AFP).

- Radiotherapy is most important as adjuvant treatment for early stage I and IIA seminomas.

- Stage I seminomas require radical inguinal orchiectomy followed by observation, para-aortic radiotherapy, or single-agent chemotherapy.

- Primary tumors >4 cm and tumors with rete testis invasion may not be appropriate for observation. Stage IIA/B seminomas with regional lymph nodes ≤5 cm require adjuvant para-aortic and pelvic radiotherapy or chemotherapy and are not eligible for observation.

- Lymph nodes larger than 5 cm are associated with a high risk of distant metastases. These patients should be treated with inguinal orchiectomy and adjuvant multiagent systemic chemotherapy without radiotherapy.

- Following multiagent chemotherapy, residual disease measuring less than 3 cm in size may be observed.

- At 5 years, overall survival for stage I, stage II, and stage III seminoma is 100%, 97%, and 85%, respectively.

- For stage I seminoma, treat with 20 Gy in 2 Gy fractions. For stage II seminomas, treat the entire field to 20 to 25 Gy, followed by a boost to a higher dose for positive nodes to total of 30–36 Gy. Alternative fractionation schemes can also be used.

REVIEW QUESTIONS

1. The NCCN guidelines recommend pelvic imaging with CT or MRI in clinically localized prostate cancer when the probability of lymph node involvement is greater than
   A. 5%
   B. 10%
   C. 15%
   D. 20%

2. A bone scan is recommended in which of the following scenarios?
   A. T1c and PSA 15
   B. Gleason 4+3
   C. T2b
   D. T2 and PSA 11

3. What are the usual prescription doses for prostate brachytherapy (monotherapy) using I-125 and Pd-103, respectively?
   A. 125 Gy and 145 Gy
   B. 110 Gy and 90 Gy
   C. 145 Gy and 125 Gy
   D. 125 Gy and 110 Gy

4. Which radioisotope is used in HDR brachytherapy?
   A. I-125
   B. Pd-103
   C. Cs-131
   D. Ir-192

5. RTOG pelvic nodal consensus CTV contours for high-risk prostate cancer include which lymph nodes?

   A. Presacral, distal common iliac, internal and external iliac, obturator
   B. Para-aortic, presacral, distal common iliac, internal iliac, obturator
   C. Presacral, distal common iliac, internal iliac
   D. Para-aortic, presacral, distal common iliac, internal and external iliac

6. What is the next most appropriate management for a patient who has had a cystoscopy with biopsies revealing an incompletely resected muscle-invasive bladder carcinoma in the background of diffuse carcinoma *in situ*?
   A. Intravesicular BCG
   B. Neoadjuvant chemotherapy and radical cystectomy
   C. Taxane-based chemotherapy and radiation
   D. Induction chemotherapy, followed by concurrent chemotherapy and radiation

7. What percentage of patients who survive selective bladder preservation strategies with TURBT and chemoradiation will have an intact bladder?
   A. 15%
   B. 25%
   C. 70%
   D. 80%

8. The initial pelvic radiotherapy field for a bladder cancer being treated with bladder-sparing chemoradiation is designed to include which of the following?

A. Inguinal lymph nodes, obturator lymph nodes, and prostate in men.
B. Obturator lymph nodes, proximal 2 cm of the female urethra, and common iliac lymph nodes.
C. Prostate, bladder, obturator lymph nodes, internal iliac lymph nodes, and external iliac lymph nodes.
D. External iliac lymph nodes, internal iliac lymph nodes, and common iliac lymph nodes.

9. What clinical stage is a patient with a large tumor with extension into the perivesicular tissues without invasion of adjacent organs who also has three positive lymph nodes in the obturator and internal iliac lymph nodes?
A. T2bN2
B. T3aN2
C. T3bN3
D. T4aN1a

10. Which of the following is the most appropriate next step in management for a patient who has had a TURBT revealing a high-grade papillary urothelial carcinoma without muscle invasion?
A. Observation
B. CT of the abdomen to look for nodal disease
C. Intravesicular mitomycin C
D. Intravesicular BCG

11. A 20-year-old man presents with a painless unilateral swelling. Inguinal orchiectomy reveals a 1-cm seminoma without rete testis invasion. CT of the abdomen demonstrates three 2-cm lymph nodes in the para-aortic chain. There are no visceral metastases noted and no lymph nodes above the diaphragm. Which of the following is the best course of management? The patient wishes to conceive with his fiancée in the near future, so he is concerned about fertility.
A. Observation with CT scans of the chest, abdomen, and pelvis every 4 months.
B. Single-agent carboplatin with follow-up imaging to monitor for resolution of positive nodes.
C. Retroperitoneal lymph node dissection to prevent radiation toxicity and chemotoxicity to the remaining testis.
D. Radiotherapy to the para-aortic and pelvic lymph nodes, and sperm banking.

12. A 40-year-old man who had a 4-cm pure seminoma with rete testis invasion and several enlarged para-aortic lymph nodes underwent chemotherapy. Two months after treatment, CT abdomen and pelvis reveals residual 1.5 cm retroperitoneal lymph node. Serum AFP and β-HCG were normal. Which of the following is the most appropriate management option?
A. Retroperitoneal lymph node dissection if the disease is PET positive
B. Observation
C. Consolidative radiotherapy to the residual disease with a 1 cm margin
D. Two additional cycles of chemotherapy

13. What is the risk of nodal relapse for patients with stage I seminoma who opt for observation after a radical inguinal orchiectomy?
A. <5%
B. 15%
C. 40%
D. 80%

14. Which of the following is true regarding studies comparing 20 versus 30 Gy adjuvant radiotherapy for patients treated with inguinal orchiectomy for stage 1 seminoma?
A. Patients who underwent radiotherapy with 30 Gy had a higher risk of late side effects, including fatigue.
B. Patients who underwent radiotherapy with 30 Gy had a lower risk of pelvic relapse, compared to patients treated with 20 Gy.
C. Patients were treated with para-aortic radiotherapy only in both arms.
D. The relapse rate at 2 years exceeded 5% in the 20 Gy arm.

15. What is the Royal Marsden staging classification for a 3-cm seminoma with rete testis invasion and a β-HCG level of 6000?
A. Stage I
B. Stage IB
C. Stage III
D. Stage IS

ANSWERS

1. B The NCCN recommends pelvic imaging for any patients with localized prostate cancer who have clinical risk factors that incur a 10% or higher probability for micrometastatic disease outside the prostate gland (i.e., pelvic lymph nodes or distant metastasis). Pelvic imaging can be done with either CT or MRI. Reference: National Comprehensive Cancer Network.

Prostate Cancer (Version 3.2020). www.nccn.org/professionals/physician_gls/pdf/prostate.pdf.

2. D A bone scan is recommended in the initial evaluation of patients who are at risk for skeletal metastases. Patients who are considered to have such increased risk include intermediate-risk (T2 and PSA >10), high-risk, very-high-risk localized prostate cancer, or symptomatic patients. Bone scan often refers to technetium-99m-MDP bone

scan in which technetium is taken up by bone that is turning over. Sites of increased uptake suggest accelerated bone turnover/remodeling, which could indicate metastatic disease. Based on one large North American population-based study, the sensitivity of bone scans in detecting osseous metastasis was 90.8% and specificity was 76.3%. Reference: Preisser F, Mazzone E, Nazzani S, et al. North American population-based validation of the National Comprehensive Cancer Network Practice Guideline Recommendations for locoregional lymph node and bone imaging in prostate cancer patients. *Br J Cancer.* 2018;119(12):1552–1556.

3. C   The ABS recommends prescription doses of 145 Gy (per TG-43) for I-125, and 125 Gy for Pd-103 (per NISTG-99) as monotherapy. For Cs-131, a prescription dose of 115 Gy is recommended as monotherapy. For combination therapy, an external beam radiotherapy dose of 40–50 Gy is combined with implantation of I-125 (100–110 Gy), Pd-103 (90–100 Gy), or Cs-131 (85 Gy). References: Nag S, Beyer D, Friedland J, et al. American Brachytherapy Society (ABS) recommendations for transperineal permanent brachytherapy of prostate cancer. *Int J Radiat Oncol Biol Phys.* 1999;44(4):789–799 and Bice WS, Prestidge BR, Kurtzman SM, et al. Recommendations for permanent prostate brachytherapy with (131)Cs: a consensus report from the Cesium Advisory Group. *Brachytherapy.* 2008;7(4):290–296.

4. D   High-dose rate (HDR) brachytherapy involves dose rates ranging greater than 12.0 Gy per hour. Ir-192 is often used during HDR brachytherapy. LDR brachytherapy includes dose rates ranging between 0.4 and 2.0 Gy per hour while MDR includes dose rates between 2.0 and 12.0 Gy/h. I-125, Pd-103, and Cs-131 are often used during LDR brachytherapy. Reference: Chassagne D, Dutreix A, Almond P, Burgers JMV, Busch M, Joslin CA. Report 38. *ICRU.* 1985;20(1). https://doi.org/10.1093/jicru/os20.1.Report38

5. A   Based on RTOG consensus guidelines, the pelvic lymph node clinical target volume (CTV) includes distal common iliac, presacral lymph nodes (S1–S3), external iliac lymph nodes, internal iliac lymph nodes, and obturator lymph nodes. This CTV volume includes the vessels (artery and vein) and a 0.7cm radial margin without extending into bowel, bladder, bone, and muscle. Pelvic lymph node CTV typically begins at the L4/L5 vertebral interspace (recommended per RTOG 0924) and end at the superior aspect of the pubic bone. Reference: Lawton CA, Michalski J, El-Naqa I, et al. RTOG GU Radiation oncology

specialists reach consensus on pelvic lymph node volumes for high-risk prostate cancer. *Int J Radiat Oncol Biol Phys.* 2009;74(2):383–387.

6. B   For patients with muscle-invasive bladder cancer in the background of diffuse carcinoma *in situ*, the next appropriate management would be neoadjuvant chemotherapy. There is an approximately 5% overall survival benefit with neoadjuvant chemotherapy used prior to radical cystectomy. More than half of patients will demonstrate notable downstaging after completing neoadjuvant chemotherapy, with more than a quarter of patients demonstrating a complete response. While responders to chemotherapy may have higher overall survival, they still require definitive therapy (cystectomy or chemoradiation). Dose-dense MVAC (methotrexate, vinblastine, doxorubicin, cisplatin) or gemcitabine/cisplatin are options for neoadjuvant chemotherapy. Reference: Neoadjuvant chemotherapy in invasive bladder cancer: a systematic review and meta-analysis. *Lancet (London, England).* 2003;361(9373):1927–1934 and Roberts JT, von der Maase H, Sengeløv L, et al. Long-term survival results of a randomized trial comparing gemcitabine/cisplatin and methotrexate/vinblastine/doxorubicin/cisplatin in patients with locally advanced and metastatic bladder cancer. *Ann Oncol.* 2006;17 Suppl 5:v118–122.7.

7. C   Quality of life after selective bladder preservation (TURBT and chemoradiation) is excellent. About 30% of patients requiring salvage cystectomy after selective bladder preservation; thus, 70% of patients will have an intact bladder. Of patients with retained bladder, over 75% of patients have been reported to retain normal urinary function by urodynamic studies, and over 85% of patients had no bothersome urinary adverse effects. Reference: Efstathiou JA, Bae K, Shipley WU, et al. Late pelvic toxicity after bladder-sparing therapy in patients with invasive bladder cancer: RTOG 89-03, 95-06, 97-06, 99-06. *J Clin Oncol.* 2009;27(25):4055–4061 and Zietman AL, Sacco D, Skowronski U, et al. Organ conservation in invasive bladder cancer by transurethral resection, chemotherapy and radiation: results of a urodynamic and quality of life study on long-term survivors. *J Urol.* 2003;170(5):1772–1776.

8. D   The whole pelvic field used during bladder-sparing chemoradiation includes the external and internal iliac lymph nodes, obturator lymph nodes, entire bladder, and prostate (men) or the proximal 2 cm of urethra (women). The common iliac lymph nodes are not targeted; therefore, the superior border of all fields in the

four-field box is at the mid-sacroiliac joint (S2-3 vertebral interspace). The inferior border is at the bottom of the obturator foramen or 2 cm below the tumor, whichever is lower. The posterior border of the lateral fields is 2 cm posterior to the bladder/internal iliac lymph nodes with up to half the rectum blocked. The anterior border is 1–2 cm anterior to the bladder/external iliac lymph nodes. The lateral border of the anterior/posterior fields should be 1.5–2 cm beyond the pelvic inlet. Reference: Videtic GM, Woody NM. *Handbook of Treatment Planning in Radiation Oncology.* 2nd Edition ed. New York, New York: Demos Medical Publishing, L.L.C., 2015.

9. B Per American Joint Committee on Cancer staging guideline (8th edition), the clinical stage could be T3aN2. Perivesicular tissue involvement without invasion to adjacent organs would designate give a T3 designation. Involvement of multiple (three) regional lymph nodes in the true pelvis would qualify an N2 designation. Reference: Amin MB GD, Vega LR, Edge SB, et al. *AJCC Cancer Staging Manual.* 8th Edition. Chicago, IL: American College of Surgeons; 2018.

10. D For superficial (Tis), papillary tumors (Ta) or tumors confined to the mucosa (T1), weekly intravesicular BCG for 6 weeks is the preferred therapy it has demonstrated to have reduced recurrence rates compared to intravesicular mitomycin C. Mitomycin C can be used for low grade, Ta tumors. Reference: Brake M, Loertzer H, Horsch R, et al. Long-term results of intravesical bacillus Calmette-Guérin therapy for stage T1 superficial bladder cancer. *Urology.* 2000;55(5):673–678.

11. D Because CT abdomen demonstrates three 2 cm suspicious lymph nodes along the para-aortic chain, this patient has stage 2A seminoma. Following diagnostic and therapeutic orchiectomy, adjuvant treatment with multi-agent chemotherapy or RT is recommended. Radiation therapy for stage 2 seminoma would be 20–25.5 Gy to the para-aortic and ipsilateral iliac lymph nodes (dog-leg field) followed by a boost to 30 Gy (to lymph nodes <2 cm) or 36 Gy (to lymph nodes 2–5 cm). Observation or single-agent carboplatin is recommended for stage I seminomas. Retroperitoneal lymph node dissection is generally not recommended since seminoma is very sensitive to either chemotherapy or radiation. Reference: National Comprehensive Cancer Network. Testicular Cancer (Version 1.2021). https://www.nccn.org/professionals/physician_gls/pdf/testicular.pdf

12. B Many patients with seminoma (especially with bulky involved lymph nodes) will have residual disease after chemotherapy. Patients with residual mass less than 3 cm after chemotherapy should be observed. A surgical series demonstrated that none of the patients with residual mass less than 3 cm who had retroperitoneal lymph node dissection following chemotherapy had viable tumor. Approximately 50% of residual masses regress on surveillance, and patients are encouraged to have follow-up imaging until residual retroperitoneal mass resolves. Furthermore, consolidative radiotherapy to residual masses following chemotherapy has not consistently shown to decrease rates of relapse. References: Horwich A, Paluchowska B, Norman A, et al. Residual mass following chemotherapy of seminoma. *Ann Oncol.* 1997;8(1):37–40.

13. B Based on several studies, early-stage patients with seminoma who are observed after inguinal orchiectomy have a 15%–25% risk of relapse in 5 years. Observation is an attractive option given the excellent outcomes from salvage therapeutic options. Reference: Groll RJ, Warde P, Jewett MA. A comprehensive systematic review of testicular germ cell tumor surveillance. *Crit Rev Oncol Hematol.* 2007;64(3):182–197 and Mortensen MS, Lauritsen J, Gundgaard MG, et al. A nationwide cohort study of stage I seminoma patients followed on a surveillance program. *Eur Urol.* 2014;66(6):1172–1178.

14. C The most notable randomized data comparing 20 versus 30 Gy adjuvant radiotherapy for stage 1 seminoma after inguinal orchiectomy is from MRC TE-18 trial. In this trial, 20 Gy in 10 fractions or 30 Gy in 15 fractions to the para-aortic strip from T11 to L5. From this trial, patients who underwent 30 Gy did not develop higher incidence of late side effects. The relapse rate in both arms were low (3% vs. 4%, respectively), and there was no difference in relapse rates on longer follow-up. Reference: Jones WG, Fossa SD, Mead GM, et al. Randomized trial of 30 versus 20 Gy in the adjuvant treatment of stage I Testicular Seminoma: a report on Medical Research Council Trial TE18, European Organisation for the Research and Treatment of Cancer Trial 30942 (ISRCTN18525328). *J Clin Oncol.* 2005;23(6):1200–1208.

15. A A patient with only a 3-cm seminoma with rete testis invasion without clinical evidence of lymph node involvement who has stage I seminoma according to the Royal Marsden staging classification. Reference: Horwich A. Testicular cancer. In: Horwich A, ed. *Oncology–A Multidisciplinary Textbook.* London: Chapman and Hall, 1995:485–498.

REFERENCES

1. Siegel RL, Miller KD, Jemal A. Cancer statistics, 2020. *CA Cancer J Clin.* 2020;70(1):7–30.
2. Etzioni R, Tsodikov A, Mariotto A, et al. Quantifying the role of PSA screening in the US prostate cancer mortality decline. *Cancer Causes Control.* 2008;19(2):175–181.
3. Etzioni R, Gulati R, Falcon S, et al. Impact of PSA screening on the incidence of advanced stage prostate cancer in the United States: a surveillance modeling approach. *Med Decis Making.* 2008;28(3):323–331.
4. Butler SS, Muralidhar V, Zhao SG, et al. Prostate cancer incidence across stage, NCCN risk groups, and age before and after USP-STF Grade D recommendations against prostate-specific antigen screening in 2012. *Cancer.* 2020;126(4):717–724.
5. Golimbu M, Morales P, Al-Askari S, et al. Extended pelvic lymphadenectomy for prostatic cancer. *J Urol.* 1979;121(5):617–620.
6. Levin-Epstein R, Qiao-Guan G, Juarez JE, et al. Clinical assessment of prostate displacement and planning target volume margins for stereotactic body radiotherapy of prostate cancer. *Front Oncol.* 2020;10:539.
7. de Crevoisier R, Tucker SL, Dong L, et al. Increased risk of biochemical and local failure in patients with distended rectum on the planning CT for prostate cancer radiotherapy. *Int J Radiat Oncol Biol Phys.* 2005;62(4):965–973.
8. Tøndel H, Solberg A, Lydersen S, Jensen CA, Kaasa S, Lund J. Rectal volume variations and estimated rectal dose during 8 weeks of image-guided radical 3D conformal external beam radiotherapy for prostate cancer. *Clin Transl Radiat Oncol.* 2019;15:113–117.
9. Zietman AL, Bae K, Slater JD, et al. Randomized trial comparing conventional-dose with high-dose conformal radiation therapy in early-stage adenocarcinoma of the prostate: long-term results from proton radiation oncology group/american college of radiology 95-09. *J Clin Oncol.* 2010;28(7):1106–1111.
10. Kuban DA, Levy LB, Cheung MR, et al. Long-term failure patterns and survival in a randomized dose-escalation trial for prostate cancer. Who dies of disease? *Int J Radiat Oncol Biol Phys.* 2011;79(5):1310–1317.
11. Kishan AU, Dang A, Katz AJ, et al. Long-term outcomes of stereotactic body radiotherapy for low-risk and intermediate-risk prostate cancer. *JAMA Network Open.* 2019;2(2):e188006.
12. Kalbasi A, Li J, Berman A, et al. Dose-escalated irradiation and overall survival in men with nonmetastatic prostate cancer. *JAMA Oncol.* 2015;1(7):897–906.
13. Ávila M, Patel L, López S, et al. Patient-reported outcomes after treatment for clinically localized prostate cancer: a systematic review and meta-analysis. *Cancer Treat Rev.* 2018;66:23–44.
14. Hoffman KE, Penson DF, Zhao Z, et al. Patient-reported outcomes through 5 years for active surveillance, surgery, brachytherapy, or external beam radiation with or without androgen deprivation therapy for localized prostate cancer. *Jama.* 2020;323(2):149–163.
15. Naji L, Randhawa H, Sohani Z, et al. Digital rectal examination for prostate cancer screening in primary care: a systematic review and meta-analysis. *Ann Fam Med.* 2018;16(2):149–154.
16. Scattoni V, Zlotta A, Montironi R, Schulman C, Rigatti P, Montorsi F. Extended and saturation prostatic biopsy in the diagnosis and characterisation of prostate cancer: a critical analysis of the literature. *Eur Urol.* 2007;52(5):1309–1322.
17. Roehl Kimberly A, Antenor Jo Ann V, Catalona William J. Serial biopsy results in prostate cancer screening study. *J Urol.* 2002;167(6):2435–2439.
18. Djavan B, Ravery V, Zlotta A, et al. Prospective evaluation of prostate cancer detected on biopsies 1, 2, 3 and 4: when should we stop? *J Urol.* 2001;166(5):1679–1683.
19. Rastinehad AR, Turkbey B, Salami SS, et al. Improving detection of clinically significant prostate cancer: magnetic resonance imaging/transrectal ultrasound fusion guided prostate biopsy. *J Urol.* 2014;191(6):1749–1754.
20. Rosenkrantz AB, Verma S, Choyke P, et al. Prostate magnetic resonance imaging and magnetic resonance imaging targeted biopsy in patients with a prior negative biopsy: a consensus statement by AUA and SAR. *J Urol.* 2016;196(6):1613–1618.
21. Schoots IG, Roobol MJ, Nieboer D, Bangma CH, Steyerberg EW, Hunink MG. Magnetic resonance imaging-targeted biopsy may enhance the diagnostic accuracy of significant prostate cancer detection compared to standard transrectal ultrasound-guided biopsy: a systematic review and meta-analysis. *Eur Urol.* 2015;68(3):438–450.
22. Fütterer JJ, Verma S, Hambrock T, et al. High-risk prostate cancer: value of multi-modality 3T MRI-guided biopsies after previous negative biopsies. *Abdom Imaging.* 2012;37(5):892–896.
23. Cooperberg MR, Pasta DJ, Elkin EP, et al. The University of California, San Francisco Cancer of the Prostate Risk Assessment score: a straightforward and reliable preoperative predictor of disease recurrence after radical prostatectomy. *J Urol.* 2005;173(6):1938–1942.
24. Cooperberg MR, Davicioni E, Crisan A, Jenkins RB, Ghadessi M, Karnes RJ. Combined value of validated clinical and genomic risk stratification tools for predicting prostate cancer mortality in a high-risk prostatectomy cohort. *Eur Urol.* 2015;67(2):326–333.
25. Nguyen PL, Haddad Z, Ross AE, et al. Ability of a genomic classifier to predict metastasis and prostate cancer-specific mortality after radiation or surgery based on needle biopsy specimens. *Eur Urol.* 2017;72(5):845–852.
26. Zhao SG, Chang SL, Spratt DE, et al. Development and validation of a 24-gene predictor of response to postoperative radiotherapy in prostate cancer: a matched, retrospective analysis. *Lancet Oncol.* 2016;17(11):1612–1620.
27. Kim HL, Li P, Huang HC, et al. Validation of the Decipher Test for predicting adverse pathology in candidates for prostate cancer active surveillance. *Prostate Cancer Prostatic Dis.* 2019;22(3):399–405.
28. Spratt DE, Zhang J, Santiago-Jiménez M, et al. Development and validation of a novel integrated clinical-genomic risk group classification for localized prostate cancer. *J Clin Oncol.* 2018;36(6):581–590.
29. Den RB, Yousefi K, Trabulsi EJ, et al. Genomic classifier identifies men with adverse pathology after radical prostatectomy who benefit from adjuvant radiation therapy. *J Clin Oncol.* 2015;33(8):944–951.
30. Freedland SJ, Choeurng V, Howard L, et al. Utilization of a genomic classifier for prediction of metastasis following salvage radiation therapy after radical prostatectomy. *Eur Urol.* 2016;70(4):588–596.
31. Karnes RJ, Choeurng V, Ross AE, et al. Validation of a genomic risk classifier to predict prostate cancer-specific mortality in men with adverse pathologic features. *Eur Urol.* 2018;73(2):168–175.
32. Cuzick J, Stone S, Fisher G, et al. Validation of an RNA cell cycle progression score for predicting death from prostate cancer in a conservatively managed needle biopsy cohort. *Br J Cancer.* 2015;113(3):382–389.
33. Cooperberg MR, Simko JP, Cowan JE, et al. Validation of a cell-cycle progression gene panel to improve risk stratification in a contemporary prostatectomy cohort. *J Clin Oncol.* 2013;31(11):1428–1434.
34. Tosoian JJ, Chappidi MR, Bishoff JT, et al. Prognostic utility of biopsy-derived cell cycle progression score in patients with National Comprehensive Cancer Network low-risk prostate cancer undergoing radical prostatectomy: implications for treatment guidance. *BJU Int.* 2017;120(6):808–814.
35. Klein EA, Cooperberg MR, Magi-Galluzzi C, et al. A 17-gene assay to predict prostate cancer aggressiveness in the context of Gleason grade heterogeneity, tumor multifocality, and biopsy undersampling. *Eur Urol.* 2014;66(3):550–560.
36. Eggener S, Karsh LI, Richardson T, et al. A 17-gene panel for prediction of adverse prostate cancer pathologic features: prospective clinical validation and utility. *Urology.* 2019;126:76–82.
37. Blume-Jensen P, Berman DM, Rimm DL, et al. Development and clinical validation of an in situ biopsy-based multimarker assay for risk stratification in prostate cancer. *Clin Cancer Res.* 2015;21(11):2591–2600.
38. Hu JC, Tosoian JJ, Qi J, et al. Clinical utility of gene expression classifiers in men with newly diagnosed prostate cancer. *JCO Precis Oncol.* 2018(2):1–15.

39. Marascio J, Spratt DE, Zhang J, et al. Prospective study to define the clinical utility and benefit of Decipher testing in men following prostatectomy. *Prostate Cancer Prostatic Dis.* 2020;23(2):295–302.

40. Amin MB GD, Vega LR, Edge SB, Greene FL, Byrd DR, Brookland RK, Washington MK, Comptom CC. *AJCC Cancer Staging Manual 8th Edition.* Chicago, IL: American College of Surgeons; 2018.

41. Terris MK, Stamey TA. Determination of prostate volume by transrectal ultrasound. *J Urol.* 1991;145(5):984–987.

42. Stock C, Hruza M, Cresswell J, et al. Transrectal ultrasound-guided biopsy of the prostate: development of the procedure, current clinical practice, and introduction of self-embedding as a new way of processing biopsy cores. *J Endourol.* 2008;22(6):1321–1329.

43. Hricak H, Dooms GC, Jeffrey RB, et al. Prostatic carcinoma: staging by clinical assessment, CT, and MR imaging. *Radiology.* 1987;162(2):331–336.

44. Wolf JS, Cher M, Dall'Era M, Presti Joseph C, Hricak H, Carroll Peter R. Prostate cancer: the use and accuracy of cross-sectional imaging and fine needle aspiration cytology for detection of pelvic lymph node metastases before radical prostatectomy. *J Urol.* 1995;153(3S):993–999.

45. Sato C, Naganawa S, Nakamura T, et al. Differentiation of noncancerous tissue and cancer lesions by apparent diffusion coefficient values in transition and peripheral zones of the prostate. *J Magn Reson Imaging.* 2005;21(3):258–262.

46. Ikonen S, Karkkainen P, Kivisaari L, et al. Magnetic resonance imaging of clinically localized prostatic canceR. *J Urol.* 1998;159(3): 915–919.

47. Cornud F, Flam T, Chauveinc L, et al. Extraprostatic spread of clinically localized prostate cancer: factors predictive of pT3 tumor and of positive endorectal MR imaging examination results. *Radiology.* 2002;224(1):203–210.

48. Sala E, Akin O, Moskowitz CS, et al. Endorectal MR imaging in the evaluation of seminal vesicle invasion: diagnostic accuracy and multivariate feature analysis. *Radiology.* 2006;238(3):929–937.

49. Perrotti M, Kaufman Ronald P, Jennings Timothy A, et al. Endorectal coil magnetic resonance imaging in clinically localized prostate cancer: is it accurate? *J Urol.* 1996;156(1):106–109.

50. Somford DM, Hamoen EH, Fütterer JJ, et al. The predictive value of endorectal 3 Tesla multiparametric magnetic resonance imaging for extraprostatic extension in patients with low, intermediate and high risk prostate cancer. *J Urol.* 2013;190(5):1728–1734.

51. Heck MM, Souvatzoglou M, Retz M, et al. Prospective comparison of computed tomography, diffusion-weighted magnetic resonance imaging and [11C]choline positron emission tomography/computed tomography for preoperative lymph node staging in prostate cancer patients. *Eur J Nucl Med Mol Imaging.* 2014;41(4):694–701.

52. Preisser F, Mazzone E, Nazzani S, et al. North American population-based validation of the National Comprehensive Cancer Network Practice Guideline Recommendations for locoregional lymph node and bone imaging in prostate cancer patients. *Br J Cancer.* 2018;119(12):1552–1556.

53. Wondergem M, van der Zant FM, van der Ploeg T, et al. A literature review of 18F-fluoride PET/CT and 18F-choline or 11C-choline PET/CT for detection of bone metastases in patients with prostate cancer. *Nucl Med Commun.* 2013;34(10):935–945.

54. Langsteger W, Balogova S, Huchet V, et al. Fluorocholine (18F) and sodium fluoride (18F) PET/CT in the detection of prostate cancer: prospective comparison of diagnostic performance determined by masked reading. *Q J Nucl Med Mol Imaging.* 2011;55(4):448–457.

55. Schuster DM, Nieh PT, Jani AB, et al. Anti-3-[(18)F]FACBC positron emission tomography-computerized tomography and (111) In-capromab pendetide single photon emission computerized tomography-computerized tomography for recurrent prostate carcinoma: results of a prospective clinical trial. *J Urol.* 2014;191(5): 1446–1453.

56. Odewole OA, Tade FI, Nieh PT, et al. Recurrent prostate cancer detection with anti-3-[(18)F]FACBC PET/CT: comparison with CT. *Eur J Nucl Med Mol Imaging.* 2016;43(10):1773–1783.

57. Perera M, Papa N, Christidis D, et al. Sensitivity, specificity, and predictors of positive (68)ga-prostate-specific membrane antigen positron emission tomography in advanced prostate cancer: a systematic review and meta-analysis. *Eur Urol.* 2016;70(6):926–937.

58. Fendler WP, Calais J, Eiber M, et al. Assessment of 68Ga-PSMA-11 PET accuracy in localizing recurrent prostate cancer: a prospective single-arm clinical trial. *JAMA Oncol.* 2019;5(6):856–863.

59. Calais J, Ceci F, Eiber M, et al. 18F-fluciclovine PET-CT and 68Ga-PSMA-11 PET-CT in patients with early biochemical recurrence after prostatectomy: a prospective, single-centre, single-arm, comparative imaging trial. *Lancet Oncol.* 2019;20(9):1286–1294.

60. Rowe S, Gorin M, Pienta K, et al. Results from the OSPREY trial: A prospective phase 2/3 multi-center study of 18F-DCFPyL PET/CT imaging in patients with prostate cancer-examination of diagnostic accuracy. *J Nucl Med.* 2019;60(supplement 1):586–586.

61. Gleason DF, Mellinger GT. Prediction of prognosis for prostatic adenocarcinoma by combined histological grading and clinical staging. *J Urol.* 1974;111(1):58–64.

62. Epstein JI, Egevad L, Amin MB, Delahunt B, Srigley JR, Humphrey PA. The 2014 International Society of Urological Pathology (ISUP) consensus conference on Gleason grading of prostatic carcinoma: definition of grading patterns and proposal for a new grading system. *Am J Surg Pathol.* 2016;40(2):244–252.

63. Kryvenko ON, Epstein JI. Changes in prostate cancer grading: Including a new patient-centric grading system. *Prostate.* 2016; 76(5):427–433.

64. Epstein JI, Zelefsky MJ, Sjoberg DD, et al. A contemporary prostate cancer grading system: a validated alternative to the gleason score. *Eur Urol.* 2016;69(3):428–435.

65. Chism DB, Hanlon AL, Troncoso P, Al-Saleem T, Horwitz EM, Pollack A. The gleason score shift: score four and seven years ago. *Int J Radiat Oncol Biol Phys.* 2003;56(5):1241–1247.

66. Carter HB, Albertsen PC, Barry MJ, et al. Early detection of prostate cancer: AUA Guideline. *J Urol.* 2013;190(2):419–426.

67. Benson MC, Whang IS, Olsson CA, et al. The use of prostate specific antigen density to enhance the predictive value of intermediate levels of serum prostate specific antigen. *J Urol.* 1992;147(3 Pt 2): 817–821.

68. Catalona WJ, Partin AW, Slawin KM, et al. Use of the percentage of free prostate-specific antigen to enhance differentiation of prostate cancer from benign prostatic disease: a prospective multicenter clinical trial. *Jama.* 1998;279(19):1542–1547.

69. Carter HB, Pearson JD, Metter EJ, et al. Longitudinal evaluation of prostate-specific antigen levels in men with and without prostate disease. *Jama.* 1992;267(16):2215–2220.

70. Bussemakers MJ, van Bokhoven A, Verhaegh GW, et al. DD3: a new prostate-specific gene, highly overexpressed in prostate cancer. *Cancer Res.* 1999;59(23):5975–5979.

71. Hessels D, Klein Gunnewiek JM, van Oort I, et al. DD3(PCA3)-based molecular urine analysis for the diagnosis of prostate cancer. *Eur Urol.* 2003;44(1):8–15; discussion 15–16.

72. Bill-Axelson A, Holmberg L, Garmo H, et al. Radical prostatectomy or watchful waiting in early prostate cancer. *N Engl J Med.* 2014;370(10):932–942.

73. Wilt TJ, Jones KM, Barry MJ, et al. Follow-up of prostatectomy versus observation for early prostate cancer. *N Engl J Med.* 2017;377(2):132–142.

74. Klotz L, Vesprini D, Sethukavalan P, et al. Long-term follow-up of a large active surveillance cohort of patients with prostate cancer. *J Clin Oncol.* 2015;33(3):272–277.

75. Hamdy FC, Donovan JL, Lane JA, et al. 10-year outcomes after monitoring, surgery, or radiotherapy for localized prostate cancer. *N Engl J Med.* 2016;375(15):1415–1424.

76. Cooperberg MR, Broering JM, Carroll PR. Time trends and local variation in primary treatment of localized prostate cancer. *J Clin Oncol.* 2010;28(7):1117–1123.

77. Sanda MG, Dunn RL, Michalski J, et al. Quality of life and satisfaction with outcome among prostate-cancer survivors. *N Engl J Med.* 2008;358(12):1250–1261.

78. Donovan JL, Hamdy FC, Lane JA, et al. Patient-reported outcomes after monitoring, surgery, or radiotherapy for prostate cancer. *N Engl J Med.* 2016;375(15):1425–1437.

79. Vernooij RWM, Cremers R, Jansen H, et al. Urinary incontinence and erectile dysfunction in patients with localized or locally advanced prostate cancer: a nationwide observational study. *Urol Oncol.* 2020;38(9):735.e717–735.e725.

80. Kishan AU, Cook RR, Ciezki JP, et al. radical prostatectomy, external beam radiotherapy, or external beam radiotherapy with brachytherapy boost and disease progression and mortality in patients with gleason score 9-10 prostate cancer. *Jama.* 2018;319(9):896–905.

81. Roach M, III, Pickett B, Rosenthal SA, et al. Defining treatment margins for six field conformal irradiation of localized prostate cancer. *Int J Radiat Oncol Biol Phys.* 1994;28(1):267–275.

82. Pilepich MV, Winter K, Lawton CA, et al. Androgen suppression adjuvant to definitive radiotherapy in prostate carcinoma--long-term results of phase III RTOG 85-31. *Int J Radiat Oncol Biol Phys.* 2005;61(5):1285–1290.

83. Bolla M, Van Tienhoven G, Warde P, et al. External irradiation with or without long-term androgen suppression for prostate cancer with high metastatic risk: 10-year results of an EORTC randomised study. *Lancet Oncol.* 2010;11(11):1066–1073.

84. D'Amico AV, Chen MH, Renshaw A, et al. Long-term follow-up of a randomized trial of radiation with or without androgen deprivation therapy for localized prostate cancer. *Jama.* 2015;314(12):1291–1293.

85. Hanks GE, Pajak TF, Porter A, et al. Phase III trial of long-term adjuvant androgen deprivation after neoadjuvant hormonal cytoreduction and radiotherapy in locally advanced carcinoma of the prostate: the Radiation Therapy Oncology Group Protocol 92-02. *J Clin Oncol.* 2003;21(21):3972–3978.

86. Bolla M, de Reijke TM, Van Tienhoven G, et al. Duration of androgen suppression in the treatment of prostate cancer. *N Engl J Med.* 2009;360(24):2516–2527.

87. Zapatero A, Guerrero A, Maldonado X, et al. High-dose radiotherapy with short-term or long-term androgen deprivation in localised prostate cancer (DART01/05 GICOR): a randomised, controlled, phase 3 trial. *Lancet Oncol.* 2015;16(3):320–327.

88. Widmark A, Klepp O, Solberg A, et al. Endocrine treatment, with or without radiotherapy, in locally advanced prostate cancer (SPCG-7/SFUO-3): an open randomised phase III trial. *Lancet.* 2009;373(9660):301–308.

89. Nabid A, Carrier N, Martin A-G, et al. Duration of androgen deprivation therapy in high-risk prostate cancer: a randomized phase III trial. *Eur Urol.* 2018;74(4):432–441.

90. Jones CU, Hunt D, McGowan DG, et al. Radiotherapy and short-term androgen deprivation for localized prostate cancer. *N Engl J Med.* 2011;365(2):107–118.

91. Shipley WU, Seiferheld W, Lukka HR, et al. Radiation with or without antiandrogen therapy in recurrent prostate cancer. *N Engl J Med.* 2017;376(5):417–428.

92. Carrie C, Hasbini A, de Laroche G, et al. Salvage radiotherapy with or without short-term hormone therapy for rising prostate-specific antigen concentration after radical prostatectomy (GETUG-AFU 16): a randomised, multicentre, open-label phase 3 trial. *Lancet Oncol.* 2016;17(6):747–756.

93. Spratt DE, Dess RT, Efstathiou JA, et al. Two years of anti-androgen treatment increases other-cause mortality in men receiving early salvage radiotherapy: a secondary analysis of the NRG oncology/RTOG 9601 randomized phase III trial. *Int J Radiat Oncol Biol Phys.* 2019;105(3):680.

94. Sathya JR, Davis IR, Julian JA, et al. Randomized trial comparing iridium implant plus external-beam radiation therapy with external-beam radiation therapy alone in node-negative locally advanced cancer of the prostate. *J Clin Oncol.* 2005;23(6):1192–1199.

95. Hoskin PJ, Rojas AM, Bownes PJ, Lowe GJ, Ostler PJ, Bryant L. Randomised trial of external beam radiotherapy alone or combined with high-dose-rate brachytherapy boost for localised prostate cancer. *Radiother Oncol.* 2012;103(2):217–222.

96. Hsu ICJ, Rodgers J, Shinohara K, et al. Long-term results of NRG oncology/RTOG 0321 a phase II trial of combined high dose rate brachytherapy and external beam radiotherapy for adenocarcinoma of the prostate. *Int J Radiat Oncol Biol Phys.* 2019;105(1):S57.

97. Burri RJ, Stone NN, Unger P, et al. Long-term outcome and toxicity of salvage brachytherapy for local failure after initial radiotherapy for prostate cancer. *Int J Radiat Oncol Biol Phys.* 2010;77(5):1338–1344.

98. Nguyen PL, Chen RC, Clark JA, et al. Patient-reported quality of life after salvage brachytherapy for radio-recurrent prostate cancer: a prospective Phase II study. *Brachytherapy.* 2009;8(4): 345–352.

99. Jabbari S, Hsu IC, Kawakami J, et al. High-dose-rate brachytherapy for localized prostate adenocarcinoma post abdominoperineal resection of the rectum and pelvic irradiation: Technique and experience. *Brachytherapy.* 2009;8(4):339–344.

100. Yamada Y, Kollmeier MA, Pei X, et al. A phase II study of salvage high-dose-rate brachytherapy for the treatment of locally recurrent prostate cancer after definitive external beam radiotherapy. *Brachytherapy.* 2014;13(2):111–116.

101. Rana ZH, D'Andrea V, Cox BW, et al. Salvage brachytherapy for recurrent prostate cancer after definitive radiation treatment and factors that may impact outcomes. *Int J Radiat Oncol Biol Phys.* 2019;105(1):E583.

102. Babaian RJ, Donnelly B, Bahn D, et al. Best practice statement on cryosurgery for the treatment of localized prostate cancer. *J Urol.* 2008;180(5):1993–2004.

103. Chin JL, Al-Zahrani AA, Autran-Gomez AM, et al. Extended followup oncologic outcome of randomized trial between cryoablation and external beam therapy for locally advanced prostate cancer (T2c-T3b). *J Urol.* 2012;188(4):1170–1175.

104. Robinson JW, Donnelly BJ, Siever JE, et al. A randomized trial of external beam radiotherapy versus cryoablation in patients with localized prostate cancer: quality of life outcomes. *Cancer.* 2009;115(20):4695–4704.

105. de Castro Abreu AL, Bahn D, Leslie S, et al. Salvage focal and salvage total cryoablation for locally recurrent prostate cancer after primary radiation therapy. *BJU Int.* 2013;112(3):298–307.

106. Li YH, Elshafei A, Agarwal G, Ruckle H, et al. Salvage focal prostate cryoablation for locally recurrent prostate cancer after radiotherapy: initial results from the cryo on-line data registry. *Prostate.* 2015;75(1):1–7.

107. Guillaumier S, Peters M, Arya M, et al. A multicentre study of 5-year outcomes following focal therapy in treating clinically significant nonmetastatic prostate cancer. *Eur Urol.* 2018;74(4):422–429.

108. Siddiqui KM, Billia M, Arifin A, Li F, Violette P, Chin JL. Pathological, oncologic and functional outcomes of a prospective registry of salvage high intensity focused ultrasound ablation for radiorecurrent prostate cancer. *J Urol.* 2017;197(1):97–102.

109. McLaughlin PW, Troyer S, Berri S, et al. Functional anatomy of the prostate: implications for treatment planning. *Int J Radiat Oncol Biol Phys.* 2005;63(2):479–491.

110. Lattanzi J, McNeely S, Hanlon A, Das I, Schultheiss TE, Hanks GE. Daily CT localization for correcting portal errors in the treatment of prostate cancer. *Int J Radiat Oncol Biol Phys.* 1998;41(5):1079–1086.

111. Lattanzi J, McNeeley S, Pinover W, et al. A comparison of daily CT localization to a daily ultrasound-based system in prostate cancer. *Int J Radiat Oncol Biol Phys.* 1999;43(4):719–725.

112. Sandler HM, Bree RL, McLaughlin PW, et al. Localization of the prostatic apex for radiation therapy using implanted markers. *Int J Radiat Oncol Biol Phys.* 1993;27(4):915–919.

113. Vigneault E, Pouliot J, Laverdière J, et al. Electronic portal imaging device detection of radioopaque markers for the evaluation of prostate position during megavoltage irradiation: a clinical study. *Int J Radiat Oncol Biol Phys.* 1997;37(1):205–212.

114. Litzenberg DW, Willoughby TR, Balter JM, et al. Positional stability of electromagnetic transponders used for prostate localization and continuous, real-time tracking. *Int J Radiat Oncol Biol Phys.* 2007;68(4):1199–1206.

115. Willoughby TR, Kupelian PA, Pouliot J, et al. Target localization and real-time tracking using the Calypso 4D localization system in patients with localized prostate cancer. *Int J Radiat Oncol Biol Phys.* 2006;65(2):528–534.

116. Kupelian PA, Langen KM, Willoughby TR, et al. Image-guided radiotherapy for localized prostate cancer: treating a moving target. *Semin Radiat Oncol.* 2008;18(1):58–66.

117. Ten Haken RK, Forman JD, Heimburger DK, et al. Treatment planning issues related to prostate movement in response to differential filling of the rectum and bladder. *Int J Radiat Oncol Biol Phys.* 1991;20(6):1317–1324.

118. Dawson LA, Litzenberg DW, Brock KK, et al. A comparison of ventilatory prostate movement in four treatment positions. *Int J Radiat Oncol Biol Phys.* 2000;48(2):319–323.

119. Litzenberg D, Dawson LA, Sandler H, et al. Daily prostate targeting using implanted radiopaque markers. *Int J Radiat Oncol Biol Phys.* 2002;52(3):699–703.

120. Bayley AJ, Catton CN, Haycocks T, et al. A randomized trial of supine vs. prone positioning in patients undergoing escalated dose conformal radiotherapy for prostate cancer. *Radiother Oncol.* 2004;70(1):37–44.

121. Diaz A, Roach M, 3rd, Marquez C, et al. Indications for and the significance of seminal vesicle irradiation during 3D conformal radiotherapy for localized prostate cancer. *Int J Radiat Oncol Biol Phys.* 1994;30(2):323–329.

122. Kestin L, Goldstein N, Vicini F, Yan D, Korman H, Martinez A. Treatment of prostate cancer with radiotherapy: should the entire seminal vesicles be included in the clinical target volume? *Int J Radiat Oncol Biol Phys.* 2002;54(3):686–697.

123. Lawton CA, DeSilvio M, Roach M, 3rd, et al. An update of the phase III trial comparing whole pelvic to prostate only radiotherapy and neoadjuvant to adjuvant total androgen suppression: updated analysis of RTOG 94-13, with emphasis on unexpected hormone/radiation interactions. *Int J Radiat Oncol Biol Phys.* 2007;69(3):646–655.

124. Wang D, Lawton C. Pelvic lymph node irradiation for prostate cancer: who, why, and when? *Semin Radiat Oncol.* 2008;18(1):35–40.

125. Roach M, 3rd, DeSilvio M, Valicenti R, et al. Whole-pelvis, "mini-pelvis," or prostate-only external beam radiotherapy after neoadjuvant and concurrent hormonal therapy in patients treated in the Radiation Therapy Oncology Group 9413 trial. *Int J Radiat Oncol Biol Phys.* 2006;66(3):647–653.

126. Calais J, Kishan AU, Cao M, et al. Potential impact of (68) Ga-PSMA-11 PET/CT on the planning of definitive radiation therapy for prostate cancer. *J Nucl Med.* 2018;59(11):1714–1721.

127. Lawton CAF, Michalski J, El-Naqa I, et al. Variation in the definition of clinical target volumes for pelvic nodal conformal radiation therapy for prostate cancer. *Int J Radiat Oncol Biol Phys.* 2009;74(2):377–382.

128. Lawton CA, Michalski J, El-Naqa I, et al. RTOG GU Radiation oncology specialists reach consensus on pelvic lymph node volumes for high-risk prostate cancer. *Int J Radiat Oncol Biol Phys.* 2009;74(2):383–387.

129. Lin CC, Gray PJ, Jemal A, et al. Androgen deprivation with or without radiation therapy for clinically node-positive prostate cancer. *J Natl Cancer Inst.* 2015;107(7):7.

130. Rusthoven CG, Carlson JA, Waxweiler TV, et al. The impact of definitive local therapy for lymph node-positive prostate cancer: a population-based study. *Int J Radiat Oncol Biol Phys. 2014;* 88(5):1064–1073.

131. Langen KM, Jones DT. Organ motion and its management. *Int J Radiat Oncol Biol Phys.* 2001;50(1):265–278.

132. Zelefsky MJ, Happersett L, Leibel SA, et al. The effect of treatment positioning on normal tissue dose in patients with prostate cancer treated with three-dimensional conformal radiotherapy. *Int J Radiat Oncol Biol Phys.* 1997;37(1):13–19.

133. Cahlon O, Hunt M, Zelefsky MJ. Intensity-modulated radiation therapy: supportive data for prostate cancer. *Semin Radiat Oncol.* 2008;18(1):48–57.

134. Zelefsky MJ, Levin EJ, Hunt M, et al. Incidence of late rectal and urinary toxicities after three-dimensional conformal radiotherapy and intensity-modulated radiotherapy for localized prostate cancer. *Int J Radiat Oncol Biol Phys.* 2008;70(4):1124–1129.

135. Roach M, 3rd, Nam J, Gagliardi G, El Naqa I, Deasy JO, Marks LB. Radiation dose-volume effects and the penile bulb. *Int J Radiat Oncol Biol Phys.* 2010;76(3 Suppl):S130–S134.

136. Ryu JK, Winter K, Michalski JM, et al. Interim report of toxicity from 3D conformal radiation therapy (3D-CRT) for prostate cancer on 3DOG/RTOG 9406, level III (79.2 Gy). *Int J Radiat Oncol Biol Phys.* 2002;54(4):1036–1046.

137. Kuban DA, Tucker SL, Dong L, et al. Long-term results of the M. D. Anderson randomized dose-escalation trial for prostate cancer. *Int J Radiat Oncol Biol Phys.* 2008;70(1):67–74.

138. Talcott JA, Rossi C, Shipley WU, et al. Patient-reported long-term outcomes after conventional and high-dose combined proton and photon radiation for early prostate cancer. *Jama.* 2010;303(11):1046–1053.

139. Michalski JM, Moughan J, Purdy J, et al. Effect of standard vs dose-escalated radiation therapy for patients with intermediate-risk prostate cancer: the NRG oncology RTOG 0126 randomized clinical trial. *JAMA Oncol.* 2018;4(6):e180039–e180039.

140. Dearnaley DP, Khoo VS, Norman AR, et al. Comparison of radiation side-effects of conformal and conventional radiotherapy in prostate cancer: a randomised trial. *Lancet.* 1999;353(9149):267–272.

141. Pollack A, Walker G, Horwitz EM, et al. Randomized trial of hypofractionated external-beam radiotherapy for prostate cancer. *J Clin Oncol.* 2013;31(31):3860–3868.

142. Lee WR, Dignam JJ, Amin MB, et al. Randomized phase III noninferiority study comparing two radiotherapy fractionation schedules in patients with low-risk prostate cancer. *J Clin Oncol.* 2016;34(20):2325–2332.

143. Dearnaley D, Syndikus I, Mossop H, et al. Conventional versus hypofractionated high-dose intensity-modulated radiotherapy for prostate cancer: 5-year outcomes of the randomised, non-inferiority, phase 3 CHHiP trial. *Lancet Oncol.* 2016;17(8): 1047–1060.

144. Arcangeli S, Strigari L, Gomellini S, et al. Updated results and patterns of failure in a randomized hypofractionation trial for high-risk prostate cancer. *Int J Radiat Oncol Biol Phys.* 2012; 84(5):1172–1178.

145. Catton CN, Lukka H, Gu C-S, et al. Randomized trial of a hypofractionated radiation regimen for the treatment of localized prostate cancer. *J Clin Oncol.* 2017;35(17):1884–1890.

146. Wang WGA, Yan D, Ye H, et al. Outcomes and toxicity from a prospective study of moderate hypofractionated radiation therapy for prostate cancer. *Int J Radiat Oncol Biol Phys.* 2016;96(2):E241.

147. Miles EF, Lee WR. Hypofractionation for prostate cancer: a critical review. *Semin Radiat Oncol.* 2008;18(1):41–47.

148. Ritter M. Rationale, conduct, and outcome using hypofractionated radiotherapy in prostate cancer. *Semin Radiat Oncol.* 2008;18(4): 249–256.

149. Madsen BL, Hsi RA, Pham HT, Fowler JF, Esagui L, Corman J. Stereotactic hypofractionated accurate radiotherapy of the prostate (SHARP), 33.5 Gy in five fractions for localized disease: first clinical trial results. *Int J Radiat Oncol Biol Phys.* 2007;67(4):1099–1105.

150. King CR, Freeman D, Kaplan I, et al. Stereotactic body radiotherapy for localized prostate cancer: pooled analysis from a multi-institutional consortium of prospective phase II trials. *Radiother Oncol.* 2013;109(2):217–221.

151. Katz A, Formenti SC, Kang J. Predicting biochemical disease-free survival after prostate stereotactic body radiotherapy: risk-stratification and patterns of failure. *Front Oncol.* 2016;6(168)3–5.

152. Meier R, Beckman A, Henning G, et al. Five-year outcomes from a multicenter trial of stereotactic body radiation therapy for low- and intermediate-risk prostate cancer. *Int J Radiat Oncol Biol Phys.* 2016;96(2):S33–S34.

153. Thompson IM, Tangen CM, Paradelo J, et al. Adjuvant radiotherapy for pathological T3N0M0 prostate cancer significantly reduces risk of metastases and improves survival: long-term followup of a randomized clinical trial. *J Urol.* 2009; 181(3):956–962.

154. Bolla M, van Poppel H, Tombal B, et al. Postoperative radiotherapy after radical prostatectomy for high-risk prostate cancer: long-term results of a randomised controlled trial (EORTC trial 22911). *Lancet (London, England).* 2012;380(9858):2018–2027.

155. Wiegel T, Bartkowiak D, Bottke D, et al. Adjuvant radiotherapy versus wait-and-see after radical prostatectomy: 10-year follow-up of the ARO 96-02/AUO AP 09/95 trial. *Eur Urol.* 2014; 66(2):243–250.

156. Eisenberg ML, Davies BJ, Cooperberg MR, et al. Prognostic implications of an undetectable ultrasensitive prostate-specific antigen level after radical prostatectomy. *Eur Urol.* 2010;57(4):622–629.

157. Stephenson AJ, Shariat SF, Zelefsky MJ, et al. Salvage radiotherapy for recurrent prostate cancer after radical prostatectomy. *Jama.* 2004;291(11):1325–1332.

158. Stephenson AJ, Scardino PT, Kattan MW, et al. Predicting the outcome of salvage radiation therapy for recurrent prostate cancer after radical prostatectomy. *J Clin Oncol.* 2007;25(15):2035–2041.

159. Stish BJ, Pisansky TM, Harmsen WS, et al. Improved metastasis-free and survival outcomes with early salvage radiotherapy in men with detectable prostate-specific antigen after prostatectomy for prostate cancer. *J Clin Oncol.* 2016;34(32):3864–3871.

160. Kneebone A, Fraser-Browne C, Delprado W, et al. A phase III multi-centre randomised trial comparing adjuvant versus early salvage radiotherapy following a radical prostatectomy: results of the TROG 08.03 and ANZUP "RAVES" trial. *Int J Radiat Oncol Biol Phys.* 2019;105(1):S37–S38.

161. Sargos P, Chabaud S, Latorzeff I, et al. Adjuvant radiotherapy versus early salvage radiotherapy plus short-term androgen deprivation therapy in men with localised prostate cancer after radical prostatectomy (GETUG-AFU 17): a randomised, phase 3 trial. *Lancet Oncol.* 2020;21(10):1341–1352.

162. Vale CL, Fisher D, Kneebone A, et al. Adjuvant or early salvage radiotherapy for the treatment of localised and locally advanced prostate cancer: a prospectively planned systematic review and meta-analysis of aggregate data. *The Lancet.* 1427.

163. Poortmans P, Bossi A, Vandeputte K, et al. Guidelines for target volume definition in post-operative radiotherapy for prostate cancer, on behalf of the EORTC Radiation Oncology Group. *Radiother Oncol.* 2007;84(2):121–127.

164. Michalski JM, Lawton C, El Naqa I, et al. Development of RTOG consensus guidelines for the definition of the clinical target volume for postoperative conformal radiation therapy for prostate cancer. *Int J Radiat Oncol Biol Phys.* 2010;76(2):361–368.

165. Sidhom MA, Kneebone AB, Lehman M, et al. Post-prostatectomy radiation therapy: consensus guidelines of the Australian and New Zealand Radiation Oncology Genito-Urinary Group. *Radiother Oncol.* 2008;88(1):10–19.

166. Sella T, Schwartz LH, Swindle PW, et al. Suspected local recurrence after radical prostatectomy: endorectal coil MR imaging. *Radiology.* 2004;231(2):379–385.

167. Miralbell R, Vees H, Lozano J, et al. Endorectal MRI assessment of local relapse after surgery for prostate cancer: a model to define treatment field guidelines for adjuvant radiotherapy in patients at high risk for local failure. *Int J Radiat Oncol Biol Phys.* 2007;67(2):356–361.

168. Boreta L, Gadzinski AJ, Wu SY, et al. Location of recurrence by Gallium-68 PSMA-11 PET scan in prostate cancer patients eligible for salvage radiotherapy. *Urology.* 2019;129:165–171.

169. Calais J, Fendler WP, Eiber M, et al. Impact of (68)Ga-PSMA-11 PET/CT on the management of prostate cancer patients with biochemical recurrence. *J Nucl Med.* 2018;59(3):434–441.

170. King CR, Kapp DS. Radiotherapy after prostatectomy: is the evidence for dose escalation out there? *Int J Radiat Oncol Biol Phys.* 2008;71(2):346–350.

171. Ost P, Fonteyne V, Villeirs G, Lumen N, Oosterlinck W, De Meerleer G. Adjuvant high-dose intensity-modulated radiotherapy after radical prostatectomy for prostate cancer: clinical results in 104 patients. *Eur Urol.* 2009;56(4):669–675.

172. Tandberg DJ, Oyekunle T, Lee WR, Wu Y, Salama JK, Koontz BF. Postoperative radiation therapy for prostate cancer: comparison of conventional versus hypofractionated radiation regimens. *Int J Radiat Oncol Biol Phys.* 2018;101(2):396–405.

173. Macchia G, Siepe G, Capocaccia I, et al. Hypofractionated postoperative IMRT in prostate carcinoma: a phase I/II study. *Anticancer Res.* 2017;37(10):5821–5828.

174. Papagikos MA, Rossi PJ, Urbanic JJ, et al. A simple model predicts freedom from biochemical recurrence after low-dose rate prostate brachytherapy alone. *Am J Clin Oncol.* 2007;30(2):199–204.

175. Chin J, Rumble RB, Kollmeier M, et al. Brachytherapy for patients with prostate cancer: American Society of Clinical Oncology/Cancer Care Ontario joint guideline update. *J Clin Oncol.* 2017;35(15):1737–1743.

176. Carlton CE Jr, Scardino PT. Combined interstitial and external irradiation for prostatic cancer. *Prog Clin Biol Res.* 1987;243b:141–169.

177. Zelefsky MJ, Whitmore WF, Jr. Long-term results of retropubic permanent 125iodine implantation of the prostate for clinically localized prostatic cancer. *J Urol.* 1997;158(1):23–29; discussion 29–30.

178. Blasko JC, Grimm PD, Ragde H. Brachytherapy and organ preservation in the management of carcinoma of the prostate. *Semin Radiat Oncol.* 1993;3(4):240–249.

179. Ling CC. Permanent implants using Au-198, Pd-103 and I-125: radiobiological considerations based on the linear quadratic model. *Int J Radiat Oncol Biol Phys.* 1992;23(1):81–87.

180. Wallner K, Merrick G, True L, Sutlief S, Cavanagh W, Butler W. 125I versus 103Pd for low-risk prostate cancer: preliminary PSA outcomes from a prospective randomized multicenter trial. *Int J Radiat Oncol Biol Phys.* 2003;57(5):1297–1303.

181. Bice WS, Prestidge BR, Kurtzman SM, et al. Recommendations for permanent prostate brachytherapy with (131)Cs: a consensus report from the Cesium Advisory Group. *Brachytherapy.* 2008;7(4):290–296.

182. Nath R, Anderson LL, Luxton G, Weaver KA, Williamson JF, Meigooni AS. Dosimetry of interstitial brachytherapy sources: recommendations of the AAPM Radiation Therapy Committee Task Group No. 43. American Association of Physicists in Medicine. *Med Phys.* 1995;22(2):209–234.

183. Williamson JF, Coursey BM, DeWerd LA, et al. Recommendations of the American Association of Physicists in Medicine on 103Pd interstitial source calibration and dosimetry: implications for dose specification and prescription. *Med Phys.* 2000;27(4):634–642.

184. Stock RG, Stone NN, Tabert A, et al. A dose-response study for I-125 prostate implants. *Int J Radiat Oncol Biol Phys.* 1998;41(1):101–108.

185. Nag S, Beyer D, Friedland J, et al. American Brachytherapy Society (ABS) recommendations for transperineal permanent brachytherapy of prostate cancer. *Int J Radiat Oncol Biol Phys.* 1999;44(4):789–799.

186. Martinez AA, Gustafson G, Gonzalez J, et al. Dose escalation using conformal high-dose-rate brachytherapy improves outcome in unfavorable prostate cancer. *Int J Radiat Oncol Biol Phys.* 2002;53(2):316–327.

187. Pisansky TM, Gold DG, Furutani KM, et al. High-dose-rate brachytherapy in the curative treatment of patients with localized prostate cancer. *Mayo Clin Proc.* 2008;83(12):1364–1372.

188. Hsu IC, Bae K, Shinohara K, et al. Phase II trial of combined high-dose-rate brachytherapy and external beam radiotherapy for adenocarcinoma of the prostate: preliminary results of RTOG 0321. *Int J Radiat Oncol Biol Phys.* 2010;78(3):751–758.

189. Yamada Y, Rogers L, Demanes DJ, et al. American Brachytherapy Society consensus guidelines for high-dose-rate prostate brachytherapy. *Brachytherapy.* 2012;11(1):20–32.

190. Hoskin PJ, Colombo A, Henry A, et al. GEC/ESTRO recommendations on high dose rate afterloading brachytherapy for localised prostate cancer: an update. *Radiother Oncol.* 2013;107(3):325–332.

191. D'Amico AV, Whittington R, Malkowicz SB, et al. Pretreatment nomogram for prostate-specific antigen recurrence after radical prostatectomy or external-beam radiation therapy for clinically localized prostate cancer. *J Clin Oncol.* 1999;17(1):168–172.

192. Kattan MW, Zelefsky MJ, Kupelian PA, Scardino PT, Fuks Z, Leibel SA. Pretreatment nomogram for predicting the outcome of three-dimensional conformal radiotherapy in prostate cancer. *J Clin Oncol.* 2000;18(19):3352–3359.

193. Kattan MW, Zelefsky MJ, Kupelian PA, et al. Pretreatment nomogram that predicts 5-year probability of metastasis following three-dimensional conformal radiation therapy for localized prostate cancer. *J Clin Oncol.* 2003;21(24):4568–4571.

194. Ray ME, Levy LB, Horwitz EM, et al. Nadir prostate-specific antigen within 12 months after radiotherapy predicts biochemical and distant failure. *Urology.* 2006;68(6):1257–1262.

195. Roach M 3rd, Hanks G, Thames H Jr, et al. Defining biochemical failure following radiotherapy with or without hormonal therapy in men with clinically localized prostate cancer: recommendations of the RTOG-ASTRO Phoenix Consensus Conference. *Int J Radiat Oncol Biol Phys.* 2006;65(4):965–974.

196. Kuban DA, Levy LB, Potters L, et al. Comparison of biochemical failure definitions for permanent prostate brachytherapy. *Int J Radiat Oncol Biol Phys.* 2006;65(5):1487–1493.

197. Pickles T, Kim-Sing C, Morris WJ, et al. Evaluation of the Houston biochemical relapse definition in men treated with prolonged neoadjuvant and adjuvant androgen ablation and assessment of follow-up lead-time bias. *Int J Radiat Oncol Biol Phys.* 2003;57(1):11–18.

198. Abramowitz MC, Li T, Buyyounouski MK, et al. The Phoenix definition of biochemical failure predicts for overall survival in patients with prostate cancer. *Cancer.* 2008;112(1):55–60.

199. Buyyounouski MK, Hanlon AL, Horwitz EM, et al. Interval to biochemical failure highly prognostic for distant metastasis and prostate cancer-specific mortality after radiotherapy. *Int J Radiat Oncol Biol Phys.* 2008;70(1):59–66.

200. Denham JW, Steigler A, Wilcox C, et al. Time to biochemical failure and prostate-specific antigen doubling time as surrogates for prostate cancer-specific mortality: evidence from the TROG 96.01 randomised controlled trial. *Lancet Oncol.* 2008;9(11):1058–1068.

201. D'Amico AV, Moul JW, Carroll PR, Sun L, Lubeck D, Chen MH. Surrogate end point for prostate cancer-specific mortality after radical prostatectomy or radiation therapy. *J Natl Cancer Inst.* 2003;95(18):1376–1383.

202. Lawton CA, Hunt D, Lee WR, et al. Long-term results of a phase II trial of ultrasound-guided radioactive implantation of the prostate for definitive management of localized adenocarcinoma of the prostate (RTOG 98-05). *Int J Radiat Oncol Biol Phys.* 2011;81(1):1–7.

203. Giberti C, Chiono L, Gallo F, et al. Radical retropubic prostatectomy versus brachytherapy for low-risk prostatic cancer: a prospective study. *World J Urol.* 2009;27(5):607–612.

204. Morris WJ, Tyldesley S, Rodda S, et al. Androgen Suppression Combined with Elective Nodal and Dose Escalated Radiation Therapy (the ASCENDE-RT Trial): an analysis of survival endpoints for a randomized trial comparing low-dose-rate brachytherapy boost to dose-escalated external beam boost for high- and intermediate-risk prostate cancer. *Int J Radiat Oncol Biol Phys.* 2017;98(2):275–285.

205. Guix I, Bartrina JM, Tello JI, et al. Dose escalation with high-dose-3D-conformal/IMRT (HD-3D-CRT/IMRT) compared with low-dose 3D-conformal/IMRT plus HDR brachytherapy (LD-3D-CRT/IMRT+HDR-B) for intermediate- or high-risk prostate cancer: Disease control, survival, and toxicity. *J Clin Oncol.* 2018;36(6_suppl):169–169.

206. Stein JP, Lieskovsky G, Cote R, et al. Radical cystectomy in the treatment of invasive bladder cancer: long-term results in 1,054 patients. *J Clin Oncol.* 2001;19(3):666–675.

207. Herr HW. Conservative management of muscle-infiltrating bladder cancer: prospective experience. *J Urol.* 1987;138(5):1162–1163.

208. Herr HW, Jakse G, Sheinfeld J. The T1 bladder tumor. *Semin Urol.* 1990;8(4):254–261.

209. Herr HW. Tumour progression and survival in patients with T1G3 bladder tumours: 15-year outcome. *Br J Urol.* 1997;80(5):762–765.

210. Brake M, Loertzer H, Horsch R, et al. Long-term results of intravesical bacillus Calmette-Guérin therapy for stage T1 superficial bladder cancer. *Urology.* 2000;55(5):673–678.

211. Shelley M, Court JB, Kynaston H, Wilt TJ, Fish R, Mason M. Intravesical Bacillus Calmette-Guérin in Ta and T1 bladder cancer. *Cochrane Database Syst Rev.* 2000(4):16.

212. Wo JY, Shipley WU, Dahl DM, et al. The results of concurrent chemo-radiotherapy for recurrence after treatment with bacillus Calmette-Guérin for non-muscle-invasive bladder cancer: is immediate cystectomy always necessary? *BJU Int.* 2009;104(2):179–183.

213. Weiss C, Wolze C, Engehausen DG, et al. Radiochemotherapy after transurethral resection for high-risk T1 bladder cancer: an alternative to intravesical therapy or early cystectomy? *J Clin Oncology.* 2006;24(15):2318–2324.

214. Rödel C, Grabenbauer GG, Kühn R, et al. Combined-modality treatment and selective organ preservation in invasive bladder cancer: long-term results. *J Clin Oncol.* 2002;20(14):3061–3071.

215. Herr HW, Faulkner JR, Grossman HB, et al. Surgical factors influence bladder cancer outcomes: a cooperative group report. *J Clin Oncol.* 2004;22(14):2781–2789.

216. Pollack A, Zagars GK, Cole CJ, Dinney CP, Swanson DA, Grossman HB. The relationship of local control to distant metastasis in muscle invasive bladder cancer. *J Urol.* 1995;154(6):2059–2063; discussion 2063–2054.

217. Neoadjuvant chemotherapy in invasive bladder cancer: a systematic review and meta-analysis. *Lancet (London, England).* 2003;361(9373):1927–1934.

218. Roberts JT, von der Maase H, Sengeløv L, et al. Long-term survival results of a randomized trial comparing gemcitabine/cisplatin and methotrexate/vinblastine/doxorubicin/cisplatin in patients with locally advanced and metastatic bladder cancer. *Ann Oncol.* 2006;17 Suppl 5:v118–v122.

219. Ruggeri EM, Giannarelli D, Bria E, et al. Adjuvant chemotherapy in muscle-invasive bladder carcinoma: a pooled analysis from phase III studies. *Cancer.* 2006;106(4):783–788.

220. Huncharek M, Muscat J, Geschwind JF. Planned preoperative radiation therapy in muscle invasive bladder cancer; results of a meta-analysis. *Anticancer Res.* 1998;18(3b):1931–1934.

221. Baumann BC, Guzzo TJ, He J, et al. Bladder cancer patterns of pelvic failure: implications for adjuvant radiation therapy. *Int J Radiat Oncol Biol Phys.* 2013;85(2):363–369.

222. Zaghloul MS, Christodouleas JP, Smith A, et al. Adjuvant sandwich chemotherapy plus radiotherapy vs adjuvant chemotherapy alone for locally advanced bladder cancer after radical cystectomy: a randomized phase 2 trial. *JAMA Surg.* 2018;153(1):e174591.

223. Zaghloul MS, Awwad HK, Akoush HH, Omar S, Soliman O, el Attar I. Postoperative radiotherapy of carcinoma in bilharzial bladder: improved disease free survival through improving local control. Int J Radiat Oncol Biol Phys. 1992;23(3):511–517.

224. Baumann BC, Sargos P, Eapen LJ, et al. The rationale for post-operative radiation in localized bladder cancer. *Bladder Cancer.* 2017;3(1):19–30.

225. Reisinger SA, Mohiuddin M, Mulholland SG. Combined pre- and postoperative adjuvant radiation therapy for bladder cancer--a ten year experience. *Int J Radiat Oncol Biol Phys.* 1992;24(3):463–468.

226. Spera JA, Whittington R, Littman P, et al. A comparison of preoperative radiotherapy regimens for bladder carcinoma. The University of Pennsylvania experience. *Cancer.* 1988;61(2):255–262.

227. Shimko MS, Tollefson MK, Umbreit EC, Farmer SA, Blute ML, Frank I. Long-term complications of conduit urinary diversion. *J Urol.* 2011;185(2):562–567.

228. Zaghloul MS, Christodouleas JP, Smith A, et al. Adjuvant sandwich chemotherapy and radiation versus adjuvant chemotherapy alone for locally advanced bladder cancer. *Int J Radiat Oncol Biol Phys.* 2016;96(2):S94.

229. Gospodarowicz MK, Hawkins NV, Rawlings GA, et al. Radical radiotherapy for muscle invasive transitional cell carcinoma of the bladder: failure analysis. *J Urol.* 1989;142(6):1448–1453; discussion 1453–1444.

230. Duncan W, Quilty PM. The results of a series of 963 patients with transitional cell carcinoma of the urinary bladder primarily treated by radical megavoltage X-ray therapy. *Radiother Oncol.* 1986;7(4):299–310.

231. Pollack A, Zagars GZ. Radiotherapy for stage T3b transitional cell carcinoma of the bladder. *Semin Urol Oncol.* 1996;14(2):86–95.

232. De Neve W, Lybeert ML, Goor C, et al. Radiotherapy for T2 and T3 carcinoma of the bladder: the influence of overall treatment time. *Radiother Oncol.* 1995;36(3):183–188.

233. Mameghan H, Fisher R, Mameghan J, et al. Analysis of failure following definitive radiotherapy for invasive transitional cell carcinoma of the bladder. *Int J Radiat Oncol Biol Phys.* 1995; 31(2):247–254.

234. Gospodarowicz MK, Quilty PM, Scalliet P, et al. The place of radiation therapy as definitive treatment of bladder cancer. *Int J Urol.* 1995;2 Suppl 2:41–48.

235. Housset M, Maulard C, Chretien Y, et al. Combined radiation and chemotherapy for invasive transitional-cell carcinoma of the bladder: a prospective study. *J Clin Oncol.* 1993;11(11):2150–2157.

236. Mak RH, Hunt D, Shipley WU, et al. Long-term outcomes in patients with muscle-invasive bladder cancer after selective bladder-preserving combined-modality therapy: a pooled analysis of Radiation Therapy Oncology Group protocols 8802, 8903, 9506, 9706, 9906, and 0233. *J Clin Oncol.* 2014;32(34):3801–3809.

237. Efstathiou JA, Bae K, Shipley WU, et al. Late pelvic toxicity after bladder-sparing therapy in patients with invasive bladder cancer: RTOG 89-03, 95-06, 97-06, 99-06. *J Clin Oncol.* 2009;27(25):4055–4061.

238. Zietman AL, Sacco D, Skowronski U, et al. Organ conservation in invasive bladder cancer by transurethral resection, chemotherapy and radiation: results of a urodynamic and quality of life study on long-term survivors. *J Urol.* 2003;170(5):1772–1776.

239. Huddart RA, Hall E, Hussain SA, et al. Randomized noninferiority trial of reduced high-dose volume versus standard volume radiation therapy for muscle-invasive bladder cancer: results of the BC2001 trial (CRUK/01/004). *Int J Radiat Oncol Biol Phys.* 2013;87(2):261–269.

240. Miyamoto DT, Drumm MR, Clayman RH, et al. Outcomes and tolerability of selective bladder preservation by combined modality therapy for invasive bladder cancer in elderly patients. *Int J Radiat Oncol Biol Phys.* 2017;99(2):S120.

241. Hafeez S, McDonald F, Lalondrelle S, et al. Clinical outcomes of image guided adaptive hypofractionated weekly radiation therapy for bladder cancer in patients unsuitable for radical treatment. *Int J Radiat Oncol Biol Phys.* 2017;98(1):115–122.

242. Duchesne GM, Bolger JJ, Griffiths GO, et al. A randomized trial of hypofractionated schedules of palliative radiotherapy in the management of bladder carcinoma: results of medical research council trial BA09. *Int J Radiat Oncol Biol Phys.* 2000;47(2):379–388.

243. Tunio MA, Hashmi A, Qayyum A, et al. Whole-pelvis or bladder-only chemoradiation for lymph node-negative invasive bladder cancer: single-institution experience. *Int J Radiat Oncol Biol Phys.* 2012;82(3):e457–e462.

244. Baumann BC, Bosch WR, Bahl A, et al. Development and validation of consensus contouring guidelines for adjuvant radiation therapy for bladder cancer after radical cystectomy. *Int J Radiat Oncol Biol Phys.* 2016;96(1):78–86.

245. Aetiology of testicular cancer: association with congenital abnormalities, age at puberty, infertility, and exercise. United Kingdom Testicular Cancer Study Group. *BMJ (Clinical research ed).* 1994;308(6941):1393–1399.

246. Jemal A, Ward EM, Johnson CJ, et al. Annual report to the nation on the status of cancer, 1975–2014, featuring survival. *J Natl Cancer Inst.* 2017;109(9).

247. International Germ Cell Consensus Classification: a prognostic factor-based staging system for metastatic germ cell cancers. International Germ Cell Cancer Collaborative Group. *J Clin Oncol.* 1997;15(2):594–603.

248. Groll RJ, Warde P, Jewett MA. A comprehensive systematic review of testicular germ cell tumor surveillance. *Crit Rev Oncol Hematol.* 2007;64(3):182–197.

249. Mortensen MS, Lauritsen J, Gundgaard MG, et al. A nationwide cohort study of stage I seminoma patients followed on a surveillance program. *Eur Urol.* 2014;66(6):1172–1178.

250. Soper MS, Hastings JR, Cosmatos HA, Slezak JM, Wang R, Lodin K. Observation versus adjuvant radiation or chemotherapy in the management of stage I seminoma: clinical outcomes and prognostic factors for relapse in a large US cohort. *Am J Clin Oncol.* 2014;37(4):356–359.

251. Jones G, Arthurs B, Kaya H, et al. Overall survival analysis of adjuvant radiation versus observation in stage I testicular seminoma: a surveillance, epidemiology, and end results (SEER) analysis. *Am J Clin Oncol.* 2013;36(5):500–504.

252. Gray PJ, Lin CC, Sineshaw H, Paly JJ, Jemal A, Efstathiou JA. Management trends in stage I testicular seminoma: Impact of race, insurance status, and treatment facility. *Cancer.* 2015;121(5):681–687.

253. Warde P, Specht L, Horwich A, et al. Prognostic factors for relapse in stage I seminoma managed by surveillance: a pooled analysis. *J Clin Oncol.* 2002;20(22):4448–4452.

254. Aparicio J, Maroto P, García Del Muro X, et al. Prognostic factors for relapse in stage I seminoma: a new nomogram derived from three consecutive, risk-adapted studies from the Spanish Germ Cell Cancer Group (SGCCG). *Ann Oncol.* 2014;25(11):2173–2178.

255. Oliver RT, Mead GM, Rustin GJ, et al. Randomized trial of carboplatin versus radiotherapy for stage I seminoma: mature results on relapse and contralateral testis cancer rates in MRC TE19/EORTC 30982 study (ISRCTN27163214). *J Clin Oncol.* 2011;29(8):957–962.

256. Warde P, Gospodarowicz M, Panzarella T, et al. Management of stage II seminoma. *J Clin Oncol.* 1998;16(1):290–294.

257. Gospodarowicz MK, Sturgeon JF, Jewett MA. Early stage and advanced seminoma: role of radiation therapy, surgery, and chemotherapy. *Semin Oncol.* 1998;25(2):160–173.

258. Abratt RP, McAdam GL, Pontin AR, et al. Primary chemotherapy for stage 2 testis cancer. *S Afr J Surg.* 1997;35(4):203–205; discussion 205–206.

259. Flechon A, Bompas E, Biron P, et al. Management of post-chemotherapy residual masses in advanced seminoma. *J Urol.* 2002;168(5):1975–1979.

260. Duchesne GM, Stenning SP, Aass N, et al. Radiotherapy after chemotherapy for metastatic seminoma--a diminishing role. MRC Testicular Tumour Working Party. *Eur J Cancer (Oxford, England : 1990).* 1997;33(6):829–835.

261. Horwich A, Paluchowska B, Norman A, et al. Residual mass following chemotherapy of seminoma. *Ann Oncol.* 1997;8(1):37–40.

262. von der Maase H, Specht L, Jacobsen GK, et al. Surveillance following orchidectomy for stage I seminoma of the testis. *Eur J Cancer (Oxford, England : 1990).* 1993;29a(14):1931–1934.

263. Warde PR, Gospodarowicz MK, Goodman PJ, et al. Results of a policy of surveillance in stage I testicular seminoma. *Int J Radiat Oncol Biol Phys.* 1993;27(1):11–15.

264. Dosoretz DE, Shipley WU, Blitzer PH, et al. Megavoltage irradiation for pure testicular seminoma: results and patterns of failure. *Cancer.* 1981;48(10):2184–2190.

265. Fosså SD, Aass N, Kaalhus O. Radiotherapy for testicular seminoma stage I: treatment results and long-term post-irradiation morbidity in 365 patients. *Int J Radiat Oncol Biol Phys.* 1989;16(2):383–388.

266. Fosså SD, Horwich A, Russell JM, et al. Optimal planning target volume for stage I testicular seminoma: A Medical Research Council randomized trial. Medical Research Council Testicular Tumor Working Group. *J Clin Oncol.* 1999;17(4):1146.

267. Capelouto CC, Clark PE, Ransil BJ, et al. A review of scrotal violation in testicular cancer: is adjuvant local therapy necessary? *J Urol.* 1995;153(3 Pt 2):981–985.

268. Marks LB, Anscher MS, Shipley WU. Radiation therapy for testicular seminoma: controversies in the management of early-stage disease. *Oncology (Williston Park).* 1992;6(6):43–48; discussion 51–42.

269. Warde P, Gospodarowicz MK, Panzarella T, et al. Stage I testicular seminoma: results of adjuvant irradiation and surveillance. *J Clin Oncol.* 1995;13(9):2255–2262.

270. Wilder RB, Buyyounouski MK, Efstathiou JA, et al. Radiotherapy treatment planning for testicular seminoma. *Int J Radiat Oncol Biol Phys.* 2012;83(4):e445–e452.

271. Jones WG, Fossa SD, Mead GM, et al. Randomized trial of 30 versus 20 Gy in the adjuvant treatment of stage I testicular seminoma: a report on Medical Research Council Trial TE18, European Organisation for the Research and Treatment of Cancer Trial 30942 (ISRCTN18525328). *J Clin Oncol.* 2005;23(6):1200–1208.

272. Warde PR, Chung P, Sturgeon J, et al. Should surveillance be considered the standard of care in stage I seminoma? *J Clin Oncol.* 2005;23(16_suppl):4520–4520.

273. Vallis KA, Howard GC, Duncan W, et al. Radiotherapy for stages I and II testicular seminoma: results and morbidity in 238 patients. *Br J Radiol.* 1995;68(808):400–405.

274. Classen J, Schmidberger H, Meisner C, et al. Radiotherapy for stages IIA/B testicular seminoma: final report of a prospective multicenter clinical trial. *J Clin Oncol.* 2003;21(6):1101–1106.

275. Mencel PJ, Motzer RJ, Mazumdar M, Vlamis V, Bajorin DF, Bosl GJ. Advanced seminoma: treatment results, survival, and prognostic factors in 142 patients. *J Clin Oncol.* 1994;12(1):120–126.

276. Schmoll HJ, Souchon R, Krege S, et al. European consensus on diagnosis and treatment of germ cell cancer: a report of the European Germ Cell Cancer Consensus Group (EGCCCG). *Ann Oncol.* 2004;15(9):1377–1399.

277. Travis LB, Curtis RE, Storm H, et al. Risk of second malignant neoplasms among long-term survivors of testicular cancer. *J Natl Cancer Inst.* 1997;89(19):1429–1439.

278. Zwahlen DR, Martin JM, Millar JL, et al. Effect of radiotherapy volume and dose on secondary cancer risk in stage I testicular seminoma. *Int J Radiat Oncol Biol Phys.* 2008;70(3):853–858.

279. Davis BJ, Horwitz EM, Lee WR, et al. American Brachytherapy Society consensus guidelines for transrectal ultrasound-guided permanent prostate brachytherapy. *Brachytherapy.* 2012;11(1):6–19.

280. Kaufman DS, Winter KA, Shipley WU, et al. Phase I-II RTOG study (99-06) of patients with muscle-invasive bladder cancer undergoing transurethral surgery, paclitaxel, cisplatin, and twice-daily radiotherapy followed by selective bladder preservation or radical cystectomy and adjuvant chemotherapy. *Urology.* 2009;73(4):833–837.

281. Fernando SA, Sandler HM. Organ preservation in muscle-invasive bladder cancer. *Oncology (Williston Park).* 2005;19(3):334–339; discussion 339–340, 345, 349, 350–333.

282. James ND, Hussain SA, Hall E, et al. Radiotherapy with or without Chemotherapy in Muscle-Invasive Bladder Cancer. *N Engl J Med.* 2012;366(16):1477–1488.

11 Gynecologic Malignancies

Aaron B. Simon, Daniel R. Simpson, Loren K. Mell, Dominique Rash, Jyoti Mayadev, Arno J. Mundt, and Catheryn M. Yashar

INTRODUCTION

Gynecologic cancers arise from organs throughout the female reproductive tract, including the ovaries, uterus, cervix, vagina, and vulva. Gynecologic cancers represent the fourth most common malignant tumors diagnosed in women in the United States each year, with approximately 113,500 cases expected in 2020.[1] Worldwide, gynecologic cancers represent approximately 15% of all cancers in woman, and 7% of all cancers, with approximately 1.3 million cases per year.[2] Radiation therapy (RT) occupies an important role in the treatment of nearly all gynecologic malignancies. Radiation is the backbone of definitive treatment for locoregionally advanced cervical, vulvar, and vaginal cancers and an important component of adjuvant treatment for uterine cancers. It is also frequently used to palliate patients when cure is not possible.

This chapter provides an overview of the role of RT in the treatment of gynecologic malignancies, with a focus on the planning of various radiotherapeutic approaches used in these patients, including external-beam RT and brachytherapy. Technologies to be discussed include intensity-modulated RT (IMRT), image-guided RT (IGRT), and image-guided brachytherapy.

RADIOTHERAPEUTIC MANAGEMENT

Cervical Cancer

Radiation is commonly used in the treatment of nearly all stages of cervical cancer; however, how it is used in combination with other local and systemic therapies is highly stage dependent. It is important to note that the International Federation of Gynecology and Obstetrics (FIGO) updated its staging system in 2018 to reflect recent advances both in diagnostic and staging technology and in therapeutic strategies.[3] The most significant change in the staging workup is that imaging technologies such as magnetic resonance imaging (MRI), positron emission tomography (PET), and computed tomography (CT) as well as pathological findings may be used to determine stage. The new staging nomenclature reflects an understanding of the significance of certain staging features. As a result, the stages included in many of the seminal trials of RT in cervical cancer may not be reflective of the stage assignment currently in use. In this chapter, we will use the FIGO 2018 staging convention throughout, even when referring to trials that employed the older staging convention. A table is included (Table 11.1) demonstrating the 2018 FIGO staging system.

Selected early (microscopic) tumors (stage IA) are treated primarily with surgery; however, when these patients are unable to undergo surgery due to advanced age and/or significant comorbidities, RT can be used and is associated with excellent results.[4] Early-stage patients with small but macroscopic disease (stages IB1-2 and IIA1) are managed well with either radical surgery or definitive RT, with cure rates exceeding 80% following either approach.[5] The choice of surgery versus radiation in early-stage cervical cancer depends on a number of factors, including patient age, comorbidities, and various tumor characteristics. Older women, particularly those with multiple comorbidities, are generally treated with RT whereas younger women receive surgery. A common reason for favoring surgery in young women is the ability to preserve ovarian function. However, it may be possible to preserve ovarian function in premenopausal patients by performing an ovarian transposition prior to RT.[6] Another oft-stated reason for favoring surgery in young women is the commonly held belief that sexual function would be less adversely affected. However, analyses of prospective quality of life have found equivalent sexual function following surgery compared to RT.[7] In general, RT is recommended over surgery in early-stage cervical cancer patients as lesion size and parametrial/vaginal involvement increase. As tumor diameter exceeds 4 cm (stages IB3 and IIA2), there is increased likelihood of tumor spread to surrounding organs and regional lymph nodes, necessitating the need for adjuvant RT following surgery. Randomized trials conducted by the Gynecologic Oncology Group (GOG) and other cooperative groups have found that postoperative RT is beneficial in many patients with cervical cancer, following surgery. GOG 92 noted an improved 2-year recurrence-free survival rate

TABLE 11.1	FIGO staging system for Cervical Cancer 2018	
Stage	**Description**	**Notes**
IA	Invasive carcinoma that can be diagnosed only by microscopy, with maximum depth of invasion <5 mm	Horizontal extent no longer considered
IA1	Measured stromal invasion <3 mm in depth	
IA2	Measured stromal invasion ≥3 mm and <5 mm in depth	
IB	Invasive carcinoma with measured deepest invasion ≥5 mm, limited to the cervix uteri	IB1 and IB2 were previously combined as IB1, IB3 was previously IB2
IB1	Invasive carcinoma ≥5 mm depth and <2 cm in greatest dimension	
IB2	Invasive carcinoma <4 cm in greatest dimension	
IB3	Invasive carcinoma ≥4 cm in greatest dimension	
IIA	Involvement limited to the upper two thirds of the vagina but without parametrial involvement	
IIA1	Invasive carcinoma <4 cm in greatest dimension	
IIA2	Invasive carcinoma ≥4 cm in greatest dimension	
IIB	With parametrial involvement but not up the pelvic wall	3D imaging (e.g., MRI) can be used to assess for parametrial involvement
IIIA	The carcinoma involves the lower third of the vagina, with no extension to the pelvic wall	
IIIB	Extension to the pelvic wall and or hydronephrosis or nonfunctioning kidney not due to another cause	3D imaging may assess sidewall involvement and/or hydroureter
IIIC	Involvement of pelvic and/or paraaortic lymph nodes	Can use 3D imaging (indicated by r) or surgical staging (indicated by p)
IIIC1	Pelvic lymph node involvement only	
IIIC2	Paraaortic lymph node involvement	
IVA	Spread to adjacent organs	
IVB	Spread to distant organs	

Adapted from Bhatla N, et al., Cancer of the cervix uteri. *Int J Gynecol Obstet*. 2018;143:22–36.

(88% vs. 79%, $p = 0.008$) comparing adjuvant RT versus no further therapy in node-negative patients with high-risk features (deep stromal invasion, bulky primary disease, and/or lymphovascular invasion [LVI])[8] as well as a trend toward an increase in overall survival.[9] GOG 109 compared adjuvant pelvic RT versus pelvic RT plus chemotherapy in women found to have involved pelvic nodes, parametrial invasion, and/or positive margins and noted a superior 4-year overall survival (81% vs. 71%, $p = 0.007$) with the combined approach.[10] Whether concomitant chemoradiotherapy is superior to RT alone in node-negative patients with high-risk features is currently being evaluated by the NRG Oncology Group, GOG 263, whereas the benefit of adjuvant chemotherapy following chemoradiotherapy in high-risk node-positive patients is the subject of GOG 0724. These studies are anticipated to complete data collection by the end of 2021.

While a treatment option in early-stage patients, radiation has long been the cornerstone of treatment in cervical cancer patients with locally advanced (stages IIB to IVA) disease. In these women, radiation is combined with concomitant chemotherapy after multiple prospective randomized trials demonstrated a survival advantage to the combined approach.[11–13] Surgery is typically not utilized in patients with locally advanced disease, albeit some investigators have advocated pelvic exenteration in cases with bladder and/or rectal invasion (stage IVA).[14] Metastatic (stage IVB) patients may also undergo RT, particularly those with a good response to chemotherapy or those requiring palliative treatment due to uncontrolled vaginal bleeding.

Definitive RT in cervical cancer is administered with a combination of pelvic RT and brachytherapy, except in earliest-stage patients in whom brachytherapy alone is sufficient.[4] Early-stage patients (stage IB1-2) may be treated with radiation alone as none of the previously mentioned trials included these patients, although there are gynecologic oncologists who recommend combined therapy. Early-stage patients with bulky (>4 cm) tumors (stage IB3) are treated with a combination of pelvic RT and chemotherapy.[15] Of note, adjuvant hysterectomy was commonly employed in the era when this trial was conducted, with the goal of improving local control due to an inability to have an adequate dose distribution with a standard brachytherapy applicator.[16] This technique is no longer considered standard unless anatomical or pathological factors preclude adequate coverage by brachytherapy.[17] When delivered adjuvantly, most patients receive pelvic RT with or without chemotherapy. In women with locally advanced disease, pelvic fields are also used, except in those with documented paraaortic lymph node involvement in whom extended field RT (EFRT) is administered. In the past, there was considerable interest in *prophylactic* paraaortic RT in locally advanced patients, following the superior survival rates reported on the Radiation Therapy Oncology Group (RTOG) trial using this approach.[18] However, the combination of chemotherapy to pelvic RT was subsequently shown to be superior to EFRT alone for women with locoregionally advanced disease.[11] There has not been a trial comparing chemoradiation with EFRT versus chemoradiation with pelvic RT. Nonetheless, EFRT with chemotherapy is frequently considered for those with multiple positive pelvic nodes, especially if the nodal disease is bulky or bilateral or extends to the common iliac nodes. For patients with lower vaginal involvement, radiation fields are extended to include the inguinal lymph nodes, and for patients with significant parametrial involvement and/or gross nodal disease, an additional external-beam RT dose is often delivered in the form of a boost.

Brachytherapy is standard in conjunction with pelvic RT for patients with cervical cancer undergoing definitive treatment.[19] In the adjuvant setting, brachytherapy is less commonly performed, except when patients are treated preoperatively. If brachytherapy is prescribed, most patients receive intracavitary brachytherapy (ICB); however, there is increasing evidence that with modern image guidance, adaptive brachytherapy employing a hybrid approach with both intracavitary and interstitial brachytherapy (ISB) may improve outcomes for women with unfavorable anatomy or bulky disease.[19,20] Completing chemoradiation and brachytherapy in ≤56 days continues to be an important goal in the definitive treatment of cervical cancer.[19] See Radiotherapy Techniques later for a full discussion of the various RT techniques used in patients with cervical cancer.

Uterine Cancer

Although radiation was historically delivered prior to surgery for many patients with uterine cancer,[21] the majority of patients today undergo upfront surgery, consisting of total hysterectomy, bilateral salpingo-oophorectomy (TH-BSO), plus/minus lymph node assessment, with RT delivered postoperatively to selected patients based on pathologic features in the surgical specimen. Historically, lymph node evaluation involved comprehensive pelvic and paraaortic lymph node dissection; however, increasingly, sentinel lymph node mapping is gaining acceptance as a method of reducing the morbidity associated with lymph node evaluation without compromising its prognostic and predictive function.[22] In addition, with low-risk features the nodal evaluation may not be done at the discretion of the gynecologic oncologist.

The most common pathologic features used to determine the need for adjuvant RT in early-stage (stages I to II) uterine cancer are tumor grade, histology, depth of myometrial invasion (MI), LVI, and cervical involvement. More advanced age has also consistently been an adverse risk factor. Some investigators also use tumor size and lower uterine segment (LUS) involvement; however, the prognostic significance of such features, particularly in the absence of other more established adverse features,

remains unclear.[19] Multiple randomized trials have been performed by the GOG and other groups demonstrating that adjuvant RT in early-stage uterine cancer patients with adverse pathologic features significantly reduces locoregional failure.[23–26] Whether it improves survival, however, remains a matter of intense debate. PORTEC I, a prospective randomized trial with sufficient power to answer the question, did not demonstrate improved survival. By contrast, two large Surveillance Epidemiology and End Results (SEER) studies do suggest a survival benefit.[27–29]

At many centers today, low-risk early-stage uterine cancer patients (stage I, grade 1, no or minimal MI) are treated with surgery alone. For many stage I patients with grade 1–2 disease and deep (>50%) MI or grade 3 disease with superficial (<50%) invasion, vaginal brachytherapy (VBT) is considered sufficient adjuvant therapy based on the results of the PORTEC-2 study, which compared adjuvant VBT to pelvic EBRT in this population.[30] While the 10-year results of this study did show a significant increase in pelvic recurrence (6.3% vs. 0.9%) with VBT, isolated pelvic failure rates were not significantly different (2.5% vs. 0.5%), nor were rates of vaginal cuff failure, distant failure, or overall survival. Subset analysis of this study suggested that patients with substantial lymph-vascular space invasion (LVSI), L1CAM expression, or *TP53* mutation, who are otherwise good candidates for VBT might benefit from EBRT in terms of pelvic control.[31] For patients with stage I disease and multiple high-risk features (grade 3, deep invasion, LVSI), the optimum treatment strategy is less certain. Two large randomized trials addressing this population were published in 2019. GOG 249 was a superiority study evaluating pelvic EBRT against VBT followed by carboplatin/paclitaxel chemotherapy. The chemotherapy arm was not found to be superior as the study found no difference in vaginal or distant recurrence between the two treatment strategies but increased pelvic failures in the group that received VBT and chemotherapy.[32] In addition, the chemotherapy and VBT arm demonstrated greater acute toxicity. PORTEC-3 also included patients in this group but combined with higher stage patients and compared pelvic EBRT against pelvic EBRT with concurrent and adjuvant chemotherapy. This study showed improved overall survival and failure-free survival with the addition of chemotherapy, especially in stage III and serous patients.[33] Taken together, these studies suggest that pelvic EBRT alone may be an appropriate adjuvant treatment strategy for selected high-risk stage I patients. PORTEC-3 also evaluated patients based on molecular staging and found that patients with p53 mutations had improved relapse-free survival with the addition of chemotherapy and those that were POLE ultramutated did well in either arm. This study demonstrates that utility of molecular staging in selecting adjuvant therapy.[34] Stage II patients, those with cervical stromal invasion, represent a smaller group of patients and have been less well studied in isolation. These patients are often treated with pelvic EBRT as they were excluded from the PORTEC-2 trial and included in PORTEC-3 and GOG 249. However, large multi-institutional series have shown low rates of pelvic and distant metastatic failure in select patients with grade 1–2 disease and without macroscopic cervical involvement who received adjuvant VBT alone, suggesting this may be adequate therapy for select stage II patients without other high-risk uterine pathologic factors.[35] For early-stage uterine cancer patients unable to undergo surgery due to advanced age and/or multiple comorbidities, adiation can be used with curative intent and typically consists of a combination of brachytherapy with pelvic RT in patients with deep myometrial or cervical invasion and brachytherapy alone in those with grade 1–2 disease and minimal MI.[36] Pelvic MRI may be helpful in these women to evaluate MI and extrauterine spread.

For stage III and IVA uterine cancers, the standard approach was historically surgery followed by adjuvant RT, using a variety of techniques including pelvic RT, EFRT, or whole abdominal RT (WART). Following the publication of GOG 122, which randomized stage III to IV patients to either WART or chemotherapy and noted a superior 5-year survival (55% vs. 42%) with adjuvant chemotherapy but inferior pelvic control,[37] multiagent chemotherapy became an important component of adjuvant therapy for advanced state patients. However, the question remained whether adjuvant RT plays a role in conjunction with chemotherapy. Patterns of failure studies suggested that it does, given the high risk of locoregional recurrence in women undergoing surgery and chemotherapy[38] and both in clinical practice and on cooperative group studies, stage III and selected stage IV patients are often treated with chemotherapy combined with limited volume RT (pelvic RT, EFRT, and/or VBT based on pathologic features), an approach known as "tumor volume–directed" RT.[39] The recently published GOG 258 trial, which randomized patients with III–IVA endometrial carcinoma to receive adjuvant chemoradiation, followed by four cycles of carboplatin and paclitaxel versus six cycles of carboplatin and paclitaxel alone, sought to define the role of radiation therapy in this setting. For the primary endpoint of relapse-free survival, it found no difference between chemoradiotherapy and chemotherapy (59% vs. 58%); however, it did find differences in vaginal recurrence (2% vs. 7%), pelvic and paraaortic recurrence (11% vs. 20%) and distant recurrence (27% vs. 21%).[40] In addition, subset analysis of PORTEC-3 (described earlier) found a benefit to chemoradiotherapy in stage III endometrial carcinoma and those with serous cancers.[33] Ongoing work continues to define the optimum sequencing and combination of chemotherapy and RT in these patients. Strategies such as "sandwich" chemotherapy-radiation-chemotherapy remain an area of active investigation.[41]

The role of RT in the treatment of patients with unfavorable histologies, notably papillary serous and clear cell tumors, is controversial. However, RT may help reduce the risk of locoregional recurrence in such patients who receive adjuvant chemotherapy following surgery.[42] Of note, early-stage clear cell and papillary serous patients were included in PORTEC-3, GOG 258, and GOG 249. While the relatively low numbers of these patients on each trial make definitive conclusions challenging to derive, PORTEC-3 did demonstrate an advantage to chemoradiation over radiation alone for this population.[33] In addition, most serous cancers have p53 mutations, and molecular analysis of patients in PORTEC-3 supports chemoradiotherapy.[34] Patients with early-stage uterine sarcomas, except those with low-grade endometrial stromal sarcoma, are considered for treatment with adjuvant pelvic RT for local control, although data suggest that with leiomyosarcoma distant failure is as common as local failure. Carcinosarcoma, now thought to be a dedifferentiated carcinoma, is treated more similar to high-grade carcinomas as described earlier. This is demonstrated by the superior outcomes for patients with carcinosarcoma undergoing chemotherapy compared to WART on the GOG 150 trial.[43] Nonetheless, adjuvant RT still remains a consideration in these patients, particularly in older women and others who are unable to undergo adjuvant chemotherapy. See the Radiotherapy Techniques later for a full discussion of the various RT techniques used in patients with uterine cancer.

Ovarian Cancer

For many years, RT occupied an important role in the treatment of ovarian cancer. Following upfront surgery, consisting of an omentectomy, TAH-BSO, peritoneal sampling, and cytoreduction of extra-ovarian disease throughout the abdomen and pelvis, and often pelvic and paraaortic lymph node dissection, adjuvant RT was routinely delivered in the form of intraperitoneal ^{32}P in high-risk early-stage and WART in locally advanced disease patients. Today, chemotherapy has largely replaced RT in the treatment of ovarian carcinoma in the United States except for focal palliative radiation. Nevertheless, it is of interest to note that both ^{32}P[44,45] and WART[46] have been found in prospective, randomized trials to compare favorably with chemotherapy in this setting.

RT is occasionally used in the management of patients with nonepithelial ovarian cancers. Given its exquisite radiosensitivity, ovarian dysgerminoma may be treated with RT; however, in these patients as well, the standard practice today is adjuvant chemotherapy, particularly in those desiring fertility-sparing treatment. As in other gynecologic cancers, RT has an important role in the palliative treatment of patients with ovarian cancer.[47] See Radiotherapy Techniques later for a discussion of the various RT techniques used in ovarian cancer.

Vulvar Cancer

The treatment of vulvar cancer consists of upfront surgery, typically radical vulvectomy or radical wide local excision in selected patients with small well-lateralized tumors,[48] with RT delivered adjuvantly in patients with high-risk features including large size, LVI, tumor invasion >5 mm, surgical margins <8 mm, grade 3 disease, and positive margins.[49,50] Most patients also undergo lymph node evaluation, which in the modern era may be limited to sentinel lymph node biopsy (SLNB) rather than inguinal-femoral dissection in clinically node-negative patients.[51,52] In the GROningen International Study on Sentinel nodes in Vulvar cancer (GROINSS-V) I study, early-stage, unifocal, clinically node-negative patients underwent radical excision of the primary and SLNB. Node-negative patients were observed while node-positive patients underwent inguinofemoral lymphadenectomy, with adjuvant radiation to the groin and pelvis employed for patients with >1 node-positive or extranodal extension (ENE).[51] SLNB-negative patients were found to have a low rate of isolated groin recurrence (2.5%). In the follow-up GROINSS-V-II study, investigators asked whether radiotherapy was a safe alternative to inguinofemoral lymphadenectomy in similar patients with a positive SLNB.[53] The study was amended to exclude patients with involved nodal metastases measuring >2 mm or ENE due to evidence of increased risk of groin recurrence with omission of lymphadenectomy in this group. Early results suggest lymphadenectomy may be safe to omit for patients with an SLN metastasis measuring ≤2 mm and without ENE who receive adjuvant radiotherapy.[53]

In women with locally advanced but resectable disease, surgery is typically performed, followed by adjuvant radiation or chemoradiation. Over 20 years ago, the GOG completed a landmark trial (GOG 37) comparing adjuvant RT versus pelvic node dissection in patients found to have involved inguinal nodes at the time of surgery.[54] A significantly higher survival rate was noted in the RT group, with the greatest benefit seen in women with clinically suspicious and/or ≥2 pathologically involved nodes. Moreover, adjuvant RT significantly reduced the risk of recurrence in the inguinal nodes (5% vs. 24%, $p = 0.02$). This trial established adjuvant RT as the treatment of choice in these patients. Although commonly used in many other gynecologic cancers, *prophylactic* nodal irradiation is rarely used to treat clinically negative regional lymph nodes in vulvar cancer without further investigation of the surgical nodal status. This practice is based on the GOG 88 trial, which compared prophylactic inguinofemoral RT versus lymphadenectomy in clinically node-negative patients and found a significantly higher rate of recurrence ($p = 0.03$) and death ($p = 0.04$) in the RT group.[55] See Radiotherapy Techniques later for critique of this influential study.

In patients with unresectable vulvar cancer, RT has been used preoperatively with promising results.[56,57] Considerable interest has been focused on further augmenting these results by combining RT with chemotherapy.[49,58,59] GOG 101 evaluated preoperative chemoradiotherapy in locally advanced unresectable patients and found that nearly all patients (97%) became resectable, with only 16% ultimately failing locally.[60] GOG 205 increased the dose of radiation to 57.6 Gy from 47.6 Gy and eliminated the twice-daily radiation and planned treatment break used in GOG 101. This resulted in an increase in the clinical complete response (CCR) rate from 48% to 64% and in the pathological CR rate from 31% to 50%.[61] The ongoing GOG 279 study will assess whether adding gemcitabine to cisplatin chemoradiation further improves outcomes for these patients.

Adjuvant RT in vulvar cancer is delivered using a variety of techniques, ranging from small electron fields directed solely at the primary site to generous fields encompassing the primary, pelvis plus one or both groins. The most common approach, however, is pelvic-inguinal irradiation, delivered with or without a midline block. Brachytherapy has a limited role in vulvar cancer, apart from patients with a positive vaginal margin or in medically inoperable patients in whom high doses are required to control the primary tumor. However, at most centers, high-dose central boosts are delivered in such patients using external-beam techniques. A description of the various RT techniques used in vulvar cancer is provided later (see Radiotherapy Techniques).

Vaginal Cancer

The treatment of choice in all stages of vaginal cancer is definitive RT. However, selected early-stage patients, such as those with small-volume disease limited to the upper vagina, can be treated with a variety of surgical approaches, including partial or radical vaginectomy.[62]

Early-stage vaginal cancer patients typically receive brachytherapy alone or combined with external beam when tumors invade the paravaginal tissues.[63,64] Some investigators advocate the use of combined external beam and brachytherapy even in patients without paravaginal invasion.[65] Overall, definitive RT is associated with excellent outcomes in most early-stage vaginal cancer patients, particularly in those with stage I disease in whom locoregional control rates exceed 85%.[63] Patients with locally advanced disease undergo pelvic RT and brachytherapy.[63–65] Extrapolating from cervical cancer studies, chemotherapy may be delivered concomitantly in these patients in an effort to improve tumor control and potentially survival. While this strategy has not been definitively tested in a randomized trial, its growing acceptance is reflected in cooperative group trials, such as NRG GY006, which include patients with vaginal cancer and designate chemoradiation as the standard treatment arm.

Brachytherapy in early-stage vaginal cancer typically involves ICB, but in women with >0.5 cm tumor invasion or thickness, ISB is recommended. Some investigators favor ISB combined with ICB even in patients with superficial tumors to reduce the total vaginal dose and, in distal vaginal tumors, the rectal dose.[65] If external beam is also delivered, patients with vaginal cancer receive either pelvic irradiation, or in cases involving the lower one-third of the vagina, pelvic-inguinal RT. See Radiotherapy Techniques next for a discussion of the various RT techniques used in patients with vaginal cancer.

RADIOTHERAPY TECHNIQUES

External-Beam Therapy

Whole Pelvic Radiotherapy

Pelvic RT is used in many gynecologic cancers to irradiate multiple target tissues within the pelvis, including the uterus/cervix (or the postoperative bed), the upper vagina, paracervical/parametrial tissues, and the pelvic (internal, external, and common iliac) lymph nodes. Pelvic RT fields were historically designed using fluoroscopic simulation based on bony landmarks and delivered with either two-field (opposed anterior–posterior:posterior–anterior [APPA] fields) or four-field (APPA plus opposed lateral fields) techniques (Fig. 11.1). Today, it is considered standard practice to employ CT-based treatment planning and either 3D conformal or intensity-modulated

radiation therapy (IMRT), with targets defined anatomically based on the gross tumor volume (GTV), clinical target volume (CTV), and planning target volume (PTV) per convention established in the International Commission on Radiation Units (ICRU) Reports 50 and 62.[17,66,67] However, the considerations involved in the development of conventional pelvic radiation fields have heavily influenced the design of modern radiation treatment volumes and so are described here.

For many years, the superior border of the pelvic RT field was placed at the L5–S1 interspace; however, this shifted to the L4–L5 interspace to include the common iliac lymph nodes, especially in cervical carcinoma. It is important to note, however, common iliac lymph nodes in some patients may extend considerably higher, requiring an upper border as high as L2–L3 to ensure their full coverage when contouring based on anatomy rather than bony landmarks. The lower pelvic RT border was conventionally placed at the inferior obturator foramen, while the lateral borders were set 1 to 1.5 cm beyond the pelvic brim. The anterior border of the lateral field was at (or 1 cm anterior) to the pubic symphysis to ensure coverage of the external iliac nodes; the posterior border was at the S2–S3 interspace.[68] Various modifications could be made to the traditional pelvic RT fields, depending on the clinical scenario. In cervical or uterine cancer patients with significant vaginal involvement, the lower border could be extended to the introitus, ensuring irradiation of the entire vaginal canal. In such cases, a radiopaque marker should be placed at the most inferior extent of disease. The superior border could be extended superiorly to fully

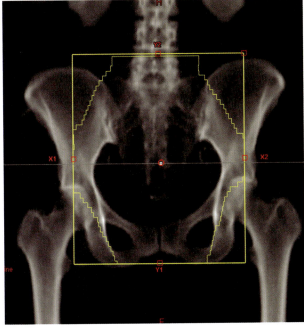
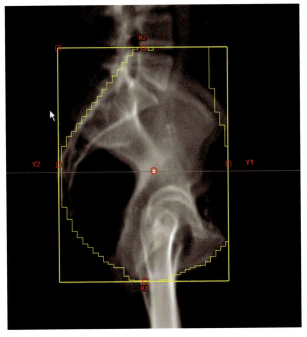

A   **B**

FIGURE 11.1. Anterior–posterior (AP) (**A**) and lateral fields (**B**) in a representative patient with gynecologic cancer undergoing whole pelvic radiation therapy.

encompass the common iliac lymph nodes, particularly in women with involvement of the external iliac lymph nodes, or could be lowered to the L5–S1 interspace in patients who underwent surgical lymph node evaluation and were found to have negative pelvic nodes. The posterior border of the lateral field could also be moved posterior to the sacrum in cervical cancer patients with bulky disease, whereas the anterior border could be moved anteriorly in women with an anteverted uterus and/or bulky external iliac nodes. Then, as now, customized blocking was added to each field using either cerrobend or multileaf collimation to reduce dose to the surrounding normal tissues, including the small bowel and rectum. Oral and/or intravenous contrast may be administered at simulation to aid in contouring and in the design of blocks.

Despite the meticulous design of these traditional fields, multiple investigators have demonstrated that this approach may underdose the target tissues and/or inadequately shield surrounding normal tissues in many patients.[69,70] Finlay et al. assessed the adequacy of nodal coverage of conventional pelvic RT fields in 43 patients with cervical cancer.[70] Pelvic vessels were contoured following CT simulation and used as surrogates for the pelvic lymph nodes. In 41 patients (95%), conventional fields inadequately covered various lymph node groups. Of note, in 24 patients (56%), conventional fields and blocks were found to be too generous. Others have similarly used three-dimensional (3D) imaging and found that conventional fields and blocking may result in inadequate target coverage in up to 50% of patients, particularly with the placement of the posterior field border of the lateral pelvic field at S2–S3.[69] These results strongly supported the design of pelvic RT field using CT simulation, which, as mentioned earlier, is now the preferred approach if advanced imaging is available.

At many centers, patients undergoing pelvic RT are immobilized and simulated in the supine position. Prone positioning with a "belly board" is favored by some investigators to help reduce the volume of small bowel irradiated. Similarly, at some centers, patients are simulated and treated with a full bladder to displace small bowel. Whatever approach is used, it is important to strive for consistent bladder and rectal filling throughout treatment, given that the volume of these organs may impact the position of the cervix/uterus (or vaginal cuff) and the organs at risk (OAR).[71,72]

Conventional pelvic RT fields were typically delivered using moderate–high energy (≥10 MV) photon beams. However, lower energies could be used in selected thin patients. Wedges could be added to the lateral fields to reduce "hot spots" in the treatment plan. As an example, a pelvic RT plan is shown in Figure 11.2. Total doses prescribed typically range from 39.6 to 50.4 Gy delivered in 1.8 to 2 Gy/fractions, the higher doses used in patients undergoing external beam alone and lower doses in those treated with both external beam and brachytherapy.

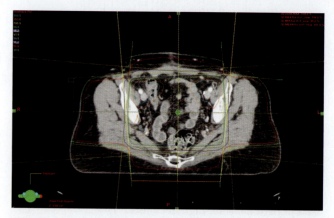

FIGURE 11.2. Treatment plan with isodose lines in a representative gynecologic cancer patient treated with whole pelvic radiation therapy.

In the past, there was considerable interest in the use of altered fractionation schedules in patients with gynecologic cancer, including accelerated hyperfractionated RT as a means of escalating the pelvic radiation dose. However, the RTOG 88–05 trial using this approach in locally advanced cervical cancer patients failed to demonstrate a benefit in terms of tumor control or complications.[73] Others have also reported high complication rates using a hyperfractionated approach.[74] Moreover, twice-daily treatment in an effort to boost the cervical tumor prior to brachytherapy has also been associated with increased complications.[75] In contrast, hypofractionated approaches, for example, 2.5- to 3-Gy daily fractions (total doses 30–35 Gy), have been used successfully in patients treated with palliative intent. Higher dose per fraction (up to 10 Gy) palliative regimens have also been explored.[75,76]

Various blocks can be added to the conventional pelvic RT field. At some centers, a midline block is utilized, allowing a higher proportion of the total dose to be delivered by brachytherapy in patients with cervical cancer, typically placed after approximately 20 Gy.[77] A midline block may also be placed following brachytherapy in cervical cancer patients with significant parametrial involvement and/or involved pelvic lymph nodes allowing an additional boost to be delivered, typically 10 to 12 Gy in five to six fractions.

At many centers, midline blocks are often standardized, but at others the midline block may be customized based on the brachytherapy isodose distributions (Fig. 11.3). In 1997, Wolfson et al. performed a survey of GOG institutions and reported that the percentages of centers using standard and customized midline blocks were 76% and 21%, respectively, at that time.[78] Only 3% utilized step-wedge blocks as popularized by Perez et al.[77] The width of the midline block should fully encompass the ovoids (colpostats) on the anterior radiograph plus a margin since narrow midline blocks inadequately shield the ureters and are associated with increased complications.[79] The

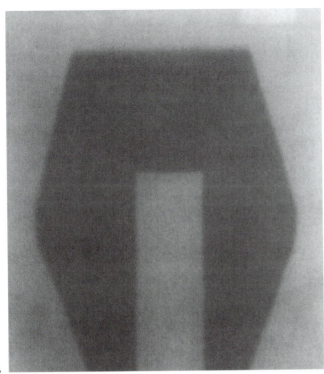
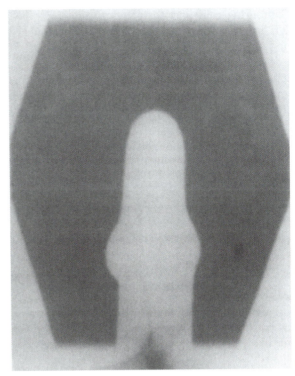

A

B

FIGURE 11.3. Example midline blocks used in patients with cervical cancer: (**A**) standard block and (**B**) customized block based on brachytherapy isodose distribution. (Adapted from Wolfson AH, et al. A quantitative assessment of standard versus customized midline shield construction for invasive cervical carcinoma. *Int J Radiat Oncol Biol Phys.* 1997;37:237–242.)

inferior edge of the block should be coincident with the lower border of the pelvic field. However, various superior block edges can be used. In the GOG survey, the upper border of the midline block was set at the top of the pelvic field, the tip of the tandem plus a 1- to 2-cm margin, or the level of the sacroiliac joint by 29%, 38%, and 33% of respondents, respectively.[78]

IMRT is increasingly used in the treatment of gynecologic cancers. Investigators at the University of Chicago were the first to compare conventional and IMRT lanning in patients with gynecologic cancer undergoing pelvic RT and found that IMRT reduced the volume of small bowel irradiated by a factor of two and the volume of both the bladder and rectum irradiated by 23%.[75] Others have confirmed these results, with reductions up to 70% seen with IMRT planning in terms of the volume of small bowel receiving the prescription dose.[79,80] Recently, the dosimetric improvements associated with IMRT were validated by the publication of the RTOG 1203 trial.[81] This trial randomized women undergoing postoperative pelvic radiation for endometrial or cervical cancer to receive either standard four-field radiation or IMRT. It found that IMRT caused significantly less acute patient-reported GI and urinary toxicity than four field RT, with 33.7% versus 51.9% of study participants reporting frequent or almost constant diarrhea in each arm, respectively.

In addition to reducing GI toxicity, IMRT planning has been shown to be an effective means of reducing the volume of pelvic bone marrow irradiated in patients undergoing pelvic RT, an appealing approach particularly in patients receiving concomitant chemotherapy.[82] The clinical benefit of this was recently demonstrated by the INTERTECC-2 trial,[83] which was a multicenter single-arm phase II trial that treated patients with stage IB-IVA cervical cancer with IMRT and concurrent weekly cisplatin followed by brachytherapy. It found an occurrence rate of 26.5% for grade 3 or above neutropenia or clinically significant GI toxicity, a rate that was significantly lower than the historical rate of 40%.

Patients undergoing pelvic IMRT are typically immobilized in the supine position and undergo CT simulation with thin (2.5-5 mm) slices, although at selected centers prone positioning is favored.[84] Contrast may be administered to aid in the delineation of the target and normal tissues; intravenous contrast is particularly useful since the pelvic vasculature is used as a surrogate for the lymph nodes in the planning process.

Following simulation, a GTV and CTV are contoured on the planning CT scan, based on ICRU 50 guidelines.[66] The GTV should include all demonstrable diseases, including involved regional lymph nodes. A variety of imaging modalities can be used to aid in target design, with growing attention on PET and MRI.[85] Modern cooperative group trials often recommend fusing PET/CT and/or MRI with the simulation CT scan to aid in target delineation.

Contouring guidelines for patients undergoing pelvic IMRT have been developed for both the postoperative setting (Fig. 11.4) and the definitive setting for cervical cancer[86–88] (Fig. 11.5) and are now employed by many cooperative group trials. Specific target volumes depend on the disease site, clinical and pathologic features, and treatment setting; however, in general, the CTV consists of the upper half of the vagina, uterus/cervix (if present), parametria, presacral region, and pelvic lymph nodes (internal, external, and either lower or entire common iliac nodes). Guidelines for contouring pelvic nodes are based, in part, on the work of Taylor et al., who mapped pelvic lymph node regions using iron oxide-enhanced MRI, a method to visualize benign lymph nodes.[89] In an analysis of 20 patients using this technique, a modified margin of 7 mm around the major pelvic vessels was found to encompass 99% of the visualized lymph nodes. The CTV is typically divided into sub-CTVs to facilitate the differential PTV expansions needed for each structure based on its setup reproducibility. Normal tissues are contoured as well, including the small bowel, bladder, rectum, and, at some centers, the sigmoid colon. The pelvic bones are used as a surrogate for the pelvic bone marrow in patients undergoing chemoradiotherapy. In the past, only the iliac crests were contoured; however, recent data suggest that the pelvic bones are a better surrogate for the bone marrow in the optimization process, with PET-guided active bone marrow sparing also being studied on the INTERTECC trials.[83,84]

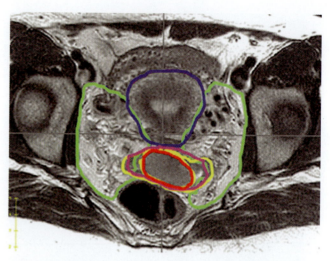

FIGURE 11.5. Axial view of a T2-weighted magnetic resonance (MR) images illustrating contours of the gross tumor volume (GTV) (*red*), cervix (*pink*), vagina (*yellow*), parametria (*green*), and uterus (*blue*) in a patient with intact cervical cancer undergoing intensity-modulated radiation therapy (IMRT) based on the Radiation Therapy Oncology Group (RTOG) consensus conference. (Adapted from Lim K, et al. Consensus guidelines for delineation of clinical target volume for intensity-modulated pelvic radiotherapy for the definitive treatment of cervical cancer. *Int J Radiat Oncol Biol Phys.* 2011;79:348–355.)

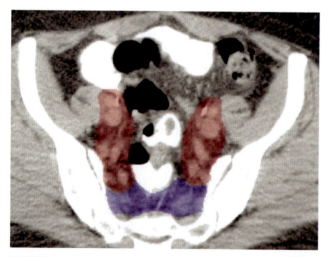

FIGURE 11.4. Mid-pelvic computed tomography (CT) image illustrating a clinical target volume (CTV) delineated in a patient with cervical cancer treated postoperatively based on guidelines developed for the Radiation Therapy Oncology Group (RTOG) 0418 trial. Upper external and internal iliac (*red*) and presacral region (*blue*). (Adapted from Small W Jr, et al. Consensus guidelines for delineation of clinical target volume for intensity-modulated pelvic radiotherapy in postoperative treatment of endometrial and cervical cancer. *Int J Radiat Oncol Biol Phys.* 2008;71:428–434.)

The next step in the IMRT planning process involves the expansion of the CTV to generate a PTV, accounting for patient setup uncertainty and organ motion. The optimal PTV expansion is an area of active research, particularly in patients with intact cervical cancer in which there may be considerable organ motion.[71,72,90] A reasonable approach is to provide generous expansions around the cervical tumor (definitive patients) and the vaginal cuff (postoperative patients) on the order of 1.5 to 2 cm. Tighter expansions can be placed around the CTV in the upper pelvis (0.5–1 cm), depending on the use of daily image guidance. Daily in-room IGRT techniques, notably cone-beam CT (CBCT) imaging, help ensure adequate coverage of the target tissues on a daily basis.[72,91,92]

No consensus exists regarding many IMRT planning parameters used in patients with gynecologic cancer . At many centers, seven to nine equally spaced 6 MV beams are used; however, others favor volumetric-modulated arc or tomotherapy approaches. As in conventional RT, the total dose prescribed is a function of the tumor site, stage, and treatment volume. Most investigators deliver 45 Gy in 1.8-Gy daily fractions, particularly in women getting concurrent chemotherapy and subsequently undergoing brachytherapy. Higher doses (50.4 Gy) can be used in postoperative patients treated with pelvic IMRT alone.[84] For patients with grossly positive nodes, a simultaneous integrated boost (SIB) may be employed to dose escalate areas of macroscopic disease while sparing normal tissues.[93–96] Series have shown a low rate of nodal failure in patients for whom this approach was employed, and cooperative groups have incorporated an SIB to grossly involved nodes into modern trial protocols.[96]

Given the potential ability to safely deliver higher and potentially more efficacious doses, some investigators have explored using IMRT as a substitute for brachytherapy in cervical cancer.[97,98] Investigators at the Princess Margaret Hospital presented a case study of a stage IIB cervical cancer patient unsuitable for brachytherapy treated with an IMRT boost.[99] Using MRI guidance, a GTV was delineated consisting of the cervix and LUS. The GTV was expanded by a 10-mm margin (7 mm posteriorly) generating the CTV, which was subsequently expanded by 5 mm (10 mm anteriorly) to generate the PTV. Six static 6 MV fields were used to deliver 25.2 Gy in 1.8-Gy daily fractions to the PTV. The resultant treatment plan was highly conformal; average doses delivered to 50% of the rectum, bladder, and small bowel were 21 Gy, 13 Gy, and 5 Gy, respectively. Treatment was tolerated well without significant sequelae. Given the paucity of data using IMRT in lieu of brachytherapy, this approach should be considered experimental at the present time and only used in women unable to undergo brachytherapy. Additionally, a recent phase II trial assessing a related technique, stereotactic body RT, as a potential alternative to brachytherapy found a concerning safety signal, as will be discussed in greater detail later.[100]

The optimal dose–volume constraints for normal tissues in gynecologic cancer patients undergoing pelvic IMRT remain an area of active investigation, though guidelines have been established for trial protocols.[83,101] In recent years, detailed normal tissue complication probability (NTCP) studies have been performed in gynecologic cancer patients undergoing pelvic IMRT, which shed light on the optimal dose–volume constraints for various normal tissues (Fig. 11.6).[102–104] In an update of the combined University of Chicago/University of California San Diego experience, the small bowel volume receiving ≥45 Gy was constrained to 250 cc, and the volume of pelvic bone marrow (defined as entire pelvic bones) receiving ≥10 Gy and ≥20 Gy were constrained to receive ≤90% and ≤75%, respectively.[105] The normal tissue dose constraints used in the previously mentioned INTERTECC trial were small bowel volume receiving >45 Gy (V45) ≤250 cc; maximum dose <115%, rectum maximum dose <115% of the prescription dose, and bone marrow volume receiving 10 Gy and 2 Gy <90% and 75%, respectively. The normal tissue planning goals were small bowel volume receiving V45 ≤200 cc; V40 <30%; maximum dose <50 Gy, rectum V45 <50%; V30 <60%; maximum dose <50 Gy, bone marrow V10 <80%; V20 <66%; bladder V45 <50%; maximum dose <50 Gy, femoral head V30 <15%; maximum dose <50 Gy.[83]

Preliminary clinical outcome studies in patients with gynecologic cancer undergoing pelvic IMRT have been extremely promising, with lower rates of acute and

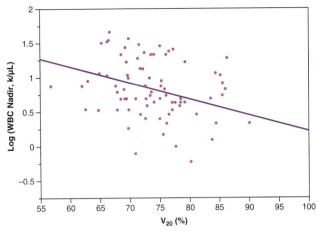

FIGURE 11.6. Plot of white blood cell count log (WBC nadir) versus bone marrow volume receiving 20 Gy or more (V_{20}) in a cohort of cervical cancer patients treated with combined chemoradiotherapy, supporting the use of bone marrow V_{20} as a constraint in the optimization process. Pelvic bones were used as a surrogate for pelvic bone marrow in this analysis. Regression coefficient (b) = –0.021 k/mL/%, $p = 0.002$. (Adapted from Rose BS, et al. Normal tissue complication probability modeling of acute hematologic toxicity in cervical cancer patients treated with chemoradiotherapy. *Int J Radiat Oncol Biol Phys.* 2010;78:912–919.)

chronic toxicities reported compared to conventional techniques.[13,105–109] Outcome studies have also reported excellent tumor control rates in both cervical[105,110] and uterine[111] cancers. Recently, data from prospective trials have supported the potential for toxicity reduction with pelvic IMRT. The favorable outcomes reported using adjuvant pelvic IMRT on the RTOG 0418 prospective clinical trial[112] were confirmed by the RTOG 1203 randomized trial, which showed decreased patient-reported GI and urinary toxicity in patients who received IMRT versus four-field pelvic radiation.[81] In addition, the INTERTECC 2 trial showed a reduction in ≥ grade 3 neutropenia and clinically significant GI toxicity in patients receiving pelvic IMRT compared with historical controls. Intriguingly, within that trial, patients who received PET-based image-guided IMRT with the goal of sparing active bone marrow demonstrated a reduction in ≥ grade 3 neutropenia compared with those who received IMRT without PET-guided bone marrow contouring, suggesting the potential for greater toxicity reduction with advanced IMRT planning incorporating functional imaging.[83]

Extended Field Radiotherapy

EFRT is used to treat the pelvic and paraaortic regions. A variety of techniques are currently utilized. At some centers, the entire volume is treated with large opposed APPA fields, extending from pelvis to the T12–L1 interspace. The paraaortic portion of these fields is typically 8 to 10 cm wide, depending on the patient's anatomy and disease extent. CT or PET/CT-based planning is helpful to ensure coverage of all enlarged lymph nodes while blocking the kidneys. To reduce the small bowel dose, some favor using four-field approaches (APPA plus opposed laterals). However, when using such approaches, care needs to be taken to minimize the dose to the kidneys with variable weightings between the APPA and lateral fields ensuring a maximum kidney dose of 18 Gy or less. At some centers, the pelvis and paraaortic regions are treated separately with a "gap" between fields to prevent dose overlap. Selected patients may need to be treated at an extended distance, given the length of the fields treated.

Whichever field arrangement is used, moderate–high energy beams (≥10 MV) are indicated, except in selected thin women; all patients are simulated and treated in the supine position. Prescribed doses range from 39.6 to 45 Gy delivered in 1.8 to 2 Gy per fractions. In women with involved paraaortic nodes, a 5- to 10-Gy boost may be delivered via reduced fields. Selected involved sites may be treated to 60 Gy or higher; however, care needs to be given to minimize the dose to the surrounding bowel, duodenum, and other normal tissues, including kidneys and spinal cord.

Multiple centers have explored the use of IMRT planning in patients with gynecologic cancer undergoing EFRT.[96,113–115] Compared to an APPA approach,

investigators at Washington University noted that RTIMRT EFRT (IM-EFRT) reduced the volume of small bowel, bladder, and rectum receiving the prescription dose by 61%, 96%, and 71%, respectively.[115] Compared to a four-field approach, corresponding reductions were 60%, 93%, and 56%, respectively. The following normal tissue constraints were used in the IM-EFRT planning: small bowel (<50% to receive ≥30 Gy), kidneys (<33% to receive ≥10 Gy), and spinal cord (<5% to receive ≥45 Gy). Lian et al. compared 3D conformal EFRT plans in 10 endometrial cancer patients to IMRT and helical tomotherapy (HT) plans.[114] The following constraints were used in the IMRT and HT optimization process: bladder (<50% to receive ≥40 Gy), rectum (<40% to receive ≥40 Gy), bowel (<35% to receive ≥35 Gy), kidneys (<35% to receive 16 Gy), and spinal cord (maximum dose, 40 Gy). Overall, both IMRT and HT resulted in superior target coverage and significantly reduced normal tissue doses compared to 3D conformal planning; however, the HT achieved the best normal tissue sparing (Fig. 11.7).

A potentially important role for IMRT in patients with gynecologic cancer undergoing EFRT is the ability to safely deliver higher-than-conventional doses to involved paraaortic lymph nodes. Using conventional techniques,

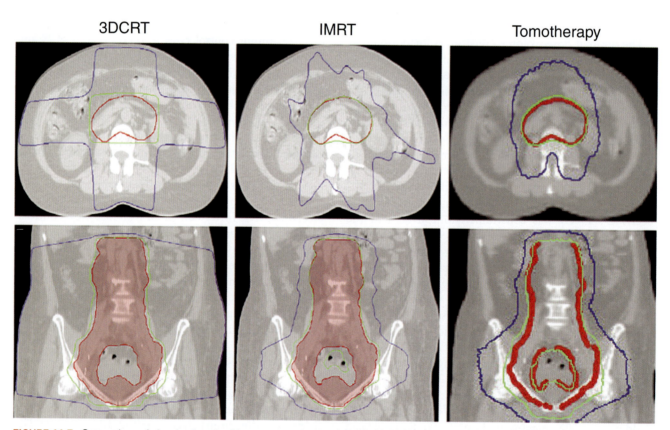

| 3DCRT | IMRT | Tomotherapy |

FIGURE 11.7. Comparison of planning target volume coverage by the 95% (*green line*) in three-dimensional conformal radiotherapy (3DCRT), intensity-modulated radiotherapy (IMRT), and helical tomotherapy (HT) plans in a stage IIIC uterine cancer patient undergoing extended field irradiation. *Blue* indicates the 50% isodose line; *red line* or *red area* indicates planning target volume. (Adapted from Lian J, et al. Assessment of extended-field radiotherapy for stage IIIC endometrial cancer using three-dimensional conformal radiotherapy, intensity-modulated radiotherapy, and helical tomotherapy. *Int J Radiat Oncol Biol Phys.* 2008;70:935–943.)

doses above 60 Gy, except in patients with small-volume disease, are difficult to deliver. However, the likelihood of controlling bulky paraaortic nodes with such doses is quite low. Multiple investigators have demonstrated that higher doses may be possible using SIB IMRT approaches in patients with involved paraaortic lymph nodes. Two different approaches have been proposed. Some investigators recommend that the entire paraaortic region be treated with conventional fraction sizes (1.8 Gy/day, 45 Gy total dose) and an SIB technique used to irradiate the involved nodes with *higher*-than-conventional fraction size, for example 2.4 Gy/day, 60 Gy total dose[95] or 2.2 Gy/day, 55 Gy total dose.[96] Alternatively, conventional fractions can be used for the SIB portion (1.8 Gy/day, 59.4 Gy total dose) and *lower* than conventional fractions used to treat the paraaortic region (1.53 Gy/day, 50.4 Gy total dose).[93] Care must be taken to calculate the duodenal dose with EFRT EBRT as MDACC reported that limiting the V55 to less than 15 cm^3 reduced the risk of complications.[116]

Limited outcome data exist using IM-EFRT. Salama et al. treated 13 women to a total dose of 45 Gy in 1.8-Gy fractions.[117] While 84% of patients experienced acute grade 2 bowel toxicity, no grade 3 or higher bowel or bladder sequelae were noted. Using the SIB approach with higher-than-conventional daily fractions (2.2 Gy/day, 55 Gy total dose) to PET-defined paraaortic nodes, investigators at the University of Pittsburgh noted acute grade 2 and 3 bowel sequelae in 10% and 0% of patients, respectively.[118] The University of Pittsburgh group also published an expanded experience using IM-ERFT with the same SIB technique in 61 consecutive women, either with PET-positive paraaortic disease or with PET-positive pelvic nodes alone, citing a false-negative rate of FDG-PET for paraaortic metastases of approximately 20%–25%. In this series, at a mean follow-up time of 29 months, 8 patients experienced recurrence. However, 10 patients (16.3%) had persistent or recurrent local disease, 3 (4.9%) involving the regional nodes, and 14 patients (23%) progressed distantly. The rate of paraaortic failure in patients with pelvic-only PET-positive nodes was 2.5%. Grade 3+ adverse events developed in only two patients (4%). Du et al. randomized 60 cervical cancer patients with involved paraaortic nodes to either IMRT or conventional RT to the paraaortic region.[94] While the IMRT patients received a higher prescribed dose (58 to 68 Gy vs. 45 to 50 Gy) than the conventional RT patients, they experienced less acute and chronic toxicity. Moreover, IMRT patients had a superior 3-year survival (36.4% vs. 15.6%, $p = 0.016$) compared to the conventional RT patients.

Pelvic-Inguinal Radiotherapy

In women with vulvar cancer and other gynecologic cancer patients involving the lower vagina, pelvic-inguinal irradiation is used to irradiate the pelvis, vagina, vulva, and bilateral inguinofemoral regions. Such patients are immobilized and simulated supine in the "frog-leg" position to minimize skin folds and thus the risk of acute perineal toxicity. Moderate–high energy beams (≥10 MV) are used for conventional radiation techniques.

The upper border of the conventional pelvic-inguinal field differs between institutions and is based on the disease extent. In patients with vulvar cancer, some advocate the treatment of reduced pelvic fields ("true pelvis") with the upper border placed inferior to the sacroiliac joints. Others place the upper border at the L5–S1 or L4–L5 interspace. In a survey of members of the Gynecologic Cancer Intergroup (GCIG), the most common upper border was L5–S1, followed by L4–L5.[49] In women with upper pelvic adenopathy, the upper border may need to be even higher. The lower border is typically placed approximately 5 cm inferior to the vulva/perineum to ensure coverage of the inguinofemoral lymph nodes.

A variety of treatment approaches have been used in patients undergoing pelvic-inguinal RT. One traditional approach is to use opposed APPA fields, with a "wide" AP field encompassing the pelvis and groin regions and a "narrow" PA field treating only the pelvis. Supplemental electron fields are used to treat the groins, reducing the dose received by the femoral heads. Alternatively, APPA fields can be equally wide, with partial transmission blocks placed on the PA field minimizing dose to the femoral heads. A third approach is to prescribe high-energy photons (10–24 MV) for the PA field and low-energy photons (4–6 MV) for the AP field. A novel modified segmental boost technique has been developed using a wide AP field, narrow PA field, and two angled photon fields encompassing the bilateral groins.[119] Whichever technique is used, attention needs to be given to avoid underdosing the vulvar region, particularly in patients treated preoperatively. Bolus is typically used with doses confirmed via thermoluminescence dosimetry (TLD). Total prescribed doses in patients undergoing pelvic-inguinal RT range from 45 to 50.4 Gy in 1.8- to 2-Gy daily fractions. Additional boosts may be delivered to the inguinal region in patients with involved lymph nodes. In the GCIG survey, the mean pelvic and groin node doses were 48.1 Gy and 49.9 Gy, respectively.[49]

When treating the inguinal lymph nodes with electrons, care needs to be taken to ensure the proper selection of beam energy. Routine use of low-energy electron beams will likely underdose the groin nodes in a significant number of patients, particularly obese women. The depth of treatment should be tailored to the individual patient based on CT imaging, since the depth of the inguinofemoral nodes is highly variable, with an average depth of 6.1 cm reported in one study.[120] The high rate of nodal failures observed in the RT patients treated on GOG 88 comparing prophylactic RT versus lymphadenectomy in clinically node-negative vulvar cancer patients was likely due, at least in part, to the fact that the groins were treated via a single anterior field prescribed to a depth of

3 cm.[55] Such an approach would significantly underdose the inguinal nodes in many patients. Prophylactic groin irradiation in clinically node-negative patients has been shown to be highly effective if properly planned and delivered.[121] Care must also be taken to ensure an adequate volume is irradiated, given inguinal nodal metastases can occur throughout the groin region. Thus, small volume fields designed to irradiate the vessels with a limited margin are not recommended.

Considerable controversy exists regarding the use of a midline block in vulvar cancer patients undergoing pelvic-inguinal RT. In one highly quoted report, Dusenbery et al. noted a 48% central recurrence rate in 26 women treated with a midline block.[122] However, all patients in this study had pathologically positive lymph nodes, and many did not have wide negative margins. Of note, central recurrences were rare in the GOG 37 trial despite the use of a midline block.[54] Thus, in the properly selected patient, a midline block may be reasonable, particularly in older, frail patients who are at high risk of requiring treatment breaks due to perineal toxicity if treated without a midline block.

IMRT is increasingly utilized for patients with gynecologic cancer undergoing pelvic-inguinal RT, and consensus contouring and treatment planning guidelines for vulvar cancer have been published.[123] Reported outcomes have been favorable with this technique. Beriwal et al. compared IMRT and conventional planning in terms of normal tissue sparing in 15 patients with vulvar cancer.[124] Various IMRT techniques were used, with a median number of seven beams (range 5–8). Normal tissue planning constraints included small bowel (<35% to receive ≥35 Gy), rectum (<40% to receive ≥40 Gy), and bladder (<40% to receive ≥30 Gy). The plans were considered acceptable if <5% of the PTV received <100% of the prescribed dose and <10% received >110%. Mean preoperative and postoperative prescribed doses were 46.4 and 50.4 Gy, respectively. IMRT planning resulted in better sparing of the small bowel, rectum, and bladder; however, no significant difference was seen in volume of the femoral heads irradiated. Treatment was well tolerated, with only one patient experiencing acute grade 3 toxicity and none developing a grade ≥3 late toxicity. Two patients ultimately recurred locally; both were treated postoperatively.

Investigators at the University of Pittsburgh also reported their experience with preoperative chemotherapy and intensity-modulated pelvic-inguinal RT in 18 vulvar cancer patients.[125] IMRT was delivered twice daily during the first and last treatment weeks. Overall, treatment was well tolerated with no grade ≥3 late toxicities. Moreover, no recurrences were seen in the nine patients achieving a pathologic CTRC, whereas three of five partial responders failed locally.

Stereotactic Body Radiotherapy

Stereotactic body radiotherapy (SBRT) is a treatment approach used to deliver high, ablative doses of radiation in a limited number of fractions (typically three to five) to extracranial targets. Popularity is rapidly growing for this technique in the treatment of primary and metastatic tumors, particularly in the liver, lung, and spine tumors,[126] and prospective data is emerging, indicating that aggressive local therapy may improve survival for patients with oligometastatic disease.[127] Initially delivered on conventional linear accelerators, SBRT today is currently delivered using specialized machines, such as the Cyberknife (Accuray, Inc., Sunnyvale, CA), Novalis (BrainLab AG, Feldkirchen, Germany), and the Trilogy or TrueBeam (Varian Medical Systems, Palo Alto, CA). Moreover, while originally developed using stereotactic localization methods, most SBRT approaches today instead rely on image guidance, using either planar- or volumetric-based imaging techniques.[128]

In recent years, several investigators have begun exploring the potential of SBRT in gynecologic cancers. Choi et al. reported their experience using SBRT to treat recurrent paraaortic lymph nodes with the Cyberknife system.[128] A total of 30 patients were treated with 33 to 45 Gy in three fractions, prescribed to the 73% to 87% isodose line. Prior to treatment, fiducial markers were placed in adjacent vertebral pedicles and used for online image guidance. In all patients, the GTV consisted of the involved lymph node defined by either CT or PET/CT imaging and was expanded by 2 mm to generate the PTV. Treatment was well tolerated with few acute and chronic sequelae. Local control was excellent, particularly in small volume (≤17 cc) disease. A treatment plan in a representative patient from this series is shown in Figure 11.8. Additional clinical series assessing the efficacy of SBRT in the setting of oligometastatic gynecological cancer have been published, with favorable reported local control and toxicity.[129,130] It is likely that as treatment planning and delivery techniques continue to improve and data from prospective trials accumulates, SBRT will play an increasing role in the management of oligometastatic gynecological malignancies.

The use of SBRT as a possible alternative to brachytherapy in the definitive treatment of gynecological malignancies has also been investigated, though to date, published results do not support its routine use in that setting. Molla et al. showed promising results in a small cohort of patients with either endometrial or cervical cancer treated with an SBRT boost in place of ICB.[131,132] However, a recently published phase II trial assessing the use of SBRT as alternative to brachytherapy for locally advanced cervical cancer was closed early due to concern for toxicity.[100] In this study grade ≥3 was 26.7% and was predominantly due to rectal ulcer or fistula. Two-year local control was also lower than expected at 70.1%. Patients enrolled on the study generally had large primary tumors and significant comorbidities, which the authors hypothesized might have contributed to the poorer than anticipated outcomes.[100]

Brachytherapy

Intracavitary Brachytherapy

ICB in patients with gynecologic cancer was initially performed by placing radioactive sources directly within the

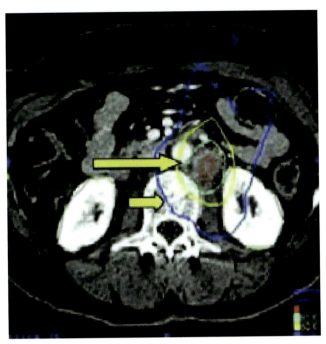

FIGURE 11.8. Treatment plan of a gynecologic cancer patient with an isolated paraaortic recurrence treated with stereotactic body radiation therapy (SBRT). The gross tumor volume (GTV) was defined as the visible tumor in the paraaortic lymph node region on computed tomography (CT) (*innermost red line*). The radiation dose was prescribed to the 81% isodose line of the maximum dose to cover the GTV + 2-mm margin (*sky-blue line* indicated by the *long arrow*). The outermost line is the 30% isodose line (*blue line* indicated by the *short arrow*). (Adapted from Choi CW, et al. Image-guided stereotactic body radiation therapy in patients with isolated paraaortic lymph node metastases from uterine cervical and corpus cancer. *Int J Radiat Oncol Biol Phys.* 2009;74:147–153.)

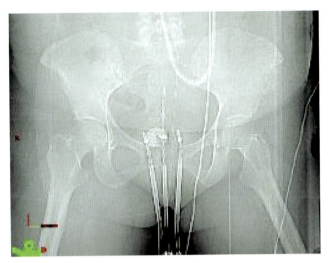

FIGURE 11.9. Tandem and ovoid applicator used for high dose rate (HDR) brachytherapy in patients with intact cervical cancer.

vagina and/or uterus. However, by the 1960s, *afterloading* techniques were introduced, whereby an applicator was first positioned within the patient while the sources were placed at a later time, typically after the patient had been transferred to an isolated (and often shielded) hospital room. Using this approach, radioactive sources were initially inserted manually but, more recently, remote-afterloading techniques have been developed, significantly reducing the exposure of the radiation oncologist and staff.

Various ICB applicators have been used in patients with gynecologic cancer, depending on the specific clinical scenario. In patients with cervical cancer treated with an intact uterus, the Fletcher–Suit–Delclos device based on the original Manchester system[133] is typically used, consisting of a curved tandem inserted into the uterus and two colpostats (ovoids) placed in the vaginal fornices. Various tandem lengths and colpostat diameters are available; most colpostats used today include shielding along the medial aspects of the anterior and posterior colpostat faces, reducing dose to the bladder and rectum (Fig. 11.9). A popular variation of the traditional tandem and ovoid

system consists of a tandem and ring, a system particularly useful in patients with asymmetric fornices. Another ICB applicator used in the treatment of cervical cancer is the Henschke device.[134] Interstitial applicators include the Vienna combined intracavitary and interstitial devices,[135] the Syed–Neblett template.[136] The Venezia applicator,[137] and the Martinez Universal Perineal Interstitial Template (MUPIT).[138]

While medically inoperable uterine cancer patients were historically treated with intrauterine Heyman-Simon capsules,[139] newer applicators have been developed, including the dual-tandem Rotte "Y" device.[140] In patients treated postoperatively, a variety of applicators can be placed within the vagina, typically either a vaginal cylinder or colpostats. The MIRALVA vaginal applicator consists of two ovoid sources and a central tandem.[141] The Capri vaginal applicator is a multichannel balloon applicator that consists of a single central channel surrounded by two concentric arrays of channels.[142]

Patients with gynecologic cancer undergoing ICB can be treated using either low dose rate (LDR) or high dose rate (HDR) techniques. According to the ICRU Report 38, LDR is defined as dose rates ranging from 0.4 to 2 Gy/h while HDR utilizes dose rates of >12 Gy/h, with modern HDR systems capable of delivering dose rates exceeding 400 Gy/h.[143] A variety of radioactive sources are used; however, the most popular are Cesium-137 (^{137}Cs) for LDR and high-activity Iridium-192 (^{192}Ir) for HDR. Unlike LDR, which is delivered in the hospital over several days, HDR is performed in the outpatient setting, obviating the need for hospitalization and prolonged bed rest. Other advantages of HDR include increased ability to optimize treatment plans, reduced radiation exposure of personnel, and better stability of the applicator during treatment. Disadvantages include increased number of treatment sessions and greater equipment cost. While some have argued that LDR is radiobiologically superior to HDR in terms of normal tissue effects, particularly in patients with an intact uterus,[144] prospective randomized trials have demonstrated that the two techniques are similar in terms of both tumor control and toxicity.[145–147] Some investigators favor the use of pulsed dose rate (PDR) brachytherapy, whereby intermittent "pulses" of radiation (10-30 minutes/h) are delivered using a machine similar to an afterloading HDR system. Proponents argue that PDR combines the logistic advantages of HDR with the potential radiobiological advantages of LDR.[148–150] Others have explored the use of HDR electronic brachytherapy in patients with gynecologic cancer.[151]

Various doses and prescription points have been used for HDR and LDR ICB. In patients with intact cervical cancer, dose was historically prescribed to a reference point known as Point A. In the original Manchester formulation,[133] Point A was defined as 2 cm lateral to the center of the intrauterine canal and 2 cm superior to the mucosal surface of the lateral fornix, presumably at the medial edge of the broad ligament, where the uterine artery crosses the ureter. In the early 1950s, however, the definition of Point A was modified to be 2 cm superior to the external cervical os and 2 cm lateral to the intrauterine canal. A second specified reference point in the Manchester system was Point B (3 cm lateral to Point A), which was felt to represent the location of the obturator lymph nodes, although CT-based studies reveal that this is rarely the case.[152] Importantly, the Manchester system was based on a system of 2D radiographic image guidance, which permitted visualization of the boney anatomy of the pelvis as well as the brachytherapy applicator but did not permit accurate visualization of a patient's soft-tissue anatomy. Today the American Brachytherapy Society (ABS) recommends adoption of the volume-based guidelines for contouring, treatment planning, and dose reporting that were originally developed by the Groupe Européen Curiethérapie-European Society of Therapeutic Radiation Oncology (GEC-ESTRO).[153,154] These guidelines are based on 3D rather than 2D radiographic image guidance for brachytherapy, which permits the prescription of dose to a target volume rather than to a point, and permits significantly greater customization of treatment planning to an individual patient's anatomy. In postoperative cervical or uterine cancer patients or patients with very superficial vaginal cancer, ICB is still standardly prescribed to either the vaginal surface or at 0.5 cm depth. In patients with uterine cancer treated with an intact uterus (either preoperatively or definitively), ICB was previously prescribed to 2 cm from the midpoint of the intrauterine sources[155]; however, the ABS has also recently developed guidelines for volumetric target delineation and treatment planning to reflect improvements in 3D volumetric imaging, in particular MRI.[36]

OAR were historically defined by surrogate reference points that could be visualized on a pair of orthogonal radiographs. The bladder point was defined on planar orthogonal radiographs as the point on the surface of the Foley balloon (pulled snugly into the bladder trigone) receiving the highest dose, although volumetric studies have demonstrated that this point consistently fails to capture the true maximum bladder dose.[156] The rectal reference point was defined 0.5 cm posterior to the posterior vaginal wall, which was itself inferred from the positions of the applicator and packing in the vagina.

The ABS recommends that intact cervical cancer patients undergoing LDR ICB be treated with two separate insertions to allow for reduction in tumor size and better coverage with the second insertion,[157] although comparable tumor control and complication rates have been reported with a single insertion, particularly in early-stage patients.[158] The ABS recommends that the first insertion be performed during the fourth to sixth weeks of pelvic RT; the second 1 to 2 weeks later. Care should be taken to complete the entire course of treatment within 8 weeks, since more protracted courses have been associated with poorer outcomes.

Intact cervical cancer patients undergoing HDR typically receive four to six insertions. Given the increased number of fractions, HDR may necessitate interdigitating pelvic RT and the initial HDR insertions to ensure that treatment is completed within 8 weeks, with the first treatment typically delivered in week 4 or 5 to allow for reduction in tumor size with chemoradiation, which improves brachytherapy coverage. It is recommended that patients are not treated with both ICB and external-beam RT or chemotherapy on the same day. For postoperative cervical and uterine cancers, vaginal cancer, and medically inoperable uterine cancer, ICB is delivered with one to two LDR or three to five HDR insertions.

For patients undergoing point-directed LDR brachytherapy, given the limited overall number of source activities and positions, treatment planning is typically performed manually by varying the various source activities and positions, focusing on the doses to Point A, as well as normal tissues. Many radiation oncologists typically start with a "standard" loading, for example, 15–10–10 milligram radium equivalents (mg-Ra-eq) in the tandem and 10 to 15 mg-Ra-eq in both colpostats in a patient with intact cervical cancer. The goal in this setting is to deliver a total Point A dose (including the pelvic RT) of approximately 80 to 85 Gy for small tumors and 85 to 90 Gy for bulky tumors, while limiting the rectal and bladder doses to <80% of the Point A dose. Different investigators have recommended different maximum acceptable rectal and bladder doses, typically <75 to 80 Gy for the bladder and <70 to 75 Gy for the rectum. Dose rates of 40 to 60 cGy/h to Point A are used at most centers. Care must be taken not only to optimize the doses and dose rates at the various reference and normal tissue points but also to review the isodose distributions themselves in an effort to obtain a classic "pear shape." Patients treated postoperatively to the vaginal cuff are typically treated with surface dose rates of 80 to 100 cGy/h or 50 to 80 cGy/h to 0.5 cm. Dose distributions in these patients should conform to the shape of the cylinder.

Given the increased number of potential dwell positions and times, HDR brachytherapy optimization lends itself to more sophisticated optimization approaches. As mentioned earlier, the ABS now recommends volume-directed rather than point-directed dose prescription and optimization. In this setting, the coverage goal, including the contribution from EBRT, is to deliver at least 80 Gy to at least 90% of the high-risk CTV (HR-CTV), as defined by the GEC-ESTRO working group,[153] for patients with residual disease less than 4 cm, and 85 to 90 Gy to at least 90% of the HR-CTV for patients with bulkier residual tumors.[159] Note that by requiring that the minimum dose to 90% (D_{90}) of the HR-CTV meet a coverage goal, the dose to point A becomes variable. The ABS still recommends reporting the point A dose in this setting but not optimizing to it. Note also that the doses specified are reported as biologically equivalent doses in 2-Gy fractions (EQD2) that also take into account the contribution from EBRT. Conversion of dose from the physical dose to EQD2 is performed according to the linear-quadratic model. A worksheet for performing this conversion is available for download on the ABS website (https://www.americanbrachytherapy.org/resources/for-professionals/physics-corner/). When employing volume-directed HDR brachytherapy, the ABS recommends optimizing the dose distribution to keep the minimum dose to the hottest 2 cc (D_{2cc}) of bladder ≤90 Gy EQD2, D_{2cc} rectum ≤75 Gy EQD2, and D_{2cc} sigmoid ≤75 Gy EQD2.[159] On their current protocol, EMRACE 2, the GEC-ESTRO recommends more stringent planning aims, with goal D_{2cc} of <80 Gy EQD2, <65 Gy EQD2, and <70 Gy EQD2 for bladder, rectum, and sigmoid, respectively.[101] On this protocol, the hard constraints are consistent with the ABS guidelines. When optimizing dose for volume-directed HDR brachytherapy, the ABS recommends that one not simply optimize dose to meet the constraints as defined by the D_{2cc} and D_{90} as these metrics do not provide information about potential hot or cold spots in both the target regions and in non-contoured regions, such as the vagina, connective tissues, nerves, vessels, or ureters. Careful inspection of the 3D dose distribution is recommended in all cases.[159]

A variety of dose–fractionation schemes have been used for patients with gynecologic cancer undergoing LDR and HDR brachytherapy. The ABS has published guidelines for LDR and HDR ICB for both cervical and uterine cancers (Tables 11.2–11.5).[157,159–163] The ABS has also published guidelines for ISB for vaginal cancer and recurrent endometrial cancer, which will be discussed in a later section.[160,161]

As described earlier, there is increasing interest in volumetric image-based treatment planning for intact cervical cancer patients. The GEC-ESTRO has pioneered MRI-based approaches in these patients. T2-weighted MRI using a pelvic coil provides excellent soft-tissue resolution and differentiation between tumor and normal tissues, allowing more accurate assessment of parametrial

TABLE 11.2		American Brachytherapy Society Guidelines Definitive Radiation Therapy for Cervical Cancer LDR Intracavitary Brachytherapy			

Stage	External-Beam Irradiation (Gy)			LDR Brachytherapy (Gy)	
	Pelvis	**Pelvic Wall**	**PMB**	**Point A Dose**	**Total Point A**
IA1	0	0	0	50–60	50–60
IA2	0	0	0	50–60	50–60
Selected IB1[a]	0	0	0	60–70	60–70
IB1	19.8 or 45	50.4 or 45	0	55 or 30–35	75 or 75–80
IB2, IIA[b]	45	45	0	40	85
IIB	45	45	9–15	40	85
III	45–50	45–50	9–15	40	85–90
IIB, IIIB, IVc	50	50	9–15	40	90

[a]Superficial ulceration less than 1 cm in diameter or involving fewer than two quadrants.
[b]Alternative approach is to increase brachytherapy contribution to point A by delivering pelvic radiotherapy of 19.8 to 30.6 Gy, followed by pelvic radiotherapy with a step-wedge midline shield for an additional 19.8 to 30.6 Gy and intracavitary brachytherapy, bringing point A to the recommended total dose levels.
[c]Poor pelvic anatomy, patient not readily treated with intracavitary insertions (barrel-shaped cervix not regressing, inability to locate external os).

LDR, low-dose rate.

Adapted from Nag et al.[163] and Lee et al.[157]

TABLE 11.3		American Brachytherapy Society Guidelines Definitive Radiation Therapy for Cervical Cancer HDR Intracavitary Brachytherapy	

EBRT (Gy)a	No. of HDR Fractions	HDR Dose (Gy)/Fraction	EQD2 (Gy)[b] to tumor
45	4	7	83.9
45	5	5.5	79.8
45	5	6	81.8
45	6	5	84.3

[a]Delivered at 1.8 Gy/fraction.
[b]Assuming an α/β ratio of 10

HDR, high dose rate; EBRT, external-beam radiotherapy.

Adapted from Viswanathan et al.[159]

and uterine tumor extension[164,165] and improved sparing of the bladder and rectum.[166] Controversy exists, however, whether MRI is needed at every insertion or whether CT imaging during subsequent insertions is sufficient.

TABLE 11.4	American Brachytherapy Society Guidelines Postoperative Radiation Therapy for Uterine Cancer HDR Intracavitary Brachytherapy		
EBRT (Gy)[a]	No. of HDR Fractions	Dose (Gy)/ Fraction	Dose-Specific Point
Brachytherapy Alone			
N/A	3	7.0	0.5-cm depth
N/A	6	2.5	0.5-cm depth
N/A	5	6	Vaginal surface
N/A	6	4	Vaginal surface
EBRT + Brachytherapy			
45	3	6	Vaginal surface
50.4	2	6	Vaginal surface

[a]Delivered at 1.8 Gy/fraction.

HDR, high dose rate; EBRT, external-beam radiation therapy.

Adapted from Small et al.[160]

TABLE 11.5	American Brachytherapy Society Guidelines Radiation Therapy for Inoperable Uterine Cancer HDR Intracavitary Brachytherapy		
EBRT (Gy)[a]	No. of HDR Fractions	Dose (Gy)/ Fraction	EQD2 (Gy)
Brachytherapy Alone			
N/A	4	8.5	52.4
N/A	5	7.3	52.6
N/A	6	6	48
N/A	6	6.4	52.5
N/A	9-10	5	50-62.5
EBRT + Brachytherapy			
45	2	8.5	70.5
45	3	6.3	69.9
45	3	6.5	71.1
45	4	5.2	70.6
45	5	5	75
50.4	2	6	65.6
50.4	6	3.75	75.3

[a]Delivered at 1.8 Gy/fraction.

HDR, high dose rate, EBRT, external-beam radiation therapy.

Adapted from Schwarz et al.[36]

Comparison studies have demonstrated that CT may overestimate tumor width[167–169] (Fig. 11.10). However, if MRI with each implant is not feasible, MRI may be used at the first insertion with CT-based planning at subsequent implants for normal tissue delineation, relying on the initial MRI for tumor delineation, especially in small tumors treated with ICB.

The ABS has adopted the recommendations of the GEC-ESTRO for contouring, image-based treatment planning, and dose reporting in cervical cancer[153,154] (Fig. 11.11). GEC-ESTRO recommendations are to contour the GTV, high-risk CTV (HR-CTV), intermediate-risk CTV, (IR-CTV), and normal tissues, including the bladder, rectum, sigmoid colon, and small bowel. The HR-CTV includes the entire cervix, as well as any macroscopic disease that persists in the parametria, uterus, rectum, bladder, or vagina (but not to cross these anatomic boundaries without clear rationale). The coverage goal is 80 to 95 Gy to the HR-CTV. The IR-CTV includes the HR-CTV with a safety margin of 5 to 15 mm, with the intent to deliver 60 Gy to this volume.

Recommendations for reporting and quality assurance in patients undergoing MRI-guided brachytherapy include calculation and reporting of the minimum D_{90} and 100% of the contoured target volume (D_{90}, D_{100}). In addition, for evaluation within a single treatment scheme, the volume encompassed by the 100% isodose line (V_{100}) should also be determined. For the normal tissues, reporting of the ICRU reference bladder and rectal points should continue for comparison with the dose–volume (DVH) data. The minimum dose received by the maximally irradiated contiguous 0.1, 1, and 2 cm^3 of the bladder, rectum, sigmoid and small bowel, respectively, should also be calculated and reported.

The GEC-ESTRO has now published numerous studies assessing the efficacy and toxicity of the MRI-guided brachytherapy approach for cervical cancer. They have demonstrated excellent rates of local control with this approach, with 3 year local control rates of >94% for small residual HR-CTVs (20 cc), >93% for intermediate HR-CTVs (30 cc), and >86% for large HR-CTVs (70 cc).[170] Intriguingly, their results suggested that increased HR-CTV size could be overcome with increased dose, with an estimated 5 Gy needed to maintain local control for each additional 10 cc volume,[170] though investigators at the University of Pittsburgh were not able to replicate this result.[171] With improvements in local control, the GEC-ESTRO investigators have found a shift in the pattern of failure for patients with cervical cancer, from predominately pelvic with conventional brachytherapy to predominately systemic in their RetroEMBRACE series.[172] These studies have also yielded important information about dose volume-effect relationships for predicting late toxicity after brachytherapy. On the prospective EMBRACE (IntErnational MRI-guided BRAchytherapy in CErvical cancer) study, the risk of rectal fistula was found to be 12.5% for patients who received a rectal $D_{2cc} \geq 75$ Gy EQD2 versus 0% to 2.7% for patients who received a lower dose. The risk of proctitis was found to be two times lower in patients who received a rectal $D_{2cc} < 65$ Gy compared with those who received a higher dose.[173] With data from

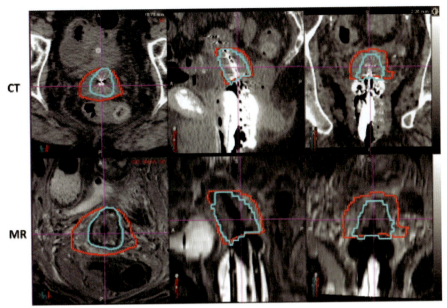

FIGURE 11.10. Potential differences between computed tomography (CT) and magnetic resonance imaging (MRI)-based target delineation for intact cervix brachytherapy. The top row shows axial, sagittal, and coronal CT views, for an example case of tandem and ovoid brachytherapy. The bottom row shows the corresponding MRI views for the same case. The MRI and CT-based clinical target volumes are shown in light blue and red, respectively. (Adapted from Viswanathan AN, et al. Comparison and consensus guidelines for delineation of clinical target volume for CT- and MR-based brachytherapy in locally advanced cervical cancer. *Int J Radiat Oncol Biol Phys.* 2014;90(2):9.)

the EMBRACE study, the GEC-ESTRO has also published data related to vaginal, bladder, bowel, and ureteral toxicity.[174–177] With the currently enrolling EMBRACE II study, the GEC-ESTRO hopes to benchmark a new standard for local control and toxicity by employing modern IGRT external beam and brachytherapy techniques.[101]

Interstitial Brachytherapy

ISB involves implanting radioactive sources directly within the target tissues. Unlike ICB, interstitial implants may be temporary, whereby sources are removed after the treatment, or permanent with limited half-life sources left in place. In gynecologic cancer patients undergoing ISB, the great majority are treated with temporary implants. Similar to patients undergoing ICB, ISB was previously performed using "live" sources but is now performed primarily using afterloading techniques. As noted in the ICB section, afterloading approaches significantly reduce the radiation exposure of the medical and ancillary staff, particularly when performed using remote afterloading techniques.

While the great majority of gynecology patients undergoing brachytherapy receive ICB,[178] ISB is recommended in women in whom ICB would result in suboptimal dose distributions,[154] and data from the retroEMBRACE study suggest a local control benefit for patients with bulky cervical tumors who receive combined ICB/ISB over ICB alone.[179] ISB should also be considered in patients with extensive parametrial involvement, bulky primary tumors,

narrow or distal vaginal involvement, post-hysterectomy central recurrence, or a history of prior RT. Other indications are distal or extensive vaginal involvement (>0.5 cm thickness) or persistent disease following external-beam RT and ICB. The ABS has published guidelines describing potential candidates and proper techniques for ISB in various gynecologic malignancies, including vaginal cancer, vulvar cancer, and vaginal recurrence.[160,180]

Multiple afterloading commercial applicators are currently available for ISB, the most popular of which are the MUPIT and the Syed–Neblett template. The MUPIT consists of two acrylic cylinders, an acrylic template with an array of equally spaced holes through which hollow needles are inserted and a cover plate.[138] The Syed–Neblett template is comprised of a vaginal cylinder, 2 lucite plates with 38 holes through which hollow needles are introduced; 6 additional needles can be inserted into groves along the vaginal cylinder.[136] The Vienna ring applicator allows placement of interstitial needles along with ICB brachytherapy (Fig. 11.12).[135,181] The Venezia applicator combines the tandem and ring with interstitial needles with a perineal plate for more lateral interstitial needles.[137]

Pre-planning using CT and/or MRI can be used in patients undergoing ISB to help determine source number and placement, particularly in patients treated with LDR techniques, which required ordering of radioactive seeds and/or wires. However, at the time of implant with the patient under anesthesia, physical examination should be performed to determine optimal applicator and needle

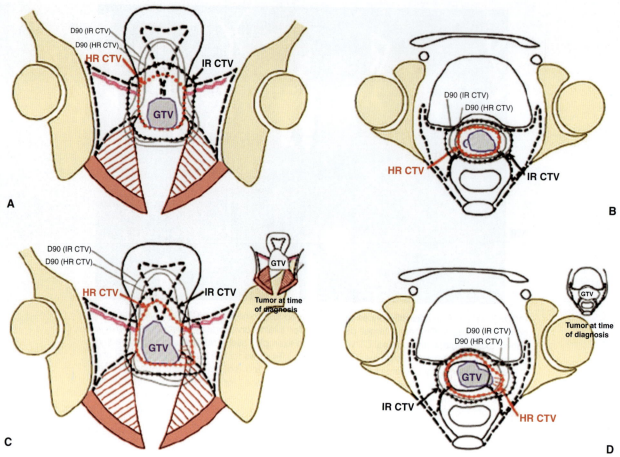

FIGURE 11.11. Group Européen de Curiethérapie–European Society for Therapeutic Radiology and Oncology (GEC-ESTRO) working group concepts and terms used for image-guided brachytherapy. Schematic diagram with coronal (**A, C**) and transverse (**B, D**) sections of an optimized treatment plan for limited (**A, B**) and advanced (**C, D**) disease with partial remission after external irradiation. GTV, gross tumor volume; HR CTV, high-risk clinical target volume; IR CTV, intermediate-risk clinical target volume. (Adapted from Haie-Meder C, et al. Recommendations from Gynaecological (GYN) GEC-ESTRO Working Group (1): concepts and terms in 3D image based 3D treatment planning in cervix cancer brachytherapy with emphasis on MRI assessment of GTV and CTV. *Radiother Oncol.* 2005;74:235–245.)

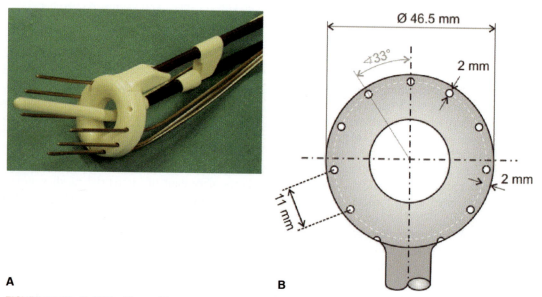

FIGURE 11.12. (**A,B**) The Vienna Ring applicator that allows placement of interstitial needs in patients with residual parametrial involvement in conjunction with intracavitary brachytherapy. (Adapted from Kirisits C, et al. The Vienna applicator for combined intracavitary and interstitial brachytherapy of cervical cancer: design, application, treatment planning, and dosimetric results. *Int J Radiat Oncol.* 2006;65(2):624–630.)

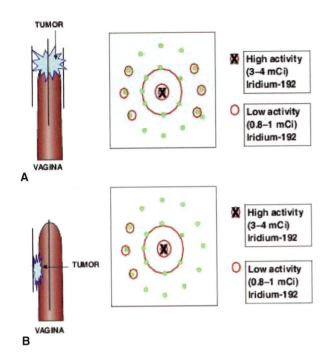

FIGURE 11.13. Example customized implant plans for uterine cancer patients with (**A**) a vaginal vault recurrence and (**B**) recurrence in the right lateral vaginal wall. (Redrawn from Nag S, et al. Interstitial brachytherapy for salvage treatment of vaginal recurrences in previously unirradiated endometrial cancer patients. *Int J Radiat Oncol Biol Phys*. 2002;54:1153–1159.)

placement, based on the patient's individual anatomy and tumor extent[180,182] (Fig. 11.13). Care needs to be taken to avoid perforation of adjacent organs, including the small bowel, bladder, and rectum. Intraoperative digital transrectal palpation is recommended not only to assess tumor extent but also to help avoid implanting needles into the rectum. Interstitial implants are performed at many centers under image and/or laparoscopic guidance.[183–185] Care should be taken to avoid excessive doses to the vaginal mucosa. If needles are inserted along the periphery of the central cylinder of a Syed–Neblett template, vaginal dose can be reduced with the placement of a sleeve over the cylinder.[183]

As with ICB, ISB can be delivered using LDR, HDR, or PDR techniques (see earlier section on ICB for a discussion of the advantages and disadvantages of each approach). [192]Ir is the most common isotope currently used, with high activity sources used for HDR. Limited data are available using permanent [198]Au or [103]Pd interstitial implants in gynecologic cancer patients.[186,187]

Various doses and prescription points have been used for ISB in gynecologic cancer patients. However, growing interest is focused on MRI-based treatment planning using the GEC-ESTRO guidelines in patients undergoing ISB,[188,189] and the current ABS contouring and treatment planning guidelines for ISB reflect this volume-directed approach.[180]

Computerized dosimetry is useful to ensure dose homogeneity throughout the implant. As with ICB, doses to 0.1 cc, 1 cc, 2 cc of OARs, including bladder, urethra, rectum,

sigmoid, and bowel, should be carefully inspected and recorded. Dose constraints for normal tissues are consistent with those used for ICB.[180] Given the high potential for hotspots with interstitial implants, special attention should be payed to the volume receiving >150% of the prescription dose, and effort should be made to limit this to the area adjacent to the individual needles or within the vaginal obturator.

Given the invasive nature of ISB, an effort is made to minimize the number of implants performed. Most patients undergoing LDR ISB are treated with a single insertion, which requires several days of bed rest in the hospital. Patients undergoing HDR ISB undergo one to three implants, often with multiple fractions delivered during each implant. If multiple implants are performed in patients with intact cervical cancer, it is recommended to initiate brachytherapy during external-beam RT to avoid unnecessary treatment protractions.[159] As with ICB, ISB should not be performed on the same day as either external-beam RT or chemotherapy. The ABS published guidelines on appropriate dose–fractionation schedules to be used for gynecologic cancer patients receiving HDR ISB with cumulative EQD2 doses ranging from 71.5 to 81.5 Gy delivered with a combinations of EBRT and 3 to 10 HDR fractions (Table 11.6).[180] Modern series employing 3D ISB

TABLE 11.6 American Brachytherapy Society Guidelines Interstitial HDR Brachytherapy for Gynecologic Cancer

Dose of EBRT (Gy)	HDR Dose to CTV (Gy)	EQD2 to CTV
36/18 fx[a]	5 × 6	72.9
	5.5 × 6	78.0
39.6/22 fx[a]	5 × 6	76.4
	5.5 × 6	81.5
45/25 fx	3 × 9	73.6
	3 × 10	76.8
	4.5 × 5	71.5
	5 × 5	75.5
	5.5 × 5	79.8
	7 × 3	74.1
50.4/28 fx	4 × 5	72.9
	4.5 × 5	76.8
	5 × 5	80.9
	7 × 3	79.4

[a]Total pelvic dose to 50.4 Gy with midline block after 36e 39.6 Gy.

HDR, high dose rate; EBRT, external-beam radiation therapy; CTV, clinical target volume; EQD2, equivalent dose in 2-Gy fractions.

Adapted from Viswanathan AN, Beriwal S, De Los Santos J, Demanes DJ, Gaffney D, Hansen J, et al. The American Brachytherapy Society Treatment Recommendations for Locally Advanced Carcinoma of the Cervix Part II: High Dose-Rate Brachytherapy. *Brachytherapy*. 2012;11(1):47–52.

for vaginal cancer show good local control of approximately 80% to 90% and low rates of high-grade toxicity.[190,191]

FUTURE DIRECTIONS

Treatment approaches in gynecologic cancer are rapidly evolving, reflecting the rapid pace of development both in technology and in our understanding of gynecologic malignancies. In endometrial cancer, recent genomic studies have demonstrated four molecular subtypes: POLE, which has an excellent prognosis; microsatellite unstable and copy number-low, which have intermediate prognoses; and copy number-high, which has a poor prognosis.[192] Other important molecular determinants of prognosis, such as TP53 mutation or L1CAM overexpression, have also been uncovered.[31] In the currently enrolling PORTEC-4a study, the ability to tailor adjuvant treatment for high-intermediate risk, stage I endometrial cancer based on a patient's molecular profile will be tested. Patients in this study will be randomized after surgery to receive either standard of care VBT or treatment based on molecular profile. For those in the experimental arm, patients with favorable profiles (e.g., POLE mutation) will be observed, patients with intermediate-risk profiles (e.g., microsatellite unstable) will receive brachytherapy, and patients with high-risk profiles (e.g., TP53 or L1CAM) will receive EBRT.[193]

Technological development may also influence radiation treatment strategies in the coming years. With the development of integrated MRI-linear accelerators (linacs), it is now feasible to treat patients with real-time image guidance with good soft-tissue contrast and to employ daily adaptive treatment planning techniques. Already, case reports have been published describing the treatment of patients with intact cervical cancer on an MRI-linac platform employing PTV margins of as little as 5 mm.[194]

There is also considerable interest in the development of technologies that permit daily adaptive radiotherapy with cone-beam CT-based image guidance.[195] Should such technologies prove safe, effective, and scalable, they could have a significant impact on the toxicity associated with definitive treatment of advanced cervical cancer in the coming years.

Finally, advancements in immunotherapy, in particular in the checkpoint inhibitors, may change the paradigm for treatment of many gynecological malignancies. In cervical cancer, the phase I study GOG 9929, which assessed the addition of the CTLA-4 inhibitor ipilimumab to definitive chemoradiation and brachytherapy for para-aortic node-positive cervical cancer reported a promising 1 year progression-free survival of 81% with a tolerable side effect profile.[196] There are currently multiple ongoing clinical trials in locally advanced cervical cancer exploring the use of concurrent and/or sequential checkpoint inhibition in addition to chemoradiation therapy (e.g., NCT03738228, NCT03830866, NCT04221945), including both early-phase and phase III trials. There is also considerable interest in investigating the role of checkpoint inhibitors in endometrial cancer, particularly in patients with microsatellite unstable subtypes. Pembrolizumab, a PD-1 inhibitor, has been shown to have efficacy in metastatic microsatellite unstable cancers that have progressed on prior therapy, regardless of site of origin.[197] For this, it was granted the first tissue-site agnostic approval by the FDA. At this time, it remains unknown how these novel radiotherapeutic, pharmaceutic, and genomic technologies will be integrated into treatment paradigms for gynecological malignancies; however, together they paint the picture of an exciting future, in which cancer treatments are more effective, less toxic, and delivered to the most appropriate patients.

KEY POINTS

- Radiation forms the backbone of definitive therapy for many advanced gynecological malignancies and can be an important adjuvant therapy after surgery for early-stage disease.

- RT is recommended over surgery in early-stage cervical cancer patients as lesion size and vaginal involvement increase. As tumor diameter exceeds 4 cm, there is increased likelihood of tumor spread to surrounding organs and regional lymph nodes, which would necessitate adjuvant RT following surgery.

- In patients with locally advanced (stages IIB to IVA) cervix cancer, radiation is combined with concomitant chemotherapy: multiple prospective randomized

trials have demonstrated a survival advantage to the combined approach.

- Definitive RT in cervical cancer is administered with a combination of pelvic RT and brachytherapy, except in earliest-stage patients for whom brachytherapy or surgery alone is sufficient.

- The majority of patients with early-stage uterine cancer undergo upfront surgery, consisting of total hysterectomy and bilateral salpingo-oophorectomy (TH-BSO), with RT delivered postoperatively to select patients based on pathologic features in the surgical specimen, including depth of invasion, tumor grade, LVI, and cervical involvement.

- Following publication of GOG 122, chemotherapy took on an important role in the adjuvant treatment of stages III to IV endometrial cancer. GOG 258 and PORTEC-3 have provided important data about the role of radiotherapy in this setting, though additional study may be needed to find the optimal combination and sequencing of chemotherapy and radiation for these patients.

- Treatment of vulvar cancer consists of upfront surgery (radical vulvectomy or radical wide local excision in selected patients with small, well-lateralized tumors), with RT delivered adjuvantly in patients with high-risk features, including LVI, tumor invasion >5 mm, surgical margins <8 mm, grade 3 disease, and microscopic-positive margins.

- IMRT is playing an increasing role in RT for gynecological malignancies, including cervical, endometrial, and vulvar cancer. Data continues to accumulate, demonstrating decreased toxicity, including GI, GU, and hematologic toxicity, with IMRT compared with conventional RT.

- Brachytherapy plays a critical role in the management of intact cervical cancer. In recent years, 3D image-guided brachytherapy has gained increasing acceptance, both in the United States and internationally. 3D image guidance has significantly changed the paradigm for brachytherapy treatment planning, and increasing evidence supports its ability to improve local control and decrease toxicity compared with conventional brachytherapy techniques. The ongoing EMBRACE II trial will provide an important benchmark for treatment outcomes with this technique.

- ISB should be considered in patients with extensive parametrial involvement, bulky primary tumors, narrow or distal vaginal involvement, post-hysterectomy central recurrence, or a history of prior RT.

? REVIEW QUESTIONS

1. What structures comprise the CTV for stage IIIA cervical cancer when using definitive IMRT?
   A. GTV, cervix, uterus, and parametria, including the ovaries
   B. GTV, cervix, uterus, and parametria, excluding the ovaries
   C. GTV, cervix, uterus, parametria, excluding the ovaries and entire vagina
   D. GTV, cervix, uterus, parametria, including the ovaries and entire vagina

2. Which examination best delineates the high-risk CTV when performing image-based contouring with IV contrast for cervical cancer brachytherapy?
   A. CT scan before the implant only
   B. CT scan before and at the time of the implant
   C. MRI before the implant only
   D. MRI before and at the time of the implant

3. What is considered to be a close surgical margin in fixed tissue for carcinoma of the vulva?
   A. 8 mm
   B. 10 mm
   C. 15 mm
   D. 18 mm

4. When treating cervical cancer with EBRT and HDR brachytherapy, the EQD2 D2 cc for the bladder (the minimum dose in the MOST irradiated 2 cm^3 normal tissue volume) should not exceed
   A. 60 Gy
   B. 70 Gy
   C. 90 Gy
   D. 100 Gy

5. For patients with high-intermediate and high-risk early-stage endometrial cancer, compared with pelvic EBRT, combined chemotherapy and VBT were found to do which of the following on GOG 249?
   A. Reduce acute toxicity
   B. Increase overall survival
   C. Increase recurrence-free survival
   D. None of the above

ANSWERS

1. D   The CTV includes the entire GTV as determined by the intermediate/high signal seen in T2-weighted MR images; the entire cervix if not included within the GTV contour; the entire uterus; the entire parametrium including ovaries. The entire mesorectum should be included if the uterosacral ligament is involved; for the vagina, if there is minimal or no vaginal extension of disease, include the upper half; if there is upper vaginal involvement, include the upper two-thirds, and if there is extensive vaginal involvement, then include the entire vagina.

Reference

1.   Lim K, Small W, Portelance L, et al. Consensus guidelines for delineation of clinical target volume for intensity-modulated pelvic radiotherapy for the definitive treatment of cervix cancer. *Int J Radiat Oncol Biol Phys.* 2011;79(2):348–355.

2. D   The advantage of MRI compared to CT with IV contrast is that MRI allows for distinction between the corpus and the cervix.
CT with IV contrast can delineate the cervico-uterine junction at the intersection of the uterine vessels and the cervix, which allows demarcation of the upper border of the cervix. However, only MRI before and at the time of brachytherapy can accurately delineate the superior border of the HR-CTV for patients with tumors extending beyond the cervix. If MRI is unavailable, the initial tumor extension into the corpus, or the entire canal, must be contoured to ensure that the CTV covers the entire extent of the areas at risk. Delineation of the HR-CTV and IR-CTV is also best informed by gynecological examination with drawings at the initial evaluation and at the time of brachytherapy.

Reference

1.   Viswanathan AN, Dimopoulos J, Kirisits C, et al. Computed tomography versus magnetic resonance imaging based contouring in cervical cancer brachytherapy: results of a prospective trial and preliminary guidelines for standardized contours. *Int J Radiation Oncology Biol Phys.* 2007;68(2):491–498.

3. A   Surgical margin is the most powerful predictor of local vulvar recurrence. Combining factors in a stepwise logistical regression does not significantly improve this predictive value. Accounting for specimen preparation and fixation, a 1-cm tumor-free surgical margin on the vulva results in a high rate of local control, whereas a margin less than 8 mm is associated with a 50% chance of recurrence.

These data come from a series of 135 patients with vulvar squamous cell carcinoma treated at UCLA and City of Hope Medical Centers between 1957 and 1985. Sixty-two cases were stage I, 48, stage II; 18, stage III; and 7 stage IV. Twenty-one patients developed a local vulvar recurrence after primary radical resection. Ninety-one patients had a surgical tumor-free margin ≥8 mm on tissue section, and none had a local vulvar recurrence. Forty-four patients had a margin less than 8 mm, 21 had a local recurrence, and 23 did not ($p \leq 0.0001$).

Reference

1.   Heaps JM, Fu YS, Montz FJ, et al. Surgical-pathologic variables predictive of local recurrence in squamous cell carcinoma of the vulva. *Gynecol Oncol.* 1990;38(3):309.

4. C   The EQD2 D2 cc constraint for bladder is <90 Gy. Modern protocols may specify 80 Gy as a soft planning goal.

Reference

1.   Viswanathan, Beriwal S, De Los Santos JF, et al. American Brachytherapy Society consensus guidelines for locally advanced carcinoma of the cervix. Part II: High-dose-rate brachytherapy. *Brachytherapy.* 2012;11(1):47–52.

5. D   GOG 249 was a superiority study designed to determine if VBT and chemotherapy could increase recurrence-free survival in patients with high-intermediate and high-risk early-stage endometrial cancer in comparison with pelvic EBRT. No improvement in recurrence-free survival or overall survival was found, and there were more frequent pelvic and paraaortic node failures in the VBT arm (9% vs. 4%). There was increased acute toxicity on the VBT arm.

Reference

1. Randall ME, Filiaci V, McMeekin DS, Gruenigen V von, Huang H, Yashar CM, et al. Phase III Trial: Adjuvant Pelvic Radiation Therapy Versus Vaginal Brachytherapy Plus Paclitaxel/Carboplatin in High-Intermediate and High-Risk Early Stage Endometrial Cancer. *J Clin Oncol.* 2019 Apr 17.

REFERENCES

1. Siegel RL, Miller KD, Jemal A. Cancer statistics, 2020. *CA Cancer J Clin*. 2020;70(1):7–30.
2. Global Cancer Observatory [Internet]. https://gco.iarc.fr/. Accessed September 26, 2020.
3. Bhatla N, Aoki D, Sharma DN, Sankaranarayanan R. Cancer of the cervix uteri. *Int J Gynecol Obstet*. 2018;143:22–36.
4. Grigsby PW, Perez CA. Radiotherapy alone for medically inoperable carcinoma of the cervix: stage IA and carcinoma in situ. *Int J Radiat Oncol Biol Phys*. 1991;21(2):375–378.
5. Landoni F, Maneo A, Colombo A, et al. Randomised study of radical surgery versus radiotherapy for stage Ib-IIa cervical cancer. *Lancet Lond Engl*. 1997;350(9077):535–540.
6. Bloemers MCWM, Portelance L, Legler C, Renaud MC, Tan SL. Preservation of ovarian function by ovarian transposition prior to concurrent chemotherapy and pelvic radiation for cervical cancer. A case report and review of the literature. *Eur J Gynaecol Oncol*. 2010;31(2):194–197.
7. Bergmark K, Avall-Lundqvist E, Dickman PW, Henningsohn L, Steineck G. Vaginal changes and sexuality in women with a history of cervical cancer. *N Engl J Med*. 1999;340(18):1383–1389.
8. Sedlis A, Bundy BN, Rotman MZ, Lentz SS, Muderspach LI, Zaino RJ. A randomized trial of pelvic radiation therapy versus no further therapy in selected patients with stage IB carcinoma of the cervix after radical hysterectomy and pelvic lymphadenectomy: a Gynecologic Oncology Group Study. *Gynecol Oncol*. 1999;73(2):177–183.
9. Rotman M, Sedlis A, Piedmonte MR, et al. A phase III randomized trial of postoperative pelvic irradiation in stage IB cervical carcinoma with poor prognostic features: follow-up of a gynecologic oncology group study. *Int J Radiat Oncol*. 2006;65(1):169–176.
10. Peters WA, Liu PY, Barrett RJ, et al. Concurrent chemotherapy and pelvic radiation therapy compared with pelvic radiation therapy alone as adjuvant therapy after radical surgery in high-risk early-stage cancer of the cervix. *J Clin Oncol Off J Am Soc Clin Oncol*. 2000;18(8):1606–1613.
11. Eifel PJ, Winter K, Morris M, et al. Pelvic irradiation with concurrent chemotherapy versus pelvic and para-aortic irradiation for high-risk cervical cancer: an update of radiation therapy oncology group trial (RTOG) 90-01. *J Clin Oncol Off J Am Soc Clin Oncol*. 2004;22(5):872–880.
12. Whitney CW, Sause W, Bundy BN, et al. Randomized comparison of fluorouracil plus cisplatin versus hydroxyurea as an adjunct to radiation therapy in stage IIB-IVA carcinoma of the cervix with negative para-aortic lymph nodes: a Gynecologic Oncology Group and Southwest Oncology Group study. *J Clin Oncol Off J Am Soc Clin Oncol*. 1999;17(5):1339–1348.
13. Rose PG, Ali S, Watkins E, et al. Long-term follow-up of a randomized trial comparing concurrent single agent cisplatin, cisplatin-based combination chemotherapy, or hydroxyurea during pelvic irradiation for locally advanced cervical cancer: a Gynecologic Oncology Group Study. *J Clin Oncol Off J Am Soc Clin Oncol*. 2007;25(19):2804–2810.
14. Ungar L, Palfalvi L, Novak Z. Primary pelvic exenteration in cervical cancer patients. *Gynecol Oncol*. 2008;111(2 Suppl):S9-S12.
15. Keys HM, Bundy BN, Stehman FB, et al. Cisplatin, radiation, and adjuvant hysterectomy compared with radiation and adjuvant hysterectomy for bulky stage IB cervical carcinoma. *N Engl J Med*. 1999;340(15):1154–1161.
16. Keys HM, Bundy BN, Stehman FB, et al. Radiation therapy with and without extrafascial hysterectomy for bulky stage IB cervical carcinoma: a randomized trial of the Gynecologic Oncology Group. *Gynecol Oncol*. 2003;89(3):343–353.
17. NCCN Clinical Practice Guidelines in Oncology (NCCN Guidelines): Cervical Cancer [Internet]. https://www.nccn.org/professionals/physician_gls/pdf/cervical_blocks.pdf. Accessed September 26, 2020.
18. Rotman M, Pajak TF, Choi K, et al. Prophylactic extended-field irradiation of para-aortic lymph nodes in stages IIB and bulky IB and IIA cervical carcinomas. Ten-year treatment results of RTOG 79-20. *JAMA*. 1995;274(5):387–393.
19. Holschneider CH, Petereit DG, Chu C, et al. Brachytherapy: a critical component of primary radiation therapy for cervical cancer: from the Society of Gynecologic Oncology (SGO) and the American Brachytherapy Society (ABS). *Brachytherapy*. 2019;18(2):123–132.
20. Pötter R, Georg P, Dimopoulos JCA, et al. Clinical outcome of protocol based image (MRI) guided adaptive brachytherapy combined with 3D conformal radiotherapy with or without chemotherapy in patients with locally advanced cervical cancer. *Radiother Oncol*. 2011;100(1):116–123.
21. Kinsella TJ, Bloomer WD, Lavin PT, Knapp RC. Stage II endometrial carcinoma: 10-year follow-up of combined radiation and surgical treatment. *Gynecol Oncol*. 1980;10(3):290–297.
22. Holloway RW, Abu-Rustum NR, Backes FJ, et al. Sentinel lymph node mapping and staging in endometrial cancer: a Society of Gynecologic Oncology literature review with consensus recommendations. *Gynecol Oncol*. 2017;146(2):405–415.
23. Keys HM, Roberts JA, Brunetto VL, et al. A phase III trial of surgery with or without adjunctive external pelvic radiation therapy in intermediate risk endometrial adenocarcinoma: a Gynecologic Oncology Group study. *Gynecol Oncol*. 2004;92(3):744–751.
24. ASTEC/EN. 5 Study Group, Blake P, Swart AM, Orton J, Kitchener H, Whelan T. Adjuvant external beam radiotherapy in the treatment of endometrial cancer (MRC ASTEC and NCIC CTG EN.5 randomised trials): pooled trial results, systematic review, and meta-analysis. *Lancet Lond Engl*. 2009;373(9658):137–146.
25. Creutzberg CL, van Putten WL, Koper PC, et al. Surgery and postoperative radiotherapy versus surgery alone for patients with stage-1 endometrial carcinoma: multicentre randomised trial. PORTEC Study Group. Post Operative Radiation Therapy in Endometrial Carcinoma. *Lancet Lond Engl*. 2000;355(9213):1404–1411.
26. Aalders J, Abeler V, Kolstad P, Onsrud M. Postoperative external irradiation and prognostic parameters in stage I endometrial carcinoma: clinical and histopathologic study of 540 patients. *Obstet Gynecol*. 1980;56(4):419–427.
27. Wright JD, Fiorelli J, Kansler AL, et al. Optimizing the management of stage II endometrial cancer: the role of radical hysterectomy and radiation. *Am J Obstet Gynecol*. 2009;200(4):419.e1-7.
28. Lee CM, Szabo A, Shrieve DC, Macdonald OK, Gaffney DK. Frequency and effect of adjuvant radiation therapy among women with stage I endometrial adenocarcinoma. *JAMA*. 2006;295(4):389–397.
29. Creutzberg CL, Nout RA, Lybeert MLM, et al. Fifteen-year radiotherapy outcomes of the randomized PORTEC-1 trial for endometrial carcinoma. *Int J Radiat Oncol*. 2011;81(4):e631–e638.
30. Nout R, Smit V, Putter H, et al. Vaginal brachytherapy versus pelvic external beam radiotherapy for patients with endometrial cancer of high-intermediate risk (PORTEC-2): an open-label, non-inferiority, randomised trial. *The Lancet*. 2010;375(9717):816–823.
31. Wortman BG, Creutzberg CL, Putter H, et al. Ten-year results of the PORTEC-2 trial for high-intermediate risk endometrial carcinoma: improving patient selection for adjuvant therapy. *Br J Cancer*. 2018;119(9):1067–1074.
32. Randall ME, Filiaci V, McMeekin DS, et al. Phase III trial: adjuvant pelvic radiation therapy versus vaginal brachytherapy plus paclitaxel/carboplatin in high-intermediate and high-risk early stage endometrial cancer. *J Clin Oncol*. 2019. doi:10.1200/JCO.18.01575
33. de Boer SM, Powell ME, Mileshkin L, et al. Adjuvant chemoradiotherapy versus radiotherapy alone for women with high-risk endometrial cancer (PORTEC-3): final results of an international, open-label, multicentre, randomised, phase 3 trial. *Lancet Oncol*. 2018;19(3):295–309.
34. León-Castillo A, de Boer SM, Powell ME, et al. Molecular classification of the PORTEC-3 trial for high-risk endometrial cancer: impact on prognosis and benefit from adjuvant therapy. *J Clin Oncol*. 2020;JCO2000549.
35. Harkenrider MM, Martin B, Nieto K, et al. Multi-institutional analysis of vaginal brachytherapy alone for women with stage II endometrial carcinoma. *Int J Radiat Oncol*. 2018;101(5):1069–1077.

36. Schwarz JK, Beriwal S, Esthappan J, et al. Consensus statement for brachytherapy for the treatment of medically inoperable endometrial cancer. *Brachytherapy*. 2015;14(5):587–599.

37. Randall ME, Filiaci VL, Muss H, et al. Randomized phase III trial of whole-abdominal irradiation versus doxorubicin and cisplatin chemotherapy in advanced endometrial carcinoma: a Gynecologic Oncology Group Study. *J Clin Oncol*. 2006;24(1):36-44.

38. Mundt AJ, McBride R, Rotmensch J, Waggoner SE, Yamada SD, Connell PP. Significant pelvic recurrence in high-risk pathologic stage I-IV endometrial carcinoma patients after adjuvant chemotherapy alone: implications for adjuvant radiation therapy. *Int J Radiat Oncol Biol Phys*. 2001;50(5):1145–1153.

39. Homesley HD, Filiaci V, Gibbons SK, et al. A randomized phase III trial in advanced endometrial carcinoma of surgery and volume directed radiation followed by cisplatin and doxorubicin with or without paclitaxel: a Gynecologic Oncology Group Study. *Gynecol Oncol*. 2009;112(3):543–552.

40. Matei D, Filiaci V, Randall ME, et al. Adjuvant chemotherapy plus radiation for locally advanced endometrial cancer. *N Engl J Med*. 2019;380(24):2317–2326.

41. Gao H, Zhang Z. Sequential chemotherapy and radiotherapy in the sandwich method for advanced endometrial cancer. *Medicine (Baltimore)*. 2015;94(16). https://www.ncbi.nlm.nih.gov/pmc/articles/PMC4602698/. Accessed September 27, 2020.

42. Murphy KT, Rotmensch J, Yamada SD, Mundt AJ. Outcome and patterns of failure in pathologic stages I-IV clear-cell carcinoma of the endometrium: implications for adjuvant radiation therapy. *Int J Radiat Oncol Biol Phys*. 2003;55(5):1272–1276.

43. Wolfson AH, Brady MF, Rocereto T, et al. A gynecologic oncology group randomized phase III trial of whole abdominal irradiation (WAI) vs. cisplatin-ifosfamide and mesna (CIM) as post-surgical therapy in stage I-IV carcinosarcoma (CS) of the uterus. *Gynecol Oncol*. 2007;107(2):177–185.

44. Young RC, Walton LA, Ellenberg SS, et al. Adjuvant therapy in stage I and stage II epithelial ovarian cancer. Results of two prospective randomized trials. *N Engl J Med*. 1990;322(15):1021–1027.

45. Young RC, Brady MF, Nieberg RK, et al. Adjuvant treatment for early ovarian cancer: a randomized phase III trial of intraperitoneal 32P or intravenous cyclophosphamide and cisplatin—A gynecologic oncology group study. *J Clin Oncol Off J Am Soc Clin Oncol*. 2003;21(23):4350–4355.

46. Smith JP, Rutledge FN, Delclos L. Postoperative treatment of early cancer of the ovary: a random trial between postoperative irradiation and chemotherapy. *Natl Cancer Inst Monogr*. 1975;42:149–153.

47. Dinniwell R, Lock M, Pintilie M, et al. Consolidative abdominopelvic radiotherapy after surgery and carboplatin/paclitaxel chemotherapy for epithelial ovarian cancer. *Int J Radiat Oncol Biol Phys*. 2005;62(1):104–110.

48. Burke TW, Stringer CA, Gershenson DM, Edwards CL, Morris M, Wharton JT. Radical wide excision and selective inguinal node dissection for squamous cell carcinoma of the vulva. *Gynecol Oncol*. 1990;38(3):328–332.

49. Gaffney DK, Du Bois A, Narayan K, et al. Patterns of care for radiotherapy in vulvar cancer: a Gynecologic Cancer Intergroup Study. *Int J Gynecol Cancer Off J Int Gynecol Cancer Soc*. 2009;19(1):163–167.

50. Heaps JM, Fu YS, Montz FJ, Hacker NF, Berek JS. Surgical-pathologic variables predictive of local recurrence in squamous cell carcinoma of the vulva. *Gynecol Oncol*. 1990;38(3):309–314.

51. te Grootenhuis NC, van der Zee AGJ, van Doorn HC, et al. Sentinel nodes in vulvar cancer: long-term follow-up of the GROningen INternational Study on Sentinel nodes in Vulvar cancer (GROINSS-V) I. *Gynecol Oncol*. 2016;140(1):8–14.

52. Levenback CF, Ali S, Coleman RL, et al. Lymphatic mapping and sentinel lymph node biopsy in women with squamous cell carcinoma of the vulva: a gynecologic oncology group study. *J Clin Oncol*. 2012;30(31):3786–3791.

53. Oonk MHM, Slomovitz B, Baldwin P, et al. Radiotherapy instead of inguinofemoral lymphadenectomy in vulvar cancer patients with a metastatic sentinel node: results of GROINSS-V II. *Int J Gynecol Cancer*. 2019;29(Suppl 4):A14.

54. Homesley HD, Bundy BN, Sedlis A, Adcock L. Radiation therapy versus pelvic node resection for carcinoma of the vulva with positive groin nodes. *Obstet Gynecol*. 1986;68(6):733–740.

55. Stehman FB, Bundy BN, Thomas G, et al. Groin dissection versus groin radiation in carcinoma of the vulva: a Gynecologic Oncology Group Study. *Int J Radiat Oncol Biol Phys*. 1992;24(2):389–396.

56. Boronow RC. Combined therapy as an alternative to exenteration for locally advanced vulvo-vaginal cancer: rationale and results. *Cancer*. 1982;49(6):1085–1091.

57. Acosta AA, Given FT, Frazier AB, Cordoba RB, Luminari A. Preoperative radiation therapy in the management of squamous cell carcinoma of the vulva: preliminary report. *Am J Obstet Gynecol*. 1978;132(2):198–206.

58. Thomas G, Dembo A, DePetrillo A, et al. Concurrent radiation and chemotherapy in vulvar carcinoma. *Gynecol Oncol*. 1989;34(3):263–267.

59. Landoni F, Maneo A, Zanetta G, et al. Concurrent preoperative chemotherapy with 5-fluorouracil and mitomycin C and radiotherapy (FUMIR) followed by limited surgery in locally advanced and recurrent vulvar carcinoma. *Gynecol Oncol*. 1996;61(3):321–327.

60. Moore DH, Thomas GM, Montana GS, Saxer A, Gallup DG, Olt G. Preoperative chemoradiation for advanced vulvar cancer: a phase II study of the Gynecologic Oncology Group. *Int J Radiat Oncol Biol Phys*. 1998;42(1):79–85.

61. Moore DH, Ali S, Koh W-J, et al. A phase II trial of radiation therapy and weekly cisplatin chemotherapy for the treatment of locally-advanced squamous cell carcinoma of the vulva: a gynecologic oncology group study. *Gynecol Oncol*. 2012;124(3):529–533.

62. Gallup DG, Talledo OE, Shah KJ, Hayes C. Invasive squamous cell carcinoma of the vagina: a 14-year study. *Obstet Gynecol*. 1987;69(5):782–785.

63. Perez CA, Korba A, Sharma S. Dosimetric considerations in irradiation of carcinoma of the vagina. *Int J Radiat Oncol Biol Phys*. 1977;2(7–8):639–649.

64. Chyle V, Zagars GK, Wheeler JA, Wharton JT, Delclos L. Definitive radiotherapy for carcinoma of the vagina: outcome and prognostic factors. *Int J Radiat Oncol Biol Phys*. 1996;35(5):891–905.

65. Frank SJ, Jhingran A, Levenback C, Eifel PJ. Definitive radiation therapy for squamous cell carcinoma of the vagina. *Int J Radiat Oncol Biol Phys*. 2005;62(1):138–147.

66. Jones D. ICRU report 50—prescribing, recording and reporting photon beam therapy. *Med Phys*. 1994;21(6):833–834.

67. Landberg T, Chavaudra J, Dobbs J, et al. Report 62. *J Int Comm Radiat Units Meas*. 1999;os32(1):NP-NP.

68. Chao KSC, Williamson JF, Grigsby PW, Perez CA. Uterosacral space involvement in locally advanced carcinoma of the uterine cervix. *Int J Radiat Oncol*. 1998;40(2):397–403.

69. Zunino S, Rosato O, Lucino S, Jauregui E, Rossi L, Venencia D. Anatomic study of the pelvis in carcinoma of the uterine cervix as related to the box technique. *Int J Radiat Oncol Biol Phys*. 1999;44(1):53–59.

70. Finlay MH, Ackerman I, Tirona RG, Hamilton P, Barbera L, Thomas G. Use of CT simulation for treatment of cervical cancer to assess the adequacy of lymph node coverage of conventional pelvic fields based on bony landmarks. *Int J Radiat Oncol Biol Phys*. 2006;64(1):205–209.

71. Beadle BM, Jhingran A, Salehpour M, Sam M, Iyer RB, Eifel PJ. Cervix regression and motion during the course of external beam chemoradiation for cervical cancer. *Int J Radiat Oncol Biol Phys*. 2009;73(1):235–241.

72. Tyagi N, Lewis JH, Yashar CM, et al. Daily online cone beam computed tomography to assess interfractional motion in patients with intact cervical cancer. *Int J Radiat Oncol*. 2011;80(1):273–280.

73. Grigsby P, Winter K, Komaki R, et al. Long-term follow-up of RTOG 88-05: twice-daily external irradiation with brachytherapy for carcinoma of the cervix. *Int J Radiat Oncol Biol Phys*. 2002;54(1):51–57.

74. MacLeod C, Bernshaw D, Leung S, Narayan K, Firth I. Accelerated hyperfractionated radiotherapy for locally advanced cervix cancer. *Int J Radiat Oncol Biol Phys*. 1999;44(3):519–524.

75. Kavanagh BD, Gieschen HL, Schmidt-Ullrich RK, et al. A pilot study of concomitant boost accelerated superfractionated radiotherapy for stage III cancer of the uterine cervix. *Int J Radiat Oncol Biol Phys.* 1997;38(3):561–568.

76. Carrascosa LA, Yashar CM, Paris KJ, Larocca RV, Faught SR, Spanos WJ. Palliation of pelvic and head and neck cancer with paclitaxel and a novel radiotherapy regimen. *J Palliat Med.* 2007;10(4):877–881.

77. Perez CA, Grigsby PW, Chao KS, Mutch DG, Lockett MA. Tumor size, irradiation dose, and long-term outcome of carcinoma of uterine cervix. *Int J Radiat Oncol Biol Phys.* 1998;41(2):307–317.

78. Wolfson AH, Abdel-Wahab M, Markoe AM, et al. A quantitative assessment of standard vs. customized midline shield construction for invasive cervical carcinoma. *Int J Radiat Oncol Biol Phys.* 1997;37(1):237–242.

79. Heron DE, Gerszten K, Selvaraj RN, et al. Conventional 3D conformal versus intensity-modulated radiotherapy for the adjuvant treatment of gynecologic malignancies: a comparative dosimetric study of dose-volume histograms. *Gynecol Oncol.* 2003;91(1):39–45.

80. Ahamad A, D'Souza W, Salehpour M, et al. Intensity-modulated radiation therapy after hysterectomy: comparison with conventional treatment and sensitivity of the normal-tissue-sparing effect to margin size. *Int J Radiat Oncol Biol Phys.* 2005;62(4):1117–1124.

81. Klopp AH, Yeung AR, Deshmukh S, et al. Patient-reported toxicity during pelvic intensity-modulated radiation therapy: NRG Oncology–RTOG 1203. *J Clin Oncol.* 2018;36(24):2538–2544.

82. Mell LK, Tiryaki H, Ahn K-H, Mundt AJ, Roeske JC, Aydogan B. Dosimetric comparison of bone marrow-sparing intensity-modulated radiotherapy versus conventional techniques for treatment of cervical cancer. *Int J Radiat Oncol Biol Phys.* 2008;71(5):1504–1510.

83. Mell LK, Sirák I, Wei L, et al. Bone marrow-sparing intensity modulated radiation therapy with concurrent cisplatin for stage IB-IVA cervical cancer: an international multicenter phase II clinical trial (INTERTECC-2). *Int J Radiat Oncol.* 2017;97(3):536–545.

84. Mell LK, Kochanski JD, Roeske JC, et al. Dosimetric predictors of acute hematologic toxicity in cervical cancer patients treated with concurrent cisplatin and intensity-modulated pelvic radiotherapy. *Int J Radiat Oncol Biol Phys.* 2006;66(5):1356–1365.

85. Simpson DR, Lawson JD, Nath SK, Rose BS, Mundt AJ, Mell LK. Utilization of advanced imaging technologies for target delineation in radiation oncology. *J Am Coll Radiol JACR.* 2009;6(12):876–883.

86. Small W, Mell LK, Anderson P, et al. Consensus guidelines for delineation of clinical target volume for intensity-modulated pelvic radiotherapy in postoperative treatment of endometrial and cervical cancer. *Int J Radiat Oncol Biol Phys.* 2008;71(2):428–434.

87. Lim K, Small W, Portelance L, et al. Consensus guidelines for delineation of clinical target volume for intensity-modulated pelvic radiotherapy for the definitive treatment of cervix cancer. *Int J Radiat Oncol.* 2011;79(2):348–355.

88. Small W, Bosch WR, Harkenrider MM, et al. NRG oncology/RTOG consensus guidelines for delineation of clinical target volume for intensity modulated pelvic radiation therapy in postoperative treatment of endometrial and cervical cancer: an update. *Int J Radiat Oncol.* 2021;109(2):413–424.

89. Taylor A, Rockall AG, Reznek RH, Powell MEB. Mapping pelvic lymph nodes: guidelines for delineation in intensity-modulated radiotherapy. *Int J Radiat Oncol Biol Phys.* 2005;63(5):1604–1612.

90. Khan A, Jensen LG, Sun S, et al. Optimized planning target volume for intact cervical cancer. *Int J Radiat Oncol Biol Phys.* 2012;83(5):1500–1505.

91. Chen VE, Gillespie EF, Manger RP, et al. The impact of daily bladder filling on small bowel dose for intensity modulated radiation therapy for cervical cancer. *Med Dosim Off J Am Assoc Med Dosim.* 2019;44(2):102–106.

92. Williamson CW, Green G, Noticewala SS, et al. Prospective validation of a high dimensional shape model for organ motion in intact cervical cancer. *Int J Radiat Oncol Biol Phys.* 2016;96(4):801–807.

93. Mutic S, Malyapa RS, Grigsby PW, et al. PET-guided IMRT for cervical carcinoma with positive para-aortic lymph nodes-a dose-escalation treatment planning study. *Int J Radiat Oncol Biol Phys.* 2003;55(1):28–35.

94. Du X, Sheng X, Jiang T, et al. Intensity-modulated radiation therapy versus para-aortic field radiotherapy to treat para-aortic lymph node metastasis in cervical cancer: prospective study. *Croat Med J.* 2010;51(3):229–236.

95. Ahmed RS, Kim RY, Duan J, Meleth S, De Los Santos JF, Fiveash JB. IMRT dose escalation for positive para-aortic lymph nodes in patients with locally advanced cervical cancer while reducing dose to bone marrow and other organs at risk. *Int J Radiat Oncol Biol Phys.* 2004;60(2):505–512.

96. Vargo JA, Kim H, Choi S, et al. Extended field intensity modulated radiation therapy with concomitant boost for lymph node–positive cervical cancer: analysis of regional control and recurrence patterns in the positron emission tomography/computed tomography era. *Int J Radiat Oncol.* 2014;90(5):1091–1098.

97. Roeske JC, Lujan A, Rotmensch J, Waggoner SE, Yamada D, Mundt AJ. Intensity-modulated whole pelvic radiation therapy in patients with gynecologic malignancies. *Int J Radiat Oncol Biol Phys.* 2000;48(5):1613–1621.

98. Low DA, Grigsby PW, Dempsey JF, et al. Applicator-guided intensity-modulated radiation therapy. *Int J Radiat Oncol Biol Phys.* 2002;52(5):1400–1406.

99. Chan PM, Paterson J. Cervical cancer not suitable for brachytherapy: case study. In: Mundt AJ, Roeske JC, eds. *Intensity Modulated Radiation Therapy: A Clinical Perspective.* Hamilton, Canada: BC Decker Inc; 2005:518–522.

100. Albuquerque K, Tumati V, Lea J, et al. A phase II trial of stereotactic ablative radiation therapy as a boost for locally advanced cervical cancer. *Int J Radiat Oncol.* 2020;106(3):464–471.

101. Pötter R, Tanderup K, Kirisits C, et al. The EMBRACE II study: the outcome and prospect of two decades of evolution within the GEC-ESTRO GYN working group and the EMBRACE studies. *Clin Transl Radiat Oncol.* 2018;9:48–60.

102. Roeske JC, Bonta D, Mell LK, Lujan AE, Mundt AJ. A dosimetric analysis of acute gastrointestinal toxicity in women receiving intensity-modulated whole-pelvic radiation therapy. *Radiother Oncol J Eur Soc Ther Radiol Oncol.* 2003;69(2):201–207.

103. Simpson DR, Song WY, Moiseenko V, et al. Normal tissue complication probability analysis of acute gastrointestinal toxicity in cervical cancer patients undergoing intensity modulated radiation therapy and concurrent cisplatin. *Int J Radiat Oncol Biol Phys.* 2012;83(1):e81-e86.

104. Rose BS, Aydogan B, Liang Y, et al. Normal tissue complication probability modeling of acute hematologic toxicity in cervical cancer patients treated with chemoradiotherapy. *Int J Radiat Oncol Biol Phys.* 2011;79(3):800–807.

105. Hasselle MD, Rose BS, Kochanski JD, et al. Clinical outcomes of intensity-modulated pelvic radiation therapy for carcinoma of the cervix. *Int J Radiat Oncol Biol Phys.* 2011;80(5):1436–1445.

106. Brixey CJ, Roeske JC, Lujan AE, Yamada SD, Rotmensch J, Mundt AJ. Impact of intensity-modulated radiotherapy on acute hematologic toxicity in women with gynecologic malignancies. *Int J Radiat Oncol Biol Phys.* 2002;54(5):1388–1396.

107. Mundt AJ, Mell LK, Roeske JC. Preliminary analysis of chronic gastrointestinal toxicity in gynecology patients treated with intensity-modulated whole pelvic radiation therapy. *Int J Radiat Oncol Biol Phys.* 2003;56(5):1354–1360.

108. Liang Y, Messer K, Rose BS, et al. Impact of bone marrow radiation dose on acute hematologic toxicity in cervical cancer: principal component analysis on high dimensional data. *Int J Radiat Oncol Biol Phys.* 2010;78(3):912–919.

109. Mundt AJ, Lujan AE, Rotmensch J, et al. Intensity-modulated whole pelvic radiotherapy in women with gynecologic malignancies. *Int J Radiat Oncol Biol Phys.* 2002;52(5):1330–1337.

110. Kidd EA, Siegel BA, Dehdashti F, et al. Clinical outcomes of definitive intensity-modulated radiation therapy with fluorodeoxyglucose-positron emission tomography simulation in patients with locally advanced cervical cancer. *Int J Radiat Oncol Biol Phys.* 2010;77(4):1085–1091.

111. Beriwal S, Jain SK, Heron DE, et al. Clinical outcome with adjuvant treatment of endometrial carcinoma using intensity-modulated radiation therapy. *Gynecol Oncol.* 2006;102(2):195–199.

112. Jhingran A, Winter K, Portelance L, et al. A phase II study of intensity modulated radiation therapy to the pelvis for postoperative patients with endometrial carcinoma: radiation therapy oncology group trial 0418. *Int J Radiat Oncol Biol Phys.* 2012;84(1):e23-e28.

113. Hermesse J, Devillers M, Deneufbourg J-M, Nickers P. Can intensity-modulated radiation therapy of the paraaortic region overcome the problems of critical organ tolerance? *Strahlenther Onkol Organ Dtsch Rontgengesellschaft Al.* 2005;181(3):185–190.

114. Lian J, Mackenzie M, Joseph K, et al. Assessment of extended-field radiotherapy for stage IIIC endometrial cancer using three-dimensional conformal radiotherapy, intensity-modulated radiotherapy, and helical tomotherapy. *Int J Radiat Oncol Biol Phys.* 2008;70(3):935–943.

115. Portelance L, Chao KS, Grigsby PW, Bennet H, Low D. Intensity-modulated radiation therapy (IMRT) reduces small bowel, rectum, and bladder doses in patients with cervical cancer receiving pelvic and para-aortic irradiation. *Int J Radiat Oncol Biol Phys.* 2001;51(1):261–266.

116. Verma J, Sulman EP, Jhingran A, et al. Dosimetric predictors of duodenal toxicity after intensity modulated radiation therapy for treatment of the para-aortic nodes in gynecologic cancer. *Int J Radiat Oncol.* 2014;88(2):357–362.

117. Salama JK, Mundt AJ, Roeske J, Mehta N. Preliminary outcome and toxicity report of extended-field, intensity-modulated radiation therapy for gynecologic malignancies. *Int J Radiat Oncol Biol Phys.* 2006;65(4):1170–1176.

118. Gerszten K, Colonello K, Heron DE, et al. Feasibility of concurrent cisplatin and extended field radiation therapy (EFRT) using intensity-modulated radiotherapy (IMRT) for carcinoma of the cervix. *Gynecol Oncol.* 2006;102(2):182–188.

119. Moran MS, Castrucci WA, Ahmad M, et al. Clinical utility of the modified segmental boost technique for treatment of the pelvis and inguinal nodes. *Int J Radiat Oncol Biol Phys.* 2010;76(4):1026–1036.

120. Koh WJ, Chiu M, Stelzer KJ, et al. Femoral vessel depth and the implications for groin node radiation. *Int J Radiat Oncol Biol Phys.* 1993;27(4):969–974.

121. Petereit DG, Mehta MP, Buchler DA, Kinsella TJ. Inguinofemoral radiation of N0, N1 vulvar cancer may be equivalent to lymphadenectomy if proper radiation technique is used. *Int J Radiat Oncol Biol Phys.* 1993;27(4):963–967.

122. Dusenbery KE, Carlson JW, LaPorte RM, et al. Radical vulvectomy with postoperative irradiation for vulvar cancer: therapeutic implications of a central block. *Int J Radiat Oncol Biol Phys.* 1994;29(5):989–998.

123. Gaffney DK, King B, Viswanathan AN, et al. Consensus recommendations for radiation therapy contouring and treatment of vulvar carcinoma. *Int J Radiat Oncol.* 2016;95(4):1191–1200.

124. Beriwal S, Heron DE, Kim H, et al. Intensity-modulated radiotherapy for the treatment of vulvar carcinoma: a comparative dosimetric study with early clinical outcome. *Int J Radiat Oncol Biol Phys.* 2006;64(5):1395–1400.

125. Beriwal S, Coon D, Heron DE, et al. Preoperative intensity-modulated radiotherapy and chemotherapy for locally advanced vulvar carcinoma. *Gynecol Oncol.* 2008;109(2):291–295.

126. Pan H, Simpson DR, Mell LK, Mundt AJ, Lawson JD. A survey of stereotactic body radiotherapy use in the United States. *Cancer.* 2011;117(19):4566–4572.

127. Palma DA, Olson RA, Harrow S, et al. Stereotactic ablative radiation therapy for the comprehensive treatment of oligometastatic tumors (SABR-COMET): results of a randomized trial. *Int J Radiat Oncol.* 2018;102(3):S3–S4.

128. Choi CW, Cho CK, Yoo SY, et al. Image-guided stereotactic body radiation therapy in patients with isolated para-aortic lymph node metastases from uterine cervical and corpus cancer. *Int J Radiat Oncol Biol Phys.* 2009;74(1):147–153.

129. Park HJ, Chang AR, Seo Y, et al. Stereotactic body radiotherapy for recurrent or oligometastatic uterine cervix cancer: a cooperative study of the Korean Radiation Oncology Group (KROG 14-11). *Anticancer Res.* 2015;35(9):5103–5110.

130. Laliscia C, Fabrini MG, Delishaj D, et al. Clinical outcomes of stereotactic body radiotherapy in oligometastatic gynecological cancer. *Int J Gynecol Cancer.* 2017;27(2):396–402.

131. Mollà M, Escude L, Nouet P, et al. Fractionated stereotactic radiotherapy boost for gynecologic tumors: an alternative to brachytherapy? *Int J Radiat Oncol Biol Phys.* 2005;62(1):118–124.

132. Jorcano S, Molla M, Escude L, et al. Hypofractionated extracranial stereotactic radiotherapy boost for gynecologic tumors: a promising alternative to high-dose rate brachytherapy. *Technol Cancer Res Treat.* 2010;9(5):509–514.

133. Tod MC, Meredith WJ. A dosage system for use in the treatment of cancer of the uterine cervix. *Br J Radiol.* 1938;11(132):809–824.

134. Henschke UK. "Afterloading" applicator for radiation therapy of carcinoma of the uterus. *Radiology.* 1960;74:834.

135. Dimopoulos JCA, Kirisits C, Petric P, et al. The Vienna applicator for combined intracavitary and interstitial brachytherapy of cervical cancer: clinical feasibility and preliminary results. *Int J Radiat Oncol Biol Phys.* 2006;66(1):83–90.

136. Fleming P, Nisar Syed AM, Neblett D, Puthawala A, George FW, Townsend D. Description of an afterloading 192Ir interstitial-intracavitary technique in the treatment of carcinoma of the vagina. *Obstet Gynecol.* 1980;55(4):525–530.

137. Fredman E, Muenkel J, Traughber B, et al. Dosimetric Analysis Using the Venezia Applicator, and Comparison with the Split Ring Applicator, in Combined Intracavitary/Interstitial High Dose Rate Brachytherapy for Cervix Cancer. *Brachytherapy.* 2019;18(3):S95.

138. Martinez A, Cox RS, Edmundson GK. A multiple-site perineal applicator (MUPIT) for treatment of prostatic, anorectal, and gynecologic malignancies. *Int J Radiat Oncol Biol Phys.* 1984;10(2):297–305.

139. Heyman J, Reuterwall O, Benner S. The radiumhemmet experience with radiotherapy in cancer of the corpus of the uterus. *Acta Radiol.* 1941;22(1–2):11–98.

140. Coon D, Beriwal S, Heron DE, et al. High-dose-rate Rotte "Y" applicator brachytherapy for definitive treatment of medically inoperable endometrial cancer: 10-year results. *Int J Radiat Oncol Biol Phys.* 2008;71(3):779–783.

141. Perez CA, Slessinger E, Grigsby PW. Design of an afterloading vaginal applicator (MIRALVA). *Int J Radiat Oncol Biol Phys.* 1990;18(6):1503–1508.

142. Park S-J, Chung M, Demanes DJ, Banerjee R, Steinberg M, Kamrava M. Dosimetric comparison of 3-dimensional planning techniques using an intravaginal multichannel balloon applicator for high-dose-rate gynecologic brachytherapy. *Int J Radiat Oncol Biol Phys.* 2013;87(4):840–846.

143. Chassagne D, Dutreix A, Almond P, Burgers JMV, Busch M, Joslin CA. Report 38. *J Int Comm Radiat Units Meas.* 1985;os20(1):NP-NP.

144. Eifel PJ. High-dose-rate brachytherapy for carcinoma of the cervix: high tech or high risk? *Int J Radiat Oncol Biol Phys.* 1992;24(2):383–386; discussion 387-388.

145. Patel FD, Sharma SC, Negi PS, Ghoshal S, Gupta BD. Low dose rate vs. high dose rate brachytherapy in the treatment of carcinoma of the uterine cervix: a clinical trial. *Int J Radiat Oncol Biol Phys.* 1994;28(2):335–341.

146. Hareyama M, Sakata K, Oouchi A, et al. High-dose-rate versus low-dose-rate intracavitary therapy for carcinoma of the uterine cervix: a randomized trial. *Cancer.* 2002;94(1):117–124.

147. Lertsanguansinchai P, Lertbutsayanukul C, Shotelersuk K, et al. Phase III randomized trial comparing LDR and HDR brachytherapy in treatment of cervical carcinoma. *Int J Radiat Oncol.* 2004;59(5):1424–1431.

148. Brenner DJ, Hall EJ. Conditions for the equivalence of continuous to pulsed low dose rate brachytherapy. *Int J Radiat Oncol Biol Phys.* 1991;20(1):181–190.

149. Fowler J, Mount M. Pulsed brachytherapy: the conditions for no significant loss of therapeutic ratio compared with traditional low dose rate brachytherapy. *Int J Radiat Oncol Biol Phys.* 1992;23(3):661–669.

150. Davidson SE, Hendry JH, West CM. Point: why choose pulsed-dose-rate brachytherapy for treating gynecologic cancers? *Brachytherapy*. 2009;8(3):269–272.

151. Dooley WC, Thropay JP, Schreiber GJ, et al. Use of electronic brachytherapy to deliver postsurgical adjuvant radiation therapy for endometrial cancer: a retrospective multicenter study. *OncoTargets Ther*. 2010;3:197–203.

152. Lee LJ, Sadow CA, Russell A, Viswanathan AN. Correlation of point B and lymph node dose in 3D-planned high-dose-rate cervical cancer brachytherapy. *Int J Radiat Oncol Biol Phys*. 2009;75(3):803–809.

153. Haie-Meder C, Pötter R, Van Limbergen E, et al. Recommendations from Gynaecological (GYN) GEC-ESTRO Working Group (I): concepts and terms in 3D image based 3D treatment planning in cervix cancer brachytherapy with emphasis on MRI assessment of GTV and CTV. *Radiother Oncol J Eur Soc Ther Radiol Oncol*. 2005;74(3):235–245.

154. Viswanathan AN, Thomadsen B, American Brachytherapy Society Cervical Cancer Recommendations Committee, American Brachytherapy Society. American Brachytherapy Society consensus guidelines for locally advanced carcinoma of the cervix. Part I: general principles. *Brachytherapy*. 2012;11(1):33–46.

155. Nag S, Erickson B, Parikh S, Gupta N, Varia M, Glasgow G. The American Brachytherapy Society recommendations for high-dose-rate brachytherapy for carcinoma of the endometrium. *Int J Radiat Oncol Biol Phys*. 2000;48(3):779–790.

156. Patil VM, Patel FD, Chakraborty S, Oinam AS, Sharma SC. Can point doses predict volumetric dose to rectum and bladder: a CT-based planning study in high dose rate intracavitary brachytherapy of cervical carcinoma? *Br J Radiol*. 2011;84(1001):441–448.

157. Lee LJ, Das IJ, Higgins SA, et al. American Brachytherapy Society consensus guidelines for locally advanced carcinoma of the cervix. Part III: low-dose-rate and pulsed-dose-rate brachytherapy. *Brachytherapy*. 2012;11(1):53–57.

158. Rotmensch J, Connell PP, Yamada D, Waggoner SE, Mundt AJ. One versus two intracavitary brachytherapy applications in early-stage cervical cancer patients undergoing definitive radiation therapy. *Gynecol Oncol*. 2000;78(1):32–38.

159. Viswanathan AN, Beriwal S, De Los Santos J, et al. The American Brachytherapy Society treatment recommendations for locally advanced carcinoma of the cervix Part II: high dose-rate brachytherapy. *Brachytherapy*. 2012;11(1):47–52.

160. Small W, Beriwal S, Demanes DJ, et al. American Brachytherapy Society consensus guidelines for adjuvant vaginal cuff brachytherapy after hysterectomy. *Brachytherapy*. 2012;11(1):58–67.

161. Beriwal S, Demanes DJ, Erickson B, et al. American Brachytherapy Society consensus guidelines for interstitial brachytherapy for vaginal cancer. *Brachytherapy*. 2012;11(1):68–75.

162. Stitt JA, Fowler JF, Thomadsen BR, Buchler DA, Paliwal BP, Kinsella TJ. High dose rate intracavitary brachytherapy for carcinoma of the cervix: the Madison system: I. Clinical and radiobiological considerations. *Int J Radiat Oncol Biol Phys*. 1992;24(2):335–348.

163. Nag S, Chao C, Erickson B, et al. The American Brachytherapy Society recommendations for low-dose-rate brachytherapy for carcinoma of the cervix. *Int J Radiat Oncol Biol Phys*. 2002;52(1):33–48.

164. Mitchell DG, Snyder B, Coakley F, et al. Early invasive cervical cancer: tumor delineation by magnetic resonance imaging, computed tomography, and clinical examination, verified by pathologic results, in the ACRIN 6651/GOG 183 Intergroup Study. *J Clin Oncol Off J Am Soc Clin Oncol*. 2006;24(36):5687–5694.

165. Dimopoulos JCA, Schard G, Berger D, et al. Systematic evaluation of MRI findings in different stages of treatment of cervical cancer: potential of MRI on delineation of target, pathoanatomic structures, and organs at risk. *Int J Radiat Oncol Biol Phys*. 2006;64(5):1380–1388.

166. Wachter-Gerstner N, Wachter S, Reinstadler E, et al. Bladder and rectum dose defined from MRI based treatment planning for cervix cancer brachytherapy: comparison of dose-volume histograms for organ contours and organ wall, comparison with ICRU rectum and bladder reference point. *Radiother Oncol J Eur Soc Ther Radiol Oncol*. 2003;68(3):269–276.

167. Nesvacil N, Pötter R, Sturdza A, Hegazy N, Federico M, Kirisits C. Adaptive image guided brachytherapy for cervical cancer: a combined MRI-/CT-planning technique with MRI only at first fraction. *Radiother Oncol J Eur Soc Ther Radiol Oncol*. 2013;107(1):75–81.

168. Eskander RN, Scanderbeg D, Saenz CC, Brown M, Yashar C. Comparison of computed tomography and magnetic resonance imaging in cervical cancer brachytherapy target and normal tissue contouring. *Int J Gynecol Cancer Off J Int Gynecol Cancer Soc*. 2010;20(1):47–53.

169. Viswanathan AN, Erickson B, Gaffney D, et al. Comparison and consensus guidelines for delineation of clinical target volume for CT- and MR-based brachytherapy in locally advanced cervical cancer. *Int J Radiat Oncol Biol Phys*. 2014;90(2):9.

170. Tanderup K, Fokdal LU, Sturdza A, et al. Effect of tumor dose, volume and overall treatment time on local control after radio-chemotherapy including MRI guided brachytherapy of locally advanced cervical cancer. *Radiother Oncol J Eur Soc Ther Radiol Oncol*. 2016;120(3):441–446.

171. Horne ZD, Karukonda P, Kalash R, et al. Single-institution experience in 3D MRI-based brachytherapy for cervical cancer for 239 women: can dose overcome poor response? *Int J Radiat Oncol*. 2019;104(1):157–164.

172. Tan L-T, Pötter R, Sturdza A, et al. Change in patterns of failure after image-guided brachytherapy for cervical cancer: analysis From the RetroEMBRACE study. *Int J Radiat Oncol Biol Phys*. 2019;104(4):895–902.

173. Mazeron R, Fokdal LU, Kirchheiner K, et al. Dose–volume effect relationships for late rectal morbidity in patients treated with chemoradiation and MRI-guided adaptive brachytherapy for locally advanced cervical cancer: Results from the prospective multicenter EMBRACE study. *Radiother Oncol*. 2016;120(3):412–419.

174. Kirchheiner K, Nout RA, Lindegaard JC, et al. Dose-effect relationship and risk factors for vaginal stenosis after definitive radio(chemo)therapy with image-guided brachytherapy for locally advanced cervical cancer in the EMBRACE study. *Radiother Oncol J Eur Soc Ther Radiol Oncol*. 2016;118(1):160–166.

175. Fokdal L, Tanderup K, Pötter R, et al. Risk factors for ureteral stricture after radiochemotherapy including image guided adaptive brachytherapy in cervical cancer: results from the EMBRACE studies. *Int J Radiat Oncol Biol Phys*. 2019;103(4):887–894.

176. Jensen NBK, Pötter R, Kirchheiner K, et al. Bowel morbidity following radiochemotherapy and image-guided adaptive brachytherapy for cervical cancer: physician- and patient reported outcome from the EMBRACE study. *Radiother Oncol J Eur Soc Ther Radiol Oncol*. 2018;127(3):431–439.

177. Fokdal L, Pötter R, Kirchheiner K, et al. Physician assessed and patient reported urinary morbidity after radio-chemotherapy and image guided adaptive brachytherapy for locally advanced cervical cancer. *Radiother Oncol J Eur Soc Ther Radiol Oncol*. 2018;127(3):423–430.

178. Erickson B, Eifel P, Moughan J, Rownd J, Iarocci T, Owen J. Patterns of brachytherapy practice for patients with carcinoma of the cervix (1996-1999): a patterns of care study. *Int J Radiat Oncol Biol Phys*. 2005;63(4):1083–1092.

179. Fokdal L, Sturdza A, Mazeron R, et al. Image guided adaptive brachytherapy with combined intracavitary and interstitial technique improves the therapeutic ratio in locally advanced cervical cancer: analysis from the retroEMBRACE study. *Radiother Oncol J Eur Soc Ther Radiol Oncol*. 2016;120(3):434–440.

180. Beriwal S, Demanes DJ, Erickson B, et al. American Brachytherapy Society consensus guidelines for interstitial brachytherapy for vaginal cancer. *Brachytherapy*. 2012;11(1):68–75.

181. Kirisits C, Lang S, Dimopoulos J, Berger D, Georg D, Pötter R. The Vienna applicator for combined intracavitary and interstitial brachytherapy of cervical cancer: Design, application, treatment planning, and dosimetric results. *Int J Radiat Oncol*. 2006;65(2):624–630.

182. Nag S, Yacoub S, Copeland LJ, Fowler JM. Interstitial brachytherapy for salvage treatment of vaginal recurrences in previously unirradiated endometrial cancer patients. *Int J Radiat Oncol Biol Phys*. 2002;54(4):1153–1159.

183. Weitmann HD, Knocke TH, Waldhäusl C, Pötter R. Ultrasound-guided interstitial brachytherapy in the treatment of advanced vaginal recurrences from cervical and endometrial carcinoma. *Strahlenther Onkol Organ Dtsch Rontgengesellschaft Al.* 2006;182(2):86–95.

184. Nag S, Martínez-Monge R, Ellis R, et al. The use of fluoroscopy to guide needle placement in interstitial gynecological brachytherapy. *Int J Radiat Oncol Biol Phys.* 1998;40(2):415–420.

185. Erickson B, Albano K, Gillin M. CT-guided interstitial implantation of gynecologic malignancies. *Int J Radiat Oncol Biol Phys.* 1996;36(3):699–709.

186. Brabham JG, Cardenes HR. Permanent interstitial reirradiation with 198Au as salvage therapy for low volume recurrent gynecologic malignancies: a single institution experience. *Am J Clin Oncol.* 2009;32(4):417–422.

187. Randall ME, Evans L, Greven KM, McCunniff AJ, Doline RM. Interstitial reirradiation for recurrent gynecologic malignancies: results and analysis of prognostic factors. *Gynecol Oncol.* 1993;48(1):23–31.

188. Yoshida K, Yamazaki H, Takenaka T, et al. A dose-volume analysis of magnetic resonance imaging-aided high-dose-rate image-based interstitial brachytherapy for uterine cervical cancer. *Int J Radiat Oncol Biol Phys.* 2010;77(3):765–772.

189. Glaser SM, Beriwal S. Brachytherapy for malignancies of the vagina in the 3D era. *J Contemp Brachytherapy.* 2015;4:312–318.

190. Dimopoulos JCA, Schmid MP, Fidarova E, Berger D, Kirisits C, Pötter R. Treatment of locally advanced vaginal cancer with radiochemotherapy and magnetic resonance image-guided adaptive brachytherapy: dose-volume parameters and first clinical results. *Int J Radiat Oncol Biol Phys.* 2012;82(5):1880–1888.

191. Beriwal S, Rwigema J-CM, Higgins E, et al. Three-dimensional image-based high-dose-rate interstitial brachytherapy for vaginal cancer. *Brachytherapy.* 2012;11(3):176–180.

192. Cancer Genome Atlas Research Network, Kandoth C, Schultz N, Cherniack AD, et al. Integrated genomic characterization of endometrial carcinoma. *Nature.* 2013;497(7447):67–73.

193. Wortman BG, Bosse T, Nout RA, et al. Molecular-integrated risk profile to determine adjuvant radiotherapy in endometrial cancer: evaluation of the pilot phase of the PORTEC-4a trial. *Gynecol Oncol.* 2018;151(1):69–75.

194. Boldrini L, Chiloiro G, Pesce A, et al. Hybrid MRI guided radiotherapy in locally advanced cervical cancer: case report of an innovative personalized therapeutic approach. *Clin Transl Radiat Oncol.* 2019;20:27–29.

195. Archambault Y, Boylan C, Bullock D, et al. Making on-line adaptive radiotherapy possilbe using artificial intelligence and machine learning for efficient daily re-planning. *Med Phys Int J.* 2020;8(2):77–86.

196. Mayadev JS, Enserro D, Lin YG, et al. Sequential ipilimumab after chemoradiotherapy in curative-intent treatment of patients with node-positive cervical cancer. *JAMA Oncol.* 2020;6(1):92–99.

197. Le DT, Uram JN, Wang H, et al. PD-1 blockade in tumors with mismatch-repair deficiency. *N Engl J Med.* 2015; 372(26):2509–2520.

12 The Lymphomas

John P. Plastaras, Stefan Both, and Ima Paydar

INTRODUCTION

The role of radiotherapy (RT) in the treatment of lymphomas has evolved significantly in recent decades. Once a mainstay of curative treatment for lymphoma, the role of radiation had become complementary to multiagent chemotherapy for the majority of patients diagnosed with lymphoma. Many of the studies over time have been aimed at reducing radiation doses and volumes treated. In addition, many studies have also investigated how to eliminate radiation altogether by appropriate use of risk stratification and/or response to treatment. Modern RT for lymphoma is thus aimed at maintaining efficacy while limiting toxicity as much as possible.

The lymphomas are broadly divided between Hodgkin lymphomas (HLs) and non-Hodgkin lymphomas (NHLs). The WHO has classified 83 subtypes of lymphoma, largely based on the implementation of immunotyping, with recognition of borderline categories and entities associated with certain age groups.[1] This list was further revised in 2016 to refine the diagnostic criteria as well as the genetic and molecular landscape of lymphoid neoplasms.[2] HLs are broadly divided based on histologic subtype into (1) classic HL (nodular sclerosing, mixed cellularity, lymphocyte rich, and lymphocyte depleted) and (2) non-classic HL (nodular lymphocyte predominant).

NHLs are divided into B-cell and T-cell/NK-cell categories. Treatment approaches depend not only on histologic subtype but also on the stage, patient factors, and predicted clinical behavior. In practice, clinicians often categorize lymphomas as indolent, aggressive, or highly aggressive, but true aggressiveness may not always track precisely with pathologic subclassification. This behavior can range broadly from indolent lymphomas that can take decades to become clinically significant to highly aggressive lymphomas that can progress within weeks. For diffuse large B-cell lymphoma (DLBCL), the most commonly diagnosed NHL, subclassification using genetic profiling is frequently used to divide lymphomas into germinal center B-cell-like and activated B-cell-like.[3] Surface markers can be used as a surrogate to classify using the Hans classification system. In addition, alterations in c-MYC paired with Bcl-2 or Bcl-6, resulting in so-called double-hit lymphomas, are associated with particularly poor responses to standard therapy.[4] Regardless, observation of the actual clinical course is a still key factor in making treatment decisions. Although radiation alone is sometimes used, such as for limited-stage, low-grade follicular lymphomas and extranodal marginal zone lymphomas, most lymphomas will be treated with chemotherapy first. RT timing, volume treated, and dose are highly dependent on the type, effectiveness, and response to chemotherapy. When patients are treated with radiation alone, relapses tend to occur outside of the RT fields. When patients are treated with chemotherapy alone, relapses tend to occur at sites of prior disease. Combining radiation and chemotherapy allows for an opportunity to truncate both modalities, which minimizes toxicities that are primarily dose dependent—without sacrificing cure. Therefore, initial multidisciplinary integration is a key for effectively and safely treating patients with lymphoma.

STAGING AND PROGNOSIS

The staging system most commonly used for HL and NHL has been the Ann Arbor Staging System; however, the Lugano Classification, based on an international working group, has refined the approach to staging, especially with respect to the use of ^{18}F-FDG PET/CT.[5] For nodal lymphomas, patients are grouped into three general categories based on general treatment approaches: (1) limited stage, (2) stage II bulky, or (3) advanced stage (Table 12.1). The definition of "bulky" has been modified based on histology, with a recommendation to designate the longest measurement by CT scan, omitting the term X. For HL, a single nodal mass of 10 cm or greater than a third of the transthoracic diameter by CT is considered bulky by the Ann Arbor staging system, but 7 cm in any direction has been shown to increase risk for local recurrence.[6] For DLBCL, 7.5 cm is a clinically relevant cutoff used in the RICOVER-60[7] and UNFOLDER (unpublished) clinical trials. The designation of A or B is based on the presence of B symptoms, which are unexplained fevers, night sweats, and unexplained weight loss of >10% over a 6-month period. In the revised Lugano Classification, B symptoms are now assigned only to HL patients.

TABLE 12.1	Revised Staging System for Primary Nodal Lymphomas from the Lugano Classification

Stage	Involvement	Extranodal (E) Status
Limited		
I	One node or a group of adjacent nodes	Single extranodal lesion without nodal involvement
II	Two or more nodal groups on the same side of the diaphragm	Stage I or II by nodal extent with limited contiguous extranodal involvement
II bulky[a]	II as above with "bulky" disease	Not applicable
Advanced		
III	Nodes on both sides of the diaphragm; nodes above the diaphragm with spleen involvement	Not applicable
IV	Additional noncontiguous extralymphatic involvement	Not applicable

[a]Whether stage II bulky disease is treated as limited or advanced disease may be determined by histology and a number of prognostic factors.

Extent of disease is determined by positron emission tomography–computed tomography for avid lymphomas and computed tomography for nonavid histologies. Tonsils, Waldeyer ring, and spleen are considered nodal tissue.

Source: Cheson BD, et al. Recommendations for initial evaluation, staging, and response assessment of Hodgkin and non-Hodgkin lymphoma: the Lugano classification. *J Clin Oncol.* 2014.

For limited stage HL, prognosis and intensity of treatment are based on factors that divide patients into favorable or unfavorable risk categories. If a patient has any one of the risk factors, they are considered unfavorable. The factors that have been used have varied slightly according to each cooperative or guideline group (Table 12.2). For advanced stage patients, the International Prognostic Score (IPS) can be used to predict prognosis, with higher scores portending worse progression-free survival.[8] One point is assigned for each of the seven factors: male sex, age $\geq$45 years, stage IV, hemoglobin <10^5 g/L, WBC count $\geq15 \times 10^9$/L, lymphocyte count <0.6×10^9/L or <8% of differential albumin <40 g/L. Although the IPS can predict the chance of relapse and has been used to define high-risk patients in clinical trials, it has not been frequently used to justify the use of consolidative radiation.

For NHL, there are scoring systems based on clinical factors that can predict outcomes. For DLBCL, the International Prognostic Index (IPI) uses a point system similar to the IPS with a point assigned for each negative prognostic factor (elevated LDH, age >60 years, ECOG performance status >1, Stage III/IV, >1 extranodal sites).[9] The original IPI was developed before the introduction of rituximab, but the same factors in the rituximab era, the "R-IPI," identifies prognostic groups with 4-year progression-free survival ranges of 53%, 80%, and 94% for the three risk groups.[10] Separate IPI scoring systems have been developed for follicular lymphoma and mantle cell lymphoma to account for the different prognoses of these NHL subtypes.

In HL, one of the most powerful and consistent predictors of outcome is interim PET scans performed partway through chemotherapy.[11–13] However, the value of interim PET scanning in DLBCL appears less consistent, showing a correlation in some studies,[14–17] but not in others.[18–20] When RT was consistently added to chemotherapy, a

TABLE 12.2	Factors for Limited-Stage, Unfavorable-Risk Disease

	GHSG	EORTC	NCIC	NCCN
Age (yr)	—	$\geq$50	$\geq$40	
Histology	—	—	Mixed cellularity or lymphocyte depleted	
ESR/B symptoms	>30 mm with any B, >50 mm without B	>30 mm with any B, >50 mm without B	>50 mm or any B sx	$\geq$50 mm or any B sx
Mediastinal mass	MMR[a] >0.33	MTR[b] >0.35	MMR >0.33	MMR >0.33
No. of nodal sites	$\geq$3	$\geq$4	$\geq$4	$\geq$4
Extranodal	Present	—	—	
Bulky				>10 cm

[a]MMR = Mediastinal mass ratio, maximum width of mass/maximum intrathoracic diameter.
[b]MTR = Mediastinal thoracic ratio, maximum width of mediastinal mass/intrathoracic diameter at T5–6.

positive interim PET scan did not predict for relapse.[21] In a separate study, an interim positive PET scan was associated with relapse only in patients treated with chemotherapy alone, but not in those treated with combined modality therapy.[22]

INDICATIONS FOR TREATMENT

In the treatment of lymphomas, the radiation technique depends on the clinical context and indications for treatment. It is important to determine first and foremost whether the intent of treatment is curative or palliative. Unlike most solid cancers where *Stage IV* is nearly synonymous with incurable disease, advanced stage lymphomas can frequently be cured by chemotherapy with or without radiation. *Consolidative radiation* is the term used for radiation given after a complete response following chemotherapy as a strategy to sterilize potential sites of relapse. This can be part of the initial therapy or for relapsed or refractory lymphoma. Although the chances of cure are certainly less in the relapsed/refractory circumstance, more aggressive treatments, including high-dose chemotherapy with autologous stem cell rescue, can often still result in cure. *Salvage* RT refers to the treatment of relapsed or refractory disease with curative intent, usually given along with other systemic therapy. When radiation alone is used for cure, this is termed *definitive* radiation. Finally, when radiation is used purely to relieve symptoms without an attempt to alter survival, this is termed *palliative*. Due to the radiosensitivity of most lymphomas, even extraordinarily low doses of radiation can often accomplish goals of symptom control. Because an ever-evolving slate of biologic therapies are being developed to target hematologic malignancies, it is hard to always know if a patient is actually incurable even when their disease is refractory to cytotoxic chemotherapy. For example, chimeric antigen receptor (CAR) T cell therapy can lead to long-term survival in patients with NHL who have progressed through standard systemic therapies.[23–25] Close discussion with medical oncology colleagues is critical to understand the overall prognosis and what role radiation needs to play in each patient.

Combined Modality for Hodgkin Lymphoma

Combined modality therapy is a standard for limited stage HL in both favorable and unfavorable risk patients. There are many who prefer a chemotherapy-only approach for limited stage patients. NCCN Guidelines and ACR Appropriateness Criteria for HL are frequently updated and reflect the ongoing debate between these approaches with a focus on matching the right intensity of treatment for each patient. One approach to determining the intensity of treatment is based on prognostic factors at the time of diagnosis (Table 12.2). The German Hodgkin Study Group trials HD10 and HD11 trials both studied combined modality approaches with an aim to find the correct intensity of treatment using a 2 by 2 randomization. In the HD10 trial of favorable risk patients, chemotherapy intensity was studied, ABVD × 2 versus ABVD × 4, along with involved field radiotherapy (IFRT) to 20 Gy versus 30 Gy.[26] Reduced intensity therapy with ABVD × 2 and 20 Gy had equivalent freedom from failure compared to the other arms and has thus emerged as a standard of care for favorable risk patients. The HD11 trial studied unfavorable risk patients who were randomized between ABVD × 4 versus BEACOPP (standard) and 20 Gy versus 30 Gy.[27] In this study, ABVD × 4 was much less toxic than BEACOPP (standard), but had similar efficacy. Although there was no difference between 20 and 30 Gy when combined with BEACOPP (standard), there were more relapses when 20 Gy was used with the less intense ABVD regimen compared to 30 Gy. Thus, ABVD × 4 and 30 Gy remained a standard for unfavorable risk patients following the results of that trial. Rather than using only prognostic factors to determine treatment, the field has evolved to use response-adapted treatments. Several trials have tested the use of FDG-PET/CT response to chemotherapy to drive RT decisions with mixed results. The EORTC/LYSA/FIL H10 trial found that omitting radiation based on interim PET scans leads to an increased risk of relapse.[28] The RAPID trial enrolled subjects with early stage HL without bulky mediastinal disease. Those who had a negative PET scan after three cycles of ABVD were randomized to observation or consolidative radiation.[29] Although these results have been interpreted in different ways, based on their predetermined statistical goals, the authors were unable to show a noninferiority of the no-radiation arm versus the radiation arm. Similarly, the HD16 trial of early favorable patients showed that omission of RT after ABVD × 2 cycles in PET-negative subjects was associated with unacceptably high rates of progression.[30] The HD17 trial tested whether a negative PET after four cycles of more aggressive chemotherapy could be used to direct the omission RT in subjects with early unfavorable HL. This study stands out as a successful example of using PET to direct therapy intensity as the arms were not significantly different.

The role of RT in advanced stage HL is very selective. It is usually reserved for large-volume residual disease after chemotherapy.[31] The decision to use radiation in advanced stage patients also depends on the intensity of the chemotherapy. For example, the HD15 trial, which studied different schedules of the relatively intense BEACOPP regimen, only gave radiation to PET-positive residual masses that were 2.5 cm or larger.[32] The use of RT in advanced stage HL therefore remains controversial, but it is generally considered after a partial response to chemotherapy or for bulky disease. Ongoing clinical trials may help clarify the role more precisely, especially with newer agents such as brentuximab (anti-CD30 monoclonal antibody) or immune checkpoint inhibitors.

Combined Modality for Non-Hodgkin Lymphoma

A common role for combined modality therapy is for limited stage DLBCL. Two randomized trials performed prior to the introduction of rituximab have demonstrated value for the addition of radiation to multiagent chemotherapy. The ECOG 1484 study evaluated the role of adding radiation to complete responders after eight cycles of CHOP chemotherapy.[33] In this setting, radiation improved disease-free survival but not overall survival. The SWOG 8736 study showed that radiation combined with limited chemotherapy (CHOP × 3) had improved progression-free and overall survival compared to eight cycles of CHOP alone.[34] Although a subsequent report with longer follow-up showed that significant differences diminished over time, limited chemotherapy with radiation is still considered a standard of care for carefully selected patients. However, there have been several other studies that have not shown a benefit for radiation in the pre-rituximab era.[35,36] Retrospective data and results from the nonrandomized prospective study (RICOVER-60) have suggested that patients who get radiation, especially for initially bulky DLBCL, have superior outcomes.[7,36,37] Other indications for consolidative RT include skeletal involvement and incomplete metabolic response (Deauville Score 4) after "full course chemotherapy."[38]

Radiation Alone

Although radiation alone has been used in the past with curative intent for both HL and NHL, the use of combination chemotherapy has been shown to be more effective for classic HL and aggressive NHL histologies. However, radiation alone is still used to cure limited stage nonclassic HL (nodular lymphocyte predominant) and limited stage low-grade NHL. Radiation alone for low-grade, limited stage follicular lymphoma results in a sizable minority of patients with long-term disease control.[39] Limited stage extranodal marginal zone (MALT) lymphomas of the stomach, thyroid, lung, salivary glands, and orbit can all be effectively controlled with doses ranging from 24 to 30 Gy.[40,41] Primary cutaneous B cell lymphomas of the skin can be frequently controlled with low doses under 12 Gy.[42] Radiation alone is also commonly used in the palliative setting. Very low dose RT (2 Gy × 2) is effective in low-grade histologies [43] and can result in meaningful palliative responses. Hypofractionated RT with lower doses can be effective as well even in aggressive histologies.[44] Although such low doses are effective for palliation, especially in patients with multiple sites of involvement, higher doses are still recommended for the curative setting.[45]

Relapsed/Refractory Setting

With the trend of chemotherapy alone being used for initial therapy, there has been an increased fraction of patients referred only after chemotherapy has failed. There is still hope for cure in patients who have persistent disease after initial standard therapy or when lymphoma relapses after first remission. For both HL and NHL, high-dose chemotherapy with stem cell rescue can result in cure. When RT can be incorporated with salvage therapy, there appears to be improved outcomes in both HL and DLBCL as summarized in the International Lymphoma Radiation Oncology Group (ILROG) guidelines on relapsed/refractory disease.[46,47] The appropriate volumes and doses to treat in the relapsed/refractory setting are unknown and a matter of judgment. Typically, larger elective volumes are considered with higher doses given to refractory foci of disease, but each patient should be highly customized based on prior distributions of disease and subsequent responses to each line of therapy. Similar questions remain when combining immunotherapy and RT. A recent development has involved incorporating RT with CAR T-cell therapy for relapsed/refractory lymphomas. Early studies suggest safety and feasibility of RT as bridging therapy to CAR T-cell therapy, though more data will be necessary to determine whether RT improves oncologic outcomes or reduces toxicity.[48-50] The optimal dose and fractionation schema for these patients remains to be clarified; however, given the timing constraints between leukapheresis and infusion of lymphocytes, close collaboration with medical oncology is critical when planning RT for these patients.

RADIATION THERAPY TECHNIQUES

History of Field Design

The history of the treatment of lymphoma paralleled the early history of RT itself. While curative treatment for HL was being developed, we also saw the introduction of the linear accelerator by Henry Kaplan, the concept of treating microscopic disease in the hopes of cures, and the use of customized blocks to shape fields to minimize toxicity. Originally, radiation fields were designed using 2-dimensional (2D) planning, based on anatomical landmarks visible on plain x-ray film or fluoroscopy. When RT was used as the primary modality for cure, very large treatment volumes were employed, with the attempt to treat all nodal tissue. As effective multiagent chemotherapy was developed, trials demonstrated that fields could be reduced from total nodal radiation, subtotal nodal irradiation, extended field, mantle, inverted-Y, and then IFRT (Figs. 12.1 and 12.2). The 2D definitions for IFRT were canonized in a 2002 review by Drs. Yahalom and Mauch.[51] For some time, IFRT was incorporated in a standard manner into combined modality lymphoma trials.[26,27,34] Most of these 2D fields used anterior–posterior/posterior–anterior (AP/PA) field arrangements. As three-dimensional (3D) planned conformal radiation therapy and intensity modulated radiation therapy (IMRT) became standard in other disease sites, their application in lymphoma appeared.[52,53] The application and comparison of volumetric treatment-planning techniques obviously required delineation of treatment volumes, which

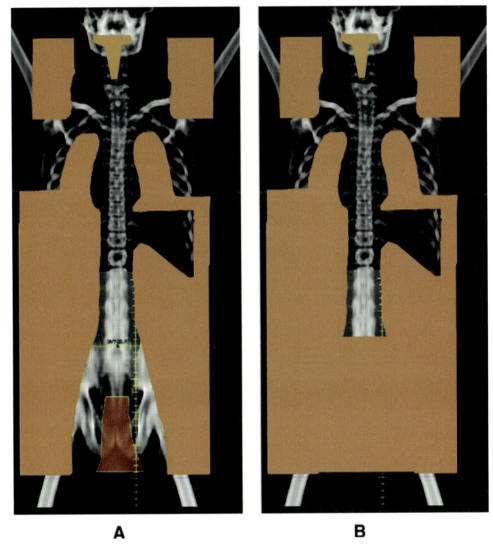

FIGURE 12.1. Historical very large radiation fields used in the treatment of lymphoma based on 2D landmarks. (**A**) Total nodal irradiation (TNI). (**B**) Subtotal nodal lymph node irradiation (STLNI). (Reproduced from Hill-Kayser CE et al. The case for combined-modality therapy for limited-stage Hodgkin's disease. *Oncologist*. 2012;17:8.)

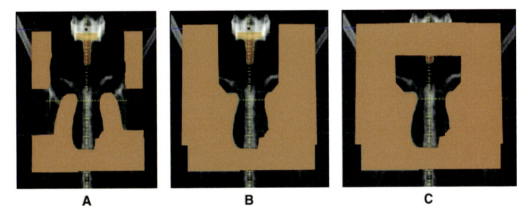

FIGURE 12.2. Historical limited radiation fields for mediastinal lymphoma based on 2D landmarks. (**A**) The classic mantle field consisted of treatment to the bilateral neck, supraclavicular regions, axillae, hilae, mediastinum, and pericardial nodes. (**B**) The "Modified mantle" that blocks the axillary regions reduces breast cancer risk[109] and pulmonary toxicity. (**C**) IFRT for mediastinal lymphoma based on Yahalom and Mauch[51] blocks the high neck and reduces dose to the carotid arteries, salivary glands, and dentition. (Reproduced from Hill-Kayser CE, et al. The case for combined-modality therapy for limited-stage Hodgkin's disease. *Oncologist*. 2012;17:8.)

was more conceivable in the IFRT era.[54,55] Different groups varied on exactly how to contour the target volumes based on the IFRT concept, but having specific targets enabled technique development to keep dose to organs-at-risk (OAR) below predefined limits.[56] Concurrently, with the advent of volumetric planning for lymphoma, some centers adopted more limited radiation volumes, using the "involved node radiotherapy" (INRT) concept. The INRT concept involves treating only the areas of previously abnormal disease with margin, but not attempting to treat any elective nodal volumes. Single-institution and pooled results have shown that the risk of failure in regions that would have been treated using IFRT was rare.[57] The EORTC–GELA group adopted INRT, described how to define these volumes, and reported on excellent outcomes using this technique.[28,58,59] Central to the precise definition of these limited radiation volumes was the use of PET/CT in the treatment planning position to ensure accuracy; however, this is difficult to achieve in practice outside of a clinical trial. Smaller target volumes inevitably result in lower dose to OARs, in particular heart, lung, breast, and thyroid.[60] In addition, compared to IFRT, INRT is predicted to have a lower risk of secondary cancers.[61] In practice, it is challenging to coordinate the staging PET/CT in the treatment position prior to starting chemotherapy, but not impossible.

Involved Site Radiotherapy

In order to take into account the reality of poor fusions, the concept of "involved site radiotherapy" (ISRT) has been advocated by the ILROG for HL and NHL.[62,63] Essentially, the concept entails using volume-based RT techniques according to the International Commission on Radiation Units and Measurements (ICRU) without any elective nodal radiation when chemotherapy has been effective. Volumes are expanded to account for inaccuracies in fusion and uncertainty when trying to interpret how lymphomas shrink during chemotherapy. When lymphomas shrink during chemotherapy, the postchemotherapy volume is used to define the clinical target volume radially, but the prechemotherapy volume is generally used superior-inferiorly.[64]

Extranodal Lymphomas

Extranodal lymphomas pose a particular challenge when determining the radiation volumes. The ILROG has published guidelines for a variety of extranodal sites.[65] According to ILROG guidelines, if an orbital lymphoma only involves the conjunctiva or eyelid, the entire conjunctival reflection to the fornices is usually treated, but not the entire orbit. However, if the lymphoma involves the retrobulbar region, lacrimal gland, or is a deep conjunctival lesion, the entire orbit is usually treated. A small but poignant series demonstrated that partial orbital radiation leads to a high ipsilateral relapse rate.[66] Thus, lower doses of radiation are advocated to decrease toxicity rather than geometric attempts to avoid periorbital

OARs.[67] Other challenging locations are the nasal/paranasal sinuses. For aggressive NHL of the sinuses, the large majority of which turn out to be DLBCL, induction chemotherapy with R-CHOP is commonly employed. The consolidative radiation volume should include the entirety of the affected sinus and any sinuses that are breached, but uninvolved sinuses need not be included in the CTV in the era of modern imaging and combined modality therapy.[65] Extranodal NK/T cell lymphomas, nasal type, are a particular subtype of NHL that requires special attention. For limited stage extranodal NK/T cell lymphomas, primary RT, with or without concurrent or sequential chemotherapy to high doses (≥ 50 Gy), can result in cure.

Cutaneous lymphomas also pose challenges in determining the appropriate radiation volume, technique, and dose. First and foremost, an understanding of the dermatopathology is key to determining the appropriate treatment. The ILROG has published general guidelines for treatment of cutaneous lymphomas.[68] When limited to a localized distribution, certain lymphomas such as primary cutaneous follicle center lymphoma, primary cutaneous marginal zone lymphoma, and primary cutaneous anaplastic large-cell lymphoma can be cured with RT alone using a margin of 1 to 1.5 cm for CTV. En face electrons can be an ideal technique for cutaneous lymphomas, and these margins should be incorporated into the design of customized blocks. Primary cutaneous diffuse large B-cell lymphoma, leg-type, has a somewhat worse prognosis and is generally treated with combined modality therapy (R-CHOP) followed by radiation with 1- to 2-cm expansion to CTV. Cutaneous T-cell lymphoma (mycosis fungoides) can be treated with RT depending on the situation. If diffuse control is required when topicals and other systemic therapies fail, total skin electron therapy may be a durable palliative treatment, particularly when intractable pruritus is present. Implementation of total skin electron therapy requires special commissioning, treatment stands to allow the patient to adopt various positions, and close attention from physicists to ensure homogenous and tolerable treatment.[69] There has been a trend toward lower total skin electron therapy doses for cutaneous T-cell lymphoma, typically 10 to 12 Gy.[70] For focal palliation of CTCL, limited en face electron fields can be used, but somewhat higher doses than the 4 Gy used for low-grade B cell lymphomas are required for a reliable response. Compared to a 30% response rate for 4 Gy (2 Gy × 2), 8 Gy (4 Gy × 2) results in a response rate of over 90%.[71]

Simulation Techniques

In planning lymphoma cases, patient positioning and immobilization depend on the site of treatment. For head and neck and mediastinal lymphomas, thermoplastic masks can allow for limited PTV expansions by reducing interfraction setup errors. In certain situations, five-point thermoplastic masks can be used to restrict rigidly the relationship between the neck, clavicles, and mediastinal structures (Fig. 12.3A). The face can be cut out to allow for breath-hold devices (Fig. 12.3B). The position of the arms depends on the treatment volume as well as the technique. While arms up may better reproduce the prechemotherapy PET/CT allowing better image fusion, it limits the potential use of lateral beam angles to approach the neck and/or Waldeyer ring. Arms down may limit certain lateral beam angles for thoracic volumes. The position of the arms does alter the position of axillary nodes, which should be considered if they need to be treated. Ultimately, the decision to treat arms up, down, or akimbo is patient- and technique specific. Putting female patients on an incline board can move the breasts and heart away from the upper mediastinum, potentially decreasing dose to the structures.[72] For inguinal lymphomas, "frog-leg" positions can alleviate skin folds as a measure to reduce skin toxicity. In addition, these positions allow for more freedom to move the penis/scrotum away from intended fields or to use a "clamshell" to reduce dose to the testicles. Ideally, CT-compatible mock clamshells can be used to position optimally the patient when testicular shielding is desired (Fig. 12.4). One half of a mock clamshell can also be used to contain and immobilize the scrotum when testicular RT is performed.

In addition to fusion with PET/CT scans, intravenous contrast-enhanced CT scans can be helpful in delineating nodes. Small PET-negative nodes that are present on prechemotherapy scans that disappear are highly suspicious for involvement by lymphoma, but are difficult to discern without contrast.[58] When using the ISRT paradigm, exclusion of normal structures is greatly aided by intravenous contrast, especially around the heart and great vessels.[62,63] If cardiac substructures are to be preferentially avoided using ultra-conformal techniques, then contrast is also helpful.[73] In particular, delineation of the left main coronary artery, left anterior descending artery, aortic valve, and left ventricle can help shape highly conformal RT plans and keep these structures limited to specific doses, as outlined in the ILROG guidelines.[74] Oral contrast is appropriate for certain abdominal lymphomas, particularly those in the mesentery. Barium can be used, but it can cause some small errors in photon dose-distributions if the Hounsfield units are not overridden to water-equivalent prior to planning. If proton therapy is used, any structures with contrast must be overridden due to profound effects on the dose distribution, but the best approach would be to acquire noncontrast and contrast scans at the time of simulation.[75] Alternative low attenuation oral contrast agents, such as VoLumen or milk,[76] with low Hounsfield units, can reduce this issue, but delineating bowel using "negative contrast agents" can be challenging when bowel is intimately involved with tumor (Fig. 12.5A and B). The addition of intravenous contrast to negative contrast agents improves the ability to distinguish bowel as the bowel wall is enhanced (Fig. 12.5C and D).

Motion Management

With the advent of highly conformal radiation for lymphoma, close attention to motion becomes increasingly relevant. In the mediastinum and abdomen, where respiratory motion predominates, gated four-dimensional (4D) CT scans can be acquired to ascertain actual target and OAR movement. The ISRT guidelines call for use of

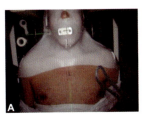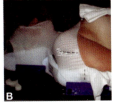

FIGURE 12.3. Thermoplastic immobilization mask. (**A**) For optimal stabilization of the cervical and thoracic spine with respect to clavicle position, a five-point mask that encompasses the shoulders can be used. (**B**) If breath-hold devices are used, the face can be cut out to accommodate the mouthpiece and goggles.

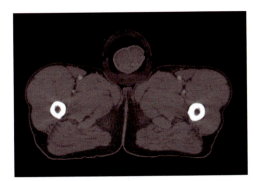

FIGURE 12.4. CT-compatible testicular shield. The high-density "clamshell" used during treatment creates artifact that compromises CT-based radiation contouring and planning. A mock testicular shield made from CT-compatible material is shown in axial cross-section that allows for accurate body positioning.

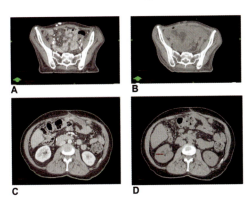

FIGURE 12.5. High-density and low-density oral contrast agents with or without intravenous contrast in CT simulation of abdomen and pelvis. (**A**) High-density barium oral contrast with intravenous contrast in the pelvis. Contrast shows clear delineation of small bowel and blood vessels, which may need to be overridden during RT planning. (**B**) Low-density oral contrast, VoLumen *without* intravenous contrast in the pelvis. Delineation of bowel and vessel is more difficult. (**C**) VoLumen *with* intravenous contrast in the abdomen shows small bowel more clearly with enhancement of the bowel wall. (**D**) VoLumen *without* intravenous contrast in the abdomen.

volumes as described by the ICRU Report 83 (GTV, CTV, PTV) and Report 62, which delineate the internal target volume (ITV).[62,63] Large anterior mediastinal masses, even those remaining after chemotherapy, tend to "pancake out" laterally when patients are supine compared to when upright. These large masses can move significantly during the breathing cycles, as shown in Figure 12.6. During the exhale phase, mediastinal masses can extend laterally, which can lead to increased dose to the lungs and breast tissues, especially when AP/PA field arrangements are used. During the inhale phase, masses elongate cranio-caudally, but show a narrower profile laterally. This narrowing of the mediastinum can be accentuated with deep (maximum or near maximum) inspiratory breath hold (Fig. 12.7).

Deep inspiratory breath-hold (DIBH) techniques have become increasingly standard for mediastinal lymphomas.[77–81] A Phase II study of DIBH was conducted where free-breathing and DIBH PET/CT scans were acquired in the treatment position prior to initiation of chemotherapy as well as postchemotherapy scans. Of the 22 eligible patients, 19 were preferentially treated with DIBH based on more favorable lung, heart, and breast dosimetry.[79] In this study, which used the RPM system with video/goggle guidance, they found that the DIBH on average could decrease the mean dose and V20 of the heart and

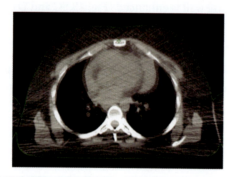

FIGURE 12.6. Effect of respiration on lateral dimensions of mediastinal lymphomas. Fused CT images of axial slices in maximal inspiration (more narrow) and maximal expiration (wider) from a planning 4D CT scan of a patient with a residual mass after chemotherapy for Hodgkin lymphoma.

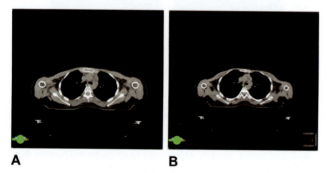

A   **B**

FIGURE 12.7. Effect of deep inspiratory breath hold on mediastinal width. Axial CT slices of a patient with residual anterior mediastinal lymphoma imaged at the level of the carina using either free-breathing (**A**) or at deep inspiratory breath hold (**B**).

lung without an effect on female breast dose. An alternate approach, using moderate DIBH with active breathing control, also decreased mean lung and heart doses, but actually showed increased dose to the breasts.[80] DIBH can reduce heart and lung doses beyond what can be achieved by IMRT alone.[77,78] In practice, the use of DIBH is more practical for patients with lymphoma than for patients with lung cancer as they are usually healthy enough to participate in the rigorous demands of this technique.[79] DIBH with IMRT rivals the impact of proton therapy for OAR sparing, with the optimal sparing achieved with a combination of DIBH and proton therapy.[82,83]

On-Board Imaging

The use of daily IGRT for patients with lymphoma can help minimize PTV expansions required. Alignment to bony anatomy with orthogonal kilovoltage on-board imaging may be satisfactory for the majority of cases, especially when optimized immobilization devices are employed. Volumetric daily imaging, such as cone beam (CBCT) or CT-on-rails, can be employed for confirmation of DIBH position and when using highly conformal techniques, such as IMRT or volumetric modulated arc therapy (VMAT).[84] When using proton therapy, variations in patient positioning can result in alterations in the dose distribution, so particular care is required for highly accurate and reproducible setup. Close attention is paid to the position of the clavicles, which are notoriously prone to motion that is independent of the thoracic spine. CBCT is becoming increasingly available in proton therapy centers, but verification of offline 4D CT scans can help assess whether RT is robustly delivered. Treatment of the entire stomach poses a special challenge, typically in the setting of gastric MALT lymphomas. Spatial resolution of soft tissue in the abdomen is challenging with CBCT, with only moderate inter-observer correlation for the stomach.[85] Keeping patients' stomachs empty prior to treatment, including encouraging patients to avoid eating after midnight prior to daily treatment, can ensure more reproducible gastric targets. DIBH can be useful in treating the stomach by both limiting motion and increasing the space between the heart and the target.[86] Customization of IGRT approaches for each patient will depend on the treatment location, modality, and patient factors.

Radiotherapy Planning Techniques

When ICRU standardized target volumes are used for lymphoma radiation, comparative radiation planning can help determine the best method for OAR-sparing with good coverage. Three-dimensional CRT plans using customized beam arrangements other than AP/PA can selectively spare OARs. IMRT can be used to spare particular OARs, but this can be at the expense of larger volumes of lung and/or breast receiving low doses. As in other thoracic sites, beam angles can substantially drive the quality of IMRT plans for mediastinal lymphomas. Equally spaced coaxial IMRT beam angles are likely to result in high volumes of lung and breast tissue treated with low–moderate doses compared to limited beams, such as the "butterfly" technique.[84] VMAT plans for mediastinal lymphomas that concentrically treat patients[81,87] will deliver excessive dose to lung and breast compared to optimized limited arcs.[88] It is imperative to use carefully selected beam angles or partial arcs to create optimal photon plans. Mesenteric lymphomas can be similarly targeted with conformal radiation, with IMRT beam angles or arcs optimized based on location.[89]

Critical to successful implementation of IMRT/VMAT inverse planning is the formulation of the target coverage goals and OAR dose constraints that reflect a balance relative to important OARs. Typically for mediastinal lymphomas, the balance between lung, heart, and breast dose depends on the patient and their personal and family medical history, and tighter constraints than QUANTEC may be appropriate.[74] Pulmonary toxicity can manifest either as subacute radiation pneumonitis or as late pulmonary fibrosis. Radiation pneumonitis is relatively uncommon, with rates ranging from 3% to 10% undergoing initial treatment.[90–93] Pneumonitis is more common (25%–35%) when radiation is combined with autologous stem cell transplant in the relapsed/refractory setting.[90,92] Lung dosimetric parameters are strong predictors of risk, with MLD over 13.5 to 14 Gy and V20 of over 30% to 36% predicting for higher rates of pulmonary toxicity.[90,92,93] Pinnix et al.[90] specifically studied patients treated with IMRT, and found that V5 over 55% was the strongest dosimetric predictor with this technique. The heart dose–volume constraints are particularly important because of the high incidence of cardiac disease noted in survivors of HL. In a large study from the Netherlands Cancer Institute examining cardiovascular risk in over 2,500 patients treated for HL with a median follow-up of 20 years, patients treated before the age of 25 were found

to have cumulative incidences at age 60 or older of 20%, 31%, and 11%, respectively, for coronary heart disease (CHD), valvular heart disease (VHD), and heart failure (HF) as first events. The hazard ratios for CHD, VHD, and HF were 2.7, 6.6, and 2.7, respectively, for those who received mediastinal RT compared to those who did not.

Of course, given their long follow-up, these studies examining 20-year risk of cardiac disease included many patients treated with relatively high doses of radiation with large outdated mantle fields in which much of the heart would have been irradiated. With a trend in RT practice over the last three decades toward lower doses and smaller fields, one would expect that the incidence of future cardiac events for patients receiving current state-of-the-art radiation would be lower. Using a dosimetric risk-modeling approach, Maraldo et al.[94] predicted a substantially lower risk in cardiac disease risk in patients INRT compared to mantle fields.

Dose constraints vary by institution, but the ILROG has proposed the constraints listed in Table 12.3 based on published literature.[74] In practice, delineation of cardiac substructures may be tedious, but may help preferentially spare regions when highly conformal radiation is used (Fig. 12.8). Although all of the dose constraints proposed by ILROG are not currently backed by specific literature, medical common sense supports that cardiac substructures should be preferentially spared in addition to mean heart dose.[95]

There is not a strong consensus on a dose parameter for breast tissue in order to reduce the risk of breast cancer. Travis et al.[96] found an increased risk of breast cancer in all radiation dose categories of 4 Gy or more in young patients. This study found that risk increased with increasing dose to the location in the breast in which the subsequent tumor developed, with up to an eightfold increased risk for doses >40 Gy. A similar conclusion regarding a dose response for breast cancer was reached by Van Leewen et al.[97] The model that appears to best fit these

TABLE 12.3 Organs-at-Risk Target Planning Parameters for Mediastinal Lymphomas as Suggested by ILROG (reproduced with permission)

Structures	Ideal	Optimize technique	Optimize field (consider field reduction)	Unacceptable	Avoid maximum dose landing in
Heart: left ventricle, coronary arteries, valves	Mean <5 Gy	Mean, 5–15 Gy	Mean >15 Gy	Mean >30 Gy	Coronary vessels
Breast (age dependent)*	Mean <4 Gy	Mean, 4–15 Gy	Mean >15 Gy	Mean >30 Gy	Glandular tissue
Lung	V_5<55%	V_5, 55%–60%	—	V_5>60%	
	V_{20}<30%	Mean, 10–13.5 Gy		Mean >13.5 Gy	
	Mean <10 Gy				
Thyroid	V_{25}<62.5%	V_{25}<62.5%			Whole thyroid

*The importance of adhering to breast-dose restrictions is inversely related to patient age.

Source: Dabaja BS, et al. Proton therapy for adults with mediastinal lymphomas: the International Lymphoma Radiation Oncology Group guidelines. *Blood.* 2018.

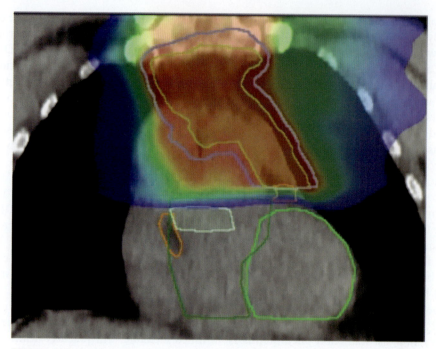

FIGURE 12.8. IMRT to spare cardiac substructures. Late cardiovascular risk was of importance in this 48-year-old man with stage II classic Hodgkin lymphoma with a bulky anterior mediastinal mass who had a complete metabolic response after six cycles of ABVD. Cardiac substructure sparing, especially left and right main coronary arteries (*orange*), left ventricle (*green*), and the aortic valve (*light green*), was prioritized over coverage of the ITV (*green*) and PTV (*purple*) using IMRT.

clinically observed rates of breast cancer was developed by Sachs and Brenner and takes into account cellular repopulation by proliferation that takes place during fractionated RT.[98] Using this model, Hodgson et al.[99] estimated the risk of breast cancer in patients treated with radiation and predicted that 35 Gy IFRT would reduce the 20-year excess relative risk of breast by 63% compared with 35 Gy mantle RT and that low-dose (20 Gy) IFRT would reduce the risk by 77%. There are patient data supporting these theoretical predictions, with one study from the Netherlands showing that women with HL treated with mediastinal irradiation (without axillae) had a substantially lower risk of developing breast cancer than those treated with mantle field irradiation that would have included the bilateral axillae.[100] Based on these data and given that even very low doses of radiation may result in second cancers, the ALARA (as low as reasonably achievable) principle is generally followed along with using the smallest volume of breast tissue that is feasible when doing treatment planning in females receiving mediastinal irradiation.

Proton beam therapy (PBT) for lymphomas is a modality, which delivers a low integral dose and has the potential to lower dose to specific OARs. For example, posterior proton fields can be used to spare glandular breast exposure in patients with axillary involvement (Fig. 12.9). This beam-stopping depth-dose characteristic of PBT is governed by the Bragg peak. Although having virtually no exit dose can result in dosimetrically superior plans as shown in a treatment planning system, the depth of penetration depends

entirely on what tissue has been traversed by the beam. The sensitivity of PBT deposition to uncertainties, and in particular to the range and setup, increases the potential for error in actual delivery and needs to be accounted for carefully. Several dosimetric studies comparing PBT to conventional 3D conformal photon therapy in patients with mediastinal lymphomas have demonstrated significantly reduced radiation dose to breast, lung, heart, and total body.[101] The relative benefit to PBT increases as the target volume dips lower into the chest, beyond the level of the left main coronary artery (similar to the T7 vertebral body).[74,102] In addition, the National Comprehensive Cancer Network (NCCN) guidelines for HL version 1.2021 state that therapy with either photons or protons is acceptable as significant dose reduction to organs at risk (e.g., lung, heart, and breasts) can be achieved. Because ISRT volumes are based on the unique distributions of lymphomas, PBT beam arrangements need to be customized to the individual patient. A young woman with axillary disease and upper mediastinal disease may be best treated with a combination of anterior and posterior beams, whereas a young man with an anterior mediastinal mass that drapes over the heart may be best treated with only anterior beams. In general, AP/PA proton beam arrangements are avoided since they do not exploit the beam stopping advantage of PBT. Both double-scatter (DS) and PBS PBT may be used for lymphoma, and each has its advantages and disadvantages. DS PBT is less conformal than PBS, especially in the proximal edge of the target volume. However, due to the necessity of using physical

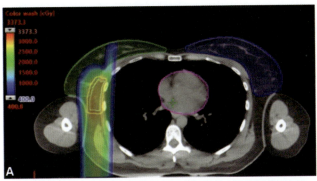

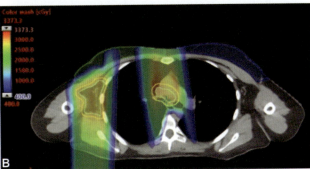

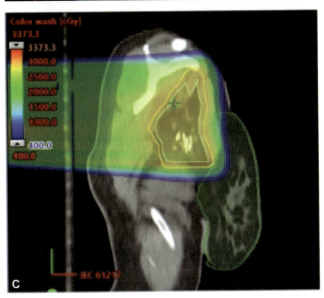

FIGURE 12.9. Pencil beam scanned PBT plan with axillary involvement. Both anterior and posterior-based PBT beams were used to treat this young woman with unfavorable risk stage IIA classic Hodgkin lymphoma involving the right axilla, right infraclavicular nodes, and mediastinum treated with ABVD × 3 cycles per the EORTC H10 trial. Axial (**A** and **B**) and sagittal (**C**) CT-slices with dose color wash with the ITV (*green*), PTV (*yellow*), and breast (*dark green and blue*) displayed.

compensators with DS, conformality distal to the target degrades with DS when the depth of the target changes drastically over a short distance. This transition typically occurs from the upper mediastinum to the lower mediastinum when there is disease anterior to the heart. This issue can be mitigated by splitting fields into upper and lower fields that use different compensators and half-beam blocking, but this can be cumbersome. PBS PBT offers high 3D dose conformality and can handle sharply changing target

volumes even using a single large field. The conformality of PBS PBT depends in part by the size of the spot, which is expressed in terms of "sigma." The distance between the snout and the patient, known as the "air gap," will impact the spot size as in general, range shifters are employed to cover superficial areas of the target. The closer the snout can get to the patient, the smaller the spot size, and the more conformal the plan can be. Therefore, positioning of the patient with their chin hyperextended can help decrease the air gap and improve conformality. PBS PBT has been shown to be dosimetrically superior to DS PBT, IMRT, and 3D CRT with respect to mean heart and lung dose and is the preferred mode of PBT.[103] However, PBS is not a continuous beam and delivers the dose to the target spot by spot, layer by layer with technical specifications that vary among manufacturers. Therefore, the dose distribution is more sensitive to the interplay effect generated by the beam delivery in conjunction with respiratory-induced target motion. Plan robustness of PBS plans has been confirmed through exhaustive modeling studies on 4D CT scans taken through a course of radiation.[104] Robustness of target coverage relative to respiratory motion can be improved by techniques such as dose "repainting," use of larger spot sizes, breath hold, increased air gap, or robust treatment planning optimization. A rule of thumb to maintain robust ITV coverage is to use a spot with sigma about twice as large as the degree of motion perpendicular to the beam direction and a single repainting of PBS PBT[104] as robust treatment plan delivery and repainting may not always be available. Meijers et al. evaluated treatment robustness by means of 4D dose reconstruction and accumulation for lymphoma and lung patients treated with robustly optimized treatment plans, delivered with five-times rescanning in a fractionated regimen.[105] No clinically relevant loss of target dose homogeneity was found. Lastly, fractionation itself can help smear out interplay problems. Compared to IMRT, both DS and PBS PBT tend to be less conformal in the high-dose region around the target volume. The relationship between the target and a sensitive OAR, such as the left anterior descending coronary artery, will affect which modality dosimetrically is best for an individual patient.

Individualized Patient Care

For lymphomas, there are multiple ways to achieve cure, which can involve all chemotherapy, all radiation therapy, or combined modality approaches. Patient preference, proximity to facilities, comorbidities, family history, tolerance of chemotherapy, and PET-based responses can all inform treatment decisions. Multidisciplinary clinics can help select which patients will benefit from RT, which is still a powerful tool in the treatment of lymphoma.

ACKNOWLEDGMENTS

The authors would like to thank Angela Natale and Bridget Bieda for help in figure preparation.

KEY POINTS

- There are many different subtypes of lymphoma based on histologic appearance, surface markers, and specific genetic changes. These differences may impact radiotherapeutic management in addition to prognosis and systemic options for treatment.

- Imaging with ^{18}F-FDG PET/CT is critical to the management of lymphomas, with respect to both initial staging and after therapy.

- Although PET/CT responses can help define patients with lymphoma with good prognosis, combined modality therapy results in the highest disease-free survival, which should be balanced with the predicted risk of significant treatment-related toxicity. Radiation therapy for lymphomas has evolved significantly with lower doses and smaller fields when effective chemotherapy has been delivered. Elective nodal treatment may be appropriate when radiation alone is used or in the relapsed/refractory setting. ISRT has been the standard of care since 2014.

- Palliation of lymphomas requires an understanding of the overall prognosis in order to integrate with evolving systemic therapies.

- Very low doses, in the range of 4 to 8 Gy, can be effective for palliation of lymphomas.

- Radiation therapy planning requires target volume definition based on careful review of prechemotherapy PET/CT scans and postchemotherapy scans to allow volumetric radiation planning using the ISRT paradigm.

- Highly conformal radiation techniques such as IMRT, VMAT, and proton therapy can be employed to optimize target coverage and OAR avoidance. When treating patients with excellent prognosis, strict OAR constraints should be used, customized to individual patients and scaled to the prescription dose.

REVIEW QUESTIONS

1. What are the average dosimetric differences between deep inspiratory breath-hold and free-breathing techniques for mediastinal lymphomas?
   A. Deep breath hold decreases dose to spinal cord
   B. Deep breath hold decreases dose to lungs and heart
   C. Deep breath hold decreases dose to female breasts
   D. Deep breath hold decreases the PTV margin required for setup error

2. When treating patients with lymphoma with an ISRT paradigm, how are previously noninvolved lymph node regions incorporated into target volumes?
   A. Previously noninvolved regions are omitted when chemotherapy was effective
   B. Previously noninvolved regions are omitted even when chemotherapy was ineffective
   C. Previously noninvolved regions are treated to a lower dose when chemotherapy was effective
   D. Previously noninvolved regions are treated to the full dose unless there is overlap with OARs

3. What are the average dosimetric differences between AP–PA beam arrangements and IMRT when treating mediastinal lymphomas?
   A. IMRT lowers mean heart dose and lung V5.
   B. IMRT increases mean heart dose and lung V5.
   C. IMRT lowers mean heart dose and increases lung V5.
   D. IMRT increases mean heart dose and lowers lung V5.

4. The risk of radiation pneumonitis in patients with lymphoma is most dependent on which factor?
   A. Cumulative dose of bleomycin
   B. History of smoking
   C. History of allergic reaction to antibody therapy
   D. Mean lung dose over 13.5 Gy
   E. RT given in newly diagnosed setting

5. RT treatment planning using INRT or ISRT focuses on what parameters for field design and daily alignment?
   A. Customized radiation plans based on pre- and postchemotherapy volumes and daily positioning based on structures with a fixed relationship to the target volumes
   B. Templated blocks with borders based on patient size positioned daily based on surface anatomy
   C. Customized blocks with borders based on easy-to-identify bony anatomy and positioned daily based on surface anatomy

ANSWERS

1. **B** DIBH decreases the dose to the lung in most mediastinal lymphoma cases by expanding the lung, thereby increasing the volume of the structure. This improves the DVH parameters. In addition, by narrowing the mediastinum, the target is narrower which can also decrease lung dose. The decreased dose to the heart is thought to result from displacing the heart inferiorly away from the target volumes.[77,78]

2. **A** ISRT is similar to the INRT concept, except that it allows for additional uncertainty in CTV delineation based on suboptimal registration between prechemotherapy and simulation scans. When combined with effective chemotherapy in the upfront setting, only previously involved nodes/lesions are treated. With the ISRT concept, elective nodal volumes may be treated when RT alone is used with curative intent (e.g., limited stage nodular lymphocyte predominant HL or low-grade NHL) or in the relapsed/refractory setting.[46,47,62,63]

3. **C** The use of intelligently arranged IMRT beams ("butterfly" or partial arcs) can improve DVH metrics for the heart. In addition to the mean heart dose, IMRT can be used to spare cardiac substructures. There is usually a compensatory increase in the V5 lung parameter.[77] The risk of radiation pneumonitis is still low if the V5 can be kept below 55%.[90]

4. **D** Radiation pneumonitis risk increased with dose to the lung, including mean lung dose as well as the V5 (volume receiving 5 Gy or higher).[90] Patients treated in the relapsed/refractory setting have a historically higher rate of radiation pneumonitis (17%–24%).[92] It is unclear if this is due to more cumulative exposure to chemotherapy, but bleomycin dose has not been correlated with higher rates. Interestingly, the use of PBT in the relapsed/refractory setting was associated with a relatively low rate of pneumonitis (12.8%), suggesting that keeping the lung dose as low as possible in this setting can potentially limit morbidity.[106]

5. **A** A key aspect of ISRT and INRT is the use of ICRU-defined target volumes, which has allowed more conformal radiation techniques to be used. The historical use of bony landmarks to define fields to treat nodal groups is clearly outdated and is not consistent with modern RT. The use of on-board imaging for patients with lymphoma has allowed for smaller PTV expansions, which in turn can help limit dose to OARs. Whether orthogonal x-rays or CBCT is used should be customized to individual patients and RT plans.[107]

REFERENCES

1. Campo E, Swerdlow SH, Harris NL, Pileri S, Stein H, Jaffe ES. The 2008 WHO classification of lymphoid neoplasms and beyond: evolving concepts and practical applications. *Blood*. 2011.
2. Swerdlow SH, et al. The 2016 revision of the World Health Organization classification of lymphoid neoplasms. *Blood*. 2016.
3. Alizadeh AA, et al. Distinct types of diffuse large B-cell lymphoma identified by gene expression profiling. *Nature*. 2000.
4. Horn H, et al. MYC status in concert with BCL2 and BCL6 expression predicts outcome in diffuse large B-cell lymphoma. *Blood*. 2013.
5. Cheson BD, et al. Recommendations for initial evaluation, staging, and response assessment of Hodgkin and non-Hodgkin lymphoma: the Lugano classification. *J Clin Oncol*. 2014.
6. Kumar A, et al. Definition of bulky disease in early stage Hodgkin lymphoma in computed tomography era: prognostic significance of measurements in the coronal and transverse planes. *Haematologica*. 2016.
7. Held G, et al. Role of radiotherapy to bulky disease in elderly patients with aggressive b-cell lymphoma. *J Clin Oncol*. 2014.
8. Hasenclever D, et al. A prognostic score for advanced Hodgkin's disease. *N Engl J Med*. 1998.
9. A predictive model for non-Hodgkin's lymphoma. *N Engl J Med*. 1994.
10. Sehn LH, et al. The revised International Prognostic Index (R-IPI) is a better predictor of outcome than the standard IPI for patients with diffuse large B-cell lymphoma treated with R-CHOP. *Blood*. 2007.
11. Gallamini A, et al. The predictive value of positron emission tomography scanning performed after two courses of standard therapy on treatment outcome in advanced stage Hodgkin's disease. *Haematologica*. 2006.
12. Hutchings M, Mikhaeel NG, Fields PA, Nunan T, Timothy AR. Prognostic value of interim FDG-PET after two or three cycles of chemotherapy in Hodgkin lymphoma. *Ann Oncol*. 2005.
13. Hutchings M, et al. FDG-PET after two cycles of chemotherapy predicts treatment failure and progression-free survival in Hodgkin lymphoma. *Blood*. 2006.
14. Safar V, et al. Interim [18F]fluorodeoxyglucose positron emission tomography scan in diffuse large B-cell lymphoma treated with anthracycline-based chemotherapy plus rituximab. *J Clin Oncol*. 2012.
15. Yang DH, et al. Prognostic significance of interim 18F-FDG PET/CT after three or four cycles of R-CHOP chemotherapy in the treatment of diffuse large B-cell lymphoma. *Eur J Cancer*. 2011.
16. Mikhaeel NG, Hutchings M, Fields PA, O'Doherty MJ, Timothy AR. FDG-PET after two to three cycles of chemotherapy predicts progression-free and overall survival in high-grade non-Hodgkin lymphoma. *Ann Oncol*. 2005.
17. Haioun C, et al. [18F]fluoro-2-deoxy-D-glucose positron emission tomography (FDG-PET) in aggressive lymphoma: an early prognostic tool for predicting patient outcome. *Blood*. 2005.
18. Pregno P, et al. Interim 18-FDG-PET/CT failed to predict the outcome in diffuse large B-cell lymphoma patients treated at the diagnosis with rituximab-CHOP. *Blood*. 2012.
19. Cashen AF, Dehdashti F, Luo J, Homb A, Siegel BA, Bartlett NL. 18F-FDG PET/CT for early response assessment in diffuse large B-cell lymphoma: poor predictive value of international harmonization project interpretation. *J Nucl Med*. 2011.
20. Yoo C, et al. Limited role of interim PET/CT in patients with diffuse large B-cell lymphoma treated with R-CHOP. *Ann Hematol*. 2011.
21. Halasz LM, et al. Combined modality treatment for PET-positive non-Hodgkin lymphoma: favorable outcomes of combined

modality treatment for patients with non-Hodgkin lymphoma and positive interim or postchemotherapy FDG-PET. *Int J Radiat Oncol Biol Phys.* 2012.

22. Dabaja BS, et al. Positron emission tomography/computed tomography findings during therapy predict outcome in patients with diffuse large B-cell lymphoma treated with chemotherapy alone but not in those who receive consolidation radiation. *Int J Radiat Oncol Biol Phys.* 2014.

23. Locke FL, et al. Long-term safety and activity of axicabtagene ciloleucel in refractory large B-cell lymphoma (ZUMA-1): a single-arm, multicentre, phase 1–2 trial. *Lancet Oncol.* 2019.

24. Schuster SJ, et al. Tisagenlecleucel in adult relapsed or refractory diffuse large B-cell lymphoma. *N Engl J Med.* 2019.

25. Abramson JS, et al. Lisocabtagene maraleucel for patients with relapsed or refractory large B-cell lymphomas (TRANSCEND NHL 001): a multicentre seamless design study. *Lancet.* 2020.

26. Engert A, et al. Reduced treatment intensity in patients with early-stage Hodgkin's lymphoma. *N Engl J Med.* 2010.

27. Eich HT, et al. Intensified chemotherapy and dose-reduced involved-field radiotherapy in patients with early unfavorable Hodgkin's lymphoma: final analysis of the German Hodgkin study group HD11 trial. *J Clin Oncol.* 2010.

28. André MPE, et al. Early positron emission tomography response-adapted treatment in stage I and II Hodgkin lymphoma: final results of the randomized EORTC/LYSA/FIL H10 trial. *J Clin Oncol.* 2017.

29. Radford J, et al. Results of a trial of PET-directed therapy for early-stage Hodgkin lymphoma. *N Engl J Med.* 2015.

30. Fuchs M, et al. Positron emission tomography-guided treatment in early-stage favorable Hodgkin lymphoma: final results of the international, randomized phase III HD16 trial by the German Hodgkin Study Group. *J Clin Oncol.* 2019.

31. Borchmann P, et al. Eight cycles of escalated-dose BEACOPP compared with four cycles of escalated-dose BEACOPP followed by four cycles of baseline-dose BEACOPP with or without radiotherapy in patients with advanced-stage Hodgkin's lymphoma: final analysis of the HD12 trial of the German Hodgkin Study Group. *J Clin Oncol.* 2011.

32. Engert A, et al. Reduced-intensity chemotherapy and PET-guided radiotherapy in patients with advanced stage Hodgkin's lymphoma (HD15 trial): a randomised, open-label, phase 3 non-inferiority trial. *Lancet.* 2012.

33. Horning SJ, et al. Chemotherapy with or without radiotherapy in limited-stage diffuse aggressive non-Hodgkin's lymphoma: Eastern Cooperative Oncology Group Study 1484. *J Clin Oncol.* 2004.

34. Miller TP, et al. Chemotherapy alone compared with chemotherapy plus radiotherapy for localized intermediate- and high-grade non-Hodgkin's lymphoma. *N Engl J Med.* 1998.

35. Bonnet C, et al. CHOP alone compared with CHOP plus radiotherapy for localized aggressive lymphoma in elderly patients: a study by the Groupe d'Etude des Lymphomes de l'Adulte. *J Clin Oncol.* 2007.

36. Phan J, et al. Benefit of consolidative radiation therapy in patients with diffuse large B-cell lymphoma treated with R-CHOP chemotherapy. *J Clin Oncol.* 2010.

37. Dabaja BS, et al. Radiation for diffuse large B-cell lymphoma in the rituximab era: analysis of the national comprehensive cancer network lymphoma outcomes project. *Cancer.* 2015.

38. Ng AK, Dabaja BS, Hoppe RT, Illidge T, Yahalom J. Re-examining the role of radiation therapy for diffuse large B-cell lymphoma in the modern era. *J Clin Oncol.* 2016.

39. Mac Manus MP, Hoppe RT. Is radiotherapy curative for stage I and II low-grade follicular lymphoma? Results of a long-term follow-up study of patients treated at Stanford University. *J Clin Oncol.* 1996.

40. Goda JS, et al. Localized orbital mucosa-associated lymphoma tissue lymphoma managed with primary radiation therapy: efficacy and toxicity. *Int J Radiat Oncol Biol Phys.* 2011.

41. Tsang RW, et al. Stage I and II malt lymphoma: results of treatment with radiotherapy. *Int J Radiat Oncol Biol Phys.* 2001.

42. Akhtari M, et al. Primary cutaneous B-cell lymphoma (non-leg type) has excellent outcomes even after very low dose radiation as single-modality therapy. *Leuk Lymphoma.* 2016.

43. Haas RLM, et al. High response rates and lasting remissions after low-dose involved field radiotherapy in indolent lymphomas. *J Clin Oncol.* 2003.

44. Wong J, et al. Efficacy of palliative radiation therapy (RT) for diffuse large B-cell lymphoma: a population-based retrospective review. *Int J Radiat Oncol.* 2018.

45. Hoskin PJ, et al. 4 Gy versus 24 Gy radiotherapy for patients with indolent lymphoma (FORT): a randomised phase 3 non-inferiority trial. *Lancet Oncol.* 2014.

46. Constine LS, et al. The role of radiation therapy in patients with relapsed or refractory Hodgkin lymphoma: guidelines from the International Lymphoma Radiation Oncology Group. *Int J Radiat Oncol Biol Phys.* 2018.

47. Ng AK, et al. Role of radiation therapy in patients with relapsed/refractory diffuse large B-cell lymphoma: guidelines from the International Lymphoma Radiation Oncology Group. *Int J Radiat Oncol Biol Phys.* 2018.

48. Sim AJ, et al. Radiation therapy as a bridging strategy for CAR T cell therapy with axicabtagene ciloleucel in diffuse large B-cell lymphoma. *Int J Radiat Oncol Biol Phys.* 2019.

49. Wright CM, et al. Bridging radiation therapy before commercial chimeric antigen receptor T-cell therapy for relapsed or refractory aggressive B-cell lymphoma. *Int J Radiat Oncol Biol Phys.* 2020.

50. Pinnix CC, et al. Bridging therapy prior to axicabtagene ciloleucel for relapsed/refractory large B-cell lymphoma. *Blood Adv.* 2020.

51. Yahalom J, Mauch P. The involved field is back: issues in delineating the radiation field in Hodgkin's disease. *Ann Oncol.* 2002.

52. Goodman KA, Toner S, Hunt M, Wu EJ, Yahalom J. Intensity-modulated radiotherapy for lymphoma involving the mediastinum. *Int J Radiat Oncol Biol Phys.* 2005.

53. MacDonald S, Bernard S, Balogh A, Spencer D, Sawchuk S. Electronic compensation using multileaf collimation for involved field radiation to the neck and mediastinum in non-Hodgkin's lymphoma and Hodgkin's lymphoma. *Med Dosim.* 2005.

54. Yahalom J. Transformation in the use of radiation therapy of Hodgkin lymphoma: new concepts and indications lead to modern field design and are assisted by PET imaging and Intensity Modulated Radiation Therapy (IMRT). *Eur J Haematol.* 2005.

55. Girinsky T, Pichenot C, Beaudre A, Ghalibafian M, Lefkopoulos D. Is intensity-modulated radiotherapy better than conventional radiation treatment and three-dimensional conformal radiotherapy for mediastinal masses in patients with Hodgkin's disease, and is there a role for beam orientation optimization and dose constraints assigned to virtual volumes? *Int J Radiat Oncol Biol Phys.* 2006.

56. Ghalibafian M, Beaudre A, Girinsky T. Heart and coronary artery protection in patients with mediastinal Hodgkin lymphoma treated with intensity-modulated radiotherapy: dose constraints to virtual volumes or to organs at risk? *Radiother Oncol.* 2008.

57. Campbell BA, et al. Involved-nodal radiation therapy as a component of combination therapy for limited-stage Hodgkin's lymphoma: a question of field size. *J Clin Oncol.* 2008.

58. Girinsky T, et al. The conundrum of Hodgkin lymphoma nodes: to be or not to be included in the involved node radiation fields. the EORTC-GELA lymphoma group guidelines. *Radiother Oncol.* 2008.

59. Girinsky T, et al. Involved-node radiotherapy (INRT) in patients with early Hodgkin lymphoma: concepts and guidelines. *Radiother Oncol.* 2006.

60. Weber DC, Peguret N, Dipasquale G, Cozzi L. Involved-node and involved-field volumetric modulated arc vs. fixed beam intensity-modulated radiotherapy for female patients with early-stage supra-diaphragmatic Hodgkin lymphoma: a comparative planning study. *Int J Radiat Oncol Biol Phys.* 2009.

61. Weber DC, Johanson S, Peguret N, Cozzi L, Olsen DR. Predicted risk of radiation-induced cancers after involved field and involved node radiotherapy with or without intensity modulation for early-stage Hodgkin lymphoma in female patients. *Int J Radiat Oncol Biol Phys.* 2011.

62. Specht L, et al. Modern radiation therapy for Hodgkin lymphoma: field and dose guidelines from the International Lymphoma Radiation Oncology Group (ILROG). *Int J Radiat Oncol Biol Phys.* 2014.

63. Illidge T, et al. Modern radiation therapy for nodal non-Hodgkin lymphoma—Target definition and dose guidelines from the

International Lymphoma Radiation Oncology Group. *Int J Radiat Oncol Biol Phys*. 2014.

64. Wirth A. et al. Involved site radiation therapy in adult lymphomas: an overview of International Lymphoma Radiation Oncology Group guidelines. *Int J Radiat Oncol Biol Phys*. 2020.

65. Yahalom J, et al. Modern radiation therapy for extranodal lymphomas: field and dose guidelines from the International Lymphoma Radiation Oncology Group. *Int J Radiat Oncol Biol Phys*. 2015.

66. Pfeffer MR, Rabin T, Tsvang L, Goffman J, Rosen N, Symon Z. Orbital lymphoma: is it necessary to treat the entire orbit? *Int J Radiat Oncol Biol Phys*. 2004.

67. Fasola CE, Jones JC, Huang DD, Le QT, Hoppe RT, Donaldson SS. Low-dose radiation therapy (2 Gy × 2) in the treatment of orbital lymphoma. *Int J Radiat Oncol Biol Phys*. 2013.

68. Specht L, Dabaja B, Illidge T, Wilson LD, Hoppe RT. Modern radiation therapy for primary cutaneous lymphomas: field and dose guidelines from the International Lymphoma Radiation Oncology Group. *Int J Radiat Oncol Biol Phys*. 2015.

69. Wilson LD, Kacinski BM, Jones GW. Local superficial radiotherapy in the management of minimal stage IA cutaneous T-cell lymphoma (Mycosis Fungoides). *Int J Radiat Oncol Biol Phys*. 1998.

70. Chowdhary M, Song A, Zaorsky NG, Shi W. Total skin electron beam therapy in mycosis fungoides—A shift towards lower dose? *Chin Clin Oncol*. 2019.

71. Neelis KJ, Schimmel EC, Vermeer MH, Senff NJ, Willemze R, Noordijk EM. Low-dose palliative radiotherapy for cutaneous B- and T-cell lymphomas. *Int J Radiat Oncol Biol Phys*. 2009.

72. Dabaja BS, et al. Radiation for Hodgkin's lymphoma in young female patients: a new technique to avoid the breasts and decrease the dose to the heart. *Int J Radiat Oncol Biol Phys*. 2011.

73. Hoppe BS, et al. Effective dose reduction to cardiac structures using protons compared with 3DCRT and IMRT in mediastinal Hodgkin lymphoma. *Int J Radiat Oncol Biol Phys*. 2012.

74. Dabaja BS, et al. Proton therapy for adults with mediastinal lymphomas: the International Lymphoma Radiation Oncology Group Guidelines. *Blood*. 2018.

75. Bradford JPP, Hoppe S, Flampouri S, Hill-Kayser C. *Target Volume Delineation and Treatment Planning for Particle Therapy, A Practical Guide*. New York: Springer; 2018:369-379.

76. Chi WK, Shah-Patel LR, Baer JW, Frager DH. Cost-effectiveness and patient tolerance of low-attenuation oral contrast material: milk versus volumen. *Am J Roentgenol*. 2008.

77. Kriz J. et al. Breath-hold technique in conventional APPA or intensity-modulated radiotherapy for Hodgkin's lymphoma. *Strahlentherapie und Onkol*. 2015.

78. Aznar MC, et al. Minimizing late effects for patients with mediastinal Hodgkin lymphoma: deep inspiration breath-hold, IMRT, or both? *Int J Radiat Oncol Biol Phys*. 2015.

79. Petersen PM, et al. Prospective phase II trial of image-guided radiotherapy in Hodgkin lymphoma: benefit of deep inspiration breath-hold. *Acta Oncol (Madr)*. 2015.

80. Charpentier AM, et al. Active breathing control for patients receiving mediastinal radiation therapy for lymphoma: impact on normal tissue dose. *Pract Radiat Oncol*. 2014.

81. Schneider U, Sumila M, Robotka J, Weber D, Gruber G. Radiation-induced second malignancies after involved-node radiotherapy with deep-inspiration breath-hold technique for early stage Hodgkin lymphoma: a dosimetric study. *Radiat Oncol*. 2014.

82. Rechner LA, et al. Life years lost attributable to late effects after radiotherapy for early stage Hodgkin lymphoma: the impact of proton therapy and/or deep inspiration breath hold. *Radiother Oncol*. 2017.

83. Moreno AC, et al. Effect of Deep Inspiration Breath Hold on Normal Tissue Sparing With Intensity Modulated Radiation Therapy Versus Proton Therapy for Mediastinal Lymphoma. *Adv Radiat Oncol*. 2020.

84. Voong KR, et al. Dosimetric advantages of a "butterfly" technique for intensity-modulated radiation therapy for young female patients with mediastinal Hodgkin's lymphoma. *Radiat Oncol*. 2014.

85. Matoba M, Oota K, Toyoda I, Kitadate M, Watanabe N, Tonami H. Usefulness of 4D-CT for radiation treatment planning of gastric MZBCL/MALT. *J Radiat Res*. 2012.

86. Choi SH, Park SH, Lee JJB, Baek JG, Kim JS, Yoon H. Combining deep-inspiration breath hold and intensity-modulated radiotherapy for gastric mucosa-associated lymphoid tissue lymphoma: dosimetric evaluation using comprehensive plan quality indices. *Radiat Oncol*. 2019.

87. Maraldo MV, et al. Estimated risk of cardiovascular disease and secondary cancers with modern highly conformal radiotherapy for early-stage mediastinal Hodgkin lymphoma. *Ann Oncol*. 2013.

88. Filippi AR, et al. Optimized volumetric modulated arc therapy versus 3d-crt for early stage mediastinal Hodgkin lymphoma without axillary involvement: a comparison of second cancers and heart disease risk. *Int J Radiat Oncol Biol Phys*. 2015.

89. Yoder AK, et al. Rainbow IMRT and Volumetric Imaging for Anterior Mesenteric Targets. *Pract Radiat Oncol*. 2019.

90. Pinnix CC, et al. Predictors of radiation pneumonitis in patients receiving Intensity Modulated Radiation Therapy for Hodgkin and non-Hodgkin lymphoma. *Int J Radiat Oncol Biol Phys*. 2015.

91. Cella L, et al. Pulmonary damage in Hodgkin's lymphoma patients treated with sequential chemo-radiotherapy: predictors of radiation-induced lung injury. *Acta Oncol (Madr)*. 2014.

92. Fox AM, et al. Predictive factors for radiation pneumonitis in Hodgkin lymphoma patients receiving combined-modality therapy. *Int J Radiat Oncol Biol Phys*. 2012.

93. Koh ES, et al. Clinical dose-volume histogram analysis in predicting radiation pneumonitis in Hodgkin's lymphoma. *Int J Radiat Oncol Biol Phys*. 2006.

94. Maraldo MV, et al. Risk of developing cardiovascular disease after involved node radiotherapy versus mantle field for Hodgkin lymphoma. *Int J Radiat Oncol Biol Phys*. 2012.

95. Van Nimwegen FA, et al. Radiation dose-response relationship for risk of coronary heart disease in survivors of Hodgkin lymphoma. *J Clin Oncol*. 2016.

96. Travis LB, et al. Breast cancer following radiotherapy and chemotherapy among young women with Hodgkin disease. *J Am Med Assoc*. 2003.

97. van Leeuwen FE, et al. Roles of radiation dose, chemotherapy, and hormonal factors in breast cancer following Hodgkin's disease. *J Natl Cancer Inst*. 2003.

98. Sachs RK, Brenner DJ. Solid tumor risks after high doses of ionizing radiation. *Proc Natl Acad Sci USA*. 2005.

99. Hodgson DC, et al. Individualized estimates of second cancer risks after contemporary radiation therapy for Hodgkin lymphoma. *Cancer*. 2007.

100. De Bruin ML, et al. Breast cancer risk in female survivors of Hodgkin's lymphoma: lower risk after smaller radiation volumes. *J Clin Oncol*. 2009.

101. Tseng YD, et al. Evidence-based review on the use of proton therapy in lymphoma from the Particle Therapy Cooperative Group (PTCOG) Lymphoma Subcommittee. *Int J Radiat Oncol Biol Phys*. 2017;99:4.

102. Ntentas G, et al. Clinical intensity modulated proton therapy for Hodgkin lymphoma: which patients benefit the most? *Pract Radiat Oncol*. 2019.

103. Zeng C, et al. Proton pencil beam scanning for mediastinal lymphoma: treatment planning and robustness assessment. *Acta Oncol (Madr)*. 2016;55:9-10.

104. Zeng C, et al. Proton pencil beam scanning for mediastinal lymphoma: the impact of interplay between target motion and beam scanning. *Phys Med Biol*. 2015;60:7.

105. Meijers A, et al. Evaluation of interplay and organ motion effects by means of 4D dose reconstruction and accumulation. *Radiother Oncol*. 2020.

106. Tseng YD, et al. Risk of Pneumonitis and Outcomes After Mediastinal Proton Therapy for Relapsed/Refractory Lymphoma: A PTCOG and PCG Collaboration. *Int J Radiat Oncol Biol Phys*. 2020.

107. Mikhaeel NG, et al. The optimal use of imaging in radiation therapy for lymphoma: Guidelines from the International Lymphoma Radiation Oncology Group (ILROG). *Int J Radiat Oncol Biol Phys*. 2019.

108. Hill-Kayser CE, Plastaras JP, Tochner Z, Glatstein E. The case for combined-modality therapy for limited-stage Hodgkin's disease. *Oncologist*. 2012;17:8.

109. Swerdlow AJ, et al. Breast cancer risk after supradiaphragmatic radiotherapy for Hodgkin's lymphoma in England and Wales: a national cohort study. *J Clin Oncol*. 2012.

13 Cancers of the Skin, Including Mycosis Fungoides

Zhe (Jay) Chen, James C. L. Chow, Alexander Sun, Himanshu Nagar, Kenneth R. Stevens Jr., and Jonathan P. S. Knisely

INTRODUCTION

The superiority of and justification for radiotherapy for cancers of the skin derive from its ability to cure while preserving normal tissues, thereby achieving both aesthetic and functional outcomes. To achieve such an outcome, radiation therapy planning and implementation must be tailored to the anatomic site and specific tumor characteristics, any previous treatment, along with some consideration of the patient's age and performance status.

Contemporary radiotherapy treatment for skin cancer can be delivered with superficial, kilovoltage, or orthovoltage radiotherapy, electron beam therapy, or isotope or electronic brachytherapy. Not all centers will have every radiation treatment modality that may be potentially useful for a given clinical indication. Therefore, critical and careful use of the available treatment modalities is mandatory to assure that optimal treatment results will be achieved. Indeed, good judgment may indicate that certain patients should be referred to alternate centers where specialized equipment or techniques and the expertise to employ them deftly may be available.

Treatment planning and implementation are usually straightforward, because the cancer can be directly visualized, palpated, and observed directly during each treatment setup. The treatment volume is frequently little more than a superficial thin slab requiring a single direct beam collimated by a simple field-defining device placed on or near the skin. However, anatomical complexities and the need for individualization of treatment may make these cases among the most complex encountered by many centers.

The steps in planning irradiation for skin cancer are as follows:

1. Define the extent and size of the cancer (staging).
2. Determine what radiotherapy treatment technique may best address the disease that needs to be treated.
3. Prescribe the treatment, including beam type, energy, daily fraction size, and total dose, including, when appropriate, specification of patient immobilization devices, beam filters, bolus, attenuator, and shielding devices.
4. Design and create any necessary field-defining device, accounting for margins.
5. Design and create device for blocking exit beam when appropriate.
6. Supervise and approve initial irradiation setup.
7. Document setup with photographs of the gross lesion, lesion with shields in place, and with both machine and shields in place.

GENERAL PRINCIPLES

Staging and Target Volume Determination

It is generally accepted that cancer staging assists in selection of therapies and provides prognostic information. In addition, for skin cancer, accurate staging can assist with radiotherapy treatment planning, augmenting its importance. The Union for International Cancer Control and the American Joint Commission on Cancer have published staging systems for squamous and basal cell carcinomas, Merkel cell carcinoma, melanoma, and cutaneous T-cell lymphoma (CTCL).[1]

There are anatomic and histopathologic high-risk features for staging of basal and squamous cancers that can be of value in assessing patients for possible radiotherapeutic treatment. For example, in differentiating between T1 and T2 tumors, high-risk histopathologic features should be assessed, including differentiation, thickness and depth of invasion, and whether perineural infiltration is seen. Also important is anatomic location, with tumors arising on the ear or lip deemed to be high-risk features.

There is also a designated TNM staging system for carcinomas of the eyelid that reflects the unique anatomic features and importance of the eyelid and ocular adnexae in protecting the eye. Knowledge of these staging systems can assist with advocating for patients receiving appropriate radiation therapy and in optimizing radiotherapy treatment parameters for these patients.

Despite the fact that skin cancers can be visualized and palpated before planning treatment and on each day at treatment setup, geographic miss is the most common cause of failure. Most of these cancers arise on the face or neck, are detected early, grow slowly, and present with a small tumor volume. The gross dimensions are usually readily determined by visual examination with adequate lighting to aid inspection for edema and by palpation to determine the extent of induration and fixation. Visual magnification is often useful to define the peripheral-most margin of the gross tumor. Occult extension of cancer beyond the gross margins is generally limited to a few millimeters, but this varies.

In certain circumstances, special imaging may be extraordinarily valuable in assuring the high-dose volume completely covers the skin cancer. This may be useful for cancers with clinically indistinct margins or high histologic grade, for sclerosing basal cell carcinomas, and for those cancers classified as recurrences following surgery or irradiation. Patients with signs or symptoms of perineural involvement or regional nodal metastases, fixity to bone, as well as lesions greater than 5 cm in diameter may also benefit from specialized imaging.

It should be remembered that basal cell carcinomas arising on skin closely overlying bone may spread along the periosteum. Tumors in the medial canthal region, overlying the cranial vault, the malar eminences, and the upper half of the nose are examples of such sites. Tumors arising at or near periauricular and nasomalar embryonic fusion planes may have occult deep extension, also meriting careful radiologic workup to accurately determine the target volume extent. These diagnostic evaluations are fortunately not required for the majority of skin carcinomas.

The deep margin of the tumor should be encompassed by at least the 90% isodose surface. Field margins for <2-cm primary keratinocyte tumors should be 1 to 1.5 cm; for tumors >2 cm, field margins should be 1.5 to 2 cm.[2] Caution should be exercised in planning and treating skin cancers over the calvarium to minimize, when feasible, dose to cortical brain. The use of CT scan–based treatment planning for small skin lesions may introduce more errors than if a simpler technique of using transparency to determine the field size and shape is used. However, for larger, more complex lesions that are deeply invading and are in contiguity to critical structures, CT simulation, with appropriate use of multimodal image fusion, has improved the ability to accurately plan treatments that will achieve tumor control and normal-tissue sparing.

Many skin cancers arising on the face and neck are managed with primary surgical excision, and detection of palpable recurrences within the relevant regional lymph node basins may prompt the first discussion of radiation as a management approach with the patient. These nodal recurrences, if not accompanied by cutaneous recurrences, may be managed appropriately with the same approaches used for managing head and neck cancer nodal recurrences, using IMRT or VMAT to achieve conformality and normal tissue sparing (see Chapter 6).

In patients with basal cell carcinoma or cutaneous squamous cell carcinoma who are not candidates for surgery, definitive radiotherapy should be considered a first-line treatment. The American Society for Radiation Oncology has published evidence-based guidelines for the use of radiation therapy as definitive and postoperative management of patients with basal and squamous carcinomas of the skin.[3]

RADIATION DELIVERY MODALITIES

Commissioning and Calibration

For all radiotherapy equipment, careful commissioning, calibration, and appropriately detailed and frequent quality assurance are mandatory to avoid underdosing or overdosing patients. Measurement and review of each treatment machine's central axis percent depth-dose and cross-sectional isodose curves, based on the type of radiation, energy, and field size should be routine. A lack of familiarity with routine, manufacturer-specified usage guidelines, and therapeutic directives, which are developed for the safe use of the equipment, is neither in the best interest of the patient nor of the responsible physician, physicists, and therapy staff.

Superficial, Kilovoltage, and Orthovoltage Therapy

Superficial, kilovoltage, and orthovoltage therapy refer to using low-energy photon beams in the range of 50 to 150 kVp for surface lesions and 150 to 500 kVp for lesions deep to the skin. Although Grenz ray (<20 kVp) and contact therapy (40–50 kVp) are no longer used for invasive skin cancer due to their low penetration depth, superficial and orthovoltage therapy are still popular because of their simple and effective treatment administration. Superficial and orthovoltage therapy are delivered with X-ray treatment units that are less complicated and easier to set up than electron therapy delivered from a linear accelerator. Since kV photon beams are used to treat superficial skin carcinomas and keloids at the skin surface, 3-dimensional (3D) treatment planning with image modalities such as computed tomography or magnetic resonance is required only when the extent of deep tumor infiltration and invasion needs to be assessed and accounted for.

Skin irradiation with superficial, kilovoltage, or orthovoltage therapy therefore commonly only needs a clinical markup followed by a beam-on time or monitor unit calculation at the first treatment fraction. Regarding dosimetric characteristics, though electron beams have a sharper falloff of depth-dose to spare critical tissue deeper than the lesion, small-field, low-energy photon beams have a sharper penumbra and superior flatness and are therefore more suitable to treat small lesions. However, low-energy photon beams will deliver a higher dose to bone than to soft tissues at the same depth.[4]

Superficial and Orthovoltage Treatment Units

Nowadays, most kV X-ray treatment units can produce low-energy photon beams ranging from the superficial and kilovoltage into the orthovoltage range. Superficial and kilovoltage therapy is commonly delivered with circular collimators between 2 and 10 cm in diameter at a source-to-surface distance (SSD) of 20 cm and orthovoltage therapy at an SSD of 50 cm with square applicators ranging from 4×4 cm^2 to 10×10 cm^2. Some square applicators are closed at the bottom using a piece of flat polymethyl methacrylate plate. Such closed applicators help to maintain a nonvaried treatment distance from the patient's skin.

A typical kV X-ray unit (Fig. 13.1) contains a standalone transformer, control console, treatment couch, and a floor-mounted tube stand and comes with the aforementioned circular and square collimators. The treatment head of the unit contains the X-ray tube, primary collimator, filter, transmission ionization chamber, and the applicator (Fig. 13.2). The filters, made of copper or aluminum, remove low-energy photons and are designed and specified for different photon beam energies, applicators, and specific (e.g., 20 and 50 cm) SSDs. More recent treatment unit models have an internal transmission ionization chamber linked to the control console. The application of monitor units instead of beam-on time avoids error due to the shutter effect in dose delivery.

Relative Exposure and Backscatter Factors

In superficial, kilovoltage, and orthovoltage therapy of skin cancer, the irradiated area may be tailored by a lead cutout placed on the skin in conjunction with an appropriately sized circular or square applicator. The collimator selected should be approximately 1 cm larger in diameter than the maximal size of the cutout, and the lead should, of course, be large enough that any inadvertent patient motion after a given day's setup has been achieved will not result in unwanted exposure of normal tissue.

In calculating the monitor units from the daily prescription dose, relative exposure and backscatter factors (BSFs) are selected based on variations in applicator and cutout size for the treatment. Relative exposure factor is the dose ratio of an applicator to a reference applicator measured using the same SSD. The reference circular applicator has a diameter of 5 cm while the reference square applicator has a dimension of 10×10 cm^2. Since absolute dose calibrations are carried out using the reference circular and square applicators, the relative exposure factor reflects the change in dose dependent on applicator selection. The relative exposure factor varies with the applicator size and photon beam energy and increases as applicator size increases.

BSF is a ratio of the dose at the depth of maximum dose in water to that in air without water. A special case of the tissue–air ratio is when the depth of the ratio is equal to the depth of maximum dose. When the applicator type and size are selected for skin therapy with lesion depth equaling zero, the BSF for the corresponding applicator reflects the percentage change in dose between the surfaces of the skin compared to the dose in air. BSF is normally larger than one due to the contribution of electron backscatter in water, and the factor depends on the field size and photon beam energy. For skin irradiation, since the lesion is outlined by a cutout made of lead, the BSF is a function of the field size (cutout) covering the lesion with a margin. In monitor unit calculations, BSF varies with the field size and photon beam energy delivered through the applicator.

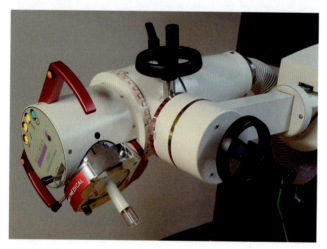

FIGURE 13.1. An example of a modern orthovoltage X-ray unit.

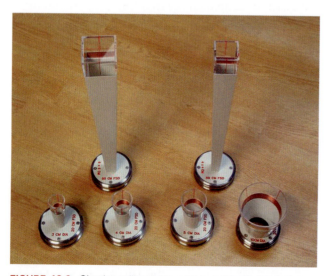

FIGURE 13.2. Circular collimators and square applicators of varying sizes for the orthovoltage unit shown in Figure 10.1 are shown.

Stand-In/Off and Attenuator Correction

For skin lesions close to the bridge or tip of the nose, the irradiated area may be curved toward (in) or away (off) from the applicator. The SSD is therefore decreased or increased and a correction is needed in the monitor unit calculation based on the inverse square/cube law. From dosimetric measurements, the output of a treatment unit is known to vary as a function of the inverse square of the distance for the open applicator, and inverse cube of the distance for the closed applicator. The radiotherapist measures the stand-in or stand-off distance in the clinical markup. In the stand-in case (e.g., tip of nose), the lesion is curved in from the bottom of the applicator. As the SSD is decreased, a correction is needed to reduce the monitor units. Similarly, more monitor units are needed when the lesion is curved off from the bottom of the applicator, leading to a larger SSD in the stand-off case (e.g., bridge of nose).

When the lesion is at the bridge or tip of nose, an attenuator may be used to correct the dose distribution due to the surface curvature. For superficial or orthovoltage energies, the nose bridge or tip attenuator is made of a stack of either aluminum or copper foils, with thickness of each foil equaling 0.5 mm. Each attenuator contains five layers of aluminum/copper foil, each cut to progressively smaller or larger areas to compensate for the dose variation from the differences in SSD and oblique beam entry as a result of the skin surface curvature (Fig. 13.3). The attenuator for the tip of the nose is therefore shaped like a ziggurat, while that for the bridge of nose is shaped similarly, like a terraced mountain ridge.

Recently, creating personalized tissue-equivalent material build up, field defining devices, and shielding has become faster and more convenient, as these processes take advantage of novel 3D printing technologies. These include fabrication of 3D patient-specific boluses for nonmelanoma skin cancer, including skin cancers involving ocular canthi treated with electron therapy,[5] boluses for treatment of squamous cell carcinoma of the nasal septum and basal cell carcinoma of the posterior pinna employing superficial/orthovoltage therapy,[6] and shielding for the treatment of superficial lesions using electrons.[7] Studies are in progress concerning the clinical workflow and dosimetry of these water-equivalent printing materials.

Monitor Unit Calculation

The monitor units required for photon therapy are calculated by the following equation:

$$\text{Monitor Unit} = (\text{Prescribed Dose(cGy)} \times \text{Standoff Correction})/((1\ \text{cGy})/\text{Monitor Unit}) \times \text{Backscatter Factor} \times \text{Relative Exposure Factor} \times \text{Attenuation Factor} \times (\text{PDD}/100))$$

Absolute dose calibration to deliver 1 cGy per monitor unit is done using the reference applicator with a specific SSD. The BSF depends on the field size and photon beam energy while the relative output factor depends on the size of applicator. An attenuation factor is used in the calculation to reflect the beam attenuation when a compensator is used in treatment. The attenuation factor used is smaller than one. Percentage depth-dose (PDD) is needed when the lesion is at a depth from the patient's surface. When the lesion depth is set to zero, the value of PDD is equal to 100 in the previously mentioned equation. The stand-off correction needs a measurement of the stand-in or stand-off distance in the clinical markup and then the application of the inverse square/cube law. For monitor unit calculation, tables of BSF, relative output factor, attenuation factor, and PDD are all incorporated. The calculation is carried out by two radiotherapists individually with the result further approved by a medical physicist.

With advances of the Internet of Things within the hospital setting, online monitor unit calculators apps have been developed for use in skin radiotherapy.[8] Based on the specific dosimetric data of the superficial/orthovoltage unit, monitor unit calculations can be performed automatically after the radiation staff inputs the required treatment variables such as prescribed dose, number of fractions, beam energy, and cone size to the app. The calculation result can be shared within the treatment group including the therapists, physicists, and oncologists in the cancer center/hospital for QA purposes. The institutional internet security system ensures safe transfer and exchange of information, and this data is readily included in the electronic medical record.

Electron Beam Therapy

Electron beam therapy, delivered with a linear accelerator, has become increasingly commonly used to treat superficial skin cancers, in part because of some of the dosimetric advantages of charged particle therapy, and in part because many radiotherapy departments no longer have access to superficial, kilovoltage, and orthovoltage therapy units, as older units have broken down and have not been replaced.

Static electron beam fields are easily employed for lesions on relatively smooth surfaces where the beam may enter orthogonal to the skin surface. A single direct electron field is employed at a nominal SSD of 100 cm and provides control rates for appropriately selected lesions

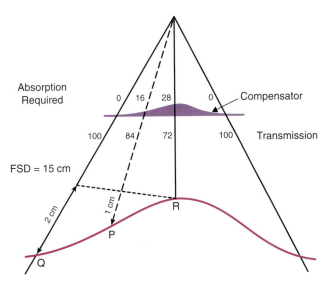

FIGURE 13.3. Cross-sectional schematic of an attenuator (compensator) used for 100 kV therapy for bridge of nose cancers. Attenuators are best suited for kV X-ray therapy and should be avoided in electron therapy where unwanted scatter may enlarge the field.

that do not differ substantially from those achieved with X-ray therapy. Electron beam therapy can provide relatively uniform dose from the surface to a defined depth (up to approximately 5–6 cm) and dose rapidly falls off to near zero thereafter. This can be a major advantage in sparing tissues deep to the cancer, particularly if large fields need to be irradiated.

The dose specification for treatment is commonly given at a depth that lies at, or beyond, the distal margin of the disease; the energy chosen for the treatment depends on the depth of the lesion to be treated. The relative biologic effectiveness (RBE) of electrons in cancer treatment is 10% to 20% less than that of superficial or orthovoltage X-rays. This can be simply addressed by prescribing electron beam therapy to the 90% isodose surface (as opposed to D_{max}). The therapeutic range is defined as the depth of the 90% isodose curve, and is, in centimeters, roughly calculated as one-fourth of the electron energy in MeV. The therapeutic range of available electron beam energies must be considered (together with the thickness of bolus required to bring the skin dose up to full dose) when considering what energy (and bolus thickness) to specify in prescribing treatment. The therapeutic range of the electron energy chosen should reach the deep edge of the planning target volume.

Because the dose falls off so rapidly for electron beam therapy (Fig. 13.4), the guiding principle is to select the next-higher electron energy if there is concern that the 90% isodose surface is not covering the deep edge of the planning target volume. This may require a reevaluation of the thickness of bolus employed as the prescription is being written. The approximate range of the depth of the 90% isodose line for electron beam energies is shown in Table 13.1. The depth and shape of the isodose lines should be determined for each treatment machine at various energies and field sizes.

TABLE 13.1	Range of Depth of 90% Isodose Lines of Electron Beams		
Electron Beam (MeV)	Minimum Depth (cm)	Maximum Depth (cm)	Depth of 5.0% Dose (cm)
6	0.6–1.0	1.7	3.0
9	0.4–1.0	2.7	4.5
12	0 (Skin surface)	3.5	6.0
16	0 (Skin surface)	4.5	9.0
20	0 (Skin surface)	5.5	12.0

Electron-beam depth-dose data depend greatly on the collimation system employed by the accelerator. These data must be measured specifically for the given machine (field size, 8 cm²; source-to-surface distance, 100 cm).

Electron beam depth doses have extremely important changes that are dependent on both field size and treatment energy. The loss of lateral electronic equilibrium in smaller electron beam fields can significantly affect central axis dose, and this will lead to the 90% isodose surface shifting to a shallower depth and an increased level of dose deposition in the skin.[9] It is very important to check and double-check small electron field output factors. Microchambers, thermoluminescent dosimeters (TLDs), or film dosimetry should be used to confirm the proper output factor. The output factor for radiation fields of 2 to 3 cm in diameter is ~0.90 cGy/MU at 100 cm (SSD). Significant dosage errors can occur if the output factor is not correct. Output factors that are significantly greater or less than 0.90 should be critically reviewed and double-checked.

For oblique beam entry, the effects on dose deposition can be quite complex. Increasing degrees of obliquity beyond ~20° are associated with a shallower D_{max} and significant changes to the depth–dose curves.[9] Equations to permit calculation of point doses for oblique beam entry on irregular surfaces have been developed; Monte Carlo techniques can also be used to better understand the effects of beam obliquity and irregular surface contours.[9–11] Misunderstanding and neglecting the effect of beam obliquity, when calculating dose per MU for an oblique electron beam with an irregular field, would lead to a significant dosimetric deviation.

Several additional particular characteristics of electron beam isodose curves that should be remembered when considering electron beam therapy include the lateral bulging of lower isodose curves that arises from larger scattering angles of the electrons in tissue as they lose energy, the lateral constriction of the higher isodose curves (>80%) at energies >15 MeV, and the fact that electron beams <12 MeV are associated with skin sparing, which requires the use of bolus material to raise the skin dose to acceptably high levels (Table 13.1 and Fig. 13.4). This added thickness must, of course, be included in beam selection and depth-dose calculation.

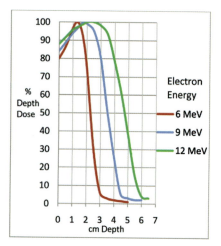

FIGURE 13.4. Isodose curves for 6-, 9-, and 12-MeV electrons, 8 × 8-cm field, showing greater skin sparing for lower energy electron beams.

Bolus is frequently applied directly to the skin in electron beam therapy to increase the surface dose to near 100% and to limit the dose delivered to deep tissues beyond the planning target volume. Superflab (Mick Radio-Nuclear Instruments, Mt. Vernon, NY) is a well-regarded bolus material, because it is nearly tissue equivalent, transparent, and easy to shape. It is available in 3-, 5-, and 10-mm thickness. This bolus, of course, blurs or masks the outline of the treatment field. For this reason, it is helpful during the treatment setup to align the patient and machine as for irradiation but with a gap to permit bolus placement. The correctness of the position of the treatment field should be visually confirmed. The bolus is then slipped into place. The minimum thickness of bolus to achieve maximum dose at the surface varies with the energy of the electron beam (Table 13.1). Although 5- and 10-mm thick boluses are commonly used for 6- and 9-MeV electrons, based on the percent depth-dose data, an 8-mm thick bolus (e.g., a combination of 5- and 3-mm thickness) may be more appropriate. Bolus can also flatten out irregular surfaces and reduce the effects of beam obliquity. CT treatment planning may permit the construction of a customized 3D wax bolus that achieves the goals of decreasing beam obliquity, decreasing dose to tissues deep to the target, and bringing the surface dose to an adequately high level.

Field Defining Devices, Field Shaping, and Protection from Exit Beam

For superficial and orthovoltage photon therapy, an applicator cone and a lead shield of a few millimeter thickness are adequate to protect the skin adjacent to the radiotherapy portal. Field shaping for electron beam therapy is considerably different from photon therapy. Electron applicators are always used to decrease the penumbra from electron scattering in the linac head and in air, and additional customized lead or Cerrobend field shaping devices may be placed on the applicator, as close as possible to the patient. To decrease the dose to the patient to below 5% beneath lead shielding, it needs to be approximately one-tenth as thick as the practical range (R_p) of the electron beam being used (Table 13.2). A rule of thumb for estimating the thickness of shielding of lead in millimeters to decrease the dose to below 5% is to divide the energy of the beam in MeV by 2 to give the number of mm of lead shielding required.

When shielding is placed upon the patient surface, as opposed to being mounted on the applicator, it must be constructed of multiple layers of thin lead, thick lead cut with a saw, or molded from Cerrobend. With such a surface shield, a zone of increased dose develops just deep to the edge of the cutout. The magnitude of this dose increases with beam energy. At lower energies, this effect is commonly disregarded. Concern for this effect, the need for bolus, and the ease of block construction encourage the practice of fixing the field-defining device for the

TABLE 13.2	Minimum Cerrobend Thickness to Block 95% of Electron Treatment Beam (10 × 10 cm field size)
Electron Energy (MeV)	Cerrobend Thickness (mm)
6	2.3
9	4.4
12	8.5
16	18.0
20	25.0

The thickness of lead required for *electron beam* blocking is approximately given by (*E*/2) mm Pb, where *E* is the incident electron energy; for example, blocking of an 6-MeV electron beam requires lead of at least 3-mm thick.

Source: From Purdy JA, Choi MC, Feldman A. Lipowitz metal shielding thickness for dose reduction of 6–20 MeV electrons. *Med Phys*. 1980;7:251–253, with permission.

electron beam on the end of an electron cone several centimeters from the skin.

A sequence of steps for fabricating customized shielding for photon or electron beam therapy of skin cancer may be adapted from these recommendations:

1. Overlay the skin surface with a clear plastic sheet that readily conforms to undulations of the surface.
2. Trace the field outline on the plastic.
3. Overlay the lead with the plastic. Then, with the point of a knife or awl, punch the outline through the plastic onto the surface of the lead. Another technique is to draw the field outline on the skin with a ballpoint pen. Overlay clear adhesive tape on the skin. The tape will pick up the ink outline. Place the clear adhesive tape with outline on lead sheet and proceed with the next step.

Cut out the lead sheet target field outline with a knife and smooth the edges of the cutout. Adhesive tape placed over the cutout's edges will prevent any sharp edges from causing problems when the lead is shaped to the patient's contour. Thin lead can be shaped with the fingers. For thicker lead or for shaping sharply undulating surfaces, such as the medial canthus, the lead can be pressed or hammered lightly to conform to a facial or other plaster cast created specifically for this purpose. The hammering must not appreciably thin the lead.

Wrapping the patient's custom-tailored shielding lead with low-density polyethylene cling film will prevent heavy metal exposure to the patient's skin. Disposable gloves used for protection from exposure to pathogens in patient care may also be used to prevent lead exposure, but because visibility of the shielding device is compromised, this protection may be better used only for exit beam shielding.

The protection of normal tissues from exit beam irradiation is important to consider. A thin layer of lead will protect tissues distal to the target from further direct irradiation. Because of the potential for electron backscattering from the high-Z material of the shielding, a 3-mm layer of wax, which will absorb any backscattered electrons, is often used to cover a 1-mm lead shield. This wax will also protect the patient from exposure to the heavy metals used to fabricate the internal shielding. Such a device will adequately protect for energies up to 12 MeV. The final thickness of the shielding may lead to difficulty with internal shielding placement or decreased patient tolerance of the shielding during therapy. Care should be taken when using internal eye shields—those made for photon therapy are inadequate for electron beam therapy—the transmitted and scattered dose will be high enough to produce cataracts.[12,13]

Electron Arc therapy

For treating large superficial lesions on a curved surface such as the chest wall, electron arc therapy is an option. Electron arc therapy uses an electron field rotating around the isocenter to provide a homogeneous dose distribution to the target. The prediction of dose distribution is complex as it is related to the beam energy, field size, SSD, patient curvature, and depth of the isocenter. Since the source-to-axis setup technique is used, an electron applicator provided by the manufacturer for the SSD setup is not needed. The electron field for electron arc therapy is defined by using a custom-made applicator with a rectangular cutout. Electron arc therapy has been found to be efficient to treat large superficial lesions of the nasal cavity; postmastectomy chest wall; and reconstructed breast, torso, and limbs, which are difficult to irradiate with a static electron or kV X-ray field. In this section, the electron beam setup, dosimetry, and monitor unit calculations are discussed.

Electron Beam Geometry and Setup
Since source-to-axis distance setup is used in electron arc therapy, the distance between the cutout and isocenter should be large enough to include the patient's body. Normally, a distance of 35 cm is used with the applicator height equal to about 15 cm. The cutout is usually made to produce a rectangular field, for example, with physical size equal to 2.6×21 cm^2 and is inserted at the bottom of a custom-made applicator. This applicator is attached to the block tray holder on the treatment head of the linear accelerator. Dosimetry calibration and measurement are carried out using cubic and cylindrical solid water phantoms with the accelerator gantry rotating to produce an electron arc.

Monitor Unit Calculation
The monitor unit for electron arc therapy is calculated by the equation:

$$\text{Monitor Unit} = \frac{\text{Prescribed Dose (cGy)}}{\dfrac{1\,\text{cGy}}{\text{Monitor Unit}} \times \text{Dwell Factor}} \\ \times \text{Relative Output Factor} \\ \times \text{Inverse Square Law Factor}$$

The dwell factor is defined as follows[14]:

$$DF = \frac{\dfrac{\text{Ionization}}{\text{MU}} \text{ for the electron arc with the electron cutout}}{\dfrac{\text{Ionization}}{\text{MU}} \text{ for the static field with the electron cutout}}$$

This factor accounts for the dosimetric variation when the static electron beam changes to rotating status in the arc therapy. The relative output factor is defined as the dose ratio of the electron arc cutout to the reference 10×10 cm^2 cutout. Measurement of the relative output factor is performed at SSD equal to 100 cm and at a depth of reference (e.g., 2 cm for the 9-MeV electron beam) in water. This factor corrects the single-beam dose from the absolute calibration to electron arc. The inverse square law factor is used to correct the monitor unit with a variation of SSD that differs from 100 cm in the electron arc delivery. For monitor unit calculation in electron arc therapy, the dwell factor, relative output factor, and inverse square law factor can be determined by measurements or Monte Carlo simulations.[14]

Electronic and Radioisotope Brachytherapy

There has been recent interest in using low-energy photons in new electronic and radioisotope brachytherapy devices and techniques. Remote afterloading high-dose rate (HDR) brachytherapy devices were initially used in locally irradiating intracavitary locations such as gynecologic malignancies and breast operative sites.[15] Their use subsequently expanded to include irradiation of small superficial cancers, including skin cancer such as Kaposi sarcoma.[16] The specialized Leipzig and Valencia applicators were developed by investigators in Germany and Spain to facilitate brachytherapy of superficial (e.g., cutaneous) tumor sites with these radiation sources.

HDR surface brachytherapy places an iridium-192 source in close proximity to the target lesion using a computer-controlled remote afterloader that houses a radioactive source that may be precisely delivered using specialized catheters or applicators. The choice of applicator is commonly dependent on the size and depth of the target. Small, superficial tumors (up to 2.5 cm in diameter and 0.5 cm in thickness) may be readily treated using vendor-specific Leipzig or Valencia skin applicators, and applicators of even greater diameter are commercially available; the risk of a poor cosmetic outcome may be unacceptably high for hypofractionated regimens delivered to larger volumes.[17] Prefabricated silicone rubber sheets with parallel catheter channels that permit a known distance between the catheters and the skin surface may be used for more extensive skin lesions on uncovered body parts with infiltration depth less than 1 cm, and in addition, special, customized applicators may be prepared for complex geometries.[18]

The dosimetry of some specialized applicators may be nonuniform because of the nonisotropic radiation dose distribution of the HDR source and because of special geometric considerations as the radiation is delivered to curved surfaces. Care is warranted in assuring acceptable dosimetry for nonstandard settings; dose delivered cannot be recovered.

The development of kV radiation sources that mimic the functionality of the remote afterloading HDR brachytherapy devices has been followed by vendor adaptation of the Leipzig and Valencia applicators. These devices may be useful in treating small superficial skin cancers that will fit well within the applicator selected and have a thickness of less than 3 or 4 mm. Circular treatment cones of a range of sizes up to 50 mm in diameter may be used. The Valencia applicator has a flattening filter, so although the dose rate is lower than for the Leipzig applicator, the flattening filter does achieve its goal of greater dose uniformity through the target volume.[19] The target/source to skin distance is 2 to 3 cm, resulting in a rapid decrease in radiation dose with increasing depth from the cone applicator and skin surface. The percent depth-doses for a 50-keV beam at these treatment distances are approximately 58% to 66% at 4 mm depth, and 51% to 60% at 5 mm depth. Some treatment cones use a step filter to provide a flatter isodose curve.

Not unexpectedly, these relatively novel radiotherapy devices harbor the potential for misadministration and misunderstanding of directives, but the process is amenable to standardization.[20] There is limited clinical information regarding the efficacy of these devices for treatment of skin cancers at this time, but a significant number of patients have been reported from Leipzig, where a complete response rate of 91% for over 500 patients with a variety of conditions was observed.[21] The Valencia group has reported a much smaller series of patients with nonmelanoma skin cancer and report 98% local control at 4 years.[22] A task force report from the Groupe Européen de Curiethérapie (GEC) and the European Society for Radiotherapy (GEC-ESTRO) and the American Association of Physicists in Medicine (AAPM) on the use of innovative brachytherapy devices and applications draws attention to a number of important factors, including the important role of a medical physicist, that should be considered carefully in the use of novel brachytherapy products and in brachytherapy's use in novel clinical applications so as to minimize the risk of problems.[23] The American Brachytherapy Society has also promulgated recommendations for skin cancer brachytherapy.[24,25]

There is, as yet, too little reported experience with electronic brachytherapy to merit more than a mention here.[15,26] Several vendors have begun to market these devices, not only to radiation oncologists, but also to dermatologists as well. It may be hoped that with appropriate case selection and careful attention to treatment-related parameters, successful treatments will be reported in an adequately detailed fashion to permit determination of this approach's suitability for continued use in treating skin cancer. The American Brachytherapy Society has recommended electronic brachytherapy's use for basal

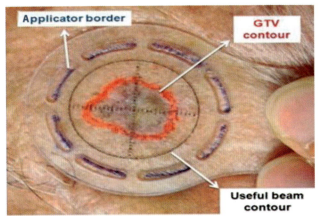

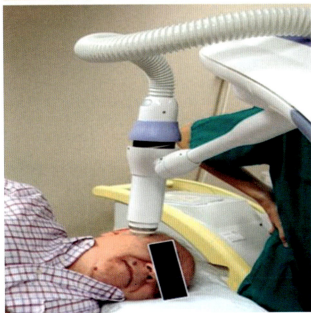

FIGURE 13.5. An example of electronic brachytherapy using an Esteya applicator. A template (specific for each applicator size) is placed on the patient's lesion and the external diameter of the applicator is drawn on the patient using the template's open areas. The arm of the device with the specific applicator is then placed in contact with the patient's skin surface. (Adapted with permission from Pons-Llanas O, Ballester-Sánchez R, Celada-Álvarez FJ, et al. Clinical implementation of a new electronic brachytherapy system for skin brachytherapy. *J Contemp Brachytherapy*. 2015;6:417–423.)

cell and squamous cell carcinomas be limited to patients enrolled in clinical trials or within registries in light of uncertainties about the ultimate efficacy and safety of these devices.[25] Figure 13.5 shows an electronic brachytherapy applicator and a treatment setup.

Selected Aspects of Treatment Setup

Because the lateral radiation margins are often narrow, the importance of effective patient immobilization and precision in cutout positioning cannot be overemphasized. Immobilization techniques used for irradiating head and neck cancers are used for skin cancers of the face and neck. The surface of the treatment field should be as nearly perpendicular to the treatment beam axis as is practical.

With an orthovoltage photon beam, dose inhomogeneities because of irregular surface contours can usually be diminished to acceptable levels by increasing the SSD. Lead cutout positioning and fixation are facilitated if the shield conforms closely to the contours of the region and the tape fixes the cutout to the patient. When the cutout can be fixed to the skin, the treatment beam breadth should exceed that of the cutout area by about 1 cm, minimizing the effect of patient movement. Of course, the width of the lead must exceed that of the treatment beam. Frequent clinical physician visualization of the treatment setup is very important to confirm that the treatment field is properly aligned relative to the tumor.

Fractionation Schedules

The National Comprehensive Cancer Network (NCCN) has published recommended dose-fractionation schedules for curative treatment of skin cancers with orthovoltage and has included recommendations for prescription modifications for electron beam treatment.[2] The dose-fractionation recommendations are the same for both squamous and basal cell carcinomas. There are recommendations for definitive and postoperative treatment of nodal metastatic disease included in the recommendations for squamous cell skin carcinoma. Additional orthovoltage radiotherapy prescriptions with dose-fractionation schedules are shown in Tables 10.3 and 10.4. As stated earlier, because of a difference in the RBE between photons and electrons, the prescription for electrons should be to the 90% isodose surface to ensure an adequate dose to the tumor.

The NCCN has also published recommendations for postsurgical and definitive radiation therapy management of Merkel cell carcinoma.[27] These guidelines acknowledge the lack of good data supporting radiotherapy dosing recommendations. It appears that locoregional control with radiotherapy as a definitive management strategy is only ~75% to 80% of that when surgery precedes irradiation. Adjuvant irradiation with wide field margins, including draining lymph nodes if involvement is suspected, is indicated in patients with any of the following risk factors: a primary tumor ≥1 cm in maximum dimension, a head and neck primary, positive or limited surgical resection margins, lymphovascular invasion, or an immunocompromised host.[28] Survival advantages appear to accrue to adjuvant irradiation in patients with stage I or II disease, but not more advanced-stage disease.[29] Trials of immune checkpoint inhibition have shown benefit for advanced-stage and chemotherapy-refractory disease; as yet it is uncertain how this will affect the management (including radiotherapy dose-fractionation) of earlier stage presentations.[30]

For melanoma, the NCCN has also published dose-fractionation recommendations, but they also acknowledge that optimal doses are not well fractionation recommendations, but again, the lack of substantive data to support their promulgated recommendations is acknowledged.[31]

TABLE 13.3		Recommended Orthovoltage Dose and Fractionation Schedule	
Total Dose (Gy)	No. of Fractions	Duration of Treatment	Comments
40	10	2 weeks	Less satisfactory cosmetic results but used when treatment course must be short or for <1.0-cm lesion away from nose, ear, or eyelids
30	5	1 week	
20	1	1 day	
45	15	3 weeks	Moderate-size (5 × 5 cm) lesion away from nose, ears, or lids
50	20	4 weeks	<1.5-cm thin lesion of nose, ears, eyelids, or canthi
55	30	6 weeks	Moderate-size (5 × 5 cm) lesion of nose, ear, canthi, or eyelid
60	33	7 weeks	Large lesion with minimal or suspected involvement of bone or cartilage
65	36	7 weeks	Large lesion recurrent or with cartilage or bone involved

Electron beam doses should be 10% to 20% greater for equivalent effect.

Fractions given 5 days a week unless indicated otherwise.

Source: Reprinted from Mendenhall WM, Million RR, Mancuso AM, et al. Carcinoma of the skin. In: Million RR, Cassisi NJ, eds. *Management of Head and Neck Cancer*. Philadelphia, PA: JB Lippincott Co.; 1994:672, with permission.

Clinical judgment and experience are necessary to give the appropriate radiation dose. The total radiation dose ultimately delivered may vary from the planned prescribed dose. The lesion at the completion of treatment should show evidence of significant regression, and a moist reaction and surface crusting on the skin may be present. It is important for the radiation oncologist to closely observe the reaction of the surface of the tumor and the surface of the surrounding normal skin, particularly toward the end of the planned time of completion of the irradiation. The desired radiation response may require a break in the treatments, and an up- or down-titration in the number of planned treatments and the ultimate total radiation dose, to achieve the desired result of tumor control without normal tissue necrosis.

TABLE 13.4	Recommended Orthovoltage Dose and Fractionation Schedule		
Area Size	Total Dose (Gy)	No. of Fractions	Duration of Treatment (days)
Small areas (<5 × 5 cm)	20	1–2	1–2
	30	5	5–7
(Less satisfactory cosmetic results with large dose or fraction)	40	10–16	16–20
Larger areas	45	15–18	21–30
	50	20–25	28–35
	60	20–30	28–40

Electron beam doses should be 10% to 20% greater for equivalent effect.

Source: Reprinted from Solan MJ, Brady LW, Binnick SA. Skin. In: Perez CA, Brady LW, eds. *Principles of Radiation Oncology*. Philadelphia, PA: JB Lippincott Co., 1992:486, with permission.

Cutaneous Basal and Squamous Cell Carcinomas

Basal and squamous cell carcinomas of the skin are most commonly diagnosed in patients over the age of 50, are related to earlier sun exposure, and are often optimally treated with radiation therapy. Many patients with small tumors are not referred for consultative opinions, and patients referred for radiation are often those that have neglected skin cancers that are too locally advanced to be considered for attempts at radical resection or are locally recurrent, potentially involving regional nodal chains, or with evidence of other metastatic spread after possibly multiple ineffective local procedures by other caregivers.

Basal cell carcinomas appear to arise in embryonic fusion plate regions with a higher frequency than elsewhere on the face.[32] Both basal and squamous skin cancers have a linkage to a sun exposure history. One important difference between basal and squamous cancers is that basal cell carcinomas, though locally invasive and destructive, metastasize extremely rarely, so that looking for metastatic disease is not generally appropriate, though imaging to assist with local radiotherapy portal design is often valuable. For squamous cell carcinomas, appropriate management with surgery, radiation, or both of the primary site and of any regional nodal metastases is critical to a good outcome.

For small basal and squamous cell carcinomas of the skin, good results have been published for superficial and orthovoltage photon therapy and electron beam therapy. Field margins for <2-cm primary keratinocytic tumors should be 1 to 1.5 cm; for tumors >2 cm, field margins should be 1.5 to 2 cm.[2] In practice, 1-cm lateral margins

for photon fields applied to lesions ≤2 cm in diameter produce control rates greater than 90%, and it is conceivable that higher local control rates can be achieved through meticulous attention to planning and delivering treatment. A review of isodose curves reveals that lateral margins for fields irradiated with electron beams should be wider compared to orthovoltage beams for similar-sized cancers, but these margins have been less well defined. If a lesion is <2 cm in diameter and a 1-cm margin is to be given a minimum of 90% of D_{max}, the lateral margin for the electron beam field needs to be almost 1.5 cm. This requirement for a larger electron beam field size can be a major disadvantage in treating lesions of the eyelids and canthi. Generous lateral margins of 2 cm or more should be strongly considered for larger lesions (7–8 cm diameter), infiltrating lesions, and lesions at high risk for occult extension.

The deep margin of the cancer should always be well-included within the planning target volume; this may preclude use of electronic brachytherapy or isotope brachytherapy treatment of some tumors because of the shallow depth-dose characteristics of these low-energy sources and the limited applicator sizes.

Perineural invasion occurs in 2% to 6% of cutaneous basal and squamous cell carcinomas of the head and neck and is associated with midface location, recurrent tumors, high histologic grade, and increasing tumor size.[33] The cranial nerves most commonly involved are named branches of the trigeminal and facial nerves. Cranial nerve involvement may portend a worse prognosis, with tumor extension and recurrence along the cranial nerves and metastases to adjacent lymph nodes often also seen. Surgical resection should be considered for the primary if the tumor is considered to be resectable, but the risk of perineural spread beyond the excision margin should lower the threshold for definitive adjuvant irradiation. It can sometimes be difficult to know whether treatment portals should include both the distribution of the trigeminal and facial nerves, but careful consideration of the location of the primary lesion and clinical symptomatology may help refine radiotherapy portal design.

University of Florida investigators recommend elective regional irradiation of first-echelon lymph nodes for patients with clinical (symptomatic) perineural invasion and for those with squamous cell carcinoma with microscopic perineural invasion. Patients with involvement of named branches of cranial nerves should have radiation volumes that include the involved cranial nerve to the base of the skull.[33,34] Planning for these volumes requires careful clinical examination, high-resolution CT and MR imaging, and conformal radiation treatment planning and delivery, for which intensity-modulated techniques may permit normal tissue sparing to a greater degree than 3D conformal techniques.

University of Michigan investigators have detailed the pathways of recurrent tumor for skin squamous cell carcinomas involving the trigeminal and facial cranial nerves.[35] They identified the auriculotemporal nerve and the greater superficial petrosal nerves as the pathways of tumor spreading between those nerves. They recommend that for tumors involving cranial nerve VII, the auriculotemporal nerve and V3 are at risk; and for tumors involving V2, the greater superficial petrosal and cranial nerve VII are at risk. They advocate that these at-risk volumes should be included in the planning target volume when these nerves are involved.

Cutaneous Melanoma

Radiotherapy Indications

Surgical resection is the most common treatment of cutaneous melanoma; primary irradiation is rarely used in the treatment of primary melanoma, but there are well-defined roles for radiation in the locoregional management of melanoma.[36,37]

Lentigo maligna, also known as melanoma in situ (Clark level 1, stage 0 melanoma) or Hutchinson melanotic freckle, is very well treated by primary irradiation.[36,38,39] Margins of 5 mm are recommended for surgical management, but an Australian report on in vivo confocal microscopy described subclinical tumor extending beyond 5 mm from the lesion in most patients.[40] The ability of radiotherapy fields to be extended to cover larger margins is an advantage for this condition, where skin flaps or skin grafts may be required to obtain adequate wound closures, and facial cosmesis may be compromised permanently.

For resected melanomas of the head and neck, where anatomical constraints on radical resection exist and ideal surgical margins are difficult to obtain, adjuvant irradiation decreases locoregional recurrences. The NCCN recommends adjuvant treatment of the primary tumor site with radiation for selected patients with factors including, but not limited to, deep desmoplastic melanoma with narrow margins, extensive neurotropism, or locally recurrent disease. A wide range of radiation dose/fractionation schedules is effective, but hypofractionated regimens may increase the risk for long-term complications.

Radiotherapy to regional nodal basins (48 Gy in 20 fractions) or observation after therapeutic nodal dissection significantly decreases locoregional recurrence, though survival is not affected.[41] Adjuvant radiotherapy's benefits must be weighed against the increased probability of long-term skin and regional toxicities and potential reduced quality of life.

Radiation Therapy Technique

An adjuvant radiotherapy technique was developed at the University of Texas, MD Anderson Cancer Center that covered the primary site, nodal operative site, and regional lymph nodes using shaped electron beams of 9 to 16 MeV to deliver 30 Gy in five fractions (6 Gy per fraction) over 2.5 weeks, Monday and Thursday, or Tuesday and Friday. Dose is calculated at D_{max}. The central

nervous system (brain and spinal cord) must be spared and should be treated to a maximum of 24 Gy in four fractions.[42,43] This radiotherapy technique has also been extended to treat metastatic nodal disease of the axilla and inguinal regions. IMRT may be used to cover some of these same volumes as effectively with the use of bolus to assure adequate skin dose.

Merkel Cell Carcinoma

Merkel cell carcinoma is a rare cutaneous malignancy with a roughly 25% mortality rate and a high propensity of regional and distant tumor spread. There is no class I data evaluating radiotherapy's role in the management of this disease. The published literature appears to show an improvement in locoregional control when radiotherapy is added to management of the primary site and nodal beds, particularly when surgical margins are compromised.[44–50]

Because of the high incidence of nodal metastases, the regional lymphatics should be electively treated with surgery and/or radiation in all patients with apparently localized disease, The addition of radiation to surgically managed regional nodes, even if sentinel nodes are negative, appears to be of value.[51,52] If nodal disease is found at surgery, postoperative irradiation should be given. The radiation doses are similar for squamous cell carcinomas of the head and neck: primary tumor–negative margins, 60 Gy in 30 fractions over 6 weeks; microscopically positive margins, 66 Gy in 33 fractions over 6.5 weeks; and gross disease, 70 Gy in 35 fractions over 7 weeks. Elective irradiation of subclinical disease in a nonresected neck would be 50 Gy in 25 fractions over 5 weeks. Radiation fields should be generous (>3-cm margins) around the primary site because of the propensity of cutaneous in-transit tumor spread. The location of the primary site in relation to regional nodal basins may preclude including these nodal stations in the same radiotherapy portals. It has been stated, "For some patients, you can't treat a radiation field big enough."

Mycosis Fungoides

Mycosis fungoides (MF) is a low-grade, non-Hodgkin T-cell lymphoma that has its primary clinical manifestations within the skin. It can also involve lymph nodes, blood, and visceral organs in patients with advanced cutaneous disease.[53] MF primarily affects adults over the age of 40, with approximately 1,400 new cases per year in the United States.[54] Approximately 50% of all CTCL cases are MF.

MF may start as a scaly, red rash in areas that usually are not exposed to the sun (premycotic phase) and progress to patch phase (with thin, reddened, eczema-like rash), plaque phase (with small, raised bumps or hardened lesions on the skin), and tumor phase (with tumors formed on the skin). Patients present with tumors or erythroderma (with patches and/or plaques covering >80% body surface area) are at high risk for extracutaneous dissemination to lymph nodes, viscera, and blood.

Early-stage MF consists of patches and/or plaques on the skin with no (stage IA and IB) or limited (stage IIA) lymph node involvement and no visceral involvement. Patients present with advanced skin lesions (e.g., tumors, generalized erythroderma) or extracutaneous disease are classified as having advanced-stage MF (stages IIB–IV).[1]

Radiation Therapy Indications

Early-stage MF is typically managed with skin-directed therapies, which include topical corticosteroids, topical chemotherapy (nitrogen mustard or carmustine), phototherapy (psoralen plus ultraviolet A, PUVA and ultraviolet B, UVB), and radiation therapy among others.[55] For patients with disease limited to the skin, skin-directed therapy alone can usually produce high rates of remission and even cure.[54] Serial administration of skin-directed therapies may be needed to achieve and/or maintain long-term disease control. When skin-directed therapies fail to control the disease, systemic therapy may be used. Systemic therapy is used either alone or in combination with skin-directed therapies for patients with advanced-stage disease. There are investigators exploring the use of immunomodulatory agents either alone or together with total skin electron beam (TSEB) for MF, and monoclonal antibodies against cell surface markers are also entering the therapeutic armamentarium.[56]

Although skin-directed therapies other than radiation are often provided initially at earlier stages of the disease, radiation therapy remains one of the most effective strategies in the management of MF due to its high sensitivity to ionizing radiation.[52,55] For patients with unilesional or localized MF (involving <10% of body surface area), local irradiation is typically used with efficient disease clearance. For patients with extended or advanced diseases, total-skin electron therapy (TSET) is used in either primary or adjuvant settings. TSET monotherapy provides rapid and effective palliation, with high complete response rates.[57] For patients with more advanced cutaneous and/or visceral disease, TSET monotherapy is rarely curative; it is often administered to induce cutaneous remission followed by adjuvant systemic and/or topical therapy to prolong remission. Some patients may be candidates for a second course of total-skin electron irradiation for recurrent MF.[53,57]

Radiation Treatment Techniques

Key factors to consider in planning radiation therapy for MF include the spatial extent of the lesions (i.e., the depth below and the lateral spread over the skin surface), the dose required to control the lesions, and the radiation impact on normal tissue and critical structures. The lesion depth dictates the type and the energy of radiation to be used. Because the primary targets of MF are mostly superficial, radiation modalities that can deliver dose to only the affected skin layers are ideal. For this reason,

electrons are preferred over photons as electrons stop at a finite penetration depth in tissue. The penetration depth can be controlled by tuning the electron energy or adding tissue-equivalent bolus at the beam entrance, to confine the radiation dose to a desired skin layer with little radiation to deeper-seated normal tissues. The lateral spread of the lesions over the skin surface determines the size of radiation field(s) and the irradiation technique to be used. When total-skin irradiation is required, only electron beams can be used because the whole-body dose from a photon-based technique would be unacceptable. Treatment planning considerations for using localized and total-skin irradiation are discussed further in the following section.

Local Radiation Therapy. Local irradiation is highly effective for MF with localized lesions or with limited skin involvement. Kilovoltage X-rays (e.g., 120 kVp) and electron beams have both been used in the treatment of localized MF lesions. Despite the recent proliferation of proton beam therapy centers, there are still no reports evaluating the use of protons for MF in the medical literature. While kilovoltage X-rays deposit maximum dose at the skin surface, they are inherently more penetrating compared to electron beams. Unwanted irradiation of deep-seated normal tissues along the beam path is unavoidable. Because a kilovoltage X-ray unit is relatively simple to maneuver for complicated setups, it is still being used in some institutions for localized MF tumors with deep disease infiltration and/or for boost irradiation of skin areas that could not receive sufficient dose in the total-skin electron treatment, such as the perineum and soles of feet.

Treatment planning considerations for local radiation therapy using electrons (or kilovoltage X-rays) are similar to those discussed in the earlier sections of this chapter for other superficial lesions. Beam energy selection is dictated by the desired treatment depth. Because the energy of available electron beams is limited on commonly used linear accelerators, custom bolus may be used to modulate beam penetration and/or ensure adequate dose to skin surface. Typically, a 6-MeV electron beam with 1 cm bolus may be sufficient. Radiation field aperture is typically designed with a field margin of 1 to 2 cm beyond the visible (or palpable) clinical lesion, although the exact size and shape are often influenced by the location of the lesions and their proximity to sensitive normal tissues. When abutting fields are used, the field junctions should be shifted during the course of treatment to improve dose homogeneity in the abutting region.

For treatment of an isolated lesion with localized superficial radiotherapy, the optimal treatment dose is ≥30 Gy delivered in 1.2 to 2.0 Gy per fraction,[57,58] although a total dose of 15 to 25 Gy delivered over 1 to 3 weeks is usually effective in long-term control of localized disease. In a dose response analysis of 110 biopsy-proven MF lesions treated to doses ranging from 6 to 40 Gy, a complete response to treatment was noted in all lesions receiving >20 Gy.[58] Among the lesions having a complete response, an infield recurrence rate of 42% was noted for those treated to a total dose of ≤10 Gy, 32% for 10.01 to 20 Gy, 21% for 20.01 to 30 Gy, and 0% for >30 Gy.[45] While radiation treatment is highly effective in local control, new lesions can develop outside of the treated field. Skin-directed maintenance therapy such as topical nitrogen mustard or topical corticosteroids may be used after local radiation therapy. If indicated, it is also appropriate to administer local radiation therapy either before or following a course of total-skin electron treatment (to be discussed next in the following section).

Treatment-related toxicity from local radiation therapy is dependent upon the radiation dose used and the location of the lesion. Typical side effects include erythema and hair loss.[55]

Total-Skin Electron Therapy

For patients with extended or advanced MF, TSET is the most effective single-agent treatment.[55,57] The dosimetric goal of TSET is to deliver a sufficient dose to the superficial skin layer of the entire body with a minimum or no dose to the normal tissues inside.[53,59] For example, the Cutaneous Lymphoma Project Group of the European Organization for Research and Treatment of Cancer recommends a desired therapeutic treatment depth of at least 4 mm below the skin surface with <0.7-Gy whole-body dose from photon contamination at the level of the bone marrow (to avoid hematologic sequelae).[60,61] Technical challenges in fulfilling this dosimetric goal arise primarily from the unusual target volume shape, which wraps around the body amid ever-changing curvatures and unavoidable self-shielding among the body structures. Use of custom shielding to overdosed or sensitive skin surfaces (e.g., fingernails, hands, lips, and eyes) and supplemental patch treatments to underdosed skin surfaces (e.g., perineum, soles of feet, scalp, and behind pendulous tissue) are necessary.[61]

Conventional TSET treatments are prescribed with a total dose of at least 26 Gy to a depth of 4 mm in truncal skin (approximately 31–36 Gy to the skin surface).[61] Treatments at this dose level are every effective at inducing complete cutaneous response.[53,57] Treatment-related toxicities are generally limited to the skin, hair, and nails.[62] In a retrospective review of 82 patients receiving 30 to 36 Gy of TSET, the most common acute adverse effects noted were erythema and dry desquamation (76%), blisters (52%), hyperpigmentation (50%), and skin pain (48%).[63] Skin infection which required antibiotics occurred in 32% of patients while no patient had grade 4/5 toxicities.[63] Other toxicities such as alopecia (potentially irreversible with doses of >25 Gy), temporary loss of fingernails and toenails, hypo- or anhidrosis, and chronically dry skin which requires the regular use of emollients have also been reported.[62] Because toxicity increases with cumulative dose, TSET given with the conventional dose

often limits its use again on patients with disease relapse. To minimize the risk of adverse events and increase the opportunity of retreatment in cases of disease recurrence, TSET given with lower total dose (<30 Gy), at standard dose per fraction, has recently been tested and utilized clinically.[64,65] Institutional studies and prospective trials have shown that TSET given with 12 Gy produced similar response rates, overall survival and symptomatic relief, albeit at the cost of complete response.[65] The impact of different TSET dosing schemes on the clinical outcomes of MF has been reviewed by Chowdhary et al.[64,65]

Modern TSET techniques are all based on electron beams produced by medical linear accelerators. The beam uniformity of an ideal TSET beam should be within 10% across clinically useful vertical and lateral dimensions.[61] The basic geometry typically involves a horizontally directed electron beam with the patient standing at 3 to 7 m away from the radiation source.[59,61] By positioning the patient at an extended distance, a large electron beam is realized at the location of the patient. For example, at an SSD of 7 m, a 3-mm diameter electron pencil beam at the accelerator's exit window will broaden into an electron beam of about 180 cm in diameter due to electron scattering within air.[66] In linear accelerator vaults not large enough to permit this extended SSD, it is still generally possible to position the patient at a shorter SSD (e.g., 3–4 m), and a composite dual-field beam can be used, which consists of two horizontally directed beams with one angled slightly toward the patient's head and the other toward the patient's feet,[67] resulting in an effective uniform beam covering patient from head to toe (Fig. 13.6). The use of dual-field beam is due primarily to the limitations of accelerator design (e.g., maximum achievable dose rate) and/or the size of accelerator vault.

The first linear accelerator-based method reported by Stanford University used a dual-field beam with the patient irradiated in two treatment positions: one facing the beam source and the other facing away from the source, equivalent to an AP-PA treatment setup.[67] Following the basic treatment planning principles, the lateral dose uniformity around the patient's circumference can be improved by using increasingly more beams equally spaced around the patient.[68] Indeed, a treatment equivalent to using infinite number of beams around the patient can be achieved by rotating the patient at a constant speed about the patient's vertical axis while the radiation is turned on.[59] Phantom studies suggest that such a rotation technique provides the best dose uniformity over large portions of the body surface, although using eight beams has proved to be almost as good.[59] Detailed information on the physical aspects of rotation technique may be found, for example, in the paper by Podgorsak et al.[69] Stanford ultimately settled on a six-field technique in which patients stand in six different orientations with respect to the dual-field beam: anterior, posterior, right and left anterior oblique, and right and left posterior oblique.[68] Although less than optimal, it provides considerably better circumferential dose

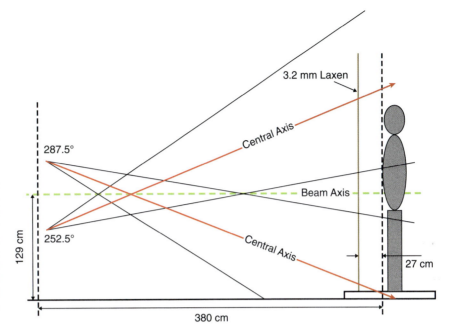

FIGURE 13.6. Illustration of a dual-field beam TSET setup currently used at Yale University. Note the beam axis for the dual-field coincides with the central axis of a horizontally directed beam. (Adapted with permission from Chen Z, Agostinelli AG, Wilson LD, et al. Matching the dosimetry characteristics of a dual-field Stanford technique to a customized single-field Stanford technique for total-skin electron therapy. *Int J Radiat Oncol Biol Phys.* 2004;59:872–885.)

uniformity than the two- or four-field techniques and is relatively simpler to carry out.[59]

While the rotation technique has been used clinically in a few selected institutions, most clinical TSET programs utilize the Stanford six-field technique, using either a single-field or a composite dual-field beam.[66] Figure 13.6 depicts a dual-field beam setup currently used in the Yale TSET program. With a patient standing at 3.8 m from the radiation source and a 3.2-mm Lexan attenuate or scatter screen placed in front of the patient, the dual-field beam is made up of two fields with the accelerator head rotated 17.5° above and below the horizontal direction toward the patient. The Lexan screen is used to attenuate and scatter the 6-MeV incident electrons produced from a Varian TrueBeam linear accelerator using the high-dose rate total-skin electron (HDTSe) mode. The mean energy of the electrons reaching patient's skin surface is approximately 3.9 MeV. For total-skin treatment, the patient is irradiated in six specific treatment positions to maximize skin unfolding and lateral dose uniformity (Fig. 13.7). Traditionally, the treatment of six positions is delivered over the course of a 2-day treatment cycle. On day one, the anterior, right posterior oblique, and left posterior oblique positions are treated. On day two, the posterior, right anterior oblique, and left anterior oblique positions are treated.

Figure 13.8 compares the depth-dose curves of a complete treatment cycle (all six positions) to a single position (e.g., anterior) at the level of beam axis. Due to the obliquity of incident electrons from the neighboring irradiation positions, the depth-dose curve of a complete treatment cycle is shifted toward the skin surface, with the dose maximum at ~1 mm, the 80% isodose line at ~6 mm, and the 20% isodose line at ~12 mm.[66] Figure 13.9 demonstrates a relatively uniform dose delivered by this setup

to the skin surface at the level of umbilicus with no electron dose to the deeper-seated tissues inside the body. The total X-ray contamination was approximately 1.2% of the skin dose, well within the acceptable limit.[61]

For conventional TSET treatment (Table 13.5), the effective dose delivered over the 2-day treatment cycle is typically 2 Gy to the skin surface. Patient receives treatment 4 days (2 cycles) per week, with a total dose of 36 Gy delivered over 9 weeks. A 1-week break may be given after a dose of 18 Gy has been delivered to provide relief from the generalized skin erythema associated with treatment. For low-dose TSET treatment, the total dose is reduced while keeping the same dose per fraction. Although the six treatment positions are designed to maximize skin unfolding and minimize self-shielding, overdose may occur to certain structures such as hands and ankles due to high convexity and radiation exposure from more than three positions. Under dose could also occur to areas such as the top of the scalp, the perineum, the underside of the breasts, panniculus folds, and the soles of the feet due to self-shielding.[59] Customized shielding and supplemental irradiation are used to bring the dose to these areas close to the desired value. In addition, some critical structures (such as the lens of the eyes) and radiosensitive structures (such as the nail beds and lips) may need additional shielding to prevent unnecessary radiation injury. Detailed dosimetric measurements (on phantom and in vivo) are required to determine the most appropriate shielding regimen or supplemental treatment for a particular treatment arrangement and patient geometry.[59,66] In vivo dosimetry is also useful in routine verification of dose delivered to key skin areas for patients receiving TSET treatments.[70]

Table 13.5 lists the nominal shielding and supplemental treatment regimen used at Yale-New Haven Hospital.[66] Individualized adjustments are made by the radiation

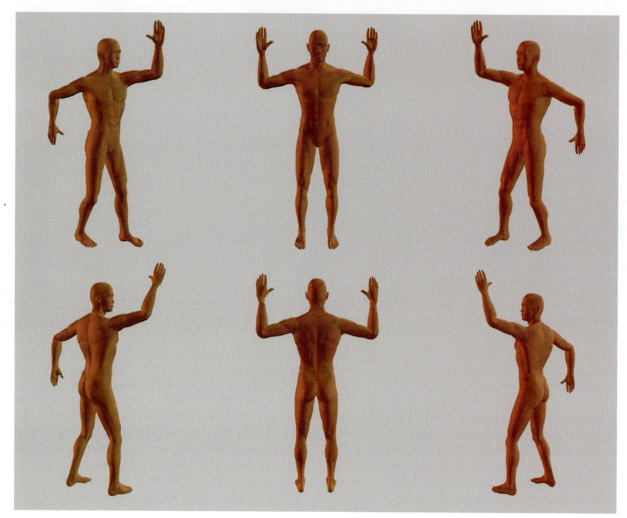

FIGURE 13.7. Illustration of the six-treatment positions used in the Stanford total-skin electron therapy. (Reprinted with permission from Smith BD, Wilson LD. Cutaneous lymphomas. *Semin Radiat Oncol*. 2007;17:158–168.)

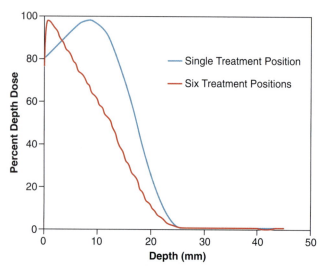

FIGURE 13.8. Comparison of percent depth-dose curves for a single-position irradiation and a six-position treatment. (Adapted with permission from Chen Z, Agostinelli AG, Wilson LD, et al. Matching the dosimetry characteristics of a dual-field Stanford technique to a customized single-field Stanford technique for total-skin electron therapy. *Int J Radiat Oncol Biol Phys*. 2004;59:872–885.)

oncologist based on the conditions of specific patients and clinical judgment. The eyes and lenses are shielded with a combination of internal and external eye shields. Because of the increased backscatter dose from the internal shield to the eyelid, use of internal eye shield throughout the treatment course would have overdosed the eyelid. External eye shields made of lead sheets or Cerrobend block casted in swimming goggles are used to prevent eyelids from overexposure. It is appropriate to start treatment with internal eye shields and switch to external eye shields during the later portion of the treatment course; or use internal and external shields in alternating treatment cycles. To prevent severe reaction to the fingers, hands, lips, and feet, lead-lined mitts, lead sheet-based custom shields, and shielding blocks can be used to reduce the dose to these areas.

Both electron beam and kilovoltage X-rays can be used for supplemental treatment to underdosed areas. One can use 120 kVp, HVL of 4.2 mm Al, X-rays to deliver patch treatments to the soles of feet (14 Gy in 14 fractions on treatment days of 1–7 and 30–36) and perineum (18 Gy in

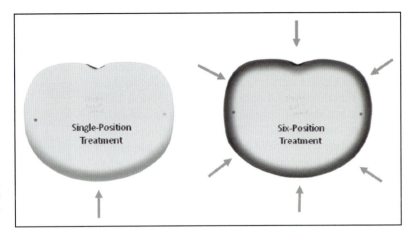

FIGURE 13.9. A representation of single-position and six-position treatment setups. The six-position treatment setup can deliver a relatively uniform dose to the surface while minimizing delivery of dose to deep tissues.

TABLE 13.5	Standard TSET Treatment Protocol at Yale-New Haven Hospital
Treatment Cycle	
Day 1	AP, RPO, LPO treatment positions
Day 2	PA, RAO, LAO treatment positions
Dose	
Dose per cycle	2 Gy
Cycles per week	2
Total cycles	18
Total dose	36 Gy
Boosts	
Perineum	1 Gy/day, first 9 and last 9 treatment days
Soles of feet	1 Gy/day, first 7 and last 7 treatment days
Shielding	
External eye shields	First 11 cycles
Internal eye shields	Last 7 cycles
Lip shield	Cycles 1–4
Lead mitt for hands	Every other cycle
Fingernail shield	Every other cycle, alternating with mitts
Foot block	Cycles 1–3, 5, 7, 9, 11, 13, 15, 17, 18
Testicular shield	Used with perineal boost only

AP, anteroposterior; LAO, left anterior oblique; LPO, left posterior oblique; PA posteroanterior; RAO, right anterior oblique; RPO, right posterior oblique; TSET, total-skin electron therapy.[44,50]

Source: *Adapted from* Chen Z, Agostinelli AG, Wilson LD, et al. Matching the dosimetry characteristics of a dual-field Stanford technique to a customized single-field Stanford technique for total skin electron therapy. *Int J Radiat Oncol Biol Phys*. 2004;59: 872–885; Ghadjar P, Kaanders JH, Poortmans P, et al. The essential role of radiotherapy in the treatment of Merkel cell carcinoma: a study from the rare cancer network. *Int J Radiat Oncol Biol Phys*. 2011;81:e583–e591; Smith BD, Wilson LD. Cutaneous lymphomas. *Semin Radiat Oncol*. 2007;17:158–168.

18 fractions on treatment days of 1–9 and 28–36). Caution should be exercised in giving >20 Gy to the soles of the feet because of the limited tolerance of the skin of the sole.[61] The scalp dose can be supplemented with either orthovoltage patches (6–20 Gy over 1–3 weeks) or with an electron reflector mounted above the patient's head.[66] Other areas of potential underdosing include the ventral penis, the upper medial thighs, inframammary folds, folds under any pannus, and the lateral and flatter regions of the face and trunk. Supplemental patch fields, as guided by in vivo dosimetry or clinical suspicion, are appropriate for these regions to ensure that the surface dose is at least 50% of the prescribed TSET dose.[57] When determining the total dose given in patch treatments, dose to areas such as the feet and perineum may be reduced as clinically indicated, provided such areas are uninvolved.[57] For tumors having a thickness greater than 6 mm (e.g., for patients with bleeding, weeping, or painful tumors at presentation), an initial or concurrent boost of 10 Gy in five fractions using either 6- to 16-MeV electrons or kilovoltage X-rays has been effective.[57] Asymptomatic plaques and tumors that persist at the end of treatment may receive a similar boost to ensure adequate dose delivery at depth.

TSET has been proven as an effective and well-tolerated treatment for MF.[53,57] However, it remains as a complex and very specialized radiation treatment technique. It requires nonstandard dosimetric measurements as well as knowledge and use of proper patient positioning to optimally expose all skin surfaces to large electron beams. Significant medical physics effort is required to set up and maintain such a technique.[59] A team of experienced radiation oncology physicians, medical physicists, medical dosimetrists, and radiation therapists must be in place to properly plan and deliver optimal TSET treatments. Recent advancements in Monte Carlo simulation for TSET treatments demonstrated that Monte Carlo can accurately simulate the percent depth-dose of TSET beams with better than 3%/mm agreement to the measured values.[71,72] The feasibility of Monte Carlo simulation of a CT-based anthropomorphic phantom for a full TSET treatment using six dual-field beams has also been demonstrated in literature with generally good agreements with the corresponding measured data.[72] These advancements indicate that Monte Carlo simulation can be a promising tool not only for initial setup and optimization of a clinical TSET technique but also for detailed and systematic dosimetric analysis of dose delivered to TSET patients. Coupled with the developments in in vivo dosimetry,[70] it can potentially make the TSET technique a little easier to setup while delivering more consistent treatments for MF patients.

CLINICAL CONSIDERATIONS

Examples of Treated Patients

Case 1: Squamous Cell Carcinoma of Lip
(Figs. 13.10–13.14)

An 87-year-old woman had a destructive squamous cell carcinoma of the right side of her upper lip. Because of her age and difficulty in arranging transportation, she was treated with 300 cGy/day to the 90% line in three fractions per week, with 6 MeV electrons, with 5 mm of gel bolus over the lip and a lead shield between the upper lip and the upper alveolar ridge. Following eight fractions, she was given a 13-day break because of an intense radiation reaction on the surface of the tumor and the surrounding skin, and then she returned for an additional eight fractions. Her tumor was subsequently totally controlled with good cosmetic result with a total dose of 4,800 cGy in 16 fractions over 42 elapsed days.

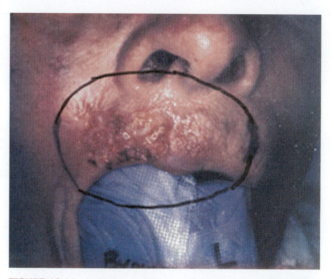

FIGURE 13.11. At the time of fourth radiation treatment with 6-MeV electrons, 5-mm gel bolus on the skin, black line, is edge of radiation field as defined by Cerrobend cutout, treated at 300 cGy per day to 90% line, three fractions per week. A lead shield enclosed in a folded glove is placed between the upper lip and the upper alveolar ridge.

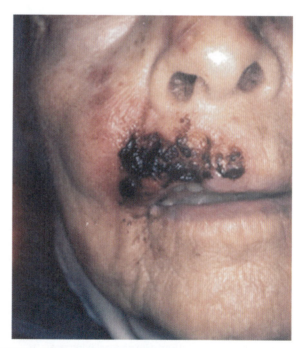

FIGURE 13.12. At seventh radiation fraction, 2,100 cGy to the 90% isodose surface. Following the eighth treatment (2,400 cGy), a 13-day treatment break was needed because of the intense symptomatic radiation reaction over the tumor surface.

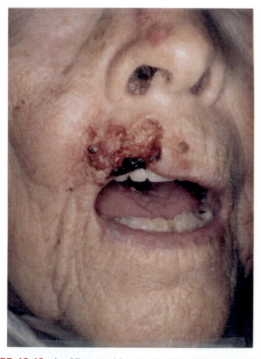

FIGURE 13.10. An 87-year-old woman with squamous cell carcinoma of right side of upper lip (prior to irradiation).

Case 2: Squamous Cell Carcinoma of the Left Ala Nasi
(Figs. 13.15–13.18)

This 79-year-old man had a very large ulcerated 4 × 4 × 3.5–cm squamous carcinoma that involved and distorted the left ala nasi blocking the left nostril (Fig. 13.15). The treatment planning CT scan and the radiation treatments were performed with the patient immobilized in a

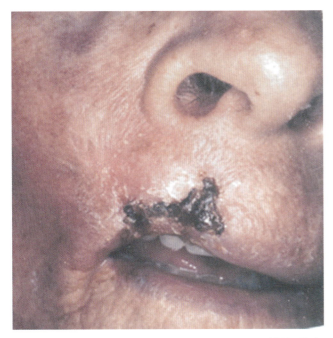

FIGURE 13.13. At completion of radiation treatments, 4,800 cGy in 16 fractions, 3 fractions per week, over 42 elapsed days. Eight fractions followed by a 13-day break, followed by eight more fractions.

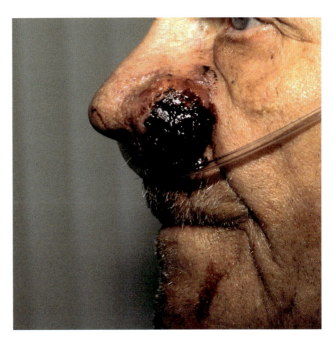

FIGURE 13.15. 4 × 4 × 3.5–cm ulcerated and bleeding squamous cell carcinoma of left ala nasi, prior to treatment.

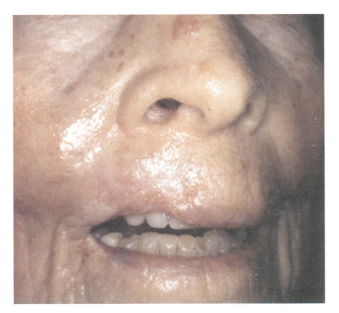

FIGURE 13.14. Six weeks following completion of irradiation. No evidence of tumor. There is slight deformity of the right side of the upper lip because of prior destruction from the tumor. Considering the original tumor appearance, this is a very good functional and cosmetic result.

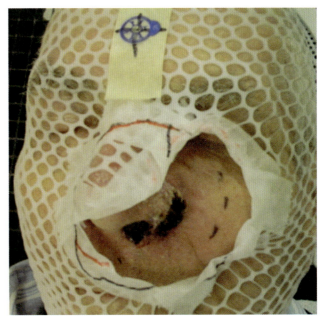

FIGURE 13.16. Photo taken at 3,000 cGy, original field is marked in *black ink* and reduced field is marked in *red ink;* treatment continued to total of 4,800 cGy.

thermoplastic mask (Fig. 13.16). The CT scan showed the depth of the tumor involvement. He was initially treated with a combination of 12-MeV electrons (70% weighting) and 16-MeV electrons (30% weighting). The shaped left anterior oblique field (Cerrobend cutout in electron cone) included a 1-cm peripheral margin. He received a total of 5,100 cGy to the 90% line in 17 fractions over 30 days, treating 4 days/week. The final 1,800 cGy was given with a reduced field size and with 12-MeV electrons because

the tumor depth had decreased by that time. No bolus was used because the 90% isodose line (green line) of the 12- and 16-MeV electron beams was at the tumor surface (Fig. 13.17). Excellent tumor control and cosmesis was provided (Fig. 13.18).

Cancer of the ala nasi commonly invades and destroys the underlying cartilage. Laterally, the lesion may extend to the embryonic fusion planes of the nasolabial fold. This permits deep infiltration. Although not used in this

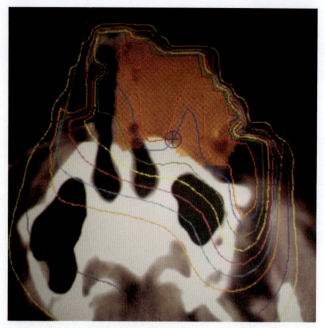

FIGURE 13.17. Isodose lines of treatment with combination of left anterior oblique 12 and 16 MeV electrons, treatment prescription calculated to green 90% isodose surface, which surrounded tumor volume and also included tumor surface. No bolus was used. Colors and percent isodose surfaces: *red* 105%, *blue* 100%, *green* 90%, *yellow* 80%, *magenta* 70%, *light blue* 60%, *orange* 50%, *purple* 30%, *light yellow* 20%.

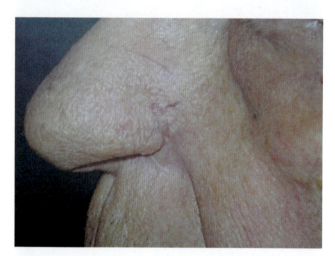

FIGURE 13.18. Two months following the completion of radiation treatment, no visible tumor, slight skin distortion, excellent cosmetic result considering initial tumor appearance.

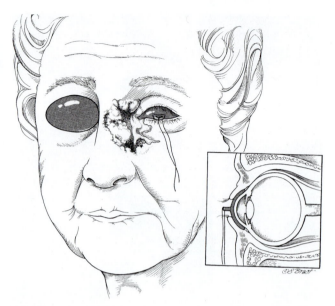

FIGURE 13.19. An internal (Gougelman) eye shield is in place in the anesthetized left eye. An external eye shield covers the right eye.

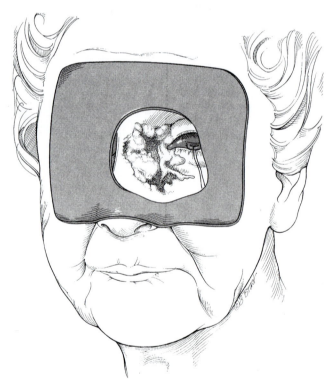

FIGURE 13.20. A lead cutout and the eye shields are in place.

patient; exit beam shields of lead, coated with paraffin, and then slipped into the left nostril or anterior to the upper gum may be used. When the tumor is close to the orbits, extra eye shields are used.

Case 3: Basal Cell Carcinoma of the Left Medial Canthus and Bridge of Nose with Extension into the Left Lower Eyelid (Figs. 13.19 and 13.20)

Cancers near the eye may invade the bone or soft tissues of the orbit. When there is any question of deep invasion, imaging studies through this level may provide useful information. Such invasion was not present in this patient. Gross margins were otherwise readily determined. The relatively small size of the treatment field, together with the problems of dose distribution and use of a lead eye shield of appropriate thickness for the electron beam, made the X-ray beam preferable.[12,13,72] The contour across the treatment field was irregular. (The bridge of the nose was ~1.5 to 2 cm anterior to the canthus.) The resulting variation in surface dose was decreased by increasing SSD of the X-ray beam to 50 cm rather than the usual 20 to 30 cm.

A 200-keV X-ray beam of half-value layer (HVL) 1-mm copper at 50-cm SSD is appropriate. The field diameter, allowing at least 1 cm of lateral margin around the lesion, was 4.5 cm. A lead cutout of 1-mm thickness was constructed and shaped. Figure 13.19 shows that before it was taped in place, an eye shield of 2-mm-thick lead was inserted on the surface of the anesthetized left eye and the closed right eye was covered with an additional 1-mm-thick shield to block radiation that might be transmitted to the right lens through the lead of the cutout. The lead cutout was then taped in place (Fig. 13.20). After each treatment, an eye patch is worn until sensation returns to the cornea.

Fractionation and total dose schedules, chosen to produce minimum fibrosis, telangiectasia, and edema of eyelids and adjacent skin, were 54 Gy given in 27 fractions. Obviously, larger and more deeply infiltrating lesions require consideration of electron beam techniques, some requiring 12- to 22-MeV electron beams.[8] In such patients, loss of vision or even of the eye may be unavoidable if the cancer is to be cured.

Case 4: Nodular Squamous Cell Carcinoma (Figs. 13.21 and 13.22)

This 93-year-old woman with a nodular squamous cell carcinoma overlying her malar eminence (Fig. 13.21) was treated with 45 Gy in 10 fractions over 2 weeks using 250-kV photons with an orthovoltage unit and applicators akin to those shown in Figures 13.1 and 13.2. At age 100, at 7-year follow-up, the patient was alert and well and had

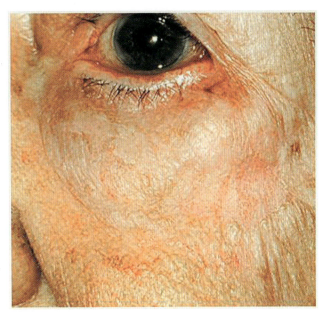

FIGURE 13.22. At age 100, at 7-year follow-up, the patient was alert and well, with a sustained complete response to treatment and an excellent cosmetic result.

maintained a clinical complete remission with excellent cosmesis (Fig. 13.22).

Case 5: Squamous Cell Carcinoma of the Bridge of the Nose (Figs. 13.23–13.25)

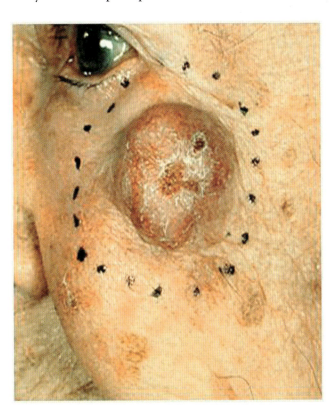

FIGURE 13.21. This 93-year-old woman with nodular squamous cell carcinoma was treated with 45 Gy in 10 fractions over 2 weeks using 250 kV photons. The black dotted lines indicate (Figs. 13.21 and 13.23) where the radiotherapy shielding (and radiotherapy portal) should be placed on the patient to comply with the physician's prescription. At the time of designing the radiotherapy treatment plan, the physician places those dotted lines on the patient's skin with a permanent magic marker.

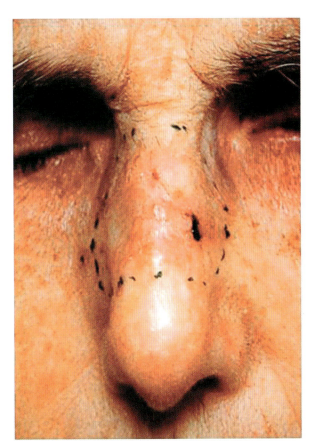

FIGURE 13.23. Basal cell carcinoma, wrapping over the bridge of the nose, prior to irradiation.

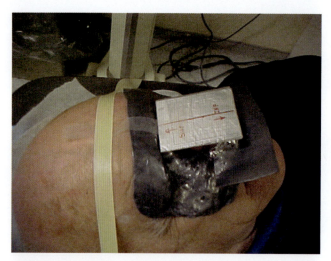

FIGURE 13.24. Clinical setup photograph showing the use of an aluminum foil attenuator and customized lead cutout shielding to protect normal tissues. The attenuator is placed to provide compensation for the missing tissue on each side of the bridge of the nose.

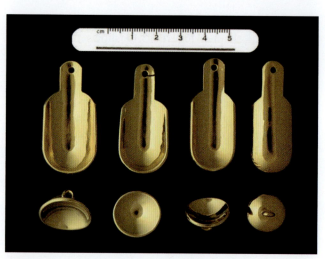

FIGURE 13.26. Gold eye shields for superficial or orthovoltage therapy can shield one or both eyelids. The spade-shaped shields can be placed to have the "handle" overlying either the upper or lower eyelid to help shield it from the therapy beam, and the spherical shields can be placed below both eyelids.

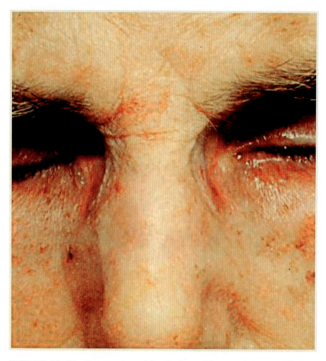

FIGURE 13.25. Regression of the lesion with complete reepithelialization is present at 3 months time. This treatment approach minimizes irradiation of tissues deep to the skin.

Figure 13.23 shows a gentleman with a basal cell carcinoma of the bridge of the nose (delineated by dotted black line) and shows the difficulty that can be encountered with complex surface changes. An aluminum foil attenuator (Fig. 13.3) was used to provide dose homogeneity at the surface and relevant superficial depths across the curved contour of the nasal bridge (Fig. 13.24). He was treated with 45 Gy in 10 fractions using 100-kV X-rays over 2 weeks time, and the cosmetic result at 3 months is shown in Figure 13.25.

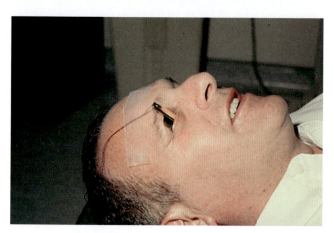

FIGURE 13.27. This gentleman was treated with 50 Gy in 20 fractions over 4 weeks' time using 100-kV X-rays for a basal cell carcinoma of the right lower eyelid. An internal gold eye shield was placed below the lower eyelid to protect the globe and upper eyelid.

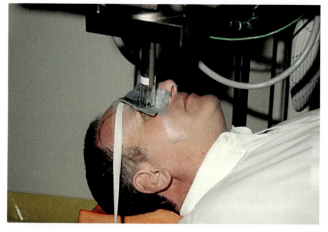

FIGURE 13.28. Treatment setup that includes additional lead cutout shielding to help protect the patient from incidental scattered irradiation.

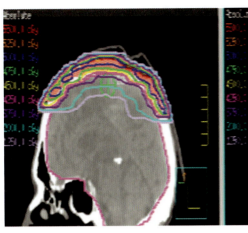
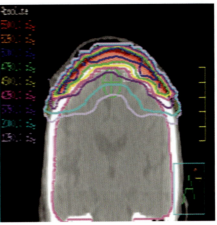

FIGURE 13.29. An example of a multi-beam IMRT plan showing that reasonable whole-scalp coverage is achievable with acceptable sparing of intracranial contents. Multiple beams are arranged to tangentially irradiate the scalp without unacceptable over- or underlap. Dose-volume histogram is shown with whole brain (*pink line*) receiving a low-dose relative to scalp (*red line*). Fatigue may be observed in the elderly thus treated.

KEY POINTS

- Skin cancer is currently most often treated with surgery, but radiotherapy remains an important therapeutic modality, especially for locations where R0 resections with acceptable cosmetic outcomes are unlikely to be achieved.

- Not every skin cancer should be treated with the same approach. The selective use of advanced imaging can help identify ostensibly normal areas that are involved with a recurrent or deeply infiltrating tumor that might have been undertreated with a simple approach.

- Normal tissue protection is as important for skin cancer radiotherapy as it is for other tumor sites. The selection of treatment techniques and the design and use of shielding, attenuators, and bolus, as well as assuring that all are being appropriately used is incumbent on the physician prescribing the treatment.

REVIEW QUESTIONS

1. Which of these skin cancers is least likely to spread to regional nodes?
   - **A.** Lentigo maligna
   - **B.** Squamous cell carcinoma
   - **C.** Merkel cell carcinoma
   - **D.** Basal cell carcinoma

2. What is the appropriate radial margin to use when prescribing orthovoltage irradiation for a 2.1-cm, moderately differentiated squamous cell carcinoma of the skin of the shoulder that recurred after a community dermatologist performed a shave excision?
   - **A.** 1.0 to 1.3 cm
   - **B.** <1.5 cm
   - **C.** >2.0 cm
   - **D.** 1.3 cm
   - **E.** 1.5 to 2.0 cm

3. What is the appropriate radial margin on the primary tumor site when treating a surgically excised Merkel cell carcinoma, where the surgeon informs you that to achieve closure, she could not achieve recommended margins of 1 to 2 cm? The pathology report indicates that the primary tumor was 1.5 cm in diameter and there was no evidence of nodal spread on the sentinel lymph node biopsy by H&E staining.
   - **A.** 2 cm
   - **B.** 3 cm
   - **C.** 4 cm
   - **D.** 5 cm

4. How many millimeters of lead must be used to protect normal tissues from an 8-MeV electron beam?
   - **A.** 2.5 mm
   - **B.** 3 mm
   - **C.** 4 mm
   - **D.** 5 mm

ANSWERS

1. **A** Although metastatic spread to regional nodes is often seen with melanoma, squamous cell carcinoma, and Merkel cell carcinoma, it is also seen, albeit very rarely, in patients with basal cell carcinoma. Lentigo maligna is a noninvasive malignancy, and therefore, has no risk of nodal metastatic spread.

2. **E** NCCN guidelines for radiotherapy margins for nonmelanoma skin cancer indicate that for lesions <2 cm, a radial margin of 1 to 1.5 cm is adequate. For lesions >2 cm, a margin of 1.5 to 2 cm is needed. If electron beam therapy is being used, even larger margins are required because of the wider penumbra, and the prescription should be written to include bolus if the full dose would not be delivered to the skin surface when an energy is chosen that will cover the deepest component of the tumor by the 90% isodose surface.

3. **D** Merkel cell carcinoma has a high propensity for occult involvement of tissues beyond any clinically apparent disease. Surgical margins of 1 to 2 cm are, therefore, recommended in the NCCN guidelines, and the prompt initiation of radiotherapy to the resection bed is well recognized to decrease local recurrence rates. In fact, the risk of occult involvement of draining lymphatics is significant enough that irradiation of nodal basins is recommended by many, with in-transit skin also included in the radiotherapy portals, if feasible, to further improve locoregional control. The addition of radiotherapy to the primary site and regional nodal volumes has not been shown with class I data to improve survival, but the relative rarity of this disease may prevent such studies from being performed.

4. **C** The "rule of thumb" for calculating the thickness of lead-equivalent shielding to protect normal tissues from incident electron beam therapy is that the thickness in millimeters of lead required is one-half the incident electron energy. This does not apply well for electron energies beyond approximately 9 MeV.

REFERENCES

1. American Joint Committee on Cancer. AJCC Cancer Staging Manual, 8th Edition. 2016.
2. NCCN Clinical Practice Guidelines in Oncology (Squamous Cell Skin Cancer, Basal Cell Skin Cancer). www.nccn.org/professionals/physician_gls. Accessed November 17, 2020.
3. Likhacheva A, Awan M, Barker CA, et al. Definitive and postoperative radiation therapy for basal and squamous cell cancers of the skin: executive summary of an American Society for Radiation Oncology Clinical Practice Guideline. *Pract Radiat Oncol.* 2020;10:8–20.
4. Chow JCL, Jiang R. Bone and mucosal dosimetry in skin radiation therapy: a Monte Carlo study using kilovoltage photon and megavoltage electron beams. *Phys Med Biol.* 2012;57:3885–3899.
5. Canters RA, Lips IM, Wendling M, et al. Clinical implementation of 3D printing in the construction of patient specific bolus for electron beam radiotherapy for non-melanoma skin cancer. *Radiother Oncol.* 2016;121(1):148–153.
6. Albantow C, Hargrave C, Brown A, Halsall C. Comparison of 3D printed nose bolus to traditional wax bolus for cost-effectiveness, volumetric accuracy and dosimetric effect. *J Med Rad Sci.* 2020;67(1):54–63.
7. Craft DF, Lentz J, Armstrong M, et al. 3D-printed on-skin radiation shields using high-density filament. *Pract Radiat Oncol.* 2020;S1879-8500(20)30100-4.
8. Pearse J, Chow JCL. An Internet of Things app for monitor unit calculation in superficial and orthovoltage skin therapy. *IOP SciNotes.* 2020;1:014002.
9. Strydom W, Parker W, Olivares M. Electron beams: physical and clinical aspects. Radiation oncology physics: a handbook for teachers and students. *Vienna:* IAEA. 2005:273–299.
10. Khan F, Doppke K, Hogstrom K, et al. Clinical Electron-Beam Dosimetry (AAPM Report No. 32). 1991.
11. Chow JCL, Grigorov GN. Effect of electron beam obliquity on lateral buildup ratio: a Monte Carlo dosimetry evaluation. *Phys Med Biol.* 2007;52:3965–3977.
12. Shiu AS, Tung SS, Gastorf RJ, et al. Dosimetric evaluation of lead and tungsten eye shields in electron beam treatment. *Int J Radiat Oncol Biol Phys.* 1996;35:599–604.
13. Amdur RJ, Kalbaugh KJ, Ewald LM, et al. Radiation therapy for skin cancer near the eye: kilovoltage x-rays versus electrons. *Int J Radiat Oncol Biol Phys.* 1992;23:769–779.
14. Chow JCL, Jiang R. Monte Carlo calculation of monitor unit for electron arc therapy. *Med Phys.* 2010;37:1571–1578.
15. Park CC, Yom SS, Podgorsak MB, et al. American Society for Therapeutic Radiology and Oncology (ASTRO) emerging technology committee report on electronic brachytherapy. *Int J Radiat Oncol Biol Phys.* 2010;76:963–972.
16. Evans MD, Podgorsak EB, Pla M, et al. Dosimetric characteristics of surface applicators for high dose-rate brachytherapy (Abstract). *Med Phys.* 1995;22:671.
17. Guix B, Finestres F, Tello J, et al. Treatment of skin carcinomas of the face by high-dose-rate brachytherapy and custom-made surface molds. *Int J Radiat Oncol Biol Phys.* 2000;47:95–102.
18. Sabbas AM, Kulidzhanov FG, Presser J, et al. HDR brachytherapy with surface applicators: technical considerations and dosimetry. *Technol Cancer Res Treat.* 2004;3:259–267.
19. Granero D, Pérez-Calatayud J, Gimeno J, et al. Design and evaluation of a HDR skin applicator with flattening filter. *Med Phys.* 2008;35:495–503.
20. Sayler E, Eldredge-Hindy H, Dinome J, et al. Clinical implementation and failure mode and effects analysis of HDR skin brachytherapy using Valencia and Leipzig surface applicators. *Brachytherapy.* 2015;14:293–299.
21. Köhler-Brock A, Prager W, Pohlmann S, et al. The indications for and results of HDR afterloading therapy in diseases of the skin and mucosa with standardized surface applicators (the Leipzig applicator). *Strahlenther Onkol.* 1999;175:170–174.
22. Tormo A, Celada F, Rodriguez S, et al. Non-melanoma skin cancer treated with HDR Valencia applicator: clinical outcomes. *J Contemp Brachytherapy.* 2014;6:167–172.

23. Nath R, Rivard MJ, DeWerd LA, et al. Guidelines by the AAPM and GEC-ESTRO on the use of innovative brachytherapy devices and applications: Report of Task Group 167. *Med Phys.* 2016;43:3178-3205.

24. Ouhib Z, Kasper M, Perez Calatayud J, et al. Aspects of dosimetry and clinical practice of skin brachytherapy: the American Brachytherapy Society working group report. *Brachytherapy.* 2015;14:840-858.

25. Shah C, Ouhib Z, Kamrava M, et al. The American Brachytherapy society consensus statement for skin brachytherapy. *Brachytherapy.* 2020;19:415-426.

26. Pons-Llanas O, Ballester-Sánchez R, Celada-Álvarez FJ, et al. Clinical implementation of a new electronic brachytherapy system for skin brachytherapy. *J Contemp Brachytherapy.* 2015;6:417–423.

27. NCCN Clinical Practice Guidelines in Oncology (Merkel Cell Carcinoma). www.nccn.org/professionals/physician_gls. Accessed November 17, 2020.

28. Tai P, Park SY, Nghiem PT. Staging, treatment, and surveillance of Merkel cell carcinoma. In: Stern RS, Robinson JK, Atkins MB, eds. *UpToDate.* Waltham, MA: UpToDate. https://www.uptodate.com/contents/staging-treatment-and-surveillance-of-merkel-cell-carcinoma? Accessed September 27, 2020.

29. Bhatia S, Storer BE, Iyer JG, et al. Adjuvant radiation therapy and chemotherapy in Merkel cell carcinoma: survival analyses of 6908 cases from the National Cancer Data Base. *J Natl Cancer Inst.* 2016;108:djw042.

30. Barrios DM, Do MH, Phillips GS, et al. Immune checkpoint inhibitors to treat cutaneous malignancies. *J Am Acad Dermatol.* 2020;83:1239-1253.

31. NCCN Clinical Practice Guidelines in Oncology (Melanoma). www.nccn.org/professionals/physician_gls. Accessed November 17, 2020.

32. Newman JC, Leffell DJ. Correlation of embryonic fusion planes with the anatomical distribution of basal cell carcinoma. *Dermatol Surg.* 2007;33:957–964; discussion 965.

33. Mendenhall WM, Amdur RJ, Hinerman RW, et al. Skin cancer of the head and neck with perineural invasion. *Am J Clin Oncol.* 2007;30:93–96.

34. Garcia-Serra A, Hinerman RW, Mendenhall WM, et al. Carcinoma of the skin with perineural invasion. *Head Neck.* 2003;25:1027–1033.

35. Gluck I, Ibrahim M, Popovtzer A, et al. Skin cancer of the head and neck with perineural invasion: defining the clinical target volumes based on the pattern of failure. *Int J Radiat Oncol Biol Phys.* 2009;74:38–46.

36. Oxenberg J, Kane JM 3rd. The role of radiation therapy in melanoma. *Surg Clin North Am.* 2014;94:1031–1047.

37. Berk LB. Radiation therapy as primary and adjuvant treatment for local and regional melanoma radiobiology of melanoma. *Cancer Control.* 2008;15:233–238.

38. Hedblad MA, Mallbris L. Grenz ray treatment of lentigo maligna and early lentigo maligna melanoma. *J Am Acad Dermatol.* 2012;67:60–68.

39. Drakensjö IRT, Rosen E, Nilsson MF, Girnita A. Ten-year follow-up study of Grenz ray treatment for lentigo maligna and early lentigo maligna melanoma. *Acta Derm Venereol.* 2020;100:adv00282.

40. Guitera P, Moloney FJ, Menzies SW, et al. Improving management and patient care in lentigo maligna by mapping with in vivo confocal microscopy. *JAMA Dermatol.* 2013;149:692–698.

41. Burmeister BH, Henderson MA, Ainslie J, et al. Adjuvant radiotherapy versus observation alone for patients at risk of lymph-node field relapse after therapeutic lymphadenectomy for melanoma: a randomised trial. *Lancet Oncol.* 2012;13:589–597.

42. Ballo MT, Ang KK. Radiation therapy for malignant melanoma. *Surg Clin North Am.* 2003;83:323–342.

43. Ballo MT, Ang KK. Radiotherapy for cutaneous malignant melanoma: rationale and indications. *Oncology* (Williston Park). 2004;18:99–107; discussion 107–110, 113–114.

44. Boyer JD, Zitelli JA, Brodland DG, et al. Local control of primary Merkel cell carcinoma: review of 45 cases treated with Mohs micrographic surgery with and without adjuvant radiation. *J Am Acad Dermatol.* 2002;47:885–892.

45. Mortier L, Mirabel X, Fournier C, et al. Radiotherapy alone for primary Merkel cell carcinoma. *Arch Dermatol.* 2003;139:1587–1590.

46. Longo MI, Nghiem P. Merkel cell carcinoma treatment with radiation: a good case despite no prospective studies. *Arch Dermatol.* 2003;139:1641–1643.

47. Medina-Franco H, Urist MM, Fiveash J, et al. Multimodality treatment of Merkel cell carcinoma: case series and literature review of 1024 cases. *Ann Surg Oncol.* 2001;8:204–208.

48. McAfee WJ, Morris CG, Mendenhall CM, et al. Merkel cell carcinoma: treatment and outcomes. *Cancer.* 2005;104:1761–1764.

49. Clark JR, Veness MJ, Gilbert R, et al. Merkel cell carcinoma of the head and neck: is adjuvant radiotherapy necessary? *Head Neck.* 2007;29:249–257.

50. Ghadjar P, Kaanders JH, Poortmans P, et al. The essential role of radiotherapy in the treatment of Merkel cell carcinoma: a study from the rare cancer network. *Int J Radiat Oncol Biol Phys.* 2011;81:e583–e591.

51. Hoeller U, Mueller T, Schubert T, et al. Regional nodal relapse in surgically staged Merkel cell carcinoma. *Strahlenther Onkol.* 2015;191:51–58.

52. Jouary T, Leyral C, Dreno B, et al. Adjuvant prophylactic regional radiotherapy versus observation in stage I merkel cell carcinoma: a multicentric prospective randomized study. *Ann Oncol.* 2012;23:1074–1080.

53. Hoppe RT. Mycosis fungoides: radiation therapy. *Dermatol Ther.* 2003;16:347–354.

54. Smith BD, Wilson LD. Management of mycosis fungoides: part 2. Treatment. *Oncology* (Williston Park). 2003;17:1419–1428; discussion 1430, 1433.

55. Hoppe RT, Kim YH, Horwitz S. Treatment of early stage (IA to IIA) mycosis fungoides. In: Kuzel TM, Zic, JA eds. *UpToDate.* Waltham, MA: UpToDate Inc. https://www.uptodate.com/contents/treatment-of-early-stage-ia-to-iia-mycosis-fungoides?topicRef=4759&source=see_link. Accessed September 27, 2020.

56. Elsayad K, Stadler R, Steinbrink K, Eich HT. Combined total skin radiotherapy and immune checkpoint inhibitors: a promising potential treatment for mycosis fungoides and Sezary syndrome. *J Dtsch Dermatol Ges.* 2020;18:193–197.

57. Smith BD, Wilson LD. Cutaneous lymphomas. *Semin Radiat Oncol.* 2007;17:158–168.

58. Cotter GW, Baglan RJ, Wasserman TH, et al. Palliative radiation treatment of cutaneous mycosis fungoides—A dose response. *Int J Radiat Oncol Biol Phys.* 1983;9:1477–1480.

59. Karzmark C, Anderson J, Fessenden P, et al. Total skin electron therapy: technique and dosimetry. *AAPM Report #23.* 1988.

60. Trump J, Wright K, Evans W, et al. High energy electrons for the treatment of extensive superficial malignant lesions. *Am J Roentgenol Radium Ther Nucl Med.* 1953;69:623–629.

61. Jones GW, Kacinski BM, Wilson LD, et al. Total skin electron radiation in the management of mycosis fungoides: consensus of the European Organization for Research and Treatment of Cancer (EORTC) Cutaneous Lymphoma Project Group. *J Am Acad Dermatol.* 2002;47:364–370.

62. Desai KR, Pezner RD, Lipsett JA, et al. Total skin electron irradiation for mycosis fungoides: relationship between acute toxicities and measured dose at different anatomic sites. *Int J Radiat Oncol Biol Phys.* 1988; 15:641-645.

63. Lloyd, S, Chen Z, Foss FM, et al. Acute toxicity and risk of infection during total skin electron beam therapy for mycosis fungoides. *J Am Acad Dermatol.* 2013;69:537-543.

64. Chowdhary, M, Chhabra AM, Kharod S, Marwaha G. Total skin electron beam therapy in the treatment of mycosis fungoides: a review of conventional and low-dose regimens. *Clin Lymphoma Myeloma Leuk.* 2016;16:662-671.

65. Chowdhary M, Song A, Zaorsky NG, Shi W. Total skin electron beam therapy in mycosis fungoides-a shift towards lower dose? *Chin Clin Oncol.* 2019;8:9.

66. Chen Z, Agostinelli AG, Wilson LD, et al. Matching the dosimetry characteristics of a dual-field Stanford technique to a customized single-field Stanford technique for total skin electron therapy. *Int J Radiat Oncol Biol Phys.* 2004;59:872–885.

67. Karzmark CJ, Loevinger R, Steele RE, et al. A technique for large-field, superficial electron therapy. *Radiology.* 1960;74:633–644.

68. Page V, Gardner A, Karzmark CJ. Patient dosimetry in the electron treatment of large superficial lesions. *Radiology*. 1970;94:635–641.

69. Podgorsak EB, Pla C, Pla M, et al. Physical aspects of a rotational total skin electron irradiation. *Med Phys*. 1983;10:159–168.

70. Guidi G, Gottardi G, Ceroni P, Costi T. Review of the results of the in vivo dosimetry during total skin electron beam therapy. *Rep Pract Oncol Radiother*. 2013;19:144–150.

71. Pavón EC, Sánchez-Doblado F, Leal A, et al. Total skin electron therapy treatment verification: Monte Carlo simulation and beam characteristics of large non-standard electron fields. *Phys Med Biol*. 2003;48:2783–2796.

72. Nevelsky A, Borzov E, Daniel S, Bar-Deroma R. Validation of total skin electron irradiation (TSEI) technique dosimetry data by Monte Carlo simulation. *J Appl Clin Med Phys*. 2016;17:418–429.

14 Pediatric Malignancies

Myrsini Ioakeim–Ioannidou, Shannon M. MacDonald, and Nancy J. Tarbell

INTRODUCTION

There are several special aspects to consider for radiation treatment planning for children. Pediatric radiation oncology differs from other radiation subspecialties in that it involves knowledge of all anatomic locations. Tolerances for organs at risk differ from adults due to growth and development. There is also greater variability in patient size and the ability of young patients to cooperate during planning and treatment. Pediatric malignancies are relatively rare. For this reason, the pediatric radiation oncology community relies greatly on the collective experience of our specialty and the collaboration with colleagues around the world. Forums and guidelines exist through Children's Oncology Group (COG) and the Pediatric Radiation Oncology Society (PROS).[1,2] These websites help to provide general radiation guidelines and also the ability to communicate with other subspecialists in pediatric oncology, enabling pediatric oncologists to benefit from the experience of others. Given that approximately 80% of pediatric cancer patients will go on to be long-term survivors, it is of paramount importance that radiation treatment plans are devised with great care to ensure the best possible local control with the lowest possible risk of long-term side effects.[3] Survivorship clinics now exist for adults who have survived the childhood malignancies to provide ongoing care for late effects of therapy and these patients help motivate pediatric oncologists to continually strive to maintain excellent cancer outcomes with less morbidity.[4]

Radiation Delivery for Children

Modern radiation planning and delivery for pediatrics take advantage of many of the same technological advances in imaging, planning software systems, and radiation modalities used for the adult population. Nearly all treatments are planned using three-dimensional (3D) imaging and cutting edge modalities such as proton radiation, carbon-ion radiotherapy, and intensity-modulated radiation to provide maximal normal tissue sparing. Advances in imaging have allowed for more precise definition of structures and areas at risk and radiation guidelines over time have allowed for smaller margins due to improved delineation of tumors and minimization of setup error.

Immobilization

Immobilization is often a challenge for young children. They may be fearful of the therapy or treatment room and may lack the ability to understand the importance of remaining still for treatment. For young children or those unable to tolerate treatment without sedation, anesthesia is necessary. It is crucial for the pediatric radiation oncology team to have a good working relationship with the pediatric anesthesia team to ensure optional positioning so that treatments may be delivered safely and efficiently. Children do not generally require deep sedation for radiation therapy as the purpose of anesthesia is to keep the patient from moving; therefore, the use of a conscious sedative rather than full general anesthetic requiring intubation is preferred at most institutions. Propofol is generally used at our institution due to ease of administration and rapid recovery. Intravenous access is required for this type of sedation.[5] A portacath is the most common mode of access and many patients will have a portacath for chemotherapy administration; some may have a Broviac catheter device that can also be used.[6,7] Children with a portacath can be accessed on Mondays prior to treatment and have the access removed on Fridays following treatment. While positioning is optimized for RT delivery, a good airway will supersede this for children under anesthesia. Most children need only an oxygen mask, but a few will require a laryngeal mask airway (LMA) or nasal trumpet to maintain a good airway. Prone positioning is the most challenging for achieving and maintaining a good airway, but this is still possible for the vast majority of patients. Older children, generally over the age of 6, can usually tolerate treatment without sedation. Music or a video may be helpful for soothing anxiety or providing distraction. Select children that cannot initially tolerate treatment without anesthesia often respond to coaching by nurses, child life specialists, and even other pediatric patients going through a similar treatment. The ability to avoid anesthesia allows for maintenance of a regular meal schedule, thereby limiting impact on weight loss or gain, and decreases the amount of time spent in the radiation oncology department, permitting greater preservation of the child's routine or "normal" life. In addition, avoidance of anesthesia limits the strain on hospital resources, including nursing and anesthesia staff while also reducing time on radiation treatment machines, and decreases the cost of a radiation course.

Some immobilization devices may be uncomfortable for children or difficult to use, as most were manufactured for adults and later adapted for use in children. Immobilization for the treatment of brain or head and neck tumors is usually accomplished with a molded thermoplastic mask. Metallic markers can be placed on the mask to help with localization. Some stereotactic treatments require a more rigid frame, often with a bite block. These systems are sometimes only feasible for a single-fraction treatment and usually too difficult for children to tolerate without sedation. Treatment to the trunk of the body or extremities will require the placement of permanent "tattoos" to help with the accuracy of the daily setup and it is very important to review with parents and children the placement and permanency of these tattoos. The placement of tattoos for children can be difficult as they are fearful of needles and more difficult for parents to accept. Some institutions use nonpermanent marks, but care must be taken to ensure these marks will last for the entire treatment course. Vac-loc bags, leg immobilizers, or custom-made immobilization devices are used depending upon treatment site and patient anatomy. Respiratory gating or a four-dimensional computed tomography (4D CT) to determine the margin needed to account for respiratory motion is appropriate for some thoracic and abdominal locations. Image-guided radiation therapy with daily KV quality images or cone-beam CT is generally used to allow for a small setup margin and to improve accuracy. The dose of radiation from setup imaging is small but may need to be discussed with parents in the era of a more heightened awareness of diagnostic radiation exposure for pediatric patients.[8–10]

Three-Dimensional Treatment Planning

Three-dimensional (3D) planning should be used for most, if not all, pediatric radiation treatments. Most departments obtain a CT scan in the treatment position and fuse diagnostic magnetic resonance imaging (MRI), CT, and/or positron emission tomography (PET)/CT sequences for treatment planning. Some radiation departments utilize MRI or PET/CT treatment planning scanners. As our imaging techniques have improved, margins for error around this volume can be made smaller, thereby allowing for full coverage of the tumor with improved avoidance of the surrounding healthy tissues.

Intensity-Modulated Radiation Therapy

Intensity-Modulated Radiation Therapy (IMRT) allows for the most conformal photon plan with high-dose isodose lines closely surrounding the target volume. While IMRT plans decrease high and moderate dose to nearby structures, these plans typically result in the delivery of low-dose radiation to a larger volume of tissue outside of the target. While this may be a little consequence in terms of function, second malignancy is a risk for even low-dose radiation and is a greater concern for the pediatric population.[11] Despite this concern, recent data with reasonably long follow-up indicate that the risk of second malignancy for pediatric patients treated with IMRT may still be low.[12] Longer follow-up with these techniques will be important to accurately assess the risk of a second malignancy in this cohort.

Proton Radiation

Proton radiation is a form of particle radiation that allows for complete sparing of tissue beyond the target volume for a given beam and often decreased dose proximal to the target compared to photon radiation.[13] Proton therapy decreases both high- and low-dose regions outside of the target volume. Pediatric tumors are considered one of the best indications for this type of treatment given the importance of sparing developing tissue from radiation. Proton radiation can be delivered using 3D conformal proton radiation (3DCPT), also referred to as double-scattered proton technique. For this treatment, individual proton beams of the required energies are stacked to create a modulated beam or Spread Out Bragg Peak (SOBP). This beam is passed through a brass aperture to shape the beam to the outline of the tumor and a Lucite compensator to allow the beam to conform to the distal edge of the tumor. Further developments in proton beam irradiation allow for delivery of protons with a scanning or pencil beam technique. Using this technique, several small pencil beams of proton radiation are scanned in layers across the target. Intensity-modulated proton therapy (IMPT) using pencil beam scanning (PBS) is a proton treatment planning and delivery method that allows for increased dose conformity and increased degrees of freedom in dose-shaping capabilities.[14] Additionally, it allows for larger treatment field sizes and may constitute a more robust delivery technique for treatments such as craniospinal irradiation (CSI), compared to passive scattering (PS), which, due to field size limitations, requires longitudinal field conjunctions, which are potentially sensitive to set-up errors. Those advances in proton therapy and improvements in immobilization and set-up verification now allow for delivery of proton CSI with substantial sparing of the vertebral bodies for fully grown children and are being studied for children that have not yet reached full height (NCT03281889). Vertebral body sparing (VBS) techniques allow for minimal

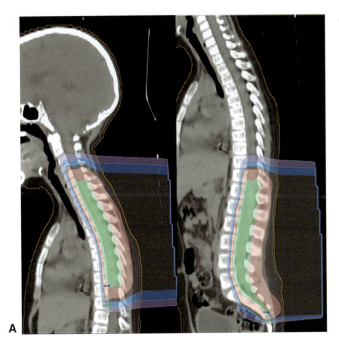

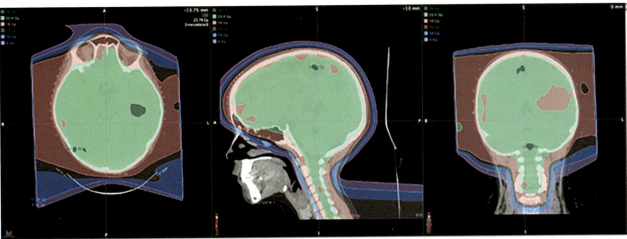

FIGURE 14.1. Pencil Beam Scanning technique for VBS CSI including matched PA spine fields (**A**) and two oblique fields for whole brain (**B**). CSI, craniospinal irradiation; PA; VBS, vertebral body sparing.

to no exit dose to thyroid, esophagus anterior to vertebral body and spare more bone and bone marrow, which may allow for additional growth and greater tolerance to chemotherapeutic regimens. Risks for growing children include a greater growth of the anterior vertebral column compared to the posterior vertebral column but clinical data available indicate no clinical sequalae from this treatment and a compensatory disc hypertrophy posteriorly[15] (Fig. 14.1).

The physical properties of protons result in superior sparing of tissues compared to photons and for a given dose in Gray-Radiobiological Equivalent (Gy(RBE)), it is considered to be biologically equivalent to photons. While clinical experience for protons is still limited relative to photon experience, many publications have supported disease outcomes that are comparable to favorable

to photons and suggest that morbidity is less.[16–21] Some tumors, such as chordoma or osteosarcoma, require a proton component to achieve the degree of sparing necessary to avoid toxicity to critical structures. Given that protons are dependent on tissue density, care must be taken when surgical hardware is in the treatment field. Often, for these cases, a combination of proton therapy and photon therapy is useful. Figure 14.2 shows a cervical spine chordoma for which beam angles with protons were limited due to metallic hardware. A volumetric-modulated arc therapy (VMAT) component was utilized for a portion of the plan to allow for the best conformity and a more robust plan. At the time of this writing, 31 proton centers exist, and many others are in either construction or planning phases despite the high capital costs involved with building a center and the higher operational costs.[22]

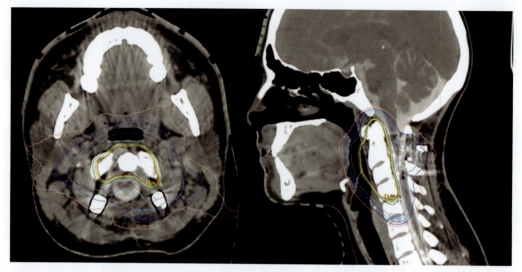

FIGURE 14.2. Mixed proton–photon plan with VMAT and PBS for upper cervical spine chordoma with limited proton beam angles due to metallic hardware used for posterior spinal stabilization. CT myelogram is a useful tool in radiation planning to better define the spinal cord in treatment position. CT, computed tomography; PBS, pencil beam scanning; VMAT, volumetric-modulated arc therapy.

Carbon Ion Radiotherapy

Similar to proton radiation, carbon ion radiotherapy (CIRT) presents a new promising treatment option for tumors, which are resistant to conventional radiotherapy. Radiobiologically, carbon-ion beams result in two to three times the relative biological effect (RBE; the ratio of the doses required by two radiation types to cause the same level of effect) of proton and photon radiation, while they exhibit a larger energy loss. In contrast to conventional radiotherapy, CIRT does not show an oxygen effect, repair of potentially lethal damage, and has less radiosensitivity throughout the cell cycle.[23]

Although, CIRT is not available in the United States, 11 cancer therapy centers worldwide offer CIRT, with the majority of these being located in Asia and a few in Europe. Until 2016, approximately 21,580 patients were recorded to have been treated with CIRT internationally.[24]

Radiation-resistant bone and soft-tissue tumors, including osteosarcomas, chordomas, chondrosarcomas, and soft-tissue sarcomas resistant to systemic therapy, have been effectively treated with CIRT.[25–27]

PEDIATRIC DISEASE SITES OR TREATMENT PLANNING

Medulloblastoma

Medulloblastoma is the most common embryonal tumor arising in the posterior fossa. The World Health Organization (WHO) has recently reclassified CNS tumors subclassifying medulloblastoma by either molecular or histological definitions.[28] Patients usually present with headaches, nausea or vomit, and ataxia, symptoms suggestive of cerebrospinal fluid flow obstruction due to mass effect. Workup includes MRI of the brain that characteristically shows a mass in the cerebellum filling the fourth ventricle and causing obstructive hydrocephalus. Maximal safe resection is recommended and additional workup includes MRI of the spine (preferably presurgical or 10–14 days after surgery) and a lumbar puncture to obtain cerebrospinal fluid (CSF) (10–14 days after surgery; CSF should be obtained by LP and should not be performed prior to surgery due to risk of herniation). As tumor size is not prognostic, the status of metastatic disease is predominantly used for staging. At present, a risk stratification system based on clinical factors divides patients into two risk groups, "high-risk" and "standard-risk", with standard-risk defined as children over the age of 3 with ≤1.5 cm^2 of residual disease following surgery and no metastatic disease (grossly or in CSF) and all others considered high risk. In recent years, diffuse anaplastic histology has been found to portend a poor prognosis and these patients should be considered for high-risk therapy regimens.[29] Molecular profiles will likely supersede current staging and histological risk stratification, but at present, these profiles are used to dictate treatment only in the setting of a clinical trial.[30–33] Accepted radiation treatment for standard-risk disease is 23.4 CSI followed by a whole posterior fossa or involved field (IF) boost to 54 Gy. A recent COG trial (ACNS 0331) showed that standard-risk patients can be treated with an IF boost to the resection bed plus margin rather than the whole posterior fossa boost without any difference in disease outcome.[34] However, reduced dose CSI of 18 Gy resulted in inferior overall survival and leptomeningeal control when compared with 23.4 Gy CSI.[34] Lower CSI doses have and are being investigated for young children (<8 years old) and for molecularly favorable profiles.[35] Standard treatment for high-risk disease includes CSI to 36 Gy followed by whole posterior fossa or involved-field boost to 54 Gy. Any sites of initial metastatic disease in the spine should receive 45 Gy and metastatic lesions in the brain should receive at least 45 Gy, sometimes a higher dose depending on location and the perceived risk-benefit ratio. Management for children under the age of 3 is a bit more heterogeneous and generally consists of maximal safe resection followed by high-dose chemotherapy with stem cell rescue followed by delayed and usually localized radiation therapy.[36–38] In these very young children that present with disseminated or refractory disease, low-dose CSI may be considered following chemotherapy depending on patient age and parental wishes. Disease-free survival for a patient with standard-risk disease treated with chemotherapy and radiation exceeds 80%.[29] Cure rates for high-risk disease are less favorable but fall between 50% and 70%.[39] Children with standard-risk disease with anaplastic histology have a disease-free survival in between these two groups of approximately 73%.[29] Future subgroup-specific trials will introduce risk-stratified therapies aiming to reduce adverse effects, while achieving excellent tumor control.

Central Nervous System Embryonal Tumors Not Otherwise Specified (Formerly Supratentorial PNETS)

These tumors are histologically similar to medulloblastoma but are located outside of the posterior fossa in any location of the supratentorial brain. They are highly malignant small round blue cell tumors that have a propensity to spread through the CSF. While treatment regimens differ, intensive treatment with surgery, radiation, and chemotherapy is indicated for all embryonal tumor subtypes for the best chance of disease control and survival. Pineoblastoma is a subset of formerly Supratentorial PNETs (SPNETs). The prognosis for patients with this disease is worse than medulloblastoma even in the absence of dissemination. All patients with these tumors are therefore considered to have "high-risk" disease, regardless of whether or not disease is metastatic at diagnosis, and standard CSI doses for localized or metastatic disease is 36 Gy. A dose of 54 Gy is recommended to the tumor bed plus a margin of approximately 1 cm within anatomical boundaries. For children under the age of 3, involved-field radiation to 50.4–54 Gy is generally recommended. Similar to medulloblastoma, management for children under the age of three is maximal safe resection followed by chemotherapy followed by delayed, and usually localized, radiation therapy.[40,41]

Atypical teratoid rhabdoid tumors (ATRT) are rare malignancies that typically affect very young children. These tumors arise most frequently in the posterior fossa or the cerebrum. ATRTs look similar to medulloblastoma but have a mutation that results in a deficiency of INI-1 protein.[42] The prognosis for ATRT is inferior to that for medulloblastoma; however, with more aggressive chemotherapy, 2-year progression-free and overall survival rates of 53% and 70%, respectively, can be achieved.[43] The

treatment of ATRT includes maximal resection of primary disease, intense induction chemotherapy including intrathecal chemotherapy, high-dose chemotherapy followed by stem cell rescue (HDCSCR), and radiation therapy. For children under the age of 3, localized radiation is recommended. For older children, CSI followed by additional IF radiation is favored due to risk of dissemination and poor prognosis.[44] Multiple studies have found that age greater than 3 years old is associated with better prognosis.[44–46] In the last COG study, ACNS0333 delivered IF RT for all children with localized disease, regardless of age and age-modified CSI for those with disseminated disease.[47] Fifty-four of 65 patients were <36 months of age. The 4-year EFS and OS were 37% and 43%, respectively. Although there is limited data on effective CSI dose, given the more aggressive nature of this disease, 36 Gy is most standard for CSI. A dose of 50.4 to 54 Gy is recommended to the IF.

Embryonal tumors are highly radiosensitive tumors. As a result, the technical quality of radiation delivery significantly influences the risk of recurrence. Treatment planning, especially CSI, must be planned with utmost care. The craniospinal volume includes the entire brain and spine. Care should be taken to ensure coverage of the cribriform plate and to give a margin of at least one vertebral body below the thecal sac, which is typically located near S2, but can vary. Adequate margin lateral to the thecal sac is also required. It is best to confirm the location of these regions with a neuroradiologist to ensure coverage. Most CSI treatments are delivered with the patient in the prone position with arms down, although supine CSI treatment is now being delivered in the supine position at several institutions. There was some reluctance to deliver CSI in the supine position, as clinical verification that matched spinal fields is only possible in the prone position. However, there is also a possibility that overconcern regarding field overlap could lead to "colder" cold spots potentially increasing the risk of relapse. The neck is hyperextended so that spine fields do not exit through the patient's mouth for photon therapy. For protons, this is not a concern due to lack of exit dose. The spinal field is typically too long to treat with just one field and typically 2 to 3 fields are necessary. Fields are matched anterior to the spinal cord, which creates a small area of underdosing in the cord but avoids any areas of overlap or hot spots in the cord. (Fig. 14.3) Care should be taken to minimize these areas of slight under and overdosing and fields should be "feathered" (match point varied during treatment) to minimize these areas and decrease uncertainty. Patients receiving CSI with volumetric arc therapy may be higher risk of developing secondary malignancies compared to patients treated with 3D conformal therapy.[48] The use of IMRT and scanning proton techniques allow for treatment without field matching of fields and because of the lack of exit dose protons avoids exit dose to the thyroid, heart, lungs, abdominal organs, and ovaries. The intracranial compartment includes all of CSF space surrounding the brain. The posterior fossa volume extends from the

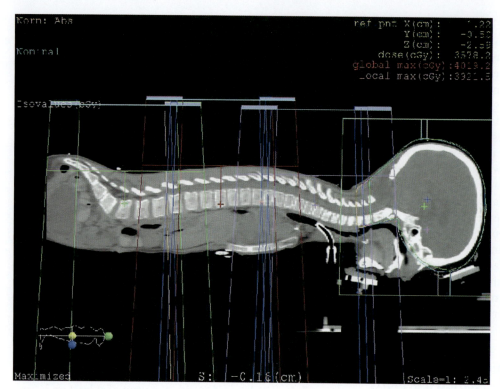

FIGURE 14.3. Craniospinal irradiation requires spinal fields to be matched. Fields should be matched anterior to spinal cord, which creates a small cold spot within the cord. To minimize this slightly underdosed area and to minimize the uncertainty associated with matched fields, fields are "feathered" so that this match is moved to different locations during treatment.

tentorium superiorly to C1 inferiorly. Laterally, the posterior fossa volume includes the entire cerebellum and extends to the bony occiput, and anteriorly, this volume includes the brainstem and lower midbrain (as defined by COG guidelines). The IF volume GTV should include the tumor bed (anything in contact with the initial tumor prior to surgery) and any residual gross disease. Care should be taken to ensure coverage of anything touched by the initial tumor and also to account for anatomical shifts following surgery. An expansion of 1 to 1.5 cm is typically used to form the CTV for the IF boost, limited by bony anatomy and the tentorium.

Ependymoma

Intracranial ependymomas are brain tumors that originate from ependymal cells lining the ventricles or from ependymal cell rests located in the brain parenchyma. The majority (approximately two thirds) occurs in the posterior fossa/fourth ventricle and the remainder occurs in the supratentorial brain.[49] According to the WHO, there are three histopathological groups with several subcategories. The WHO CNS fourth edition has updated those subclassifications recognizing the first molecular ependymoma variant, the RELA fusion-positive subtype.[28] The cIMPACT-NOW panel has recently revised grading of myxopapillary ependymoma to grade II (applicable to spinal ependymoma).[50] Diagnostic workup includes MRI of the brain and spine and CSF sampling, though CSF is rarely positive when MRIs show no evidence of metastatic

disease.[51] Intracranial ependymomas have been defined as classic/differentiated (WHO grade II) or anaplastic (WHO grade III) by histology, but this may change in the future as molecular profiles seem more indicative of prognosis. RELA fusion subtype comprises 70% of supratentorial ependymomas.[52] Infratentorial ependymomas are classified as EPN_PFA or EPN_PFB. The initial treatment for intracranial ependymoma is maximal safe resection. Removal of the entire tumor is critical for a favorable outcome and this has been demonstrated clearly in both small and large series. For localized disease, the 3- to 5-year progression-free survival rates range from 51% to 88% for gross total resection and from 0% to 54% for subtotal resection.[16,53] If complete removal is achieved, radiation to the tumor bed plus a margin is recommended. If resection is incomplete, a short course of chemotherapy followed by a second look surgery in attempt to achieve a gross total resection prior to radiation is generally favored. In the largest prospective trial so far (COG ACNS0121), survival rates in very young children treated with immediate postoperative radiation therapy were more than twice that of children treated using strategies that delayed the use of irradiation.[54] The 5-year EFS was 37.2% for patients with an STR and 68.5% for patients with an NTR/GTR. Anaplastic histology and 1q gain were significant adverse prognostic factors. Chemotherapy has not shown benefit for this disease and cannot be used in place of RT; it is unclear if chemotherapy adds benefit over surgery and radiation alone, but this is being investigated in a randomized fashion on the current

COG protocol, ACNS0831. Off protocol, maximal resection and radiation remain standard. Although there are concerns about radiating very young children, localized radiation has been proven safe and effective for children as young as 12 months of age.

Treatment planning should start with a careful review of all images with a neuroradiologist to determine any areas of residual disease and review all surfaces contacted by initial tumor. Infratentorial ependymomas are notorious for extension through the foramina of Luschka and Magendie. It is critical to determine original tumor extension into these regions and treat these surfaces. Contouring the preoperative volume to become familiar with both the anatomical location of the tumor as well as ependymal and CNS structures in contact with the tumor may be useful. Care should be taken to adjust this volume for anatomical shifts following surgery. The GTV should include any surface contacted by the original tumor as well as any gross residual disease. The CTV expansion should be approximately 5 mm with constraints for anatomical boundaries. The recommended dose to this volume is 54 to 59.4 Gy in 30 to 33 fractions. The recently closed and current COG protocols (ACNS0121 and ACNS0831, respectively) prescribe a total dose of 59.4 Gy, but ACNS0831 requires that critical structures (the spinal cord and optics) outside of the area of highest risk be blocked after 54 Gy. It should be recognized that brainstem tolerance is considered 54 Gy and that doses in excess of this may increase the risk of brainstem necrosis. Many do however feel that the risk of local recurrence after radiation warrants this additional risk. Children under the age of 18 months or with known brainstem injury should not receive a total dose in excess of 54 Gy. Off protocol, our institution generally favors a dose of 54 Gy for patients who have undergone a gross total resection and have infratentorial disease that are being treated with proton therapy. Adjuvant radiation to a total dose of 54 to 59.4 Gy is indicated for grade III or subtotal resected supratentorial tumors. Again, care should be taken to define GTV as any residual tumor and areas of the cerebrum in contact with presurgical tumor. Due to shifts in the brain parenchyma, this is sometimes challenging and sulci/gyri of the brain in contact with the initial tumor should be reviewed with a neuroradiologist. Figure 14.4 shows an IMRT plan for a patient with an infratentorial ependymoma. Although supratentorial WHO Grade II tumors that are completely resected have been observed without radiation on protocol, all patients off study should receive RT. Limited data exist for patients with metastatic ependymoma and outcomes are very poor. Most patients are treated with CSI to 36 Gy followed by a localized boost to 54 to 59.4 Gy. For patients with recurrence following radiation, re-irradiation has been explored and may allow for long-term survival for some patients, but, in general, this treatment is considered palliative.

Spinal cord ependymomas are most commonly low-grade tumors that are relatively rare in pediatric

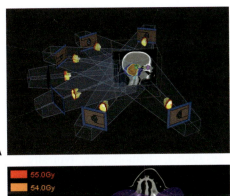

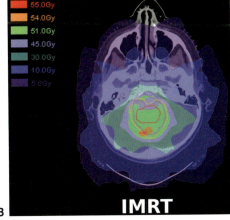

FIGURE 14.4. Intensity modulated radiation therapy (IMRT) is one advanced technique used for the treatment of pediatric malignancies. It shows beam arrangement and intensity modulation of fields for an infratentorial ependymoma (**A**) and an axial image of plan and doses (**B**).

population. MRI of the brain and the entire axis along with CSF cytology is required for any patient with anaplastic disease or other concern for dissemination. Adjuvant radiation is often recommended after subtotal or piecemeal resection of myxopapillary or grade II ependymomas aiming to achieve better local control; however, several studies suggest radiation in the setting of recurrence.[55,56] If nondisseminated disease, radiation to a cumulative dose of 50.4 to 54 Gy is delivered to the tumor bed and any residual disease. CSI to a dose of 36 Gy should be considered for patients with disseminated or metastatic disease.

Low-Grade Glioma

Though the most common pediatric brain tumor, low-grade gliomas can be cured with surgery alone if they occur in a location amenable to surgery with acceptable morbidity, and therefore, many do not require radiation. Tumors that occur in the hypothalamus, thalamus, tectum, optics, and brainstem often require radiation, as surgical morbidity may be unacceptable in these locations. Histological subtypes of pediatric low-grade gliomas include pilocytic (WHO grade I) and diffuse (WHO grade II), with pilocytic astrocytoma accounting for the majority of tumors in young children. Younger patients are often treated with chemotherapy to delay radiation and for children with NF-1 chemotherapy alone may be sufficient and spontaneous regression has been reported. Packer et al. reported a 68% 3-year progression-free survival rate for children treated with carboplatin and vincristine.[57] Additional chemotherapeutic agents have since been studied and also shown efficacy, but second- and third-line regiments tend to lead to less efficacious and less durable results. For most children with low-grade glioma, chemotherapy typically delays progression, but radiation is often required for definitive treatment. Overall survival rates are excellent for most of the low-grade gliomas, with 20-year overall survival up to 87%.[58,59] When determining the appropriate therapy, one must also consider the cumulative morbidity of multiple regimens and risks of functional loss from progression of tumor. Data also indicate that young children are more likely to respond and have a durable response than older children. Radiation provides durable control. Merchant et al. report 10-year progression-free survival rates of 74% for conformal focal radiation.[60,61] A prospective study by Marcus et al. evaluated the efficacy of stereotactic radiotherapy, as up-front or salvage treatment, for small (less than 5 cm) tumors and they concluded that this approach offers excellent local control with 5- and 8-year PFS rates being 82.5% and 65%, respectively, supporting the use of limited margins to lower the risk of radiation-related toxicities.[62] In the same study, the overall survival was 97.8% at 5 years and 82% at 8 years.[62] The recent COG phase II study (ACNS0221) evaluated conformal radiation for pediatric low-grade glioma and reported 5-year PFS and OS rates of 71% and 93% respectively, with no marginal failures.[63] In addition, as evidenced by a few retrospective studies, proton therapy seems to provide similar tumor control to photons while reducing the low/intermediate dose to developing brain tissue.[64,65]

Because these tumors are not highly infiltrative, only a small volume expansion is necessary around visible tumors. The GTV should include enhancing and non-enhancing or cystic tumor plus a small margin, typically 3 to 5 mm. A dose of 50.4 to 54 Gy is recommended. If tumors contain a cystic component, it is important to monitor the cystic component for changes during radiation therapy and adjust the plan as needed. Although it is relatively rare for low-grade gliomas to disseminate, for these cases, the treatment plan is individualized. Radiation volumes may encompass the entire craniospinal axis to a dose of 36 Gy followed by IF treatment to 45–54 Gy depending on tumor location. Pseudo-progression enhancement and/or enlargement of tumor may occur following treatment, most frequently at 6 to 12 months following delivery of radiation.[64,66,67] Care should be taken to consider this in order to avoid unnecessary treatment or assume tumor progression or transformation to a more malignant process.

High-Grade Glioma

High-grade gliomas of the supratentorial brain are seen much less frequently in the pediatric population, than the adult population. Most high-grade gliomas are localized. Maximal safe resection followed by radiation is standard. Macdonald et al. found a 5-year overall survival of only 24% in pediatric patients with high-grade glioma treated with conventional radiation of 59.4 Gy.[68] Chemotherapy has been studied, but without great success and temozolomide seems less efficacious for children than adults, perhaps due to the relatively low frequency of MGMT deletion for childhood tumors.[69] Despite this, at present, temozolomide is often used as a first-line chemotherapy concurrent with RT and following RT due to absence of a more effective agent and the still relatively poor prognosis of high-grade gliomas in children. The COG phase II study ACNS0423 concluded that the addition of lomustine to temozolomide was associated with significantly improved outcome compared with the preceding COG ACNS0126 study in which participants received temozolomide alone, but outcomes were still poor.[70,71] Despite a less favorable prognosis compared with many other pediatric brain tumors, long-term survival is attainable for some children, especially the very young, and some pediatric patients with high-grade gliomas will be long-term survivors.[72] The use of targeted agents is being investigated in several ongoing studies.

For treatment planning, one must be careful to include areas of contrast enhancement and T2 FLAIR signal abnormality for the initial GTV. Again, review of all MRI sequences with pediatric neuroradiologist should be done. The GTV plus a generous margin of approximately 1 to 1.5 cm is usually treated to 45 Gy. The enhancing area plus a margin should receive a boost dose to bring this region to a dose of 54 to 59.4 Gy. While anatomical boundaries such as bone and tentorium should be respected when defining the CTV, these tumors often cross white matter tracts and it is important to consider this when defining tumor margins to account for microscopic spread of disease.

Diffuse Pontine Glioma

Diffuse infiltrating pontine gliomas (DIPG) are high-grade tumors that arise from the pons. These tumors have a characteristic appearance on MRI of a non-enhancing T2 bright lesion that expands the pons. Biopsy is not necessary when this classic radiographic appearance is evident; however, more recently and for clinical trials, pathology is obtained for molecular profiling and sometimes drug selection.[73] Radiation is palliative but indicated to the tumor with a small margin to a dose of approximately 54 Gy. Symptoms almost always improve promptly with treatment, but sadly, duration of resolution or improvement of presenting symptoms is relatively short, on the order of months. This disease is almost uniformly fatal and the median survival is approximately 1 year. Dose escalations of radiation, altered fractionation, and chemotherapy have all been explored and have failed to improve DFS or OS.[74,75] No effective treatment exists for recurrence following RT, and time to death after relapse is approximately 3 months.[76] The use and benefit of reirradiation have been reported in progressive DIPG with a median survival of 5 to 7 months following the second course of RT and without any complications, with the majority of the patients being treated with conventional RT at doses of 20 to 36 Gy.[77] Molecular targets are currently under investigation for this tumor, but to date, no successful systemic agent has been defined.

Germinoma/Non-Germinomatous Germ Cell Tumors

Pediatric intracranial germ cell tumors are rare and usually occur in adolescents. The most common locations for these tumors are in the pineal gland and infundibulum/suprasellar region. Rarely, they occur in other locations of the brain, with the third most common location being the basal ganglia. Bifocal or metachronous tumors are present in 5% to 25% of all cases.[78,79] When a GCT is suspected by MRI findings, serum tumor markers, α-fetoprotein (AFP), and β Human Chorionic Gonadotropin (β-HCG) should be obtained. If a lumbar puncture can be safely performed, CSF should be obtained for cytology and tumor markers. MRI of the spine is also standard to rule out disseminated disease. Pathology is subdivided into two broad categories: pure germinomas (PG) and non-germinomatous germ cell tumors (NGGCT).[80,81]

"Pure" germinomas are highly curable tumors with DFS rates in excess of 90% for both localized and disseminated disease. In the United States, chemotherapy followed by response-based reduced-dose radiation is usually recommended for children to eliminate late side effects of radiation. Two to four cycles of platinum-based therapy, usually carboplatin and etoposide are delivered. If a complete response is achieved, a dose of 21 Gy to the whole ventricles followed by a boost to 30 to 40 Gy to the primary tumor region is delivered, as most of the relapses occur within the ventricular system.[82] If a complete response is not achieved, a second-look surgery is recommended (if this can be safely performed) to ensure that a non-germinomatous component is not present and/or higher doses of radiation may be recommended. Some studies have explored the use of chemotherapy followed by involved-field radiation to 30 to 40 Gy. Early reports showed promising results, but higher rates of ventricular relapse were later reported by Alapetite and colleagues, resulting in a shift back to a larger low-dose volume, whole-ventricular RT, first followed by an involved-field boost.[82,83] The most recent COG protocol, ACNS1123 investigated the use of pre-RT chemotherapy with four

cycles of carboplatin and etoposide followed by very low-dose whole-ventricular radiation to 18 Gy and a boost to a total of 30 Gy to the primary tumor for localized PG following a complete response to four cycles of carboplatin and etoposide. Results of this study arm are anticipated in the near future. For rare cases of PG arising in the basal ganglia, whole-brain radiation is favored over whole-ventricular radiation.

The prognosis for non-germinomatous germ cell tumors is inferior to PG. The standard chemotherapeutic regimen in the United States consists of 6 cycles of alternating carboplatin/etoposide and ifosfamide/etoposide followed by radiation. Patients who do not have a complete response to chemotherapy should undergo a second look surgery and those who have viable tumors remaining have been shown to have an inferior prognosis. For these unfortunate patients, high-dose chemotherapy followed by stem cell rescue should be considered.[84] The ACNS0122 COG protocol delivered CSI to 36 Gy followed by a boost to the tumor volume to 54 Gy after 6 cycles of chemotherapy. The 5-year event-free and overall survival rates, of 84% and 93%, respectively, have been published.[85] Stratum 1 of ACNS1123, which used a limited RT field for patients with localized NGGCT delivering 30.6 Gy to the whole ventricles followed by a dose of 54 Gy to the IF following CR or PR to chemotherapy, identified a similar PFS and OS as ACN 0122 though at earlier follow-up.[86] ACNS1123 also showed that a lower dose of 30.6 Gy (as opposed to 36 Gy) was successful for the treatment of microscopic disease as there were no failures seen in the ventricles. Nonetheless, this study closed due to an excess of failures in the spine. The next NGGCT trial led by COG and open to young adults through the national NCI Clinical Trials Network (NCTN) program, ACNS2021, will investigate the use of whole ventricle and spine irradiation to 30.6 Gy f/b a boost to the primary tumor to 54 Gy in attempt to decrease neurocognitive effects of the whole-brain component of CSI to 36 Gy while decreasing the rate of spinal relapse compared to WVRT alone.

It is critical that the IF volume is determined at the time of planning CSI or whole-ventricle treatment planning to ensure the CTV boost volume receives full dose. The whole-ventricular CTV should include the whole ventricles plus the CTV for the boost volume. Germ cell tumors can involve the optic nerves and hypothalamus in areas that are not part of classic CSI or whole-ventricle volumes and the CTV volume for pineal gland tumors may extend outside of the whole-ventricle volume, especially for infiltrating tumors. Guidelines to assist in contouring the whole-ventricular volume, a somewhat challenging and tedious volume, are demonstrated in Figure 14.5. Endoscopic third ventriculostomy (ETV) tracts may be included in the whole-ventricular volume if tumor biopsy is performed via ETV as reports of ETV tract recurrence have been reported.[87–89]

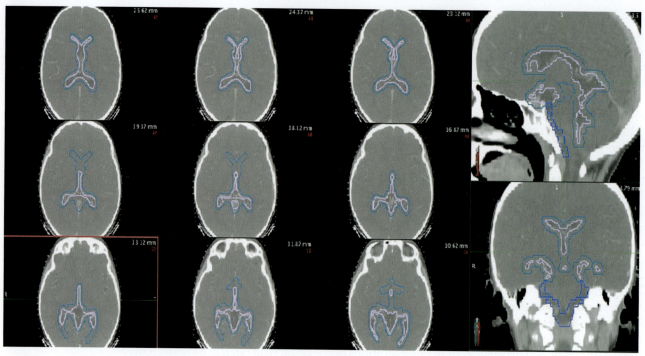

FIGURE 14.5. The whole-ventricle volume is used for treatment of microscopic disease for germinomas. This figure shows contours in axial, sagittal, and coronal views.

CRANIOPHARYNGIOMA

Craniopharyngioma is considered a "benign" tumor and highly curable. However, these children can suffer great morbidity from tumor progression and/or treatment.[90,91] These tumors are most often located in the suprasellar area but they tend to expand in different directions.[92] The most common type of craniopharyngiomas, adamantinomatous histology, is often difficult to separate surgically from adjacent critical structures preventing a curative complete surgical resection. Treatment with biopsy and cyst decompression or minimal excision followed by radiation is usually favored as a less morbid treatment. The standard GTV for craniopharyngiomas includes both solid and cystic components. A small margin of 3 to 5 mm around the GTV should be given for the CTV volume. A dose of 50.4 to 54 Gy at daily fractions of 1.8 Gy is recommended. IMRT and VMAT allow a highly conformal high-dose volume,[93,94] while IMPT can offer the same along with low-volume low dose.[95,96] Figure 14.6 (new image from Ch 78 CNS Tumors).

Given the high likelihood of survival, minimizing late morbidity is of paramount importance and modern modalities are recommended for treatment in attempt to decrease long-term morbidity. Intracavitary radiation may be used for the cystic recurrence.[97,98] Because of limited penetration, this treatment is not useful for treatment of the solid component of craniopharyngioma.

For any tumors that have a cystic component, cyst growth or change in position may occur during radiation therapy. Since the cystic portion of the tumor is also targeted in treatment, it is crucial to make appropriate adjustments in the radiation plan during the course of radiation. It is also important to recognize that dose to organs at risk may also be altered by cystic change. CT or T2-weighted non-contrast MRI every 7 to 14 days or daily cone-beam CT for cyst monitoring should be strongly considered.

Wilms Tumor and Other Renal Malignancies

Wilms tumor or nephroblastoma is the most common abdominal malignancy in children. These children generally present with an abdominal mass but are otherwise healthy. The North American standard is to perform surgical resection as the initial treatment for therapeutic treatment as well as for diagnosis, staging, and determination of subsequent therapy. COG radiation therapy guidelines are based on both stage and pathology. Flank radiation is recommended for patients with stage I–III unfavorable histologies (diffuse anaplasia, focal anaplasia, CCSK, CCSK—stage II and III) and for stage III FH. In addition to anaplastic subtype, loss of heterozygosity (LOH) in 1p and 16q is worse prognostic factor.[99] The standard dose is 10.8 Gy in fractions of 1.8 Gy following complete removal of tumor, but higher doses are recommended for recurrent disease, stage III DA, and sometimes for children diagnosed at an older age. An additional 10.8 Gy is advised for gross residual disease. Although

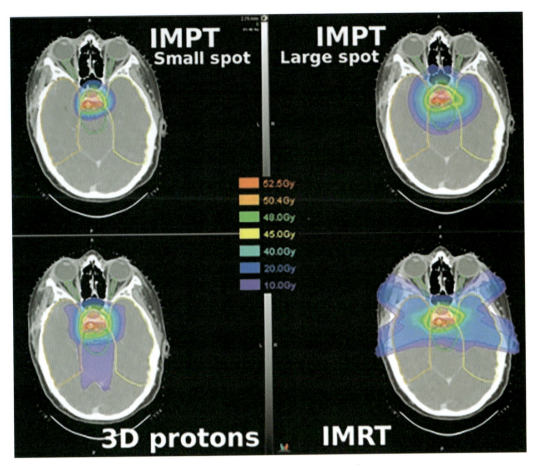

FIGURE 14.6. Modern modalities for localized treatment of craniopharyngioma. IMPT, intensity-modulated proton therapy; IMRT, intensity-modulated radiation therapy.

three-dimensional planning is useful for delineation of the tumor bed and gross residual disease if present, guidelines are still based in large part on bony landmarks. Respiratory motion should be considered and a 4D CT may be useful for planning. Respiratory gating is not typically employed, but margins for respiratory motion are added. The initial tumor should be reproduced on planning CT scan. Care should be taken to include or evenly dose the entire vertebral body and to spare the contralateral kidney and ovaries for females. AP/PA fields are typically used, but oblique fields may be of benefit for contralateral renal sparing in some cases. Whole-abdominal radiation (WART) to a dose of 10.5 Gy at 1.5 Gy per fraction is recommended for positive cytology, diffuse spillage, prior biopsy, or peritoneal seeding. If feasible, RT should be started by postoperative day 9 if and no later than postoperative day 14. Whole-lung irradiation (WLI) to 10.5 Gy is recommended for patients with pulmonary metastases that do not resolve following chemotherapy and for patients with pulmonary metastases at diagnosis with LOH for 1p16q.[100] Brain, liver, and bone irradiation is indicated when metastases are present. Other high-risk renal malignancies such as rhabdoid tumors require RT.

For patients with clear cell sarcoma of the kidney, all but Stage I tumors receive radiation.

Neuroblastoma

Neuroblastoma is the most common solid non-CNS malignancy. Neuroblastoma occurs in very young children and usually originates from the adrenal gland or paraspinal ganglia. Children often present with and abdominal mass but in contrast to Wilms tumor, the other common abdominal malignancy in children, these children are typically very ill due to systemic involvement, as more than 50% of patients are found to have metastatic disease at the time of diagnosis. The International Neuroblastoma Staging System (INSS) is based on the extent of both the tumor and the resection, while the International Neuroblastoma Risk Groups Staging System (INRGSS) utilizes additional prognostic factors including age at diagnosis, histology, MCYCN amplification, and DNA ploidy.

Radiation therapy is not used for favorable disease and is recommended mainly for patients with high-risk disease or rarely for children with intermediate-risk disease refractory to chemotherapy. At present, children with high-risk disease are treated with chemotherapy, high-dose chemotherapy followed by stem cell rescue, immunotherapy, and usually surgery and radiation for local control.[101] Many children with high-risk disease have primary tumors that cannot be resected at diagnosis and surgery is performed after 5 or 6 cycles of systemic therapy. The standard dose of RT recommended to the post-chemotherapy presurgical volume in 21.6 Gy. This volume should include a tumor bed (GTV) that encompasses all areas touched by this disease but accounts for shifts in organs following surgical resection. For children with residual disease following surgery, a total dose of 36 Gy is recommended to areas of gross disease. Organ toxicity within the radiation field should have resolved prior to initiating radiation course. The INRGSS guides the current phase III COG study ANBL1531 that uses novel therapies during induction based on MIBG and ALK status while external beam RT remains post-consolidation.

Advanced radiation techniques such as IMRT, intraoperative radiation, and proton radiation should be considered to minimize dose to the kidneys, liver, lung, developing bone, and other normal structures.[102] Although the dose of radiation is relatively low compared with other disease sites, children are usually very young, and volumes may be quite large. Figure 14.7A demonstrates various treatment techniques for a child with high-risk neuroblastoma with proton therapy for a fully-grown child. Note the gradient seen over the vertebral body. If this plan were devised for a growing child contours or plan should be devised, the entire vertebral body receives a relatively homogeneous dose. Figure 14.7B shows a proton planning volume that includes the vertebral body to ensure homogeneous dose delivery. Radiation therapy to a dose of 21.6 Gy is also advised for any metastatic sites persistent following induction chemotherapy. Metastatic sites requiring RT are typically present in the bone. Figure 14.8 shows a bony metastatic site treated with protons. Note the low dose achieved to both the pelvis and femoral head growth plates. This would not be possible with an alternative modality. In the setting of multiple metastatic sites still positive after induction chemotherapy, consideration must be given to the amount of tissue to be irradiated and typically children are re-evaluated after further chemotherapy and an attempt is made to limit the number of metastatic sites receiving radiation to three to five. Additional indications for radiation for neuroblastoma are in an emergent setting and include radiation to the liver for liver metastases, in infants to relieve respiratory distress after other measures have failed, and radiation for spinal cord compression if surgical decompression is not feasible. A dose of 1.5 Gy for 3 fractions is recommended to a portion of the liver and is generally promptly effective. Care should be taken to shield the ovaries for females. For spinal cord compression, a decision should be made

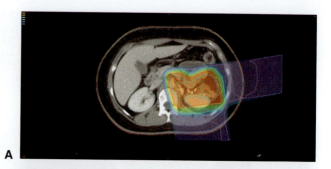

A

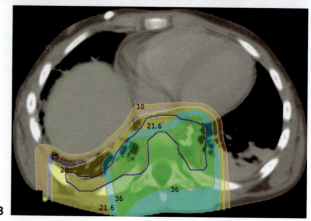

B

FIGURE 14.7. Proton plan for neuroblastoma. (**A**) A plan for a fully grown 17-year-old child with no effort made to include the whole vertebral body. (**B**) A plan for a young child, which intentionally includes the whole vertebral body. It is important to be aware of even doses to the vertebral bodies/bone. When using advanced techniques, it may be necessary to adjust contours in order to facilitate homogeneous dosing.

regarding dose based on additional risk factors and plans for subsequent radiation.

Hodgkin's disease

Hodgkin's disease is a highly curable lymphoma often cured with chemotherapy alone, but sometimes requiring radiation. Historically, high-dose radiation therapy was deployed with good therapeutic outcomes but significant adverse effects.[103–105] At present, most patients are treated with risk-adapted therapy dictating amount of chemotherapy and/or radiation therapy based on response to chemotherapy.[106] The radiation treatment of this disease has evolved over many decades from large volume extended field radiation to involved-field radiation and now to involved-site or involved-node radiation therapy.[107] Defining these nodal areas requires the use of both pre- and post-chemotherapy imaging according to the EORTC-GELA.[108] Ideally, a PET-CT in the treatment position at the time of diagnosis should be obtained, but often this is not feasible to obtain. Information regarding the initial nodal disease and use of fusion of PET or PET/CT to treatment-planning CT should be performed. Though these fusions must be carefully evaluated if PET/

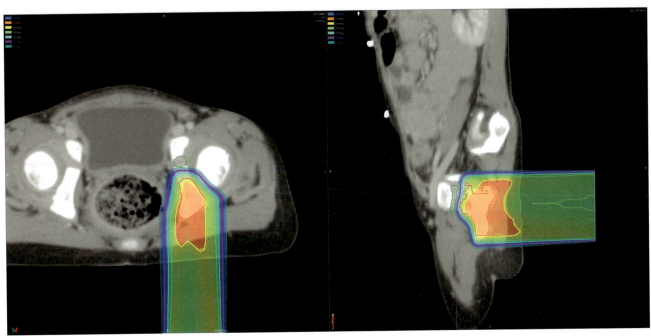

FIGURE 14.8. Treatment of a bone metastasis for a child with neuroblastoma with proton radiation. Protons allow for excellent sparing of nearby growth plates.

CT is not acquired in the same position as the planning CT and shifts in organs will likely occur due to disease response. The location of nodal disease should be carefully reviewed with radiology to assist in design of the GTV and CTV. Motion should be accounted for by use of a 4DCT and/or additional margin for motion. Most pediatric patients are treated if they present with initial bulky disease or do not achieve a rapid early response. The most commonly used dose is 21 Gy at 1.5 Gy per fraction. The COG study AHOD0031, a randomized phase III study in pediatric intermediate-risk Hodgkin lymphoma, showed that involved-field radiation did not improve outcomes, as 40% to 50% of relapses occurred inside the radiation field.[109] Given the very high cure rates seen in this disease, extreme care must be taken to avoid long-term morbidity from this disease and cooperative trial groups continue to determine how to minimize radiation dose and volume for this disease.[110,111]

Leukemia

In spite of the frequency of leukemia in children, modern chemotherapy radiation is seldom necessary. For acute lymphocytic leukemia (ALL), radiation is employed in the setting of high-risk disease, refractory disease, or at relapse. For patients with T-cell, ALL current guidelines indicate radiation for patients with the following high-risk features: WBC >50 × 10^9, CNS3 disease (>5 WBC/l or blasts in the CSF), Ph+ALL, or other high-risk disease that are "slow responders" with poor response to induction chemotherapy. Cranial radiation to a dose of 12 to 18 Gy, more often 12 Gy, at 1.5 Gy per fraction, is the recommended CNS dose for this disease.[112] Testicular radiation is other site for which radiation may be necessary, but it is now used only in the setting of refractory or recurrent disease. The recommended dose for testicular radiation for leukemia is 20 to 24 Gy.[113]

Rhabdomyosarcoma

Rhabdomyosarcoma is the most common soft-tissue sarcoma of childhood. Two main histologies exist, embryonal and alveolar, and these tumors may occur in any location of the body. Currently, the COG studies stratify patients into three risk groups (low, intermediate, and high) on the basis of site, stage, histology, and group, but TNM staging is also used. In the current COG study, ARST1431, PAX-FOXO1 fusion status is used to determine risk groups and doses.[114] Risk stratification is highly complex but in general risk groups include (1) low risk: embryonal non-metastatic favorable sites and embryonal group 1 or 2 unfavorable sites; (2) intermediate-risk: embryonal group III unfavorable sites and non-metastatic alveolar RMS at any site; and (3) high risk: metastatic disease.

The Intergroup Rhabdomyosarcoma Studies (IRS) enabled marked improvement in therapy and outcomes for this disease over the past several decades.[115] At present, combined modality risk-stratified therapy is used for children with rhabdomyosarcoma and this represents another disease site that requires multidisciplinary discussion regarding best management. Radiation treatment depends on several prognostic factors and feasibility of surgery with organ preservation. Surgery is performed upfront for resectable tumors and may be attempted following chemotherapy if tumors become resectable usually with the goal of decreasing radiation dose and sometimes volume.

Contemporary treatment and the existing COG rhabdomyosarcoma trials require three-dimensional treatment planning to allow for full visualization of areas at risk and target volumes. Radiation is omitted only for patients with completely resected favorable histology disease. Thirty-six Gy is recommended for microscopic disease following surgical resection and nodal disease is treated to a dose of 41.4 Gy. Patients with gross disease receive a dose of 50.4 Gy. Target volumes delineate pre-chemotherapy volume as the gross tumor volume. A margin of 1 cm around this volume respecting anatomical boundaries is recommended to encompass microscopic disease. The recent low-risk COG study, ARST0331, examined simultaneous reduction in alkylating chemotherapy and radiotherapy dose for pediatric orbital embryonal rhabdomyosarcoma. Ermoian et al.[116] found that the de-escalated radiation dose of 45 Gy was insufficient for patients with orbital RMS who failed to achieve a complete response to induction chemotherapy. There is currently an open intermediate-risk COG study evaluating experimental dose escalation and reduction (NCT02567435).

Ewing Sarcoma and Osteosarcoma

Pediatric bone tumors require multidisciplinary treatment approach including systemic chemotherapy, surgery, and/or radiation. Ewing's sarcoma follows rhabdomyosarcoma in its frequency in the pediatric population. When complete surgical resection can be achieved without unacceptable morbidity, this is the preferred treatment and radiation is not required. Radiation therapy is indicated for inoperable or either partially resected tumors.[117,118] Local failure rates after primary RT range from 10% to 25%. Radiation dose to 50.4–55.8 Gy to the involved area of bone with a margin for microscopic disease is standard. The initial extent of disease should be treated to a dose of approximately 45 Gy adjusting for the shifting of organs or tissues after regression of the soft-tissue portion of the tumor following chemotherapy, but not the bony component of tumor. A margin of approximately 1.5 cm should be used around this volume to form the CTV. Gross disease at the time of treatment along with initially involved bone with a margin of approximately 1.5 cm should receive an additional dose of 10.8 Gy to total 55.8 Gy with the exception of tumors located in the vertebral body, which may receive a total dose of 45 Gy to 55.8 depending on location and ability to avoid the spinal cord due to spinal cord tolerance.

For osteosarcoma, en bloc resection of the tumor with negative margins is the gold standard. Adjuvant radiation is typically indicated in the setting of positive margins or for patients at high risk for local relapse.[119] Definitive radiation up to 76 Gy is the preferred dose for inoperable tumors, while microscopic disease should be treated with >64.8 Gy. Margins are dependent on location and anatomic constraints. With the development of RT techniques and the incorporation of particle-based treatment, including proton RT and CIRT, unresectable or incompletely resected osteosarcomas can be safely and effectively treated (Fig. 14.9).[119–121]

Retinoblastoma

Retinoblastoma is a rare disease almost always diagnosed in infants or children under the age of three. Approximately

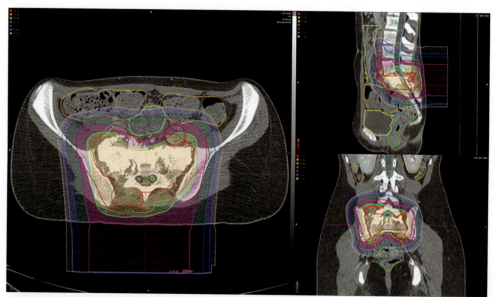

FIGURE 14.9. Representative axial, sagittal, and coronal slices for unresectable chondrogenic osteosarcoma of the sacrum receiving 72 Gy with PBS. PBS, pencil beam scanning.

60% of patients will have a nonhereditary and unilateral form of the this disease and the remainder of patients will have the hereditary form of retinoblastoma with a high propensity for bilateral disease as well as subsequent malignancies, some radiation induced and some that occur in children that have not received radiation.[122] Radiation is largely avoided because of the fear of radiation-induced malignancies and because of the young age of these patients and bony growth abnormalities that will occur in the irradiated bone following RT.[123–125] Radiation is generally reserved for disease refractory to alternative therapies (cryotherapy, laser therapy, intra-arterial chemotherapy, intra-vitreal chemotherapy, and systemic chemotherapy) in an eye with useful vision while enucleation is advised if it is thought that there is no meaningful visual potential. The most common indication for treatment of the intact eye is vitreous seeding. Postoperative radiation is delivered for advanced disease following enucleation. A dose of 45 Gy is standard for all indications. Treatment of the entire retina is most standard. For very localized tumors, the area of the involved retina may be considered if alternative options exist for anterior retinal tumor occurrence (i.e., cryotherapy or laser therapy). In the postoperative setting, the orbit and up to the optic chiasm is necessary in cases of frank orbital disease and high-risk pathology features (trans-scleral extension or tumor involvement of the cut end of the optic nerve). Plaque brachytherapy may be an option for unifocal tumors that are located in the peripheral retina. Radiation does provide an excellent chance at durable control of disease but carries risks of facial hypoplasia and radiation-induced malignancies. Proton radiation is an excellent option for this disease to reduce exposure of tissue at risk for a radiation-induced malignancy and to avoid severe bony growth abnormalities.[18,20] Referral to a proton center with expertise in retinoblastoma should be considered.[18] Figure 14.10 shows a treatment setup utilizing an eye cup to ensure eye

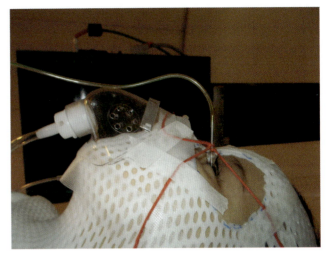

FIGURE 14.10. Retinoblastoma treatment. A suction eye cup is used to provide reproducible eye positioning for a child under anesthesia.

immobilization in addition to an aquaplast face mask to ensure immobilization of the head. A cup similar to a contact lens with a metal post is placed on the eye following sedation. A small amount of suction allows for the eye to be positioned. The metallic post can be imaged with KV X-rays for daily setup. Figure 14.11 shows a representative proton plan in a patient with bilateral disease.

Chordomas and Chondrosarcomas

Chordomas and low-grade chondrosarcomas are rare slow-growing tumors located in the base of skull and the axial skeleton. Although they are considered low-grade neoplasms, these tumors have a very high rate of recurrence after surgery and are locally destructive. The mainstay of treatment for primary and recurrent chordomas and chondrosarcomas is maximal resection

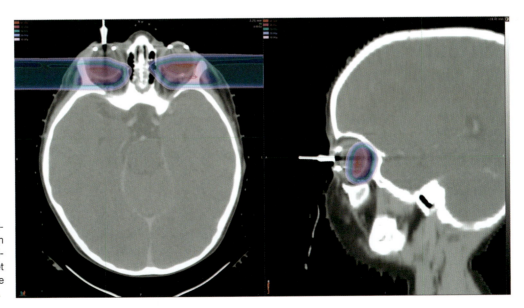

FIGURE 14.11. Representative proton radiotherapy plan in a patient with bilateral retinoblastoma. Clinical target volume is confined to the tumor in the posterior retina.

with minimal morbidity followed by high-dose radiation therapy. The treatment efficacy of conventional radiation is not satisfactory due to the close proximity to critical structures, namely the brainstem, the spinal cord, temporal lobes, and the optic pathway and the inability to deliver a therapeutic dose to the tumor while avoiding life-altering and life-threatening side effects. Therefore, charged-particle radiotherapy, taking advantage of its excellent physical dose distribution, has been widely used for the treatment of these radio-resistant solid tumors.[126,127]

In our institution, for chordoma, radiation to a cumulative dose of 76 Gy(RBE) is delivered to the GTV in 38 fractions, while chondrosarcoma patients are treated with 70 Gy(RBE) in 35 fractions. The GTV should include the tumor bed (anything in contact with the initial tumor prior to surgery) and any residual gross disease, whereas the CTV should contain the target volume and an additional margin for microscopic extension of disease of about 2 mm. The dose to target volumes should be delivered in such a manner as to respect constraints on adjacent normal structures. These constraints are as follows: The maximum dose to the surface of the spinal cord or brain stem shall not exceed 67 Gy(RBE), and the dose to the center of the spinal cord or brain stem should not be higher than 55 Gy(RBE). The maximum dose to the optic chiasm and both optic nerves should not exceed 62 Gy(RBE). Figure 14.12 shows a proton plan in a pediatric patient with classic chordoma of the base of the skull. Patients with low-grade chondrosarcoma usually have a better long-term survival than those with chordoma and can achieve a curable effect. Despite improvements made in the past decade in our knowledge of chordoma biology, systemic therapies still offer a limited benefit. Thus, patients with progressive disease should be encouraged to participate in clinical trials when and where available.

CONCLUSIONS

The field of radiation oncology is evolving rapidly both technologically as well as biologically and we see much improved cancer outcomes and survival rates than we did just a few decades ago. As malignancies become more curable and as life expectancies following the diagnosis of cancer become prolonged, the impact of our treatments on quality of life or even secondary risks of life-threatening complications become more apparent. We have learned a great deal from our childhood cancer survivors. In no other subset of patients are the late effects of treatment more apparent. Though we debate the absolute benefit of these technological advances in adults, there has been little argument against utilizing advanced technology for our children in order to protect healthy tissues from the adverse effects of radiation, even though costs may be greater and families may need to travel to receive more advanced radiation therapy. As we continue to learn from our experience with childhood malignancies and advance with biological treatments, radiation treatments will without doubt evolve and change with continued goals of providing curative treatment while minimizing side effects and allowing our patients to experience a good quality of life following the diagnosis of cancer. We hope that new treatment guidelines will include lower-dose and smaller volume radiation treatments combined with less toxic biological agents. In the future, we may see a decreased role for radiation as some pediatric malignancies become curable with less radiation, whereas our role for others may increase as a broadly curative modality rather than a specifically or primarily palliative measure. In the meantime, we should continue to provide the most targeted treatment possible by delineating proper target volumes and using the appropriate technology to deliver radiation with the optimal therapeutic ratio.

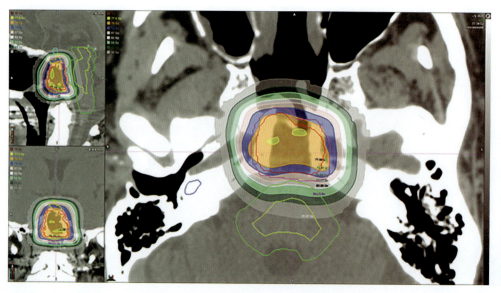

FIGURE 14.12. PBS plan for chordoma of the base of the skull treated with 76 Gy. Protons provide excellent sparing of tissues outside of the target area. PBS, pencil beam scanning.

KEY POINTS

- Highly conformal therapy is indicated in the treatment of pediatric tumors given the importance of sparing developing tissue from radiation. Advanced treatment modalities, such as proton therapy, should be considered.

- Medulloblastoma is the most common malignant brain tumor of childhood. Currently, to achieve high cure rates, surgery, chemotherapy, and radiation therapy are all part of standard treatment for this tumor.

- Intracranial germ cell tumors are a heterogeneous group of lesions that mostly occur in adolescents. Chemotherapy and radiation therapy are both required to give the best outcome and the least long-term side effects.

- Wilms tumor and neuroblastoma are common tumors in children, often presenting with an abdominal mass. Advanced radiation techniques should be considered to minimize dose to the surrounding organs at risk.

- Radiation for Hodgkin's lymphoma has evolved over time. Children are now treated with risk-adapted involved involved-site or involved-node radiation therapy to relatively low doses (21 Gy).

- IRS studies guide treatment management for rhabdomyosarcoma. Radiation is generally given to Groups II and III following cytotoxic chemotherapy regimens.

- Ewing sarcoma and osteosarcoma require multidisciplinary treatment approach including systemic chemotherapy, surgery, and/or high-dose radiation therapy.

- Retinoblastoma is the most common primary intraocular malignancy in children. Radiation is used for disease resistant to alternative therapies (cryotherapy, laser, and chemotherapy) or for metastatic disease.

- Childhood tumors generally have high cure rates and thus great care should be taken in the planning and treatment to decrease the morbidity of treatment.

REVIEW QUESTIONS

1. Approximately what percentage of pediatric cancer patients will be long–term survivors?
   A. <20%
   B. 20% to 50%
   C. 50% to 70%
   D. >70%

2. All of the following are true about ATRT except:
   A. The prognosis of ATRT is superior to that of medulloblastoma.
   B. Tumors arise in the posterior fossa and the cerebrum.
   C. The recommended dose of involved field radiation is currently 50.4 to 54 Gy.
   D. Younger age <3 years old is associated with better prognosis.

3. Which of the following is true about ependymoma?
   A. Craniospinal irradiation is used for metastatic disease.
   B. Infratentorial ependymomas often extend through the foramina of Luschka.
   C. The recommended dose of involved field radiation is currently 54 to 59.4 Gy.
   D. All of the above.

4. Which of the following is NOT true regarding pediatric low-grade gliomas?
   A. They can sometimes be cured with surgery alone.
   B. Young patients are often treated with chemotherapy to delay radiation therapy.
   C. When using radiation therapy to treat low-grade gliomas, a large margin is needed around the visible tumor.
   D. Radiation often provides durable control rates for this tumor.

5. Localized CNS germinoma is highly curable with therapy that includes
   A. 2 to 4 cycles of platinum-based therapy.
   B. Whole-ventricle RT plus a cone down to the primary tumor site.
   C. Dose of RT that is typically reduced after a complete response to chemotherapy.
   D. All of the above.

6. Which of the following is NOT true regarding pediatric skull base chordomas?
A. They are radio-resistant tumors.
B. Particle-based radiotherapy is preferred for this disease.
C. CTV should include target volume and a small margin for microscopic disease.
D. Chondrosarcomas appear to have worse survival rates than chordomas.

ANSWERS

1. D >70%
2. A The prognosis of ATRT is superior to that of medulloblastoma
3. D All of the above
4. C When using radiation therapy to treat low-grade gliomas, a large margin is needed around the visible tumor
5. D All of the above
6. D Chondrosarcomas appear to have worse survival rates than chordomas

REFERENCES

1. Breneman JC, Donaldson SS, Constine L, et al. The Children's Oncology Group radiation oncology discipline: 15 years of contributions to the treatment of childhood cancer. *Int J Radiat Oncol Biol Phys*. 2018;101(4):860–874.
2. Kortmann R-D, Freeman C, Marcus K, et al. Paediatric radiation oncology in the care of childhood cancer: a position paper by the International Paediatric Radiation Oncology Society (PROS). *Radiother Oncol*. 2016;119(2):357–360.
3. Oeffinger KC, Mertens AC, Sklar CA, et al. Chronic health conditions in adult survivors of childhood cancer. *N Engl J Med*. 2006;355(15):1572–1582.
4. Meadows AT. Pediatric cancer survivorship: research and clinical care. *J Clin Oncol*. 2006;24(32):5160–5165.
5. Fortney JT, Halperin EC, Hertz CM, Schulman SR. Anesthesia for pediatric external beam radiation therapy. *Int J Radiat Oncol Biol Phys*. 1999;44(3):587–591.
6. McFadyen JG, Pelly N, Orr RJ. Sedation and anesthesia for the pediatric patient undergoing radiation therapy. *Curr Opin Anaesthesiol*. 2011;24(4):433–438.
7. Seiler G, De Vol E, Khafaga Y, et al. Evaluation of the safety and efficacy of repeated sedations for the radiotherapy of young children with cancer: a prospective study of 1033 consecutive sedations. *Int J Radiat Oncol Biol Phys*. 2001;49(3):771–783.
8. Brenner D, Elliston C, Hall E, Berdon W. Estimated risks of radiation-induced fatal cancer from pediatric CT. *AJR Am J Roentgenol*. 2001;176(2):289–296.
9. Brenner DJ, Hall EJ. Computed tomography—an increasing source of radiation exposure. *N Engl J Med*. 2007;357(22):2277–2284.
10. Alcorn SR, Zhou XC, Bojechko C, et al. Low-dose image-guided pediatric CNS radiation therapy: final analysis from a prospective low-dose cone-beam CT protocol from a multinational pediatrics consortium. *Technol Cancer Res Treat*. 2020;19:1533033820920650.
11. Hall EJ, Wuu CS. Radiation-induced second cancers: the impact of 3D-CRT and IMRT. *Int J Radiat Oncol Biol Phys*. 2003;56(1):83–88.
12. Casey DL, Friedman DN, Moskowitz CS, et al. Second cancer risk in childhood cancer survivors treated with intensity-modulated radiation therapy (IMRT). *Pediatr Blood Cancer*. 2014.
13. MacDonald SM, DeLaney TF, Loeffler JS. Proton beam radiation therapy. *Cancer Invest*. 2006;24(2):199–208.
14. Trofimov A, Bortfeld T. Optimization of beam parameters and treatment planning for intensity modulated proton therapy. *Technol Cancer Res Treat*. 2003;2(5):437–444.
15. MacEwan I, Chou B, Moretz J, Loredo L, Bush D, Slater JD. Effects of vertebral-body-sparing proton craniospinal irradiation on the spine of young pediatric patients with medulloblastoma. *Adv Radiat Oncol*. 2017;2(2):220–227.
16. Macdonald SM, Sethi R, Lavally B, et al. Proton radiotherapy for pediatric central nervous system ependymoma: clinical outcomes for 70 patients. *Neuro-oncology*. 2013;15(11):1552–1559.
17. MacDonald SM, Trofimov A, Safai S, et al. Proton radiotherapy for pediatric central nervous system germ cell tumors: early clinical outcomes. *Int J Radiat Oncol Biol Phys*. 2011;79(1):121–129.
18. Mouw KW, Sethi RV, Yeap BY, et al. Proton radiation therapy for the treatment of retinoblastoma. *Int J Radiat Oncol Biol Phys*. 2014;90(4):863–869.
19. Rombi B, DeLaney TF, MacDonald SM, et al. Proton radiotherapy for pediatric Ewing's sarcoma: initial clinical outcomes. *Int J Radiat Oncol Biol Phys*. 2012;82(3):1142–1148.
20. Sethi RV, Shih HA, Yeap BY, et al. Second nonocular tumors among survivors of retinoblastoma treated with contemporary photon and proton radiotherapy. *Cancer*. 2014;120(1):126–133.
21. Yock TI, Bhat S, Szymonifka J, et al. Quality of life outcomes in proton and photon treated pediatric brain tumor survivors. *Radiother Oncol*. 2014;113(1):89–94.
22. Mohan R, Grosshans D. Proton therapy–present and future. *Adv Drug Deliv Rev*. 2017;109:26–44.
23. Ando K, Kase Y. Biological characteristics of carbon-ion therapy. *Int J Radiat Biol*. 2009;85(9):715–728.
24. Goetz G, Mitic M, Mittermayr T, Wild C. Health technology assessment of carbon-ion beam radiotherapy: a systematic review of clinical effectiveness and safety for 54 oncological indications in 12 tumour regions. *Anticancer Res*. 2019;39(4):1635–1650.
25. Mohamad O, Imai R, Kamada T, Nitta Y, Araki N, and Soft Tissue Sarcoma tWGfB. Carbon ion radiotherapy for inoperable pediatric osteosarcoma. *Oncotarget*. 2018;9(33).
26. Combs SE, Kessel KA, Herfarth K, et al. Treatment of pediatric patients and young adults with particle therapy at the Heidelberg Ion Therapy Center (HIT): establishment of workflow and initial clinical data. *Radiat Oncol*. 2012;7(1):170.
27. Combs SE, Nikoghosyan A, Jaekel O, et al. Carbon ion radiotherapy for pediatric patients and young adults treated for tumors of the skull base. *Cancer*. 2009;115(6):1348–1355.
28. Louis DN, Perry A, Reifenberger G, et al. The 2016 World Health Organization classification of tumors of the central nervous system: a summary. *Acta Neuropathol*. 2016;131(6):803–820.
29. Packer RJ, Gajjar A, Vezina G, et al. Phase III study of craniospinal radiation therapy followed by adjuvant chemotherapy for newly diagnosed average-risk medulloblastoma. *J Clin Oncol*. 2006;24(25):4202–4208.
30. Packer RJ, Hoffman EP. Neuro-oncology: understanding the molecular complexity of medulloblastoma. *Nat Rev Neurol*. 2012;8(10):539–540.

31. Northcott PA, Korshunov A, Witt H, et al. Medulloblastoma comprises four distinct molecular variants. *J Clin Oncol.* 2011;29(11):1408–1414.

32. Northcott PA, Shih DJ, Peacock J, et al. Subgroup-specific structural variation across 1,000 medulloblastoma genomes. *Nature.* 2012;488(7409):49–56.

33. Kool M, Korshunov A, Remke M, et al. Molecular subgroups of medulloblastoma: an international meta-analysis of transcriptome, genetic aberrations, and clinical data of WNT, SHH, Group 3, and Group 4 medulloblastomas. *Acta Neuropathol.* 2012;123(4):473–484.

34. Michalski JM, Janss A, Vezina G, et al. Results of COG ACNS0331: a phase III trial of involved-field radiotherapy (IFRT) and low dose craniospinal irradiation (LD-CSI) with chemotherapy in average-risk medulloblastoma: a report from the Children's oncology group. *Int J Radiat Oncol Biol Phys.* 2016;96(5):937–938.

35. Gajjar A, Packer RJ, Foreman NK, Cohen K, Haas-Kogan D, Merchant TE. Children's Oncology Group's 2013 blueprint for research: central nervous system tumors. *Pediatr Blood Cancer.* 2013;60(6):1022–1026.

36. Rutkowski S, Bode U, Deinlein F, et al. Treatment of early childhood medulloblastoma by postoperative chemotherapy alone. *N Engl J Med.* 2005;352(10):978–986.

37. Dhall G, Grodman H, Ji L, et al. Outcome of children less than three years old at diagnosis with non-metastatic medulloblastoma treated with chemotherapy on the "Head Start" I and II protocols. *Pediatr Blood Cancer.* 2008;50(6):1169–1175.

38. Raleigh DR, Tomlin B, Buono BD, et al. Survival after chemotherapy and stem cell transplant followed by delayed craniospinal irradiation is comparable to upfront craniospinal irradiation in pediatric embryonal brain tumor patients. *J Neuro-Oncol.* 2017;131(2):359–368.

39. Tarbell NJ, Friedman H, Polkinghorn WR, et al. High-risk medulloblastoma: a pediatric oncology group randomized trial of chemotherapy before or after radiation therapy (POG 9031). *J Clin Oncol.* 2013;31(23):2936–2941.

40. Fangusaro JR, Jubran RF, Allen J, et al. Brainstem primitive neuroectodermal tumors (bstPNET): results of treatment with intensive induction chemotherapy followed by consolidative chemotherapy with autologous hematopoietic cell rescue. *Pediatr Blood Cancer.* 2008;50(3):715–717.

41. Gururangan S, McLaughlin C, Quinn J, et al. High-dose chemotherapy with autologous stem-cell rescue in children and adults with newly diagnosed pineoblastomas. *J Clin Oncol.* 2003;21(11):2187–2191.

42. Biegel JA, Kalpana G, Knudsen ES, et al. The role of INI1 and the SWI/SNF complex in the development of rhabdoid tumors: meeting summary from the workshop on childhood atypical teratoid/rhabdoid tumors. *Cancer Res.* 2002;62(1):323–328.

43. Chi SN, Zimmerman MA, Yao X, et al. Intensive multimodality treatment for children with newly diagnosed CNS atypical teratoid rhabdoid tumor. *J Clin Oncol.* 2009;27(3):385–389.

44. Tekautz TM, Fuller CE, Blaney S, et al. Atypical teratoid/rhabdoid tumors (ATRT): improved survival in children 3 years of age and older with radiation therapy and high-dose alkylator-based chemotherapy. *J Clin Oncol.* 2005;23(7):1491–1499.

45. Hilden JM, Meerbaum S, Burger P, et al. Central nervous system atypical teratoid/rhabdoid tumor: results of therapy in children enrolled in a registry. *J Clin Oncol.* 2004;22(14):2877–2884.

46. Bartelheim K, Nemes K, Seeringer A, et al. Improved 6-year overall survival in AT/RT–results of the registry study Rhabdoid 2007. *Cancer Med.* 2016;5(8):1765–1775.

47. Reddy AT, Strother DR, Judkins AR, et al. Efficacy of high-dose chemotherapy and three-dimensional conformal radiation for atypical teratoid/rhabdoid tumor: a report from the children's oncology group trial ACNS0333. *J Clin Oncol.* 2020;38(11):1175–1185.

48. Holmes JA, Chera BS, Brenner DJ, et al. Estimating the excess lifetime risk of radiation induced secondary malignancy (SMN) in pediatric patients treated with craniospinal irradiation (CSI): conventional radiation therapy versus helical intensity modulated radiation therapy. *Pract Radiat Oncol.* 2017;7(1):35–41.

49. Tamburrini G, D'Ercole M, Pettorini BL, Caldarelli M, Massimi L, Di Rocco C. Survival following treatment for intracranial ependymoma: a review. *Childs Nerv Syst.* 2009;25(10):1303–1312.

50. Ellison DW, Aldape KD, Capper D, et al. cIMPACT-NOW update 7: advancing the molecular classification of ependymal tumors. *Brain Pathol.* 2020;30(5):863–866.

51. Fangusaro J, Van Den Berghe C, Tomita T, et al. Evaluating the incidence and utility of microscopic metastatic dissemination as diagnosed by lumbar cerebro-spinal fluid (CSF) samples in children with newly diagnosed intracranial ependymoma. *J Neurooncol.* 2011;103(3):693–698.

52. Parker M, Mohankumar KM, Punchihewa C, et al. C11orf95-RELA fusions drive oncogenic NF-κB signalling in ependymoma. *Nature.* 2014;506(7489):451–455.

53. Merchant TE, Li C, Xiong X, Kun LE, Boop FA, Sanford RA. Conformal radiotherapy after surgery for paediatric ependymoma: a prospective study. *Lancet Oncol.* 2009;10(3):258–266.

54. Merchant TE, Bendel AE, Sabin ND, et al. Conformal radiation therapy for pediatric ependymoma, chemotherapy for incompletely resected ependymoma, and observation for completely resected, supratentorial ependymoma. *J Clin Oncol.* 2019;37(12):974–983.

55. Chao ST, Kobayashi T, Benzel E, et al. The role of adjuvant radiation therapy in the treatment of spinal myxopapillary ependymomas. *J Neurosurg Spine.* 2011;14(1):59–64.

56. Pica A, Miller R, Villà S, et al. The results of surgery, with or without radiotherapy, for primary spinal myxopapillary ependymoma: a retrospective study from the rare cancer network. *Int J Radiat Oncol Biol Phys.* 2009;74(4):1114–1120.

57. Packer RJ, Lange B, Ater J, et al. Carboplatin and vincristine for recurrent and newly diagnosed low-grade gliomas of childhood. *J Clin Oncol.* 1993;11(5):850–856.

58. Wisoff JH, Sanford RA, Heier LA, et al. Primary neurosurgery for pediatric low-grade gliomas: a prospective multi-institutional study from the Children's Oncology Group. *Neurosurgery.* 2011;68(6):1548–1554; discussion 1554–1545.

59. Bandopadhayay P, Ramkissoon LA, Jain P, et al. MYB-QKI rearrangements in angiocentric glioma drive tumorigenicity through a tripartite mechanism. *Nat Genet.* 2016;48(3):273–282.

60. Merchant TE, Conklin HM, Wu S, Lustig RH, Xiong X. Late effects of conformal radiation therapy for pediatric patients with low-grade glioma: prospective evaluation of cognitive, endocrine, and hearing deficits. *J Clin Oncol.* 2009;27(22):3691–3697.

61. Merchant TE, Kun LE, Wu S, Xiong X, Sanford RA, Boop FA. Phase II trial of conformal radiation therapy for pediatric low-grade glioma. *J Clin Oncol.* 2009;27(22):3598–3604.

62. Marcus KJ, Goumnerova L, Billett AL, et al. Stereotactic radiotherapy for localized low-grade gliomas in children: final results of a prospective trial. *Int J Radiat Oncol Biol Phys.* 2005;61(2):374–379.

63. Cherlow JM, Shaw DWW, Margraf LR, et al. Conformal radiation therapy for pediatric patients with low-grade glioma: results from the Children's Oncology Group Phase 2 Study ACNS0221. *Int J Radiat Oncol Biol Phys.* 2019;103(4):861–868.

64. Indelicato DJ, Rotondo RL, Uezono H, et al. Outcomes following proton therapy for pediatric low-grade glioma. *Int J Radiat Oncol Biol Phys.* 2019;104(1):149–156.

65. Greenberger BA, Pulsifer MB, Ebb DH, et al. Clinical outcomes and late endocrine, neurocognitive, and visual profiles of proton radiation for pediatric low-grade gliomas. *Int J Radiat Oncol Biol Phys.* 2014;89(5):1060–1068.

66. Tsang DS, Murphy ES, Lucas JT, Jr., Lagiou P, Acharya S, Merchant TE. Pseudoprogression in pediatric low-grade glioma after irradiation. *J Neurooncol.* 2017;135(2):371–379.

67. Ludmir EB, Mahajan A, Paulino AC, et al. Increased risk of pseudoprogression among pediatric low-grade glioma patients treated with proton versus photon radiotherapy. *Neuro Oncol.* 2019;21(5):686–695.

68. MacDonald TJ, Arenson EB, Ater J, et al. Phase II study of high-dose chemotherapy before radiation in children with newly diagnosed high-grade astrocytoma: final analysis of Children's Cancer Group Study 9933. *Cancer.* 2005;104(12):2862–2871.

69. Lashford LS, Thiesse P, Jouvet A, et al. Temozolomide in malignant gliomas of childhood: a United Kingdom Children's Cancer Study Group and French Society for Pediatric Oncology Intergroup Study. *J Clin Oncol.* 2002;20(24):4684–4691.

70. Cohen KJ, Pollack IF, Zhou T, et al. Temozolomide in the treatment of high-grade gliomas in children: a report from the Children's Oncology Group. *Neuro Oncol.* 2011;13(3):317–323.

71. Jakacki RI, Cohen KJ, Buxton A, et al. Phase 2 study of concurrent radiotherapy and temozolomide followed by temozolomide and lomustine in the treatment of children with high-grade glioma: a report of the Children's Oncology Group ACNS0423 study. *Neuro Oncol.* 2016;18(10):1442–1450.

72. Duffner PK, Krischer JP, Burger PC, et al. Treatment of infants with malignant gliomas: the Pediatric Oncology Group experience. *J Neurooncol.* 1996;28(2–3):245–256.

73. Kaye EC, Baker JN, Broniscer A. Management of diffuse intrinsic pontine glioma in children: current and future strategies for improving prognosis. *CNS Oncol.* 2014;3(6):421–431.

74. Jalali R, Raut N, Arora B, et al. Prospective evaluation of radiotherapy with concurrent and adjuvant temozolomide in children with newly diagnosed diffuse intrinsic pontine glioma. *Int J Radiat Oncol Biol Phys.* 2010;77(1):113–118.

75. Walter AW, Gajjar A, Ochs JS, et al. Carboplatin and etoposide with hyperfractionated radiotherapy in children with newly diagnosed diffuse pontine gliomas: a phase I/II study. *Med Pediatr Oncol.* 1998;30(1):28–33.

76. Lassaletta A, Strother D, Laperriere N, et al. Reirradiation in patients with diffuse intrinsic pontine gliomas: the Canadian experience. *Pediatr Blood Cancer.* 2018;65(6):e26988.

77. Cacciotti C, Liu KX, Haas-Kogan DA, Warren KE. Reirradiation practices for children with diffuse intrinsic pontine glioma. *Neuro Oncol.* 2020.

78. Lafay-Cousin L, Millar BA, Mabbott D, et al. Limited-field radiation for bifocal germinoma. *Int J Radiat Oncol Biol Phys.* 2006;65(2):486–492.

79. Echevarria ME, Fangusaro J, Goldman S. Pediatric central nervous system germ cell tumors: a review. *Oncologist.* 2008;13(6):690–699.

80. Dearnaley DP, A'Hern RP, Whittaker S, Bloom HJ. Pineal and CNS germ cell tumors: Royal Marsden Hospital experience 1962–1987. *Int J Radiat Oncol Biol Phys.* 1990;18(4):773–781.

81. Villano JL, Propp JM, Porter KR, et al. Malignant pineal germ-cell tumors: an analysis of cases from three tumor registries. *Neuro Oncol.* 2008;10(2):121–130.

82. Alapetite C, Brisse H, Patte C, et al. Pattern of relapse and outcome of non-metastatic germinoma patients treated with chemotherapy and limited field radiation: the SFOP experience. *Neuro Oncol.* 2010;12(12):1318–1325.

83. Allen JC, DaRosso RC, Donahue B, Nirenberg A. A phase II trial of preirradiation carboplatin in newly diagnosed germinoma of the central nervous system. *Cancer.* 1994;74(3):940–944.

84. Modak S, Gardner S, Dunkel IJ, et al. Thiotepa-based high-dose chemotherapy with autologous stem-cell rescue in patients with recurrent or progressive CNS germ cell tumors. *J. Clin. Oncol.* 2004;22(10):1934–1943.

85. Goldman S, Bouffet E, Fisher PG, et al. Phase II trial assessing the ability of neoadjuvant chemotherapy with or without second-look surgery to eliminate measurable disease for nongerminomatous germ cell tumors: a Children's Oncology Group Study. *J Clin Oncol.* 2015;33(22):2464–2471.

86. Fangusaro J, Wu S, MacDonald S, et al. Phase II trial of response-based radiation therapy for patients with localized CNS non-germinomatous germ cell tumors: a Children's Oncology Group Study. *J Clin Oncol.* 2019;37(34):3283–3290.

87. Choi UK, Cha SH, Song GS, et al. Recurrent intracranial germinoma along the endoscopic ventriculostomy tract. Case report. *J Neurosurg.* 2007;107(1 Suppl):62–65.

88. Haw C, Steinbok P. Ventriculoscope tract recurrence after endoscopic biopsy of pineal germinoma. *Pediatr Neurosurg.* 2001;34:215–217.

89. Talamonti G, Ligarotti GK, Bramerio M, Imbesi F. Unusual behaviour of a pineal germinoma mimicking neurosarcoidosis

and metastasising along the endoscopic route. *BMJ Case Rep.* 2013;2013:bcr2013200278.

90. Habrand JL, Ganry O, Couanet D, et al. The role of radiation therapy in the management of craniopharyngioma: a 25-year experience and review of the literature. *Int J Radiat Oncol Biol Phys.* 1999;44(2):255–263.

91. Tan TSE, Patel L, Gopal-Kothandapani JS, et al. The neuroendocrine sequelae of paediatric craniopharyngioma: a 40-year meta-data analysis of 185 cases from three UK centres. *Eur J Endocrinol.* 2017;176(3):359–369.

92. Pan J, Qi S, Liu Y, et al. Growth patterns of craniopharyngiomas: clinical analysis of 226 patients. *J Neurosurg Pediatr.* 2016;17(4):418–433.

93. Merchant TE, Kun LE, Hua CH, et al. Disease control after reduced volume conformal and intensity modulated radiation therapy for childhood craniopharyngioma. *Int J Radiat Oncol Biol Phys.* 2013;85(4):e187–192.

94. Uto M, Mizowaki T, Ogura K, Hiraoka M. Non-coplanar volumetric-modulated arc therapy (VMAT) for craniopharyngiomas reduces radiation doses to the bilateral hippocampus: a planning study comparing dynamic conformal arc therapy, coplanar VMAT, and non-coplanar VMAT. *Radiat Oncol.* 2016;11:86.

95. Eaton BR, Yock T. The use of proton therapy in the treatment of benign or low-grade pediatric brain tumors. *Cancer J.* 2014;20(6):403–408.

96. Bishop AJ, Greenfield B, Mahajan A, et al. Proton beam therapy versus conformal photon radiation therapy for childhood craniopharyngioma: multi-institutional analysis of outcomes, cyst dynamics, and toxicity. *Int J Radiat Oncol Biol Phys.* 2014;90(2):354–361.

97. Voges J, Sturm V, Lehrke R, Treuer H, Gauss C, Berthold F. Cystic craniopharyngioma: long-term results after intracavitary irradiation with stereotactically applied colloidal beta-emitting radioactive sources. *Neurosurgery.* 1997;40(2):263–269; discussion 269–270.

98. Vanhauwaert D, Hallaert G, Baert E, Van Roost D, Okito JP, Caemaert J. Treatment of cystic craniopharyngioma by endocavitary instillation of yttrium(9)(0) radioisotope—still a valuable treatment option. *J Neurol Surg A Cent Eur Neurosurg.* 2013;74(5):307–312.

99. Grundy PE, Breslow NE, Li S, et al. Loss of heterozygosity for chromosomes 1p and 16q is an adverse prognostic factor in favorable-histology Wilms tumor: a report from the National Wilms Tumor Study Group. *J Clin Oncol.* 2005;23(29):7312–7321.

100. Dix DB, Seibel NL, Chi YY, et al. Treatment of stage IV favorable histology Wilms Tumor with lung metastases: a report from the Children's Oncology Group AREN0533 Study. *J Clin Oncol.* 2018;36(16):1564–1570.

101. Yu AL, Gilman AL, Ozkaynak MF, et al. Anti-GD2 antibody with GM-CSF, interleukin-2, and isotretinoin for neuroblastoma. *N Engl J Med.* 2010;363(14):1324–1334.

102. Hattangadi JA, Rombi B, Yock TI, et al. Proton radiotherapy for high-risk pediatric neuroblastoma: early outcomes and dose comparison. *Int J Radiat Oncol Biol Phys.* 2012;83(3):1015–1022.

103. Meadows AT, Friedman DL, Neglia JP, et al. Second neoplasms in survivors of childhood cancer: findings from the Childhood Cancer Survivor Study cohort. *J Clin Oncol.* 2009;27(14):2356–2362.

104. Zhou R, Ng A, Constine LS, et al. A comparative evaluation of normal tissue doses for patients receiving radiation therapy on the Childhood Cancer Survivor Study and Recent Children's Oncology Group Trials. *Int J Radiat Oncol Biol Phys.* 2016;95(2):707–711.

105. Moskowitz CS, Chou JF, Wolden SL, et al. Breast cancer after chest radiation therapy for childhood cancer. *J Clin Oncol.* 2014;32(21):2217–2223.

106. Nachman JB, Sposto R, Herzog P, et al. Randomized comparison of low-dose involved-field radiotherapy and no radiotherapy for children with Hodgkin's disease who achieve a complete response to chemotherapy. *J Clin Oncol.* 2002;20(18):3765–3771.

107. Hoppe BS, Hoppe RT. Expert radiation oncologist interpretations of involved-site radiation therapy guidelines in the management of hodgkin lymphoma. *Int J Radiat Oncol Biol Phys.* 2015;92(1):40–45.

108. Girinsky T, Specht L, Ghalibafian M, et al. The conundrum of Hodgkin lymphoma nodes: to be or not to be included in the involved node radiation fields. The EORTC-GELA lymphoma group guidelines. *Radiother Oncol.* 2008;88(2):202–210.

109. Dharmarajan KV, Friedman DL, Schwartz CL, et al. Patterns of relapse from a phase 3 Study of response-based therapy for intermediate-risk Hodgkin lymphoma (AHOD0031): a report from the Children's Oncology Group. *Int J Radiat Oncol Biol Phys.* 2015;92(1):60–66.

110. Donaldson SS. Finding the balance in pediatric Hodgkin's lymphoma. *J Clin Oncol.* 2012;30(26):3158–3159.

111. Metzger ML, Weinstein HJ, Hudson MM, et al. Association between radiotherapy vs no radiotherapy based on early response to VAMP chemotherapy and survival among children with favorable-risk Hodgkin lymphoma. *Jama.* 2012;307(24):2609–2616.

112. Unal S, Yetgin S, Cetin M, et al. The prognosis and survival of childhood acute lymphoblastic leukemia with central nervous system relapse. *Pediatr Hematol Oncol.* 2004;21(3):279–289.

113. Quaranta BP, Halperin EC, Kurtzberg J, Clough R, Martin PL. The incidence of testicular recurrence in boys with acute leukemia treated with total body and testicular irradiation and stem cell transplantation. *Cancer.* 2004;101(4):845–850.

114. Skapek SX, Anderson J, Barr FG, et al. PAX-FOXO1 fusion status drives unfavorable outcome for children with rhabdomyosarcoma: a children's oncology group report. *Pediatr Blood Cancer.* 2013;60(9):1411–1417.

115. Raney B, Stoner J, Anderson J, et al. Impact of tumor viability at second-look procedures performed before completing treatment on the Intergroup Rhabdomyosarcoma Study Group protocol IRS-IV, 1991–1997: a report from the children's oncology group. *J Pediatr Surg.* 2010;45(11):2160–2168.

116. Ermoian RP, Breneman J, Walterhouse DO, et al. 45 Gy is not sufficient radiotherapy dose for Group III orbital embryonal rhabdomyosarcoma after less than complete response to 12 weeks of ARST0331 chemotherapy: a report from the Soft Tissue Sarcoma Committee of the Children's Oncology Group. *Pediatr Blood Cancer.* 2017;64(9).

117. Laskar S, Mallick I, Gupta T, Muckaden MA. Post-operative radiotherapy for Ewing sarcoma: when, how and how much? *Pediatr Blood Cancer.* 2008;51(5):575–580.

118. Donaldson SS. Ewing sarcoma: radiation dose and target volume. *Pediatr Blood Cancer.* 2004;42(5):471–476.

119. Ciernik IF, Niemierko A, Harmon DC, et al. Proton-based radiotherapy for unresectable or incompletely resected osteosarcoma. *Cancer.* 2011;117(19):4522–4530.

120. Matsunobu A, Imai R, Kamada T, et al. Impact of carbon ion radiotherapy for unresectable osteosarcoma of the trunk. *Cancer.* 2012;118(18):4555–4563.

121. Tinkle CL, Lu J, Han Y, et al. Curative-intent radiotherapy for pediatric osteosarcoma: the St. Jude experience. *Pediatr Blood Cancer.* 2019;66(8):e27763–e27763.

122. Poulaki V, Mukai S. Retinoblastoma: genetics and pathology. *Int Ophthalmol Clin.* 2009;49(1):155–164.

123. Kaste SC, Chen G, Fontanesi J, Crom DB, Pratt CB. Orbital development in long-term survivors of retinoblastoma. *J Clin Oncol.* 1997;15(3):1183–1189.

124. Egbert PR, Donaldson SS, Moazed K, Rosenthal AR. Visual results and ocular complications following radiotherapy for retinoblastoma. *Arch Ophthalmol.* 1978;96(10):1826–1830.

125. Fletcher O, Easton D, Anderson K, Gilham C, Jay M, Peto J. Lifetime risks of common cancers among retinoblastoma survivors. *J Natl Cancer Inst.* 2004;96(5):357–363.

126. Lu VM, O'Connor KP, Mahajan A, Carlson ML, Van Gompel JJ. Carbon ion radiotherapy for skull base chordomas and chondrosarcomas: a systematic review and meta-analysis of local control, survival, and toxicity outcomes. *J Neuro-Oncol.* 2020;147(3):503–513.

127. Rombi B, Ares C, Hug EB, et al. Spot-scanning proton radiation therapy for pediatric chordoma and chondrosarcoma: clinical outcome of 26 patients treated at paul scherrer institute. *Int J Radiat Oncol Biol Phys.* 2013;86(3):578–584.

15 Soft Tissue and Bone Sarcoma

Kilian E. Salerno, Yen-Lin Chen, Thomas F. DeLaney, and Elizabeth H. Baldini

INTRODUCTION

Sarcomas are rare malignant tumors of mesenchymal cell origin that can arise from connective tissues throughout the body and are divided into sarcomas of soft tissues and those of bone.[1] Soft tissue and bone sarcomas account for approximately 1% of new cancer cases, 1% of adult malignancies, and 15% of pediatric malignancies.[2] In 2020, the estimated number of new soft tissue sarcoma diagnoses in the United States is 13,130 and the number of new bone sarcoma diagnoses is 3,600; with 5,350 and 1,720 estimated deaths from each respectively.[2] Five-year relative survival for each is approximately 65%.[3,4] There is a bimodal age distribution with peaks in children and young adults and in adults over 60 years of age. In patients under 40 years of age, sarcomas are among the top five leading causes of cancer death.[2]

Soft tissue sarcoma is heterogeneous and includes over 50 histopathologic subtypes, with undifferentiated pleomorphic sarcoma (UPS or formerly malignant fibrous histiocytoma), liposarcoma, and leiomyosarcoma most common.[1] Soft tissue sarcoma can arise at any anatomic site throughout the body, most commonly in the lower extremities (46%), trunk/body wall (18%), upper extremities (13%), retroperitoneum (13%), and head and neck (9%).[5] The updated eighth edition of the American Joint Committee on Cancer (AJCC) staging system reflects the importance of anatomic site with the development of new staging systems for sarcomas of the head and neck, retroperitoneum, and abdominal/visceral organs.[6] Genetic cancer syndromes arising from germline mutations with known predisposition to develop soft tissue sarcomas include TP53 mutation and Li-Fraumeni syndrome with multiple malignancies including sarcomas; familial adenomatous polyposis and desmoid fibromatosis; soft tissue and bone sarcomas in hereditary retinoblastoma; and malignant peripheral nerve sheath tumor (MPNST) in neurofibromatosis type 1. Bone sarcomas are similarly heterogenous and include osteosarcoma, chondrosarcoma, and Ewing sarcoma most commonly. Chordoma, UPS of bone, and giant cell tumor of bone are included among the bone sarcomas but uncommon.[1] Histopathologic subtypes of both soft tissue and bone sarcomas differ in their natural history and risk for local recurrence (LR) and distant metastatic spread.

Both soft tissue and bone sarcomas are rare malignancies with high potential for morbidity and mortality. Clinical outcomes are improved with multidisciplinary input from care providers with expertise in sarcoma, including radiation oncology, orthopedic oncology, surgical oncology, medical/pediatric oncology, pathology, and musculoskeletal radiology.[7-13] Given each histopathologic subtype has a unique natural history, accurate pathologic diagnosis is critical to inform appropriate clinical care.[14] Similarly, expertise in understanding the patterns of spread, local involvement, and areas at risk for regional and distant spread improves radiologic interpretation of imaging and subsequent care.[15,16] Medical or pediatric oncologists should be involved to determine whether systemic therapy may be indicated, and if so, how to sequence with local therapy. Genetics assessment and referral for fertility counseling should be considered for appropriate patients. Collaboration between all providers is necessary to determine the appropriate therapeutic modalities indicated for optimal outcomes and the sequence of such treatments. Care at high volume centers is associated with improved outcomes, with increased use of limb-sparing approaches, and overall survival.[7-10,17-19]

Treatment paradigms differ between soft tissue and bone sarcomas, in particular the relative roles for radiation and systemic therapies. Surgical resection with wide margins is the primary treatment modality. Radiation therapy (RT) improves local control and is used for preservation of limb and organ function. RT plays a central role in the management of soft tissue sarcoma in most anatomic sites and is used for bone sarcomas at sites for which resection with wide margins is challenging, such as head and neck, spine, and pelvis, or in the setting of unresectable disease. This chapter reviews the role of RT in the management of extremity and truncal soft tissue sarcoma, retroperitoneal sarcoma (RPS), bone sarcoma, unique considerations for optimal radiation treatment planning for each, and the use of stereotactic approaches for oligometastatic disease.

EXTREMITY AND SUPERFICIAL TRUNCAL SOFT TISSUE SARCOMA

Presentation and Natural History

Extremity and superficial truncal soft tissue sarcomas most commonly present as painless masses. Given the lack of associated symptoms, soft tissue sarcomas are often large in size at time of diagnosis. Rarely is pain, edema, or paresthesia present. A soft tissue mass that is new, has rapid growth, is >5 cm in size, or is with associated symptoms should raise concern for malignant etiology. Given the rarity of soft tissue sarcoma in comparison to other differential diagnoses including benign etiologies, delay in diagnosis or initial misdiagnosis is not uncommon.

Soft tissue sarcomas grow along muscle planes and connective tissues and rarely invade bone or spread beyond the compartment in which they originate. In the extremity, muscles are separated into compartments by major intermuscular septae. Within a compartment, muscles are separated by minor septae. Sarcomas tend to grow longitudinally along the axis of the compartment and radially within the confines of the major fascial barrier of the compartment, and typically do not cross into neighboring compartments until late in their natural history. It is important to recognize that the longitudinal spread of tumor is along the plane of the muscle fibers and that this may not be craniocaudal but rather diagonal (e.g., superficial truncal muscles of the back and gluteal muscles). Radially, the tumor compresses the surrounding muscles and tissue, resulting in a pseudocapsule, a zone with a mixture of sarcoma cells, atrophic muscles, and edema. This pseudocapsule is not a true barrier to microscopic spread, nor are the minor intramuscular septae between the muscles within a compartment, as microscopic spread of the sarcoma can occur well beyond the gross tumor. Oncologic resection of sarcoma, in the absence of RT, requires wide margins, often to include the major compartmental fascia, interosseous membrane, peritoneum, perineurium, or adventitia of an organ, or at least a centimeter beyond the mass into surrounding fat. Figure 15.1 demonstrates magnetic resonance imaging (MRI) images of an atypical lipomatous tumor (ALT), formerly known as well-differentiated liposarcoma (WDLPS), of the left thigh with longitudinal and radial spread within the compartment.

Unlike carcinomas, most soft tissue sarcomas of the extremity and superficial trunk do not routinely spread to lymph nodes. Specific histopathologic subtypes with greater propensity to involve lymph nodes include clear cell sarcoma, angiosarcoma, rhabdomyosarcoma, and epithelioid sarcoma.[20,21] Synovial sarcoma is no longer included with these subtypes.[22] Given the rarity of lymphotrophic spread, there is no role for elective management of regional lymph nodes. Dissection of the regional nodal basin and elective nodal irradiation is not indicated in the vast majority of patients with soft tissue sarcoma. Some have suggested that more formal evaluation of the regional nodal basins be done for those histologies with greater likelihood of nodal involvement.[23] In the setting of clinical suspicion for nodal involvement, positron emission tomography (PET) may be considered as well as biopsy confirmation.[24] Optimal management of patients with clinically involved lymph nodes or nodes highly suspicious on imaging requires multidisciplinary care to consider the role for and sequence of therapies including lymph node dissection, nodal irradiation, and systemic therapies. Involvement of lymph nodes (N1 disease) predicts worse outcomes similar to presence of distant metastatic disease.[21] The eighth edition of the AJCC staging system for extremity and truncal soft tissue sarcoma now defines N1 disease as stage IV, reflecting this worse survival.[6]

The predominant site of metastatic spread of soft tissue sarcomas is hematogenous to the lung. Specific histopathologic subtypes have additional unique patterns of spread; understanding these patterns is important for appropriate staging evaluation and imaging beyond the primary site and chest. For example, myxoid liposarcoma has a propensity to spread to the spine, abdomen, and retroperitoneum; alveolar soft part sarcoma to the brain; and angiosarcoma to the brain and liver.

Diagnostic Evaluation and Staging

When a soft tissue sarcoma is suspected, anatomic imaging of the primary site is recommended prior to biopsy or other intervention. Cross-sectional imaging using MRI with and without contrast of the primary site is recommended to evaluate the extent of local disease and relationship to critical adjacent normal tissues, including neurovascular structures, bone, and visceral organs depending on anatomic location. MRI is the preferred modality to image soft tissue sarcomas of the trunk and extremities because of superior tissue definition of tumor from individual muscles compared with computed tomography (CT).[25,26] Figure 15.2 shows axial MRI and CT images of a liposarcoma of the right proximal thigh. Note the superior tumor definition on the MR image.

Definitive diagnosis of extremity or superficial truncal sarcoma requires pathologic confirmation. Core needle biopsy, most often image guided, is the preferred method for pathologic confirmation. This method is associated with a low complication rate and high accuracy and should be done by a radiologist or surgeon with sarcoma expertise.[27] The location and path of the biopsy must be planned in coordination with anticipated subsequent surgical management with meticulous attention to hemostasis. In the unlikely situation that histologic diagnosis cannot be made on the core biopsy sample, incisional biopsy may be performed as an alternative. If incisional biopsy is performed, the orthopedic or surgical oncologist who will be performing the oncologic resection should be

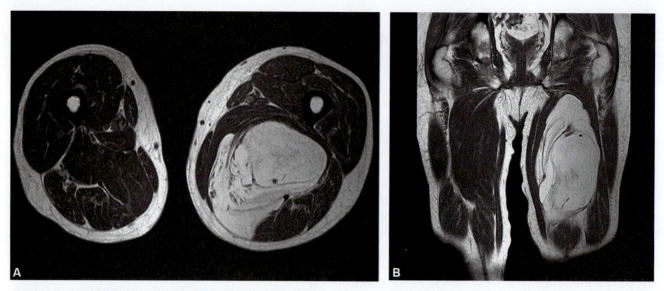

FIGURE 15.1. Axial **(A)** and coronal **(B)** MRI images of an atypical lipomatous tumor (ALT), formerly known as well-differentiated liposarcoma (WDLPS), of the left thigh demonstrating radial and longitudinal spread within the compartment.

involved in planning or performing the procedure. The incision must be oriented overlying the primary tumor site and longitudinally directed so that it may be excised at time of oncologic resection. Transverse incisions or poorly planned biopsy tracks that traverse unaffected tissues can violate compartments otherwise not likely to be involved by direct tumor extension. As sarcoma cells have a propensity for seeding, these tissues would then also be at risk, complicating subsequent local management including surgical resection and radiation. Fine needle aspiration does not provide adequate sample for histologic assessment and is not recommended for diagnosis. Excisional biopsy is generally not recommended. Such marginal excisions and unplanned excisions of soft tissue masses, when a sarcoma diagnosis is not anticipated, are non-oncologic and may complicate subsequent management. As such procedures are not performed with concern for margins, they essentially serve as "biopsies" for diagnosis and still require subsequent oncologic resections.[28] Procedural risks associated with excisional biopsies and unplanned excisions include hematomas, seeding of adjacent tissues, and poorly placed incisions that need to be resected at the time of oncologic surgery. These events can impact subsequent oncologic resection and increase risk for wound complications and need for reconstruction and complex closure.[29,30] The impact of initial unplanned excision on long-term sarcoma outcomes varies in the literature.[29–34] The biopsy approach also impacts subsequent radiation treatment planning, volume definition for areas at risk, and field design. Figure 15.3 demonstrates an example of a poorly placed transverse incision from an unplanned excision and the extent of subsequent oncologic resection required to excise the prior incision. Had the initial incision been placed longitudinally, the subsequent resection would have been much smaller.

Ideally, when soft tissue sarcoma is in the differential diagnosis, the biopsy should be performed by a team with expertise in sarcoma management, including surgery, radiology, and pathology. The important pathologic results from the biopsy are the histopathologic subtype and grade. There are over 50 different histopathologic subtypes of soft tissue sarcomas, named based on the presumed normal tissue that the tumor most closely resembles (e.g., adipocytic, fibroblastic/myofibroblastic, smooth muscle, skeletal muscle, vascular, nerve sheath, and undifferentiated).[1] The most common soft tissue sarcoma subtypes are UPS or unclassified soft tissue sarcoma (previously named malignant fibrous histiocytoma), liposarcoma, leiomyosarcoma, synovial sarcoma, and MPNST. Ancillary techniques, including molecular genetic testing, can be used to support the histologic diagnosis for some soft tissue sarcomas, such as ALT/WDLPS with MDM2 amplification, myxoid liposarcoma t(12;16)(q13;p11) involving FUS-DDIT3 gene and t(12;22)(q13;q12) involving ESWR1-DDIT3, synovial sarcoma t(X;18)(p11;q11), and dermatofibrosarcoma protuberans involving COL1A1-PDGFβ (platelet-derived growth factor). Pleomorphic liposarcoma and leiomyosarcoma have complex alterations. Individual histopathologic subtypes have unique natural histories, patterns of behavior, and risk for LR and distant metastatic spread.

Histologic grade of sarcoma is generally assigned using the French Federation of Cancer Centers Sarcoma Group (FNCLCC) system of grades 1, 2, and 3.[1] The FNCLCC grade is determined by the sum of scores for differentiation, mitotic activity, and necrosis. Grade is an integral component within the AJCC staging system.[6] High-grade best predicts risk for distant metastatic spread.[35,36] Both high- and low-grade tumors have risk for LR.

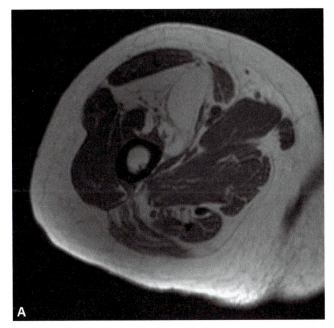

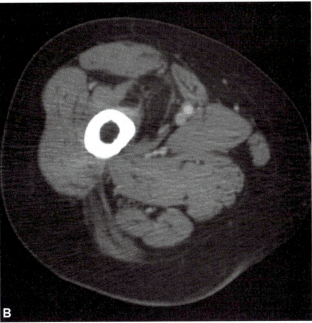

FIGURE 15.2. Axial MRI **(A)** and CT **(B)** images of a liposarcoma of the right proximal thigh. Note the superior tumor definition on the MR compared to CT image.

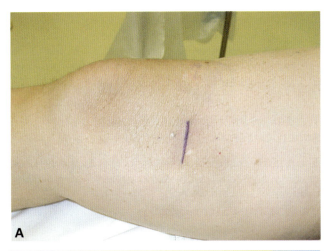

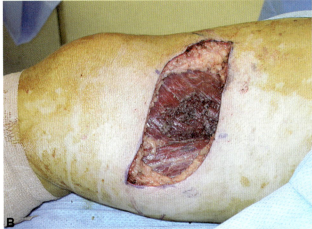

FIGURE 15.3. Images demonstrating a poorly placed transverse incision from an unplanned excision **(A)** with the purple marker delineating the prior incision. Extent of subsequent oncologic resection **(B)** required to excise the prior incision. Had the initial incision been placed longitudinally, the subsequent resection would have been much smaller.

Further evaluation, including the need for staging imaging, can be done following pathologic confirmation of soft tissue sarcoma histopathology and grade and is based on risk for local, regional, and distant spread. Staging imaging for soft tissue sarcoma most commonly includes chest imaging (either chest x-ray or chest CT based on risk, with CT commonly used for primary tumors >5 cm, deep to fascia, and intermediate/high grade). Additional site directed imaging should be determined by the patterns of spread for the individual histopathologic subtype. For example, abdominal pelvic CT and MR of the spine are recommended for myxoid liposarcoma because of risk of extrapulmonary spread.[37] PET/CT is not routinely used for staging, although some centers will use PET/CT for certain histopathologic subtypes with a significant risk of nodal involvement (e.g., epithelioid sarcoma) and to assess response to chemotherapy.[38–40]

There are important changes in the AJCC eighth edition staging system for soft tissue sarcoma. New classifications for anatomic subsites, such as retroperitoneum, head and neck, and abdomen and thoracic visceral organs, have been introduced. The T category size criteria have been updated and differ by anatomic subsite. For soft tissue sarcoma of the extremity and trunk, the T category is no longer subdivided as superficial or deep to fascia, and regional nodal involvement (N1) is now considered stage IV disease. For RPS, in the absence of distant metastases, N1 disease is stage IIIB. As reflected in the AJCC staging system, anatomic site, increasing size of the primary tumor, nodal involvement, and grade are important prognostic factors in assessing risk for LR and distant metastatic spread.[6] The AJCC eighth edition staging tumor-node-metastasis (TNM) classification system for soft tissue sarcoma of the extremity and trunk and retroperitoneum is shown in Table 15.1. The prognostic stage groups for soft tissue sarcoma of the extremity and trunk are shown in Table 15.2. The prognostic stage groups for RPS are shown in Table 15.3.

Treatment Paradigm for Extremity and Superficial Truncal Soft Tissue Sarcoma

The primary treatment modality for localized soft tissue sarcoma is resection with widely negative margins. The treatment paradigm for local therapy has evolved from radical resection (i.e., amputation for primary extremity tumors) to combined modality therapy with wide local excision and RT for most patients. Goals of therapy for localized disease include local control and preservation of function, with use of limb- or organ-sparing approaches. Resection alone may result in high rates of local control in selected patients, usually those with small, low-grade tumors for whom widely negative margins can be achieved. RT may be delivered pre- or postoperatively, definitively for unresectable disease, and palliatively. The role for systemic therapy, including chemotherapy, immunotherapy, and other targeted agents, is complex and changing, and consideration for use should be addressed by medical or pediatric oncology in appropriate patients.[41,42] Given the heterogeneity of soft tissue sarcoma, systemic therapy recommendations are increasingly tailored to histopathologic subtype. Treatment recommendations for individual patients should be determined by multidisciplinary evaluation and input from sarcoma specialists in all disciplines for optimal outcomes. Such care coordination and evaluation should be done prior to initiation of treatment.[8]

Surgical Resection

Historically, soft tissue sarcoma of the extremity was treated with amputation. In the modern era, primary amputation may still be indicated in about 5% of cases, including those for whom a functional limb after limb-conserving therapy is not feasible (e.g., severe peripheral vascular disease, diabetes, other comorbidities; involvement of a major nerve plexus or artery, involvement of multiple compartments; or near-circumferential subcutaneous involvement for which reconstruction may not be possible).[43] Figure 15.4 shows contrast-enhanced MRI and CT images of a high-grade UPS of the right proximal thigh with involvement of the neurovascular bundle, skin, and subcutaneous tissues.

With limb-sparing resections, primary tumors are excised en bloc without violating tumor and with widely negative margins. The generally recommended margin for soft tissue sarcoma in the absence of adjuvant RT is at least 1 cm, but is dependent on location, adjacent tissues and organs, and type of resection planned, and should be individualized to the patient. Excisional biopsies and

---

TABLE 15.1   AJCC Staging TNM Classification for Soft Tissue Sarcoma of the Extremity and Trunk or Retroperitoneum

TNM Classification

T Primary Tumor of the Extremity and Trunk or Retroperitoneum

T0	No evidence of primary tumor
T1	Tumor ≤5 cm in greatest diameter
T2	Tumor >5 and ≤10 cm in greatest diameter
T3	Tumor >10 and ≤15 cm in greatest diameter
T4	Tumor >15 cm in greatest diameter

N Regional Lymph Nodes

N0	No regional lymph node metastasis or unknown lymph node status
N1	Regional lymph node metastasis

M Distant Metastasis

M0	No distant metastasis
M1	Distant metastasis

G FNCLCC Histologic Tumor Grade*

G1	Total differentiation, mitotic count, and necrosis score of 2 or 3
G2	Total differentiation, mitotic count, and necrosis score of 4 or 5
G3	Total differentiation, mitotic count, and necrosis score of 6, 7, or 8

*FNCLCC histologic tumor grade = differentiation, mitotic activity, and necrosis are each scored and the summed to determine grade.

From Amin MB, Edge SB, Greene FL, et al. *AJCC Cancer Staging Manual*, 8th edition. New York: Springer; 2017 reproduced with permission of SNCSC.

TABLE 15.2   AJCC Staging Classification for Soft Tissue Sarcoma—Stage Groups for Extremity and Trunk

Stage Groups

Stage IA	T1	N0	M0	G1 or GX
Stage IB	T2, T3, or T4	N0	M0	G1 or GX
Stage II	T1	N0	M0	G2 or G3
Stage IIIA	T2	N0	M0	G2 or G3
Stage IIIB	T3 or T4	N0	M0	G2 or G3
Stage IV	Any T	N1	M0	Any G
Stage IV	Any T	Any N	M1	Any G

From Amin MB, Edge SB, Greene FL, et al. *AJCC Cancer Staging Manual*, 8th edition. New York: Springer; 2017 reproduced with permission of SNCSC.

TABLE 15.3	AJCC Staging Classification for Soft Tissue Sarcoma—Stage Groups for Retroperitoneum			
Stage Groups				
Stage IA	T1	N0	M0	G1 or GX
Stage IB	T2, T3, or T4	N0	M0	G1 or GX
Stage II	T1	N0	M0	G2 or G3
Stage IIIA	T2	N0	M0	G2 or G3
Stage IIIB	T3 or T4	N0	M0	G2 or G3
Stage IIIB	Any T	N1	M0	Any G
Stage IV	Any T	Any N	M1	Any G

From Amin MB, Edge SB, Greene FL, et al. *AJCC Cancer Staging Manual*, 8th edition. New York: Springer; 2017 reproduced with permission of SNCSC.

marginal excisions are not considered oncologic resection for soft tissue sarcoma as they do not provide appropriate margins. Resections that violate the pseudocapsule or are intralesional, piecemeal, or subtotal in nature are suboptimal and are associated with higher LR. For tumors near neurovascular structures, bones, or other critical structures, acceptable margins may be much smaller (1 to 2 mm) if the specimen is removed with the involved natural anatomic barriers such as fascia of the compartment. Such anticipated close margins are oncologically appropriate and the proximity of the tumor to critical structures often an indication for use of RT to improve local control.[44] Unanticipated positive margins are associated with increased risk for LR.[44–47] Soft tissue sarcomas generally do not cross compartmental fascia or periosteum with the exception of locally advanced cases or where violation of the barrier has occurred through biopsy or prior procedures. Major nerves are usually preserved if possible, with nerve sheath as a margin. The exception is for MPNST, which often arise within the nerve itself and where it may be necessary to resect the involved nerve to minimize risk of leaving macroscopic or diffuse microscopic disease. Major arteries involved may be resected and reconstructed, whereas veins generally are not reconstructed. Margins along abutting bone can be cleared by stripping the involved periosteum. Periosteal stripping should be limited to tumors directly abutting the periosteum, especially in weight-bearing bones such as the femur, as periosteal stripping is associated with increased risk for fracture.[48–51] If periosteal stripping is necessary for tumors directly abutting bone, some surgeons may recommend prophylactic fixation, particularly if RT is planned.

Surgical wounds may be closed primarily or require complex closure with rotational or free tissue flaps. The use of flap reconstruction does not appear to adversely affect postoperative function or health status outcomes.[52]

A multidisciplinary discussion of the surgical approach, including anticipated close margins and plan for periosteal stripping, vascular resection, and reconstruction, informs radiation treatment planning, both in the preoperative and postoperative settings.

Importance of Radiation Therapy in Limb-Sparing Approaches

The role for limb-sparing resection with RT was established by the National Cancer Institute (NCI) I prospective clinical trial. On this study, 43 patients with high-grade soft tissue sarcoma were randomized to limb salvage surgery with postoperative RT (5000 cGy to the entire anatomic area at risk and a total dose of 6000 to 7000 cGy to the tumor bed) versus amputation. Both arms received chemotherapy. At 5 years, there were four LRs in the limb-sparing group. There was no statistical difference in disease-free survival (71% vs. 78% at 5 years p = 0.75) or overall survival (83% vs. 88% p = 0.99) between the limb-sparing or the amputation groups, respectively. Positive margins were associated with increased risk for LR (p < 0.0001).[53]

The subsequent NCI II study further evaluated the role for RT in the setting of limb-sparing resections. Patients were randomized to surgery alone versus surgery and postoperative radiation. Patients with high-grade soft tissue sarcoma also received adjuvant chemotherapy. The impact of RT on LR was significant in both high-grade and low-grade sarcoma. With long-term follow-up, the rate of LR was 1.4% (n = 1) with limb-sparing surgery and RT versus 25% (n = 18) with limb-sparing surgery alone (p = 0.0001). There was no difference in rates of distant metastasis or overall survival. The results of the study also suggested that selected patients at low risk for LR may be well treated with resection alone.[54,55]

A trial of adjuvant brachytherapy versus no brachytherapy after complete excision of extremity or trunk sarcoma also demonstrated the impact of radiotherapy on local control.[56] Brachytherapy was delivered using iridium-192 implant to 4200 to 4500 cGy over 4 to 5 days. Five-year local control rate was 82% with brachytherapy versus 69% without brachytherapy (p = 0.04). For high-grade sarcoma, local control was 89% with brachytherapy versus 66% without brachytherapy (p = 0.0025). In contrast to the NCI II trial, brachytherapy did not show a statistically significant local control benefit for low-grade sarcoma (p = 0.49).[54–56] As in the NCI studies, use of adjuvant RT did not impact distant metastasis, disease-specific survival, or overall survival.[53–56]

Results of these studies demonstrate that use of RT in the setting of limb-sparing surgery improves local control without a detriment to survival. These studies established limb (or organ)-sparing resection with RT as the standard treatment approach, preserving function, and replacing amputation or radical resection for most patients.

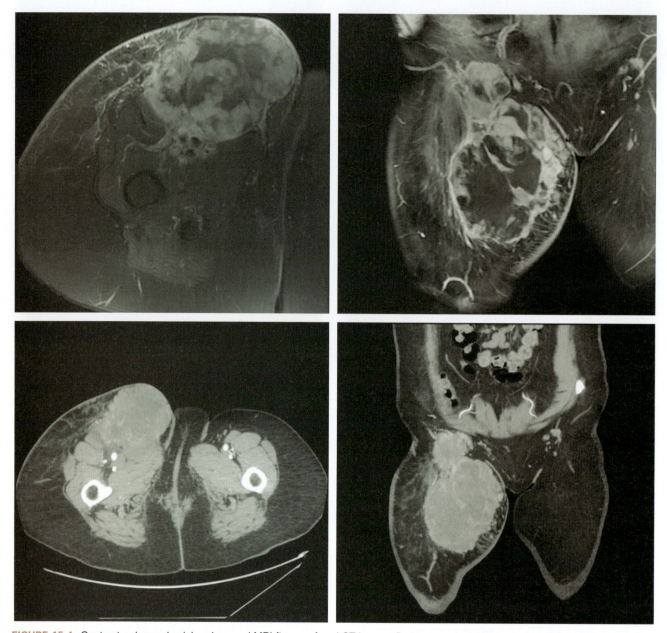

FIGURE 15.4. Contrast-enhanced axial and coronal MRI **(top row)** and CT images **(bottom row)** of a high-grade undifferentiated pleomorphic sarcoma (UPS) of the right proximal thigh with involvement of the neurovascular bundle, skin, and subcutaneous tissues. Extensive internal necrosis is present.

Factors Associated with Recurrence Risk and Indications for Radiation

Indications for addition of RT, preoperatively or postoperatively, to oncologic resection are based on evaluation of risk for LR and options for salvage in such an event. Estimation of recurrence risk is based on patient, tumor, and treatment factors including ability to achieve negative margin resection, adjacent critical normal structures, tumor grade, size, location, and histopathologic subtype.

While the relative impact of each factor varies throughout the literature, the most consistent and important prognostic risk factor for LR is a positive or uncertain surgical margin.[35,36,57–64] Macroscopic positive margins or gross residual diseases are categorized as R2 resections and are associated with significantly high rates of recurrence. Microscopically positive or close margins are R1. Close or microscopically positive margins differ in their risk for recurrence based on whether they are anticipated or planned (i.e., adjacent to a critical structure including vessel, nerve, or bone) or unanticipated, with the latter associated with higher risk.[44] Negative margin resections are R0 and are defined as no tumor on ink.[6] Given the increased risk for LR with positive margins, especially in the setting of R2 resections or unanticipated R1 margins, re-resection to obtain negative margins should be considered if possible.[65] Such clinical scenarios warrant multidisciplinary discussion and collaboration between the surgeon and radiation oncologist regarding the role for RT to improve local control. The addition of RT does not fully offset the negative impact of R2 disease or unanticipated microscopic positive margins on recurrence and outcomes, highlighting the importance of negative margin resection for soft tissue sarcoma.

The ability to obtain widely negative margins is impacted by anatomic location and size of the primary tumor. The importance of these factors is highlighted by the introduction of new classification systems for anatomic subsites with different T size categories in the AJCC eighth edition.[6] These variables are important for LR risk but are also prognostic for distant recurrence risk and outcome. Similarly, tumor grade is the key determinant for distant metastatic risk and prognosis and is a critical factor in the staging system. High-grade tumors have greater distant recurrence risk; both low- and high-grade tumors have risk for LR.

Individual histopathologic subtypes differ in their natural histories and risk for local versus distant recurrence. For example, superficial myxofibrosarcoma is highly infiltrative, particularly in subcutaneous tissues, and the extent of local involvement and microscopic spread is difficult to determine based on imaging. Myxofibrosarcoma has a propensity for multiple LRs, and lesser overall metastatic risk. Given their infiltrative spread, positive margin resection rates are not uncommon, and RT is often used to improve local control.[66–69] MPNST is also highly infiltrative, frequently with microscopic extension well beyond the disease visible on imaging. Accordingly, MPNST is associated with increased risk for LR, and also has high risk for distant metastases.[70] Myxoid liposarcomas are relatively more responsive to RT than other histopathologies. Significant volume reductions have been seen with preoperative RT, and local control rates are excellent.[71,72] The DOREMY study (Dose Reduction of Preoperative Radiotherapy in Myxoid Liposarcoma) is currently investigating preoperative dose reduction to 3600 cGy in 18 fractions in this setting (ClinicalTrials.gov Identifier: NCT02106312).

Surgery Alone for Soft Tissue Sarcoma

There is a subset of patients with soft tissue sarcoma for whom resection alone will provide high rates of local control and thus may not require RT. Large population–based studies and single institution studies suggest that some patients with T1 or low-grade tumors may not benefit from adjuvant RT.[58,73–75] In a prospective trial of selected patients with T1 soft tissue sarcoma, 84% of patients were able to have R0

resection and were treated with surgery alone with isolated LR of 10.6% at 10 years.[74] In a series of 74 patients treated with function-sparing surgery without RT, 10-year local control rate was 93%. Patients with margins <1 cm had 87% local control compared with 100% for those with margins ≥1 cm (p = 0.04), rates comparable to that reported with RT.[75] A nomogram was developed to predict LR based on 684 patients with extremity sarcoma treated with limb-sparing surgery alone that includes age, size, margin status, grade, and histology as five independent predictors of recurrence.[58] In clinical practice, surgical resection alone is reserved for select cases, often low grade, and those with small superficial tumors or small tumors that are entirely intramuscular for which widely negative margins can be achieved.

Sequencing of Radiation Therapy and Resection in Combined Modality Therapy

The studies first investigating limb-sparing approaches included resection with postoperative radiation. The role for preoperative radiation with limb-sparing resection was established by the seminal National Cancer Institute Canada (NCIC) SR2 trial. NCI Canada conducted this randomized clinical trial comparing preoperative RT versus postoperative RT in 190 patients with extremity soft tissue sarcoma, mostly intermediate or high grade. Patients were randomized to preoperative RT with 5000 cGy (with postoperative boost of 1600 to 2000 cGy if positive margins) versus postoperative RT to 6600 cGy (5000 cGy covering an initial large field covering the incision plus a 1600 to 2000 cGy reduced field to the tumor bed). The tumor volumes on both arms were 5 cm proximal and distal to the tissues at risk, followed by reduction to 2 cm around the initial tumor bed (the reduced volume boost field was only used in the preoperative arm if the surgical margins were positive). The primary endpoint was major wound healing complication within 120 days of resection. Major wound complications were defined as an operation for wound repair or other wound management such as readmission for care, including antibiotics, or persistent deep packing for 120 days or longer. A planned interim analysis found more acute wound healing complications with preoperative RT versus postoperative RT (35% versus 17% p = 0.01), and the study was terminated early.[76] Tumor size (>10 cm) and anatomic site (upper and lower legs vs. upper and lower arms) were predictors for wound complications with preoperative RT. Local control was similar with either preoperative or postoperative RT. Within the first year, the timing of RT had minimal impact on patient function, however with longer follow-up, preoperative RT was associated with less late toxicity.[77,78] Late radiation morbidity and its impact on function was assessed by the Musculoskeletal Tumor Society (MSTS) Rating Scale and the Toronto Extremity Salvage Score (TESS). Long-term follow-up demonstrated a trend toward greater rates of fibrosis (48.2% vs. 31.5%), joint stiffness

(23.2% vs. 17.8%), and edema (23.2% vs. 15.5%) in the postoperative versus preoperative groups. The presence of these late toxicities, which were more frequent in postoperative group, predicted for lower functional scores (p < 0.01). Field size, greater with postoperative RT, was a predictor of fibrosis and joint stiffness with a trend for edema (p = 0.002, p = 0.006, and p = 0.06, respectively).[78]

There are advantages and disadvantages to preoperative and postoperative RT. Compared to postoperative RT, preoperative RT allows for clear delineation of tumor and areas at risk, potential reduction of seeding, improvement in margin negative resection rates, and delivery of lower dose and treatment of smaller volumes, resulting in reduction in late effects and improved function.[76,78–80] The primary disadvantage of preoperative RT is increased risk for acute wound complications. Postoperative RT allows for evaluation of the entire tumor specimen and surgical margins, and potentially may allow omission of RT in selected cases. The primary disadvantage is higher risk for late irreversible RT-related toxicities.[78,81,82] There are no significant differences in local control or other disease outcomes between preoperative and postoperative RT.[76]

As preoperative RT delivers lower doses to smaller field sizes than postoperative RT and is associated with fewer late toxicities, for the majority of patients, the general preference is for preoperative RT over postoperative RT. This preference for preoperative RT acknowledges the associated increased risk for acute wound complications. However, wound complications, while causing disability in the short term, are usually temporary and reversible, whereas fibrosis, joint stiffness, and edema are irreversible and cause lasting impact on function.

Patient factors (e.g., age, comorbidities associated with anesthesia, operative, and wound healing risks such as obesity and diabetes, smoking), tumor characteristics (e.g., anticipated margins, anatomic site, size, and histopathologic subtype), and planned treatments (surgical approach, use of RT, and systemic therapy) should be considered for individual patients in management decisions. The sequence of irradiation and resection is optimally coordinated in a multidisciplinary manner and considers both short-term wound complication risks and long-term functional outcomes. Areas of concern for close or microscopically positive margins, type of resection, anticipated closure technique and possible reconstruction, and tentative plan for management of potential wound complications if they occur, should be discussed by the treating radiation oncologist and surgeon.

There are some exceptions to the general preference for preoperative RT. Selected patients who are at significant increased risk for major wound complications due to factors such as multiple existing medical comorbidities (e.g., obesity, diabetes, and peripheral vascular disease), smoking, and anatomic site (e.g., medial proximal thigh, anterior lower leg) may be better treated with postoperative RT after complete healing.[76,82–86] Some selected patients

with significant tumor-associated symptoms at presentation, including fungating and bleeding tumor or pain, may also be considered for resection followed by postoperative RT. In these clinical scenarios, the acute issues or risk for major wound complications would be determined to outweigh risk for late toxicities by the treating team. In circumstances when the tumor and extent of microscopic extension are difficult to determine on preoperative imaging, such that defining appropriate treatment volumes is not possible for preoperative RT, resection first may be appropriate, as may be the case with some subcutaneous myxofibrosarcomas.

Indication for Radiation Therapy with Resection

Indication for RT in addition to wide local excision for extremity and truncal soft tissue sarcoma is complex and based on assessment of risk for LR. Risk assessment considers natural history of the histopathologic subtype, anatomic site of presentation, the ability to obtain negative margins at resection, and potential consequences of a LR and options for salvage. RT is indicated when an improvement in local control is clinically important, when risks for LR are high, when the consequences of an LR are significant, and when there are limited options for management of recurrent disease.[45,46] In clinical practice, RT is indicated for most patients with stages II and III disease and is also appropriate in select patients with stages I and IV disease. When risk for recurrence is high, preoperative delivery of RT is preferred for most patients. Surgery alone is appropriate when there is no clear indication for RT at presentation and high local control with widely negative margin resection is anticipated. Some patients treated with initial resection may have unexpected adverse pathologic features discovered, such as positive margins, conversion to higher grade, significantly larger tumor extent than suspected on preoperative imaging, discontinuous spread, and nodal involvement. These patients at high risk for LR and postoperative RT are indicated to improve local control.[53–56]

Dose and Fractionation for Radiation Therapy

Preoperative RT

The majority of clinical trials establishing the role for RT in combined modality therapy for soft tissue sarcoma of the extremity and trunk have used conventional fractionation.[53,54,76,79] The preferred dose for preoperative RT is 5000 cGy as 200 cGy per fraction in 25 fractions. If chemotherapy is given concurrently or in an interdigitated manner, the total dose and dose per fraction may be reduced to minimize complications with chemosensitization (4500 to 5040 cGy in 25 to 28 fractions or 4400 cGy in 22 fractions.[87–90] Figure 15.5 demonstrates extensive internal tumor necrosis in a high-grade UPS following preoperative chemoRT.

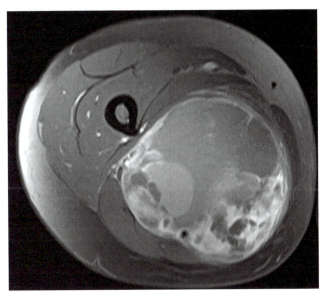

FIGURE 15.5. High-grade undifferentiated pleomorphic sarcoma (UPS) of the thigh after preoperative chemoRT showing extensive internal necrosis.

Hypofractionation

There is growing evidence for use of hypofractionated preoperative RT regimens and such courses remain a promising area of active investigation. These regimens differ by dose fractionation schema, use of concurrent systemic therapy (chemotherapy and targeted agents), and time to resection. As these hypofractionated courses have limited patient numbers and variable follow-up and toxicity assessments, no one regimen can be considered an established alternative option at this time. Furthermore, there is no randomized trial comparing these hypofractionated regimens with conventional fractionation. Most reports suggest acceptable local control rates. Representative RT regimens include 500 cGy × 5 fractions, 600 cGy × 5 fractions, 700 to 800 cGy × 5 fractions, and chemoRT 350 cGy × 5 to 8 fractions with doxorubicin and/or ifosfamide as well as 300 cGy × 10 fractions.[91–99] Initial reports suggested lower rates of R0 resections and local control with 500 cGy × 5 fractions, although a subset of patients with myxoid liposarcoma had excellent control with this regimen.[91,92]

Boost for Positive Margins or Gross Disease

In the setting of a positive margin following delivery of preoperative RT, the feasibility of re-resection for negative margins should always be addressed. If re-resection is not feasible, a radiation boost may be considered in select patients with positive margins acknowledging the efficacy of this approach is unclear. Boost doses may be delivered via various techniques including external beam RT (EBRT), intraoperative RT (IORT), and brachytherapy. Brachytherapy boost is typically 1600 cGy low-dose rate or 340 cGy twice daily for four fractions with high-dose rate. The dose

for intraoperative electron RT is 1000 to 1250 cGy in a single fraction. Use of an IORT boost in addition to EBRT is associated with high local control rates and no significant increase in acute or late morbidity.[100–104] Given the prolonged time interval between preoperative EBRT and postoperative healing, it is unclear whether a postoperative EBRT boost is beneficial for positive margins in this setting. EBRT boost dose is typically 1600 cGy for positive margins and 2000 cGy for gross residual disease. Some studies found no impact of EBRT boost on local control, while others have shown a benefit with dose escalation.[47,105–107] Given the unclear efficacy for an EBRT boost following preoperative RT, its use should be tailored to individual patients at high risk of recurrence for whom the areas of concern are well defined, and further RT is expected to be associated with minimal additional morbidity.

Postoperative RT

Total dose for postoperative RT is influenced by margin status of the resection. A larger volume encompassing the resection bed, preoperative target with margin, incision, and drain sites (when feasible), is treated to 5000 cGy as 200 cGy per fraction. Additional dose of 1000 cGy (for negative margins) or 1600 cGy (for positive margins) is delivered to a reduced volume, defined by target with margin, often the tumor bed and area of surgical clips.[53,54,76] Higher dose may be considered for gross residual disease. Traditionally, these courses have been given sequentially, but they may also be delivered concurrently using a simultaneous integrated boost.

Target Definitions for Preoperative and Postoperative Radiation Therapy

Historically, RT treatment fields were large. Targets were determined by the natural growth patterns of sarcoma, using a 5 to 10 cm longitudinal margin on tumor, reflecting the greater risk of microscopic spread of sarcomas along the axis of the involved compartment, and a 2 to 3 cm radial expansion. Treatment volumes nearly encompassed the full compartment of the limb and were designed with understanding of the anatomy of involved muscle groups, operative findings, and with intent to spare a strip limb circumference.[108] In the modern era with use of advanced imaging and planning techniques, including MRI for target definition, CT simulation, and volumetric planning, volumes have been able to be reduced.

The NCIC SR2 randomized trial provided definitions for the preoperative and postoperative volumes to be treated. The preoperative and initial postoperative irradiated volume treated to 5000 cGy was defined as the target with 5 cm longitudinal and 2 cm radial margins. For patients receiving postoperative RT or those who required a postoperative boost, a reduced target volume, including the tumor or tumor bed with 2 cm margins, was treated with an additional 1600 to 2000 cGy.[76] CT simulation and planning was encouraged. Using these target definitions and margins, the local control on this trial was high.

Increasing use of MRI has allowed for more precise target definition on imaging and subsequent reduction of these large margins. A study of patients with high-grade extremity and truncal soft tissue sarcoma correlated the extent of peritumoral edema and reactive changes on preoperative MRI with presence of tumor cells in tissue at time of resection. This study demonstrated that T1 contrast enhancement abnormalities ranged from 0 to 5.3 cm and T2 peritumoral signal abnormalities ranged from 0 to 7.1 cm beyond the gross tumor. Sarcoma cells could be identified beyond the gross tumor in 10 of 15 cases. Of these, six cases had sarcoma cells within 1 cm of the gross tumor, four cases had sarcoma cells >1 cm, and up to maximum of 4 cm from the gross tumor. The presence of microscopic spread did not correlate with tumor size or MRI peritumoral changes.[109] The information provided by this study, particularly the presence of microscopic spread up to 4 cm from the gross tumor, justified the recommended margins for preoperative RT.

A review by Haas et al. provided updated target definitions for extremity soft tissue sarcoma.[110] Longitudinal margins are oriented along the plane of the muscle fibers, and radial margins are perpendicular to the fibers. For preoperative RT, a dose of 5000 cGy in 25 fractions is prescribed to a single planning target volume (PTV). The gross tumor volume (GTV) is defined based on visible tumor seen on T1 contrast-enhanced MRI. The MRI should be fused to the planning CT when possible. The clinical target volume (CTV) includes a 4 cm longitudinal and 1.5 cm radial expansion on GTV and is adapted to encompass any suspicious peritumoral edema (when feasible). The CTV is anatomically constrained and should not expand into uninvolved bone or beyond compartmental fascia. There is no elective nodal irradiation. Figure 15.6 demonstrates an example of a CTV that has been anatomically constrained.

In patients receiving postoperative boost, the CTV is defined by the surgical bed and includes the reconstructed "GTV" from fused preoperative imaging with 2 cm longitudinal and 1.5 cm radial expansions. The boost volume is treated with an additional 1000 to 1600 cGy depending on margin status and recurrence risk.

For postoperative RT, a larger volume encompassing the resection bed, preoperative target with margin, surgical clips, incision, and drain sites (if not at significant distance from resection bed) is treated to 5000 cGy in 25 fractions. This volume, CTV1, includes the previous location of the tumor "GTV" by fusing the preoperative imaging with the simulation CT. An expansion of 4 cm longitudinally and 1.5 cm radially is added. CTV2 is a reduced volume defined by the target with margin (often the tumor bed and aided by surgical clips) with 4 cm longitudinal and 1.5 cm radial margins that have been anatomically constrained. This reduced volume CTV2 is treated with an additional 1000 to 1600 cGy.[53,54,76,110]

Higher dose may be considered for gross residual disease. Often, these courses are given sequentially but may also be treated as simultaneous integrated boost.

The recommended PTV is 0.5 to 1 cm in all directions, but the appropriate PTV for each patient should take into account the reproducibility of the setup, use of immobilization and image guidance, and institutional practice. Importantly, these volume definitions and margins are general recommendations and should not replace clinical decision-making for individual patients.

The previously mentioned target volume recommendations have been extrapolated to non-extremity sites. For subcutaneous tumors not involving fascia, it is not appropriate to employ different longitudinal and radial expansions as tumor extension is not along muscle fibers nor constrained within a defined compartment. In such circumstances, a 3 to 4 cm circumferential expansion around the subcutaneous GTV is used and constrained to 0.5 to 1 cm into underlying uninvolved muscle.

The Radiation Therapy Oncology Group (RTOG) 0630 prospective trial evaluated the use of MRI fusion and image-guided radiation therapy (IGRT) to further reduce both CTV and PTV for preoperative RT. The GTV was defined by T1 contrast-enhanced MRI sequences, ideally with registration and fusion to the planning CT. The CTV expansions on GTV differed based on grade. For high-grade tumors, the CTV was defined as GTV with 3 cm longitudinal and 1.5 cm radial expansions. For low-grade tumors, the CTV was the GTV with 2 cm longitudinal and 1 cm radial margins. The CTV was adapted to encompass any suspicious peritumoral edema and was anatomically constrained to the intact fascial barrier excluding uninvolved bone, skin, and subcutaneous tissue. IGRT, using either daily orthogonal imaging or cone beam CT (CBCT), was required for a reduced PTV of 0.5 cm.[79,111] Figure 15.7 demonstrates an example of CTV that encompasses suspicious peritumoral edema.

Companion studies to RTOG 0630 assessed the variability of preoperative GTV and CTV target volume definition and contouring of suspicious peritumoral edema among sarcoma radiation oncologists.[112,113] There was a near-perfect agreement in the GTV and CTV of a lower extremity case, but more variation in the CTV definition for an upper extremity case.[112] There was also good agreement on suspicious edema using T2-weighted MRI images of high-grade extremity sarcomas.[113] A consensus for preoperative RT GTV and CTV target definition was developed to guide target definition for the RTOG 0630 trial.[111] A deformable RTOG Consensus Atlas of Musculoskeletal Anatomy (CAMAS) of the lower extremities was developed as a part of this trial to be a useful tool for designing anatomically appropriate target volumes.[114]

High rates of local control were seen on RTOG 0630 with use of these reduced margins and daily IGRT. Out of 79 evaluable patients on the cohort treated without chemotherapy, there were five local failures. All the local failures were in field, none were marginal. Acute major

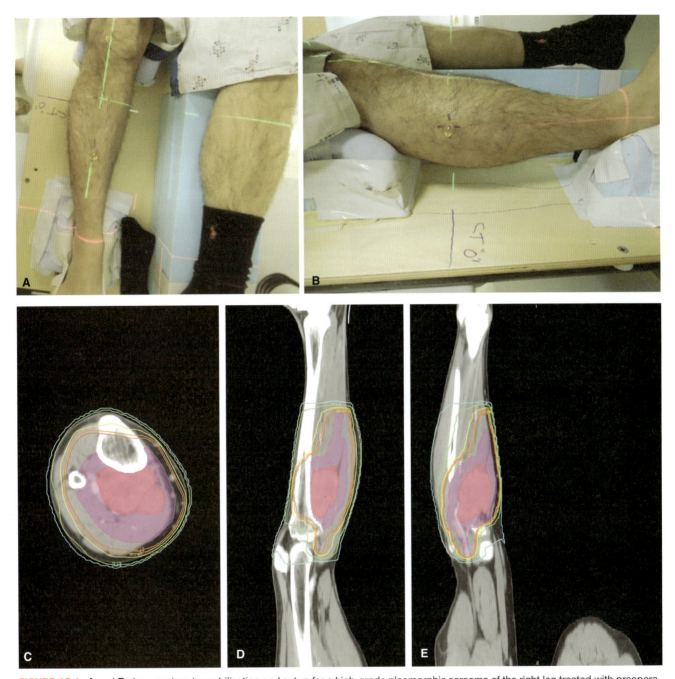

FIGURE 15.6. **A** and **B** show custom immobilization and setup for a high-grade pleomorphic sarcoma of the right leg treated with preoperative RT. Axial **(C)**, sagittal **(D)**, and coronal **(E)** images of GTV (solid red) and CTV (shaded magenta). 3D conformal photon plan. Note that the CTV is anatomically constrained and does not extend into bone or beyond the fascia into subcutaneous tissue or skin. This allows dose sparing of the uninvolved subcutaneous tissue laterally and the pretibial soft tissue anteriorly.

wound complications, as defined on the NCIC SR2 trial, occurred in 36.6% of assessable patients, all with primary tumors of the lower extremity, and included reoperation (25.4%), readmission (21.1%), and prolonged dressing changes (23.9%). Fifty-seven patients were evaluable for the primary endpoint of late toxicity (fibrosis, joint stiffness, or edema). Grade ≥2 late toxicity at 2 years was 10.5%. The authors concluded that with daily image guidance, the reduction in target volumes used on the study did not lead to higher rates of LR and resulted in reduction of late toxicities.[79]

Consistently, limb-conserving therapy with irradiation provides high local control rates with preservation of function. Similar to extent of surgical resection, for radiotherapy treatment planning, there is a balance between wide margins to reduce LR and attempts to spare surrounding normal tissues to preserve function. The margins delineated earlier have been associated with few marginal recurrences and less late RT toxicities.[79,110,115,116]

Soft tissue late effects are related to both total dose and irradiated volume. As shown in the NCIC SR2

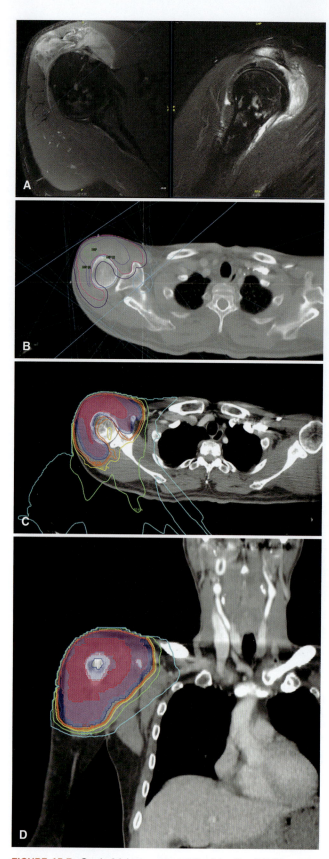

FIGURE 15.7. Grade 2 leiomyosarcoma involving the deltoid muscle. **A:** Note the extensive suspicious peritumoral edema along the deltoid muscle from origin to insertion. **B:** Target contours for a preoperative IMRT plan using daily CBCT for IGRT to allow for a 5 mm PTV (*dark purple*) around the CTV (*red*). The CTV includes the suspicious peritumoral edema. Axial **(C)** and coronal **(D)** views of the isodose distribution.

trial, late effects of fibrosis, edema, and joint stiffness were greater with postoperative RT versus preoperative RT.[76,78] The RTOG 0630 trial demonstrated reduction in late toxicities with preoperative RT with standardized target volume definitions, using MRI imaging for target definitions, reduced CTV and PTV expansions, and daily IGRT.[79] The VORTEX Trial (randomised trial of volume of post-operative radiotherapy given to adult patients with extremity soft tissue sarcoma) in the United Kingdom is a randomized controlled multicenter trial evaluating whether a smaller postoperative treatment volume can be used to improve limb function without a detriment to local control (ClinicalTrials.gov Identifier NCT 00423618). On this study, the control arm receives 5000 cGy to CTV1 (5 cm longitudinal and 2 cm radial margins) followed by 1600 cGy to CTV2 (2 cm margins). The experimental arm receives 6600 cGy to a single CTV with smaller 2 cm circumferential expansions. A separate ongoing randomized phase III clinical trial of preoperative versus postoperative intensity-modulated RT (IMRT) for extremity and truncal soft tissue sarcoma is evaluating potential dose reduction to 5000 cGy in the postoperative setting for patients with negative margins. The preoperative dose is 5000 cGy. Both arms include an optional boost of 1600 cGy for positive margins. The primary endpoint is incidence of acute wound complications (ClinicalTrials.gov Identifier: NCT02565498).

Acute and Late Effects, Organs at Risk, and Dose Constraints

Treatment planning for soft tissue sarcoma balances delivery of the prescribed dose to targets while minimizing dose to normal adjacent tissues. The sparing of normal tissues is important for both acute effects, which are generally self-limited, and late effects, which are irreversible and can impact long-term functional outcomes. As soft tissue sarcomas occur at anatomic sites throughout the body, the appropriate set of normal tissue dose constraints for treatment planning will be based on the relevant adjacent organs at risk (OARs). For extremity soft tissue sarcoma, the important OARs include the skin and subcutaneous tissues, joints, and adjacent weight bearing bone.

Acute effects of preoperative or postoperative RT include skin reactions, or dermatitis, most prominently seen within the groin or when the tumor involves skin or subcutaneous tissues. These acute reactions usually resolve with time and local skin care. Major wound healing complications are the most concerning acute toxicities associated with preoperative RT. Tumor location in the lower extremity, particularly proximally, is associated with higher acute wound complication rates compared to the upper extremity.[76,79,82,86,117,118] Treatment of tumors in medial (adductor) compartments is associated with higher rates of wound complications, reoperation, and edema.[119,120] For posterior compartment tumors, nerve damage is more frequent.[119] Tumor proximity to the skin surface <3 mm is another important predictor of major wound complications following preoperative RT.[82] Additional predictors for wound complications include patient factors such as diabetes, obesity, peripheral vascular disease, and smoking; tumor factors such as high grade, size >10 cm, and location in the proximal lower extremity; and treatment factors such as use of preoperative RT or closure with vascularized flaps or split-thickness skin grafts.[82,119]

Attention in planning to the dose delivered to skin and subcutaneous tissues can minimize acute skin reactions and major wound complications. Recommended dose constraints for RT planning include sparing a longitudinal strip of uninvolved skin and subcutaneous tissue in the extremity (no more than 50% should receive 2000 cGy), minimizing dose to skin over areas of frequent trauma (elbow, knee, anterior leg), avoidance of use of bolus, and limiting hot spots in superficial tissues.[79] In patients receiving preoperative RT, minimizing dose to the site of planned incision and cropping the PTV 3 to 5 mm from skin surface (provided this does not compromise target coverage) may be used to try to reduce wound healing complications.[82,121] Additionally, entrance or exit through the contralateral extremity should be avoided. For tumors in the upper thigh and pelvis, dose to the external genitalia or perineum and reproductive organs should be minimized. Men with proximal thigh or pelvic tumors who have interest in fertility preservation should be referred for sperm banking prior to treatment and dose to the testicles minimized. Women with proximal lower extremity, pelvic, or RPS who are interested in fertility preservation should be referred for fertility consultation prior to treatment initiation.

There are no well-defined dose constraints for joints. In clinical practice, the aim is to minimize dose to any joint as much as possible, to avoid treating the entire joint, and to try to keep <50% of the joint from receiving 5000 cGy.[122] Hip dose constraints used in the setting of gastrointestinal, genitourinary, and gynecologic malignancies can be followed as well.

Beyond concern for tissue fibrosis, joint stiffness, and chronic edema, one of the greatest causes of significant post irradiation morbidity is bone fracture. Radiation associated pathologic fractures are uncommon; however, when they occur, they frequently involve weight-bearing long bones of the lower extremity, and management is challenging with high risk for delayed union or nonunion.[48,50] Factors associated with fracture risk vary in the literature and include increasing age, female sex, tumor size and location, total radiation dose and bone dose volume parameters (including circumferential dose), RT technique, presence and extent of periosteal stripping, and use of chemotherapy.[48–50,123] Risk for fracture is increased with receipt of higher RT doses as delivered with postoperative RT.[48–51,55,124] For treatment planning, the bone contour should be the weight-bearing bone extending 2 cm beyond the PTV longitudinally. Recommended dose constraints for bone to minimize risk of fracture include V40 <64%, mean dose to bone <3700 cGy, and D_{max} <5900 cGy.[48] Additionally, no more that 50% of a weight-bearing bone should receive 5000 cGy.[79] For the femur, V50 <100% of the circumference is recommended.[50] However, target coverage should not be compromised however to spare bone. Constraining the CTV to exclude bone when there is no radiographic evidence of invasion, optimizing these dosimetric parameters including using IMRT, and consideration for prophylactic intramedullary fixation in select patients at high risk for fracture may help reduce the risk of this morbid late effect.[50,123]

Radiation Treatment Planning Considerations

Setup and Immobilization

Radiation treatment planning for truncal and soft tissue sarcoma is complex and requires careful consideration of positioning and appropriate immobilization. As sarcomas can involve many different anatomic sites, there is no one specific "sarcoma setup." Fundamental understanding of anatomy, including the compartments in the extremities, and the unique natural history of individual histopathologic subtypes is necessary when positioning the patient. CT simulation with slice thickness ≤3 mm for volumetric conformal planning is recommended. Relevant diagnostic imaging should be fused to the simulation CT for target delineation.

The most important initial steps in RT simulation and planning are thoughtful positioning and immobilization for setup reproducibility. In particular, the extremities have significant potential for mobility and rotation. The patient should be simulated in a comfortable neutral position. Use of a supine position is generally preferred to maximize comfort and reproducibility; however, prone, akimbo, swimmer's and frog leg positions all may be the optimal choice for select patients. Use of custom immobilization has been shown to reduce setup time and improve reproducibility, allowing for smaller PTV margins.[125] Practices differ across institutions and a variety of devices may be used including thermoplastic molds, vacuum pillows, and adaptable baseplate.[125,126] Immobilization across the joints adjacent to the involved portion of the extremity, similar to casting in the setting of bone fractures, can minimize movement and rotation. Use of thermoplastic molds distally at the hand or foot is helpful to immobilize the remainder of ipsilateral extremity. Whenever possible, the immobilization should minimize soft tissue distortion of the affected portion of the limb. Figure 15.8 shows the treatment setup and plan for a proximal lower extremity soft tissue sarcoma.

During simulation, for patients who have had prior excision or surgical resection, the surgical incision should be wired. Any drain sites, if present should be marked. A wide variety of radio-opaque markers and wires can be used. Delineation of these areas is important for target

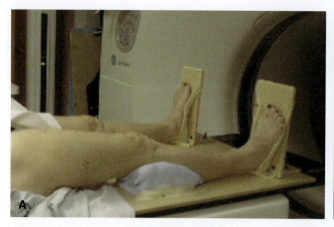
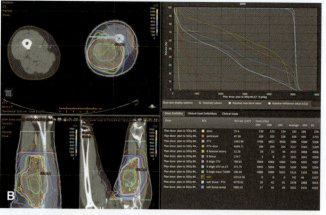

FIGURE 15.8. **A:** Treatment setup for high-grade sarcoma of the proximal lower extremity. Custom Accuform cushion, thermoplast foot mold, and foot plate allow for reproducible immobilization for daily treatment. **B:** The IMRT plan for treatment. Prescribed dose (in *orange*) covers the CTV, which was anatomically constrained to the affected compartmental fascia and does not extend into the femur. Planning objectives limited dose to the femur, uninvolved soft tissue, and a strip of subcutaneous tissue and skin laterally.

definition in planning as they are potential sites of seeding. Photographic documentation of setup and any markers placed should be done to facilitate planning and subsequent daily treatment delivery. Figure 15.9 demonstrates examples of simulation for postoperative RT with vacuum bags for immobilization and wires overlying the incisions.

For tumors involving the proximal medial thigh, frog-leg position and displacement of external genitalia to the contralateral side using a scrotal sling can help reduce skin folds and dose to the scrotum/perineum. There should be maximal separation between the legs. In some cases, the ipsilateral leg can be in a neutral position and the contralateral leg in a frog-leg position, while in other cases, the ipsilateral leg may be in the frog-leg position. For tumors of the posterior thigh, the prone position may be preferable to avoid deforming the tumor and target area. One should consider potential beam arrangements at the time of the immobilization so the desired dose can be delivered as conformally as possible to the target and the uninvolved limb can be positioned to avoid exit dose or clearance problems with the gantry head. When 3-dimensional conformal RT (3D CRT) is planned for the sarcomas occupying the near entirety of the anterior or posterior compartment, elevation of the contralateral leg may allow for opposed lateral beams. However, for tumors in the medial/lateral compartments, IMRT usually results in superior dose conformality and in such cases, the contralateral leg may be best left in the neutral position.

For patients with primary tumors in the upper extremity, both supine and prone positions may be used. The arm may be placed akimbo, away from the trunk, or elevated above the head. At simulation, the patient often needs to be positioned off center to fit through the CT bore and to reduce risk of gantry interference when on the treatment couch. Supination or pronation may affect tumor position

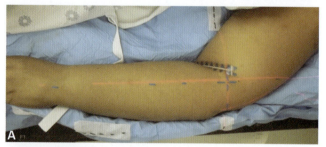
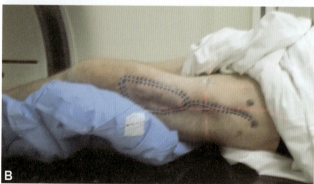

FIGURE 15.9. Images of patients simulated for postoperative RT for sarcomas of the upper extremity **(A)** and lower extremity **(B)** demonstrating use of vacuum bags for immobilization, wires overlying the incisions, and BBs marking drain sites.

within the forearm and optimal beam arrangements to spare joints and a strip of skin and subcutaneous tissue. For tumors of the hands and feet, thermoplastic molds are helpful and occasionally custom bolus may be built into the immobilization if dose build-up is required.

Figures 15.10 and 15.11 demonstrate setup, immobilization, and treatment plans for soft tissue sarcomas of the hand and foot, respectively.

For truncal tumors, both supine and prone positions may be appropriate. Devices such as alpha cradles and vacuum bags can be used for immobilization. The arm(s)

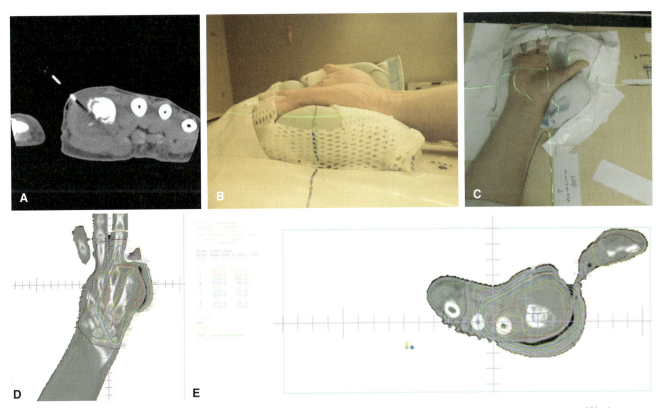

FIGURE 15.10. CT-guided biopsy of a high-grade fibrosarcoma of the second metacarpal (**A**). Lateral view (**B**) and AP view (**C**) of a custom aquaplast immobilization device. Coronal (**D**) and axial (**E**) isodose distributions for a 3D CRT plan.

should be moved away from the involved area to allow for beam entry and exit. The setup and immobilization for each patient must be individualized to optimize treatment planning.

Radiation Treatment Planning

Radiation treatment planning advancements from the 2D era to 3D planning and more conformal planning using IMRT have improved the ability to deliver the prescription dose to target and better spare OARs. Initial experiences using IMRT for preoperative and post-operative RT in extremity soft tissue sarcoma showed reduced volume of adjacent soft tissues receiving prescription dose and reduced dose to bone compared to 3D CRT.[127–129] Despite initial concerns that more conformal dose distribution might lead to increased local failures or marginal recurrences, a study of patients treated with either 3D CRT or IMRT showed improvement in local control in the IMRT cohort. This comparison of IMRT versus EBRT in 319 patients showed higher local control at 5 years (92% vs. 85%, p = 0.05) despite higher-grade lesions and more close/positive margins, and less-grade ≥2 radiation dermatitis (31.5% vs. 48.7%, p = 0.002) with use of IMRT.[129] A separate comparison of IMRT versus

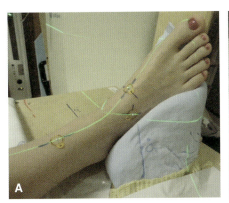
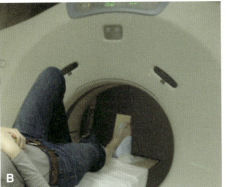
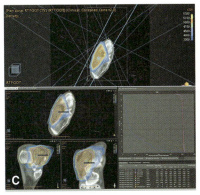

FIGURE 15.11. Treatment setup and plans for a soft tissue sarcoma of the right foot. Immobilization using a supportive ankle mold (**A** and **B**). An IMRT plan showing avoidance of high dose to the uninvolved weight-bearing bones of the foot (**C**).

adjuvant LDR brachytherapy for high-grade extremity soft tissue sarcoma found local control was better with IMRT (92% vs. 81%, p = 0.04) and that IMRT was the only predictor of improved local control on multivariate analysis despite worse clinical features (positive/close margins <1 mm, large tumors >10 cm, and bone/nerve stripping/resection) in the IMRT group.[130] A separate analysis of expected fracture risk demonstrated that the improved sparing of bone with IMRT, especially sparing the entire circumference of the femur from full dose, resulted in a reduction in femoral fracture risk. In this report, the observed fracture rate was 6.5% compared to the expected fracture rate of 25.6% estimated using a scoring system developed to predict radiation-associated fracture risk.[49,123] Combined, these studies demonstrate that the dosimetric advantages in normal tissue sparing with use of IMRT translated into a reduction in late toxicity including a reduction in fracture risk without decline in local control.

Given the increased risk for major wound complications with preoperative radiation, a prospective phase II study aimed to use image guided IMRT to try to reduce acute effects and morbidity by delivering more conformal dose, minimize dose to normal tissues (i.e., skin flaps for wound closure, bone, or other uninvolved tissue) in patients with lower extremity soft tissue sarcoma. While there was no significant reduction in the acute wound complication rate (30.5%) compared to the NCIC SR2 trial, there were increased rates of primary closure and fewer reoperations with IMRT. No fractures were observed. With a median follow-up of 49 months, the LR rate was low (6.8%).[121]

The use of IMRT, including volumetric-modulated arc therapy (VMAT), to improve tumor coverage while better sparing normal tissues versus 3D conformal RT has been expanded for treatment of anatomic sites beyond the proximal lower extremity. IMRT is considered a standard, and often preferred, planning technique for soft tissue sarcoma similar to its use in radiation treatment of other malignancies. In upper thigh/groin sarcomas close to the pelvis, IMRT may significantly reduce dose to external genitalia, perineum, anus, rectum, and femoral heads. At the shoulder girdle, IMRT may help reduce dose to the brachial plexus. For paraspinal and other truncal sarcomas, IMRT may be helpful for reduction of dose to spinal cord, lung, heart, esophagus, and other OARs.

There may be clinical circumstances in which 3D CRT plans provide comparable or improved dosimetry compared to IMRT. In soft tissue sarcoma involving the distal parts of the extremities (i.e., forearm, leg, hands, and feet) use of block edge to spare a strip of skin and subcutaneous tissue may be preferable. To minimize acute wound complications when using 3D CRT in the preoperative treatment setting, it is important to use caution regarding the location of the hotspots in the treated volumes, in particular to avoid the skin and subcutaneous tissues at the site of planned incision and or reconstruction. Collaboration

with the surgical or orthopedic oncologist to define which tissue will be critical to wound closure may also be helpful. Ultimately, the choice of treatment modality should be individualized for each patient to best provide target coverage and spare OARs.

Use of Bolus

The routine use of bolus is discouraged, especially for preoperative RT, as it increases risk for wound complications. The RTOG 0630 and phase II IMRT studies specified that bolus not be used (barring the rare exception of a situation where the biopsy incision will not be resected).[79,121] Generally, even for CTVs close to but not involving superficial subcutaneous tissue or skin, it is not necessary to bring full dose to cover the PTV expansion to skin. Use of bolus should be limited to cases where skin or superficial spread may be a concern (e.g., cutaneous angiosarcoma or superficial myxofibrosarcoma involving the subcutaneous tissues). For postoperative RT, bolus may be considered in selected patients with involvement of skin or subcutaneous tissue and concern for margins. The incidence of scar or drain site recurrences are low and therefore do not justify use of bolus for these indications in most circumstances.

Treatment Setup and Uncertainties and Use of Image Guidance

Even with custom immobilization, proper positioning for extremity sarcomas can be challenging. Robust processes and use of image guidance are necessary to ensure the accurate setups needed for reduction in PTV margins and use of highly conformal planning techniques. The appropriate PTV margin for individual patients should take into account the likelihood of interval tumor changes during the treatment course, the frequency of image guidance, and institutional practice to address systematic and random setup errors. Figure 15.12 shows an example of orthogonal KV images for alignment to bone.

A study registered planning CTs with CBCTs and an optical localization system to measure interfractional and intrafractional motion in 31 patients with lower extremity soft tissue sarcoma receiving preoperative IMRT. This study found that a uniform 5 mm PTV margin was necessary and sufficient for setup when using image guidance with IMRT.[131] The same study evaluated immobilization and intrafractional errors in patients with upper extremity soft tissue sarcoma.[132] Large errors, especially rotational, were observed and were not able to be offset by a specific immobilization technique. The authors noted that improved positioning strategies are needed for upper extremity sites and reduction of PTV margin as used in lower extremity tumors may not be appropriate.[132] A similar analysis of setup uncertainties evaluated 236 treatments in 15 patients with extremity sarcoma to assess whether surface imaging could improve patient positioning and reduce the necessary PTV.[133] The intrafraction motion was small (the mean 3D vector shift was 2.1 mm

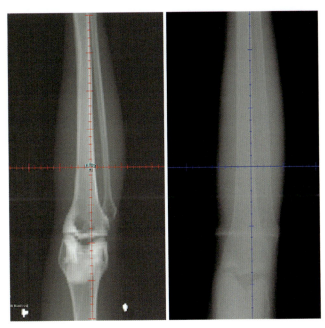

FIGURE 15.12. Daily orthogonal KV images for alignment to bone.

and systematic and random errors were ≤1.3 mm). However, the mean interfraction error was 7.6 mm and systematic and random errors were 3 to 4 mm in all directions. The required PTV margins would have been 10 mm, 12 mm, and 13 mm in the anterior–posterior, superior–inferior, and lateral directions, respectively. The use of surface imaging reduced setup errors to within the tolerance of a 5 mm PTV. The institutional practice of the

authors of this reference is to use daily surface imaging with weekly CBCT.[133]

The RTOG 0630 trial required daily image guidance, with either daily kV or MV orthogonal imaging or CBCT, to use the reduced PTV margin of 5 mm.[79] This reduced PTV of 5 mm is not adequate to account for setup uncertainties when only weekly imaging is used, and a larger PTV expansion of at least 1 cm is required. A secondary analysis of the patient positioning data revealed that daily shifts were large when alignment to bone was used, necessitating daily IGRT when the smaller 5 mm PTV expansion is used. Without daily IGRT, a CTV to PTV margin of 15 mm is required.[134] Figure 15.13 shows a comparison of CBCT and surface image for daily alignment for a sarcoma involving the shoulder girdle.

Interval anatomic and volume changes in the primary sarcoma may occur during the course of preoperative therapy and plan adaptation may be necessary in some circumstances.[135,136] Both enlargement and shrinkage can be observed on imaging after preoperative RT. In a study of preoperative RT for borderline resectable soft tissue sarcoma, tumor volumes increased in 20% of cases; however, all of these cases had R0 resections and no LR. In the other 80% of tumors, maximal diameter was reduced by 13.5% and median volume reduction was 33%.[137] Another study quantified tumor volume on MRI imaging using T1 gadolinium-enhanced sequences and tried to correlate with pathologic response; median decrease in tumor volume was 13.8% for non-myxoid low-grade sarcomas, 82.1% for myxoid liposarcomas, and

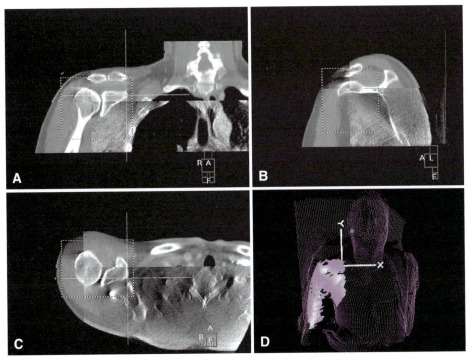

FIGURE 15.13. Comparison of CBCT and surface imaging for daily treatment alignment for a sarcoma of the shoulder girdle. In this case, the CBCT was superior to surface imaging for setup verification. Coronal **(A)**, sagittal **(B)**, and axial **(C)** images based on CBCT alignment compared to surface imaging **(D)**.

<1% for high-grade sarcomas, despite a variety of pathologic responses.[138]

Assessment of potential changes in tumor size can be done by clinical examination and measurement of the circumference of the limb at the site of the tumor, evaluation of larger than expected changes in patient setup, or review of surface or CBCT used for image guidance. Target coverage from the initial treatment plan should be re-evaluated in the setting of interval changes, and plan adaptation or re-planning may be required for some patients. A study evaluated 982 CBCTs for interval change in 99 patients with extremity soft tissue sarcoma receiving preoperative RT. The CTV to PTV expansion used for treatment planning was 1 cm. Action levels based on extremity contour change and tumor change on daily imaging were developed that required physician review. In 41 patients, no action levels were required. For the 59 patients with substantial change, most change was accounted for within the PTV; however, eight patients were required plan adaptation.[136]

Other Radiation Modalities

Brachytherapy and IORT

The role for brachytherapy in the management of soft tissue sarcoma to improve local control is well established. Brachytherapy can be used as adjuvant treatment or boost.[56] However, there are no randomized comparisons between EBRT and brachytherapy as monotherapy, or EBRT and EBRT with brachytherapy boost. Some appealing features of brachytherapy compared to EBRT, especially prior to the availability of 3D conformal and IMRT techniques, include direction visualization of the surgical bed, the dose distribution and rapid dose fall off, normal tissue sparing, low integral dose, and short treatment times. The American Brachytherapy Society consensus statement for sarcoma brachytherapy provides a comprehensive guide to the use of this technique in soft tissue sarcomas.[139] This comprehensive guide provides specific details regarding use of brachytherapy delivery for soft tissue sarcoma.

Brachytherapy is most often accomplished as interstitial implants at the time of resection. Hollow needles are placed through the skin and soft tissue at least 1 to 2 cm away from the wound incision. The catheters are placed in parallel 1 to 1.5 cm apart, away from critical structures, and exiting the body such that they are not easily distorted. Placement of the catheters may be either parallel or perpendicular to the incision depending on the curvature of the extremity. The CTV should encompass the entire area at risk, usually defined by surgical clips, as either a single plane or multiple planes. Catheters are then sutured and anchored to the external skin with fixation buttons. Tissue expanders, gel foam, drains, or inflatable material may be used to protect normal tissues. Catheters are numbered for correct identification, and the positions of the catheters at the skin are marked to ensure consistent depth between fractions. Patients are planned postoperatively using CT simulation with "dummy ribbons" which help identify potential source positions. The quality of implant is measured as D90 (dose to 90% of the CTV), V100 (percent of CTV receiving 100% of the prescribed dose), and V150 (percent of CTV receiving 150% of the prescribed dose). Dose to the OARs (i.e., the surgical incision, nerves, bones, vessels) is limited to <100% of the prescription dose unless at high risk. Skin dose should be less than two third of the prescribed dose, and source loading should not be closer than 0.5 cm from the skin surface.

Brachytherapy for extremity soft tissue sarcoma is most commonly delivered using an iridium-192 source. For planar IORT implants, dose is often prescribed to a depth. Complex implants should use CT-based 3D planning. To minimize wound healing complications, brachytherapy should be delayed until after final wound closure and not started until after postoperative Day 5 for adjuvant monotherapy. The recommended prescription doses and fractionation vary by treatment type (i.e., low dose rate (LDR), pulsed dose rate (PDR), high dose rate (HDR), or IORT) and whether brachytherapy is being given alone or with EBRT.

For LDR or PDR, the prescription is delivered to the lowest continuous isodose rate line covering CTV (usually 5 mm from the plane of the implant) at a dose of 4500 to 5000 cGy over 4 to 6 days at 45 to 50 cGy/hr, or 1500 to 2500 cGy over 2 to 4 days at 45 to 50 cGy/hr with 4500 to 5000 cGy of EBRT. Pulse dose rate is a way to use remote after-loading to deliver dose in short bursts at hourly doses that are radiobiologically comparable to LDR. For HDR, the recommended prescription dose is 3000 to 5000 cGy over 4 to 7 days at 200 to 400 cGy twice daily (BID), or 1200 to 2000 cGy over 2 to 3 days at 200 to 400 cGy BID. BID treatments should be delivered >6 hours apart. Intraoperative RT is given as 1000 to 2000 cGy in 1 fraction at the time of resection with 4500 to 5000 cGy EBRT.

The American Brachytherapy Society guidelines on brachytherapy for soft tissue sarcoma suggest brachytherapy monotherapy may be optimal for small high-grade primary tumors, re-irradiation, and in pediatric patients or frail older patients. The guidelines conclude brachytherapy boost offers local control benefit with EBRT for patients at high risk for recurrence (>10 cm, recurrent disease, or close margins).[139] As with all therapies for soft tissue sarcoma, multidisciplinary evaluation and collaboration are important for optimal outcomes and coordination between the surgeon and radiation oncologist is necessary for planning and delivery of brachytherapy.

Proton Radiotherapy

There are no randomized trials comparing proton and photon RT for adult extremity and truncal sarcoma. Most available data using proton RT for sarcoma arise from treatment of pediatric patients with rhabdomyosarcoma or from treatment of primary bone tumors including Ewing sarcoma, osteosarcoma, chondrosarcoma, and chordoma. Rationale for use of protons includes the ability to deliver lower integral dose and absence of exit dose, resulting in smaller volumes irradiated. The ability to spare normal tissues using either protons and photons is dependent on the patient, anatomic site, and dose delivery method (3D CRT or IMRT). Protons can be considered and are accepted on most protocols for children with soft tissue sarcomas. Young adults with hip/truncal sarcoma may also benefit from proton beam therapy to spare reproductive, pelvic, or other normal tissues, but long-term benefits remain unproven. On a prospective study of proton re-irradiation for recurrent and secondary soft tissue sarcoma in 23 patients, median re-irradiation doses of 5000 cGy (CGE) preoperatively, 6840 cGy (CGE) postoperatively, and 7470 cGy (CGE) definitively were delivered with no reported grade 4 or 5 toxicities.[140]

Definitive Radiation for Unresectable Disease

For patients for whom limb-sparing resection is not feasible but amputation is unacceptable or for patient who cannot undergo surgery due to medical comorbidities, definitive RT may be considered for local therapy, albeit with low rates of local control compared to approaches that include resection.[141,142] A study of 112 patients treated with RT to a median dose of 6400 cGy for gross unresected disease reported 5-year local control of 45%. The local control differed based on size: 51% for tumors <5 cm; 45% for tumors 5 to 10 cm; and only 9% for tumors >10 cm. Doses >6300 cGy were associated with better local control; however, doses >6800 cGy were associated with higher complication rates (27% versus <8% for dose <6800 cGy).[142] As these patients were treated between 1970 and 2001, it is possible that modern radiation techniques may allow for dose escalation with lower rates of toxicity. Figure 15.14 shows an example of a definitive RT plan for local control in the setting of a high-grade sarcoma involving multiple compartments of the thigh in an older patient with medical comorbidities for whom hemipelvectomy was not recommended. Other strategies that have been used in the setting of unresectable disease include particle and heavy ion radiotherapy.[143]

Re-Irradiation for Local Recurrence

Management of isolated LR following prior radiation includes surgical resection when feasible. In the extremity, treatment of a recurrence after prior limb-sparing therapy often may involve an amputation. If a recurrence is amenable to wide local excision and yet remains at high risk for subsequent LR, or when radical resection is not possible or declined, re-irradiation with resection may be considered in select cases.[144] Repeat attempts at combined modality therapy (and limb preservation in patients with

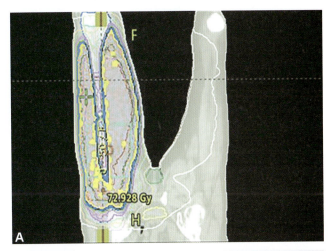
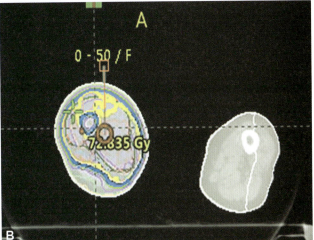
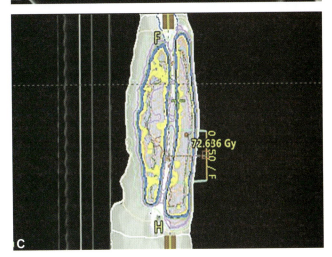

FIGURE 15.14. Coronal **(A)**, axial **(B)**, and sagittal **(C)** images from a definitive RT plan for local control in the setting of a high-grade sarcoma involving multiple compartments of the thigh in an older patient with medical comorbidities for whom hemipelvectomy was not recommended. Note the attempt to spare the length of femur from the prescription dose.

extremity primaries) can achieve local control although with significant risk for wound complications.[145–148] Management of the wound complications themselves may ultimately require amputation.[145] Many of the available reports on re-irradiation have included brachytherapy (either alone or in combination with EBRT), and more recently proton RT, to try to spare adjacent normal tissues further dose.[140,145–148] On the previously discussed prospective study of proton re-irradiation for recurrent and secondary soft tissue sarcoma, limb preservation was possible in 7 of 10 patients with extremity soft tissue sarcoma.[140] When considering re-irradiation for recurrent soft tissue sarcoma, one must carefully balance the higher risk of complications with the anticipated functional outcomes of a limb or organ-sparing approach versus radical resection including amputation. The challenges of such salvage treatment confirm the importance of optimizing initial management.

RETROPERITONEAL SARCOMA

RPS comprises approximately 15% of all soft tissue sarcoma and different histopathologic subtypes, each with unique characteristics and patterns of behavior.[1,5] Similar to soft tissue sarcoma of the trunk and extremity, RPS are often quite large at presentation and may not have attributable symptoms. As for all soft tissue sarcoma, multidisciplinary input from care providers with expertise in sarcoma is recommended prior to initiation of treatment for optimal outcomes.[9,10,18] Local therapy options should be assessed by both surgical and radiation oncology. Medical oncology input regarding the role of systemic therapy is advisable, especially for high-grade tumors and specific histologies (e.g., leiomyosarcoma).

The primary treatment for RPS is surgical resection. Given the complex anatomy of the retroperitoneal space and numerous adjacent critical normal tissues, achieving widely negative margins at resection is often impossible. Preservation of organ function is a key consideration in local therapy decision-making, including extent of resection. Satisfactory margins may require en-bloc removal of tumor with adjacent viscera.[149,150] Incomplete (R2) resections are not curative. LR is frequent even with complete macroscopic resection.[149–154] Risk for distant metastatic spread is high and a determinant of survival. The pattern of distant spread differs from extremity and truncal sarcoma, as the liver and peritoneum, in addition to lung, are common sites of metastasis. Histopathologic subtype significantly influences natural history and risk for LR and hematogenous metastatic spread.[151–155] For RPS, uncontrolled locoregional disease is a source of significant morbidity and mortality. As many deaths from RPS are related to uncontrolled locoregional disease, improvements in local control could improve overall survival. This potential local control benefit is the rationale for use of RT in the treatment of RPS.

The addition of RT to surgery in the management of RPS remains controversial. There are few prospective randomized studies to inform decision-making. Both preoperative and postoperative of RT have been used. Non-randomized prospective studies, retrospective reports, and large database-derived series have shown conflicting results regarding the role of RT. Some report increased local control with surgery and RT versus surgery alone, while others have shown no benefit.[45,156–162]

The NCI conducted a trial in 35 patients randomized to receive postoperative EBRT (5000 to 5500 cGy as 3500 to 4000 cGy extended field RT + 1500 cGy boost) or electron IORT (2000 cGy) and postoperative EBRT (3500 to 4000 cGy).[163] There were fewer LRs in the IORT + EBRT arm (6 of 15) versus the higher-dose EBRT arm (16 of 20) (p < 0.001). Significant radiation-related enteritis was more common in patients receiving postoperative EBRT alone; peripheral neuropathy rates were higher in the IORT + EBRT group. As both arms included EBRT, this study cannot address the question of whether to add radiation to surgery versus surgery alone. Two prospective randomized studies that aimed to better inform the benefit of addition of preoperative RT to surgery alone closed prematurely due to poor accrual (RTOG 0124 NCT00017160 and American College of Surgeons Oncology Group (ACOSOG) Z9031 NCT00091351).

The STRASS trial (European Organization for Research and Treatment of Cancer (EORTC) 62092) is a randomized controlled trial of preoperative RT (5040 cGy) and surgery versus surgery alone.[162] Surgery involved multivisceral en-bloc resection with intent for macroscopic negative margins. The primary outcome was abdominal recurrence-free survival (ARFS), defined as local/abdominal or distant progressive disease during RT, tumor or patient becoming inoperable, peritoneal metastases found at surgery, R2 resection, or local relapse. With a median follow-up of 43.1 months, the trial did not show a difference in 3-year ARFS between the two arms: 60% (95% CI: 51% to 68%) for RT + surgery versus 59% (95% CI 50% to 67%) for surgery alone (HR 1.01, log rank 0.95). Unplanned sensitivity analyses were recommended with local progression during RT excluded as an ARFS event when a macroscopically complete resection was performed. The authors concluded that preoperative RT should not be considered standard of care for RPS. A post hoc analysis by histopathologic subtype and grade suggested that there may be an improvement in ARFS with the addition of preoperative RT in liposarcoma and low-grade sarcoma. There did not appear to be a similar benefit for leiomyosarcoma and high-grade sarcoma. A caveat is that the follow-up is relatively short, especially for liposarcoma.

The decision regarding whether to add RT to surgery should be based on multidisciplinary evaluation and assessment of risk for LR. When RT is planned in addition to surgery, preoperative RT is favored. Postoperative RT is generally not recommended as the appropriate treatment dose (6000 to 6600 cGy) exceeds small bowel, kidney, liver, and spinal cord tolerance. Furthermore, the postoperative irradiated volume is typically large given the need to encompass the initial extent of disease and the entire surgical bed, and often contains multiple loops of bowel (see Figure 15.15). The presence of postoperative adhesions may lower bowel mobility, potentially resulting in greater dose to fixed loops of bowel than for mobile loops that could move in and out of the treatment field in the preoperative setting. As a result, many sarcoma experts do not routinely offer postoperative RT and favor close surveillance after resection. At time of recurrence, preoperative RT would be considered prior to resection. However, in circumstances where a recurrence would be associated with significant morbidity or when there are limited options for surgical salvage, selective use of postoperative RT may be considered. In such cases, coordination between the surgeon and radiation oncologist is important for treatment planning. If postoperative RT is planned, displacement of bowel out of the anticipated treatment field with omentum or other spacers should be considered.[164]

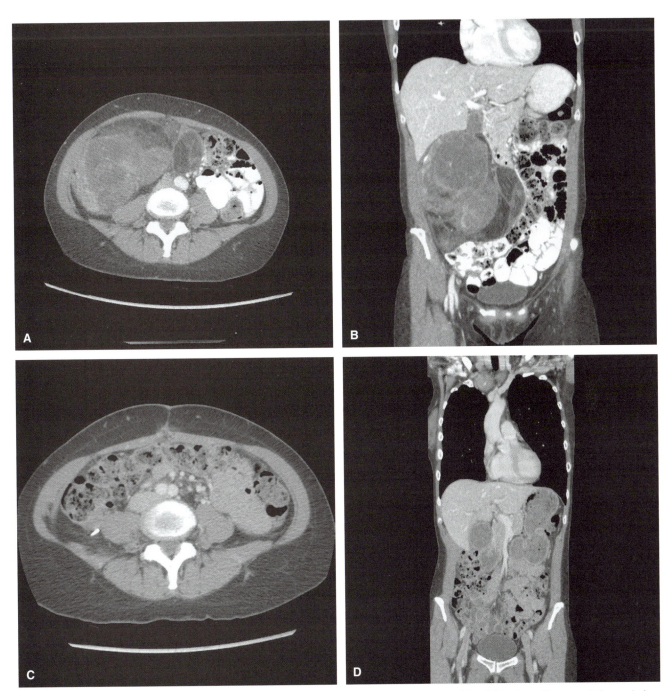

FIGURE 15.15. Axial and coronal CT images of a patient with a dedifferentiated liposarcoma of the right retroperitoneum at diagnosis (top row) and post resection (bottom row). Note the displacement of bowel by tumor in the axial **(A)** and coronal **(B)** preoperative images. After resection, multiple loops of bowel are present in the anatomic region previously occupied by tumor. Delivery of postoperative radiation in this setting would be challenging given the large volume of bowel that would be in field as shown in the axial **(C)** and coronal **(D)** postoperative images.

Advantages for preoperative RT include improved target delineation with the tumor in place, displacement of small bowel out of the treatment volume by the tumor itself, less toxicity, and reduced risk of tumor seeding and intraperitoneal dissemination at surgery. Potential disadvantages of preoperative RT include limited histologic sampling and delay to time of surgery.

When preoperative RT is used, the patient must have a localized tumor with intent for macroscopic complete resection, have no symptoms requiring urgent immediate resection (e.g., bowel obstruction), and be judged a suitable candidate to tolerate RT (defined by the ability to meet normal tissue constraints) with acceptable toxicity. The plan for surgery, especially anticipated nephrectomy or partial hepatic resection, should be discussed by the surgeon and radiation oncologist as the extent of resection impacts RT planning and dose constraints.[165] The dose for preoperative RT is 5000 to 5040 cGy using conventional fractionation.[159,162,165] Attempts at dose escalation in the preoperative setting have used brachytherapy, intraoperative RT, and dose painting to provide higher dose to selected volumes deemed at greater risk for recurrence. These areas of concern should be defined by the surgeon and radiation oncologist jointly.

Simulation and Planning Considerations

For preoperative RT, patients should be immobilized in a comfortable and reproducible position, most often in the supine position with arms elevated and supported over the head. CT simulation with slice thickness ≤3 mm is recommended for volumetric planning. Oral and/or IV contrast can be useful for delineating target and normal tissues. Registration and fusion to diagnostic imaging (CT and/ or MRI with contrast) aids in target definition. As upper abdominal tumors and organs can move significantly with respiration, 4D CT simulation is recommended for tumors above the iliac crest or pelvic brim.[165,166–168] When significant motion is noted, use of a respiratory control technique is recommended.

For RT planning, the GTV is defined by diagnostic CT or MRI T1 plus contrast images.[165,169] An iGTV is created from the GTV incorporating internal motion for tumors above the iliac crest. A symmetric 1.5 cm expansion on the GTV or iGTV is applied to create the CTV, which is anatomically constrained. If 4D motion is not assessed for tumors located in the upper abdomen, larger CTV expansions of 2 to 2.5 cm craniocaudally and 1.5 to 2 cm radially are required. The CTV/internal target volume (ITV) is edited at the bone, renal, and hepatic interfaces (0 mm), bowel and air cavity (5 mm), and under the surface of the skin (3 to 5 mm). The CTV is expanded fully into retroperitoneal muscles but not beyond the peritoneal compartment or intact fascia. For RPS extending into the inguinal canal, a 3 cm margin is used inferiorly below the GTV and a 1.5 cm radial margin is used in the

thigh. This CTV does not extend beyond the compartment, intact fascia, or into uninvolved bone similar to the expansions used in treatment of extremity soft tissue sarcoma.[165] A PTV of 5 mm is appropriate when frequent volumetric IGRT will be used. In the absence of volumetric imaging for guidance, a PTV of 9 to 15 mm is needed.[165,170] Volumetric imaging with at least weekly CBCT scans has demonstrated changes in tumor size and position over the course of treatment and is important for positional verification and assessing the need for adaptive replanning.[170]

Studies have evaluated treating only a high-risk posterior target volume or delivering a dose-escalated boost to the high-risk volume.[171,172] This target volume is defined by locations at high risk for positive margins and includes the tumor margin along posterior abdominal wall or retroperitoneal musculature, ipsilateral pre- and paravertebral space, major vessels, and organs that will be left in situ at time of surgery. The potential benefit of dose escalation to the high-risk target volume requires careful selection of patients most at risk for isolated LR and without multifocal disease.[173] The high-risk target volume is defined as 1.5 cm of the GTV abutting the anticipated positive margin, expanded 5 to 10 mm into the tissues at risk.[174,175] On a study investigating the use of preoperative IMRT (5000 cGy) to a limited CTV encompassing the posterior abdominal wall region at higher risk for relapse, 2 of 18 patients had LR at 27-month median follow-up.[171] A separate investigation delivered dose-painted, dose-escalated preoperative IMRT of 4500 cGy to a standard risk volume and 5750 cGy to the high-risk posterior retroperitoneal margin where surgical margins were predicted to be positive.[172] The actuarial risk of LR at 2 years was 20%. A phase I trial of preoperative RT using intensity-modulated proton RT with image guidance delivered a simultaneous integrated boost to high-risk margins to doses of 6020 cGy RBE, 6160 cGy RBE, and 6300 cGy RBE. Dose escalation was feasible to 6300 cGy RBE without acute dose-limiting toxicity.[175] This approach is being further evaluated on a prospective multi-institutional phase II trial using protons or IMRT to treat the high-risk margin to 6300 cGy and 5040 cGy to the entire target simultaneously (ClinicalTrials.gov Identifier: NCT01659203). Figure 15.16 shows an example of a preoperative RT plan with simultaneous integrated boost to the high-risk margin.

The recommended treatment dose for preoperative RT is 5000 to 5040 cGy using conventional fractionation.[159,162,165] IMRT, including VMAT, is preferred over 3D CRT as a treatment planning technique given the complex anatomy and many adjacent OARs.[165] Normal tissue dose constraints should be used for planning. 3D CRT may be used when a comparable plan can achieve similar dose to target and all constraints for OARs can be met. On a dosimetric study of IMRT and 3D CRT plans, small bowel mean dose and volume of small bowel

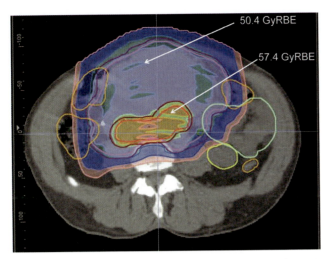

FIGURE 15.16. Preoperative RT plan with a simultaneous integrated boost to the high-risk margin. Standard clinical risk target volume (CTV1) and high-risk boost region (CTV2) in a patient with undifferentiated pleomorphic sarcoma (UPS) of the retroperitoneum receiving preoperative radiation to 5040 cGy RBE to CTV1 and 5740 cGy RBE to CTV2 with scanned beam protons.

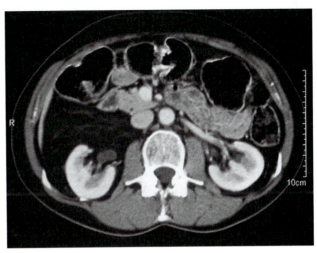

FIGURE 15.17. Axial image from a contrast-enhanced CT demonstrating a retroperitoneal well-differentiated liposarcoma. Note the fat density tumor surrounding right kidney. Confirmation of plan for nephrectomy and evaluation for adequate contralateral renal function are necessary prior to preoperative radiotherapy planning.

receiving >3000 cGy were reduced and target coverage was improved with IMRT.[176] A comparative analysis of VMAT and IMRT demonstrated similar PTV coverage, homogeneity, and OAR sparing with both techniques; however, VMAT plans had shorter delivery times.[177]

Preservation of renal and hepatic function is important in treatment of RPS. The extent of planned resection, specifically whether ipsilateral nephrectomy or partial hepatic resection is anticipated, should be discussed by the surgeon and treating radiation oncologist as both impact radiation planning (see Figure 15.17). Assessment of adequate renal function is essential if the ipsilateral kidney will be resected and can be done by various means, including differential renal function scan or assessment of contrast clearance on diagnostic CT in addition to renal function bloodwork. The contralateral (remaining) kidney should be maximally spared dose and a dose constraint of V18 <15% followed.[165] When partial hepatic resection is planned, the remaining liver should similarly be spared with mean dose <2600 cGy.[165] Dose constraints for small and large bowel depend on the method contoured (i.e., bowel bag or individual loops). Following dose constraints used in the treatment of gynecologic and genitourinary malignancies, a bowel bag constraint of V45 ≤195 cm^3 has been used.[165] A study evaluating bowel dose and toxicity patients with RPS treated with preoperative RT found low rates of significant acute gastrointestinal toxicity despite exceeded bowel dose constraints. This suggests that this bowel bag dose-volume parameter may be too conservative and warrants further evaluation.[178] The displacement of bowel out of the field by the in situ tumor may permit higher tolerance doses.

Image guidance with volumetric imaging is recommended to verify accuracy of the setup and to evaluate for interval changes in targets during the course of RT. A study investigating spatial and volumetric changes during preoperative RT using CBCT showed initial volumetric increase followed by subsequent decrease. Internal margins of 8.6 mm lateral, 15 mm anterior/posterior, and 15 mm superior/inferior directions would be necessary to account for these changes. The authors also noted that the extent of respiratory motion was greater in tumors more superiorly located in the abdomen.[170]

BONE SARCOMA

Primary bone sarcomas are rare, accounting for less than 0.2% of all cancers.[2] In 2020, an estimated 3600 new cases will be diagnosed and 1720 estimated deaths will occur.[2,4] These tumors are uncommon, have significant heterogeneity, and present at anatomic locations throughout the body. Successful treatment with good functional outcome most often requires specialized surgical expertise, including complex reconstructive techniques, aggressive multiagent chemotherapy, and, in selected cases, sophisticated radiation techniques. Accordingly, management by experienced multidisciplinary sarcoma teams is preferred.

Common histologic subtypes include osteosarcomas (35%), chondrosarcomas (30%), and Ewing sarcoma (15%).[1] Other histologic variants accounting for less than 5% of primary bone tumors include high-grade UPS of bone, fibrosarcoma, chordoma, and giant cell tumor of bone (GCTB).[1] Similar to sarcomas of soft tissue, bone sarcomas are named by presumed tissue of origin, osteosarcoma from bone, chondrosarcoma from cartilage, and chordoma from notochordal tissue.[1] Osteosarcoma can be associated with Li-Fraumeni syndrome with germline mutation in TP53, occur in patients with retinoblastoma, and arise as a secondary radiation-associated cancer.

TABLE 15.4 AJCC Staging TNM Classification for Bone

TNM Classification

T Primary Tumor of Appendicular Skeleton, Trunk, Skull, and Facial Bones

T0	No evidence of primary tumor
T1	Tumor ≤8 cm in greatest dimension
T2	Tumor >8 cm in greatest dimension
T3	Discontinuous tumors in the primary bone site

T Primary Tumor of Spine

T0	No evidence of primary tumor
T1	Tumor confined to one vertebral segment or two adjacent vertebral segments
T2	Tumor confined to three adjacent vertebral segments
T3	Tumor confined to four or more adjacent vertebral segments, or any nonadjacent vertebral segments
T4	Extension into the spinal canal or great vessels
	T4a extension into the spinal canal
	T4b evidence of gross vascular invasion or tumor thrombus in the great vessels

T Primary Tumor of Pelvis

T0	No evidence of primary tumor
T1	Tumor confined to one pelvic segment with no extraosseous extension
	T1a tumor ≤8 cm in greatest dimension
	T1b tumor >8 cm in greatest dimension
T2	Tumor confined to one pelvic segment with extraosseous extension or two segments without extraosseous extension
	T2a tumor ≤8 cm in greatest dimension
	T2b tumor >8 cm in greatest dimension
T3	Tumor spanning two pelvic segments with extraosseous extension
	T3a tumor ≤8 cm in greatest dimension
	T3b tumor >8 cm in greatest dimension
T4	Tumor spanning three pelvic segments or crossing the sacroiliac joint
	T4a tumor involves the sacroiliac joint and extends medial to the sacral neuroforamen
	T4b tumor encasement of external iliac vessels or presence of gross tumor thrombus in the major pelvic vessels

TNM Classification

N Regional Lymph Nodes

N1	No regional lymph node metastasis
N2	Regional lymph node metastasis

M Distant Metastasis

M0	No distant metastasis
M1	Distant metastasis
	M1a lung
	M1b bone or other distant sites

G Histologic Tumor Grade

G1	Well differentiated, low grade
G2	Moderately differentiated, high grade
G3	Poorly differentiated, high grade

From Amin MB, Edge SB, Greene FL, et al. *AJCC Cancer Staging Manual*, 8th edition. New York: Springer; 2017 reproduced with permission of SNCSC.

TABLE 15.5 AJCC Staging Classification for Bone—Stage Groups for Appendicular Skeleton, Trunk, Skull, and Facial Bones

Stage Groups

Stage IA	T1	N0	M0	G1 or GX
Stage IB	T2 or T3	N0	M0	G1 or GX
Stage IIA	T1	N0	M0	G2 or G3
Stage IIB	T2	N0	M0	G2 or G3
Stage III	T3	N0	M0	G2 or G3
Stage IVA	Any T	N0	M1a	Any G
Stage IVB	Any T	N1	Any M	Any G
	Any T	Any N	M1b	Any G

From Amin MB, Edge SB, Greene FL, et al. *AJCC Cancer Staging Manual*, 8th edition. New York: Springer; 2017. reproduced with permission of SNCSC.

The 8th edition of the AJCC staging TNM classification for primary tumors of bone is provided in Table 15.4. The updated staging system includes separate classifications based on primary site: appendicular skeleton, trunk, skull, and facial bones; spine; and pelvis. The prognostic stage groups for bone sarcoma of the appendicular skeleton, trunk, skull, and facial bones are shown in Table 15.5. The prognostic stage groups do not apply for spine and pelvic sites.[6]

Multiagent chemotherapy is a critical component of treatment for all patients with Ewing sarcoma and most patients with intermediate and high-grade osteosarcomas. In contrast, for chondrosarcomas and chordomas, chemotherapy is not commonly used as a component of primary treatment, though systemic therapy with targeted agents can play a role.

Margin negative resection is the preferred treatment for the primary site and results in very high rates of local control in patients with extremity bone tumors. Limb-sparing resections are preferred when feasible and assessment should be done by orthopedic oncologists to determine appropriate resection and ability to preserve function. In the case of primary extremity osteosarcoma, for example, the rate of local control with chemotherapy and surgical resection is over 90%.[179] In contrast, for osteosarcoma of the head and neck, spine, and pelvis, local control with surgery and chemotherapy is less favorable reflecting the challenges in obtaining wide margins in certain anatomic sites.[180–185]

The role for radiotherapy in the treatment of bone sarcoma is less than for soft tissue sarcoma. Radiation can be delivered pre or postoperatively, definitively as the primary local therapy in unresectable disease, and for palliation. Indications for use of RT are dependent on the histology, anatomic site of tumor, ability to obtain margin negative resection and preserve function, and the efficacy of chemotherapy. RT is not routinely used when resection with wide negative margins can be performed. RT may be considered in patients at high risk for LR and can help improve local control in unfavorable sites, including the pelvis, sacrum, spine, and craniofacial region.[180–185] Preoperative RT can be delivered prior to resection of spine or pelvic sarcomas.[182,185] For patients with bone sarcomas, adjuvant radiation is used following resection when margins are positive or inadequate, and in other selected cases, including presentation with pathologic fracture, poor histologic response to chemotherapy, intralesional excision, or intramedullary rod placement through a radiographically or cytologically benign-appearing lesion that was later determined to be sarcoma.[184–187] Definitive radiotherapy is used as the primary local therapy without surgery for medically inoperable patients, for patients with Ewing sarcoma where surgery would compromise function, and for primary bone tumors involving anatomic sites (e.g., the upper sacrum and portions of the pelvis, the base of skull, and the ethmoid/sphenoid sinus region) where complete resection is either not technically possible or would be associated with significant morbidity.[184,185,188–192]

Ewing sarcoma is quite radiosensitive. The original description of this tumor by James Ewing noted that this radiation sensitivity was one of the features that distinguished this tumor from other bone sarcomas.[193] For Ewing sarcoma, unresected disease or gross residual disease is usually treated to 5580 cGy with chemotherapy.[188,189,194] Higher doses may be selectively considered. Microscopic residual disease is usually treated to 5040 cGy. Vertebral lesions are often treated to doses of 4500 to 5000 cGy to respect spinal cord tolerance. Further discussion of RT for Ewing sarcoma is covered in the chapter on pediatric malignancies.

Chondrosarcoma and osteogenic sarcoma require doses of approximately 6600 cGy for control of microscopic residual disease and doses >7000 cGy for control of gross residual disease.[182] Chordomas require doses of 7000 cGy for microscopic residual disease and doses of 7200 to 7800 cGy for gross residual and unresectable disease.[182,195,196] Some investigators have delivered 1980 to 5040 cGy preoperatively followed by resection and postoperative RT in an attempt to minimize tumor seeding at surgery and to limit the total volume receiving the higher postoperative dose.[197] Additional techniques used to dose escalate for local control while trying to minimize effects on normal tissues include proton RT, carbon ions and other heavy ions, and stereotactic ablative approaches.[198]

SBRT FOR SARCOMA

The most common site of metastasis for soft tissue and bone sarcomas is the lungs by hematogenous spread. Although pulmonary metastatic disease is generally incurable, selected patients with lung metastases may have long-term survival with lung metastasectomy, 5-year overall survival ranges from 15% to 20%.[199–203] Traditionally, these patients have been selected based on performance status, disease-free interval, response to chemotherapy, histology, extent of disease, and number of metastases. Not all patients are candidates for operative management however, and historically RT was used primarily with palliative intent in the metastatic setting. Increasingly, studies show stereotactic body radiation therapy (SBRT) is a feasible and effective option for local control of limited pulmonary oligometastatic disease with minimal toxicity.[204–211] The use of SBRT has been expanded for treatment of multiple oligometastatic sites outside the lung, including liver, spine, soft tissue, and lymph nodes.[212] A study of 44 patients with 56 metastases treated at two institutions with SBRT to a median dose of 5000 cGy in 4 to 5 fractions, demonstrated 1- and 2-year local control rates of 96% and 90% and overall survival rates of 64% and 46%, respectively.[207] Three grade 2 chest wall toxicities and one grade 2 pneumonitis occurred; however, no other ≥ grade 2 toxicities were seen.[207] A study of patients with sarcoma pulmonary metastases treated with SBRT to 5000 cGy in 5 fractions found 83% local control of treated lesions with no grade 3 toxicity.[209] Patients treated with SBRT had longer median overall survival than those who did not receive SBRT (2.1 yrs vs. 0.6 yrs p = 0.002). Other studies have found SBRT to be safe and effective for management of pulmonary metastases from both soft tissue and bone sarcomas.[204–206,208,210,211] Ablative doses used on a study of SBRT in patients with sarcoma included 3000 cGy in fraction for peripheral tumors ≤1 cm, 6000 cGy in 3 fractions for peripheral tumors >1 cm to ≤2 cm, and 4800 cGy in 4 fractions for larger peripheral tumors. Central tumors were treated with 6000 cGy in 8 fractions.[210] On this study, the reported 2- and 5-year local control rates were 96% and 96% and overall survival rates were 85% and 54%, respectively.[210] On a similar study of SBRT for the management of lung metastases from both soft tissue and bone sarcomas, 3000 to 6000 cGy in 3 to 8 fractions was delivered with 2-year local control of 85% and overall survival of 66% with no reported ≥grade 3 toxicities.[211] The use of SBRT for metastatic sarcoma has been expanded to sites outside the lung, including liver and spine, though the data in support are less robust. For spine, local control rates of 88% at 18 months have been reported with delivery of 1800 to 2400 cGy in 1 fraction with <5% rates of acute and late toxicity.[213] With this growing evidence, SBRT should be considered among local treatment options available for sarcoma patients

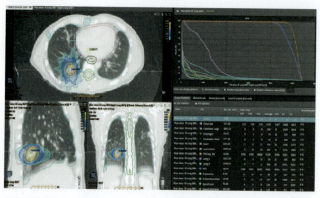

FIGURE 15.18. SBRT plan to deliver 5000 cGy in 5 fractions for a patient with a new pulmonary metastasis after prior metastasectomies who was deemed not to be a candidate for another operation.

with limited metastases. The decision to use locally ablative therapies in the setting of metastatic sarcoma should be determined in multidisciplinary consultation. Figure 15.18 shows an example of an SBRT plan for treatment of a pulmonary metastasis.

KEY POINTS

- Soft tissue and bone sarcomas are rare malignancies that can arise from connective tissue throughout the body. There is significant heterogeneity among the many different histopathologic subtypes.

- Optimal management of sarcoma involves multidisciplinary evaluation and coordination of care between oncologic providers (surgical and orthopedic oncology, radiation oncology, and medical and pediatric oncology) to jointly determine the feasibility of limb or organ-sparing resection, the role for RT and systemic therapies, and the sequence of treatment modalities.

- For extremity and truncal soft tissue sarcoma, combined modality local therapy with wide local excision and radiotherapy results in high rates of local control and good functional outcomes. Preoperative RT is generally preferred over postoperative RT for most patients as it is associated with less long-term toxicity (i.e., fibrosis, joint stiffness, and edema).

- Reproducible setup positioning, custom immobilization, and image guidance are essential for delivery of highly conformal radiotherapy, including IMRT, particularly when reduced PTV margins are used.

- For retroperitoneal sarcoma, when RT is used in addition to surgery, preoperative RT is preferred. Simultaneous integrated boost is a strategy under investigation to escalate the dose to the high-risk retroperitoneal margin.

- For bone sarcoma, RT is used in the adjuvant setting to improve local control in patients with positive or inadequate margins, as primary local therapy for unresectable disease, or to preserve function at certain anatomic sites.

- Stereotactic body radiotherapy can offer an ablative, nonsurgical option for local control in the management of oligometastases from soft tissue and bone sarcomas.

REVIEW QUESTIONS

1. What outcome(s) is/are improved with the addition of RT to limb-sparing resection for extremity soft tissue sarcoma?
   A. Local control
   B. Disease-free and overall survival
   C. Local control and disease-free survival
   D. Local control, disease-free, and overall survival

2. Which histopathologic subtype of soft tissue sarcoma is more likely to have significant volume reduction in response to preoperative RT?
   A. Leiomyosarcoma
   B. Myxofibrosarcoma
   C. Myxoid liposarcoma
   D. Undifferentiated pleomorphic sarcoma

3. For treatment of extremity soft tissue sarcoma, what is the minimum recommended PTV when daily IGRT is not used?
   A. 3 mm
   B. 5 mm
   C. 7 mm
   D. 10 mm

4. What bone constraint should be used in RT planning for extremity soft tissue sarcoma to reduce the risk for fracture?
   A. Max bone dose <6600 cGy
   B. Mean bone dose <4500 cGy
   C. V40 <64%
   D. V60 <50%

5. When RT is used for RPS, what is the preferred approach?
   A. Intraoperative RT + postoperative RT
   B. Preoperative RT
   C. Postoperative RT
   D. Stereotactic body radiotherapy

ANSWERS

1. **A** As shown in the NCI studies and adjuvant brachytherapy trial, the addition of RT to limb-sparing resection for extremity soft tissue sarcoma improves local control with no difference in disease free or overall survival.

References

1. Rosenberg SA, Tepper J, Glatstein E, et al. The treatment of soft tissue sarcomas of the extremities: prospective randomized evaluations of (1) limb-sparing surgery plus radiation therapy compared with amputation and (2) the role of adjuvant chemotherapy. *Ann Surg.* 1982;196(3):305–315.
2. Yang JC, Chang AE, Baker AR, et al. Randomized prospective study of the benefit of adjuvant radiation therapy in the treatment of soft tissue sarcomas of the extremity. *J Clin Oncol.* 1998;16(1):197–203.
3. Pisters PW, Harrison LB, Leung DH, Woodruff JM, Casper ES, Brennan MF. Long-term results of a prospective randomized trial of adjuvant brachytherapy in soft tissue sarcoma. *J Clin Oncol.* 1996 Mar;14(3):859–68.

2. **C** Myxoid liposarcomas are relatively more radio-responsive than other soft tissue histopathologic subtypes. Studies have shown significant volume reduction in response to preoperative RT with excellent local control rates.

References

1. Chung PW, Deheshi BM, Ferguson PC, et al. Radiosensitivity translates into excellent local control in extremity myxoid liposarcoma: a comparison with other soft tissue sarcomas. *Cancer.* 2009;115(14):3254–3261.
2. Guadagnolo BA, Zagars GK, Ballo MT, et al. Excellent local control rates and distinctive patterns of failure in myxoid liposarcoma treated with conservation surgery and radiotherapy. *Int J Radiat Oncol Biol Phys.* 2008;70(3):760–765.

3. **D** For treatment of extremity soft tissue sarcoma, the minimum recommended PTV is 10 mm when daily IGRT is not used. The RTOG 0630 trial required daily IGRT to use a reduced PTV margin of 5 mm.

References

1. Haas RL, Delaney TF, O'Sullivan B, et al. Radiotherapy for management of extremity soft tissue sarcomas: why, when, and where? *Int J Radiat Oncol Biol Phys.* 2012 Nov 1;84(3):572–80.
2. Wang D, Zhang Q, Eisenberg BL, et al. Significant reduction of late toxicities in patients with extremity sarcoma treated with image-guided radiation therapy to a reduced target volume: results of Radiation Therapy Oncology Group RTOG-0630 Trial. *J Clin Oncol.* 2015;33(20):2231–2238.
3. Li XA, Chen X, Zhang Q, et al. Margin reduction from image guided radiation therapy for soft tissue sarcoma: Secondary analysis of Radiation Therapy Oncology Group 0630 results. *Pract Radiat Oncol.* 2016 Jul-Aug;6(4):e135–e140.

4. C When treating extremity soft tissue sarcoma, recommended dose constraints for bone to minimize risk of fracture include V40 <64%, mean dose to bone <3700 cGy, D_{max} <5900 cGy, no more that 50% of a weight bearing bone should receive 5000 cGy, and for the femur, V50 <100% of the circumference is suggested.

References

1. Dickie CI, Parent AL, Griffin AM, et al. Bone fractures following external beam radiotherapy and limb-preservation surgery for lower extremity soft tissue sarcoma: relationship to irradiated bone length, volume, tumor location and dose. *Int J Radiat Oncol Biol Phys.* 2009;75(4):1119–1124.

2. Bishop AJ, Zagars GK, Allen PK, et al. Treatment-related fractures after combined modality therapy for soft tissue sarcomas of the proximal lower extremity: Can the risk be mitigated? *Pract Radiat Oncol.* 2016 May-Jun;6(3):194–200.
3. Wang D, Zhang Q, Eisenberg BL, et al. Significant reduction of late toxicities in patients with extremity sarcoma treated with image-guided radiation therapy to a reduced target volume: results of Radiation Therapy Oncology Group RTOG-0630 Trial. *J Clin Oncol.* 2015;33(20):2231–2238.

5. B The primary treatment for RPS is oncologic resection. The addition of RT to surgery for RPS is an area of ongoing controversy; however, when RT is used for RPS, a preoperative approach is favored. Postoperative RT is usually not recommended.

References

1. Baldini EH, Wang D, Haas RL, et al. Treatment Guidelines for Preoperative Radiation Therapy for Retroperitoneal Sarcoma: Preliminary Consensus of an International Expert Panel. *Int J Radiat Oncol Biol Phys.* 2015 Jul 1;92(3):602–12.
2. Bonvalot S, Gronchi A, Le Péchoux C, et al. Preoperative radiotherapy plus surgery versus surgery alone for patients with primary retroperitoneal sarcoma (EORTC-62092: STRASS): a multicentre, open-label, randomised, phase 3 trial. *Lancet Oncol.* 2020 Oct;21(10):1366–1377.

REFERENCES

1. Fletcher CDM, Bridge KA, Hogendoorn P, Mertens, F, eds. *World Health Organization Classification of Tumours of the Soft Tissue and Bone. Fourth Edition*, Lyon: IARC; 2013.
2. Siegel RL, Miller KD, Jemal A. Cancer statistics, 2020. *CA Cancer J Clin.* 2020 Jan;70(1):7–30.
3. Surveillance, Epidemiology, and End Results (SEER) Program (www.seer.cancer.gov), National Cancer Institute, https://seer.cancer.gov/statfacts/html/soft.html, accessed October 9, 2020.
4. Surveillance, Epidemiology, and End Results (SEER) Program (www.seer.cancer.gov), National Cancer Institute, https://seer.cancer.gov/statfacts/html/bones.html, accessed October 9, 2020.
5. Lawrence W Jr, Donegan WL, Natarajan N, et al. Adult soft tissue sarcomas. A pattern of care survey of the American College of Surgeons. *Ann Surg.* 1987;205(4):349–359.
6. Amin MB, Edge SB, Greene FL, et al. *AJCC Cancer Staging Manual*, 8th edition. New York: Springer; 2017.
7. Blay JY, Honore C, Stoeckle E, et al. Surgery in reference centers improves survival of sarcoma patients: a nationwide study. *Ann Oncol.* 2019;30(8):1407.
8. Blay JY, Soibinet P, Penel N, et al. Improved survival using specialized multidisciplinary board in sarcoma patients. *Ann Oncol.* 2017 Nov 1;28(11):2852–2859.
9. Martin-Broto J, Hindi N, Cruz J, et al. Relevance of Reference Centers in Sarcoma Care and Quality Item Evaluation: Results from the Prospective Registry of the Spanish Group for Research in Sarcoma (GEIS). *Oncologist.* 2019;24(6):e338–e346.
10. Bonvalot S, Gaignard E, Stoeckle E, et al. Survival Benefit of the Surgical Management of Retroperitoneal Sarcoma in a Reference Center: A Nationwide Study of the French Sarcoma Group from the NetSarc Database. *Ann Surg Oncol.* 2019;26(7):2286–2293.
11. Sherman KL, Wayne JD, Chung J, et al. Assessment of multimodality therapy use for extremity sarcoma in the United States. *J Surg Oncol.* 2014;109(5):395–404.
12. Wasif N, Smith CA, Tamurian RM, et al. Influence of physician specialty on treatment recommendations in the multidisciplinary management of soft tissue sarcoma of the extremities. *JAMA Surg.* 2013;148(7):632–639.
13. Sherman KL, Wayne JD, Bilimoria KY. Overcoming specialty bias: another important reason for multidisciplinary management of soft tissue sarcoma. *JAMA Surg.* 2013;148(7):640.
14. Arbiser ZK, Folpe AL, Weiss SW. Consultative (expert) second opinions in soft tissue pathology. Analysis of problem-prone diagnostic situations. *Am J Clin Pathol.* 2001;116(4):473–476.
15. Chalian M, Del Grande F, Thakkar RS, et al. Second-Opinion Subspecialty Consultations in Musculoskeletal Radiology. *AJR Am J Roentgenol.* 2016;206(6):1217–1221.
16. Rozenberg A, Kenneally BE, Abraham JA, et al. Second opinions in orthopedic oncology imaging: can fellowship training reduce clinically significant discrepancies? *Skeletal Radiol.* 2019;48(1):143–147.
17. Ray-Coquard I, Thiesse P, Ranchere-Vince D, et al. Conformity to clinical practice guidelines, multidisciplinary management and outcome of treatment for soft tissue sarcomas. *Ann Oncol.* 2004;15(2):307–315.
18. Gutierrez JC, Perez EA, Moffat FL, Livingstone AS, et al. Should soft tissue sarcomas be treated at high-volume centers? An analysis of 4205 patients. *Ann Surg.* 2007;245(6):952–958.

19. Voss RK, Chiang YJ, Torres KE, et al. Adherence to National Comprehensive Cancer Network Guidelines is Associated with Improved Survival for Patients with Stage 2A and Stages 2B and 3 Extremity and Superficial Trunk Soft Tissue Sarcoma. *Ann Surg Oncol.* 2017;24(11):3271–3278.

20. Fong Y, Coit DG, Woodruff JM, Brennan MF. Lymph node metastasis from soft tissue sarcoma in adults. Analysis of data from a prospective database of 1772 sarcoma patients. *Ann Surg.* 1993 Jan;217(1):72–7.

21. Keung EZ, Chiang YJ, Voss RK, et al. Defining the incidence and clinical significance of lymph node metastasis in soft tissue sarcoma. *Eur J Surg Oncol.* 2018 Jan;44(1):170–177.

22. Jacobs AJ, Morris CD, Levin AS. Synovial Sarcoma Is Not Associated With a Higher Risk of Lymph Node Metastasis Compared With Other Soft Tissue Sarcomas. *Clin Orthop Relat Res.* 2018 Mar;476(3):589–598.

23. Ecker BL, Peters MG, McMillan MT et al. Implications of Lymph Node Evaluation in the Management of Resectable Soft Tissue Sarcoma. *Ann Surg Oncol.* 2017 Feb;24(2):425–433.

24. Fuglo HM, Jorgensen SM, Loft A, et al. The diagnostic and prognostic value of 18F-FDG PET/CT in the initial assessment of high-grade bone and soft tissue sarcoma. A retrospective study of 89 patients. *Eur J Nucl Med Mol Imaging.* 2012 Sep;39(9):1416–1424.

25. Sundaram M, McGuire MH, Herbold DR. Magnetic resonance imaging of soft tissue masses: an evaluation of fifty-three histologically proven tumors. *Magn Reson Imaging.* 1988;6(3):237–248.

26. Demas BE, Heelan RT, Lane J, et al. Soft-tissue sarcomas of the extremities: comparison of MR and CT in determining the extent of disease. *AJR Am J Roentgenol.* 1988;150(3):615–620.

27. Strauss DC, Qureshi YA, Hayes AJ, et al. The role of core needle biopsy in the diagnosis of suspected soft tissue tumours. *J Surg Oncol.* 2010;102(5):523–529.

28. Guadagnolo BA, Xu Y, Zagars GK, Cormier JN, Pollock RE, Feig BW, Giordano S, Buchholz TA, Shih YC. A population-based study of the quality of care in the diagnosis of large (≥5 cm) soft tissue sarcomas. *Am J Clin Oncol.* 2012 Oct;35(5):455–61.

29. Smolle MA, Tunn PU, Goldenitsch E, et al. The Prognostic Impact of Unplanned Excisions in a Cohort of 728 Soft Tissue Sarcoma Patients: A Multicentre Study. *Ann Surg Oncol.* 2017 Jun;24(6):1596–1605. doi: 10.1245/s10434-017-5776-8. Epub 2017 Jan 20. PMID: 28108827; PMCID: PMC5413518.

30. Traub F, Griffin AM, Wunder JS, Ferguson PC. Influence of unplanned excisions on the outcomes of patients with stage III extremity soft-tissue sarcoma. *Cancer.* 2018 Oct 1;124(19):3868–3875.

31. Fiore M, Casali PG, Miceli R, et al. Prognostic effect of re-excision in adult soft tissue sarcoma of the extremity. *Ann Surg Oncol.* 2006 Jan;13(1):110–7.

32. Bianchi G, Sambri A, Cammelli S, et al. Impact of residual disease after "unplanned excision" of primary localized adult soft tissue sarcoma of the extremities: evaluation of 452 cases at a single Institution. *Musculoskelet Surg.* 2017 Dec;101(3):243–248.

33. Potter BK, Adams SC, Pitcher JD Jr, Temple HT. Local recurrence of disease after unplanned excisions of high-grade soft tissue sarcomas. *Clin Orthop Relat Res.* 2008 Dec;466(12):3093–100.

34. Scoccianti G, Innocenti M, Frenos F, et al. Re-excision after unplanned excision of soft tissue sarcomas: Long-term results. *Surg Oncol.* 2020 Sep; 34:212–217.

35. Zagars GK, Ballo MT, Pisters PW, et al. Prognostic factors for patients with localized soft-tissue sarcoma treated with conservation surgery and radiation therapy: an analysis of 1225 patients. *Cancer.* 2003;97(10):2530–2543.

36. Pisters PW, Leung DH, Woodruff J, et al. Analysis of prognostic factors in 1,041 patients with localized soft tissue sarcomas of the extremities. *J Clin Oncol.* 1996;14(5):1679–1689.

37. Schwab JH, Boland PJ, Antonescu C, et al. Spinal metastases from myxoid liposarcoma warrant screening with magnetic resonance imaging. *Cancer.* 2007;110(8):1815–1822.

38. Eary JF, Conrad EU, O'Sullivan J, et al. Sarcoma mid-therapy [F-18]fluorodeoxyglucose positron emission tomography (FDG PET) and patient outcome. *J Bone Joint Surg Am.* 2014;96(2):152–158.

39. Roberge D, Vakilian S, Alabed YZ, et al. FDG PET/CT in initial staging of adult soft-tissue sarcoma. *Sarcoma.* 2012; 2012:960194.

40. Schuetze SM, Rubin BP, Vernon C, et al. Use of positron emission tomography in localized extremity soft tissue sarcoma treated with neoadjuvant chemotherapy. *Cancer.* 2005;103:339–48.

41. Pervaiz N, Colterjohn N, Farrokhyar F, et al A systematic meta-analysis of randomized controlled trials of adjuvant chemotherapy for localized resectable soft-tissue sarcoma. *Cancer.* 2008 Aug 1;113(3):573–81.

42. Istl AC, Ruck JM, Morris CD, et al. Call for improved design and reporting in soft tissue sarcoma studies: A systematic review and meta-analysis of chemotherapy and survival outcomes in resectable STS. *J Surg Oncol.* 2019 Jun;119(7):824–835.

43. Erstad DJ, Ready J, Abraham J, Ferrone ML, Bertagnolli MM, Baldini EH, Raut CP. Amputation for extremity sarcoma: Contemporary indications and outcomes. *Ann Surg Oncol.* 2018;25(2):394–403.

44. O'Donnell PW, Griffin AM, Eward WC, et al. The effect of the setting of a positive surgical margin in soft tissue sarcoma. *Cancer.* 2014;120(18):2866–2875.

45. Albertsmeier M, Rauch A, Roeder F, et al. External Beam Radiation Therapy for Resectable Soft Tissue Sarcoma: A Systematic Review and Meta-Analysis. *Ann Surg Oncol.* 2018;25(3):754–767.

46. Willeumier JJ, Rueten-Budde AJ, Jeys LM, et al. Individualised risk assessment for local recurrence and distant metastases in a retrospective transatlantic cohort of 687 patients with high-grade soft tissue sarcomas of the extremities: a multistate model. *BMJ Open.* 2017;7(2):e012930.

47. Delaney TF, Kepka L, Goldberg SI, et al. Radiation therapy for control of soft-tissue sarcomas resected with positive margins. *Int J Radiat Oncol Biol Phys.* 2007;67(5):1460–1469.

48. Dickie CI, Parent AL, Griffin AM, et al. Bone fractures following external beam radiotherapy and limb-preservation surgery for lower extremity soft tissue sarcoma: relationship to irradiated bone length, volume, tumor location and dose. *Int J Radiat Oncol Biol Phys.* 2009;75(4):1119–1124.

49. Gortzak Y, Lockwood GA, Mahendra A, et al. Prediction of pathologic fracture risk of the femur after combined modality treatment of soft tissue sarcoma of the thigh. *Cancer.* 2010;116(6):1553–1559.

50. Bishop AJ, Zagars GK, Allen PK, et al. Treatment-related fractures after combined modality therapy for soft tissue sarcomas of the proximal lower extremity: Can the risk be mitigated? *Pract Radiat Oncol.* 2016 May-Jun;6(3):194–200.

51. Pak D, Vineberg KA, Griffith KA, et al. Dose–effect relationships for femoral fractures after multimodality limb-sparing therapy of soft-tissue sarcomas of the proximal lower extremity. *Int J Radiat Oncol Biol Phys.* 2012;83(4):1257–1263.

52. Davidge KM, Wunder J, Tomlinson G, et al. Function and health status outcomes following soft tissue reconstruction for limb preservation in extremity soft tissue sarcoma. *Ann Surg Oncol.* 2010;17(4):1052–1062.

53. Rosenberg SA, Tepper J, Glatstein E, et al. The treatment of soft-tissue sarcomas of the extremities: prospective randomized evaluations of (1) limb-sparing surgery plus radiation therapy compared with amputation and (2) the role of adjuvant chemotherapy. *Ann Surg.* 1982;196(3):305–315.

54. Yang JC, Chang AE, Baker AR, et al. Randomized prospective study of the benefit of adjuvant radiation therapy in the treatment of soft tissue sarcomas of the extremity. *J Clin Oncol.* 1998;16(1):197–203.

55. Beane JD, Yang JC, White D, et al. Efficacy of adjuvant radiation therapy in the treatment of soft tissue sarcoma of the extremity: 20-year follow-up of a randomized prospective trial. *Ann Surg Oncol.* 2014 Aug;21(8):2484–9.

56. Pisters PW, Harrison LB, Leung DH, Woodruff JM, Casper ES, Brennan MF. Long-term results of a prospective randomized trial of adjuvant brachytherapy in soft tissue sarcoma. *J Clin Oncol.* 1996 Mar;14(3):859–68.

57. Jebsen NL, Trovik CS, Bauer HC, et al. Radiotherapy to improve local control regardless of surgical margin and malignancy grade in extremity and trunk wall soft tissue sarcoma: a Scandinavian sarcoma group study. *Int J Radiat Oncol Biol Phys.* 2008;71(4):1196–1203.

58. Cahlon O, Brannon MF, Jia X, et al. A postoperative nomogram for local recurrence risk in extremity soft tissue sarcomas after limb-sparing surgery without adjuvant radiation. *Ann Surg*. 2012;255(2):343–347.

59. Gerrand CH, Bell RS, Wunder JS, et al. The influence of anatomic location on outcome in patients with soft tissue sarcoma of the extremity. *Cancer*. 2003;97(2):485–492.

60. Biau DJ, Ferguson PC, Chung P, et al. Local recurrence of localized soft tissue sarcoma: a new look at old predictors. *Cancer*. 2012 Dec 1;118(23):5867–77.

61. Fleming JB, Berman RS, Cheng SC, et al. Long-term outcome of patients with American Joint Committee on Cancer stage IIB extremity soft tissue sarcomas. *J Clin Oncol*. 1999 Sep;17(9):2772–80.

62. McKee MD, Liu DF, Brooks JJ, et al. The prognostic significance of margin width for extremity and trunk sarcoma. *J Surg Oncol*. 2004 Feb;85(2):68–76.

63. Alamanda VK, Crosby SN, Archer KR, et al. Predictors and clinical significance of local recurrence in extremity soft tissue sarcoma. *Acta Oncol*. 2013 May;52(4):793–802.

64. Gronchi A, Lo Vullo S, Colombo C, et al. Extremity soft tissue sarcoma in a series of patients treated at a single institution: local control directly impacts survival. *Ann Surg*. 2010 Mar;251(3):506–11.

65. Funovics PT, Vaselic S, Panotopoulos J, et al. The impact of re-excision of inadequately resected soft tissue sarcomas on surgical therapy, results, and prognosis: A single institution experience with 682 patients. *JSurg Oncol*. 2010;102(6):626–633.

66. Mutter RW, Singer S, Zhang Z, et al. The enigma of myxofibrosarcoma of the extremity. *Cancer*. 2012;118(2):518–527.

67. Haglund KE, Raut CP, Nascimento AF, et al. Recurrence patterns and survival for patients with intermediate- and high-grade myxofibrosarcoma. *Int J Radiat Oncol Biol Phys*. 2012 Jan;82(1):361–7.

68. Sanfilippo R, Miceli R, Grosso F, et al. Myxofibrosarcoma: prognostic factors and survival in a series of patients treated at a single institution. *Ann Surg Oncol*. 2011 Mar;18(3):720–5.

69. Boughzala-Bennadji R, Stoeckle E, Le Péchoux C, et al. Localized Myxofibrosarcomas: Roles of Surgical Margins and Adjuvant Radiation Therapy. *Int J Radiat Oncol Biol Phys*. 2018 Oct 1;102(2):399–406.

70. Martin, E., Coert, J. H., Flucke, U. E., et al. A nationwide cohort study on treatment and survival in patients with malignant peripheral nerve sheath tumours. *European Journal of Cancer*. 2020. 124:77–87

71. Chung PW, Deheshi BM, Ferguson PC, et al. Radiosensitivity translates into excellent local control in extremity myxoid liposarcoma: a comparison with other soft tissue sarcomas. *Cancer*. 2009;115(14):3254–3261.

72. Guadagnolo BA, Zagars GK, Ballo MT, et al. Excellent local control rates and distinctive patterns of failure in myxoid liposarcoma treated with conservation surgery and radiotherapy. *Int J Radiat Oncol Biol Phys*. 2008;70(3):760–765.

73. Al-Refaie WB, Habermann EB, Jensen EH, et al. Surgery alone is adequate treatment for early stage soft tissue sarcoma of the extremity. *Br J Surg*. 2010;97(5):707–713.

74. Pisters PW, Pollock RE, Lewis VO, et al. Long-term results of prospective trial of surgery alone with selective use of radiation for patients with T1 extremity and trunk soft tissue sarcomas. *Ann Surg*. 2007;246(4):675–681; discussion 681–682.

75. Baldini EH, Goldberg J, Jenner C, et al. Long-term outcomes after function-sparing surgery without radiotherapy for soft tissue sarcoma of the extremities and trunk. *J Clin Oncol*. 1999;17(10):3252–3259.

76. O'Sullivan B, Davis AM, Turcotte R, et al. Preoperative versus postoperative radiotherapy in soft-tissue sarcoma of the limbs: a randomised trial. *The Lancet*. 2002;359(9325):2235–2241.

77. Davis AM, O'Sullivan B, Bell RS, et al. Function and health status outcomes in a randomized trial comparing preoperative and postoperative radiotherapy in extremity soft tissue sarcoma. *J Clin Oncol*. 2002 Nov 15;20(22):4472–7.

78. Davis A, O'Sullivan B, Turcotte R, et al. Late radiation morbidity following randomization to preoperative versus postoperative radiotherapy in extremity soft tissue sarcoma. *Radiother Oncol*. 2005;75(1):48–53.

79. Wang D, Zhang Q, Eisenberg BL, et al. Significant reduction of late toxicities in patients with extremity sarcoma treated with image-guided radiation therapy to a reduced target volume: results of Radiation Therapy Oncology Group RTOG-0630 Trial. *J Clin Oncol*. 2015;33(20):2231–2238.

80. Shelby, R. D., Suarez-Kelly, L. P., Yu, P. Y., et al. Neoadjuvant radiation improves margin-negative resection rates in extremity sarcoma but not survival. *Journal of Surgical Oncology*. 2020. 121:1249–1258.

81. Zagars GK, Ballo MT, Pisters PW, et al. Preoperative vs. postoperative radiation therapy for soft tissue sarcoma: a retrospective comparative evaluation of disease outcome. *Int J Radiat Oncol Biol Phys*. 2003;56(2):482–488.

82. Baldini EH, Lapidus MR, Wang Q, et al. Predictors for major wound complications following preoperative radiotherapy and surgery for soft-tissue sarcoma of the extremities and trunk: importance of tumor proximity to skin surface. *Ann Surg Oncol*. 2013 May;20(5):1494–9.

83. Slump J, Bastiaannet E, Halka A, et al. Risk factors for postoperative wound complications after extremity soft tissue sarcoma resection: A systematic review and meta-analyses. *J Plast Reconstr Aesthet Surg*. 2019;72(9):1449–1464.

84. Moore J, Isler M, Barry J, Mottard S. Major wound complication risk factors following soft tissue sarcoma resection. *Eur J Surg Oncol*. 2014;40(12):1671–1676.

85. Karthik N, Ward MC, Juloori A, et al. Factors Associated With Acute and Chronic Wound Complications in Patients With Soft Tissue Sarcoma With Long-term Follow-up. *Am J Clin Oncol*. 2018;41(10):1019–1023.

86. Alektiar KM, Brennan MF, Singer S. Influence of site on the therapeutic ratio of adjuvant radiotherapy in soft-tissue sarcoma of the extremity. *Int J Radiat Oncol Biol Phys*. 2005;63(1):202–208.

87. Kraybill WG, Harris J, Spiro IJ, et al. Long-term results of a phase 2 study of neoadjuvant chemotherapy and radiotherapy in the management of high-risk, high-grade, soft tissue sarcomas of the extremities and body wall: Radiation Therapy Oncology Group Trial 9514. *Cancer*. 2010;116(19):4613–4621.

88. Mullen JT, Kobayashi W, Wang JJ, Harmon DC, Choy E, Hornicek FJ, Rosenberg AE, Chen YL, Spiro IJ, DeLaney TF. Long-term follow-up of patients treated with neoadjuvant chemotherapy and radiotherapy for large, extremity soft tissue sarcomas. *Cancer*. 2012 Aug 1;118(15):3758–65.

89. Edmonson JH, Petersen IA, Shives TC, et al. Chemotherapy, irradiation, and surgery for function-preserving therapy of primary extremity soft tissue sarcomas: initial treatment with ifosfamide, mitomycin, doxorubicin, and cisplatin plus granulocyte macrophage-colony-stimulating factor. *Cancer*. 2002;94(3):786–792.

90. Palassini E, Ferrari S, Verderio P, et al. Feasibility of Preoperative Chemotherapy With or Without Radiation Therapy in Localized Soft Tissue Sarcomas of Limbs and Superficial Trunk in the Italian Sarcoma Group/Grupo Espanol de Investigacion en Sarcomas Randomized Clinical Trial: Three Versus Five Cycles of Full-Dose Epirubicin Plus Ifosfamide. *J Clin Oncol*. 2015;33(31):3628–3634.

91. Kosela-Paterczyk H, Szacht M, Morysinski T, et al. Preoperative hypofractionated radiotherapy in the treatment of localized soft tissue sarcomas. *Eur J Surg Oncol*. 2014;40(12):1641–1647.

92. Koseła-Paterczyk H, Spałek M, Borkowska A, et al. Hypofractionated Radiotherapy in Locally Advanced Myxoid Liposarcomas of Extremities or Trunk Wall: Results of a Single-Arm Prospective Clinical Trial. *J Clin Med*. 2020 Aug 1;9(8):2471.

93. Kalbasi, A., Kamrava, M., Chu, F. I., et al. A Phase II Trial of 5-Day Neoadjuvant Radiotherapy for Patients with High-Risk Primary Soft Tissue Sarcoma. *Clinical Cancer Research*. 2020. 26:1829–1836.

94. Kubicek GJ, LaCouture T, Kaden M, et al. Preoperative radiosurgery for soft tissue sarcoma. *Am J Clin Oncol*. 2018 Jan;41(1):86–89.

95. Temple WJ, Temple CL, Arthur K, Schachar NS, Paterson AH, Crabtree TS. Prospective cohort study of neoadjuvant treatment in conservative surgery of soft tissue sarcomas. *Ann Surg Oncol*. 1997;4(7):586–590.

96. Eilber F, Eckhardt J, Rosen G, et al. Preoperative therapy for soft tissue sarcoma. *Heamatol Oncol Clin North Am*. 1995;9:817–23.

97. Pennington JD, Eilber FC, Eilber FR, et al. Long-term Outcomes With Ifosfamide-based Hypofractionated Preoperative Chemoradiotherapy for Extremity Soft Tissue Sarcomas. *Am J Clin Oncol*. 2018 Dec;41(12):1154–1161.

98. Meyer JM, Perlewitz KS, Hayden JB, et al. Phase I trial of preoperative chemoradiation plus sorafenib for high-risk extremity soft tissue sarcomas with dynamic contrast-enhanced MRI correlates. *Clin Cancer Res.* 2013;19:6902–11.

99. Ryan CW, Montag AG, Hosenpud JR, et al. Histologic response of dose-intense chemotherapy with preoperative hypofractionated radiotherapy for patients with high-risk soft tissue sarcomas. *Cancer.* 2008;112(11):2432–2439.

100. Azinovic I, Martinez Monge R, Javier Aristu J, et al. Intraoperative radiotherapy electron boost followed by moderate doses of external beam radiotherapy in resected soft-tissue sarcoma of the extremities. *Radiother Oncol.* 2003;67(3):331–337.

101. Calvo FA, Sole CV, Polo A, et al. Limb-sparing management with surgical resection, external-beam and intraoperative electron-beam radiation therapy boost for patients with primary soft tissue sarcoma of the extremity: a multicentric pooled analysis of long-term outcomes. *Strahlenther Onkol.* 2014;190(10):891–898.

102. Kunos C, Colussi V, Getty P, et al. Intraoperative electron radiotherapy for extremity sarcomas does not increase acute or late morbidity. *Clin Orthop Relat Res.* 2006; 446:247–252.

103. Oertel S, Treiber M, Zahlten-Hinguranage A, et al. Intraoperative electron boost radiation followed by moderate doses of external beam radiotherapy in limb-sparing treatment of patients with extremity soft-tissue sarcoma. *Int J Radiat Oncol Biol Phys.* 2006;64(5):1416–1423.

104. Roeder F, Lehner B, Saleh-Ebrahimi L, et al. Intraoperative electron radiation therapy combined with external beam radiation therapy and limb sparing surgery in extremity soft tissue sarcoma: a retrospective single center analysis of 183 cases. *Radiother Oncol.* 2015; pii:S0167–S8140(15)00619-2.

105. Al Yami A, Griffin AM, Ferguson PC, et al. Positive surgical margins in soft tissue sarcoma treated with preoperative radiation: is a postoperative boost necessary? *Int J Radiat Oncol Biol Phys.* 2010;77(4):1191–1197.

106. Pan E, Goldberg SI, Chen YL, et al. Role of post-operative radiation boost for soft tissue sarcomas with positive margins following preoperative radiation and surgery. *J Surg Oncol.* 2014;110(7):817–822.

107. Wells, S., Ager, B., Hitchcock, Y. J., Poppe, M. M. The radiation dose-response of non-retroperitoneal soft tissue sarcoma with positive margins: An NCDB analysis. *Journal of Surgical Oncology.* 2019. 120:1476–1485.

108. Tepper J, Rosenberg SA, Glatstein E. Radiation therapy technique in soft tissue sarcomas of the extremity—policies of treatment at the national cancer institute. *Int J Radiat Oncol Biol Phys.* 1982;8(2):263.273.

109. White LM, Wunder JS, Bell RS, et al. Histologic assessment of peritumoral edema in soft tissue sarcoma. *Int J Radiat Oncol Biol Phys.* 2005;61(5):1439–1445.

110. Haas RL, Delaney TF, O'Sullivan B, et al. Radiotherapy for management of extremity soft tissue sarcomas: why, when, and where? *Int J Radiat Oncol Biol Phys.* 2012 Nov 1;84(3):572–80.

111. Wang D, Bosch W, Roberge D, et al. RTOG sarcoma radiation oncologists reach consensus on gross tumor volume and clinical target volume on computed tomographic images for preoperative radiotherapy of primary soft tissue sarcoma of extremity in Radiation Therapy Oncology Group studies. *Int J Radiat Oncol Biol Phys.* 2011;81(4):e525–e528.

112. Wang D, Bosch W, Kirsch DG, et al. Variation in the gross tumor volume and clinical target volume for preoperative radiotherapy of primary large high-grade soft tissue sarcoma of the extremity among RTOG sarcoma radiation oncologists. *Int J Radiat Oncol Biol Phys.* 2011;81(5):e775–e780.

113. Bahig H, Roberge D, Bosch W, et al. Agreement among RTOG sarcoma radiation oncologists in contouring suspicious peritumoral edema for preoperative radiation therapy of soft tissue sarcoma of the extremity. *Int J Radiat Oncol Biol Phys.* 2013;86(2):298–303.

114. Finkelstein SE, Trotti A, Letson G, et al. Deformable imaging capability for the Radiation Therapy Oncology Group (RTOG) Consensus Atlas of Musculoskeletal Anatomy (CAMAS) for soft tissue sarcoma of the lower extremities. *Pract Radiat Oncol.* 2013;3(2 suppl 1):S7.

115. Kim B, Chen YL, Kirsch DG, et al. An effective preoperative three-dimensional radiotherapy target volume for extremity soft tissue sarcoma and the effect of margin width on local control. *Int J Radiat Oncol Biol Phys.* 2010;77(3):843–850.

116. Dickie CI, Griffin AM, Parent AL, et al. The relationship between local recurrence and radiotherapy treatment volume for soft tissue sarcomas treated with external beam radiotherapy and function preservation surgery. *Int J Radiat Oncol Biol Phys.* 2012 Mar 15;82(4):1528–34.

117. Gerrand CH, Wunder JS, Kandel RA, et al. The influence of anatomic location on functional outcome in lower-extremity soft-tissue sarcoma. *Ann Surg Oncol.* 2004;11(5):476–482.

118. Tseng JF, Ballo MT, Langstein HN, et al. The effect of preoperative radiotherapy and reconstructive surgery on wound complications after resection of extremity soft-tissue sarcomas. *Ann Surg Oncol.* 2006;13(9):1209–1215.

119. Rimner A, Brennan MF, Zhang Z, et al. Influence of compartmental involvement on the patterns of morbidity in soft tissue sarcoma of the thigh. *Cancer.* 2009;115(1):149–157.

120. Moore J, Isler M, Barry J, et al. Major wound complication risk factors following soft tissue sarcoma resection. *Eur J Surg Oncol.* 2014;40(12):1671–1676.

121. O'Sullivan B, Griffin AM, Dickie CI, et al. Phase 2 study of preoperative image-guided intensity-modulated radiation therapy to reduce wound and combined modality morbidities in lower extremity soft tissue sarcoma. *Cancer.* 2013;119(10):1878–1884.

122. Alektiar KM, McKee AB, Jacobs JM, McKee BJ, Healey JH, Brennan MF. Outcome of primary soft tissue sarcoma of the knee and elbow. *Int J Radiat Oncol Biol Phys.* 2002;54(1):163–169.

123. Folkert MR, Casey DL, Berry SL, Crago A, Fabbri N, Singer S, Alektiar KM. Femoral Fracture in Primary Soft-Tissue Sarcoma of the Thigh and Groin Treated with Intensity-Modulated Radiation Therapy: Observed versus Expected Risk. *Ann Surg Oncol.* 2019 May;26(5):1326–1331.

124. Holt GE, Griffin AM, Pintilie M, et al. Fractures following radiotherapy and limb-salvage surgery for lower extremity soft-tissue sarcomas. A comparison of high-dose and low-dose radiotherapy. *J Bone Joint Surg Am.* 2005 Feb;87(2):315–9.

125. Dickie CI, Parent A, Griffin A, et al. A device and procedure for immobilization of patients receiving limb-preserving radiotherapy for soft tissue sarcoma. *Med Dosim.* 2009;34(3):243–249.

126. Swinscoe JA, Dickie CI, Ireland RH. Immobilization and image-guidance methods for radiation therapy of limb extremity soft tissue sarcomas: Results of a multi-institutional survey. *Med Dosim.* 2018 Winter;43(4):377–382.

127. Alektiar KM, Hong L, Brennan MF, et al. Intensity modulated radiation therapy for primary soft tissue sarcoma of the extremity: preliminary results. *Int J Radiat Oncol Biol Phys.* 2007;68(2):458–464.

128. Alektiar KM, Brennan MF, Healey JH, et al. Impact of intensity-modulated radiation therapy on local control in primary soft-tissue sarcoma of the extremity. *J Clin Oncol.* 2008;26(20):3440–3444.

129. Folkert MR, Singer S, Brennan MF, et al. Comparison of local recurrence with conventional and intensity-modulated radiation therapy for primary soft-tissue sarcomas of the extremity. *J Clin Oncol.* 2014;32(29):3236–3241.

130. Alektiar KM, Brennan MF, Singer S. Local control comparison of adjuvant brachytherapy to intensity-modulated radiotherapy in primary high-grade sarcoma of the extremity. *Cancer.* 2011;117(14):3229–3234.

131. Dickie CI, Parent AL, Chung PW, et al. Measuring interfractional and intrafractional motion with cone beam computed tomography and an optical localization system for lower extremity soft tissue sarcoma patients treated with preoperative intensity-modulated radiation therapy. *Int J Radiat Oncol Biol Phys.* 2010;78(5):1437–1444.

132. Kim A, Kelly V, Dickie C, et al. Impact of Immobilization on Interfractional Errors for Upper Extremity Soft Tissue Sarcoma Radiation Therapy. *J Med Imaging Radiat Sci.* 2019 Jun;50(2):308–316.

133. Gierga DP, Turcotte JC, Tong LW, et al. Analysis of setup uncertainties for extremity sarcoma patients using surface imaging. *Pract Radiat Oncol.* 2014;4(4):261–266.

134. Li XA, Chen X, Zhang Q, et al. Margin reduction from image guided radiation therapy for soft tissue sarcoma: Secondary

analysis of Radiation Therapy Oncology Group 0630 results. *Pract Radiat Oncol.* 2016 Jul-Aug;6(4):e135–e140.

135. Dickie C, Parent A, Griffin AM, et al. The value of adaptive preoperative radiotherapy in management of soft tissue sarcoma. *Radiother Oncol.* 2017 Mar;122(3):458–463

136. Haas RL, van Beek S, Betgen A, et al. Substantial Volume Changes and Plan Adaptations During Preoperative Radiation Therapy in Extremity Soft Tissue Sarcoma Patients. *Pract Radiat Oncol.* 2019 Mar;9(2):115–122.

137. le Grange F, Cassoni AM, Seddon BM, Tumour volume changes following pre-operative radiotherapy in borderline resectable limb and trunk soft tissue sarcoma. *Eur J Surg Oncol.* 2014;40(4):394–401.

138. Roberge D, Skamene T, Nahal A, et al. Radiological and pathological response following pre-operative radiotherapy for soft-tissue sarcoma. *Radiother Oncol.* 2010;97(3):404–407.

139. Naghavi AO, Fernandez DC, Mesko N, et al. American Brachytherapy Society consensus statement for soft tissue sarcoma brachytherapy. *Brachytherapy.* 2017 May-Jun;16(3):466–489.

140. Guttmann DM, Frick MA, Carmona R, et al. A prospective study of proton reirradiation for recurrent and secondary soft tissue sarcoma. *Radiother Oncol.* 2017 Aug;124(2):271–276.

141. Tepper JE, Suit HD. Radiation therapy alone for sarcoma of soft tissue. *Cancer.* 1985 Aug 1;56(3):475–9.

142. Kepka L, DeLaney TF, Suit HD, et al. Results of radiation therapy for unresected soft-tissue sarcomas. *Int J Radiat Oncol Biol Phys.* 2005;63(3):852–859.

143. Demizu Y, Jin D, Sulaiman NS, et al. Particle Therapy Using Protons or Carbon Ions for Unresectable or Incompletely Resected Bone and Soft Tissue Sarcomas of the Pelvis. *Int J Radiat Oncol Biol Phys.* 2017 Jun 1;98(2):367–374.

144. Abatzoglou S, Turcotte RE, Adoubali A, et al. Local recurrence after initial multidisciplinary management of soft tissue sarcoma: is there a way out? *Clin Orthop Relat Res* 2010; 468(11):3012–8.

145. Torres MA, Ballo MT, Butler CE, et al. Management of locally recurrent soft-tissue sarcoma after prior surgery and radiation therapy. *Int J Radiat Oncol Biol Phys.* 2007;67(4):1124–1129.

146. Indelicato DJ, Meadows K, Gibbs CP Jr, et al. Effectiveness and morbidity associated with reirradiation in conservative salvage management of recurrent soft-tissue sarcoma. *Int J Radiat Oncol Biol Phys.* 2009;73(1):267–272.

147. Catton C, Davis A, Bell R, et al. Soft tissue sarcoma of the extremity. Limb salvage after failure of combined conservative therapy. *Radiother Oncol.* 1996;41(3):209–214.

148. Pearlstone DB, Janjan NA, Feig BW, et al. Re-resection with brachytherapy for locally recurrent soft tissue sarcoma arising in a previously radiated field. *Cancer J Sci Am.* 1999;5(1):26–33.

149. Gronchi A, Lo Vullo S, Fiore M, et al. Aggressive surgical policies in a retrospectively reviewed single-institution case series of retroperitoneal soft tissue sarcoma patients. *J Clin Oncol.* 2009;27(1):24–30.

150. Bonvalot S, Rivoire M, Castaing M, et al. Primary retroperitoneal sarcomas: a multivariate analysis of surgical factors associated with local control. *J Clin Oncol.* 2009;27(1):31–37.

151. Tan MC, Brennan MF, Kuk D, et al. Histology-based classification predicts pattern of recurrence and improves risk stratification in primary retroperitoneal sarcoma. *Ann Surg.* 2016;263(3):593–600.

152. Gronchi A, Strauss DC, Miceli R, et al. Variability in Patterns of Recurrence After Resection of Primary Retroperitoneal Sarcoma (RPS): A Report on 1007 Patients From the Multi-institutional Collaborative RPS Working Group. *Ann Surg.* 2016 May;263(5):1002–9.

153. Singer S, Antonescu CR, Riedel E, et al. Histologic subtype and margin of resection predict pattern of recurrence and survival for retroperitoneal liposarcoma. *Ann Surg.* 2003;238(3):358–370.

154. Stoeckle E, Coindre JM, Bonvalot S, et al. Prognostic factors in retroperitoneal sarcoma: a multivariate analysis of a series of 165 patients of the French Cancer Center Federation Sarcoma Group. *Cancer.* 2001;92(2):359–368.

155. Tseng W, Martinez SR, Tamurian RM, et al. Histologic type predicts survival in patients with retroperitoneal soft tissue sarcoma. *J Surg Res.* 2012 Jan;172(1):123–30.

156. Pawlik TM, Pisters PW, Mikula L, et al. Long-term results of two prospective trials of preoperative external beam radiotherapy for localized intermediate- or high-grade retroperitoneal soft tissue sarcoma. *Ann Surg Oncol.* 2006;13(4):508–517.

157. Le Pechoux C, Musat E, Baey C, et al. Should adjuvant radiotherapy be administered in addition to front-line aggressive surgery (FAS) in patients with primary retroperitoneal sarcoma? *Ann Oncol.* 2013;24(3):832–837.

158. Kelly KJ, Yoon SS, Kuk D, et al. Comparison of Perioperative Radiation Therapy and Surgery Versus Surgery Alone in 204 Patients With Primary Retroperitoneal Sarcoma: A Retrospective 2-Institution Study. *Ann Surg.* 2015;262(1):156–162.

159. Bishop AJ, Zagars GK, Torres KE, et al. Combined Modality Management of Retroperitoneal Sarcomas: A Single-Institution Series of 121 Patients. *Int J Radiat Oncol Biol Phys.* 2015;93(1):158–165.

160. Nussbaum DP, Speicher PJ, Gulack BC, et al. Long-term oncologic outcomes after neoadjuvant radiation therapy for retroperitoneal sarcomas. *Ann Surg.* 2015;262(1):163–170.

161. Chouliaras K, Senehi R, Ethun CG, et al. Role of radiation therapy for retroperitoneal sarcomas: An eight-institution study from the US Sarcoma Collaborative. *J Surg Oncol.* 2019 Dec;120(7):1227–1234.

162. Bonvalot S, Gronchi A, Le Péchoux C, et al. Preoperative radiotherapy plus surgery versus surgery alone for patients with primary retroperitoneal sarcoma (EORTC-62092: STRASS): a multicentre, open-label, randomised, phase 3 trial. *Lancet Oncol.* 2020 Oct;21(10):1366–1377.

163. Sindelar WF, Kinsella TJ, Chen PW, et al. Intraoperative radiotherapy in retroperitoneal sarcomas. Final results of a prospective, randomized, clinical trial. *Arch Surg.* 1993;128(4):402–410.

164. White JS, Biberdorf D, DiFrancesco LM, Kurien E, Temple W. Use of tissue expanders and pre-operative external beam radiotherapy in the treatment of retroperitoneal sarcoma. *Ann Surg Oncol.* 2007;14(2):583–590.

165. Baldini EH, Wang D, Haas RL, et al. Treatment Guidelines for Preoperative Radiation Therapy for Retroperitoneal Sarcoma: Preliminary Consensus of an International Expert Panel. *Int J Radiat Oncol Biol Phys.* 2015 Jul 1;92(3):602–12.

166. Hallman JL, Mori S, Sharp GC, et al. A four-dimensional computed tomography analysis of multiorgan abdominal motion. *Int J Radiat Oncol Biol Phys.* 2012;83(1):435–441.

167. Aruga T, Itami J, Aruga M, et al. Target volume definition for upper abdominal irradiation using CT scans obtained during inhale and exhale phases. *Int J Radiat Oncol Biol Phys.* 2000 Sep 1;48(2):465–9.

168. Brandner ED, Wu A, Chen H, et al. Abdominal organ motion measured using 4D CT. *Int J Radiat Oncol Biol Phys.* 2006 Jun 1;65(2):554–60.

169. Baldini EH, Abrams RA, Bosch W, et al. Retroperitoneal Sarcoma Target Volume and Organ at Risk Contour Delineation Agreement Among NRG Sarcoma Radiation Oncologists. *Int J Radiat Oncol Biol Phys.* 2015 Aug 1;92(5):1053–1059.

170. Wong P, Dickie C, Lee D, et al. Spatial and volumetric changes of retroperitoneal sarcomas during pre-operative radiotherapy. *Radiother Oncol.* 2014;112(2):308–313.

171. Bossi A, De Wever I, Van Limbergen E, et al. Intensity modulated radiation-therapy for preoperative posterior abdominal wall irradiation of retroperitoneal liposarcomas. *Int J Radiat Oncol Biol Phys.* 2007;67:164–170.

172. Tzeng CW, Fiveash JB, Popple RA, et al. Preoperative radiation therapy with selective dose escalation to the margin at risk for retroperitoneal sarcoma. *Cancer.* 2006;107(2):371–379.

173. McBride SM, Raut CP, Lapidus M, et al. Locoregional recurrence after preoperative radiation therapy for retroperitoneal sarcoma: adverse impact of multifocal disease and potential implications of dose escalation. *Ann Surg Oncol.* 2013 Jul;20(7):2140–7.

174. Baldini EH, Bosch W, Kane JM 3rd, et al. Retroperitoneal sarcoma (RPS) high risk gross tumor volume boost (HR GTV boost) contour delineation agreement among NRG sarcoma radiation and surgical oncologists. *Ann Surg Oncol.* 2015 Sep;22(9):2846–52.

175. DeLaney TF, Chen YL, Baldini EH, Wang D, Adams J, Hickey SB, Yeap BY, Hahn SM, De Amorim Bernstein K, Nielsen GP, Choy E, Mullen JT, Yoon SS. Phase 1 trial of preoperative image guided intensity modulated proton radiation therapy with simultaneously integrated boost to the high risk margin for retroperitoneal sarcomas. *Adv Radiat Oncol.* 2017 Jan 4;2(1):85–93.

176. Koshy M, Landry JC, Lawson JD, et al. Intensity modulated radiation therapy for retroperitoneal sarcoma: a case for dose escalation and organ at risk toxicity reduction. *Sarcoma.* 2003; 7(3–4):137–48.

177. Taggar AS, Graham D, Kurien E, Gräfe JL. Volumetric-modulated arc therapy versus intensity-modulated radiotherapy for large volume retroperitoneal sarcomas: A comparative analysis of dosimetric and treatment delivery parameters. *J Appl Clin Med Phys.* 2018 Jan;19(1):276–281.

178. Mak KS, Phillips JG, Barysauskas cm, et al. Acute gastrointestinal toxicity and bowel bag dose-volume parameters for preoperative radiation therapy for retroperitoneal sarcoma. *Pract Radiat Oncol.* 2016;6(5):360–366.

179. Bielack SS, Kempf-Bielack B, Delling G, et al. Prognostic factors in high-grade osteosarcoma of the extremities or trunk: an analysis of 1,702 patients treated on neoadjuvant cooperative osteosarcoma study group protocols. *J Clin Oncol.* 2002;20(3):776–790.

180. Ozaki T, Flege S, Kevric M, et al. Osteosarcoma of the pelvis: experience of the Cooperative Osteosarcoma Study Group. *J Clin Oncol.* 2003;21(2):334–341.

181. Ozaki T, Flege S, Liljenqvist U, et al. Osteosarcoma of the spine: experience of the Cooperative Osteosarcoma Study Group. *Cancer.* 2002;94(4):1069–1077.

182. DeLaney TF, Liebsch NJ, Pedlow FX, et al. Phase II study of high-dose photon/proton radiotherapy in the management of spine sarcomas. *Int J Radiat Oncol Biol Phys.* 2009;74(3):732–739.

183. Guadagnolo BA, Zagars GK, Raymond AK, et al. Osteosarcoma of the jaw/craniofacial region: outcomes after multimodality treatment. *Cancer.* 2009 Jul 15;115(14):3262–70.

184. Ciernik IF, Niemierko A, Harmon DC, et al. Proton-based radiotherapy for unresectable or incompletely resected osteosarcoma. *Cancer.* 2011 Oct 1;117(19):4522–30.

185. DeLaney TF, Park L, Goldberg SI, et al. Radiotherapy for local control of osteosarcoma. *Int J Radiat Oncol Biol Phys.* 2005 Feb 1;61(2):492–8.

186. Scully SP, Ghert MA, Zurakowski D, et al. Pathologic fracture in osteosarcoma: prognostic importance and treatment implications. *J Bone Joint Surg Am.* 2002;84-A(1):49–57.

187. Picci P, Sangiorgi L, Bahamonde L, et al. Risk factors for local recurrences after limb-salvage surgery for high-grade osteosarcoma of the extremities. *Ann Oncol.* 1997;8(9):899–903.

188. Yock TI, Krailo M, Fryer CJ, et al. Children's Oncology Group. Local control in pelvic Ewing sarcoma: analysis from INT-0091--a report from the Children's Oncology Group. *J Clin Oncol.* 2006 Aug 20;24(24):3838–43.

189. La TH, Meyers PA, Wexler LH et al. Radiation therapy for Ewing's sarcoma: results from Memorial Sloan-Kettering in the modern era. *Int J Radiat Oncol Biol Phys.* 2006 Feb 1;64(2):544–50.

190. Hug EB, Fitzek MM, Liebsch NJ, et al. Locally challenging osteo- and chondrogenic tumors of the axial skeleton: results of combined proton and photon radiation therapy using three-dimensional treatment planning. *Int J Radiat Oncol Biol Phys.* 1995;31(3):467–476.

191. Chen YL, Liebsch N, Kobayashi W, et al. Definitive high-dose proton based radiotherapy for unresected mobile spine and sacral chordomas. *Spine.* 2013;38:E930–E936.

192. Goda JS, Ferguson PC, O'Sullivan B, et al. High-risk extracranial chondrosarcoma: long-term results of surgery and radiation therapy. *Cancer.* 2011 Jun 1;117(11):2513–9.

193. Ewing J. Classics in oncology. Diffuse endothelioma of bone. James Ewing. Proceedings of the New York Pathological Society, 1921. *CA Cancer J Clin.* 1972;22(2):95–98.

194. Laskar S, Mallick I, Gupta T, Muckaden MA. Post-operative radiotherapy for Ewing sarcoma: when, how and how much? *Pediatr Blood Cancer.* 2008 Nov;51(5):575–80. doi: 10.1002/pbc.21657. PMID: 18561167.

195. Park L, Delaney TF, Liebsch NJ, et al. Sacral chordomas: Impact of high-dose proton/photon-beam radiation therapy combined with or without surgery for primary versus recurrent tumor. *Int J Radiat Oncol Biol Phys.* 2006 Aug 1;65(5):1514–21.

196. Kabolizadeh P, Chen YL, Liebsch N, et al. Updated Outcome and Analysis of Tumor Response in Mobile Spine and Sacral Chordoma Treated With Definitive High-Dose Photon/Proton Radiation Therapy. *Int J Radiat Oncol Biol Phys.* 2017 Feb 1;97(2):254–262.

197. Wagner TD, Kobayashi W, Dean S. Combination short-course preoperative irradiation, surgical resection, and reduced-field high-dose postoperative irradiation in the treatment of tumors involving the bone. *Int J Radiat Oncol Biol Phys.* 2009 Jan 1;73(1):259–66.

198. Patel S, DeLaney TF. Advanced-technology radiation therapy for bone sarcomas. *Cancer Control.* 2008 Jan;15(1):21–37.

199. Pastorino U, Buyse M, Friedel G, et al. Long-term results of lung metastasectomy: prognostic analyses based on 5206 cases. *J Thorac Cardiovasc Surg.* 1997;113(1):37–49.

200. Rehders A, Hosch SB, Scheunemann P, et al. Benefit of surgical treatment of lung metastasis in soft tissue sarcoma. *Arch Surg.* 2007;142(1):70–75; discussion 76.

201. Billingsley KG, Lewis JJ, Leung DH, et al. Multifactorial analysis of the survival of patients with distant metastasis arising from primary extremity sarcoma. *Cancer.* 1999;85(2):389–395.

202. Billingsley KG, Burt ME, Jara E, et al. Pulmonary metastases from soft tissue sarcoma: analysis of patterns of diseases and post-metastasis survival. *Ann Surg.* 1999;229(5):602–610; discussion 610–612.

203. van Geel AN, Pastorino U, Jauch KW, et al. Surgical treatment of lung metastases: The European Organization for Research and Treatment of Cancer-Soft Tissue and Bone Sarcoma Group study of 255 patients. *Cancer.* 1996;77(4):675–682.

204. Sharma A, Duijm M, Oomen-de Hoop E, Aerts JG, Verhoef C, Hoogeman M, Nuyttens JJ. Survival and prognostic factors of pulmonary oligometastases treated with stereotactic body radiotherapy. *Acta Oncol.* 2019 Jan;58(1):74–80.

205. Falk AT, Moreau-Zabotto L, Ouali M, et al; Groupe Sarcome FrancaisGroupe D'etude Des Tumeurs Osseuses. Effect on survival of local ablative treatment of metastases from sarcomas: a study of the French sarcoma group. *Clin Oncol (R Coll Radiol).* 2015; 27:48–55.

206. Tree AC, Khoo VS, Eeles RA, et al. Stereotactic body radiotherapy for oligometastases. *Lancet Oncol.* 2013;14:e28–e37.

207. Baumann BC, Bernstein KA, DeLaney TF, Simone CB 2nd, Kolker JD, Choy E, Levin WP, Weber KL, Muniappan A, Berman AT, Staddon A, Hartner L, Van Tine B, Hirbe A, Glatstein

E, Hahn SM, Nagda SN, Chen YL. Multi-institutional analysis of stereotactic body radiotherapy for sarcoma pulmonary metastases: High rates of local control with favorable toxicity. *J Surg Oncol.* 2020 Jun 25. doi: 10.1002/jso.26078. Epub ahead of print. PMID: 32588468.

208. Baumann BC, Nagda SN, Kolker JD, Levin WP, Weber KL, Berman AT, Staddon A, Hartner L, Hahn SM, Glatstein E, Simone CB 2nd. Efficacy and safety of stereotactic body radiation therapy for the treatment of pulmonary metastases from sarcoma: A potential alternative to resection. *J Surg Oncol.* 2016 Jul;114(1): 65–9.

209. Dhakal S, Corbin KS, Milano MT, et al. Stereotactic body radiotherapy for pulmonary metastases from soft-tissue sarcomas: excellent local lesion control and improved patient survival. *Int J Radiat Oncol Biol Phys.* 2012;82(2):940–945.

210. Navarria P, Ascolese AM, Cozzi L, et al. Stereotactic body radiation therapy for lung metastases from soft tissue sarcoma. *Eur J Cancer.* 2015;51:668–674.

211. Frakulli R, Salvi F, Balestrini D, et al. Stereotactic radiotherapy in the treatment of lung metastases from bone and soft tissue sarcomas. *Anticancer Res.* 2015;35:5581–5586.

212. Salama JK, Hasselle MD, Chmura SJ, et al. Stereotactic body radiotherapy for multisite extracranial oligometastases: final report of a dose escalation trial in patients with 1 to 5 sites of metastatic disease. *Cancer.* 2012;118:2962–2970.

213. Folkert MR, Bilsky MH, Tom AK, et al. Outcomes and toxicity for hypofractionated and single-fraction image-guided stereotactic radiosurgery for sarcomas metastasizing to the spine. *Int J Radiat Oncol Biol Phys.* 2014;88:1085–1091.

Treatment Planning: Physics and Dosimetric Principles

16 Introduction: Process, Equipment, and Personnel

Faiz M. Khan and John P. Gibbons

INTRODUCTION

Treatment planning in Radiation Oncology has evolved into a very complex and sophisticated procedure. It is through meticulous planning and careful implementation of the needed treatment that the potential benefits of radiotherapy can be realized. The ideas presented in this book pertain to the clinical, physical, and technical aspects of procedures used in radiotherapy treatment planning. Optimal planning and attention to detail will make it possible to fulfill the goal of the radiation oncology treatment, namely, to provide the best possible care for every patient with cancer.

TREATMENT PLANNING PROCESS

Treatment planning is a process that involves the determination of treatment parameters considered optimal in the management of a patient's disease. In radiotherapy, these parameters include patient positioning and immobilization, segmentation of anatomical volumes (e.g., target volume(s) and organ(s) at risk), treatment planning parameters (e.g., dose prescription and fractionation, isodose distribution), treatment machine and image guidance settings, and adjuvant therapies. The final product of this activity is a blueprint for the treatment, to be followed precisely over several weeks.

TARGET AND NORMAL TISSUE VOLUME ASSESSMENT

Treatment planning starts right after the therapy decision is made and radiotherapy is chosen as the treatment modality. The first step is to determine the tumor location and its extent. The *target volume*, as it is called, consists of a volume that includes the tumor (demonstrated through imaging or other means) and its spread to the surrounding tissues. The determination of this volume and its precise location is of paramount importance. Considering that radiotherapy is an agent for local or regional tumor control, it is logical to believe that errors in target volume assessment or its localization will cause radiotherapy failures.

Imaging modalities such as computed tomography (CT), magnetic resonance imaging (MRI), ultrasound, and positron emission tomography (PET) assist the radiation oncologist in the localization of target volume. However, what is discernible in an image may not be the entire extent of the tumor. Sufficient margins must be added to the demonstrable tumor to allow for uncertainty in imaging as well as microscopic spread, depending upon the invasive characteristics of the tumor.

Assessment of the target volume for radiotherapy is not as easy as it may sound. The first and foremost difficulty is the fact that no imaging modality at present can reveal the entire extent of the tumor with its microscopic spread. The visible tumor, or *gross tumor volume* (GTV), represents only a part of the tumor. The volume that includes the entire tumor, namely, GTV, and the invisible microscopic disease can be estimated only clinically and is therefore called the *clinical target volume* (CTV).

The estimate of CTV is usually made by giving a suitable margin around the GTV to include the occult disease. This process of assessing CTV is not precise because it is subjective and depends entirely on one's clinical judgment. Because it is an educated guess at best, one should not be overly tight in assigning these margins around the GTV. The assigned margins must be wide enough to ensure that the CTV thus designed includes the entire tumor, including both the gross and the microscopic disease. If in doubt, it is better to be more generous than too tight because missing a part of the disease, however tiny, would certainly result in treatment failure.

Added to the inherent uncertainty of CTV are the uncertainties of target volume localization in space and time. An image-based GTV, or the inferred CTV, does not have static boundaries or shape. Its extent and location can change as a function of time because of variations in patient setup, physiologic motion of internal organs, patient breathing, and positioning instability. A planning target volume (PTV) is therefore required, which should include the CTV plus suitable margins to account for the above uncertainties. The PTV, therefore, is the ultimate target volume—the primary focus of the treatment planning and delivery. Adequate dose delivered to PTV at each treatment session presumably assures adequate treatment of the entire disease-bearing volume, the CTV.

The next step in treatment planning is the localization of critical structures. Again, modern imaging is greatly helpful in providing detailed anatomic information. All relevant organs at risk (OAR) are segmented to ensure the planned treatment does not exceed the tissue tolerance of these structures. As in the case of the GTV and CTV, the OAR represents the structure at a particular instant of time. Thus, in parallel to the definition of the PTV, it is necessary to define the planning organ-at-risk volume (PRV) as the OAR plus a margin to include uncertainties in the position of the OAR during treatment.

Because of the importance of accurate determination of both target and normal tissue structures, the International Commission on Radiation Units and Measurements (ICRU) has come up with a systematic approach to the whole process, as illustrated in Figures 16.1 and 16.2. The reader is referred to ICRU Reports 50, 62, and 71 for the underlying concepts and details of the system.[1-3]

The substantial growth in the number of structures (and their respective expansions) required in any treatment plan has added to the complexity of both recording and reporting

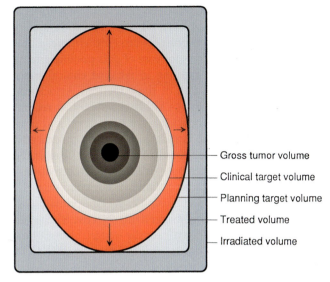

FIGURE 16.1. Schematic illustration of ICRU volumes. ICRU, the International Commission on Radiation Units and Measurements. (Modified from ICRU. *Prescribing, Recording, and Reporting Photon Beam Therapy*. ICRU Report 50. Bethesda, MD: International Commission of Radiation Units and Measurements; 1993.)

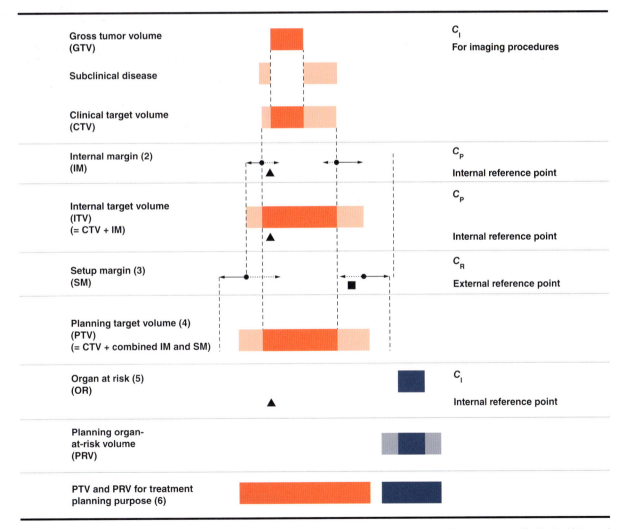

FIGURE 16.2. Schematic representation of ICRU volumes and margins. ICRU, the International Commission on Radiation Units and Measurements. (Modified from ICRU. *Prescribing, Recording, and Reporting Photon Beam Therapy [Supplement to ICRU Report 50]*. ICRU Report 62. Bethesda, MD: International Commission on Radiation Units and Measurements; 1999.)

patient treatment plans. It is thus important that a uniform nomenclature be utilized when possible to avoid variability and ambiguity when reporting results. Furthermore, a uniform nomenclature allows for ease of data pooling among those institutions participating in national clinical trials. Recently, Task Group 263 of the American Association of Physicists in Medicine (AAPM) has published recommended a detailed nomenclature for both target and non-target structures for use in radiation oncology treatments.[4] Although the details are beyond the scope of this chapter, the reader is referred to this report for additional information.

Treating the right target volume conformally with the right dose distribution and fractionation is the primary goal of radiotherapy. It does not matter if this objective is achieved with open beams or uniform-intensity wedged beams, compensators, intensity-modulated radiation therapy (IMRT), or image-guided radiation therapy (IGRT). As will be discussed in the following chapters, various technologies and methodologies are currently available, which should be selected on the basis of their ability to achieve the above radiotherapy goal for the given disease to be treated. In some cases, simple arrangements such as a single beam, parallel-opposed beams, or multiple beams, with or without wedges, are adequate, while in others IMRT or IGRT is the treatment of choice.

EQUIPMENT

Treatment planning is a process essentially of optimization of therapeutic choices and treatment techniques. This is all done in the context of available equipment. In the absence of adequate or versatile equipment, optimization of treatment plans is difficult, if not impossible. For example, if the best equipment in an institution is a cobalt unit or a traditional low-energy (4–6 MV) linear accelerator, the choice of beam energy for different patients and tumor sites cannot be optimized. If a good-quality simulator (conventional or CT) is not available, accurate design of treatment fields, beam positioning, and portal localization are not possible. Without modern imaging equipment, high accuracy is not possible in the determination of target volumes and critical structures, so that techniques that require conformal dose distributions in three dimensions cannot be optimized. Accessibility to a reasonably sophisticated computerized treatment planning system is essential to plan isodose distributions for different techniques so as to select the one that is best suited for a given patient. Therefore, the quality of treatment planning and the treatment itself depend on how well equipped the facility is with regard to treatment units, imaging equipment, and treatment planning computers.

External Beam Units

Low-Energy Megavoltage X-ray Beams

Low-energy megavoltage beams without IMRT capability (e.g., cobalt-60 and/or 4- to 6-MV X-rays) are principally used for relatively shallow or moderately deep tumors such as in the head and neck, breast, and extremities. Parallel-opposed beam arrangement should be limited to regions where the body thickness is not very large (e.g., <20 cm).

In addition to the beam energy, it is also important to have machine specifications that improve beam characteristics as well as accuracy of treatment delivery. Some example specifications, for example, may include isocentric capability with source-to-axis distance of 100 cm (not less than 80 cm for cobalt-60), field size of at least 40 × 40 cm, versatile and rigid treatment couch, asymmetrical collimators, MLCs, and other features that allow optimization of treatment techniques.

For IMRT or IGRT techniques, a 6-MV X-ray beam is sufficient so far as the energy is concerned. However, the unit must be equipped with a special collimator having dynamic multileaf collimator (MLC) or apertures suitable for these techniques. Its operation must be computer-controlled to allow for intensity-modulated beam delivery in accordance with the IMRT or IGRT treatment plans.

Medium- or High-Energy Megavoltage X-ray Beams

X-ray beams in the energy range of 10 to 25 MV allow treatment techniques for deep-seated tumors in the thorax, abdomen, or pelvis. For parallel-opposed beam techniques, the deeper the tumor, the higher the energy required to maximize the dose to the tumor, relative to the normal tissue. In addition, the dose buildup characteristics of these beams allow substantial sparing of normal subcutaneous tissue in the path of the beams.

Charged-Particle Beams

1. **Electrons**: Electron beams in the range of 6 to 20 MeV are useful for treating superficial tumors at depths of up to about 5 cm. They are often used in conjunction with X-ray beams, either as a boost or as a mixed-beam treatment, to provide a particular isodose distribution. The principal clinical applications include the treatment of skin and lip cancers, chest wall irradiation, boost therapy for lymph nodes, and the treatment of head and neck cancers.

   Depth-dose characteristics of electron beams have unique features that allow effective irradiation of relatively superficial cancers and almost complete sparing of normal tissues beyond them. The availability of this modality is essential for optimizing treatments of approximately 10% to 15% of cancers managed with radiotherapy.

2. **Protons**: Proton beam therapy has been used to treat almost all cancers that are traditionally treated with X-rays and electrons (e.g., tumors of the brain, spine, head and neck, breast, lung, gastrointestinal malignancies, prostate, and gynecologic cancers). Because of the ability to obtain a high degree of conformity of dose distribution to the target volume with practically no exit dose to the normal tissues, the proton radiotherapy is an excellent option for tumors in close proximity of

critical structures such as tumors of the brain, eye, and spine. Also, protons give a significantly less integral dose than photons and, therefore, should be a preferred modality in the treatment of pediatric tumors where there is always a concern for a possible development of secondary malignancies during the lifetime of the patient.

3. **Carbon ions**: Efficacy of charged particles heavier than protons such as nuclei of helium, carbon, nitrogen, neon, silicon, and argon has also been explored. Although carbon ions or heavier charged particles have the potential to be just as good as protons, if not better, it is debatable whether the benefits justify the high cost of such machines. As it stands, for most institutions, even the acquisition of protons is hard to justify over the far less expensive but very versatile megavoltage X-ray and electron accelerators.

Patient Load Versus Treatment Units

The number of patients treated on a given unit can be an important determinant of the quality of care. Overloaded machines and overworked staff often give rise to suboptimal techniques, inadequate care in patient setup, and a greater possibility of treatment errors. As in any other human activity, rushed jobs do not yield the best results. In radiotherapy, in which the name of the game is accuracy and precision, there is simply no room for sloppiness, which can easily creep in if the technologist's primary concern is to keep up with the treatment schedule. An assembly line type of atmosphere should never be allowed in a radiotherapy facility because it deprives the patients of their right to receive the best possible care that radiotherapy has to offer.

Staffing levels need to be appropriate for the workload of the clinic. These levels have increased over the years due to the increased complexity of both planning and executing patient treatments. The American Society for Therapeutic Radiation Oncology (ASTRO) report "Safety is No Accident: A Framework for Quality Radiation Oncology Care"[5] states that an excessive workload can lead to errors in reporting, communication, or even treatment of the patient. This issue is covered in more detail in the Patient Safety chapter of this book.

Brachytherapy Equipment

Brachytherapy is an important integral part of a radiotherapy program. Some tumors are best treated with brachytherapy, alone or in conjunction with an external beam. It is therefore important to have this modality available if optimal treatment planning is the goal. Although electrons are sometimes used as an alternative, brachytherapy continues to have an important role in treating certain tumors such as gynecologic malignancies, oral cancers, sarcomas, prostate cancer, and brain tumors.

Currently, the sources most often being used are cesium-137 tubes, iridium-192 seeds contained in ribbons, iodine-125 seeds, and palladium-103 seeds. These isotopes can be used in after-loading techniques for interstitial as well as intracavitary implantation. Numerous applicators and templates have been designed for conventional low-dose rate (LDR) brachytherapy. The institution must follow a particular system consistently with all its hardware, rules of implantation, and dose specification schemes. Remote after-loading units, LDR as well as high-dose rate (HDR), are becoming increasingly popular, especially among institutions with large patient loads for brachytherapy. Brachytherapy hardware, software, and techniques are discussed in later chapters.

Imaging Equipment

Modern treatment planning is intimately tied to imaging. Although all diagnostic imaging equipment has some role in defining and localizing target volumes, the currently most commonly used modalities are CT, MRI, and PET.

Most radiotherapy institutions have access to these machines either within their department or through diagnostic radiology departments. In the latter case, the fidelity of imaging data obtained under diagnostic conditions may be inferior when used for treatment planning. This is caused primarily by the lack of reproducibility in patient positioning. Besides appropriate modifications in the scanner equipment (e.g., flat tabletop, patient positioning aids), the patient setup should be supervised by a member of the treatment planning staff. With the growing demand for CT, 4-dimensional (4D) CT (respiration-correlated), and MRI in radiotherapy and the large number of scans that 3-dimensional (3D) treatment planning requires, dedicated scanners in radiotherapy departments are becoming the norm.

Simulator

Conventional simulators have largely been replaced by CT simulation. A conventional simulator may be useful for final verification of the field placement, but with the availability of good-quality digitally reconstructed radiographs (DRRs) and special software for CT simulation, this need no longer exists. Final field verification before treatment can be obtained with the portal imaging system available on modern linacs.

CT scanners have been used for treatment planning for many years because of their ability to image patient anatomy and gross tumor, slice by slice. These data can be processed to view images in any plane or in three dimensions. In addition, CT numbers can be correlated with tissue density, pixel by pixel, thereby allowing heterogeneity corrections in treatment planning.

A dedicated radiation therapy CT scanner, with accessories (e.g., flat table identical with those of the treatment units, lasers for positioning, immobilization, and image registration devices, etc.) to accurately reproduce treatment conditions, is called a *CT-simulator*. Many types of such units are commercially available. Some of them are designed specifically for radiation therapy with wide apertures (e.g., 85 cm diameter) to provide flexibility in patient positioning for a variety of treatment setups.

The CT image data set thereby obtained, with precise localization of patient anatomy and tissue density information, is useful not only in generating an accurate treatment plan but also in providing a reference for setting up treatment plan parameters. This process is sometimes called *virtual simulation*.

Positron Emission Tomography/Computed Tomography

The physics of PET is based on the positron–electron annihilation into photons. Although several positron-emitting radioisotopes have been used in PET imaging, the most commonly used compound is fluorodeoxyglucose (FDG). FDG incorporates ^{18}F as the positron-emitting isotope. FDG is an analog of glucose that accumulates in metabolically active cells. Because tumor cells are generally more active metabolically than normal cells, an increased uptake of FDG is positively correlated with the presence of tumor cells and their metabolic activity. When the positron is emitted by ^{18}F, it annihilates a nearby electron, with the emission of two 0.511-MeV photons in opposite directions. These photons are detected by ring detectors placed in a circular gantry surrounding the patient. From the detection of these photons, computer software (e.g., filtered back-projection algorithm) reconstructs the site of the annihilation events and the intervening anatomy. The site of increased FDG accumulation, with the surrounding anatomy, is thereby imaged with a resolution of about 4 mm.

Combining PET with CT scanning has several advantages:

1. Superior quality CT images with their geometric accuracy in defining anatomy and tissue density differences are combined with PET images to provide physiologic imaging, thereby differentiating malignant tumors from the normal tissue on the basis of their metabolic differences.
2. PET images may allow differentiation between benign and malignant lesions well enough in some cases to permit tumor staging.
3. PET scanning may be used to follow changes in tumors that occur over time and with therapy.
4. By using the same treatment table for a PET/CT scan, the patient is scanned by both modalities without moving (only the table is moved between scanners). This minimizes positioning errors in the scanned data sets from both units.
5. By fusing PET and CT images, the two modalities become complementary.

Although PET provides physiologic information about the tumor, it lacks correlative anatomy and is inherently limited in resolution. CT, on the other hand, lacks physiologic information but provides superior images of anatomy and localization. Therefore, PET/CT provides combined images that are superior to either PET or CT images alone.

Accelerator-Mounted Imaging Systems

After the treatment planning and simulation comes the critical step of accurate treatment delivery of the planned treatment. Traditionally, patients are set up on the treatment couch with the help of localization lasers and various identification marks on the patient, for example, ink marks, tattoos, or palpable bony landmarks. Sometimes identification marks are drawn on the body casts worn by the patient for immobilization. These procedures would be considered reasonable if only the patient would not move within the cast and the ink or tattoo marks did not shift with the stretch of the skin. Bony landmarks are relatively more reliable, but their location by palpitation cannot be pinpointed to better than a few millimeters. Good immobilization devices are critical in minimizing setup variations and are discussed later in the book.

With the introduction of 3D conformal radiation therapy (CRT), including IMRT and IGRT, it has become increasingly apparent that the benefit of these technologies cannot be fully realized if the patient setup and anatomy do not match the precision of the treatment plan within acceptable limits at every treatment session. As the treatment fields are made more conformal, the accuracy requirements of patient setup and the PTV coverage during each treatment accordingly have to be made more stringent. These requirements have propelled advances in the area of patient immobilization and dynamic targeting of PTV through imaging systems mounted on the accelerators themselves. Thus began the era of IGRT.

Each major linear accelerator manufacturer provides accelerator-mounted imaging systems allowing online treatment plan verification and correction (adaptive radiation therapy). Corrections may range from simple patient set-up shifts to more complex dynamic targeting or tracking, synchronized with the patient's respiratory cycle. These products come with various options, some of which may be work in progress or currently not FDA approved. The reader can get the updated information by visiting the corresponding Web sites.

The important consideration in acquiring any of these systems is dictated by the desire to provide state-of-the-art radiation therapy. While there are specialty configurations available, a general-purpose treatment delivery system is expected to have the following capabilities:

1. 3D CRT with linac-based megavoltage photon beam(s) of appropriate energy (e.g., 6–18 MV)
2. Electron beam therapy with five or six different energies in the range of 6 to 20 MeV
3. IMRT, IGRT, and gated radiation therapy capabilities
4. Accelerator-mounted imaging equipment to allow for IGRT treatments.

Typically, such a system consists of an electronic portal imaging device (EPID), a kVp source for radiographic verification of setup, an online fluoroscopic mode to permit overlaying of treatment field aperture onto the fluoroscopy image, and cone-beam CT capability for treatment plan verification. Many of these devices and their use in modern radiotherapy such as IGRT are discussed in the following chapters.

Treatment Planning Computers

Commercial treatment planning computers became available in the early 1970s. Some of the early ones such as the Spear PC, the Artronix PC-12, Rad-8, Theratronics Theraplan, and ADAC were instant hits and provided a quantum jump from manual to computerized treatment planning. They served their purpose well in providing fast and reasonably accurate 2-dimensional (2D) treatment plans. Typically, they allowed the input (through the digitizer) of external patient contours, anatomic landmarks, and outlines of the target volume and critical structures in a specified plane (usually central). Beams were modeled semiempirically from the stored beam data obtained in a water phantom. Various corrections were used to apply the water phantom data to the patient situation, presenting irregular surfaces, tissue inhomogeneities, and multiple beam angles. However, from today's standards, the old systems would be considered very limited in capability and rudimentary in the context of modern 3D treatment planning.

With the explosion of computer and imaging technologies in the last 30 years or so, the treatment planning computers and their algorithms have accordingly become more powerful and sophisticated. Systems that are currently available allow 3D treatment planning in which patient data obtained from CT scanning, MRI, PET, and so on, are input electronically. Beams are modeled with sophisticated computational algorithms, for example, pencil or point beam convolution algorithms, Monte Carlo techniques, and most recently, numerical solutions of the Boltzmann transport equations. These algorithms for photons, electrons, protons, and brachytherapy sources are discussed in later chapters.

Besides major improvements in dose computational methods, there have been revolutionary advances in software, which allow planning of complex treatments such as 3D CRT, IMRT, IGRT, and HDR brachytherapy. The addition of inverse planning algorithms allows the planner to specify the desired dose distribution and let the computer generate a plan as close to the input specifications as possible. Again, these techniques and algorithms are topics of discussion later in the book.

There are currently many 3D treatment planning systems that are commercially available including, among others, Pinnacle (www.medical.philips.com), Eclipse (www.varian.com), Monico HD (www.elekta.com), and RayStation (www.raystation.com). As these systems are constantly evolving and undergoing revisions, the reader should be mindful of the fact that an older version of any given system may not carry much resemblance to the newest version. Therefore, anyone in the market for such a system needs to do some research and check out each system with its most current version. Also, because these systems and their software are frequently revised and updated, the user is advised to carry a service contract for maintenance as well as the option of receiving future updates as they are released.

STAFFING

The ASTRO document "Safety is No Accident"[5] provides a blueprint for modern radiation oncology facilities in terms of structure, process, and personnel requirements. The basis for their recommendations is the fundamental principle that radiation oncology practice requires a team of personnel with appropriate educational and training backgrounds. Besides the physician specialists, the radiation oncologists, radiotherapy requires the services of medical physicists, dosimetrists, therapists, and nurses. The minimum level of staffing recommended is shown in Table 16.1. In the specific areas of treatment planning, the key personnel are radiation oncologists, medical physicists, and dosimetrists. The quality of treatment planning largely depends on the strength of this team.

TABLE 16.1 Minimum Personnel Requirements for Clinical Radiation Therapy[a]

Category	Staffing
Medical Director	One per practice
Radiation Oncologist	Minimum of one radiation oncologist present during treatment hours*
Physicist	Minimum of one physicist available during treatment hours*
Administrator	One per practice (in some practices this function may be filled by clinical staff)
Dosimetrist	As needed, approximately one per 250 patients treated annually[a]
Radiation Therapist	As needed, approximately one per 90 patients treated annually[a,b]
Mold Room Technologist	As needed to provide service
Other staff (e.g., nurse, social worker, dietician)	As needed to provide service

*Refers to minimum requirements for treatment to take place. The number of clinical staff required to safely provide clinical care for patients is likely to be higher.

[a]This number may be higher or lower depending upon the complexity of patients and treatments.

[b]It is recommended that a minimum of at least two qualified individuals be present for any external beam patient treatment.

From American Society for Radiation Oncology (ASTRO). *Safety is No Accident*. https://www.astro.org/clinical-practice/patient-safety/safety-book/safety-is-no-accident.aspx; 2019, with permission.

Radiation Oncologist

The radiation oncologist, who has the ultimate responsibility for the care of the patient, heads the treatment planning team. It is their responsibility to formulate the overall plan for the treatment, including dose prescription to tumor-bearing sites of the body. Details of the actual treatment technique, beam energies, beam directions, and other specific details of the treatment are finalized after a number of isodose plans have been calculated and an optimal plan has been selected. The final plan must meet the approval of the radiation oncologist in charge of the patient.

The American College of Radiology (ACR) standards require that the radiation oncologist be board-certified to practice radiation oncology. In addition, the number of radiation oncologists in a given institution must be in proportion to the patient load (Table 16.1). No more than 25 to 30 patients should be treated by a single physician. It is important to ensure that each patient receives adequate care and attention from the physician and that the treatments are not compromised because of the physician's lack of time.

Medical Physicist

No other medical specialty draws as much from physics as radiation oncology. The science of ionizing radiation is the province of physics, and its application to medicine requires the services of a physics specialist, the medical physicist. It is the collaboration between the radiation oncologist and the medical physicist that makes radiotherapy an effective treatment modality for cancer.

Ralston Paterson,[6] emphasizing this relationship, stated in 1963: "In radiotherapy the physicist who has given special study to this field is full partner with the therapist, not only in the development of the science, but in the day-to-day treatment of patients. The unit team, therefore, even for the smallest department, consists of a radiotherapist and a physicist."

The unit team of radiation oncologist and medical physicist must have a supporting cast to provide radiotherapy service effectively to all patients referred to the department. Dosimetrists, radiation therapists (previously called technologists), nurses, and service engineers are the other members of the team. It must be recognized by all concerned that without this infrastructure and adequate staffing in each area of responsibility, radiotherapy is reduced to an ineffective, if not unsafe, modality of treatment.

Adequacy of the support of physics has been spelled out in the ASTRO document.[5] The number of physicists required in a radiotherapy institution depends not only on the number of patients treated per year but also on the complexity of the radiotherapy services offered. For example, special procedures such as stereotactic radiotherapy, HDR brachytherapy, total-body irradiation for bone marrow transplantation, 3D CRT, IMRT, IGRT, SBRT, respiratory gating, TomoTherapy, CyberKnife treatments, and intraoperative radiotherapy are all physics-intensive procedures and therefore require more physicists as recommended by ASTRO.

According to the AAPM, a medical physicist involved with clinical services must have a PhD or MS degree and be board certified in the relevant specialty; in this case,

TABLE 16.2	Roles and Responsibilities of Physicists			
Equipment (teletherapy, brachytherapy and simulator)	Treatment planning (teletherapy and brachytherapy)	Dosimetry	Radiation protection	Academic and administrative
Selection and specifications	Management and QA of treatment planning computer	Dose calculation formalism	Regulatory	Teaching
Acceptance testing	Beam data management	Special treatment techniques	Radiation survey	Research
Commissioning, beam data measurement	Simulation consultation	Special dosimetry	Personnel monitoring	Developmental
Calibration	Patient data for treatment planning	In vivo dosimetry	Facility design	Administrative
Quality assurance	Technique optimization, isodose planning; plan analysis, evaluation; treatment aids; beam modifiers			

QA, quality assurance.

From Khan FM. Residency training for medical physicists. *Int J Radiat Oncol Biol Phys.* 1992;24:853–855.

radiation oncology physics. Also, most physicists in an academic setting teach and do research, and therefore a doctorate degree is more desirable for them. Such research plays a key role in the development of new techniques and in bringing about new advances to radiation oncology. Paterson[6] emphasized this role by stating "While the physicist has a day-to-day routine task in this working out or checking of cases, it is important that he has time for study of special problems. These may include the development of new X-ray techniques, the devising of special applicators to simplify or assist treatment, the critical analysis of existing techniques, or research work of a more fundamental nature."

A medical physicist's role in radiotherapy is summarized in Table 16.2. Specifically in treatment planning, the physicist has the overall responsibility of ensuring that the treatment plan is accurate and scientifically valid. That means that the physicist is responsible for testing the computer software and commissioning it for clinical use. They are also responsible for proper interpretation of the treatment plan as it relates to the dose distribution and calculation of treatment duration or monitor units.

One important role of a medical physicist that is often overlooked is that of a consultant to radiation oncologists in the design of the treatment plan. Physicians working directly with dosimetrists to generate a treatment plan without any significant input from the physicist can often be seen. This process may be operationally smooth and less costly but can be risky if serious errors go undetected and the final plan is not optimal. It must be recognized that a qualified medical physicist, by virtue of education and training, is the only professional on the radiotherapy team who is familiar with the treatment planning algorithm and can authenticate the scientific validity of a computer treatment plan. It is important that they be actively involved with the treatment planning process and that the final plan receives their careful review. Because of the tendency of some physicians to bypass the physicist, some institutions have developed the policy of having the physicist present during simulation and doing the treatment planning either personally or closely working with the dosimetrist in the generation and optimization of the treatment plan.

Dosimetrist

Historically, dosimetrists were classified as physics personnel with a Bachelor of Science degree in the physical sciences. They assisted physicists in routine clinical work such as treatment planning, exposure time calculations, dosimetry, and quality assurance. They could be called a *physicist assistant*, analogous to physician assistant.

Today the dosimetrist's role is not much different, but the educational requirements have been formalized to include certification by the Medical Dosimetrist Certification Board (MDCB), in addition to a Bachelor's Degree and graduation from an accredited Medical Dosimetry training program.

As discussed earlier, the role of a dosimetrist is traditionally to assist the physicist in all aspects of physics service. However, in some institutions, dosimetrists substitute for physicists, and/or the treatment planning procedure is made the sole responsibility of the dosimetrist with no supervision from the physicist. Whether it is done for economic or practical reasons, leaving out the physicist from the treatment planning process is not appropriate and definitely not in the best interest of the patient. The dosimetrist's role is to assist the physicist, not to replace him or her. The radiation oncologist must understand that a computer treatment plan necessitates the physicist's input and review just as much as it necessitates consultation of other medical specialists in the diagnosis and treatment of a patient.

REFERENCES

1. ICRU. *Prescribing, Recording, and Reporting Photon Beam Therapy*. ICRU Report 50. Bethesda, MD: International Commission on Radiation Units and Measurements; 1993.
2. ICRU. *Prescribing, Recording, and Reporting Photon Beam Therapy (Supplement to ICRU Report 50)*. ICRU Report 62. Bethesda, MD: International Commission on Radiation Units and Measurements; 1999.
3. ICRU. *Prescribing, Recording, and Reporting Electron Beam Therapy*. ICRU Report 71. Bethesda, MD: International Commission on Radiation Units and Measurements; 2004.
4. Mayo CS, Moran JM, Bosch W, et al. *Standardizing Nomenclatures in Radiation Oncology: The Report of AAPM Task Group 263*. Alexandria VA: AAPM; 2018.
5. American Society for Radiation Oncology (ASTRO). *Safety is No Accident: A Framework for Quality Radiation Oncology Care*. Fairfax, VA: American Society for Radiation Oncology; 2019. https://www.astro.org/ASTRO/media/ASTRO/Patient%20Care%20and%20Research/PDFs/Safety_is_No_Accident.pdf
6. Paterson R. *The Treatment of Malignant Disease by Radiotherapy*. 2nd ed. Baltimore, MD: Williams & Wilkins; 1963:527.

17 Image-Guided Radiation Therapy

Guang Li, Gig S. Mageras, Lei Dong, and Radhe Mohan

INTRODUCTION

The aim of external beam radiation therapy (EBRT) of cancer is to target localized disease noninvasively with radiation that conforms to the target while minimizing dose to surrounding organs at risk (OAR). Radiation dose is often delivered with inadequate visualization of the regions being irradiated. Therefore, imaging guidance is crucial at every step of the process, including cancer diagnosis, staging and delineation; treatment simulation and planning; patient setup, tumor localization and motion monitoring; and treatment response assessment, efficacy evaluation and strategy refinement. In fact, most of the significant advances in radiation oncology over the last three decades have been made possible by advances in medical imaging. Using three-dimensional (3D) images of patient anatomy from computed tomography (CT) and magnetic resonance imaging (MRI), as well as visualization of viable tumor extent from MR spectroscopic imaging (MRSI), positron emission tomography (PET), and single-photon-emission computed tomography (SPECT), treatment target and OARs can be delineated with precision, thus reducing the likelihood of marginal misses in tumor and minimizing the exposure of normal tissues to high radiation dose. Multimodality imaging has become an integrated component throughout the treatment process, providing the ability to localize and visualize the tumor in space and time to ensure accurate delivery of a highly conformal treatment plan.

Image-guided radiation therapy (IGRT) is composed of a multitude of major innovations in radiation oncology to address the problems arising from inter- and intra-fractional target variations. IGRT aims to deliver treatment as it is planned based on 3D images acquired at treatment simulation. These images establish a 3D reference frame of patient anatomy (with the possible inclusion of motion) for both image-based treatment planning and image-guided treatment delivery. The former process follows the exact 3D patient anatomy (the tumor and nearby OARs) for dosimetric planning, while the latter focuses mostly on tumor alignment between the planning image and images acquired at the treatment unit before and during treatment, thereby aligning to the radiation fields. The variations of tumor position in the image-guided inter-fractional setup (between treatment fractions) and intra-fractional (within a treatment fraction) patient and organ motion can be corrected for more accurate delivery. The variation of normal tissue positions is often assessed in terms of proximity to the irradiated volume in the current image-guided approach, but is also a focus of adaptive IGRT research and practice to assess dosimetric and clinical consequences under various clinical scenarios. Examples of image guidance in various stages of radiation therapy are illustrated in Figure 17.1.

Increasing evidence has shown that there are substantial inter- and intra-fractional variations, in contrast to the "snapshot" planning anatomy of a patient. The causes of such variations include voluntary motion (body shift, rotation, and deformation), involuntary motion (respiratory, cardiac, and digestive), disease-related changes (tumor growth and weight loss), and radiation-induced changes (tumor shrinkage). The variation in respiratory-induced tumor motion during treatment may substantially deviate from the one-cycle motion extent quantified by four-dimensional CT (4DCT) at simulation, owing to common breathing irregularities. These variations could have a significant impact on the outcome of treatments, as they may result in underdosing the target or overdosing the OAR.[1–3] In the current practice of treatment planning and delivery, it is assumed implicitly that the patient's anatomy remains static throughout the course of radiation therapy. To account for statistical variations, wide treatment margins derived from population-based studies are used to ensure coverage of the disease at the expense of exposing considerable OAR volumes to or near full prescribed radiation dose. A large margin limits the ability to safely deliver lethal dose to the tumor because of the increased risk of OAR toxicity, especially for hypo-fractionated stereotactic body radiotherapy (SBRT), in which the high dose per fraction exceeds the normal tissue's capacity for sublethal repair. Furthermore, the margin needed for some patients exhibiting large target variations may exceed the population-based margin, potentially leading to marginal misses, especially with the use of highly conformal treatment modalities, such as 3D conformal radiotherapy (3DCRT), intensity-modulated radiotherapy (IMRT), volumetric-modulated arc therapy (VMAT), and proton therapy.[4–6] Treatment planning and delivery techniques that do not correct for such daily volumetric variations adequately may lead to

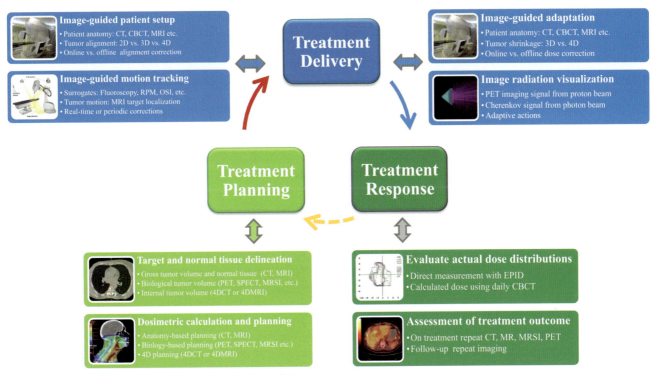

FIGURE 17.1. Image guidance at various stages of the radiotherapy process.

suboptimal treatments. These factors may, in part, be responsible for the poor outcome and high toxicity in radiation therapy for some cancers.[7] IGRT has the potential to target gross and microscopic diseases accurately, to individualize treatments to reduce population-based margins, and to allow dose escalation to higher levels with the expectation of improving local control and reducing toxicity.[8-10] Therefore, IGRT can help to improve the therapeutic ratio, namely the ratio of tumor control probability (TCP) and normal tissue complication probability (NTCP).[1,7] The recent efforts to introduce MRI, PET, and optical surface imaging (OSI) into the treatment room can further improve the ability to assess the accuracy of treatment delivery by direct viewing of the target during treatment,[11] imaging proton beam path,[12] and visualizing photon Cherenkov scattering,[13] respectively.

This chapter focuses on IGRT technologies related to treatment planning and delivery of EBRT. The "Conceptual and Practical Changes in IGRT Paradigm" section summarizes the conceptual and practical changes in the IGRT paradigm of the radiotherapy (RT) clinic. The "Inter-Fractional IGRT Imaging and Patient Setup" and "Intra-Fractional Real-Time Imaging and Motion Compensation" sections introduce various forms of IGRT technologies and their commercial implementations for inter- and intra-fractional imaging, respectively. The "IGRT Requirements and Considerations" section reviews requirements and considerations for IGRT, including quality assurance (QA). Various possible IGRT strategies, margin assessment and reduction, and clinical implications are described in the "IGRT Correction Strategies and Applications" section. Finally, the "Future Directions" section looks into the future and speculates on new processes coming into this field.

CONCEPTUAL AND PRACTICAL CHANGES IN IGRT PARADIGM

The EBRT applies a medical linear accelerator (linac) to provide a megavoltage (MV) collimated radiation beam from the gantry to irradiate an irregularly-shaped tumor within a patient's body on the treatment couch. The tumor is positioned at the linac isocenter so that no matter what are the rotation angles of the gantry, collimator, and couch, the beam always points to the tumor. The mechanical isocenter in space can be localized by the intersection point of three in-room line lasers and the radiation isocenter of treatment should be co-aligned at the same spot with a sub-millimeter (mm) uncertainty. In conventional setup, a patient is usually immobilized on the treatment couch with the tumor set at the isocenter using skin markers and the room lasers.

In the IGRT paradigm, in-room two-dimensional (2D)/3D/4D imaging sets the standard for patient setup at higher accuracy, better than the room laser system.[14,15] To apply the imaging data for patient setup, the concept of imaging isocenter is introduced and utilized for all in-room imaging modalities, in analogy of the linac radiation isocenter. When the imaging isocenter is aligned with the radiation isocenter as the origin of their coordinate systems, the in-room imaging system can provide the image-guided patient setup by visualizing the internal tumor at the treatment and aligning it to the planning CT at the higher setup accuracy.

Clinically, in-room medical imaging systems include kilovoltage (kV) and/or MV radiography, fluoroscopy, cone-beam CT (CBCT) or CT-on-rail, OSI, PET/SPECT imaging, and most recently MRI.[16] For an in-room imaging modality, to establish the isocenter congruence with the linac is paramount important in the commissioning of the imaging system and in routine calibration and QA to ensure IGRT accuracy, especially for frameless cranial stereotactic radiosurgery (SRS) and SBRT.[14,17] For instance, in frame-based SRS the accordance of the mechanical and radiation isocenter must be checked prior to the SRS treatment, including the Winston-Lutz test. However, in the image-guided frameless SRS treatment, the accordance of the imaging isocenter and radiation isocenter is checked by acquiring and analyzing the 2D/3D kV/MV imaging pairs. In addition, continuous imaging is required to monitor a patient's motion during SRS, such as OSI, whose isocenter is also verified with the MV radiation isocenter. The real-time OSI signal triggers the radiation beam to be held when motion exceeds a set tolerance and resumed when motion falls back within the tolerance, via inter-system communication with the linac, ensuring an accurate SRS treatment delivery.[17,18]

INTER-FRACTIONAL IGRT IMAGING AND PATIENT SETUP

In this section, we focus on in-room IGRT imaging modalities for daily patient setup. Images acquired immediately before treatment are used to reposition the patient to align the tumor or its surrogate (such as implanted radiopaque fiducials in or near the tumor) with the planning target. The planning CT or digitally reconstructed radiograph (DRR) images are used as the reference to align with on-site CBCT or 2DkV images, respectively, via rigid image registration with up to six degrees of freedom (DOF: three translational and three rotational shifts) and corresponding couch adjustment. This is the simplest form of IGRT without modification of the treatment plan.

2D Radiographic Imaging

Two-dimensional radiographic (projection) imaging is typically used in treatment rooms to set up the patient. The MV imaging uses therapy x-ray beams and an amorphous-silicon (a-Si) flat-panel imager, known as an electronic portal imaging device (EPID), to verify the patient's setup using the skeletal anatomy as the landmark.[19] Other uses of MV imaging are to verify treatment beam apertures before treatment and *in vivo* portal dosimetry during treatment.[20,21] Because MV imaging uses the therapy

beam, it provides direct in-field verification of treatment delivery, known as the beam eye's view (BEV), and therefore serves as a "gold standard" for validating new IGRT techniques. Disadvantages of MV imaging include higher radiation dose to the patient (typically 1–5 cGy) and poorer image quality owing to a large Compton scattering contribution from the higher x-ray energies and high-energy electrons reaching the detector.

Two general categories of 2DkV x-ray imaging are frequently used for IGRT. One is a gantry-mounted kV imaging system on a linac, orthogonal to the MV beam. The kV x-ray source and flat-panel imager are mounted on retractable arms, providing near-diagnostic quality images. The second category of kV imaging is room-mounted systems: the x-ray source and detector are mounted on the floor and ceiling, or vice versa. These systems provide an oblique orthogonal image pair for stereoscopic imaging at a wide range of treatment couch angles. Most kV x-ray imaging systems have a companion fluoroscopic imaging mode, which is useful for observing the motion of the internal anatomy or implanted fiducials. Since kV imaging systems are distinct from the MV beamline, the kV–MV isocenter coincidence must be established within a clinical tolerance through initial and periodic QA processes.

In-room kV imaging represents a major improvement over MV imaging due to its superior image quality and its low-imaging dose (0.01–0.1 cGy), facilitating its use for daily image-guided patient setup.[22] Although kV radiography is often not capable of detecting soft-tissue targets, it is more successful in aligning skeletal landmarks or implanted radiopaque fiducials as target surrogates. The different appearance of kV and MV thoracic images is shown in Figure 17.2.

Tomographic Imaging

CT imaging inside the treatment room provides 3D anatomical information and improved soft-tissue visibility, thus providing advantages over radiographic imaging with higher imaging doses.[23] In-room CT images are the standard for six DOF patient setup and can be used to estimate the delivered dose distributions based on the anatomy captured at treatment. The planning CT image is used as the reference for patient alignment on the bone, fiducials, or tumors in some disease sites. Deformable/mobile target may be localized using the centroid position of a visible gross tumor volume (GTV) in the thorax,[24] but it may differ in clinical tumor volume (CTV) alignment.[25] This is still an area of investigation and deformable image registration (DIR) will be discussed in Chapter 3.

kV Helical CT and kV Cone-Beam CT

Helical multi-slice CT systems have been widely used in diagnostic imaging and radiation treatment planning for

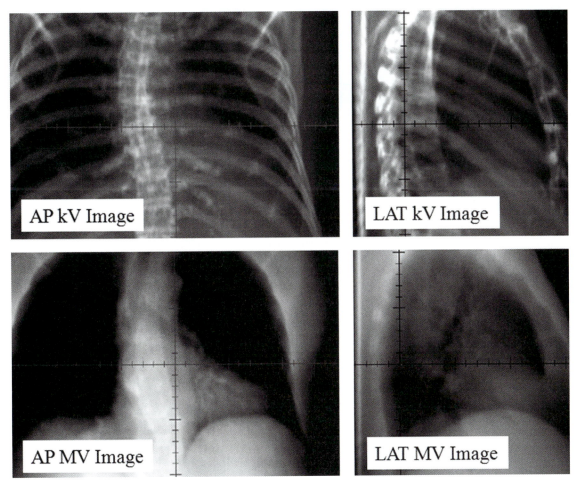

FIGURE 17.2. The appearance of anatomy kV (top row) and MV (bottom row) radiographs can be quite different. At kV x-ray energies, the bony structures are enhanced; at the therapeutic (MV) energies, the air cavity is enhanced.

many years. The first integrated CT-linac clinical system was designed for noninvasive, frameless stereotactic RT of brain and lung cancers with reduced uncertainty between fractions.[26] Another integrated CT-linac system with a rail to transport the patient between treatment and CT couches was assembled at the Memorial Sloan Kettering Cancer Center for the treatment of paraspinal lesions and prostate cancer.[27,28]

A commercial CT-linac system was introduced in the clinic in 2000.[29] It consists of a medical linac and a moveable CT scanner that slides along a pair of rails ("CT-on-Rails"). A similar "CT-on-Rails" commercial system (EXaCT™, Varian Oncology Systems, Palo Alto, CA) has a mechanical accuracy of within 0.5 mm.[30,31] The biggest advantage of an in-room CT scanner for IGRT is the similarity of image quality and field of view (FOV) with planning CT images.

Gantry-mounted kV imaging systems are capable of radiography, fluoroscopy, and CBCT, providing a versatile solution for IGRT applications.[32,33] CBCT imaging acquires projection images of the patient as the gantry rotates through an arc of ~200° total by the imaging panel. A filtered back-projection algorithm is used to reconstruct the volumetric images. Geometric calibration of the CBCT system is needed periodically to maintain image quality and geometric accuracy. Corrections on the order of 2.0 mm may be required to compensate for the gravity-induced flex in the support arms of the source, detector, and gantry. Submillimeter spatial resolution and accuracy have been demonstrated in phantom. The volumetric image with the nearly isotropic spatial resolution is useful in frameless SRS.[17]

Since 2005, major manufacturers have offered CBCT capabilities (Elekta Synergy HD and Infinity HD, Elekta Inc., Sweden; Varian On-board Imager [OBI] and TrueBeam Imaging, Palo Alto, CA), as shown in Figure 17.3. Elekta's system uses a slightly larger flat panel detector (41 × 41 cm), compared to Varian's detector (40 cm × 30 cm), which limits the scan length to 15 cm when using the full-fan scan mode. A half-fan scan method displaces the detector vertically to capture half projection images and requires 360° rotation to have the axial FOV to at least 40 cm.[34] Recently, Halcyon (Varian Oncology Systems, Palo Alto, CA) linac is also commercially available to have fast gantry rotation up to 4 rpm, so

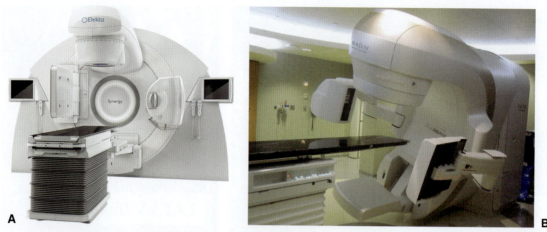

FIGURE 17.3. **A:** An Elekta Synergy® linear accelerator (Image courtesy of Elekta). **B:** A Varian TrueBeam™ unit (Image(s) courtesy of Varian Medical Systems, Inc., Palo Alto, CA. Copyright [2021]. All rights reserved). Both linear accelerators have a kV imaging system orthogonal to the therapy beam direction. Both systems provide 2D radiographic, fluoroscopic, and CBCT modes.

that CBCT can be acquired in 15 s or one breath-hold, 7 s per 2 DkV pair, and the beam-on time for VMAT/IMRT treatment is about 2 min per plan.[35,36]

Limitations of CBCT image quality include elevated x-ray scatter, which reduces image contrast and introduces cupping artifacts. Scatter can be reduced by using both anti-scatter grids and post-processing methods.[37,38] To further improve the image quality, Kim *et al.* have proposed to use orthogonal dual-source and dual-detector "in-line" with MV beam to produce 2D and 3D images with tetrahedral collimation.[39] Because of regulations on gantry (uncovered) rotation speed (1 rpm), CBCT image quality is adversely affected by the breathing motion. The IGRT setup process may add 5 min (~2 min acquisition/reconstruction and ~3 min registration/approval) to the regular treatment schedule.

MV Helical CT and MV Cone-Beam CT

Tomotherapy (Accuray Inc., Sunnyvale, CA) is an integrated technology that combines a helical MVCT with a linear accelerator (Fig. 17.4A) as an x-ray source, which is specially designed for delivering intensity-modulated radiation in a slit geometry.[40–42] Low-dose (1–2 cGy), pretreatment MVCT images are obtained from the same treatment beamline but with a nominal energy of 4 MV. The CT detector uses an array of 738 channel xenon ion chambers and a FOV of 40 cm can be reconstructed.

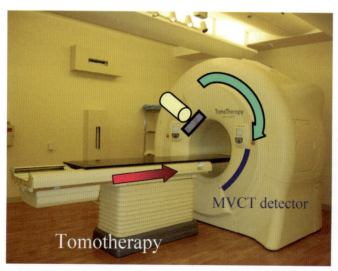
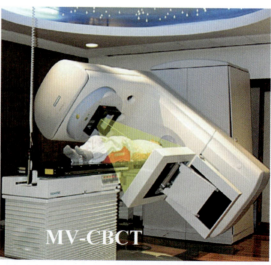

FIGURE 17.4. **A:** A picture of tomotherapy unit (Images used with permission from Accuray Incorporated). Tomotherapy is an integrated IGRT system, which combines a linear accelerator with an MVCT image guidance system. **B:** A Siemens MV CBCT imaging system using a conventional linac and a flat-panel EPID. *Source:* Reprinted from Morin O, Gillis A, Chen J, et al. Megavoltage cone-beam CT: system description and clinical applications. *Med Dosim* 2006;31:51–61.

MV CBCT uses the therapy MV x-ray and the EPID detector.[43,44] With the a-Si flat panel EPID,[45] it has become possible to rapidly acquire multiple, low-dose 2D projection images with treatment beams, as shown in Figure 17.4B. Because of the Compton interaction and lack of effective MV scatter-reduction mechanism for EPID, MV image quality and contrast are limited. The amount of scatter reaching the detector depends on the photon energy, field size, and thickness of the imaged object; however, the imaging system can be optimized by calibrating the system using site-specific phantoms.[46]

The MVCT and MV CBCT images provide sufficient contrast to verify patient position and to delineate many anatomic structures.[46,47] It is interesting to note that the MVCT numbers are linear with respect to the electron density of material imaged, yielding accurate dose calculations.[48] Another advantage is the reduced influence of implanted metal objects on image quality, in contrast to kV CT, which exhibits strong artifacts when high-Z material is present (Fig. 17.5), although the metal artifact reduction (MAR) algorithms have been available commercially to improve the CT image quality by most venders (Fig. 17.5C).

Hybrid Cone-Beam CT and Digital Tomosynthesis

A hybrid CBCT can be achieved by combining orthogonal kV and MV projection images with a partial arc gantry rotation as little as 90°[49] while maintaining projection images span an arc of 180°. The acquisition requires only 15 s, making it optimal for breath-hold imaging.[50]

Digital tomosynthesis (DTS) is a special situation of tomographic reconstruction with a limited arc (20° to 40°) of projection images.[51-53] The DTS scan has a short time (<10 s), less radiation, but sacrifices spatial resolution in the direction perpendicular to the x-ray beam. When necessary, a second DTS can be added quasi-orthogonal to the first.

Respiratory-Correlated (4D) Computed Tomography Imaging

The respiratory-induced motion should be considered in some disease sites, in which tumor motion up to 4 cm has been observed.[54] CT scans acquired synchronously with the respiratory signal can be used to reconstruct a set of

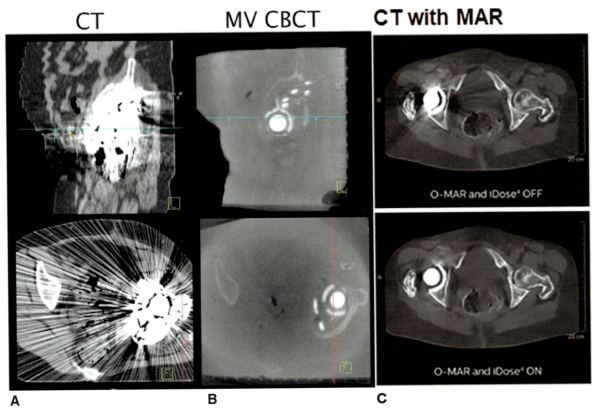

FIGURE 17.5. Metal artifacts and reduction. **A:** Images showing the artifacts due to the presence of metal objects in the conventional kV CT images. **B:** Artifact-free images were obtained with an MV CBCT. (*Source:* Reprinted from Morin O, Gillis A, Chen J, et al. Megavoltage cone-beam CT: system description and clinical applications. *Med Dosim* 2006;31:51–61.) **C:** The MAR for orthopedic implants (O-MAR) can be applied to CT reconstruction to reduce the artifact (Image courtesy by Philips Healthcare).

CT, representing 3D anatomy at typically 10 respiratory phases. This collection of 3DCT data sets is called respiratory-correlated CT (RCCT), or 4DCT, which describes the snapshots of a patient's 3D anatomy over one composite breathing cycle.

Respiratory-Correlated 4DCT

The RC 4DCT can be acquired in either cine or helical mode. In cine mode, repeat CT projections are acquired over slightly more than one respiratory cycle with the couch stationary while recording patient respiration; the couch is then incremented and the process is repeated. Following the acquisition, the images are sorted with respect to the respiratory signal, leading to a set of volume images at different respiration points in the cycle.[55,56] A helical scan uses a low pitch and adjusts the gantry rotation period such that all voxels are viewed by the CT detectors for at least one respiratory cycle.[57,58] Both techniques have been widely characterized and applied clinically for estimating the extent of moving tumors in the lung and abdomen.[59,60]

The selection of the type of respiratory signal can vary, and commercial systems commonly use one of the two types of breathing monitors. One such monitor (Real-time Position Management, RPM™, Varian Oncology Systems, Palo Alto, CA) captures the anterior–posterior motion of an infrared-reflective block placed on the patient's abdomen or chest using an infrared (IR) camera. The other is a "pneumo bellows" system (Philips Medical Systems, Milpitas, CA) that records the digital voltage signal from a differential pressure sensor wrapped around the patient's abdomen. Periodic motion is assumed in the binning approach and breathing irregularity adversely affects the quality of 4DCT images, leading to anatomical distortions.[61,62] Phase-based binning assumes repeatable breathing cycles and often produces 4DCT images with greater motion artifacts than amplitude-based binning.[63,64] Reduction of motion artifacts in 4DCT is an active area of investigation and numerous methods have been proposed.[65–67]

Respiratory-Correlated 4D CBCT

As CBCT is acquired with limited gantry speed at 1 rpm, motion artifacts are different and more pronounced in CBCT than CT. RC 4D CBCT has been developed similar to 4DCT.[68,69] A slower gantry rotation is required to acquire sufficient projections in each phase bin, resulting in scan times of 3 to 6 min. The limited number of projections per phase reduces the contrast resolution and introduces image artifacts; thus, the method is more suited to detecting high-contrast objects such as a tumor in the parenchymal lung.[68–70] RC DTS has also been reported.[53] An alternative approach is to process the CBCT images with motion correction using a patient-specific motion model.[71,72] Most of the methods use DIR to deform the images to a common

motion state. Motion-corrected CBCT allows normal scanning time and accurate tumor positioning.[73,74]

Respiratory-Gated CBCT

Gated CBCT is an alternative method to reduce respiratory motion-induced blurring for image-guided RT. It uses intermittent machine gantry rotation and image acquisition, yielding a reconstructed volume at a specified gate in the breathing cycle.[75] The anatomy is thereby depicted as it will appear in the subsequent treatment. The technique (available in Varian's TrueBeam imaging system) is applicable to free-breathing gated treatment or breath-hold treatment. An advantage is that projection images are uniformly and closely spaced, resulting in higher-quality CBCT reconstructions compared to respiration correlated 4D CBCT.

Magnetic Resonance Imaging

MRI is well-known for its non-ionization radiation imaging, flexible imaging orientation, and high soft-tissue contrast. The appearance of the soft tissue can be manipulated with different pulse sequences and contrasts, such as T1-weighted (T1w) or T2-weighted (T2w). The tumor visibility can be further enhanced by administering a contrast agent, such as a gadolinium-chelated compound. The magnetic field strength ranges from 0.2 Tesla (T) for open-field MRI to 1.5 T or 3 T for a closed-field whole-body (≤70 cm bore) MRI scanner. MRI may suffer from geometric distortion due to the non-uniformity of the magnetic field strength. This scanner-specific factor can be corrected by imaging a large grid phantom.[76] The geometric integrity is also affected by susceptibility differences at tissue interfaces.

MR-guided Radiotherapy (MRgRT)

The MR-integrated linac (MR-linac) utilizes 0.35 T in ViewRay's MRIdian System (ViewRay, Inc., Gainesville, FL) and 1.5 T for Elekta Unity System (Elekta Inc., Sweden). The MRIdian system utilized cobalt (60) as a radiation source in 2014[77] and changed to linac in 2017.[78] The Unity system was developed by Elekta and Philips, tested at the University Medical Center Utrecht in the Netherlands,[79–81] and have been used in treating cancer patients since 2017.[82] Both systems (Fig. 17.6) have the radiation beam perpendicular to the magnetic field and irradiate the tumor through a gap between two split magnets and both systems can acquire 3D motion-compensated images for patient setup and 2D cine MR images for motion monitoring during treatment. Regardless the magnetic field strength, the linac waveguide is shielded from both the magnetic field and RF signal of the MRI unit. On the other hand, the beam modifiers, such as the multi-leaf

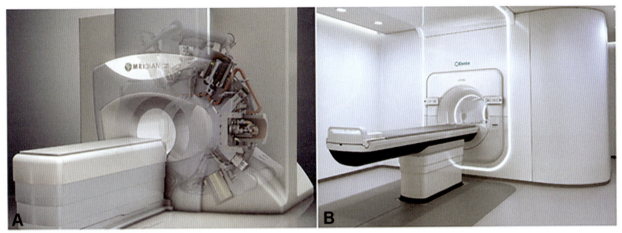

FIGURE 17.6. Two MR-integrated linacs: **A:** MRIdian (Reproduced with the permission of ViewRay Technologies, Inc. All rights reserved.) and **B:** Elekta Unity MR-Linac. (Image courtesy of Elekta).

collimator (MLC), may affect the homogeneity of the magnetic field.[83] Moreover, the magnetic field interacts with secondary electrons generated in the patient, thereby affecting the dose distribution.[84,85] The effect is most pronounced at tissue–air interfaces, where exiting electrons return to the tissue as a result of the Lorentz force and locally deposit additional dose on the surface. Clinical commissioning methods have been developed for both MR-linac systems.[86-89] There are two other MR-linac prototypes and one has been used in an animal study.[90-92]

A third clinical MRI-guided system that has been installed in Princess Margaret Cancer Center nearing clinical implementation enables a rail-mounted 1.5-T MR scanner to operate in three different rooms: MR simulation, MR-guided brachytherapy, and MR-guided RT linac.[93] Such in-room systems offer both soft-tissue-based 3D target alignment and near real-time 2D tumor motion monitoring.[80] The goals are to provide online setup and intra-fractional treatment guidance, adaptive replanning, and monitoring of treatment response.

3D MRI for Radiotherapy Planning

A 3D volumetric MR image is potentially useful for MRI-based treatment planning[94-96] with high soft-tissue contrast without ionizing radiation. It is important to minimize MRI geometric distortions[97,98] and obtain the electronic density of MRI voxels for dose calculation.[95] To create tissue electronic density using MRI images, bulk anatomy-density, atlas-based, and deep learning approaches have been applied.[99-102] The MR-based plan can be delivered either on an MR-linac with MR-MR registration for patient setup, or on a conventional lianc by generating pseudo-CT or pseudo-DRRs as reference images to align with CBCT or 2D radiographs to set up patients.[103] Clinically, MR-only treatment planning has been applied to treat brain and pelvis lesions with relatively simple anatomy and low

heterogeneity.[100,104-106] On MR-linac, adaptive planning is possible to accommodate daily patient anatomical changes or even tumor shrinkage (Fig. 17.7). Clinically, automatic organ and tumor segmentation is needed and has been an active research area.[107-112]

Respiratory-correlated and Time-resolved 4DMRI

MRI can produce 2D planar, 3D volumetric, and 4D temporal images,[113] which are scanned and reconstructed slice by slice. When a fast scan pulse sequence is applied, such as TrueFISP (true fast imaging with steady-state precession), 2DMR cine images in sagittal and/or coronal views, can be acquired at 4 to 5 fps. At this acquisition speed, respiratory-induced tumor motion can be monitored for respiratory gating or real-time tumor tracking. RC 4DMRI has been developed using a method similar to 4DCT.[114-116] Hu *et al.* introduced an amplitude-based triggering system to acquire prospective T2w 4DMRI for abdominal tumor tracking.[116] Li *et al.* compared the image quality of RC 4DMRI using simultaneous internal and external surrogates for respiratory binning.[117] Mickevicius and Paulson have developed a pulse sequence to simultaneously acquire sagittal and coronal 2D cines and applied a super-resolution method to reconstruct an isotropic resolution RC 4DMRI.[118]

Dynamic 3D cine images can be acquired to reconstruct low-resolution 4DMRI with the aid of parallel imaging with multi-channel coils and k-space approximation to achieve a temporal resolution of 1 to 2 fps.[119] This is a low-resolution time-resolved (TR) 4DMRI. Recently, Li *et al.* applied a super-resolution approach to reconstruct high-resolution TR 4DMRI by deforming a 3D breath-hold MRI image to a series of dynamic 3D cine images in free-breathing, achieving 2 Hz frame rate T1w TR 4DMRI.[120,121] The super-resolution method was extended and applied to reconstruct T2w TR-4DMRI using three MRI image sets.[122]

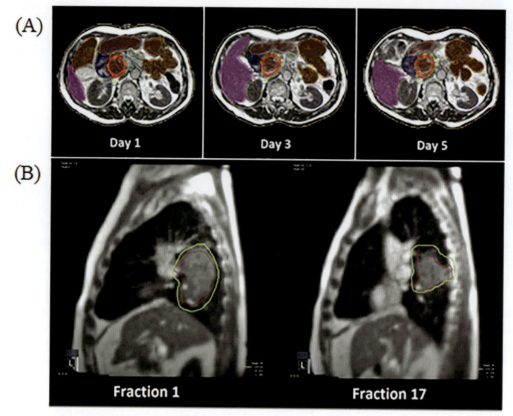

FIGURE 17.7. Two examples of patient anatomy changes during the course of radiotherapy. **A:** Daily patient anatomic changes illustrated from MR-linac requires online plan re-optimization for adaptation in a pancreatic cancer patient. **B:** Tumor shrinkage viewed by MR-linac in the course of radiotherapy of a lung cancer patient between fractions 1 and 17 needs adaptive planning. (Reproduced with the permission of ViewRay Technologies, Inc. All rights reserved).

Positron Emission Tomography

PET is used increasingly for tumor delineation in treatment planning and for assessment of tumor response to radiation treatment. Using a positron-emitting biological tracer, tumor metabolic, proliferating, or hypoxic conditions can be probed. A well-established PET tracer is ^{18}F-fluoro-deoxyglucose (^{18}F-FDG), a sugar-like molecule, which accumulates in tumor cells owing to their high-metabolic activities. In the event of positron emission, a positron annihilates with an electron in the tissue to emit a pair of 511 keV photons in opposite directions. A PET scanner with a band of scintillation detectors around the gantry detects the two coincident events and determines the event location by the times of flight of the two photons. Similarly, SPECT uses gamma-emitting tracers to image a tumor by detecting independent γ-decay events. Clinically, hybrid PET/CT, SPECT/CT, and PET/MRI scanners are used with the co-registration between the two sets of images, facilitating tumor delineation and localization.

Recently, in-room PET and SPECT have been studied as a direct means for tumor positioning and tracking for IGRT.[12,123–125] For proton therapy, PET has been applied to directly image the by-products of positron emitters, such as ^{15}O, in the beam path and assess the geometric accuracy of treatment delivery.[124]

Ultrasound Imaging

Ultrasound is useful in soft-tissue targeting in the abdomen for RT. Fontanarosa *et al.* have recently reviewed ultrasound guidance for external beam RT.[126] The ultrasound transducer is both a sound source and a detector. It transmits brief pulses that propagate into the tissues and receives the echo that is bounced back at tissue interfaces where acoustic impedance changes, owing to differences in tissue density or elasticity. The round-trip time of the pulse-echo wave is used to determine the transducer-to-object distances. A scan line converter constructs a 3D image of the patient using 1D (one-dimensional) (with sweeping) or 2D transducer. Poor ultrasound image quality, unfamiliar image appearance, and anatomy distortions due to applied pressure have limited their utility for precise image guidance. The inter- and intra-user variability are large for ultrasound-guided setup[127] and more pronounced for fiducial alignment.[128]

Optical Surface Imaging

Stereoscopic OSI provides real-time imaging, primarily used for aligning superficial tumors (the breast) or immobile tumors (the brain). A commercial OSI system (AlignRT™, VisionRT, Ltd., London, UK) is composed of three ceiling-mounted stereo-camera pods, each having two cameras and a speckle projector to provide structured light for 3D surface reconstruction with sub-millimeter accuracy.[129] Another commercial OSI system is C-RAD, producing the Catalyst using laser scanning and the Catalyst+ with a structured light approach (Catalyst). Varian Identify system (Varian Oncology Systems, Palo Alto, CA) integrated the in-room camera systems with patient palm reader to check patient identification and treatment accessories to enhance the treatment safety, in addition to surface-guided radiotherapy (SGRT) setup and motion monitoring.

Validated with x-ray imaging, OSI provides quick and non-radiologic means for SGRT setup for the breast, brain, head and neck patients, and other anatomical sites.[18,129–131] Patient SGRT setup requires to register the on-site surface image to a reference region of interest (ROI) defined on the delineated patient body surface in the planning CT. Recently, SGRT efforts to replace the conventional setup methods using skin tattoo and room lasers have been reported.[132,133]

A different type of OSI is Cherenkov video imaging to visualize radiation delivery relative to patient anatomies, such as the breast.[13,134] The optical detection is gated with the radiation pulse from a linac, providing direct evidence of radiation delivery.

Image-guided Patient Setup

With imaging guidance, the patient setup may contain two steps. A gross alignment of patients is fast with real-time guidance and can be done inside the treatment room using the OSI, which may have the potential to replace the conventional skin-tattoo-based patient alignment with room lasers. The discrepancy between the OSI and CBCT setup in brain cases is usually about 1 to 2 mm.[17]

This quick step involves patient adjustment. The second step is to align internal anatomy using 2DkV or CBCT, especially for hypofractional SBRT treatments. The patient position is corrected by shifting the treatment couch in up to six DOF (three translational and three rotational shifts) based on 2D–3D or 3D–3D image registration. The six DOF treatment couch is commercially available and commonly used for high-precision treatments, such as cranial SRS and SBRT,[135] where sub-millimeter and sub-degree precision setup is needed. For a mobile tumor, such as a lung tumor, the mean position may be acquired to match the position in the planning CT.

INTRA-FRACTIONAL REAL-TIME IMAGING AND MOTION COMPENSATION

During a treatment fraction, real-time tumor tracking allows minimizing targeting uncertainty with reduced treatment margin. Tumor tracking usually requires real-time motion monitoring (detection) and motion compensation (execution) with minimal time delay. Conventionally, implanted markers are primarily used as surrogates for target position using x-ray fluoroscopy, but markerless approaches are used in the clinic, including fluoroscopy,[136] MV-EPID imaging,[137,138] Electromagnetic position tracking,[139] optical surface imaging,[17,140] and MR-guided radiotherapy (MRgRT).[141] In the following sections, we review different approaches for real-time monitoring and tracking in photon RT.

Fluoroscopic Imaging with Implant Fiducials

Two commercially available room-mounted systems, as shown in Figure 17.8, are CyberKnife™ (Accuray Inc., Sunnyvale, CA) and ExacTrac® (BrainLAB AG, Feldkirchen, Germany). Both are integrated IGRT systems for target localization, setup correction, and the delivery of high-precision frameless SRS and SBRT. The image guidance uses two distinct imaging subsystems: kV stereoscopic x-ray imaging and real-time IR marker tracking. CyberKnife

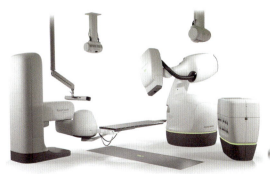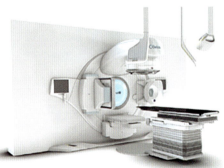

FIGURE 17.8. Two room-mounted kV image-guided IGRT real-time tracking systems. **A:** CyberKnife system (Images used with permission from Accuray Incorporated). **B:** ExacTrac system, BrainLAB AG, Feldkirchen, Germany (Photograph courtesy of BrainLAB AG.).

A   B

provides fluoroscopy for target tracking, external marker tracking, and can perform adaptive beam gating or real-time target tracking.[142] ExacTrac is designed for isocentric linacs to treat cranial SRS and SBRT. It can acquire x-ray images at nonzero couch angles to periodically verify patient position during treatment.[143] Recently, optical/thermal imaging is also added to the ExacTrac system.

Gantry-mounted kV imaging systems usually have only one kV x-ray imager and acquire an orthogonal image pair by rotating the gantry, including Varian's OBI™ and TrueBeam™ Imaging systems and Elekta's Synergy™ and Infinity™ systems. The kV imaging beamlines are orthogonal to the MV treatment beamline and its isocenter must be in accordance with the MV beam isocenter. Fluoroscopic kV imaging has been applied to intrafraction monitoring of implanted markers during VMAT delivery in the prostate,[144] and more recently in combination with MLC tracking.[145] VERO (BrainLAB AG Feldkirchen, Germany) is another gantry-mounted linac system (Fig. 17.9A), equipped with two orthogonal kV imaging and an optical tracking system.[146] It provides CBCT, simultaneous orthogonal 2DkV imaging, and fluoroscopic imaging. Fast gantry tracking by a gimbal-based gantry system has a latency of less than 50 ms.[147] Poels et al. have reported tumor tracking using both orthogonal kV and planar MV imaging to achieve 0.3 mm accuracy on phantom.[148] Clinical applications of VERO for SRS and SBRT have been reported.[146,148,149] Halcyon (Varian) is another newly introduced IGRT linac system with faster gantry rotation and MLC speeds to allow imaging with single breath-hold and accelerated treatment (Fig. 17.9B). Due to the concern of imaging radiation dose, fluoroscopic imaging is often used in conjunction with OSI and a patient-specific tumor

motion prediction model based on internal–external motion correlation.[150]

Triggered Intrafractional Imaging

An alternative method is to acquire 2DkV images at specified intervals during treatment using Varian's TrueBeam imaging system and this is referred to as triggered images. Trigger criteria can be defined based on time, monitor units, gantry angle, or respiratory gating. Projections of 3D structures from the treatment plan can be overlaid on the triggered image to aid inspection during treatment. The images can also be analyzed following treatment, for example, to assess residual target motion.[151,152] In cases where the patient has implanted fiducial markers, a capability called Intrafraction Motion Review (IMR) allows visual comparison of the fiducial with its planned position during treatment, as well as automatic fiducial detection.[153,154]

MV/kV Imaging

The MV-EPID imaging during treatment does not give the patient extra radiation but provides on-treatment target localization when patients have implanted fiducials or surgical clips. Studies have shown that EPID can capture at least one fiducial marker 40% to 95% of the time in VMAT prostate treatment, while kV imaging can be used as needed for the rest,[155,156] allowing motion monitoring during treatment. The EPID can also be used to calculate the delivered dose from the treatment.[157] The MV–kV imaging provides a possibility to acquire images during treatment with alternated beam-on time,[158–160] minimizing the scatter interference from the other x-ray source. Recently, the MV–kV has been used in the clinic

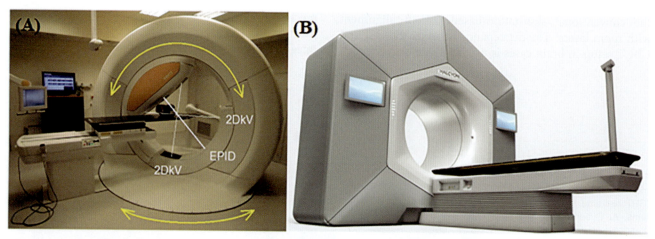

FIGURE 17.9. A: VERO system (BrainLAB AG Feldkirchen, Germany and Mitsubishi Heavy Industries, Tokyo, Japan) offers quick gantry movement aiming at a moving tumor, guided by gantry-mounted stereoscopic x-ray imaging systems. (Photograph courtesy of Dirk Verellen, PhD) and **B:** Halcyon provides IGRT to guide fast-rotating gantry and fast-moving MLC for quick treatment delivery. (Image(s) courtesy of Varian Medical Systems, Inc., Palo Alto, CA. Copyright [2021]. All rights reserved.)

to verify the target location during treatment, allowing beam hold if the fiducials move out of the tolerance.[138,161] At any selected VMAT control points, MLC leaves can be opened wide enough to show the fiducials while the extra radiation dose can be compensated through the leaf modulation at non-control-points in the arcs or by inserting low-dose "imaging" control points.[154]

Real-time Optical Surface Imaging

Surface Fiducials as Motion Surrogates

Optical tracking determines the position of an IR-emitting or reflecting marker via triangulation from two stereoscopic cameras. Owing to its clean stereoscopic marker images and simple geometric calculation, it has high spatial (0.1 mm) and temporal (<0.1 s) resolution in marker tracking. Multiple markers can be tracked simultaneously in real-time allowing continuous correction of patient position during treatment. Markers can also serve as fiducials, but variation in marker placement between simulation and treatment causes uncertainty. Meeks *et al.* have reviewed this technology in several implementations for intracranial and extracranial SBRT.[162]

Video-Based Optical Surface Imaging

OSI utilizes the same principles mentioned previously to determine the position of a surface point, which is identified with the assistance of a texture image projected onto a patient skin. High spatial resolution is achievable although the temporal resolution is limited by the substantially increased number of points to track. The speed of 3D surface image reconstruction depends on the size of the ROI and image resolution: for the facial area with high resolution, the frame rate has been increased from 2 to 3 fps to 8 to 12 fps in the latest AlignRT system (version 6.2, VisionRT Ltd, London, UK).[17,163]

For surface alignment, an ROI should be created with sufficiently reliable landscape on a reference surface, which is either an OSI image acquired at simulation or an external surface rendered from the planning CT image imported via Digital Imaging and Communications in Medicine (DICOM)-RT. The image registration algorithm is based on an iterative-closest-point method leading to an efficient and robust surface alignment of the ROI. Clinical setup time can be less than 2 min with high accuracy and reproducibility.[17] The real-time surface matching capability has been applied to head motion monitoring during SRS treatment.[17,140] Using an OSI image captured at treatment as a reference, systematic errors of the OSI system can be canceled, yielding 0.2 mm accuracy for rigid motion detection. For non-rigid anatomy, OSI-based spirometry has been reported,[164] aiming to utilize respiratory-induced torso surface motion to predict tumor motion via physical relationships.[165]

Real-Time Electromagnetic Localization and Tracking

Tracking of implanted fiducials without ionizing radiation imaging is possible with a technology that uses radiofrequency (RF) electromagnetic fields to induce and detect signals from implanted "wireless" beacon transponders (Calypso, Varian Medical Systems). The electromagnetic tracking system is integrated with Varian's Edge™ treatment machine. The system consists of a console, an optical tracking system, and a tracking station. The console is situated near the treatment couch with a magnetic array panel extended above and close to the patient's surface. The array panel contains RF source coils to excite the transponders and sensor coils to detect the transponder response signals, each at a different resonant frequency for unique identification at 10 Hz and sub-millimeter accuracy.[139,166] The Calypso system requires 1 to 3 transponders to be implanted in or near the tumor, including the lungs, for real-time motion tracking.[138,167,168]

MRI Real-Time Cine Imaging

Both commercial MRI-linac machines (Fig. 17.6) are capable of providing 4 to 5 Hz frame rate 2DMR cine imaging for near-real-time motion monitoring. MRI can track soft-tissue targets and OARs without interrupting treatment delivery. Interleaving sagittal and coronal 2D cines can be acquired to provide pseudo-3D images, but the frame rate for each is reduced by half. In these two views, major respiratory-induced motions can be visualized during treatment.[78,169] Tumor motion in many anatomic sites has been monitored with respiratory gating to reduce treatment margin, so that toxicity is reduced and a lethal dose (or near lethal dose) can be prescribed. Recently, a study has shown that 2DMR cine images can be acquired in the BEV of beams in an IMRT plan and projected with volumetric tumor contour via library matching in real-time, therefore, checking of tumor-beam conformality can be achieved directly during MRgRT.[170] This would provide the ultimate tumor motion-monitoring tool to guide respiratory gating or tumor tracking.

The 3D MR cine imaging can only provide low-spatial resolution at a 2 Hz frame rate using all available accelerated MR scanning techniques with multiple coils,[171] and the super-resolution reconstruction method improves the spatial resolution but cannot achieve real-time performance for tumor tracking.[120–122] Another approach is to use 2D cine as the guidance and RC-4DMRI as the source of volumetric anatomy data to reconstruct the volumetric TR-4DMRI via a patient-specific motion model built based on DIR with principal component analysis.[172–174] One advantage of this method, compared with the super-resolution TR-4DMRI method,[120–122] is that the online 2D cine images acquired during treatment can be used for retrospective dosimetry analysis with the online patient/organ motion information. Although more than 56 MR-linacs worldwide so far have been commissioned for clinical use, integrated MRI-linac systems are still an active area of development, including adaptive planning,[175–177] MR imaging,[122,178] MRgRT method,[179,180] hardware improvements,[181,182] and clinical investigations.[183,184]

Real-Time Tumor Motion Compensation

Real-time tumor tracking refers to a continuous adjustment of the radiation beam or patient position during treatment to follow the changing position of the tumor or its surrogate. In principle, real-time tracking provides a combination of increased normal tissue sparing relative to motion-encompassing methods by reducing the treatment margin, and more efficient treatment with near 100% duty cycle relative to gated treatment. Although the current clinical methods to manage patient motion is via respiratory gating or breath-holding, tumor tracking offers the best option to treat a mobile tumor as if it is standing still. In the following sections, we summarize three strategies in various stages of development involving motion tracking of a linac system.

Dynamic Multi-leaf Collimator Approach

Keall *et al.* have demonstrated motion tracking using dynamic MLC (DMLC) guided by real-time motion signal from the Calypso system in prostate with better than 2 mm accuracy and 220 ms system latency.[139,168] When MLC leaves move in the direction of tumor motion, the spatial resolution for tracking is <1 mm. Different strategies to optimize leaf trajectories have been studied.[185,186] Motion-tracking radiation delivery has been demonstrated using 2DMR cine for image guidance in motion phantom experiments.[187] Keall *et al.* have reported the first clinical experience on DMLC tracking of Calypso transponder for a prostate treatment.[188] Zhang *et al.* have reported a clinical feasibility study using both MLC and couch to compensate for tumor motion in pancreas and liver treatments.[189]

Mobile Treatment Couch Approach

D'Souza *et al.* have proposed the compensation of the tumor motion using a robotic couch,[190] which moves in the opposite direction of the tumor motion, so that no apparent motion in the BEV. However, there may be patient-related physical and medical concerns, including physical inertia of the patient's body, causing tissue deformation when changing motion directions, especially for obese patients. Varian 6D (six-dimensional) couch is capable of motion tracking but has not been released for clinical use, while developments on mobile couch/extension have been shown.[191] Menten *et al.* have illustrated comparable motion compensation between mobile couch tracking and DMLC tracking,[192] and Zhang *et al.* have demonstrated that it is feasible to combine both methods of motion compensation.[189]

Movable Gantry Approach

The CyberKnife[TM] has a 6D robotic arm to position a light-weighted linac and a 6D robotic couch to align a patient and provides the first clinical solution for tumor tracking[142] (Fig. 17.8A). The robotic arm can move at speeds of several centimeters per second, which makes it compatible with tracking respiratory-induced tumor motion. The VERO[TM] system is designed for image-guided tumor tracking (Fig. 17.9A). Based on a gimbaled design, the beam can rotate transversely (panned) or longitudinally (tilted) to track implanted fiducials in or near the tumor with the maximum motion range of 4.4 cm (or 2.5°) at the treatment isocenter and a latency of 50 ms for 4DRT.[147,193,194]

IGRT REQUIREMENTS AND CONSIDERATIONS

IGRT Commissioning and Quality Assurance

Commissioning and QA of IGRT-enabled technologies are essential. The American Association of Physicists in Medicine (AAPM) has issued several task group (TG) reports, covering in-room kV x-ray imaging for patient setup/target localization (TG#104),[195] QA for non-radiographic imaging for patient setup/target localization (TG#147),[196] QA for CT-based IGRT technologies (TG#179),[197] QA for medical accelerators (TG#142),[198] SBRT procedures (TG#101),[199] and management of respiratory motion (TG#76).[54] These reports provide guidelines for clinical use and QA of the IGRT imaging systems and procedures. In the following, we summarize three important aspects: geometric accuracy, image quality, and motion detection.

Coincidence of Imaging Isocenter and Treatment Isocenter

One of the most important tasks in commissioning an in-room imaging modality is to check the isocenter coincidence between the imaging isocenter and the radiation isocenter in the IGRT paradigm, as stated in "Conceptual and Practical Changes in IGRT Paradigm" section, to ensure that discrepancy is within clinically acceptable tolerances. For stereotactic procedures, the discrepancy must be within 1.0 mm; otherwise, it should be within 2.0 mm.[198] It is paramount to check the alignment of mechanical and radiation isocenters, and conventionally the room laser is used as the isocenter surrogate. In fact, the IGRT setup emphasizes imaging isocenter alignment with treatment isocenter, with higher accuracy than the room laser for stereotactic treatments. The MV-EPID system provides direct reference to the treatment beam and therefore serves as the gold standard. A calibration procedure is required to correct mechanical sagging for kV imaging and MV EPID detectors.[46,200] Customized QA phantoms have been developed for different IGRT systems, including kV and MV imaging systems of C-arm linacs,[198,201] MVCT imaging of tomotherapy units,[202] and AlignRT surface imaging in a linac and Halcyon system.[203,204] To determine the geometric accuracy of IGRT for SRS/SBRT, together with the dosimetry accuracy, an end-to-end test (from simulation to delivery) is recommended, by comparing the alignment of the center of the delivered MV dose distribution with the planned isocenter.[146,205]

Image Quality

Bissonnette *et al.* have established a QA program for CBCT image quality with Elekta Synergy and Varian OBI systems.[37,38,113] The report evaluates flat-panel detector stability, performance, and image quality of 10 linac imaging systems over 3 years. Details for correcting background (dark current) and pixel-by-pixel gain uniformity (flood-field image) of the plat-panel detector are also described. The CatPhan 500 phantom (The Phantom Laboratory, Salem, NY) is used to quantify image quality.[206] A comprehensive QA program by Yoo *et al.* describes safety, functionality, geometric accuracy, and image quality for the Varian OBI system.[207] Image quality characterization and QA procedures for EPID,[208] MV CBCT,[209] and MVCT in helical tomotherapy[202] have also been reported. A stereotactic head phantom (Model 605 Radiosurgery Head Phantom; CIRS, Norfolk, VA) or equivalent is used for imaging QA of the CyberKnife system.[210]

Motion Detection

Clinical motion management guidelines have been published in AAPM TG#76,[54] pertaining to respiratory-induced motions of the target and normal tissue. For fluoroscopic imaging, the temporal resolution should be 100 ms or less, which produces an uncertainty of <2 mm for an object moving at speeds up to 2 cm/s. Jiang *et al.* have outlined major clinical challenges in respiratory-related procedures, including respiratory gating, breath-hold, and 4DCT.[211] As external surrogates are used in many respiratory gating and breath-hold procedures, the biggest challenge is to ensure treatment accuracy. Milewski *et al.* reported that the internal–external motion correlations can be enhanced by correcting the phase shift between the two motions based on the 4DMRI data of volunteers.[212] When external monitoring is used, verification of internal–external correlation using image guidance before each treatment session is needed.

In the MR-linac system, the dynamic 2DMR cine has a 4 to 5 fps frame rate, and if orthogonal 2D cine is applied, the frame rate of each would be 2–2.5 fps.[78,174] Clinically, this technique has been applied to visually tracking the abdominal tumor,[213,214] pelvis tumor,[215,216] and thoracic tumors.[217] For real-time motion monitoring for respiratory gating or tumor tracking, sagittal and/or coronal 2D cines were applied in the clinic. Recently, Nie *et al.* proposed and studied the feasibility of using BEV 2D cine and tumor volume projected on the BEV, based on the IMRT plan beam directions and a TR-4DRI library of lung cancer patients. This technique only take 15 ms computation time, allowing real-time check of beam conformality within 1 mm.[170]

Image Registration and Fusion

In the IGRT context, image registration serves to align daily 3D or 2D patient setup images with the planning CT/3DMR or DRR/2DMR images, respectively. IGRT patient setup accuracy depends on registration accuracy, which further depends on the imaging/treatment isocenter alignment (hidden from the clinician), the registration algorithm, and the anatomic landmark. QA of the image registration and fusion methods should be performed using an appropriate phantom.[218] Based on the registration target, clinically the uncertainty can be estimated as isocenter registration error (IRE) or target registration error (TRE).[219] Uncertainty in image registration increases when the underlying anatomy changes, including motion, deformation, or physical changes. To minimize the uncertainty, image registration often focuses on the vicinity of the tumor using surrogates, such as the bone and fiducials. Visual verification with the necessary manual adjustment is essential after automatic image registration, using three orthogonal views of fused 3D images through color blending, checkerboard, or split windows. Direct evaluation of 3D volumetric images rendered by graphics processing unit (GPU)-based, real-time computation is also possible.[220,221]

Rigid Image Registration

Most image registration tools used for IGRT are rigid registration using a rigid transformation in six DOF, a cost function for evaluation, and an algorithm to determine and search for the lowest cost function iteratively in the optimization process. For multi-modality registration, the maximization of mutual information (MI) is often applied as the cost function, while the greatest descending gradience is usually used for optimization process.[222,223] In addition to deformation-related uncertainty in rigid image registration, uncertainty may also come from inter-observer variation in manual alignment and different tumor appearance in different imaging modalities.[107] The overall setup accuracy for tumor localization is determined by many factors, including registration accuracy, couch adjustment accuracy, imaging/treatment isocenter discrepancy, couch walk for non-coplanar beams, and patient motion during and after image acquisition and registration.

Deformable Image Registration

DIR is essential for contour propagation and delivered-dose estimation: it is a useful tool for adaptive IGRT. Since 2007, DIR has been intensively studied focusing on deformation algorithms, physical constraints, self-consistency, and accuracy assessment.[224,225] The uncertainty of DIR is 2 to 3 mm on average. DIR can track deformed anatomy voxel by voxel between two 3D images, producing a deformation vector field (DVF) useful in at least three IGRT areas[24,226–228]: organ motion, contour propagation, and dose estimation. Lately, machine learning methods have been applied in medical image analysis, including image registration.[229] More details on DIR can be found in Chapter 18.

Information Technology Infrastructure for IGRT

Implementation of IGRT into routine clinical workflow requires tighter integration of imaging and treatment systems and more efficient information flow. IGRT represents a shift from a traditionally static treatment planning process to a more dynamic, closed-loop process with multiple feedback check/control points, especially for intrafractional IGRT guidance. To meet the technical and logistical needs, the following infrastructure and software tools are considered important to IGRT applications:

IGRT Data Management:

- Picture Archival and Communication Systems specifically designed for radiotherapy (RT-PACS) are needed that integrate IGRT workflows, data management, user interfaces, and statistical tools among different imaging and treatment procedures.
- The Integrated Health Enterprise in Radiation Oncology (IHE-RO)[230] endeavors to specify and address specific clinical problems and ambiguities including those for IGRT. It aims to overcome the shortcomings of the DICOM in RT, which is the current industry standard.[231]
- Treatment management systems play a central role in integrating image guidance and treatment delivery systems. With more frequent use of 2D, 3D, and 4D multimodal images and possible adaptive replanning during the course of treatment, data storage requirements can increase 1 to 2 orders of magnitude.

IGRT Facilitating Tools

- Automatic tools for rigid and DIR and organ segmentation are necessary for implementing various IGRT approaches.[24,226,229,232]
- Automatic treatment planning and optimization are needed to perform online or offline plan adaptation to changing anatomy or altered target volumes.[233]
- Cross-platform treatment plan comparison tools are needed for multi-institutional studies. The computational environment for radiotherapy research (CERR)[234] and DIR for adaptive radiotherapy research (DIRART)[226] provide a common platform for treatment plan database and tools for clinical outcome research and analysis.

Selection of IGRT Technology

The selection of an appropriate image-guidance solution is a complex process that may involve a compromise among clinical objectives, product availability, existing infrastructure, manpower, and resources.[9,235] The

implementation of an IGRT technology in the clinic requires a thorough understanding of the complete clinical process and the necessary infrastructure to support data collection, analysis, and intervention. The four considerations: clinical, technical, resource, and administration, suggested by the AAPM TG#104 report,[195] may evolve with the industry trend.

Although IGRT focus on target alignment in treatment delivery, they are strongly related to treatment simulation and planning.[169,236] As mentioned before, the planning CT acquired is a snapshot of patient anatomy and may not be representative of treatment. An alternative method is to perform online (immediately before treatment) re-optimization of the treatment plan.[81,237] Clinically, online adaptive planning has been implemented and applied in MR-linac systems based on the 3DMR images of the day.[89,238] Therefore, the selection of IGRT is strongly associated with clinical needs, resources, and capacities.

IGRT in Proton Therapy

Proton (or particle) therapy offers the advantage of OAR sparing at the distal edge of the tumor from the radiation owing to the Bragg Peak of the heavy particle radiation. The abrupt drop in dose at the end of the finite range of particles makes their dose distributions more vulnerable to intra- and inter-fractional anatomy variations. Thus, there is a greater need for image guidance and more frequent adaptation of treatment plans.[239] IGRT is more critical for RT with protons than with photons and robust optimization of IMPT dose distributions is more important in light of intra- and inter-fractional variations.[240–242] To ascertain the position of the Bragg peak in patients, PET and prompt gamma imaging have been investigated.[243,244]

Recently, the studies of ultra-high dose rate deliveries have shown the potential for greater OAR sparing while keeping tumor control unchanged, leading to a potentially revolutionary change in radiation therapy.[245,246] Termed FLASH RT, dose rates beginning at 40 Gy/s[247,248] are used to complete a treatment in fractions of a second. Therefore, the accuracy and timing of patient setup and motion management become more important than any conventional dose–rate RT. Although initial biological effects have been evidenced and the FLASH technology is achievable, it may take years to gather sufficient animal and human data before clinical applications.

IGRT in Combination with Immunotherapy

The combination of image-guided SBRT and immunotherapy is a promising new development in recent years because an augmented tumor cell recognition by host immune cells can be achieved after SBRT.[249–251] Immunotherapy tries to simulate the immune system via immunogenic pathways and/or target co-inhibitory checkpoints. Cancerous cells, although malignant, belong to the host system and cannot be recognized as a target by the patient immune system under normal conditions. SBRT causes cancer cell death and tumor antigens are released in the microenvironment of the disease and activate the immune response subsequently.[252,253] Because the immune response is systematic, the abscopal effect, beyond the targeted site of radiation, can occur as the immune system attacks other metastatic sites within the patient's body. This is an on-going active area of pre-clinical and clinical research.

IGRT CORRECTION STRATEGIES AND APPLICATIONS

Online Versus Offline Corrections

The establishment of a clinical process for correcting patient position based on the data from clinical studies is referred to as a correction strategy. Strategies are broadly divided into online and offline approaches. The online approach makes adjustment to the current treatment session based on data acquired. This may be as simple as couch position adjustment or as complex as a full plan re-optimization for adaptation. The offline approach is to intervene treatment at a later time, such as weekly physician review of portal images and replanning in response to patient changes.[254] The online approach has a greater capacity to increase precision than offline strategies but at the cost of a higher workload. A hybrid correction strategy is often used clinically with different error thresholds and time allowance.[9,102,33,235]

In an accuracy-demanding procedure, such as frameless SRS[17] or MR-guided SBRT,[213,255] IGRT patient setup and motion management can take a large portion of treatment time. The overhead associated with the alignment tools, adaptive methods, and decision rules can be prohibitive unless properly integrated. The adaptive RT program at William Beaumont Hospital[256–258] was made possible only through in-house software integration efforts. For 4D tumor tracking, such as MRgRT, additional automatic tools are necessary to support online correction in the intrafractional intervention.[259,260]

Correction of Interfractional Setup Error

Various techniques have been developed for pretreatment setup corrections. Without loss of generality, we consider an in-room CT-guided IGRT system (Fig. 17.10). Following patient immobilization and alignment of skin marks with room lasers, or using OSI for alignment, a CBCT is acquired and aligned with the planning CT. The primary means of intervention is to correct translational deviations, although the six DOF correction is more desirable for stereotactic treatments, especially for treating multiple lesions with a single isocenter. The second level of intervention may be based on an online plan adaptation based on patient daily anatomic changes, which have been clinically implemented in MRgRT,[260]

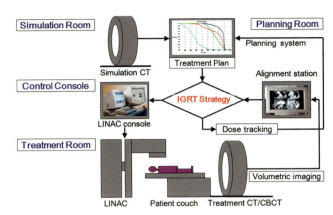

FIGURE 17.10. An in-room volumetric CT-guided radiotherapy process. CT images of a patient's setup and anatomy information are acquired and sent to an alignment workstation where the images are compared and aligned to match with the planning CT. An interventional decision is made based on the magnitude of anatomic variations to assess the need for an online or offline correction. If necessary, dose tracking may be enabled and used for replanning.

to ensure delivered dose distribution. The CBCT images of the patient's treatment anatomy make it possible to estimate the delivered dose distributions and to calculate accumulated dose offline. Accumulated dose deviations can be corrected infrequently using an offline adaptive correction scheme.[233,258]

Management of Intra-fractional Tumor Motion

In the presence of significant intra-fractional motion, additional geometric and dosimetric variations should be taken into account, which increases treatment complexity. Not surprisingly, most motion management is related to the treatment of lung and abdominal cancers.[54,113,233,261] For a mobile lung tumor, the tumor is often visible in CBCT for alignment. For abdominal lesions, localization of implanted fiducials using fluoroscopy can be achieved by aligning the track of the implanted marker with the track discerned from the reference 4DCT.

During treatment, real-time monitoring of implanted fiducials, or the tumor directly, is needed for accurate radiation gating around end-expiration. MLC motion is intermittent during gated IMRT, thereby reducing possible interplay effects between MLC and respiratory motions.[262] Audiovisual feedback may improve breathing regularity and breath-hold reproducibility[263–265] and can be used in respiratory-gated treatment. There will be a time delay from motion detection to the action of beam hold or motion tracking, usually 100 to 400 ms.[266,267] This latency can cause a targeting error of 1 to 2 mm,[155] critical to tumor tracking. A predictive model can be used to anticipate the tumor position to reduce the latency-caused error to gain sub-millimeter accuracy.[187,268] Tumor motion can be predicted using external markers based on a motion correlation model, and such a model needs initially calibration and periodic verification and update by frequent imaging measurements.[194,269] Recent advents of

MR-linac allowing direct, near real-time visualization of tumor motion have greatly improved the targeting accuracy with reduced setup and motion margin. 2DMR cine can align the target directly, increasing the dose to the target while maximally sparing nearby vital OARs.[255,270,271]

Population-Based and Individualized Margins

The relative importance of systematic and random errors in the determination of PTV margins should be considered in the design of a clinical strategy. Geometric errors in radiation field placement are typically characterized by distributions of nonzero mean and variance. The mean represents the systematic discrepancy while the variance represents the random component. The relative importance of these two categories of errors may vary in determining appropriate PTV margins.[272,273] The reported margin formula may not completely general, as the number of fractions is not concerned, especially for SBRT cases with five treatment fractions or less. In addition to 4DCT, motion simulation for ITV derivation based on 4DMRI or cine 2DMRI has been proposed and investigated.[141,274–276] However, 4DCT-based or RC-4DMRI-based motion simulation is based on single respiratory cycles and thus could be statistically unreliable.[277]

A treatment margin depends not only on the imaging modality chosen and tumor surrogate used but also on the type of patient immobilization and motion management technique employed. For respiratory motion, breath-hold, abdominal compression, respiratory gating, or motion tracking manage tumor motion at different levels. The respiratory-induced motion margin is patient-specific, as it is taken from 4DCT or 4DMRI at the simulation with an immobilization device. For instance, the motion

margin added to form the internal tumor volume (ITV) will be reduced with abdominal compression.[256,278] Due to patient breathing irregularities, it adds another level of uncertainty and complexity for the treatment of targets with respiratory-induced motion. The overall margin is the sum of all uncertainties from both inter- and intra-fractional motions.

For non-periodic organ motion, such as in prostate cases, IGRT margin reduction is one of the most dramatic examples in all anatomic sites. With in-room CT guidance, a 3-mm margin was reported adequate for prostate dose coverage, but may lose some of seminal vesicles coverage due to daily variation in rectal and bladder filling that causes local deformation.[279] A comparative study using four different IGRT setup methods, skin marks, 3D bony landmarks, 3D fiducial markers, and Calypso transponders, has shown that the last two methods can achieve 4 mm and 3 mm margin requirement, respectively.[280] A recent Calypso study has shown that a margin of 2 mm would produce sufficient CTV dose coverage based on 1,267 tracking sessions of 35 patients.[281] Figure 17.11 A demonstrates that the alignment accuracy increases along with the complexity of the alignment technology: from the skin to bone to ultrasound and CT.[8] The dosimetric result for one patient exhibiting large organ motion is shown in Figure 17.11B.

Anatomic Variations and Dosimetric Consequences

Inter- and Intra-fractional Variations in Anatomy
Substantial inter- and intra-fractional organ variations and setup uncertainties of lung, liver, diaphragm, gynecological, prostate, seminal vesicles, bladder, and

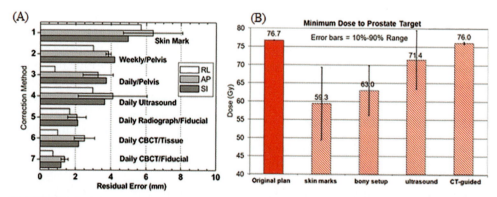

FIGURE 17.11. A: Patient setup accuracy of prostate cancer using different in-room imaging modalities. Generally, the accuracy increases with imaging frequency, dimension, and use of fiducial. The skin mark and ultrasound setup have the largest variation, as indicated by the error bars. The margin could be reduced from 8 to 2 mm based on this finding. *Source:* Reprinted with permission from Mageras GS and Mechalakos J, Planning in the IGRT context: Closing the loop, *Semin Radiat Oncol* 2007;17:268–77. **B:** Target coverage based on various types of image-guided setups for treatment. In this example, 24 treatment-time CT scans of a prostate cancer patient were used to compare the effectiveness of four alignment techniques for patient setup using a fixed-margin IMRT plan. The minimum target dose is lowest (59.3 Gy) for skin marks-based setup and highest (76.0 Gy) for the CT-guided setup. The day-to-day variations in the minimum dose (represented by the error bars) are smallest for CT-guided technique and largest for skin-mark and ultrasound-guided techniques.

rectum have been reviewed by Langen et al.[282] Even with careful immobilization and alignment of the patient, significant changes occur because of the nonrigidity of anatomy, bowel gas movement, and variable fillings of the bladder.[283] During a prostate IMRT treatment, changes in bladder filling can cause prostate and OARs to move away from the planning position, as demonstrated in Figure 17.12. Li et al. reported inter-fractional anatomic variations for all major sites based on daily CT assessment.[284] Target and OAR variations may follow certain trends, including tumor volume shrinkage up to 12 months after initial hormone treatment,[285] radiation-induced tumor shrinkage, and disease-related weight loss. Predictive treatment planning has been studied to anticipate tumor shrinkage due to radiation in lung treatment.[286] Figure 17.13 A shows a side-by-side comparison of a head and neck target volume that has shrunk significantly during the course of treatment and the skin contour no longer matches well with the immobilization mask. Changes in target volume and OAR position could have significant clinical consequences.[287,288]

Dosimetric Effects due to Inter-fractional Motion

The common approach to evaluating a delivered dose is to use the daily setup 3DCT images and actual dynamic leaf sequence from a treatment log file for dose reconstruction.[289] To generate a cumulative dose distribution over multiple fractions, dose mapping based on DIR is applied to a reference image for final dose evaluation.[228] Using MR-linac, the 2D cine data can be utilized to reconstruct 4DMRI images for more accurate dose evaluation, by incorporating intrafractional organ/tumor motions.[290,291]

In prostate cases, it is reported that 25% (8/33) of patients would have geometric or dosimetric miss without daily MVCT guidance to improve prostate localization.[292] Langen et al. have investigated the dosimetric consequences of prostate motion during helical tomotherapy for 16 patients with 515 daily MVCT scans.[293] The study finds that the mean change in target $D_{95\%}$ is 1% ± 4% and the average cumulative effect is smeared out after 5 fractions. In individual fractions, the $D_{95\%}$ may be off by up to 20%. In conventional fractionation, the dose error can be compensated statistically, but may not in hypo-fractionation SBRT treatment.[294] The adaptive re-planning based on daily volumetric MR image using MR-linac may overcome this problem.[295] For normal tissues, Chen et al. have reported that daily dose variation caused by rectal volume changes is significant and 27% of treatments would benefit from adaptive replanning.[296] Zelefsky et al. conducted a clinical study with 186 IGRT and

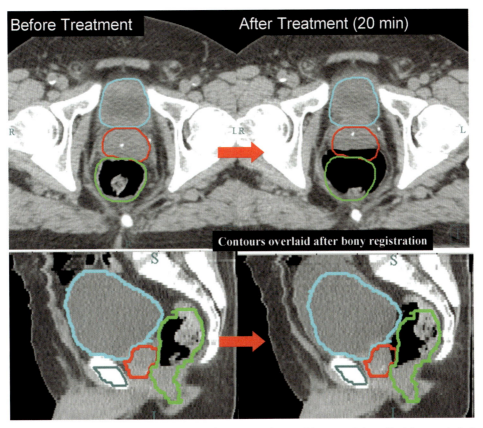

FIGURE 17.12. Intra-fractional variations of anatomy observed in a prostate patient in a period of 20 min. CT images were acquired just prior to and immediately after an IMRT treatment fraction. The contours of pelvic anatomy before treatment (left) are overlaid on the CT image of the patient acquired immediately after the treatment (right). Prostate target (red) was displaced anteriorly for >5 mm.

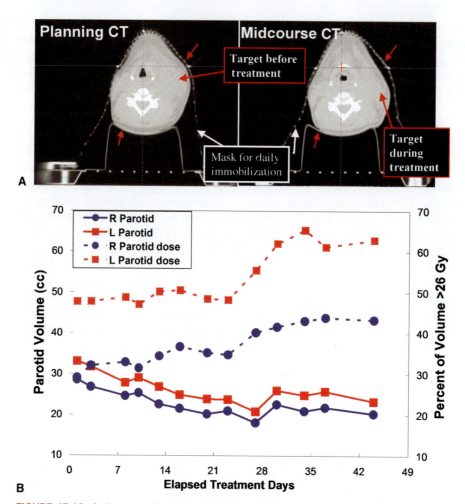

FIGURE 17.13. **A:** An example of setup error for a patient immobilized with a thermoplastic facemask due to tumor shrinkage as treatment progresses. Approximately halfway through the treatment course (right panel), the lower neck was not centered on the headrest, presumably due to the relatively "roomier" mask. **B:** Dosimetric impact of inter-fractional variations in head and neck anatomy. The solid lines show the volumes of the parotid glands (left and right) decreased as the treatment progressed. At the same time, the centers of both parotid glands also moved medially due to tumor shrinkage and weight loss. As a result, the percent of parotid volume exceeding 26 Gy increased by at least 10% over the course of radiotherapy.)

190 non-IGRT treatments and demonstrated significant improvement in biochemistry control at 3 years among high-risk prostate patients with IGRT versus non-IGRT (97% vs. 77%, p = 0.05).[297]

In head and neck treatments, it is desirable to reduce the dose to the parotid glands in order to minimize the incidence of late xerostomia.[298] Unfortunately, the parotid glands can decrease in volume and move medially during the course of treatment.[299] As a result, parotid mean dose increased by 10% and exceed 26 Gy (Fig. 17.13B). A single mid-course correction to adapt the treatment plan to the anatomical change can help reduce the dose for both parotid glands.[300] SBRT is mostly used only to treat a recurrent tumor in the head and neck.[301]

Dosimetric Effects of Intra-fractional Motion

Although the dosimetric consequence of intra-fractional breathing motion for lung tumors can be demonstrated by 4DCT-based planning, MR-linac has demonstrated its advantage in assessing the delivered dose more accurately. A tumor trailing can overcome baseline drifts of respiratory motion in liver SBRT treatments, as shown in Figure 17.14. Figure 15A shows a case study that used a free-breathing CT image to design a treatment plan with an inadequate 8-mm margin to cover the CTV (shown in yellow). The actual dose distribution does not cover the entire target volume in some of the breathing phases due to respiratory motion, which is not detected in the free-breathing CT. Using DIR, the cumulative dose distribution from the 10 individual phases is calculated and mapped to a free-breathing fast CT scan (near phase 7). The resultant cumulative dose distribution summed from the entire breathing cycle shows a dose deficiency in the CTV (red arrow), as illustrated in the bottom row of Figure 17.15B. In this case, the cumulative dose distribution when using the ITV derived from the 10-phase

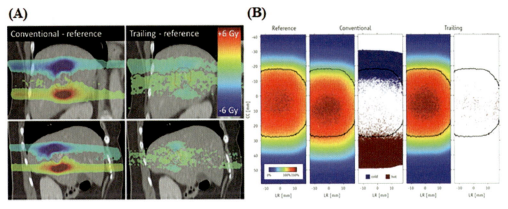

FIGURE 17.14. An example of tumor motion trailing to overcome the respiratory baseline drifts during the MRgRT of a liver cancer patient. **A:** Dose distribution differences compared between conventional and trailing reference images. **B:** Tumor dose coverage between conventional and trailing treatments. (*Source:* Reprinted with permission from Sonke, J. J. Tumor trailing for liver SBRT on the MR-Linac, *Int J Radiat Oncol Biol Phys*. 2019;103: 468–478.)

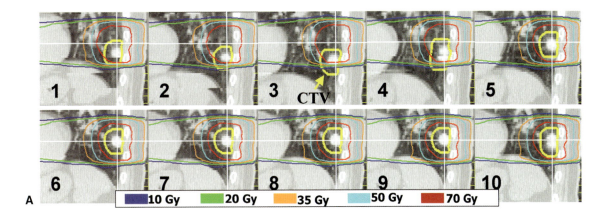

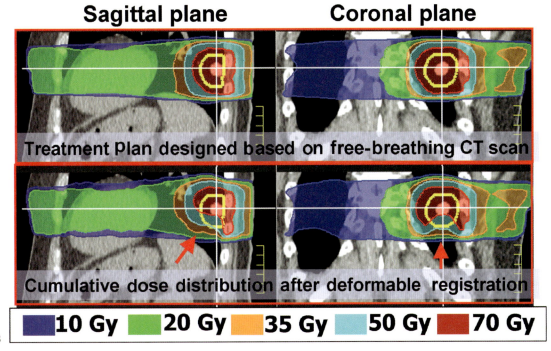

FIGURE 17.15. **A:** Potential consequence of respiratory motion on target coverage. An IMRT plan, developed using conventional CT, was applied to the patient's 4DCT. Dose distributions were calculated in each of the 10 phases of the breathing cycle. A portion of the CTV, shown in a thick yellow line, was not covered by the 70 Gy prescription dose line (red) in phases 1 through 4. **B:** Comparison of a treatment plan as perceived on a free-breathing CT (top row) and as realized after accounting for breathing motion in all 10 phases (bottom row). The latter was obtained by summing dose distributions computed on individual phases of the 4DCT image (**A**) and mapped to a reference CT image using deformable image registration (DIR).

4DCT does not underdose the target but results in treatment to a larger volume.

Adaptive Approaches for Correcting Dosimetric Deviations

The adaptive concept as applied to RT practice derives from modern informatics and control theory. William Beaumont Hospital has pioneered the adaptive RT strategy by using a purpose-built treatment planning system to facilitate offline dosimetric evaluation and replanning.[257,258] Offline adaptation has been implemented for various disease sites in various institutions,[254,302] and online replanning has been reported, with computation time within 5 to 8 min.[237] Mageras and Mechalakos have discussed treatment planning in the IGRT context and various challenges to treatment-plan adaptation strategies in various disease sites.[8] Studies from several groups have focused on implementing an automated treatment planning system[303,304] and an automatic CT simulation optimization strategy.[305] Using the MR-linac, adaptive replanning has become a clinical routine: depending on geometric deviation, online replanning can be realized as plan re-optimization with simple shift (rigid) or with recontouring and re-optimization (deformable).[81,306]

FUTURE DIRECTIONS

Image-guided RT is commonly considered in the context of treatment delivery, but it is more appropriate to broaden its scope to include imaging at other stages of the RT.[10] We, therefore, briefly discuss future directions as they apply to this broader definition.

We believe that further advances in IGRT rely on the innovation and integration of automated technologies to facilitate evaluation and decision-making processes. Automation in treatment simulation, planning, and delivery will be active areas of investigation, allowing standardization of treatment planning based on a planning library with optimal plans of all anatomical sites and planning optimization techniques. Technologies such as GPU,[220,307] cloud computing,[308,309] as well as deep machine learning[229,310,311] allow online 3D/4D image reconstruction, automatic organ/tumor segmentation, online plan re-optimization, and real-time tumor tracking. A new clinical workflow for adaptive IGRT has been implemented for MR-linac with the focus shifting from the routine planning process to personalized plan tailoring, plan QA, and treatment assessment and adaptation. Tattoo-free patient setup using OSI has emerged and potentially set a new clinical standard for SGRT setup and motion monitoring.

Further employment of multimodal imaging in both the simulation room and treatment room will be an active area of development. Functional imaging provides viable tumor volumes for planning and biological image guidance for treatment. MRI-based treatment planning has been applied in the clinic, especially with the use of MRI-linac, realizing adaptive IGRT clinically. MR-linac has visualized a moving tumor and OAR during treatment for the first time and could assist to minimize the chance of a marginal miss while maximally sparing nearby OARs. 2DMR Cine and TR 4DMRI to visualize tumor and OAR is more clinically desirable for tumor motion assessment at simulation and tumor motion monitoring during treatment. The BEV 2D cine guidance with tumor volume projection offers the ultimate check of beam conformality without interference of through-plane tumor motion.

Treatment response evaluation using multi-modality imaging will continue to be an active area of investigation. Treatment verification may be augmented with in-room PET, SPECT, MRI, or Cherenkov OSI. Due to the complexity of radiation response, a multi-level approach at the molecular, cellular, organ, and physiological levels is more likely to yield useful information. Different biological tracers could be designed to probe proper biological attributes, such as DNA double-strand breaks or cellular membrane rupture. Ideally, response assessment within the treatment course would be most beneficial for individualized treatments, while the reality is the lack of an effective assessment index even after treatment. A response-driven, biologically adaptive RT is still distant from clinical practice. However, the use of MR-linac in the clinic has made online treatment response assessment possible, and more studies are expected to emerge in this clinical research direction. The dosimetric feedback loop, which is within reach and will ensure that the treatment process goes along the intended course, can provide more reliable clinical data to tune prediction models of treatment outcome.

Radiation therapy has gone through a series of technological revolutions following multiple breakthroughs in medical imaging and RT in the past three decades. We have witnessed the growth of IGRT, which has provided improved geometric and dosimetric accuracy in radiation therapy of localized cancers. The combined SBRT with immunotherapy may have the ability to control distant metastasis, while the ultra-high dose rate FLASH has the potential to spare OAR maximally and unconventionally. We expect that more technological advances are forthcoming at all levels of IGRT, and further close the physical, biological, and clinical feedback loop for radiation therapy.

KEY POINTS

● In the application of IGRT to treatment delivery, we have a better understanding of various uncertainties, correction strategies, and technical limitations. Geometrically, a large body of evidence has shown the improved accuracy of IGRT in patient setup and motion management. Dosimetrically, IGRT improves treatment delivery in treatment plans that contain sharp dose gradients or mobile targets. Clinically, increasing evidence has revealed associations of local failure with a marginal miss and high-grade toxicity with organ motion.

● In this chapter, we have discussed the importance of image-guided radiation therapy (IGRT) and many in-room imaging modalities, which serve as visual and quantitative guidance for 3D/4D treatment simulation, accurate treatment planning, and image-guided treatment delivery. Using 2D cine imaging, 3D tomographic imaging, 4D respiratory-correlated or time-resolved imaging, the setup image before treatment is aligned to the planning image with reference to the radiation isocenter, so that the treatment can be delivered as planned. Tumor-tracking images during treatment serve to align the target with the radiation beam so that the mobile tumor is irradiated continuously or within a gating window.

● Implementation of IGRT requires various tools, QA procedures, and resources to achieve clinical objectives for radiotherapy. IGRT has been successfully implemented for all major anatomical sites and has been demonstrated to improve treatment accuracy with reduced uncertainty and margin requirements.

● In the past three decades, the evolution of IGRT has been punctuated with major technological advancements. In the future, IGRT will continue to evolve as emerging technologies and clinical challenges motivate investigations into promising new areas.

REVIEW QUESTIONS

1. On all isocentric linac machines, the kV and MV radiographic imaging are available commercially. Which of the following statements is incorrect in regard to kV and MV imaging?
   (1) The kV and MV images can be used together to produce a hybrid CBCT
   (2) The alignment of the kV and MV imaging isocenters should be periodically checked
   (3) The quality of kV imaging is better than that of MV imaging due to a large component of Compton scatters in the MV beam
   (4) The kV image quality can be improved by using a metal grid in front of the imager and post-acquisition image processing, the same techniques can be applied to MV image quality
   (5) Both kV and MV CBCT images can be used for evaluating the delivered dose, while MV CBCT has the advantage of fewer metal artifacts and no need for CT number conversion.
   A. (1)
   B. (2)
   C. (3)
   D. (4)
   E. (5)

2. A variety of in-room imaging modalities has been developed for IGRT procedures. Which of the following imaging modalities or non-imaging tools can be used for intrafractional real-time motion monitoring as a direct or indirect tumor motion surrogate?
   (1) 4DCT or 4D CBCT imaging
   (2) Gantry-mounted orthogonal 2DkV imaging
   (3) Room-mounted orthogonal 2DkV imaging
   (4) Infrared marker tracking system
   (5) Calypso electromagnetic transponder system
   A. (1) only
   B. (2) + (3)
   C. (2) + (4) + (5)
   D. (2) + (3) + (4) + (5)
   E. all above

3. A CBCT scan is acquired during a paraspinal SBRT procedure and ready for approval. However, the attending physician, who is with another patient, approves the image alignment 10 min later. The physicist on duty requests that the therapists take a verification orthogonal 2DkV image pair. Is the physicist's action correct and why?
   (1) No; there is no need for 2DkV verification since 2DkV alignment is inferior to CBCT.
   (2) No; there is no need for 2DkV verification since the physician has approved the CBCT,

(3) No; there is no need for 2DkV verification since the patient is immobilized in a mask,

(4) Yes; the 2DkV verification is necessary since the patient may have moved out,

(5) Yes; the orthogonal 2DkV images can provide six DOF registration via 2D/3D registration, so they can be used for verification of CBCT alignment.

A. (1) + (2) + (3)
B. (2) only
C. (3) only
D. (4) only
E. (4) + (5).

4. In a radiation oncology clinic, a frameless SRS (fSRS) procedure is implemented for clinical use. An end-to-end test is conducted using an anthropomorphic head phantom with inserted orthogonal films to deliver an fSRS plan and shows a 2-mm difference between the center of the delivered spherical dose distribution and the planning isocenter marked on the films. Which of the following factors could be the major causes of the observed discrepancy?

(1) A misalignment of the isocenter of the gantry-mounted kV and the MV beamlines;

(2) Couch walk that causes misalignment of the couch isocenter and radiation isocenter;

(3) Image registration error between the CBCT and planning CT;

(4) Couch sag at the setup position, since a 100-pound object was placed on the couch inferior to the phantom to mimic patient body weight;

(5) The film placed inside the head phantom with a small angle relative to the CT slices.

A. (1) + (2)
B. (1) + (3)
C. (1) + (2) + (3)
D. (1) + (2) + (3) + (5)
E. all 5.

5. When treating SBRT for a mobile tumor such as lung lesions, it is important to first align the target during patient setup and then to consider intrafractional motion management. Which of the following methods would introduce the largest uncertainty in tumor alignment?

(1) Using free-breathing CT for planning with the ITV delineated based on 4DCT and free-breathing CBCT for setup,

(2) Using respiratory-gated CT at full exhalation for both planning and CBCT setup,

(3) Using respiratory-gated CT at full inhalation for both planning and CBCT setup,

(4) Using motion-compensated mid-ventilation CT for planning and motion-compensated mid-ventilation CBCT for setup.

A. (1)
B. (2)
C. (3)
D. (4)
E. (1) and (3)

ANSWERS

1. D The MV image quality cannot be improved using the septa grid, as the MV photon can be further scattered by the metal grid, causing more scatters.

2. D (1) 4DCT or 4D CBCT are retrospectively reconstructed and cannot be used in real-time; (2) Varian and Elekta linac can only take orthogonal 2DkV one at a time, but VERO can take orthogonal fluoroscopic imaging simultaneously; (3) CyberKnife uses fluoroscopy for tumor tracking, (4) and (5) can be used as external and internal tumor tracking systems.

3. E After CBCT imaging, the alignment approval should be done immediately to avoid patient motion, even with an immobilization device. The orthogonal 2DkV imaging qualifies as a verification means to confirm the correctness of CBCT alignment.

4. C The kV and MV isocenter discrepancy and couch walk are transparent to image registration but will affect the setup accuracy. Couch sag and film angle are minor factors since they only cause rotational misalignment, which is secondary to translational misalignment.

5. C The full-inhalation phase is known to be irreproducible and therefore unreliable for tumor alignment.

REFERENCES

Uncategorized References

1. Park SS, Yan D, McGrath S, et al. Adaptive image-guided radiotherapy (IGRT) eliminates the risk of biochemical failure caused by the bias of rectal distension in prostate cancer treatment planning: clinical evidence. *Int J Radiat Oncol Biol Phys.* 2012;83(3):947–952.
2. Eisbruch A, Harris J, Garden AS, et al. Multi-institutional trial of accelerated hypofractionated intensity-modulated radiation therapy for early-stage oropharyngeal cancer (RTOG 00-22). *Int J Radiat Oncol Biol Phys.* 2010;76(5):1333–1338.
3. Tucker SL, Jin H, Wei X, et al. Impact of toxicity grade and scoring system on the relationship between mean lung dose and risk of radiation pneumonitis in a large cohort of patients with non-small cell lung cancer. *Int J Radiat Oncol Biol Phys.* 2010;77(3):691–698.
4. Leibel SA, Fuks Z, Zelefsky MJ, et al. Intensity-modulated radiotherapy. *Cancer J.* 2002;8(2):164–176.
5. Suit H. The Gray Lecture 2001: coming technical advances in radiation oncology. *Int J Radiat Oncol Biol Phys.* 2002;53(4):798–809.
6. Matuszak MM, Yan D, Grills I, Martinez A. Clinical applications of volumetric modulated arc therapy. *Int J Radiat Oncol Biol Phys.* 2010;77(2):608–616.
7. Sveistrup J, af Rosenschold PM, Deasy JO, et al. Improvement in toxicity in high risk prostate cancer patients treated with image-guided intensity-modulated radiotherapy compared to 3D conformal radiotherapy without daily image guidance. *Radiat Oncol.* 2014;9:44.
8. Mageras GS, Mechalakos J. Planning in the IGRT context: closing the loop. *Semin Radiat Oncol.* 2007;17(4):268–277.
9. van Herk M. Different styles of image-guided radiotherapy. *Semin Radiat Oncol.* 2007;17(4):258–267.
10. Greco C, Clifton Ling C. Broadening the scope of image-guided radiotherapy (IGRT). *Acta Oncol.* 2008;47(7):1193–1200.
11. Lagendijk JJ, Raaymakers BW, Raaijmakers AJ, et al. MRI/linac integration. *Radiother Oncol.* 2008;86(1):25–29.
12. Nishio T, Miyatake A, Ogino T, et al. The development and clinical use of a beam ON-LINE PET system mounted on a rotating gantry port in proton therapy. *Int J Radiat Oncol Biol Phys.* 2010;76(1):277–286.
13. Jarvis LA, Zhang R, Gladstone DJ, et al. Cherenkov video imaging allows for the first visualization of radiation therapy in real time. *Int J Radiat Oncol Biol Phys.* 2014;89(3):615–622.
14. Yamada Y, Lovelock DM, Yenice KM, et al. Multifractionated image-guided and stereotactic intensity-modulated radiotherapy of paraspinal tumors: a preliminary report. *Int J Radiat Oncol Biol Phys.* 2005;62(1):53–61.
15. Mao W, Speiser M, Medin P, et al. Initial application of a geometric QA tool for integrated MV and kV imaging systems on three image guided radiotherapy systems. *Med Phys.* 2011;38(5):2335–2341.
16. Dorsch S, Mann P, Elter A, et al. Measurement of isocenter alignment accuracy and image distortion of an 0.35 T MR-Linac system. *Phys Med Biol.* 2019;64(20):205011.
17. Li G, Ballangrud A, Kuo LC, et al. Motion monitoring for cranial frameless stereotactic radiosurgery using video-based three-dimensional optical surface imaging. *Med Phys.* 2011;38(7):3981–3994.
18. Li G, Ballangrud A, Chan M, et al. Clinical experience with two frameless stereotactic radiosurgery (fSRS) systems using optical surface imaging for motion monitoring. *J Appl Clin Med Phys.* 2015;16(4):5416.
19. Boyer AL, Antonuk L, Fenster A, et al. A review of electronic portal imaging devices (EPIDs). *Med Phys.* 1992;19(1):1–16.
20. van Elmpt W, McDermott L, Nijsten S, et al. A literature review of electronic portal imaging for radiotherapy dosimetry. *Radiother Oncol.* 2008;88(3):289–309.
21. Mans A, Remeijer P, Olaciregui-Ruiz I, et al. 3D dosimetric verification of volumetric-modulated arc therapy by portal dosimetry. *Radiother Oncol.* 2010;94(2):181–187.
22. Russo GA, Qureshi MM, Truong MT, et al. Daily orthogonal kilovoltage imaging using a gantry-mounted on-board imaging system results in a reduction in radiation therapy delivery errors. *Int J Radiat Oncol Biol Phys.* 2012;84(3):596–601.
23. Kalender WA. Dose in x-ray computed tomography. *Phys Med Biol.* 2014;59(3):R129–150.
24. Yue NJ, Kim S, Lewis BE, et al. Optimization of couch translational corrections to compensate for rotational and deformable target deviations in image guided radiotherapy. *Med Phys.* 2008;35(10):4375–4385.
25. Hugo GD, Weiss E, Badawi A, Orton M. Localization accuracy of the clinical target volume during image-guided radiotherapy of lung cancer. *Int J Radiat Oncol Biol Phys.* 2011;81(2):560–567.
26. Uematsu M, Fukui T, Shioda A, et al. A dual computed tomography linear accelerator unit for stereotactic radiation therapy: a new approach without cranially fixated stereotactic frames. *Int J Radiat Oncol Biol Phys.* 1996;35(3):587–592.
27. Yenice KM, Lovelock DM, Hunt MA, et al. CT image-guided intensity-modulated therapy for paraspinal tumors using stereotactic immobilization. *Int J Radiat Oncol Biol Phys.* 2003;55(3):583–593.
28. Hua C, Lovelock DM, Mageras GS, et al. Development of a semi-automatic alignment tool for accelerated localization of the prostate. *Int J Radiat Oncol Biol Phys.* 2003;55(3):811–824.
29. Wong JR, Cheng CW, Grimm L, Uematsu M. Clinical implementation of the world's first primatom, a combination of CT scanner and linear accelerator, for precise tumor targeting and treatment. *Phys Med.* 2001;17(4):271–276.
30. Court L, Rosen I, Mohan R, Dong L. Evaluation of mechanical precision and alignment uncertainties for an integrated CT/LINAC system. *Med Phys.* 2003;30(6):1198–1210.
31. Shiu AS, Chang EL, Ye JS, et al. Near simultaneous computed tomography image-guided stereotactic spinal radiotherapy: an emerging paradigm for achieving true stereotaxy. *Int J Radiat Oncol Biol Phys.* 2003;57(3):605–613.
32. Jaffray DA, Drake DG, Moreau M, et al. A radiographic and tomographic imaging system integrated into a medical linear accelerator for localization of bone and soft-tissue targets. *Int J Radiat Oncol Biol Phys.* 1999;45(3):773–789.
33. Siewerdsen JH, Moseley DJ, Bakhtiar B, et al. The influence of antiscatter grids on soft-tissue detectability in cone-beam computed tomography with flat-panel detectors. *Med Phys.* 2004;31(12):3506–3520.
34. Cho PS, Rudd AD, Johnson RH. Cone-beam CT from width-truncated projections. *Comput Med Imaging Graph.* 1996;20(1):49–57.
35. Lim TY, Dragojevic I, Hoffman D, et al. Characterization of the Halcyon(TM) multileaf collimator system. *J Appl Clin Med Phys.* 2019;20(4):106–114.
36. De Roover R, Crijns W, Poels K, et al. Validation and IMRT/VMAT delivery quality of a preconfigured fast-rotating O-ring linac system. *Med Phys.* 2019;46(1):328–339.
37. Stankovic U, van Herk M, Ploeger LS, Sonke JJ. Improved image quality of cone beam CT scans for radiotherapy image guidance using fiber-interspaced antiscatter grid. *Med Phys.* 2014;41(6):061910.
38. Gardner SJ, Studenski MT, Giaddui T, et al. Investigation into image quality and dose for different patient geometries with multiple cone-beam CT systems. *Med Phys.* 2014;41(3):031908.
39. Kim J, Lu W, Zhang T. Dual source and dual detector arrays tetrahedron beam computed tomography for image guided radiotherapy. *Phys Med Biol.* 2014;59(3):615–630.
40. Mackie TR, Holmes T, Swerdloff S, et al. Tomotherapy: a new concept for the delivery of dynamic conformal radiotherapy. *Med Phys.* 1993;20(6):1709–1719.
41. Ruchala KJ, Olivera GH, Schloesser EA, Mackie TR. Megavoltage CT on a tomotherapy system. *Phys Med Biol.* 1999;44(10):2597–2621.
42. Forrest LJ, Mackie TR, Ruchala K, et al. The utility of megavoltage computed tomography images from a helical tomotherapy system for setup verification purposes. *Int J Radiat Oncol Biol Phys.* 2004;60(5):1639–1644.
43. Swindell W, Simpson RG, Oleson JR, et al. Computed-tomography with a linear-accelerator with radiotherapy applications. *Med Phys.* 1983;10(4):416–420.

44. Mosleh-Shirazi MA, Evans PM, Swindell W, et al. A cone-beam megavoltage CT scanner for treatment verification in conformal radiotherapy. *Radiother Oncol.* 1998;48(3):319–328.

45. Sillanpaa J, Chang J, Mageras G, et al. Developments in megavoltage cone beam CT with an amorphous silicon EPID: reduction of exposure and synchronization with respiratory gating. *Med Phys.* 2005;32(3):819–829.

46. Pouliot J, Bani-Hashemi A, Chen J, et al. Low-dose megavoltage cone-beam CT for radiation therapy. *Int J Radiat Oncol Biol Phys.* 2005;61(2):552–560.

47. Kupelian PA, Ramsey C, Meeks SL, et al. Serial megavoltage CT imaging during external beam radiotherapy for non-small-cell lung cancer: observations on tumor regression during treatment. *Int J Radiat Oncol Biol Phys.* 2005;63(4):1024–1028.

48. Langen KM, Meeks SL, Poole DO, et al. The use of megavoltage CT (MVCT) images for dose recomputations. *Phys Med Biol.* 2005;50(18):4259–4276.

49. Yin FF, Guan H, Lu W. A technique for on-board CT reconstruction using both kilovoltage and megavoltage beam projections for 3D treatment verification. *Med Phys.* 2005;32(9):2819–2826.

50. Blessing M, Stsepankou D, Wertz H, et al. Breath-hold target localization with simultaneous kilovoltage/megavoltage cone-beam computed tomography and fast reconstruction. *Int J Radiat Oncol Biol Phys.* 2010;78(4):1219–1226.

51. Kolitsi Z, Panayiotakis G, Anastassopoulos V, et al. A multiple projection method for digital tomosynthesis. *Med Phys.* 1992;19(4):1045–1050.

52. Godfrey DJ, Yin FF, Oldham M, et al. Digital tomosynthesis with an on-board kilovoltage imaging device. *Int J Radiat Oncol Biol Phys.* 2006;65(1):8–15.

53. Santoro J, Kriminski S, Lovelock DM, et al. Evaluation of respiration-correlated digital tomosynthesis in lung. *Med Phys.* 2010;37(3):1237–1245.

54. Keall PJ, Mageras GS, Balter JM, et al. The management of respiratory motion in radiation oncology report of AAPM Task Group 76. *Med Phys.* 2006;33(10):3874–3900.

55. Low DA, Nystrom M, Kalinin E, et al. A method for the reconstruction of four-dimensional synchronized CT scans acquired during free breathing. *Med Phys.* 2003;30(6):1254–1263.

56. Pan T, Lee TY, Rietzel E, Chen GT. 4D-CT imaging of a volume influenced by respiratory motion on multi-slice CT. *Med Phys.* 2004;31(2):333–340.

57. Ford EC, Mageras GS, Yorke E, Ling CC. Respiration-correlated spiral CT: a method of measuring respiratory-induced anatomic motion for radiation treatment planning. *Med Phys.* 2003;30(1):88–97.

58. Vedam SS, Keall PJ, Kini VR, et al. Acquiring a four-dimensional computed tomography dataset using an external respiratory signal. *Phys Med Biol.* 2003;48(1):45–62.

59. Keall P. 4-dimensional computed tomography imaging and treatment planning. *Semin Radiat Oncol.* 2004;14(1):81–90.

60. Mageras GS, Pevsner A, Yorke ED, et al. Measurement of lung tumor motion using respiration-correlated CT. *Int J Radiat Oncol Biol Phys.* 2004;60(3):933–941.

61. Yamamoto T, Langner U, Loo BW, Jr., et al. Retrospective analysis of artifacts in four-dimensional CT images of 50 abdominal and thoracic radiotherapy patients. *Int J Radiat Oncol Biol Phys.* 2008;72(4):1250–1258.

62. Li G, Caraveo M, Wei J, et al. Rapid estimation of 4DCT motion-artifact severity based on 1D breathing-surrogate periodicity. *Med Phys.* 2014;41(11):111717.

63. Lu W, Parikh PJ, Hubenschmidt JP, et al. A comparison between amplitude sorting and phase-angle sorting using external respiratory measurement for 4D CT. *Med Phys.* 2006;33(8):2964–2974.

64. Abdelnour AF, Nehmeh SA, Pan T, et al. Phase and amplitude binning for 4D-CT imaging. *Phys Med Biol.* 2007;52(12):3515–3529.

65. Coolens C, Bracken J, Driscoll B, et al. Dynamic volume vs respiratory correlated 4DCT for motion assessment in radiation therapy simulation. *Med Phys.* 2012;39(5):2669–2681.

66. Hertanto A, Zhang Q, Hu YC, et al. Reduction of irregular breathing artifacts in respiration-correlated CT images using a respiratory motion model. *Med Phys.* 2012;39(6):3070–3079.

67. Thomas D, Lamb J, White B, et al. A novel fast helical 4D-CT acquisition technique to generate low-noise sorting artifact-free images at user-selected breathing phases. *Int J Radiat Oncol Biol Phys.* 2014;89(1):191–198.

68. Sonke JJ, Zijp L, Remeijer P, van Herk M. Respiratory correlated cone beam CT. *Med Phys.* 2005;32(4):1176–1186.

69. Purdie TG, Moseley DJ, Bissonnette JP, et al. Respiration correlated cone-beam computed tomography and 4DCT for evaluating target motion in Stereotactic Lung Radiation Therapy. *Acta Oncol.* 2006;45(7):915–922.

70. Li T, Xing L, Munro P, et al. Four-dimensional cone-beam computed tomography using an on-board imager. *Med Phys.* 2006;33(10):3825–3833.

71. Rit S, Wolthaus JW, van Herk M, Sonke JJ. On-the-fly motion-compensated cone-beam CT using an a priori model of the respiratory motion. *Med Phys.* 2009;36(6):2283–2296.

72. Zhang Q, Hu YC, Liu F, et al. Correction of motion artifacts in cone-beam CT using a patient-specific respiratory motion model. *Med Phys.* 2010;37(6):2901–2909.

73. Rit S, Nijkamp J, van Herk M, Sonke JJ. Comparative study of respiratory motion correction techniques in cone-beam computed tomography. *Radiother Oncol.* 2011;100(3):356–359.

74. Dzyubak O, Kincaid R, Hertanto A, et al. Evaluation of tumor localization in respiration motion-corrected cone-beam CT: prospective study in lung. *Med Phys.* 2014;41(10):101918.

75. Kincaid RE, Jr., Yorke ED, Goodman KA, et al. Investigation of gated cone-beam CT to reduce respiratory motion blurring. *Med Phys.* 2013;40(4):041717.

76. Wang D, Doddrell DM. A proposed scheme for comprehensive characterization of the measured geometric distortion in magnetic resonance imaging using a three-dimensional phantom. *Med Phys.* 2004;31(8):2212–2218.

77. Mutic S, Dempsey JF. The ViewRay system: magnetic resonance-guided and controlled radiotherapy. *Semin Radiat Oncol.* 2014;24(3):196–199.

78. Kluter S. Technical design and concept of a 0.35 T MR-Linac. *Clin Transl Radiat Oncol.* 2019;18:98–101.

79. Raaijmakers AJ, Raaymakers BW, Lagendijk JJ. Integrating a MRI scanner with a 6 MV radiotherapy accelerator: dose increase at tissue-air interfaces in a lateral magnetic field due to returning electrons. *Phys Med Biol.* 2005;50(7):1363–1376.

80. Lagendijk JJ, Raaymakers BW, Van den Berg CA, et al. MR guidance in radiotherapy. *Phys Med Biol.* 2014;59(21):R349–369.

81. Winkel D, Bol GH, Kroon PS, et al. Adaptive radiotherapy: The Elekta Unity MR-linac concept. *Clin Transl Radiat Oncol.* 2019;18:54–59.

82. Raaymakers BW, Jurgenliemk-Schulz IM, Bol GH, et al. First patients treated with a 1.5 T MRI-Linac: clinical proof of concept of a high-precision, high-field MRI guided radiotherapy treatment. *Phys Med Biol.* 2017;62(23):L41–L50.

83. Kolling S, Oborn B, Keall P. Impact of the MLC on the MRI field distortion of a prototype MRI-linac. *Med Phys.* 2013;40(12):121705.

84. Raaymakers BW, de Boer JC, Knox C, et al. Integrated megavoltage portal imaging with a 1.5 T MRI linac. *Phys Med Biol.* 2011;56(19):N207–214.

85. Woodings SJ, Bluemink JJ, de Vries JHW, et al. Beam characterisation of the 1.5 T MRI-linac. *Phys Med Biol.* 2018;63(8):085015.

86. Snyder JE, St-Aubin J, Yaddanapudi S, et al. Commissioning of a 1.5T Elekta Unity MR-linac: a single institution experience. *J Appl Clin Med Phys.* 2020;21(7):160–172.

87. Tijssen RHN, Philippens MEP, Paulson ES, et al. MRI commissioning of 1.5T MR-linac systems—a multi-institutional study. *Radiother Oncol.* 2019;132:114–120.

88. Schneider S, Dolde K, Engler J, et al. Commissioning of a 4D MRI phantom for use in MR-guided radiotherapy. *Med Phys.* 2019;46(1):25–33.

89. Elter A, Dorsch S, Mann P, et al. End-to-end test of an online adaptive treatment procedure in MR-guided radiotherapy using a phantom with anthropomorphic structures. *Phys Med Biol.* 2019;64(22):225003.

90. Keall PJ, Barton M, Crozier S, et al. The Australian magnetic resonance imaging-linac program. *Semin Radiat Oncol.* 2014;24(3):203–206.

91. Liney GP, Whelan B, Oborn B, et al. MRI-Linear Accelerator Radiotherapy Systems. *Clin Oncol (R Coll Radiol)*. 2018;30(11):686–691.

92. Fallone BG. The rotating biplanar linac-magnetic resonance imaging system. *Semin Radiat Oncol*. 2014;24(3):200–202.

93. Jaffray DA, Carlone MC, Milosevic MF, et al. A facility for magnetic resonance-guided radiation therapy. *Semin Radiat Oncol*. 2014;24(3):193–195.

94. Chen L, Price RA, Jr., Wang L, et al. MRI-based treatment planning for radiotherapy: dosimetric verification for prostate IMRT. *Int J Radiat Oncol Biol Phys*. 2004;60(2):636–647.

95. Wang C, Chao M, Lee L, Xing L. MRI-based treatment planning with electron density information mapped from CT images: a preliminary study. *Technol Cancer Res Treat*. 2008;7(5):341–348.

96. Metcalfe P, Liney GP, Holloway L, et al. The potential for an enhanced role for MRI in radiation-therapy treatment planning. *Technol Cancer Res Treat*. 2013;12(5):429–446.

97. Wang H, Balter J, Cao Y. Patient-induced susceptibility effect on geometric distortion of clinical brain MRI for radiation treatment planning on a 3T scanner. *Phys Med Biol*. 2013;58(3):465–477.

98. Weiss S, Nejad-Davarani S, Eggers H, et al. A novel and rapid approach to estimate patient-specific distortions based on mDIXON MRI. *Phys Med Biol*. 2019;64(15):155002.

99. Farjam R, Tyagi N, Veeraraghavan H, et al. Multiatlas approach with local registration goodness weighting for MRI-based electron density mapping of head and neck anatomy. *Med Phys*. 2017;44(7):3706–3717.

100. Maspero M, van den Berg CAT, Landry G, et al. Feasibility of MR-only proton dose calculations for prostate cancer radiotherapy using a commercial pseudo-CT generation method. *Phys Med Biol*. 2017;62(24):9159–9176.

101. Klages P, Benslimane I, Riyahi S, et al. Patch-based generative adversarial neural network models for head and neck MR-only planning. *Med Phys*. 2019.

102. Lei Y, Harms J, Wang T, et al. MRI-based synthetic CT generation using semantic random forest with iterative refinement. *Phys Med Biol*. 2019;64(8):085001.

103. Dowling JA, Lambert J, Parker J, et al. An atlas-based electron density mapping method for magnetic resonance imaging (MRI)-alone treatment planning and adaptive MRI-based prostate radiation therapy. *Int J Radiat Oncol Biol Phys*. 2012;83(1):e5–11.

104. Farjam R, Tyagi N, Deasy JO, Hunt MA. Dosimetric evaluation of an atlas-based synthetic CT generation approach for MR-only radiotherapy of pelvis anatomy. *J Appl Clin Med Phys*. 2019;20(1):101–109.

105. Dinkla AM, Wolterink JM, Maspero M, et al. MR-Only Brain Radiation Therapy: dosimetric Evaluation of Synthetic CTs Generated by a Dilated Convolutional Neural Network. *Int J Radiat Oncol Biol Phys*. 2018;102(4):801–812.

106. Tyagi N, Fontenla S, Zhang J, et al. Dosimetric and workflow evaluation of first commercial synthetic CT software for clinical use in pelvis. *Phys Med Biol*. 2017;62(8):2961–2975.

107. Zhang J, Srivastava S, Wang C, et al. Clinical evaluation of 4D MRI in the delineation of gross and internal tumor volumes in comparison with 4DCT. *J Appl Clin Med Phys*. 2019;20(9):51–60.

108. Zhang J, Markova S, Garcia A, et al. Evaluation of automatic contour propagation in T2-weighted 4DMRI for normal-tissue motion assessment using internal organ-at-risk volume (IRV). *J Appl Clin Med Phys*. 2018;19(5):598–608.

109. Hama Y, Tate E. Comparison of gross tumor volumes of pulmonary metastasis defined by CT and MRI in 0.345 T MRI-guided radiotherapy. *BJR Open*. 2020;2(1):20200010.

110. Gou S, Lee P, Hu P, et al. Feasibility of automated 3-dimensional magnetic resonance imaging pancreas segmentation. *Adv Radiat Oncol*. 2016;1(3):182–193.

111. Tseng CL, Stewart J, Whitfield G, et al. Glioma consensus contouring recommendations from a MR-Linac International Consortium Research Group and evaluation of a CT-MRI and MRI-only workflow. *J Neurooncol*. 2020;149(2):305–314.

112. Jiang J, Hu YC, Tyagi N, et al. Self-derived organ attention for unpaired CT-MRI deep domain adaptation based MRI segmentation. *Phys Med Biol*. 2020;65(20):205001.

113. Li G, Citrin D, Camphausen K, et al. Advances in 4D medical imaging and 4D radiation therapy. *Technol Cancer Res Treat*. 2008;7(1):67–81.

114. Cai J, Chang Z, Wang Z, et al. Four-dimensional magnetic resonance imaging (4D-MRI) using image-based respiratory surrogate: a feasibility study. *Med Phys*. 2011;38(12):6384–6394.

115. Liu Y, Yin FF, Czito BG, et al. T2-weighted four dimensional magnetic resonance imaging with result-driven phase sorting. *Med Phys*. 2015;42(8):4460.

116. Hu Y, Caruthers SD, Low DA, et al. Respiratory amplitude guided 4-dimensional magnetic resonance imaging. *Int J Radiat Oncol Biol Phys*. 2013;86(1):198–204.

117. Li G, Wei J, Olek D, et al. Direct comparison of respiration-correlated four-dimensional magnetic resonance imaging reconstructed using concurrent internal navigator and external bellows. *Int J Radiat Oncol Biol Phys*. 2017;97(3):596–605.

118. Mickevicius NJ, Paulson ES. Simultaneous acquisition of orthogonal plane cine imaging and isotropic 4D-MRI using super-resolution. *Radiother Oncol*. 2019;136:121–129.

119. Plathow C, Klopp M, Schoebinger M, et al. Monitoring of lung motion in patients with malignant pleural mesothelioma using two-dimensional and three-dimensional dynamic magnetic resonance imaging: comparison with spirometry. *Invest Radiol*. 2006;41(5):443–448.

120. Li G, Wei J, Kadbi M, et al. Novel Super-Resolution Approach to Time-Resolved Volumetric 4-Dimensional Magnetic Resonance Imaging With High Spatiotemporal Resolution for Multi-Breathing Cycle Motion Assessment. *Int J Radiat Oncol Biol Phys*. 2017;98(2):454–462.

121. Nie X, Huang K, Deasy J, et al. Enhanced super-resolution reconstruction of T1w time-resolved 4DMRI in low-contrast tissue using 2-step hybrid deformable image registration. *J Appl Clin Med Phys*. 2020;21(10):25–39.

122. Nie X, Saleh Z, Kadbi M, et al. A super-resolution framework for the reconstruction of T2-weighted (T2w) time-resolved (TR) 4DMRI using T1w TR-4DMRI as the guidance. *Med Phys*. 2020;47(7):3091–3102.

123. Yan S, Bowsher J, Yin FF. A line-source method for aligning on-board and other pinhole SPECT systems. *Med Phys*. 2013;40(12):122501.

124. Zhu X, Espana S, Daartz J, et al. Monitoring proton radiation therapy with in-room PET imaging. *Phys Med Biol*. 2011;56(13):4041–4057.

125. Fan Q, Nanduri A, Mazin S, Zhu L. Emission guided radiation therapy for lung and prostate cancers: a feasibility study on a digital patient. *Med Phys*. 2012;39(11):7140–7152.

126. Fontanarosa D, van der Meer S, Bamber J, et al. Review of ultrasound image guidance in external beam radiotherapy: I. Treatment planning and inter-fraction motion management. *Phys Med Biol*. 2015;60(3):R77–114.

127. Fuss M, Cavanaugh SX, Fuss C, et al. Daily stereotactic ultrasound prostate targeting: inter-user variability. *Technol Cancer Res Treat*. 2003;2(2):161–170.

128. Scarbrough TJ, Golden NM, Ting JY, et al. Comparison of ultrasound and implanted seed marker prostate localization methods: implications for image-guided radiotherapy. *Int J Radiat Oncol Biol Phys*. 2006;65(2):378–387.

129. Bert C, Metheany KG, Doppke K, Chen GT. A phantom evaluation of a stereo-vision surface imaging system for radiotherapy patient setup. *Med Phys*. 2005;32(9):2753–2762.

130. Djajaputra D, Li S. Real-time 3D surface-image-guided beam setup in radiotherapy of breast cancer. *Med Phys*. 2005;32(1):65–75.

131. Hoisak JDP, Pawlicki T. The Role of Optical Surface Imaging Systems in Radiation Therapy. *Semin Radiat Oncol*. 2018;28(3):185–193.

132. Jimenez RB, Batin E, Giantsoudi D, et al. Tattoo free setup for partial breast irradiation: a feasibility study. *J Appl Clin Med Phys*. 2019;20(4):45–50.

133. Zhao H, Williams N, Poppe M, et al. Comparison of surface guidance and target matching for image-guided accelerated partial breast irradiation (APBI). *Med Phys*. 2019;46(11):4717–4724.

134. Zhang R, Andreozzi JM, Gladstone DJ, et al. Cherenkoscopy based patient positioning validation and movement tracking during post-lumpectomy whole breast radiation therapy. *Phys Med Biol.* 2015;60(1):L1–14.

135. Wen N, Li H, Song K, et al. Characteristics of a novel treatment system for linear accelerator-based stereotactic radiosurgery. *J Appl Clin Med Phys.* 2015;16(4):125–148.

136. Li R, Lewis JH, Cervino LI, Jiang SB. A feasibility study of markerless fluoroscopic gating for lung cancer radiotherapy using 4DCT templates. *Phys Med Biol.* 2009;54(20):N489–500.

137. Rottmann J, Keall P, Berbeco R. Markerless EPID image guided dynamic multi-leaf collimator tracking for lung tumors. *Phys Med Biol.* 2013;58(12):4195–4204.

138. Zhang P, Hunt M, Telles AB, et al. Design and validation of a MV/kV imaging-based markerless tracking system for assessing real-time lung tumor motion. *Med Phys.* 2018;45(12):5555–5563.

139. Sawant A, Smith RL, Venkat RB, et al. Toward submillimeter accuracy in the management of intrafraction motion: the integration of real-time internal position monitoring and multileaf collimator target tracking. *Int J Radiat Oncol Biol Phys.* 2009;74(2):575–582.

140. Cervino LI, Pawlicki T, Lawson JD, Jiang SB. Frame-less and mask-less cranial stereotactic radiosurgery: a feasibility study. *Phys Med Biol.* 2010;55(7):1863–1873.

141. Tryggestad E, Flammang A, Hales R, et al. 4D tumor centroid tracking using orthogonal 2D dynamic MRI: implications for radiotherapy planning. *Med Phys.* 2013;40(9):091712.

142. Murphy MJ. Tracking moving organs in real time. *Semin Radiat Oncol.* 2004;14(1):91–100.

143. Jin JY, Yin FF, Tenn SE, et al. Use of the BrainLAB ExacTrac X-Ray 6D system in image-guided radiotherapy. *Med Dosim.* 2008;33(2):124–134.

144. Keall PJ, Aun Ng J, O'Brien R, et al. The first clinical treatment with kilovoltage intrafraction monitoring (KIM): a real-time image guidance method. *Med Phys.* 2015;42(1):354–358.

145. Keall PJ, Nguyen DT, O'Brien R, et al. The first clinical implementation of real-time image-guided adaptive radiotherapy using a standard linear accelerator. *Radiother Oncol.* 2018;127(1):6–11.

146. Solberg TD, Medin PM, Ramirez E, et al. Commissioning and initial stereotactic ablative radiotherapy experience with Vero. *J Appl Clin Med Phys.* 2014;15(2):4685.

147. Depuydt T, Verellen D, Haas O, et al. Geometric accuracy of a novel gimbals based radiation therapy tumor tracking system. *Radiother Oncol.* 2011;98(3):365–372.

148. Poels K, Depuydt T, Verellen D, et al. A complementary dual-modality verification for tumor tracking on a gimbaled linac system. *Radiother Oncol.* 2013;109(3):469–474.

149. Burghelea M, Verellen D, Gevaert T, et al. Feasibility of using the Vero SBRT system for intracranial SRS. *J Appl Clin Med Phys.* 2014;15(1):4437.

150. Hoogeman M, Prevost JB, Nuyttens J, et al. Clinical accuracy of the respiratory tumor tracking system of the cyberknife: assessment by analysis of log files. *Int J Radiat Oncol Biol Phys.* 2009;74(1):297–303.

151. Zeng C, Xiong W, Li X, et al. Intrafraction tumor motion during deep inspiration breath hold pancreatic cancer treatment. *J Appl Clin Med Phys.* 2019;20(5):37–43.

152. Llacer-Moscardo C, Riou O, Azria D, et al. Imaged-guided liver stereotactic body radiotherapy using VMAT and real-time adaptive tumor gating. Concerns about technique and preliminary clinical results. *Rep Pract Oncol Radiother.* 2017;22(2):141–149.

153. Kaur G, Lehmann J, Greer P, Simpson J. Assessment of the accuracy of truebeam intrafraction motion review (IMR) system for prostate treatment guidance. *Australas Phys Eng Sci Med.* 2019;42(2):585–598.

154. Korpics MC, Rokni M, Degnan M, et al. Utilizing the TrueBeam Advanced Imaging Package to monitor intrafraction motion with periodic kV imaging and automatic marker detection during VMAT prostate treatments. *J Appl Clin Med Phys.* 2020;21(3):184–191.

155. Yan H, Li H, Liu Z, et al. Hybrid MV-kV 3D respiratory motion tracking during radiation therapy with low imaging dose. *Phys Med Biol.* 2012;57(24):8455–8469.

156. Azcona JD, Li R, Mok E, et al. Development and clinical evaluation of automatic fiducial detection for tumor tracking in cine megavoltage images during volumetric modulated arc therapy. *Med Phys.* 2013;40(3):031708.

157. Nicolini G, Clivio A, Vanetti E, et al. Evaluation of an aSi-EPID with flattening filter free beams: applicability to the GLAaS algorithm for portal dosimetry and first experience for pretreatment QA of RapidArc. *Med Phys.* 2013;40(11):111719.

158. Nakagawa K, Haga A, Shiraishi K, et al. First clinical cone-beam CT imaging during volumetric modulated arc therapy. *Radiother Oncol.* 2009;90(3):422–423.

159. Ling C, Zhang P, Etmektzoglou T, et al. Acquisition of MV-scatter-free kilovoltage CBCT images during RapidArc or VMAT. *Radiother Oncol.* 2011;100(1):145–149.

160. Zhang P, Hunt M, Happersett L, et al. Incorporation of treatment plan spatial and temporal dose patterns into a prostate intrafractional motion management strategy. *Med Phys.* 2012;39(9):5429–5436.

161. Happersett L, Wang P, Zhang P, et al. Developing a MLC modifier program to improve fiducial detection for MV/kV imaging during hypofractionated prostate volumetric modulated arc therapy. *J Appl Clin Med Phys.* 2019;20(6):120–124.

162. Meeks SL, Tome WA, Willoughby TR, et al. Optically guided patient positioning techniques. *Semin Radiat Oncol.* 2005;15(3):192–201.

163. Li G. Commissioning and routine quality assurance of the VisionRT AlignRT system. In: Hoisak JD, Paxton A, Waghorn BJ, Pawlicki T, editors. *Surface Guided Radiation Therapy.* 1st ed. Boca Raton, FL: CRC Press, Taylor & Francis Group; 2020:157–186.

164. Li G, Huang H, Wei J, et al. Novel Spirometry based on optical surface imaging. *Med Phys.* 2015;42(4):1690.

165. Li G, Yuan A, Wei J. (ORAL) An analytical respiratory perturbation model for lung motion prediction. *Medical Phys.* 2014;41(6):473–473.

166. Balter JM, Wright JN, Newell LJ, et al. Accuracy of a wireless localization system for radiotherapy. *Int J Radiat Oncol Biol Phys.* 2005;61(3):933–937.

167. Shah AP, Kupelian PA, Waghorn BJ, et al. Real-time tumor tracking in the lung using an electromagnetic tracking system. *Int J Radiat Oncol Biol Phys.* 2013;86(3):477–483.

168. Keall PJ, Joshi S, Vedam SS, et al. Four-dimensional radiotherapy planning for DMLC-based respiratory motion tracking. *Med Phys.* 2005;32(4):942–951.

169. Kontaxis C, Bol GH, Stemkens B, et al. Towards fast online intrafraction replanning for free-breathing stereotactic body radiation therapy with the MR-linac. *Phys Med Biol.* 2017;62(18):7233–7248.

170. Nie X, Rimner A, Li G. Feasibility of MR-guided radiotherapy using beam-eye-view 2D-cine with tumor-volume projection. *Phys Med Biol.* 2021, 66, 045020.

171. Bertholet J, Knopf A, Eiben B, et al. Real-time intrafraction motion monitoring in external beam radiotherapy. *Phys Med Biol.* 2019;64(15):15TR01.

172. Harris W, Wang C, Yin FF, et al. A Novel method to generate on-board 4D MRI using prior 4D MRI and on-board kV projections from a conventional LINAC for target localization in liver SBRT. *Med Phys.* 2018;45(7):3238–3245.

173. Harris W, Ren L, Cai J, et al. A Technique for Generating Volumetric Cine-Magnetic Resonance Imaging. *Int J Radiat Oncol Biol Phys.* 2016;95(2):844–853.

174. Stemkens B, Tijssen RH, de Senneville BD, et al. Image-driven, model-based 3D abdominal motion estimation for MR-guided radiotherapy. *Phys Med Biol.* 2016;61(14):5335–5355.

175. van Timmeren JE, Chamberlain M, Krayenbuehl J, et al. Treatment plan quality during online adaptive re-planning. *Radiat Oncol.* 2020;15(1):203.

176. Liang Y, Schott D, Zhang Y, et al. Auto-segmentation of pancreatic tumor in multi-parametric MRI using deep convolutional neural networks. *Radiother Oncol.* 2020;145:193–200.

177. de Prez L, Woodings S, de Pooter J, et al. Direct measurement of ion chamber correction factors, k Q and k B, in a 7 MV MRI-linac. *Phys Med Biol.* 2019;64(10):105025.

178. Bruijnen T, van der Heide O, Intven MPW, et al. Technical feasibility of magnetic resonance fingerprinting on a 1.5T MRI-linac. *Phys Med Biol.* 2020;65, 22NT01.

179. Nie X, Rimner A, Li G. Feasibility of MR-guided radiotherapy using beam-eye-view 2D-cine with tumor-volume projection. *Phys Med Biol.* 2021;66, 045020.

180. Kurz C, Buizza G, Landry G, et al. Medical physics challenges in clinical MR-guided radiotherapy. *Radiat Oncol.* 2020;15(1):93.

181. Zijlema SE, Tijssen RHN, Malkov VN, et al. Design and feasibility of a flexible, on-body, high impedance coil receive array for a 1.5 T MR-linac. *Phys Med Biol.* 2019;64(18):185004.

182. Hoogcarspel SJ, Zijlema SE, Tijssen RHN, et al. Characterization of the first RF coil dedicated to 1.5 T MR guided radiotherapy. *Phys Med Biol.* 2018;63(2):025014.

183. Sahin B, Zoto Mustafayev T, Gungor G, et al. First 500 Fractions Delivered with a Magnetic Resonance-guided Radiotherapy System: initial Experience. *Cureus.* 2019;11(12):e6457.

184. Winkel D, Werensteijn-Honingh AM, Kroon PS, et al. Individual lymph nodes: "See it and Zap it". *Clin Transl Radiat Oncol.* 2019;18:46–53.

185. McQuaid D, Webb S. IMRT delivery to a moving target by dynamic MLC tracking: delivery for targets moving in two dimensions in the beam's eye view. *Phys Med Biol.* 2006;51(19):4819–4839.

186. McMahon R, Papiez L, Rangaraj D. Dynamic-MLC leaf control utilizing on-flight intensity calculations: a robust method for real-time IMRT delivery over moving rigid targets. *Med Phys.* 2007;34(8):3211–3223.

187. Yun J, Wachowicz K, Mackenzie M, et al. First demonstration of intrafractional tumor-tracked irradiation using 2D phantom MR images on a prototype linac-MR. *Med Phys.* 2013;40(5):051718.

188. Keall PJ, Colvill E, O'Brien R, et al. The first clinical implementation of electromagnetic transponder-guided MLC tracking. *Med Phys.* 2014;41(2):020702.

189. Zhang L, LoSasso T, Zhang P, et al. Couch and multileaf collimator tracking: a clinical feasibility study for pancreas and liver treatment. *Med Phys.* 2020;47(10):4743–4757.

190. D'Souza WD, Naqvi SA, Yu CX. Real-time intra-fraction-motion tracking using the treatment couch: a feasibility study. *Phys Med Biol.* 2005;50(17):4021–4033.

191. Buzurovic I, Yu Y, Werner-Wasik M, et al. Implementation and experimental results of 4D tumor tracking using robotic couch. *Med Phys.* 2012;39(11):6957–6967.

192. Menten MJ, Guckenberger M, Herrmann C, et al. Comparison of a multileaf collimator tracking system and a robotic treatment couch tracking system for organ motion compensation during radiotherapy. *Med Phys.* 2012;39(11):7032–7041.

193. Kamino Y, Takayama K, Kokubo M, et al. Development of a four-dimensional image-guided radiotherapy system with a gimbaled X-ray head. *Int J Radiat Oncol Biol Phys.* 2006;66(1):271–278.

194. Akimoto M, Nakamura M, Mukumoto N, et al. Predictive uncertainty in infrared marker-based dynamic tumor tracking with Vero4DRT. *Med Phys.* 2013;40(9):091705.

195. Yin F-F, Wong J, James Balter, et al. The role of in-room kV X-ray imaging for patient setup and target localization. http://wwwaapmorg/pubs/reports/RPT_104pdf 2009;(1–72):Last visited by 03/20/2015.

196. Willoughby T, Lehmann J, Bencomo JA, et al. Quality assurance for nonradiographic radiotherapy localization and positioning systems: report of Task Group 147. *Med Phys.* 2012;39(4):1728–1747.

197. Bissonnette JP, Balter PA, Dong L, et al. Quality assurance for image-guided radiation therapy utilizing CT-based technologies: a report of the AAPM TG-179. *Med Phys.* 2012;39(4):1946–1963.

198. Klein EE, Hanley J, Bayouth J, et al. Task Group 142 report: quality assurance of medical accelerators. *Med Phys.* 2009;36(9):4197–4212.

199. Benedict SH, Yenice KM, Followill D, et al. Stereotactic body radiation therapy: the report of AAPM Task Group 101. *Med Phys.* 2010;37(8):4078–4101.

200. Sharpe MB, Moseley DJ, Purdie TG, et al. The stability of mechanical calibration for a kV cone beam computed tomography system integrated with linear accelerator. *Med. Phys.* 2006;33(1):136–144.

201. Mao W, Lee L, Xing L. Development of a QA phantom and automated analysis tool for geometric quality assurance of on-board MV and kV x-ray imaging systems. *Med Phys.* 2008;35(4):1497–1506.

202. Langen KM, Papanikolaou N, Balog J, et al. QA for helical tomotherapy: report of the AAPM Task Group 148. *Med Phys.* 2010;37(9):4817–4853.

203. Paxton AB, Manger RP, Pawlicki T, Kim GY. Evaluation of a surface imaging system's isocenter calibration methods. *J Appl Clin Med Phys.* 2017;18(2):85–91.

204. Nguyen D, Farah J, Barbet N, Khodri M. Commissioning and performance testing of the first prototype of AlignRT InBore a Halcyon and Ethos-dedicated surface guided radiation therapy platform. *Phys Med.* 2020;80:159–166.

205. Wang L, Kielar KN, Mok E, et al. An end-to-end examination of geometric accuracy of IGRT using a new digital accelerator equipped with onboard imaging system. *Phys Med Biol.* 2012;57(3):757–769.

206. Bissonnette JP, Moseley DJ, Jaffray DA. A quality assurance program for image quality of cone-beam CT guidance in radiation therapy. *Med Phys.* 2008;35(5):1807–1815.

207. Yoo S, Yin FF. Dosimetric feasibility of cone-beam CT-based treatment planning compared to CT-based treatment planning. *Int J Radiat Oncol Biol Phys.* 2006;66(5):1553–1561.

208. Gopal A, Samant SS. Use of a line-pair resolution phantom for comprehensive quality assurance of electronic portal imaging devices based on fundamental imaging metrics. *Med Phys.* 2009;36(6):2006–2015.

209. Gayou O, Miften M. Commissioning and clinical implementation of a mega-voltage cone beam CT system for treatment localization. *Med Phys.* 2007;34(8):3183–3192.

210. Antypas C, Pantelis E. Performance evaluation of a CyberKnife G4 image-guided robotic stereotactic radiosurgery system. *Phys Med Biol.* 2008;53(17):4697–4718.

211. Jiang SB, Wolfgang J, Mageras GS. Quality assurance challenges for motion-adaptive radiation therapy: gating, breath holding, and four-dimensional computed tomography. *Int J Radiat Oncol Biol Phys.* 2008;71(1 Suppl):S103–107.

212. Milewski A, Olek D, Deasy JO, et al. Enhancement of long-term external-internal correlation by phase-shift detection and correction based on concurrent external bellows and internal navigator signals. *Adv Radiat Oncol.* 2019;(4(2)):377–389.

213. Kim T, Lewis BC, Price A, et al. Direct tumor visual feedback during free breathing in 0.35T MRgRT. *J Appl Clin Med Phys.* 2020;21(10):241–247.

214. Keiper TD, Tai A, Chen X, et al. Feasibility of real-time motion tracking using cine MRI during MR-guided radiation therapy for abdominal targets. *Med Phys.* 2020;47(8):3554–3566.

215. de Muinck Keizer DM, Pathmanathan AU, Andreychenko A, et al. Fiducial marker based intra-fraction motion assessment on cine-MR for MR-linac treatment of prostate cancer. *Phys Med Biol.* 2019;64(7):07NT02.

216. Menten MJ, Mohajer JK, Nilawar R, et al. Automatic reconstruction of the delivered dose of the day using MR-linac treatment log files and online MR imaging. *Radiother Oncol.* 2020;145:88–94.

217. Bainbridge H, Salem A, Tijssen RHN, et al. Magnetic resonance imaging in precision radiation therapy for lung cancer. *Transl Lung Cancer Res.* 2017;6(6):689–707.

218. Sharpe M, Brock KK. Quality assurance of serial 3D image registration, fusion, and segmentation. *Int J Radiat Oncol Biol Phys.* 2008;71(1 Suppl):S33–37.

219. Kuo HC, Lovelock MM, Li G, et al. A phantom study to evaluate three different registration platform of 3D/3D, 2D/3D, and 3D surface match with 6D alignment for precise image-guided radiotherapy. *J Appl Clin Med Phys.* 2020.

220. Li G, Xie H, Ning H, et al. A novel 3D volumetric voxel registration technique for volume-view-guided image registration of multiple imaging modalities. *Int J Radiat Oncol Biol Phys.* 2005;63(1):261–273.

221. Li G, Xie H, Ning H, et al. Accuracy of 3D volumetric image registration based on CT, MR and PET/CT phantom experiments. *J Appl Clin Med Phys.* 2008;9(4):2781.

222. Hill DL, Batchelor PG, Holden M, Hawkes DJ. Medical image registration. *Phys Med Biol.* 2001;46(3):R1–45.

223. Li G, Yang TJ, Furtado H, et al. Clinical Assessment of 2D/3D Registration Accuracy in 4 Major Anatomic Sites Using On-Board 2D Kilovoltage Images for 6D Patient Setup. *Technol Cancer Res Treat.* 2015;14(3):305–314.

224. Pluim JP, Maintz JB, Viergever MA. Mutual-information-based registration of medical images: a survey. *IEEE Trans Med Imaging.* 2003;22(8):986–1004.

225. Al-Mayah A, Moseley J, Velec M, Brock K. Toward efficient biomechanical-based deformable image registration of lungs for image-guided radiotherapy. *Phys Med Biol.* 2011;56(15):4701–4713.

226. Yang D, Brame S, El Naqa I, et al. Technical note: DIRART–A software suite for deformable image registration and adaptive radiotherapy research. *Med Phys.* 2011;38(1):67–77.

227. Saleh ZH, Apte AP, Sharp GC, et al. The distance discordance metric-a novel approach to quantifying spatial uncertainties in intra- and inter-patient deformable image registration. *Phys Med Biol.* 2014;59(3):733–746.

228. Wijesooriya K, Weiss E, Dill V, et al. Quantifying the accuracy of automated structure segmentation in 4D CT images using a deformable image registration algorithm. *Med Phys.* 2008;35(4):1251–1260.

229. Shen D, Wu G, Suk HI. Deep learning in medical image analysis. *Annu Rev Biomed Eng.* 2017.

230. Standard. IHE-RO: Integrating Healthcare Enterprise—Radiation Oncology http://wikiihenet/indexphp?title=Radiation_Oncology. 2015:Accessed by 03/20/2015.

231. Standard. DICOM: Digital Imaging and Communications in Medicine, managed by the Medical Imaging & Technology Alliance—a division of NEMA http://medicalnemaorg/standardhtml. 2015:Accessed by 03/20/2015.

232. Seo H, Badiei Khuzani M, Vasudevan V, et al. Machine learning techniques for biomedical image segmentation: an overview of technical aspects and introduction to state-of-art applications. *Med Phys.* 2020;47(5):e148-e167.

233. Yan D. Adaptive radiotherapy: merging principle into clinical practice. *Semin Radiat Oncol.* 2010;20(2):79–83.

234. Deasy JO, Blanco AI, Clark VH. CERR: a computational environment for radiotherapy research. *Med Phys.* 2003;30(5):979–985.

235. Jaffray DA. Image-guided radiation therapy: from concept to practice. *Semin Radiat Oncol.* 2007;17(4):243–244.

236. Lalondrelle S, Huddart R, Warren-Oseni K, et al. Adaptive-predictive organ localization using cone-beam computed tomography for improved accuracy in external beam radiotherapy for bladder cancer. *Int J Radiat Oncol Biol Phys.* 2011;79(3):705–712.

237. Ahunbay EE, Peng C, Godley A, et al. An on-line replanning method for head and neck adaptive radiotherapy. *Med Phys.* 2009;36(10):4776–4790.

238. Acharya S, Fischer-Valuck BW, Kashani R, et al. Online Magnetic Resonance Image Guided Adaptive Radiation Therapy: first Clinical Applications. *Int J Radiat Oncol Biol Phys.* 2016;94(2):394–403.

239. Mohan R, Sahoo N. Uncertainties in proton therapy: their impact and management. In: Paganetti H, Das I, editors. *Principles and Practice of Proton Therapy.* Madison, WI: Medical Physics Publishing, Inc.; 2015:595–622.

240. Liu W, Li Y, Li X, et al. Influence of robust optimization in intensity-modulated proton therapy with different dose delivery techniques. *Med Phys.* 2012;39(6):3089–3101.

241. Park PC, Zhu XR, Lee AK, et al. A beam-specific planning target volume (PTV) design for proton therapy to account for setup and range uncertainties. *Int J Radiat Oncol Biol Phys.* 2012;82(2):e329–336.

242. Zhang M, Zou W, Teo BK. Image guidance in proton therapy for lung cancer. *Transl Lung Cancer Res.* 2018;7(2):160–170.

243. Min CH, Zhu X, Winey BA, et al. Clinical application of in-room positron emission tomography for in vivo treatment monitoring in proton radiation therapy. *Int J Radiat Oncol Biol Phys.* 2013;86(1):183–189.

244. Hueso-Gonzalez F, Enghardt W, Fiedler F, et al. First test of the prompt gamma ray timing method with heterogeneous targets at a clinical proton therapy facility. *Phys Med Biol.* 2015;60(16):6247–6272.

245. Favaudon V, Caplier L, Monceau V, et al. Ultrahigh dose-rate FLASH irradiation increases the differential response between normal and tumor tissue in mice. *Sci Transl Med.* 2014;6(245):245ra293.

246. Esplen NM, Mendonca MS, Bazalova-Carter M. Physics and biology of ultrahigh dose-rate (FLASH) radiotherapy: a topical review. *Phys Med Biol.* 2020;65, 23TR03.

247. Zhou S, Zheng D, Fan Q, et al. Minimum dose rate estimation for pulsed FLASH radiotherapy: a dimensional analysis. *Med Phys.* 2020;47(7):3243–3249.

248. Zou W, Diffenderfer ES, Cengel KA, et al. Current delivery limitations of proton PBS for FLASH. *Radiother Oncol.* 2020;155:212–218.

249. Kumar SS, Higgins KA, McGarry RC. Emerging therapies for stage III non-small cell lung cancer: stereotactic body radiation therapy and immunotherapy. *Front Oncol.* 2017;7:197.

250. Rosati LM, Kumar R, Herman JM. Integration of stereotactic body radiation therapy into the multidisciplinary management of pancreatic cancer. *Semin Radiat Oncol.* 2017;27(3):256–267.

251. Breen WG, Leventakos K, Dong H, Merrell KW. Radiation and immunotherapy: emerging mechanisms of synergy. *J Thorac Dis.* 2020;12(11):7011–7023.

252. Sampson JH, Heimberger AB, Archer GE, et al. Immunologic escape after prolonged progression-free survival with epidermal growth factor receptor variant III peptide vaccination in patients with newly diagnosed glioblastoma. *J Clin Oncol.* 2010;28(31):4722–4729.

253. Demaria S, Golden EB, Formenti SC. Role of local radiation therapy in cancer immunotherapy. *JAMA Oncol.* 2015;1(9):1325–1332.

254. Oh S, Stewart J, Moseley J, et al. Hybrid adaptive radiotherapy with online MRI in cervix cancer IMRT. *Radiother Oncol.* 2013;110:323–328.

255. Feldman AM, Modh A, Glide-Hurst C, et al. Real-time magnetic resonance-guided liver stereotactic body radiation therapy: an institutional report using a magnetic resonance-linac system. *Cureus.* 2019;11(9):e5774.

256. Yan D, Vicini F, Wong J, Martinez A. Adaptive radiation therapy. *Phys Med Biol.* 1997;42(1):123–132.

257. Yan D, Jaffray DA, Wong JW. A model to accumulate fractionated dose in a deforming organ. *Int J Radiat Oncol Biol Phys.* 1999;44(3):665–675.

258. Yan D, Lockman D, Brabbins D, et al. An off-line strategy for constructing a patient-specific planning target volume in adaptive treatment process for prostate cancer. *Int J Radiat Oncol Biol Phys.* 2000;48(1):289–302.

259. Chen GP, Ahunbay E, Li XA. Technical Note: development and performance of a software tool for quality assurance of online replanning with a conventional Linac or MR-Linac. *Med Phys.* 2016;43(4):1713.

260. Das IJ, McGee KP, Tyagi N, Wang H. Role and future of MRI in radiation oncology. *Br J Radiol.* 2019;92(1094):20180505.

261. Riboldi M, Sharp GC, Baroni G, Chen GT. Four-dimensional targeting error analysis in image-guided radiotherapy. *Phys Med Biol.* 2009;54(19):5995–6008.

262. Chen H, Wu A, Brandner ED, et al. Dosimetric evaluations of the interplay effect in respiratory-gated intensity-modulated radiation therapy. *Med Phys.* 2009;36(3):893–903.

263. Kini VR, Vedam SS, Keall PJ, et al. Patient training in respiratory-gated radiotherapy. *Med Dosimetry.* 2003;28(1):7–11.

264. Parkhurst JM, Price GJ, Sharrock PJ, et al. Self-management of patient body position, pose, and motion using wide-field, real-time optical measurement feedback: results of a volunteer study. *Int J Radiat Oncol Biol Phys.* 2013;87(5):904–910.

265. Mageras GS, Yorke E. Deep inspiration breath hold and respiratory gating strategies for reducing organ motion in radiation treatment. *Semin Radiat Oncol.* 2004;14(1):65–75.

266. Steidl P, Haberer T, Durante M, Bert C. Gating delays for two respiratory motion sensors in scanned particle radiation therapy. *Phys Med Biol.* 2013;58(21):N295–302.

267. Poulsen PR, Cho B, Sawant A, et al. Detailed analysis of latencies in image-based dynamic MLC tracking. *Med Phys.* 2010;37(9):4998–5005.

268. Sharp GC, Jiang SB, Shimizu S, Shirato H. Prediction of respiratory tumour motion for real-time image-guided radiotherapy. *Phys Med Biol.* 2004;49(3):425–440.

269. Hoisak JD, Sixel KE, Tirona R, et al. Correlation of lung tumor motion with external surrogate indicators of respiration. *Int J Radiat Oncol Biol Phys.* 2004;60(4):1298–1306.

270. Fast M, van de Schoot A, van de Lindt T, et al. Tumor Trailing for Liver SBRT on the MR-Linac. *Int J Radiat Oncol Biol Phys.* 2019;103(2):468–478.

271. Paulson ES, Ahunbay E, Chen X, et al. 4D-MRI driven MR-guided online adaptive radiotherapy for abdominal stereotactic body radiation therapy on a high field MR-Linac: implementation and initial clinical experience. *Clin Transl Radiat Oncol.* 2020;23:72–79.

272. van Herk M. Errors and margins in radiotherapy. *Semin Radiat Oncol.* 2004;14(1):52–64.

273. van Herk M, Remeijer P, Rasch C, Lebesque JV. The probability of correct target dosage: dose-population histograms for deriving treatment margins in radiotherapy. *Int J Radiat Oncol Biol Phys.* 2000;47(4):1121–1135.

274. Tryggestad E, Flammang A, Han-Oh S, et al. Respiration-based sorting of dynamic MRI to derive representative 4D-MRI for radiotherapy planning. *Med Phys.* 2013;40(5):051909.

275. Akino Y, Oh RJ, Masai N, et al. Evaluation of potential internal target volume of liver tumors using cine-MRI. *Med Phys.* 2014;41(11):111704.

276. Grills IS, Hugo G, Kestin LL, et al. Image-guided radiotherapy via daily online cone-beam CT substantially reduces margin requirements for stereotactic lung radiotherapy. *Int J Radiat Oncol Biol Phys.* 2008;70(4):1045–1056.

277. Ge J, Santanam L, Noel C, Parikh PJ. Planning 4-dimensional computed tomography (4DCT) cannot adequately represent daily intrafractional motion of abdominal tumors. *Int J Radiat Oncol Biol Phys.* 2013;85(4):999–1005.

278. Nelson C, Balter P, Morice RC, et al. Evaluation of tumor position and PTV margins using image guidance and respiratory gating. *Int J Radiat Oncol Biol Phys.* 2010;76(5):1578–1585.

279. Melancon AD, O'Daniel JC, Zhang L, et al. Is a 3-mm intrafractional margin sufficient for daily image-guided intensity-modulated radiation therapy of prostate cancer? *Radiother Oncol.* 2007;85(2):251–259.

280. Tanyi JA, He T, Summers PA, et al. Assessment of planning target volume margins for intensity-modulated radiotherapy of the prostate gland: role of daily inter- and intrafraction motion. *Int J Radiat Oncol Biol Phys.* 2010;78(5):1579–1585.

281. Li HS, Chetty IJ, Enke CA, et al. Dosimetric consequences of intrafraction prostate motion. *Int J Radiat Oncol Biol Phys.* 2008;71(3):801–812.

282. Langen KM, Jones DT. Organ motion and its management. *Int J Radiat Oncol Biol Phys.* 2001;50(1):265–278.

283. Fokdal L, Honore H, Hoyer M, et al. Impact of changes in bladder and rectal filling volume on organ motion and dose distribution of the bladder in radiotherapy for urinary bladder cancer. *Int J Radiat Oncol Biol Phys.* 2004;59(2):436–444.

284. Li XA, Qi XS, Pitterle M, et al. Interfractional variations in patient setup and anatomic change assessed by daily computed tomography. *Int J Radiat Oncol Biol Phys.* 2007;68(2):581–591.

285. Sanguineti G, Marcenaro M, Franzone P, et al. Neoadjuvant androgen deprivation and prostate gland shrinkage during conformal radiotherapy. *Radiother Oncol.* 2003;66(2):151–157.

286. Zhang P, Yorke E, Hu YC, et al. Predictive treatment management: incorporating a predictive tumor response model into robust prospective treatment planning for non-small cell lung cancer. *Int J Radiat Oncol Biol Phys.* 2014;88(2):446–452.

287. Zhang L, Garden AS, Lo J, et al. Multiple regions-of-interest analysis of setup uncertainties for head-and-neck cancer radiotherapy. *Int J Radiat Oncol Biol Phys.* 2006;64(5):1559–1569.

288. van Kranen S, van Beek S, Rasch C, et al. Setup uncertainties of anatomical sub-regions in head-and-neck cancer patients after offline CBCT guidance. *Int J Radiat Oncol Biol Phys.* 2009;73(5):1566–1573.

289. Litzenberg DW, Hadley SW, Tyagi N, et al. Synchronized dynamic dose reconstruction. *Med Phys.* 2007;34(1):91–102.

290. Chin S, Eccles CL, McWilliam A, et al. Magnetic resonance-guided radiation therapy: a review. *J Med Imaging Radiat Oncol.* 2020;64(1):163–177.

291. Li G, Liu Y, Nie X. Respiratory-correlated (RC) versus time-resolved (TR) four-dimensional magnetic resonance imaging (4DMRI) for radiotherapy of thoracic and abdominal cancer. *Front Oncol.* 2019;9(9):1024–1032.

292. Ramsey CR, Scaperoth D, Seibert R, et al. Image-guided helical tomotherapy for localized prostate cancer: technique and initial clinical observations. *J Appl Clin Med Phys.* 2007;8(3):2320.

293. Langen KM, Lu W, Willoughby TR, et al. Dosimetric effect of prostate motion during helical tomotherapy. *Int J Radiat Oncol Biol Phys.* 2009;74(4):1134–1142.

294. Antico M, Prinsen P, Fracassi A, et al. Comparison between conventional IMRT planning and a novel real-time adaptive planning strategy in hypofractionated regimes for prostate cancer: a proof-of-concept planning study. *Healthcare (Basel).* 2019;7(4).

295. Ruggieri R, Rigo M, Naccarato S, et al. Adaptive SBRT by 1.5 T MR-linac for prostate cancer: on the accuracy of dose delivery in view of the prolonged session time. *Phys Med.* 2020;80:34–41.

296. Chen L, Paskalev K, Xu X, et al. Rectal dose variation during the course of image-guided radiation therapy of prostate cancer. *Radiother Oncol.* 2010;95(2):198–202.

297. Zelefsky MJ, Kollmeier M, Cox B, et al. Improved clinical outcomes with high-dose image guided radiotherapy compared with non-IGRT for the treatment of clinically localized prostate cancer. *Int J Radiat Oncol Biol Phys.* 2012;84(1):125–129.

298. Chao KS, Majhail N, Huang CJ, et al. Intensity-modulated radiation therapy reduces late salivary toxicity without compromising tumor control in patients with oropharyngeal carcinoma: a comparison with conventional techniques. *Radiother Oncol.* 2001;61(3):275–280.

299. Barker JL, Jr., Garden AS, Ang KK, et al. Quantification of volumetric and geometric changes occurring during fractionated radiotherapy for head-and-neck cancer using an integrated CT/linear accelerator system. *Int J Radiat Oncol Biol Phys.* 2004;59(4):960–970.

300. O'Daniel JC, Garden AS, Schwartz DL, et al. Parotid gland dose in intensity-modulated radiotherapy for head and neck cancer: is what you plan what you get? *Int J Radiat Oncol Biol Phys.* 2007;69(4):1290–1296.

301. Lee J, Kim WC, Yoon WS, et al. Reirradiation using stereotactic body radiotherapy in the management of recurrent or second primary head and neck cancer: a meta-analysis and systematic review. *Oral Oncol.* 2020;107:104757.

302. Sonke JJ, Belderbos J. Adaptive radiotherapy for lung cancer. *Semin Radiat Oncol.* 2010;20(2):94–106.

303. Zarepisheh M, Long T, Li N, et al. A DVH-guided IMRT optimization algorithm for automatic treatment planning and adaptive radiotherapy replanning. *Med Phys.* 2014;41(6):061711.

304. Olsen LA, Robinson CG, He GR, et al. Automated radiation therapy treatment plan workflow using a commercial application programming interface. *Pract Radiat Oncol.* 2014;4(6):358–367.

305. Li H, Yu L, Anastasio MA, et al. Automatic CT simulation optimization for radiation therapy: a general strategy. *Med Phys.* 2014;41(3):031913.

306. Corradini S, Alongi F, Andratschke N, et al. MR-guidance in clinical reality: current treatment challenges and future perspectives. *Radiat Oncol.* 2019;14(1):92.

307. Li R, Jia X, Lewis JH, et al. Real-time volumetric image reconstruction and 3D tumor localization based on a single x-ray projection image for lung cancer radiotherapy. *Med Phys.* 2010;37(6):2822–2826.

308. Na YH, Suh TS, Kapp DS, Xing L. Toward a web-based real-time radiation treatment planning system in a cloud computing environment. *Phys Med Biol.* 2013;58(18):6525–6540.

309. Xue H, Inati S, Sorensen TS, et al. Distributed MRI reconstruction using gadgetron-based cloud computing. *Magn Reson Med.* 2015;73:215–225.

310. Jiang J, Hu YC, Tyagi N, et al. Cross-modality (CT-MRI) prior augmented deep learning for robust lung tumor segmentation from small MR datasets. *Med Phys.* 2019;46(10):4392–4404.

311. Wang C, Tyagi N, Rimner A, et al. Segmenting lung tumors on longitudinal imaging studies via a patient-specific adaptive convolutional neural network. *Radiother Oncol.* 2019;131:101–107.

18 Deformable Image Registration

Raj Varadhan

INTRODUCTION

Image registration can be defined as determining a spatial transformation that relates positions in one image, to corresponding positions in one or more, other images. The meaning of correspondence varies and takes different significance depending on the clinical application. For example, the user may be interested in structural correspondence[1] (e.g., comparing the same anatomical structures before and after radiation treatment to detect response), functional correspondence (e.g., comparing functionally equivalent regions of the brains of a group of subjects), or structural–functional correspondence (e.g., correctly positioning functional information on a structural image). Deformable image registration (DIR) studies have been advocated to more accurately quantify these anatomical and biological variations.[2] The registration is considered deformable or nonlinear when the geometric transformation is not rigid or requires a non-affine transformation due to deformations like tissue change, shrinking, or expansion. Deformable registration is essential to map the position of each voxel to a reference Computed Tomography (CT) image for dose tracking and to ultimately practice adaptive radiotherapy.[3,4] The accuracy of deformable registration is particularly important in intensity-modulated radiation therapy (IMRT) and adaptive radiotherapy that deliver differential doses to different parts of the tumor and organs at risk (OAR), which then sum to a uniform dose.[5]

From a radiation oncology perspective, there are four broad applications of DIR: (i) identifying and correlating tumor or organ of interest across a series of medical scans (e.g., CT, Positron Emission Tomography (PET), or Magnetic Resonance Imaging (MRI)); (ii) multimodal registration that involves matching images of the same patient acquired by different imaging modalities (CT to MRI or CT to PET/CT, etc.); (iii) matching of images from different patients (inter-patient registration), which has applications in atlas-based segmentation;[6–9] and (iv) workflows in image-guided radiation therapy (IGRT) involving contour propagation, treatment response evaluation,[10] and dose accumulation for adaptive radiotherapy.

However, the basic ingredients on how a DIR algorithm is operational are the same. Any DIR algorithm has three basic components: (i) similarity measures of how well the images match, (ii) deformation model (parametric, nonparametric, or biomechanical), which specifies how a source or moving image can be made to match target or fixed image, and (iii) an optimization process that varies the parameters of a particular deformation model to maximize the matching criterion.

Deformable registration is inherently degenerate and is considered an ill-posed problem because there is generally no unique solution to a registration problem. In DIR, the geometric transformation can be spatially variant with the number of degrees of freedom that can be as large as three times the number of voxels in the source image.[11] Usually, image registration is presented as an optimization problem. Registration methods can be based on information derived from image intensities or landmark information (such as contours or points) placed on the images. Hybrid models are possible using a combination of intensities and landmarks. A review of DIR and the algorithm implementation details from the perspective of radiation oncology applications will be presented in this chapter. First, we review the classical definition of DIR as an image matching problem.

DEFORMABLE IMAGE REGISTRATION DEFINITION

DIR is an iterative process that searches for the geometric correspondence between fixed (target) and moving (source) images. This concept is illustrated in Figure 18.1. The basic idea is that at each iteration of the registration loop, the geometric transformation is updated and the moving image is deformed accordingly. The goal is to find a transformation that finds the optimal value of the similarity metric comparing the fixed and moving images. The optimizer has the function of defining the search strategy. The role of the interpolator is to resample the voxel intensity in the new coordinate system based on the geometric transformation found. This process can be mathematically written as[12]

$$\widehat{T} = \operatorname*{argmin}_{T} C\big[I_{\text{fixed}}, T\big(I_{\text{moving}}\big)\big],$$

where $\widehat{T}$ represents the geometric transformation that minimizes the cost function C, based on the similarity metric comparing the fixed image (I_{fixed}) and the moving

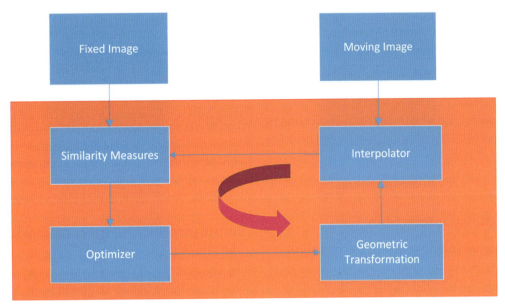

FIGURE 18.1. Flow chart illustrating iterative registration loop used in DIR algorithms. **DIR,** deformable image registration.

image (I_{moving}). "argmin" represents the optimization process, which updates the transformation T to minimize the cost function C.

The output of DIR is the deformation vector field (DVF), which is applied to the moving image. Typically, the spatially variant vector fields are constrained by regularization (e.g., smoothing with Gaussian, etc.) that prioritizes any specific properties based on the deformation model chosen and addresses the difficulty associated with the registration. Regularization and deformation models are closely related. In general, the role of regularization is to prevent sharp discontinuities in the DVF and to provide anatomically consistent registration.

SIMILARITY MEASURES

Two images that are deformably registered are never perfectly matched in reality. The quality of how well the images are matched after DIR is defined by the similarity measure. The optimal registration is the one that features a transformation, which minimizes the similarity measure. The commonly used similarity measures are discussed in the following section.

Sum of Squared Differences

The most widely used similarity metric is the sum of squared differences (SSD) measure defined as SSD = $1/N \sum_x \{T(x) - S(t(x))\}^2$, where $T(x)$ is the intensity at a position x in an image, and $S(t(x))$ is the intensity at the corresponding point given by the current estimate of the transformation $t(x)$. N is the number of voxels in the region of overlap.

SSD is very sensitive to voxels with large intensity differences (outliers), which makes SSD only applicable in single-modality registration contexts (e.g., both must be CT or MRI images, etc.) or more precisely, in cases where the images to be registered only differ by noise. The least-squares form of SSD makes the measure computationally very attractive since fast optimization schemes can be used.

Correlation Coefficient

The Correlation Coefficient (CC) metric can be written as

$$CC = \frac{\Sigma x \left(T(x) - \overline{T} \right) \times \left(S(t(x)) - \overline{S} \right)}{\sqrt{\Sigma x \left(T(x) - \overline{T} \right)^2 \Sigma x (S \left(t(x) \right) - \overline{S})^2}}$$

This metric has the advantage that it has a reduced dependence on linear scaling of image intensities. This means that two images can be registered even though one is different in image intensity from the other. However, CC is not suited for multi-modality registration since data from different imaging modalities contains inherently different pixel intensities of corresponding anatomy, and a registration metric based on simple differences or products of image intensities is not sufficient.

Mutual Information

The basic idea in mutual information (MI) is to exploit a statistically significant relationship between the intensity values of the input images. This relationship does not have to be explicitly known but rather only assumes a probabilistic relationship between intensities. MI seeks to align voxels whose values have common probabilities of being present in their respective image sets. Proper registration requires proper alignment of significant intensity value structures that lead to pronounced peaks in the joint intensity distribution detected as maxima of its MI or entropy. The MI can be defined in terms of entropies (H) of the intensity distribution as

$$\text{MI} = H_T + H_s - H_{T,S}, \text{ where } H_T = -\Sigma_i P_i \log P_i,$$
$$H_s = -\Sigma_j Q_j \log Q_j \text{ and } H_{T,S} = -\Sigma_{i,j} p_{i,j} \log p_{i,j}$$

P and Q are probability of intensity i and j occurring in target (T) and source image (S), respectively, and $p_{i,j}$ is the joint probability of both occurring at the same time.

MI has evolved into the accepted standard for similarity measures, especially in multi-modality image registration.

Normalized Mutual Information

Normalized mutual information (NMI) is defined as $\text{NMI} = (H_T + H_S)/H_{T,S}$

This metric was proposed to minimize the overlap problems occasionally seen when using the MI metric.

DEFORMATION MODELS

DIR models can be divided into those using parametric-based registration (model-based), those using nonparametric-based registration and biomechanical models. The parametric methods are characterized by featuring a transformation function that is described by a limited number of parameters. These typically include (i) radial basis functions (RBFs), (ii) elastic body splines (EBS),[13] thin plate splines (TPSs),[14] and (iii) free-form deformation (FFD) using B-splines.[15] The advantage of using parametric methods is that a change in a parameter affects the transformation in a spatially limited neighborhood while other parts of the deformation remain unchanged. Hence, with respect to image resampling, only the relevant part of the image has to be resampled, which improves the computational performance of DIR.

In contrast to this, nonparametric methods typically feature a transformation function that is based on a vector per voxel describing the displacement of the point represented by this voxel. This is converted to a continuous function by interpolation. Commonly used nonparametric methods include Demons registration,[16] optical flow methods,[17] and viscous fluid.[18]

Biomechanical model-based registration has been recently introduced in radiation oncology applications and relies on modeling the physical properties of organs that obey biomechanical laws. A summary of these deformation models and their relative merits will be discussed in the next section.

Parametric or Model-Based Deformation Models

A registration method based on a parametric transformation function is usually written as a minimization problem in which an optimal set of parameters must explicitly

be found that minimizes the chosen similarity measure. Typically, parametric-based deformation models rely on constructing a mapping function, which maps points from the moving (source) image to the corresponding landmark points in the fixed (target) image.

The matching of point features in source and target images can be done manually by a trained anatomy expert based on fiducial markers placed before image acquisition or image features extracted from images after scanning. However, this method is not fully automatic and is sometimes limited by the difficulty in finding corresponding landmarks in both source and target images.

Transformations Based on Radial Basis Functions

A generalized way to describe the geometric transformation is creating a global function based on a set of RBFs, which are functions depending only on the distance between two points. TPSs are an example of RBFs that are derived from the minimization of a smoothness measure based on the partial derivatives of the transformation.[14] The name "thin plate" refers to a physical analogy of bending a thin sheet of metal plate orthogonal to the plate such that the plate will arrange itself in a configuration where the bending is evenly distributed or producing radially symmetric transformations.

A number of other basis functions for RBF-based transformations have been proposed for image registration including EBS,[13] Wendland functions,[19] and Gaussian functions.[20]

Transformations Based on a Grid of Control Points

B-Splines

B-splines are a commonly used deformation model in radiation oncology applications. A common approach to parameterizing a transformation using basis functions is to base the transformation on some control points arranged in a regular grid and four basis functions. In short, a function is represented as a linear combination of basis functions such that

$$\vartheta(u) = \Sigma_i p_i \beta_i(u),$$

where $\vartheta(u)$ is the deformation field, p_i is a scaling factor, and $\beta(u)$ is a piecewise cubic polynomial described in the following section.

$$\beta_o(u) = (1-u)^3/6, \; \beta_1(u) = (3u^3 - 6u^2 + 4)/6, \; \beta_2(u)$$
$$= (-3u^3 + 3u^2 + 3u + 1)/6 \text{ and } \beta_3(u) = u^3/6$$

The four piecewise polynomials are shown in Figure 18.2.[21]

Using these, it is possible to develop a transformation function that is locally controlled, i.e., when a control point is moved, the points in the vicinity are transformed.

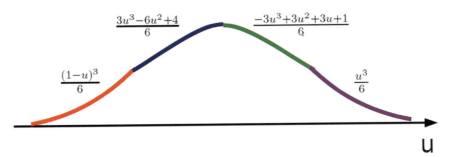

FIGURE 18.2. Graphical representation of four piecewise polynomials in cubic B-spline algorithm.

This technique is sometimes called FFD. The compact support of the B-splines means that when evaluating the effect of moving a control point, only the voxels in the vicinity of this point need to be considered. The cubic B-spline FFD transformation approach has been applied in registrations used in mammography for breast cancer.[15] The registration is based on MRI images using MI as similarity measure for creation of external forces. The B-spline approach combined with Mattes MI similarity metric has been widely used for several applications in radiotherapy.[22–24]

Mesh-Based Models

Mesh-based models perform DIR (also known as deformable mesh registration [DMR]) based on dividing the entire image into polygons (2D) or polyhedra (3D), where the subdivision follows boundaries in the images. This can be used for finite element analysis-based methods in image registration.[25,26] Registration approaches can also be based on using organ segmentations for creating a mesh of points connected by triangles (organ surface), and tetrahedra or hexahedra (entire organ volume). This method was used to verify the accuracy of automatic target registration by comparing tumor and lymph nodes delineated by an anatomy expert on weekly CT scans with those derived from mesh registration.[27]

In summary, parametric models are highly customizable with individualized constraints that can be introduced in the model. However, parameter settings are application-dependent and can potentially induce poor matching or convergence if not properly chosen.

NONPARAMETRIC DEFORMATION MODELS

Nonparametric deformation models or transformations are typically described by a field consisting of a displacement vector per voxel of the reference image. A continuous transformation function is defined by interpolation between these vectors and consequently the DVF generated in nonparametric models constitutes a vast number of degrees of freedom.

Methods for Nonparametric Registration

Deformation models in parametric approaches to some extent are regularized by the continuous nature of the parametric functions. However, regularization is crucial when using nonparametric transformations. In this section, some examples will be given of nonparametric registration methods, which rely on physical properties based on an underlying physics to guide the registration process.

Demons Algorithm

The Demons registration method was introduced by Thirion[16] and has been widely used in several radiotherapy applications.[28–30]

Optical flow is used to find a driving force at each point based on the intensity gradient of the moving image. The allowed transformations are described using a vector field where each voxel has an associated deformation vector describing where this voxel is mapped to in the reference image. The main concept is to drive the voxels of the moving image in the direction of the gradient if their intensity is higher than the corresponding intensity of voxels in fixed image and in the opposite direction if intensity is lower. To regularize the flow, a Gaussian filter is used.

The Demons algorithm defines the deformation field as

$$\vec{u}(\vec{x}) = \frac{(m-s)\vec{\Delta}s}{\left|\vec{\Delta}s\right|^2 + \left(m-s\right)^2} = \frac{\vec{F}\vec{\Delta}s}{\left|\vec{\Delta}s\right|^2 + \vec{F}^2},$$

where $(m-s)$ is the differential force $\vec{F}$ between moving and static images and $\vec{\Delta}s$ is the gradient of the static image.

Demons registration has been improved in its ability to converge by integrating an "active" force that considers moving image gradient[29] and also guaranteeing DVF invertibility. The latter algorithm is referred as diffeomorphic demons.[31] A diffeomorphism by definition also preserves the topology of objects in the image. In other words, it prevents folding of structures onto itself.

Viscous Fluid Registration

A registration method designed to handle large geometric displacements between two images is the viscous-fluid registration method by Christensen.[18] The general idea in this method is to use a motion model that is derived from continuum physics that describes the motion of a viscous fluid for regularizing the registration process.

The general equation can be described using Navier–Stokes equation namely

$$\mu \nabla^2 \vec{u}(\vec{x}) + (\mu + \lambda) \nabla [\nabla \bullet \vec{u}(\vec{x})] = \vec{f}(\vec{x}),$$

where $\vec{u}(\vec{x})$ is the displacement from the original position $\vec{x}$, ∇^2 and ∇ are, respectively, the Laplacian and gradient operators. The force field $\vec{f}(\vec{x}) = \vec{c}r(\vec{x})$. Position vector can be written as $\vec{r}(\vec{x}) = |\vec{x}| = [x_1^2 + x_2^2 + x_3^2]^{1/2}$. μ and λ are the coefficients that describe the physical properties of the materials derived from Young's modulus (E) and Poisson ratio (v) and can be written as

$$E = \frac{\mu(3\lambda + 2\mu)}{\lambda + \mu} \text{ and } v = \lambda/[2(\lambda+\mu)]$$

For an incompressible fluid, the conservation of energy, momentum, and mass leads to the Navier–Stokes equations to describe the motion of a fluid substance. In the viscous fluid model equation provided earlier, μ is set to 1 and λ to 0, resulting in the simplified equation

$$\nabla^2 \vec{u}(\vec{x}) + \nabla [\nabla \bullet \vec{u}(\vec{x})] = \vec{f}(\vec{x})$$

The driving force in the viscous-fluid registration is a body force vector field that is derived on the basis of image intensities finding the local direction of the steepest decrease of an SSD similarity measure. The method is very time-consuming because it requires an iterative solution of a partial differential equation (PDE) and in each iteration, another PDE must be solved to find a vector field of velocities.

An example of viscous-fluid registration method extended to include the use of landmark information was used in cervical cancer registration with patients with CT compatible intracavitary applicators.[32] A hybrid model is presented here in which regions of interest are converted to binary volumes. These volumes are included when body forces are calculated, which makes it easier to ensure that structures of importance in the images are matched.

Optical Flow-Based Registration Methods

The process of estimating optical flow consists of finding a mapping between the fixed and moving image that relates quantitatively how the image intensity information has changed between the two images. In theory, both images are regarded as part of one mathematical function where spatial changes have occurred in the time between acquisitions transforming one image into the other.

The optical flow is a vector field consisting of the changes in spatial coordinates. These vectors can be thought of as "optical velocity" vectors showing the direction of image intensity flow.

A well-known method for estimating optical flow is the classical Horn and Schunck algorithm.[17] The optical flow field is found by minimizing a cost function that consists of an intensity term and a term penalizing non-smooth optical flow fields. The Horn and Schunck algorithm is available to radiation oncology community through the DI-ART platform in public domain.[33] A global optimization method is performed in Horn and Schunck algorithm based on the calculus of variations and can produce very smooth transformations. This method has been used for estimating intra-thoracic tumor motion.[34] Further, the Horn and Schunck algorithm was found to be the best performing algorithm in low-contrast DIR accuracy studies using a deformable gel that played the roles of both a dosimeter and imaging study set.[35–37]

An invertibility term can be added to the Horn and Schunck method as done by Yang et al.[38] for obtaining inverse consistent registration (i.e., registration of moving image to the fixed image is the same as the inverse transformation of the fixed image to the moving image). A different approach than the global optimization performed by Horn and Schunck was taken by Lucas and Kanade,[39] which is also available to the radiation oncology community through the Deformable Image Registration and Adaptive Radiotherapy Toolkit (DI-ART) package.[33] Here, an assumption of constant flow in a window around the pixel being considered was chosen, which can be solved by the least squares method. The Lucas and Kanade method leads to a registration result, which is of a more local nature in that the information about displacements at edges does not propagate through areas of uniform intensity.

In summary, nonparametric registration methods can converge to a solution with minimal customization. However, when large deformations are involved, the registration mapping may not be optimal.

BIOMECHANICAL MODELS

Biomechanical models rely on the physical properties of registered organs. In biomechanical models, a finite element model of the organ to be deformed is generated from the segmentation. The organ deformation can then be modeled with underlying physics of increasing complexity. The simplest model is the linear elastic matching model that obeys Hooke's law. Hooke's law of elasticity describes the strain, the deformation a body undergoe when subjected to stress. Under Hooke's law, the restoring force exerted on the body, F, is given by $F = -kx$, where x is the change in length of the object, and k is the spring or force constant. Hooke's law can be rewritten, as $\sigma = E* \varepsilon$, where E is Young's modulus, σ and ε are the applied stress and strain, respectively. The deformation, x, along the axis of applied force can be expressed as

$$x = \frac{\Delta L}{L} = \frac{1}{E} * \frac{F}{A},$$

where E = Young's modulus of an organ, $\frac{F}{A}$ (force per unit area) is the applied stress, and $\frac{\Delta L}{L}$ is the fractional change in length.

In a simple 2D model, the deformation in a direction perpendicular to the direction of applied force can be written in terms of the Poisson ratio of a particular organ as follows:

$$y = \frac{\Delta H}{H} = \frac{v}{E} * \frac{F}{A},$$

where v is the poisson ratio of the individual organ defined as the ratio of transverse contraction strain to longitudinal extension strain that describes the compressibility of a material. Typical Young's modulus and poisson ratio for various anatomical organs that can be used in biomechanical DIR are discussed by Brock et al.[26]

Other biomechanical DIR models include the hyperelastic model that considers soft tissues to behave nonlinearly as a rubber-like material and the viscoelastic model that takes into consideration both viscous and elastic properties, with a time-dependent strain.

Based on the chosen biomechanical law, material properties and boundary conditions are assigned, which are then used to perform a numerical optimization (finite element analysis) to compute the resulting displacement, stress, and strain of each element of the organ. In summary, biomechanical DIR models can potentially provide complex but realistic organ deformations based on the underlying physics. However, accurate delineations along with boundary conditions and individual organ elasticity properties are required for an accurate registration.

HYBRID METHODS

There is no universal DIR method that yields a perfect solution and hence hybrid methods have been recently proposed to take advantage of the relative merits of each approach.[12] Their goal is to improve regularization, accuracy, and speed of convergence. The hybrid process can be applied either during optimization, by generating a DVF from different available information (e.g., landmark points, image intensities, or segmented structures), or afterward, by fusing the different DVFs resulting from the different methods. The idea is to compensate for errors introduced by each algorithm.[40–46]

OPTIMIZATION METHODOLOGIES

Optimization refers to the manner in which a transformation function is adjusted to improve image similarity metrics. A good optimizer can be thought of as one which finds the best possible transformation between the source and fixed images quickly and robustly. DIR as discussed before is, in general, an ill-posed problem due to lack of a singular solution. There can be many DVFs in a nonparametric registration resulting in the same deformed image and thereby resulting in the same cost value as calculated by the chosen similarity measure. Therefore, the similarity metric is usually combined with a regularization term. For parametric transformations, the regularization is often achieved using a combination of a regularization energy term on the parameters and the properties of the parameterization function itself. Other transformations (like RBFs) function as interpolators and work by providing a smooth interpolation of prescribed displacements (e.g., the matching of landmarks). For nonparametric methods, the smoothness of the resulting transformation is dependent on the regularization chosen. Most practical implementations of image registration methods utilize some kind of hierarchical coarse-to-fine approach. Several possible approaches exist as discussed in Lester et al.[47]

Multiresolution Approaches

In a multiresolution approach, the deformation is first approximated on low resolution versions of the images to be registered. The result of this coarse registration is then used as a starting point for a registration at a higher resolution. This continues until the deformation has been approximated at the highest resolution. A multiresolution strategy enables the optimizer to systematically handle modes of deformation at different scales. By finding a minimizing transformation at a low resolution, there is a better chance of avoiding local minima at a higher resolution.

It should be noted that most DIR algorithms use different registration methods of increasing complexity as part of the hierarchical approach. Almost every deformable registration method requires an initial global (rigid or affine) registration to be performed that reduces the parametric search space before the deformable model is invoked. Preprocessing the input images by extracting specific features, cropping images to limit anatomy to selected structures, and filtering the images to improve intensity consistency can also guide the DIR process to a faster convergence.

Optimization Methods for Parametric Registration Models

For parametric methods, a number of numerical methods can be used for optimization of the cost function. Gradient descents and conjugate gradients are commonly used optimizers for parametric models.

A key ingredient in efficient optimization of a cost function is how efficient it is to compute the derivative of the cost function with respect to each of its parameters. If these derivatives cannot be found analytically, they may be estimated using finite difference approximations.

Optimization Methods for Nonparametric Registration Models

The nonparametric deformation models discussed before often need a method to solve the PDEs that arise from various models (Demons, viscous fluid, etc.) There are two primary methods to solve PDEs, the finite element method and finite difference method. The finite element method solves the PDEs by approximating the solution using a mesh to describe the volume and in general leads to a better solution in more complex geometries because the mesh can be made flexible. The finite element methods are computationally more intensive.

On the other hand, the finite difference method approximates the PDEs and a solution is found by finite difference. These equations can then be solved by assigning appropriate boundary conditions applicable to a particular deformation model.

VALIDATION OF DEFORMABLE IMAGE REGISTRATION IN RADIATION ONCOLOGY

There have been many techniques proposed to validate the accuracy of various DIR algorithms.[5,29,48–55] All DIR evaluation procedures require the use of evaluation data and validation methods. Considering the evaluation data one can separate the methods into two groups: (i) those using real patient image data and (ii) those using phantom image data. In the first set of methods, the authors use real patient images that they deform artificially to create the reference and the test study. Alternately, multiple imaging acquisitions at different time intervals where changes in anatomy are clearly visible and anticipated (e.g., replanning scans or cone beam CT scans) are used. The use of deformable phantoms is attractive in DIR validation as phantoms can be scanned before and after ground truth deformations are applied, which can

then be compared to those estimated by the DIR algorithm. Physical phantoms made from balloons, sponges, bladder shapes, and 3D printers have been used in DIR validation.[56–62] However, phantoms as described earlier cannot be routinely used in most busy clinical departments because of the lack of resources and time required to build and test these phantoms. Further, it is not practical to build a phantom that will be sophisticated enough to simulate all anatomical deformations that can occur in a clinical environment. It has also been suggested that the presence of uniform intensity regions in the phantom images as opposed to more intensity gradients in clinical CT images may limit the applicability of phantom tests in DIR verification.[48] The validation methods often include using landmark points in regions of interest, as a surrogate tool in verifying accuracy of the DIR. A frequent problem with this technique is locating the landmark points, which in real patients anatomy can be time-consuming, and difficult to identify markers in low-contrast regions. The contour-based evaluation is useful qualitative verification in contour propagation and inspecting anatomical differences among images. Although contour propagation techniques seem to provide a more efficient way of validation compared to markers, including changes in shape, volume, and location of a structure, they often do not confirm that the volume within the contour has been properly registered.[5]

Numerical or digital phantoms are very attractive to DIR evaluation as they use real patient CT data and can simulate a clinically observed organ deformation, which can be then used to test the performance of a particular DIR algorithm. Both commercially available[5,63] and open-source phantom libraries[64,65] are available for testing the performance of a DIR algorithm.

Figures 18.3 to 18.5 illustrate how clinically relevant deformations observed in IGRT for prostate cancer are simulated to establish the ground truth in order to validate the performance of DIR algorithm using a commercially available digital phantom.[5]

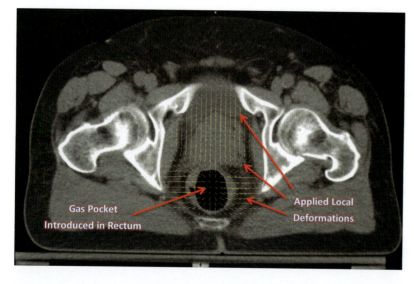

FIGURE 18.3. Axial view illustrating the local deformations introduced in the prostate and rectal region and gas pocket in the rectum.

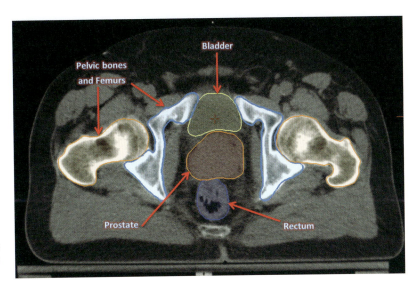

FIGURE 18.4. Axial view of the prostate CT image with original Radiotherapy (RT) structures namely bladder, prostate, rectum, and pelvic bones.

In summary, it is critical that some quantitative validation of the system accuracy of the implemented DIR algorithm and its potential limitations in the commonly encountered IGRT clinical situations exists.[11,66] DIR performance can be evaluated from a simple qualitative visual inspection to more robust quantitative methods and the various evaluation methodologies are presented in the following section.

Visual Inspection

The simplest evaluation of the performance of a DIR is by viewing a fused reference and deformed image. The alignment of common anatomical structures and other landmarks can be visually inspected between the two images. Visual representation of fusion in terms of checkerboard images and colored rendering are frequently used in aiding a qualitative inspection of the fusion accuracy. In addition, visualizing the DVF overlapped on the images as a 2D vector or a deformed grid can help to detect local irregularities. However, visual inspection methods provide no quantitative information, cannot detect small uncertainties, and hence should be used only as a starting point in the evaluation of a DIR performance.

Anatomical Correspondence

Anatomical correspondence between the original and deformed image sets can be identified using markers or contour segmentation defined by the users. This validation is important because in radiotherapy clinical applications, the tumor and OAR volume change over time and consequently, the partial volume dose received by these structures. The magnitude and location of these changes dictate the need for adaptive radiotherapy. A quantitative metric comparing the original tumor and OAR segmentation in the fixed image with those obtained from warping the RT structures with the DVF derived from DIR in the moving image is widely used. Dice similarity coefficient (DSC), Hausdorff distance (HD), and average surface

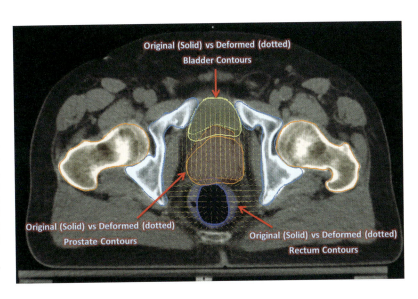

FIGURE 18.5. Contour changes in prostate, bladder, and rectum from the applied DVF when compared with original segmentation of these structures. Solid figures refer to original segmentation done by radiation oncologist on CT image, and dotted figures refer to the deformed volumes due to the applied deformation using the digital phantom. A perfect DIR algorithm will recover the original contours when DVF is applied to the deformed contours.

DIR, deformable image registration; DVF, deformation vector field.

distance are some of the commonly used metrics to evaluate the accuracy of tumor and OAR segmentation and spatial overlap index.

Dice Similarity Coefficient

DSC[67] computes the number of pixels that overlap between the two volumes and normalizes it by half the sum of the number of nonzero pixels in the two volumes. The result is a value between 0 (no overlap) and 1 (perfect overlap)

$$\text{DSC} = \frac{2* \ |A \cap B|}{|A| + |B|},$$

where A is the ground truth segmentation in fixed image, and B is the segmentation mapped from the deformably registered image. The metric is symmetric and is sensitive to both differences in scale and position. While volume overlap is a good indicator of mismatch, it is a poor indicator of shape since it is not a measure of distance and hence the following metrics are usually evaluated to assess the overall accuracy. Typically, within the contouring uncertainty of a structure, a DSC tolerance limit of 0.8 to 0.9 is considered acceptable.[11] However, DSC is typically higher for larger organs (liver, lung, etc.) compared to smaller organs (Brainstem, prostate, etc.) because of the smaller relative change in overall volume of the larger organ.

Hausdorff Distance

The Hausdorff distance (HD)[68,69] is defined as the maximum of the closest distance between two volumes where the closest distance is computed for each vertex of the two volumes. The HD $H(A,B)$ between 2 sets of points $A = \{a1, ..., am\}$ and $B = \{b1, ..., bm\}$ is given by $H(A,B) = \max(h(A,B), h(B,A))$. The metric is very sensitive to outliers since the most mismatched point is the sole determining criterion of the distance. The 95% HD (95% HD) metric is sometimes used as a threshold as the outliers are rejected in 95% HD. Figure 18.6 shows a description of HD.

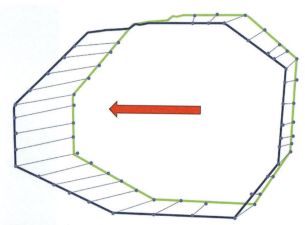

FIGURE 18.6. Hausdorff distance is the maximum perpendicular distance between closest points from two contours of registered images. Green line represents an external contour from one image and blue line represents an external contour from another image after DIR. Blue dots represent corresponding closest points between each contour. Hausdorff distance represents the distance between small circles at red arrow.

DIR, deformable image registration.

Average Surface Distance

This metric mitigates the outlier problem exhibited by the HD. The metric is the average of the absolute distance from each surface pixel in one image to its closest point on the other image.

Point-to-Point Error Comparisons

Point-to-point error or target registration error (TRE) defined as the distance between the ground truth point and the point propagated by the DVF can be used to verify the accuracy of DIR as shown in Figure 18.7.

A frequent problem with this method is that the landmark points have to be manually placed by an anatomy expert, which is very time-consuming and could be difficult to do in images with poor contrast, artifacts,

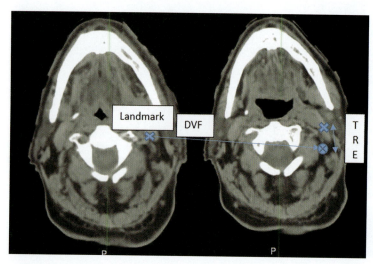

FIGURE 18.7. A set of landmark points are placed in both source and target images by the anatomy expert. The distance between the true landmark point and the point propagated by the DVF in source image is used to compute metric (TRE).

DVF, deformation vector field; TRE, target registration error.

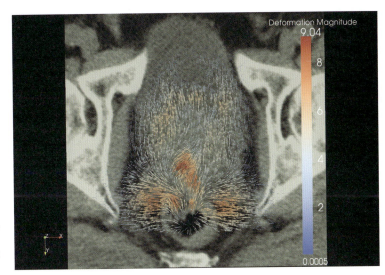

FIGURE 18.8. Forward diffeomorphic demons DVF from the DIR overlaid on the original prostate CT image illustrating the local changes due to the DVF. The field vectors are pointing outward.

DIR, deformable image registration; DVF, deformation vector field.

and noise.[55] More robust approaches based on automatic feature extractions that can identify a large number of landmark points have been proposed.[70,71] Typically, maximum voxel dimension of the order of 2 to 3 mm is considered an acceptable tolerance for TRE.[11]

Deformation Vector Field

The physical characteristics of the deformation fields should be investigated.[5] Recent applications in Adaptive Radiation Therapy (ART) have used the deformation fields arising from image registration process to warp the RT dose and display a deformed dose.[72–75] Hence, some quantitative information on the physical characteristics of the deformation fields is necessary for clinical implementation of ART. It is known that matching of structures based on their intensities alone is not a sufficient condition to produce physically achievable deformations.[76]

One of the key methods reported in the literature is the concept of inverse consistency that allows quantifying DVF consistency by comparing the results of two deformations

that have different paths.[38,77,78] Inverse consistency between two images, A and B, is evaluated as follows. Image A is deformed to match image B, and image B is separately deformed to match image A. A perfect inverse consistent algorithm will produce a true inverse DVF when the roles of source and target images are switched. However, in practice this is not the case. The inverse consistency error (ICE) between forward and inverse registration is calculated by compositive accumulation[79] of forward and inverse DVFs. The magnitude of compositive accumulation will be zero for perfectly inverse consistent algorithm. The disadvantage of the inverse consistency method is that a zero value for ICE is a necessary, but not sufficient, condition for an accurate algorithm since errors in one DVF may cancel with errors in the other to yield a net zero value during composition of two deformation maps.[77] Typically, maximum voxel dimension of the order of 2 to 3 mm is considered an acceptable tolerance for ICE.[11]

Figures 18.8 and 18.9 show the DVF arising from diffeomorphic demons registration for forward and inverse registrations using the synthetic deformations

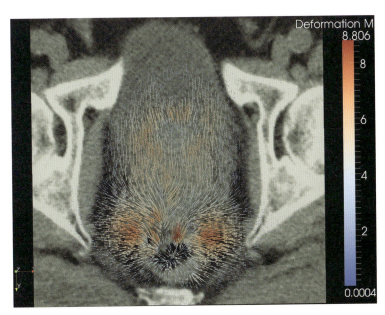

FIGURE 18.9. Inverse diffeomorphic demons DVF when the roles of source and target images were switched from previous example, overlaid on the original CT image. The field vectors are pointing inward.

DVF, deformation vector field.

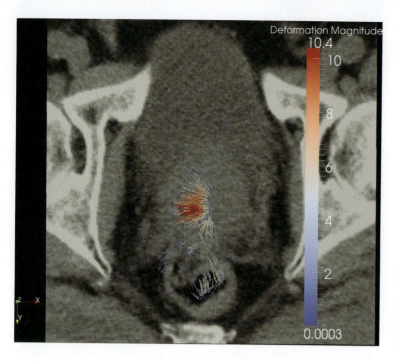

FIGURE 18.10. Compositive addition of forward and inverse demons DVF overlaid on the original CT image. If the algorithm were truly inverse consistent, this composition would yield zero, but a small resultant ICE as shown exists. DVF, deformation vector field; ICE, inverse consistency error.

described in Figure 18.3 to validate DIR performance. Figure 18.10 is the resultant ICE between the forward and inverse DVFs.

The distance discordance metric (DDM) measures the backward distances of the distributed voxels from multiple registered images to a single fixed image.[80] DDM allows the local uncertainties of DIR to be quantified based on at least four observations.[12] Target registration discrepancy (TRD) is another metric that has been proposed to compare two DIR methods from the same observation.[81] TRD is defined as the vector distance between two points warped from the same reference point by at least two DIR algorithms.

Diffeomorphism is a necessary condition for deformation fields to be physically feasible.[82] This property is related to the Jacobian of the deformation field. The Jacobian is a matrix given by the first partial derivatives of the transformation with $J_{ij} = \frac{\partial \Delta i}{\partial xj} = \partial_{ij} + \frac{\partial Di}{\partial xj}$, where ∂_{ij} is Kronecker delta $\left(\partial_{ij} = 1 \text{ if } i = j, 0 \text{ otherwise}\right)$ and D_i is the ith component of deformation field. The determinant of the Jacobian of the deformation field can be used to validate the physical behavior of deformation.[83] A negative Jacobian indicates singularities in the field and corresponds to a physically unrealistic organ deformation as organs can only be compressed and deformed but cannot undergo non-invertible spatial transformations like folding of structures.[84,85] A determinant of Jacobian greater than 1 indicates expansion at that location while a value less than 1 indicates contractions.

The harmonic energy of the deformation field can be used to quantify the regularity of the spatial transformation obtained by the deformable registration process.[86]

The harmonic energy captures the nonlinearity of the warp, i.e., deviation from an affine transformation. The harmonic energy at a voxel can be defined based on the first-order partial derivatives of the deformation field as follows:

$$HE(D) = \frac{1}{2} \int \Sigma_{i=1}^{n} \Sigma_{j=1}^{n} \left[\frac{\partial D_i}{\partial x_j}\right]^2 dv, \text{ where } v \text{ is the domain}$$

of the deformation field. The mean harmonic energy is inversely proportional to smoothness of the deformation field.

In summary, although evaluation of DVF-based approaches may fulfill the requirements of physical fidelity, the DVF may still differ from the underlying ground truth of deformation.[87] Hence, the DVF consistency check is a necessary but not sufficient condition for an accurate deformation model as it has been shown to be a poor predictor of registration errors.[88]

Image Characteristics

Mean Squared Error (MSE) can be used as a metric to define the extent of mismatch between the original image A and the deformably registered image B and is the normalized square difference between the two images A and B.[89] If $f(n)$ and $g(n)$ represent the value (intensity) of an image pixel at location n, the MSE between $f(n)$ and $g(n)$ is defined as

$$MSE = 1/N\Sigma_n \{f(n) - g(n)\}2,$$

where N is the total number of pixel locations in $f(n)$ or $g(n)$. For a perfect image match between images A and B, the MSE error is zero. However, for clinical applications, use of the MSE as image quality metric has proven to be inadequate for drawing a useful and consistent conclusion.[5] A small value of MSE indicates an overall good accuracy in the entire image voxel space but does not guarantee good accuracy of DVF inside the organs.

CLINICAL CHALLENGES IN DEFORMABLE IMAGE REGISTRATION (DIR) VALIDATION AND RECOMMENDATIONS

For the medical physicist, there are several challenges to proper evaluation of DIR in a clinical setting so that the accurate quantification of uncertainties involved can be communicated to the radiation oncologist on a patient-specific basis. Image noise is a frequent problem in clinical settings that adds intensity information not related to patient anatomy, thus hampering DIR performance and accuracy. Artifacts in images and different fields of view (FOV) between fixed and moving images can also degrade DIR performance.[90] Most DIR algorithms assume the same tissue to be present in both source and target images. However, in clinical scenarios, this is typically not the case. For example, parotid gland volume changes,[91] gas appearance and disappearance in bowel, tumor shrinkage, and empty versus full bladder are frequently observed over the course of radiotherapy. Specific methods to handle these such as preprocessing images to remove gas need to be implemented to prevent the DVF from producing unrealistic deformations. Organs that slide against each other like the brain sliding against the skull due to intraoperative brain shift, the heart sliding against the lungs throughout the cardiac cycle, the respiration-induced sliding of the lungs against the chest wall, and the abdominal organs sliding against each other are encountered during course of radiotherapy, which can potentially cause DVF discontinuities. These require more complex regularization methods[92,93] that are not typically available in commercial DIR platforms. Also, the results of DIR in uniform low-contrast anatomy (liver, abdomen, etc.) are usually poor[35] and if the results of DIR performance are solely assessed with the contrast-rich features present in clinical anatomy, the results may not be reflective of the true DIR performance in uniform low-contrast anatomy.[61]

In addition, deforming the dose with DVF (dose deformation) should be handled carefully.[94] It has been shown that dose propagation using DIR must follow the principle of energy and mass conservation,[95] which is not always obeyed in various clinical scenarios. In general, uncertainties due to dose warping are complex and difficult to quantify as they involve an interplay between spatial errors associated with the DVF and the dose gradient at that voxel. The distance to dose metric (DTD) defined as the distance to observe a given dose difference in irradiated geometry has been proposed to link geometric uncertainties with dose mapping accuracy.[96] Specifically, it indicates how large a DVF error can be, before the DVF error from DIR could introduce a predetermined maximum tolerable dose mapping error.[97]

As such, dose warping methods should not be routinely used to drive clinical decisions. However, they may be more practical to use in retreatment situations where the patient positioning was completely different (arms up vs arms down, etc.) as compared to rigid registration to assess the overlap dose.

Recommendations

Clinical physicists should follow the framework outlined in the American Association of Physicists in Medicine Task Group-132 (AAPM TG-132) report[11] for commissioning commercial DIR platforms. Digital or physical phantoms with a known ground truth deformation can be used to assess data integrity, and baseline DIR performance that can be used for periodic upgrades and end-to-end testing for any new application in the clinical environment. At very minimum, clinical physicists should have a clear understanding of the similarity measures, regularization methods, and deformation models used in a commercial DIR platform as well as understand their potential limitations. Patient-specific validation of DIR has many caveats,[97] but the adoption of a patient-specific report as suggested in TG-132 outlining the uncertainty assessment level and description is crucial for clear communication with the radiation oncologist with the ultimate goal of improving clinical efficiency and outcomes. When implementing DIR, the following elements should be communicated and clearly documented: the image sets to be registered, an understanding of the local regions of importance, the intended clinical use of DIR, and the accuracy required for final use. Some basic best practice guidelines of DIR[98] can be followed that will improve department-specific workflows with clear understanding of user role at each step of the process.

SUMMARY

There has been a significant increase in DIR applications in radiotherapy without a set of definitive practice guidelines. Despite several quantitative evaluation techniques proposed, there is no consensus on a universal quantitative measure that can be used in all DIR applications. The choice of an evaluation metric is likely application-dependent[5] and as such, a range of quantitative metrics, and qualitative QA, including visual inspection should be used in a clinical setting. Different DIR algorithms will behave differently for the same deformation observed, so the clinical physicist must understand the limitations of their algorithm before routine clinical use. It is critical to adopt a patient-specific uncertainty report as suggested in AAPM TG-132, so that accurate quantification of uncertainties involved in DIR can be communicated to the radiation oncologist on a patient-specific basis. In summary, DIR is a valuable tool; however, it must be used with caution and uncertainties must be understood and evaluated when implementing it clinically to ensure accuracy.

ACKNOWLEDGEMENTS

The author gratefully thanks Chris Overbeck MS and Sarah Way MS for careful reading of the manuscript and feedback.

KEY POINTS

- Deformable registration is inherently degenerate and is considered an ill-posed problem because there is generally no unique solution to a registration problem.

- Every DIR algorithm has three basic components: (i) similarity measures of how well the images match, (ii) deformation model (parametric, nonparametric, or biomechanical), which specifies how a source or moving image can be made to match target or fixed image, (iii) an optimization process that varies the parameters of a particular deformation model to maximize the matching criterion.

- Despite several quantitative evaluation techniques proposed to verify the accuracy of DIR, there is no consensus on a universal quantitative measure that can be used in all DIR applications. The choice of an evaluation metric is likely application dependent.

- When implementing DIR, the following elements should be communicated and clearly documented: the image sets to be registered, an understanding of the local regions of importance, the intended clinical use of DIR, and the accuracy required for final use. The use of patient-specific uncertainty report as outlined in AAPM TG-132 must be adopted.

REVIEW QUESTIONS

1. Which similarity metric is most optimal for CT/MR registration?
   A. Cross correlation
   B. Mutual information
   C. Sum of squared differences
   D. Gradient descent

2. A registration between contrast-enhanced diagnostic CT and treatment planning CT is performed for delineating target for liver metastasis. A large deformation of liver is seen between the two scans. Which of the following algorithms is best suited for DIR?
   A. B-Splines
   B. Demons
   C. Diffeomorphic Demons
   D. Biomechanical

3. Target registration error (TRE) can be described as
   A. Average surface distance between two targets in the registered image
   B. Maximum distance between two targets in the registered image
   C. The distance between the true landmark point and the point propagated by the DVF in source image.
   D. Volume mismatch between the two registered targets.

4. Which of the following metrics is most suited to evaluate DIR algorithm accuracy for clinical use during commissioning?
   A. Inverse consistency error and Jacobian of the DVF
   B. Careful visual inspection of the fused images to detect alignment of common anatomical structures and other landmarks.
   C. Anatomical correspondence as evaluated by DSC.
   D. All of the above as different DIR algorithms behave differently for a given deformation.

5. Which of the following statements are correct?
   A. Commissioning tests are not required for DIR algorithms unlike TPS commissioning.
   B. Accurate DIR performance can be evaluated by careful visual inspection alone.
   C. A patient-specific uncertainty report is required, so that accurate quantification of uncertainties involved in DIR can be communicated to the radiation oncologist.
   D. Dose deformation should not be used to drive routine clinical decisions.

ANSWERS

1. **B** When using different imaging modalities where pixel intensities of corresponding anatomy are inherently different, sophisticated metrics that use intensity statistics are required. Mutual Information (MI) is the only metric that satisfies these criteria.

2. **D** Liver is a large deforming anatomy with minimal contrast-rich features. Intensity-based registration algorithms like Demons and diffeomorphic demons are not well suited for DIR of liver. Because of the complex deformation required and lack of sufficient contrast-rich features inside the liver, biomechanical DIR will be the best performing algorithm among the given choices.

3. **C** Target registration error (TRE) can be used as one of the metrics for verifying DIR accuracy. TRE is defined as the distance between the ground truth point and the point propagated by the DVF.

4. **D** DIR is considered an ill-posed problem, as there is no one unique solution to a registration. Commercial DIR platforms available today use a wide range of DIR algorithms (B-Spline, Intensity-based, Biomechanical DIR, etc.) and each algorithm will behave differently for a given applied deformation. As such, the clinical physicist at the time of commissioning should have a clear understanding of the performance and limitations of the particular algorithm they intend to use clinically. Choice A evaluates the physical characteristics of DVF; choice B gives a qualitative accuracy in the regions of interest, while choice C quantifies the registered organ accuracy using DSC. All are needed at the time of commissioning.

5. **C & D** Commissioning tests are required for evaluating DIR as recommended in AAPM TG-132 report. One cannot fully evaluate DIR accuracy by visual inspection alone. Dose deformation should not be used routinely to drive clinical decisions as dose deformation involves a complex interplay between dose gradient at a particular voxel and spatial error associate with DVF and cannot be verified easily. It is critical that an uncertainty report associated with DIR be communicated to the radiation oncologist on a patient-specific basis.

REFERENCES

1. Crum WR, Hartkens T, Hill DL. Non-rigid image registration: theory and practice. *Br J Radiol.* 2004;77 Spec No 2:S140–S153.
2. Sarrut D. Deformable registration for image-guided radiation therapy. *Z Med Phys.* 2006;16(4):285–297.
3. Yan D, Vicini F, Wong J, Martinez A. Adaptive radiation therapy. *Phys Med Biol.* 1997;42:123–132.
4. Yan D. Adaptive radiotherapy: merging principle into clinical practice. *Semin Radiat Oncol.* 2010;20(2):79–83.
5. Varadhan R, Karangelis G, Krishnan K, Hui S. A framework for deformable image registration validation in radiotherapy clinical applications. *J Appl Clin Med Phys.* 2013;14(1):4066.
6. Acosta O, Simon A, Monge F, Commandeur F, Bassirou C, Cazoulat G, Crevoisier RD, Haigron P. Evaluation of multi-atlas-based segmentation of CT scans in prostate cancer radiotherapy. In: *2011 IEEE International Symposium on Biomedical Imaging: From Nano to Macro: 30 March–2 April 2011*; 2011:1966–1969.
7. Iglesias JE, Sabuncu MR. Multi-atlas segmentation of biomedical images: a survey. *Med Image Anal.* 2015;24(1):205–219.
8. Kim N, Chang JS, Kim YB, Kim JS. Atlas-based auto-segmentation for postoperative radiotherapy planning in endometrial and cervical cancers. *Radiat Oncol (London, England).* 2020;15(1):106.
9. Lee H, Lee E, Kim N, et al. Clinical evaluation of commercial atlas-based auto-segmentation in the head and neck region. *Front Oncol.* 2019;9:239–239.
10. Badawi AM, Weiss E, Sleeman WCT, Hugo GD. Classifying geometric variability by dominant eigenmodes of deformation in regressing tumours during active breath-hold lung cancer radiotherapy. *Phys Med Biol.* 2012;57(2):395–413.
11. Brock KK, Mutic S, McNutt TR, Li H, Kessler ML. Use of image registration and fusion algorithms and techniques in radiotherapy: report of the AAPM radiation therapy committee task group No. 132. *Med Phys.* 2017;44(7) e43–e76.
12. Rigaud B, Simon A, Castelli J, et al. Deformable image registration for radiation therapy: principle, methods, applications and evaluation. *Acta Oncol.* 2019;58(9):1225–1237.
13. Davis MH, Khotanzad A, Flamig DP, Harms SE. A physics-based coordinate transformation for 3-D image matching. *Med Imaging IEEE Trans.* 1997;16(3):317–328.
14. Bookstein FL. Principal Warps: thin-plate splines and the decomposition of deformations. *IEEE Trans Pattern Anal Mach Intell.* 1989;11(6):567–585.
15. Rueckert D, Sonoda L, Hayes C, Hill DL, Leach MO, Hawkes DJ. Nonrigid registration using free-form deformations: application to breast MR images. *IEEE Trans Med Imaging* 1999;18(8):712–721.
16. Thirion JP. Image matching as a diffusion process: an analogy with Maxwell's demons. *Med Image Anal.* 1998;2(3):243–260.
17. Horn BKP, Schunck BG. Determining optical flow. *Artif Intell.* 1981;17:185–204.
18. Christensen GE, Rabbitt RD, Miller MI. Deformable templates using large deformation kinematics. *IEEE Trans Image Process.* 1996;5(10):1435–1447.
19. Wendland H. Piecewise polynomial, positive definite and compactly supported radial functions of minimal degree. *Adv Comput Math.* 1995;4:389–396.
20. Shusharina N, Sharp G. Analytic regularization for landmark-based image registration. *Phys Med Biol.* 2012;57(6):1477–1498.

21. Deformable Image Registration Part 2. https://gray.mgh.harvard.edu/attachments/article/233/Lecture%205b.pdf

22. Lawson JD, Schreibmann E, Jani AB, Fox T. Quantitative evaluation of a cone-beam computed tomography-planning computed tomography deformable image registration method for adaptive radiation therapy. *J Appl Clin Med Phys.* 2007;8(4):2432.

23. Mattes D, Haynor DR, Vesselle H, Lewellen TK, Eubank W. PET-CT image registration in the chest using free-form deformations. *IEEE Trans Med Imaging.* 2003;22(1):120–128.

24. Schreibmann E, Fox T, Crocker I. Dosimetric effects of manual cone-beam CT (CBCT) matching for spinal radiosurgery: our experience. *J Appl Clin Med Phys.* 2011;12(3):3467.

25. Zhong H, Peters T, Siebers JV. FEM-based evaluation of deformable image registration for radiation therapy. *Phys Med Biol.* 2007;52(16):4721–4738.

26. Brock KK, Sharpe MB, Dawson LA, Kim SM, Jaffray DA. Accuracy of finite element model-based multi-organ deformable image registration. *Med Phys.* 2005;32(6):1647–1659.

27. Robertson S, Weiss E, Hugo GD. Deformable mesh registration for the validation of automatic target localization algorithms. *Med Phys.* 2013;40(7):071721. doi: 071710.071118/071721.4811105.

28. Wang H, Dong L, Lii MF, Lee AL, de Crevoisier R, Mohan R, Cox JD, Kuban DA, Cheung R. Implementation and validation of a three-dimensional deformable registration algorithm for targeted prostate cancer radiotherapy. *Int J Radiat Oncol Biol Phys.* 2005;61(3):725–735.

29. Wang H, Dong L, O'Daniel J, et al. Validation of an accelerated 'demons' algorithm for deformable image registration in radiation therapy. *Phys Med Biol.* 2005;50(12):2887–2905.

30. Wang H, Garden AS, Zhang L, et al. Performance evaluation of automatic anatomy segmentation algorithm on repeat or four-dimensional computed tomography images using deformable image registration method. *Int J Radiat Oncol Biol Phys.* 2008;72(1):210–219.

31. Vercauteren T, Pennec X, Perchant A, Ayache N. Diffeomorphic demons: efficient non-parametric image registration. *Neuroimage.* 2009;45(1 Suppl):S61–S72.

32. Christensen GE, Carlson B, Chao KS, et al. Image-based dose planning of intracavitary brachytherapy: registration of serial-imaging studies using deformable anatomic templates. *Int J Radiat Oncol Biol Phys.* 2001;51(1):227–243.

33. Yang D, Brame S, El Naqa I, et al. Technical note: DIRART: a software suite for deformable image registration and adaptive radiotherapy research. *Med Phys.* 2011;38(1):67–77.

34. Guerrero T, Zhang G, Huang TC, Lin KP. Intrathoracic tumour motion estimation from CT imaging using the 3D optical flow method. *Phys Med Biol.* 2004;49(17):4147–4161.

35. Yeo UJ, Supple J, Taylor ML, Smith RL, Kron T, Franich RD. Performance of 12 DIR algorithms in low-contrast regions for mass and density conserving deformation. *Med Phys.* 2013;40(101701).

36. Yeo UJ, Taylor ML, Dunn L, Kron T, Smith RL, Franich RD. A novel methodology for 3D deformable dosimetry. *Med Phys.* 2012;39(4):2203–2213.

37. Yeo UJ, Taylor ML, Supple JR, et al. Is it sensible to "deform" dose? 3D experimental validation of dose-warping. *Med Phys.* 2012;39(8):5065–5072.

38. Yang D, Li H, Low DA, Deasy JO, El Naqa I. A fast inverse consistent deformable image registration method based on symmetric optical flow computation. *Phys Med Biol.* 2008;53(21):6143–6165. doi: 6110.1088/0031-9155/6153/6121/6017. Epub 2008 Oct 6114.

39. Lucas BD, Kanade T. An iterative image registration technique with an application to Stereo Vision (DARPA). In: *Proceedings of the 7th International Joint Conference on Artificial Intelligence: 1981*; 1981:674–679.

40. Cazoulat G, Owen D, Matuszak MM, Balter JM, Brock KK. Biomechanical deformable image registration of longitudinal lung CT images using vessel information. *Phys Med Biol.* 2016;61(13):4826–4839.

41. Samavati N, Velec M, Brock K. A hybrid biomechanical intensity based deformable image registration of lung 4DCT. *Phys Med Biol.* 2015;60(8):3359.

42. Li M, Castillo E, Zheng X-L, et al. Modeling lung deformation: a combined deformable image registration method with spatially varying Young's modulus estimates. *Med Phys.* 2013;40(8):081902.

43. Staring M, Van Der Heide U, Klein S, Viergever M, Pluim JP. Registration of cervical MRI using multifeature mutual information. *IEEE Trans Med Imaging.* 2009;28(9):1412–1421.

44. Weistrand O, Svensson S. The ANACONDA algorithm for deformable image registration in radiotherapy. *Med Phys.* 2015;42(1):40–53.

45. Yang Y, Teo SK, Van Reeth E, Tan C, Tham I, Poh C. A hybrid approach for fusing 4D-MRI temporal information with 3D-CT for the study of lung and lung tumor motion. *Med Phys.* 2015;42(8):4484–4496.

46. Zhong H, Wen N, Gordon JJ, Elshaikh MA, Movsas B, Chetty IJ. An adaptive MR-CT registration method for MRI-guided prostate cancer radiotherapy. *Phys Med Biol.* 2015;60(7):2837.

47. Lester H, Arridge SR. A survey of hierarchical non-linear medical image registration. *Pattern Recogn.* 1999;32(1):129–149.

48. Zhong H, Kim J, Chetty IJ. Analysis of deformable image registration accuracy using computational modeling. *Med Phys.* 2010;37(3):970–979.

49. Kashani R, Hub M, Balter JM, et al. Objective assessment of deformable image registration in radiotherapy: a multi-institution study. *Med Phys.* 2008;35(12):5944–5953.

50. Schaly B, Bauman GS, Battista JJ, Van Dyk J. Validation of contour-driven thin-plate splines for tracking fraction-to-fraction changes in anatomy and radiation therapy dose mapping. *Phys Med Biol.* 2005;50(3):459–475.

51. Brock KK. Results of a multi-institution deformable registration accuracy study (MIDRAS). *Int J Radiat Oncol Biol Phys.* 2009;76(2):583–596.

52. Kaus MR, Brock KK, Pekar V, Dawson LA, Nichol AM, Jaffray DA. Assessment of a model-based deformable image registration approach for radiation therapy planning. *Int J Radiat Oncol Biol Phys.* 2007;68(2):572–580.

53. Ostergaard Noe K, De Senneville BD, Elstrom UV, Tanderup K, Sorensen TS. Acceleration and validation of optical flow based deformable registration for image-guided radiotherapy. *Acta Oncol.* 2008;47(7):1286–1293.

54. Zhang T, Chi Y, Meldolesi E, Yan D. Automatic delineation of on-line head-and-neck computed tomography images: toward on-line adaptive radiotherapy. *Int J Radiat Oncol Biol Phys.* 2007;68(2):522–530.

55. Castillo R, Castillo E, Guerra R, et al. A framework for evaluation of deformable image registration spatial accuracy using large landmark point sets. *Phys Med Biol.* 2009;54(7):1849–1870.

56. Serban M, Heath E, Stroian G, Collins DL, Seuntjens J. A deformable phantom for 4D radiotherapy verification: design and image registration evaluation. *Med Phys.* 2008;35(3):1094–1102.

57. Kashani R, Hub M, Kessler ML, Balter JM. Technical note: a physical phantom for assessment of accuracy of deformable alignment algorithms. *Med Phys.* 2007;34(7):2785–2788.

58. Kirby N, Chuang C, Pouliot J. A two-dimensional deformable phantom for quantitatively verifying deformation algorithms. *Med Phys.* 2011;38(8):4583–4586.

59. Stanley N, Glide-Hurst C, Kim J, et al. Using patient-specific phantoms to evaluate deformable image registration algorithms for adaptive radiation therapy. *J Appl Clin Med Phys.* 2013;14(6):177–194.

60. Wognum S, Heethuis S, Rosario T, Hoogeman M, Bel A. Validation of deformable image registration algorithms on CT images of ex vivo porcine bladders with fiducial markers. *Med Phys.* 2014;41(7).

61. Varadhan R, Magome T, Hui S. Characterization of deformation and physical force in uniform low contrast anatomy and its impact on accuracy of deformable image registration. *Med Phys.* 2016;43(1):52–61.

62. Chang J, Suh TS, Lee DS. Development of a deformable lung phantom for the evaluation of deformable registration. *J Appl Clin Med Phys.* 2010;11(1):281–286.

63. Loi G, Fusella M, Lanzi E, et al. Performance of commercially available deformable image registration platforms for contour propagation using patient-based computational phantoms: a multi-institutional study. *Med Phys.* 2018;45(2):748–757.

64. Castillo R, Castillo E, Fuentes D, et al. A reference dataset for deformable image registration spatial accuracy evaluation using the COPDgene study archive. *Phys Med Biol.* 2013;58(9):2861.

65. Pukala J, Meeks SL, Staton RJ, Bova FJ, Mañon RR, Langen KM. A virtual phantom library for the quantification of deformable image registration uncertainties in patients with cancers of the head and neck. *Med Phys.* 2013;40(11):-.

66. Yan D. Developing quality assurance processes for image-guided adaptive radiation therapy. *Int J Radiat Oncol Biol Phys.* 2008;71(1 Suppl):S28–S32.

67. Dice LR. Measures of the amount of ecologic association between species. *Ecology.* 1945;26:297–302.

68. Huttenlocher DP, Klanderman GA, Rucklidge WA. Comparing images using the Hausdorff distance. *IEEE Trans Pattern Anal Mach Intell.* 1993;15:850–863.

69. Oguro S, Tuncali K, Elhawary H, Morrison PR, Hata N, Silverman SG. Image registration of pre-procedural MRI and intra-procedural CT images to aid CT-guided percutaneous cryoablation of renal tumors. *Int J Comput Assist Radiol Surg.* 2011;6(1):111–117.

70. Paganelli C, Peroni M, Riboldi M, et al. Scale invariant feature transform in adaptive radiation therapy: a tool for deformable image registration assessment and re-planning indication. *Phys Med Biol.* 2013;58(2):287.

71. Yang D, Zhang M, Chang X, et al. A method to detect landmark pairs accurately between intra-patient volumetric medical images. *Med Phys.* 2017;44(11):5859–5872.

72. Janssens G, de Xivry JO, Fekkes S, et al. Evaluation of nonrigid registration models for interfraction dose accumulation in radiotherapy. *Med Phys.* 2009;36(9):4268–4276.

73. Orban de Xivry J, Janssens G, Bosmans G, et al. Tumour delineation and cumulative dose computation in radiotherapy based on deformable registration of respiratory correlated CT images of lung cancer patients. *Radiother Oncol.* 2007;85(2):232–238.

74. Rosu M, Chetty IJ, Balter JM, Kessler ML, McShan DL, Ten Haken RK. Dose reconstruction in deforming lung anatomy: dose grid size effects and clinical implications. *Med Phys.* 2005;32(8):2487–2495.

75. Schaly B, Kempe J, Bauman GS, Battista JJ, Van Dyk J. Tracking the dose distribution in radiation therapy by accounting for variable anatomy. *Phys Med Biol.* 2004;49(5):791–805.

76. Rohlfing T. Transformation model and constraints cause bias in statistics on deformation fields. *Med Image Comput Comput Assist Interv.* 2006;9(Pt 1):207–214.

77. Bender E, Tome W. The utilization of consistency metrics for error analysis in deformable image registration. *Phys Med Biol.* 2009;54:5561–5567.

78. Christensen GE, Johnson HJ. Consistent image registration. *IEEE Trans Med Imaging.* 2001;20(7):568–582.

79. Janssens G, Jacques L, Orban de Xivry J, Geets X, Macq B. Diffeomorphic registration of images with variable contrast enhancement. *Int J Biomed Imaging.* 2011;2011:891585.

80. Saleh Z, Thor M, Apte AP, et al. A multiple-image-based method to evaluate the performance of deformable image registration in the pelvis. *Phys Med Biol.* 2016;61(16):6172.

81. Qin A, Liang J, Han X, O'Connell N, Yan D. The impact of deformable image registration methods on dose warping. *Med Phys.* 2018.

82. Arsigny V, Commowick O, Pennec X, Ayache N. A log-Euclidean framework for statistics on diffeomorphisms. *Med Image Comput Comput Assist Interv.* 2006;9(Pt 1):924–931.

83. Leow AD, Yanovsky I, Chiang MC, et al. Statistical properties of Jacobian maps and the realization of unbiased large-deformation nonlinear image registration. *IEEE Trans Med Imaging.* 2007;26(6):822–832.

84. Chen M, Lu W, Chen Q, Ruchala KJ, Olivera GH. A simple fixed-point approach to invert a deformation field. *Med Phys.* 2008;35(1):81–88.

85. Rey D, Subsol G, Delingette H, Ayache N. Automatic detection and segmentation of evolving processes in 3D medical images: application to multiple sclerosis. *Med Image Anal.* 2002;6(2):163–179.

86. Jost J, ed. *Riemannian Geometry and Geometric Analysis.* New York, NY: Springer; 2005.

87. Hub M, Karger CP. Estimation of the uncertainty of elastic image registration with the demons algorithm. *Phys Med Biol.* 2013;58(9):3023–3036.

88. Rohlfing T. Image similarity and tissue overlaps as surrogates for image registration accuracy: widely used but unreliable. *IEEE Trans Med Imaging.* 2012;31(2):153–163.

89. Gonzalez RC, Woods RW. *Digital Image Processing.* New York: Addison-Weseley; 1992.

90. Zhen X, Yan H, Zhou L, Jia X, Jiang SB. Deformable image registration of CT and truncated cone-beam CT for adaptive radiation therapy. *Phys Med Biol.* 2013;58(22):7979.

91. Fiorentino A, Caivano R, Metallo V, et al. Parotid gland volumetric changes during intensity-modulated radiotherapy in head and neck cancer. *Br J Radiol.* 2012;85(1018):1415–1419.

92. Pace DF, Enquobahrie A, Yang H, Aylward SR, Niethammer M. Deformable image registration of sliding organs using anisotropic diffusive regularization. In: *2011 IEEE International Symposium on Biomedical Imaging: From Nano to Macro: 30 March–2 April 2011;* 2011:407–413.

93. Delmon V, Rit S, Pinho R, Sarrut D. Registration of sliding objects using direction dependent B-splines decomposition. *Phys Med Biol.* 2013;58(5):1303.

94. Schultheiss TE, Tome WA, Orton CG. Point/counterpoint: it is not appropriate to "deform" dose along with deformable image registration in adaptive radiotherapy. *Med Phys.* 2012;39(11):6531–6533.

95. Zhong H, Chetty IJ. Caution must be exercised when performing deformable dose accumulation for tumors undergoing mass changes during fractionated radiation therapy. *Int J Radiat Oncol Biol Phys.* 2017;97(1):182–183.

96. Saleh-Sayah NK, Weiss E, Salguero FJ, Siebers JV. A distance to dose difference tool for estimating the required spatial accuracy of a displacement vector field. *Med Phys.* 2011;38(5):2318–2323.

97. Paganelli C, Meschini G, Molinelli S, Riboldi M, Baroni G. Patient-specific validation of deformable image registration in radiation therapy: overview and caveats. *Med Phys.* 2018;45(10):e908–e922.

98. Barber J, Yuen J, Jameson M, et al. Deforming to best practice: key considerations for deformable image registration in radiotherapy. *J Med Radiat Sci.* 2020;67(4):318–332.

19 Patient Simulation

Dimitris N. Mihailidis and Niko Papanikolaou

INTRODUCTION

Treatment planning is one of the most crucial processes of radiotherapy, through which the most appropriate way to irradiate the patient is determined. The process is composed of several important steps, such as:

1. reproducible patient positioning and immobilization;
2. accurate identification of the location and shape of the tumor and neighboring critical organs;
3. selecting the most appropriate beam arrangement;
4. computing the doses to be delivered and evaluation of resulting dose distributions; and
5. transfer of the treatment planning information to the treatment delivery system;

Three-dimensional patient anatomy visualization and target definition enable planning to conform the dose to the target volume, delivering as high doses as possible, while avoiding the critical organs. In order to achieve this, a process called *treatment simulation* is necessary to be performed. Treatment simulation is, in essence, a combination of steps 1 to 3 that have been successfully performed. There are several ways to perform a simulation, each with a different level of complexity. The most common ones are:

1. When clinical treatment volume can be determined via simple radiographic and fluoroscopic images from a traditional radiotherapy simulator (1), sometimes called the *anatomical* approach (clinical setup).
2. When only a limited number of transverse computed tomography (CT) images are used for the target delineation along with radiographic planar images (as mentioned previously) in order to complete the treatment planning, sometimes called the *traditional* approach.
3. When simulation can be performed on a CT scanner via a special computer software that provides a fully 3D patient representation in the treatment planning position, a process called *CT-simulation*. Then, a complete treatment planning strategy can be designed, a process referred to as *virtual simulation*.[1,2]

Radiotherapy simulation is a very important process on which treatment planning and treatment delivery depend and are based. The accuracy of the entire radiotherapy treatment can be influenced by the quality of treatment simulation on patient-per-patient basis.

SIMULATION METHODS

Treatment simulation can also be thought of as a "feasibility study" of the patient treatment strategy. Technological advances in medical imaging and computing have brought great improvement to the simulation process and limitless capabilities.

We will describe the three most common methods of radiotherapy simulation today, which strongly depend on the treatment strategy that will be followed for the patient.

Simple Simulation—Anatomical and Traditional Approach

When the patient is necessary to be prepared for treatment in a short amount of time, or there is a simple treatment to be delivered, a conventional simulation can be performed. In this case, a radiographic simulator, which actually operates in both the radiographic and fluoroscopic mode, is used (Fig. 19.1A, B). It is an apparatus that uses a diagnostic X-ray tube with an image intensifier (Fig. 19.1C) but duplicates that radiotherapy treatment unit in terms of its geometric, mechanical, and optical properties.[3–5]

The patient is set up and immobilized on the simulator the same way that he or she will be treated on the treatment unit. The clinical borders of the treatment area are marked on the patient skin by the physician and radio-opaque markers are placed on skin on these borders. The selection of the treatment isocenter is done via fluoroscopic imaging of the area, typically with two orthogonal reference views, anterior (AP) and lateral (LAT) (Fig. 19.2). Upon selection of the isocenter, two orthogonal radiographic films (or digital images) are produced for further use and comparison with the treatment setup, and documentation purposes. Then, the beams that will be used for treatment are simulated in order to be geographically optimized, depending on the treatment site, by selecting gantry and collimator angles, treatment field sizes, etc; all in a

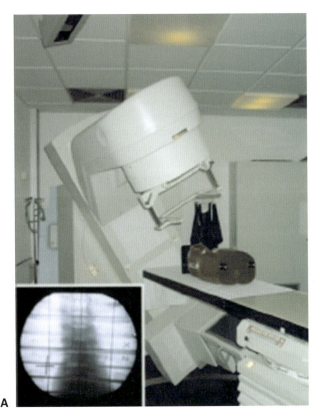

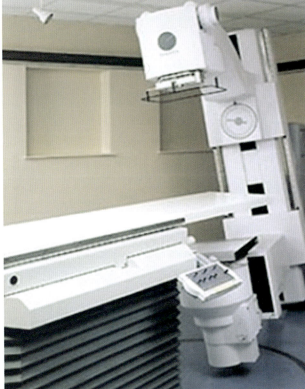

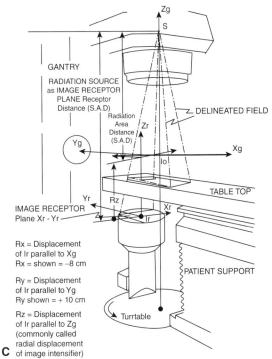

FIGURE 19.1. Typical radiotherapy simulator. Patient setup represented by a phantom **(A)**, room view **(B)**, and geometric diagram **(C)**.

relationship with externally placed markers and internal bony landmarks. A crucial step is the proper marking of the patient: like the isocenter (as a "3-point" marking) and alignment skin marks using the simulator laser system in all planes. At the same time, other necessary information

is collected to be used for setup and dosimetry such as source-to-surface distances of the simulated treatment fields, patient thickness, determination of the time-set or monitor unit calculation point relative to the isocenter (if half-blocked or heavily-blocked fields are used, as in

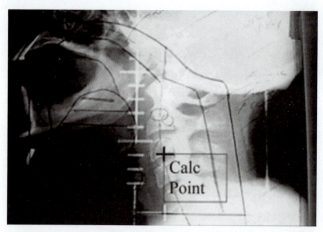

FIGURE 19.2. Typical simulation portal, lateral view for a head and neck treatment. The blocking is represented by the black marker outlines on the film and the prescription point is denoted as "Calc Point," which is off-axis related to the half-blocked central-axis.

Figure. 19.2), simple contours of the patient surface (with contour-makers) through points of dosimetric interest, and evaluation data for bolus or compensator.

Some simulators have a tomographic attachment (simulator-CT) that analyzes and reconstructs the images from the image intensifier using either analog or digital processing.[6] However, the quality of the reconstructed image is inferior to the CT-based simulation. However, it is adequate for acquiring patient contours and identifying bony landmarks. The simulator CT does provide a volumetric reconstruction of the patient's anatomy and as such could be used as a basic image data set in treatment planning. The reduced spatial resolution of such volumetric imaging renders this technique unsuitable for high-precision conformal radiotherapy planning where series of many thin slices is required for detail volume reconstruction.[7,8]

Interestingly, the concept of simulator CT has recently re-emerged and is referred to as cone-beam CT (CBCT). Cone-beam imaging is currently used in the context of image-guided radiotherapy (IGRT) for daily patient localization and setup verification prior to treatment. Those images could also be used for patient re-planning in the context of adaptive radiotherapy although for the time being this is only a research application. It is expected however that once the image quality, imaging dose to the patient, and the speed of re-planning improve that CBCT adaptive radiotherapy will become an integral part of advanced radiotherapy.

CBCT imaging can be obtained using the kilovoltage (kV) imaging system of a linear accelerator (linac; Varian, Elekta) or the megavoltage (MV) beam itself (Tomotherapy, Siemens). Regardless of the implementation, CBCT is similar to and suffers from the same characteristics as the simulator CT.

Verification Simulation

This is a simulation approach "positioned" between the earlier described approach and the virtual simulation that

will be described next. This process starts by immobilizing the patient in the treatment planning position with all the necessary devices, this time on the CT scanner flat table-top. In this case, there is no laser localization system available in the CT room. A standard treatment planning study of the patient will be obtained throughout the clinical area, after radio-radio-opaque markers are placed by the physician on the patient's skin. The simulation team will need to place a "3-point" tattoo or other types of long-lasting marker on the patient's skin. For CT purposes, the "3-point" locations and the treatment area borders will be visible on the CT images. Patient scans are typically obtained in an axial mode, 3 to 5 mm slice thickness. Smaller slice thickness can be used for small areas when higher resolution and accuracy are necessary.

The CT images are reviewed and then imported to a treatment planning system where a computer simulation will be done offline. The physician will define the volumes of interest and the isocenter might be adjusted to accommodate the target volume extensions. The coordinates of the treatment isocenter can be referenced to the original "3-point" location marked in the CT room. Next, the remaining treatment planning process is completed and the plan gets finalized. Two orthogonal (AP and LAT) digitally reconstructed radiographs (DRRs)[9,10] at the original CT point and the new isocenter will be produced at this point (Fig. 19.3). DRRs of the treatment fields will also be produced.

A verification simulation is scheduled in the conventional simulator, where the patient is immobilized and set up again in the treatment planning position. The patient then is simulated according to the approved treatment plan. A sample simulation form is shown in Figure 19.4, where all the appropriate shifts from the original CT marks to the final isocenter are implemented. An orthogonal set of setup ports, first at the original CT point ("3-point" mark) and then at the treatment isocenter will assure the proper localization, when compared to the DRRs at the same locations. The patient will be marked appropriately to insure reproducibility of setup during treatment. Further on, additional ports of the treatment fields can be obtained to increase the accuracy of the simulation setup and for documentation purposes. The orthogonal ports and treatment ports will be compared to portal images or portal films in the treatment room, especially on the first day of treatment. A diagram of the verification simulation process is shown in Figure 19.5A.

CT-Simulator and Virtual Simulation

CT or virtual simulation combines a CT scanner (or other scanning modality) with a patient support assembly into a simulator.[1,2,11–13] Both patient and treatment unit are virtual, the patient is represented by CT images and the treatment unit by model beam geometry and expected dose distributions. The simulation film is replaced by the DRRs. The DDRs are generated from the CT scan data

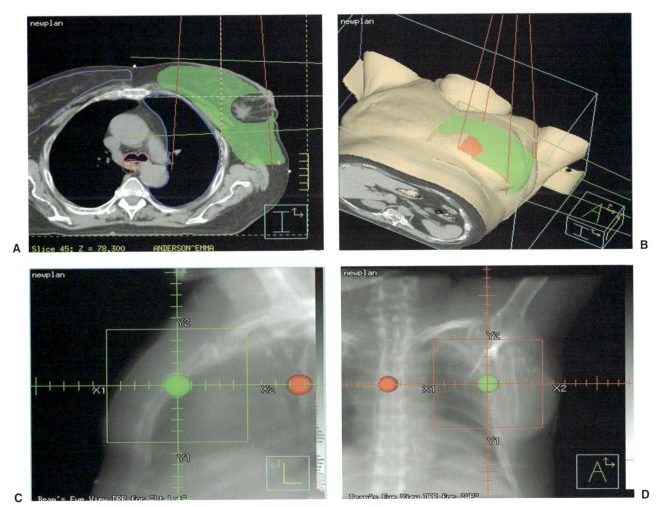

FIGURE 19.3. Breast patient CT image with two orthogonal reference fields on the treatment isocenter-GREEN point **(A)**, 3D reconstruction of the patient imaged area with the reference field **(B)**, LAT-reference field to the treatment isocenter **(C)**, AP-reference filed to the isocenter **(D)**. The RED-point is the original CT point.

by mapping average CT values computed along lines drawn from a "virtual source" to the location of the "virtual film." A DRR is essentially a calculated port film that serves as a simulator film, which contains all the useful anatomical information of the patient (Fig. 19.6). A dedicated radiation therapy CT scanner, with the previously described virtual simulation software and simulation accessories (e.g., flat table-top, immobilization devices, etc), is called a CT-simulator (Fig. 19.7A). In addition, CT-simulators are equipped with high-precision movable laser systems to mark the isocenter location on the patient during the virtual simulation process. The laser system is mounted on fixed pedestals on the floor and ceiling as shown in Figure 19.7B.

Modern radiotherapy CT-simulators are based on the most recent CT scanner technology with multi-slice (multi-detector) detector technology, axial and helical scanning mode capabilities, rapid CT acquisition time, and high image quality performance and wide bore (>75 cm diameter) to accommodate the patient immobilization devices. Further on, an option called *gating* allows the scanner to

perform "motion-correlated" scanning, a process called 4-dimensional computed tomography (4DCT) (the fourth being the time information), useful for accurate treatment planning on moving anatomy (e.g., respiratory motion in lung). The standard linac requirements, for large weight capability (up to 450–600 lb load), small sag (<2 mm), and hard table top, apply for CT-simulators, too.

A diagram that describes the CT-simulation and virtual simulation processes is shown in Figure 19.5B.

CT-Simulation Process

The patient is immobilized on the CT table and in the treatment planning position. At this initial stage, all special immobilization devices (e.g., head and neck masks, pelvic shells, breast boards, etc.) are required to be constructed and/or utilized, in order to be included in the CT image study of the patient. These devices can be indexed on the CT table top, the same way that later on will be indexed on the linac treatment table (Fig. 19.9A–C). Additional planning modifiers, such

CAMC Cancer Center
Charleston Area Medical Center
Radiation Oncology Services
In partnership with Alliance Oncology

Patient Name: _____

Physicist/Dosimetrist: _____

Plan/Simulation Name: _____

Department of Radiation Oncology

BREAST-VIRTUAL SIMULATION

SPECIAL INSTRUCTIONS:

(DRR's: SFD = _____ cm)

SET-UP PARAMETERS:

Set-up Instructions:

1. 3 point set up to CT marks. 　　　　　　　　Initial [Ant / Post] SSD: _____ cm.

2. Vertical: Shift Isocenter: _____ cm [Ant / Post]. 　　　New SSD: _____ cm.

3. Longitudinal: Shift Isocenter: _____ cm towards [Head / Foot]. 　New SSD: _____ cm.

4. Lateral: Shift Isocenter: _____ cm towards patients [Rt / Lt]. 　New SSD: _____ cm.

Final Couch Coordinates:

Vertical: _____ 　　　　Lateral: _____ 　　　　Longitudinal: _____

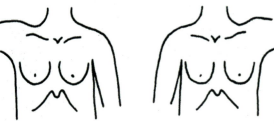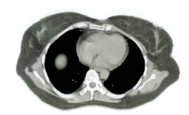

BEAM PARAMETERS:

Field Name/ Energy	Gantry Angle	Coll Angle	Table Angle	Field Size						Wedge Angle	SSD Plan	SSD Sim
				X	X1	X2	Y	Y1	Y2			

Created by: D. Mihailidis, PhD., 12/29/2005

FIGURE 19.4. Sample in-house simulation form for breast setup. Note the setup instructions and appropriate shift information from the "3-point" computed tomography (CT) mark to the treatment isocenter. Detail information on the treatment fields are entered in the following table. This form can be used for verification simulation, too.

as skin bolus may also be included. The borders of the clinical area marked by the physician on the patient can be outlined with CT radio-opaque markers (Fig. 19.8C). Sometimes, initial reference skin marks are placed in the middle of the clinical treatment area. The CT movable lasers are used to define and mark the CT reference point on the patient.

A set of AP and LAT topograms ("scout views") will assist the patient alignment on the CT table. The patient will be scanned based on a preset protocol according to

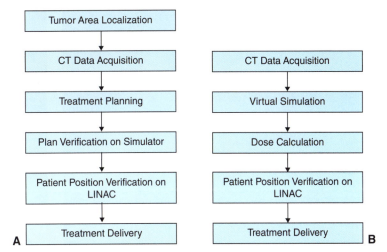

FIGURE 19.5. Verification simulation process diagram **(A)** and computed tomography (CT) simulation process **(B)**.

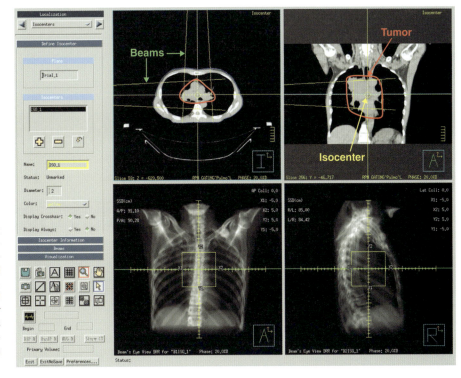

FIGURE 19.6. Virtual simulation as part of computed tomography (CT) simulation for a lung patient. The user can visualize the anatomical information that will assist appropriate placement of points, such as the treatment isocenter and the fields. In addition, tumor and other critical volumes can be outlined at this stage. This information will be eventually transferred to the treatment planning system.

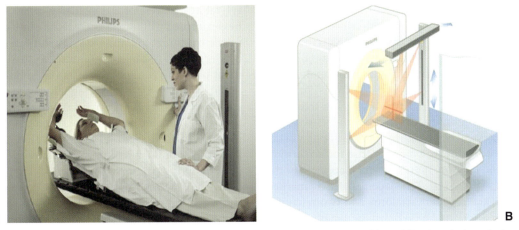

FIGURE 19.7. A large (wide) bore CT-simulator accommodates the majority of immobilization devices to be included in patient setup **(A)**. A room view of a CT-simulator with the localization laser system **(B)**.

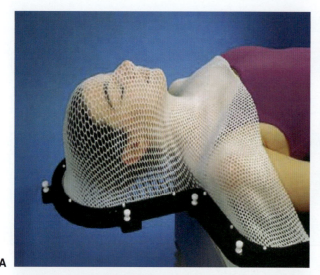
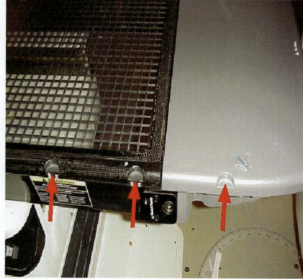
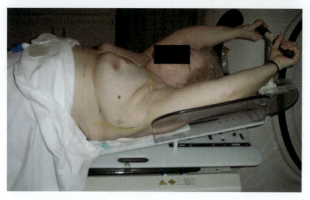

FIGURE 19.8. Patient immobilization devices as integral part of computed tomography (CT) simulation process for radiotherapy. A head and neck head holder and mask **(A)**, indexing grooves for the immobilization devices on the table top **(B)**, and **(C)** a breast patient on a breast board with reference CT radio-opaque markers ready to be CT-simulated.

the disease site and the images will be stored for virtual simulation, while the patient remains on the CT table.

Virtual Simulation Process

There are three tasks that pertain to virtual simulation. First, is the treatment isocenter localization, which is typically placed at the geometric center of the treatment volume. The second is the target and critical structures volumes delineation. And the third is to determine the treatment beam parameters via beam's-eye-view (BEVs)[14] using DRRs, including gantry, collimator and couch angles, field sizes, shielding block, etc. This last part can also be performed at a later time during the treatment planning and isodose computation process.

The CT images will be utilized to render a 3D view of the patient which will allow the more precise localization of the isocenter and later on, more efficient placement of the treatment fields (Fig. 19.9). The isocenter will be marked on the reconstructed patient anatomy and two reference fields (typically an AP and a LAT) will be assigned at that point. The DRRs (Fig. 19.10) of the reference fields will be compared with the equivalent ports films later on, the

same way simulator films have been used in the past. Having determined the isocenter, the patient is marked with the assistance of the movable lasers, one AP and two LAT marks on each side "3-point." Shifts between the original CT reference marks and the isocenter marks should be logged in patient's chart.

At this stage, the patient can be removed from the CT table. The rest of the virtual simulation process can be performed offline via the special simulation software or the treatment planning system software. Connectivity between the CT scanner's computer system and the treatment planning computer is essential to be evaluated and tested by the physicist on a frequent basis.[13] The industry standards such as the Digital Imaging and Communications in Medicine (DICOM)[15] protocol and DICOM-RT[16] (developed especially for radiation therapy) allow the transfer of imaging information between the imaging device and the treatment planning system.

In the treatment planning system, the patient's CT study and CT-simulation information (reference marks, points, reference fields, etc.) should be available for potential registration or fusion with other imaging modalities (other CT studies, magnetic resonance imaging [MRI],

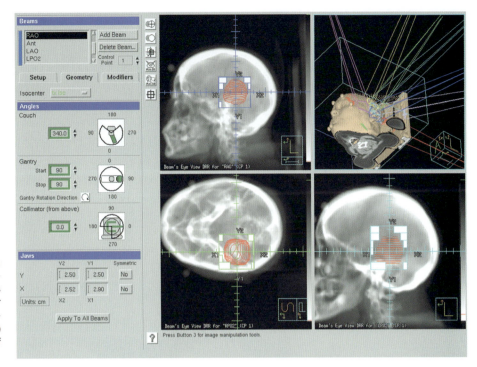

FIGURE 19.9. Virtual simulation based on 3D reconstruction allows accurate placement of treatment fields (top-right). In this brain treatment, for example, two lateral (top-left and bottom-right) and a vertex (bottom-left) treatment fields shaped by multi-leaf collimators (MLCs) are shown.

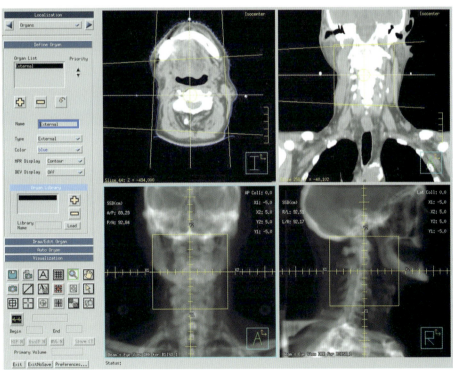

FIGURE 19.10. Isocenter placement during virtual simulation, based on reconstructed planes (top) and orthogonal DRRs (bottom) for a head and neck treatment.

positron emission tomography [PET], etc.) that, the patient might have gone through (Fig. 19.11). The information provided by the multi-imaging studies will allow the physician to outline target and other volumes more accurately.

Starting from the reference marks and setup ports, the treatment isocenter is typically selected at the center of the treatment area. Relative shifts of the isocenter from the reference CT marks are monitored for subsequent patient setup, as described previously, and shown in Figure 19.12. The physician will outline the target areas and other critical structures in a slice-by-slice process and will review the 3D representation of these volumes in three major views (axial, sagittal, and coronal). Delineation of target and critical organs is an extremely time-consuming process, in most clinical cases. Progress has been made towards computer-assisted automatic contouring, pattern recognition, and auto segmentation.[17] Figure 19.13 compares

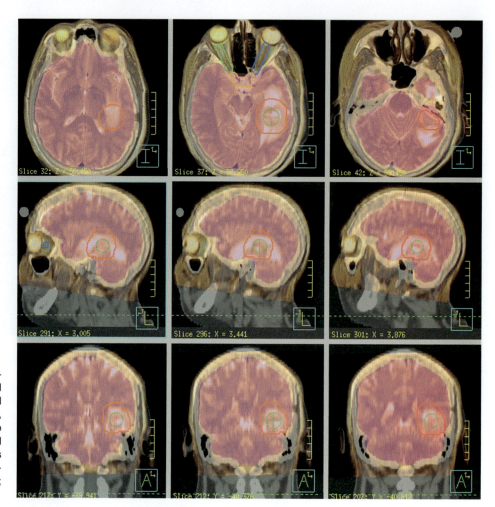

FIGURE 19.11. Multi-image registration for a brain patient. MRI and CT are aligned and fused in all three major views, axial, sagittal, and coronal. This allows the user to outline volumes that are visualized in MR images onto the CT images and proceed with treatment planning. CT, computed tomography; MRI, magnetic resonance imaging.

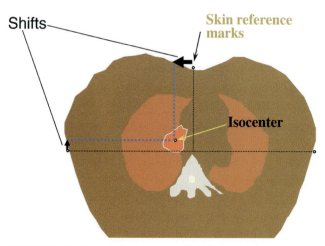

FIGURE 19.12. A diagram showing the relative shifts from the reference computed tomography (CT) marks to the treatment isocenter. Visualization of internal body structures is essential in this process.

manually outlined and auto-segmented heart volumes. However, the basic problem remains that target delineation is inherently a manual process, since the extent of target depends on tumor grade, stage, and patterns of spread to adjacent structures. Clinical evaluation of the contouring results by a radiation oncologist provides the final judgment in defining the target volume.

With all the volumes (targets and critical structures) approved by the physician, the treatment planning team can initiate the selection of the appropriate treatment fields via BEVs and 3D reconstruction of internal geometry of the patient (Fig. 19.9). Keeping in mind the clinical and setup margins to the tumor volume, as defined by the ICRU (International Commission on Radiation Units and Measurements),[18,19] appropriate blocks with multi-leaf collimators (MLCs) can be used for 3D conformal treatment planning. It is important to remember that each beam has physical penumbra where the dose varies rapidly and that the dose at the edge of the field is approximately 50% of the center dose. For this reason, to achieve adequate dose coverage of the target volume, the field penumbra should lie sufficiently beyond the target volume to offset any uncertainties in planning target volume (PTV). Beam apertures can be designed automatically or manually depending on the proximity of the critical structures and the uncertainty involved in the allowed margins to the target volume (Fig. 19.14). Clinical judgment frequently is required between sparing of critical structures and target coverage.

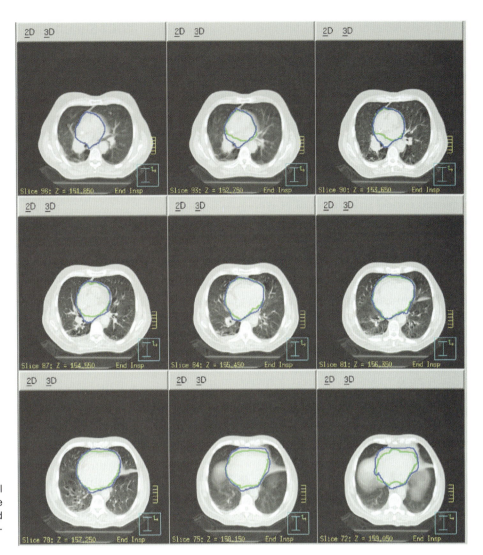

FIGURE 19.13. Subsequent CT axial images. Compare the heart volume that has been manually outlined (BLUE-line) and the result of auto-segmentation (GREEN-line).

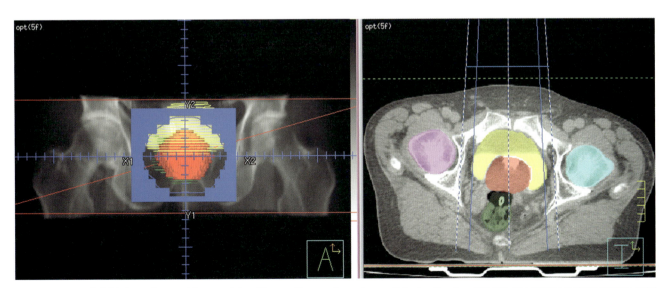

FIGURE 19.14. A field shaped around the prostate with specific margins using multi-leaf collimators (MLCs). The BEV view (left) and the axial view (right). BEV, beam's-eye-view.

All possible gantry, collimator, and couch angles can be evaluated based on target coverage and critical structures avoidance. Some commercial planning systems provide software-assisted beam geometry parameter optimization[20,21] which is important for highly conformal treatment plans. Beam directions that create greater separation between the target and critical structures are generally preferred unless other constraints such as obstructions in the beam path, gantry collisions with the treatment couch or patient, preclude those choices. Alternatively, dose–volume objectives for the target volume and critical structures can be employed to produce an inversely optimized plan, with the majority of commercial planning systems being capable of providing inverse planning optimization algorithms.[22] Final dose computations take full advantage of CT-electron density information in order to account for tissue inhomogeneities.[23] Recently, with the introduction of dual-energy CT (DECT) technology in RT,[24] more accurate CT-electron density information for photon beam dose calculations and, stopping power ratio (SPR) information for proton beam dose calculations, are possible.[25,26] The virtual simulation process, smoothly make a transition into treatment planning and treatment evaluation stage, which is beyond the purpose of this chapter.

A few points of precaution are in order when virtual simulation is performed.

- Due to precise visualization of internal organ and target volumes, one might be misled to use arbitrary small margins to the target volume in a feeling of false confidence. Thus, other important effects such as patient setup and target motion might not be properly taken into account, since patient and organ motion is not well visualized by traditional 3D virtual simulation. In absence of 4DCT imaging, an additional fluoroscopic study, in a traditional simulator, might be of great benefit to treatment planning, especially for moving targets such as lung.
- The spatial resolution is generally limited by the spacing of the axial images. Thus, within the target area, it is required that smaller scanning spacing (typically 2–3 mm) is used while a larger spacing (typically 1–2 cm) can be used further from the area of interest. One needs to keep in mind that this will affect the quality of the reconstructed DRRs.
- Limitation of CT imaging in visualizing all treatment sites can influence the clinical target volume (CTV) design, in other words, CT imaging does not always provide the best method to visualize microscopic disease. Most commonly, this is the case for brain tumors that CT imaging cannot provide clear borders of the disease. The clinician needs to keep in mind that combination (image registration process) of the treatment planning CT with other modalities, such as MR or PET, will allow a more accurate delineation of the target volume. It is important to remember that the ability to precisely conform to a target volume has limited value if the target is not determined accurately.

4DCT-Simulation Process

Modern CT scanners are capable of providing a high-resolution volumetric reconstruction of the patient's anatomy. Each image voxel has a characteristic CT number that is uniquely related to the electron (or mass) density of that voxel. The density information is used in the computation of dose and accounts for the effects of tissue inhomogeneity in treatment planning. When the anatomy that is imaged is mobile (tumor and organs move during the imaging study due to cardiac or respiratory motion), the image data are subject to motion artifacts. Consequently, the resulting volumetric reconstruction of the patient is a blurred representation of the true patient anatomy. In addition, motion artifacts will result in erroneous CT numbers and electron density values in the vicinity of the mobile anatomy. It is therefore important to minimize any motion artifact as it impacts not only the image quality and the specificity by which we can resolve anatomical changes, but also the accuracy of the calculated dose in treatment planning.

There are three different types of motion artifacts that we can observe during a CT acquisition[27]:

- If the CT scanning speed in the superior–inferior direction is much less than the tumor motion speed, then we observe a smeared image of the tumor.
- If the CT scanning speed is much faster than the tumor motion speed, then the tumor position and shape are captured on the image at an arbitrary phase of the breathing cycle.
- If the CT scanning speed is similar to the tumor motion speed, then the tumor position and shape can be significantly distorted.

It is evident that patient motion can cause significant artifacts during 3-dimensional computed tomography (3-DCT) imaging[28,29] which not only degrade the image quality and our ability to delineate anatomical structures,[30] but sometimes can even simulate the presence of disease.[31] Figure 19.15 illustrates image artifacts that are caused by superior–inferior motion during conventional CT imaging of a test sphere.[32]

Ritchie[33] proposed a high-speed (fast) scan to avoid motion artifacts that was of limited success with the third-generation CT scanners. The use of multi-slice technology[34] has significantly reduced motion artifacts in CT images when acquired in fast scanning mode. However, fast scans, although less susceptible to motion artifacts, do not portray the full extent of motion of the tumor and are therefore not of clinical use in treatment planning of mobile tumors. Multi-slice helical scanning, on the other hand, can be used with a 4DCT scanning protocol and reduce the overall scanning time while achieving the goal of capturing the temporal position of the tumor in the imaging study.

When we consider the organ motion, we have to choose an imaging technique that will minimize motion artifacts during the CT simulation. Several methods have been proposed to address this problem including:

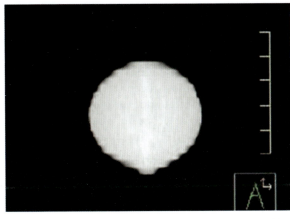 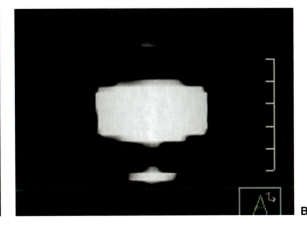

A   B

FIGURE 19.15. Illustration of image artifacts that are caused by superior–inferior (SI) motion during 3D CT imaging. **(A)** CT coronal section of a static sphere. **(B)** CT coronal section of the same sphere in oscillatory motion (range = 2 cm, period = 4 s).[32] (Vedam SS, Keall PJ, Kini VR, Mostafavi H, Shukla HP and Mohan R Acquiring a four-dimensional computed tomography dataset using an external respiratory signal. *Phys Med Biol*. 2003;48:45–62;with permission of IOP Publishing. All rights reserved.)

- A breath-hold CT simulation, where the patient is instructed to voluntarily hold their breath while the scanning beam is turned on. A similar result can be achieved using the active breathing control technique (ABC) proposed by Wong et al.[35] This technique is common in deep inspiration breath-hold (DIBH) treatments of left-sided breast treatments
- A slow CT scan where axial images are acquired at a speed of 4 s or slower per slice. A slow scan will ensure that the envelope of motion of any moving organ subject to respiratory motion will be captured in the image (typical respiratory period is 4–6 s)
- A gated CT scan where the beam is turned on only when the patient's breathing is at a certain window of the respiratory cycle (typically 30%–35% duty cycle). The respiratory-related motion is usually monitored using an external marker. In one of the commercially available implementations, this is accomplished by correlating the respiration-related tumor motion to the displacement of an external marker placed on the patient's chest as measured using an infrared camera. The user can specify which portion of the sinusoidal shaped signal obtained from the infrared camera is used to trigger the CT scanner using the cardiac gating port. This method of imaging is also known as prospective-gated image acquisition.
- A 4DCT scan where multiple scans are obtained for each location (oversampling) whereby the organ motion is captured at different sampled phases of the respiratory cycle. At the end of the scan a very large set of 3D images is produced corresponding to each of the phases in which the breathing cycle was sampled (Fig. 19.16). The collection of those 3DCT scans constitutes the 4DCT study for this patient. This method is also known as retrospective image reconstruction.

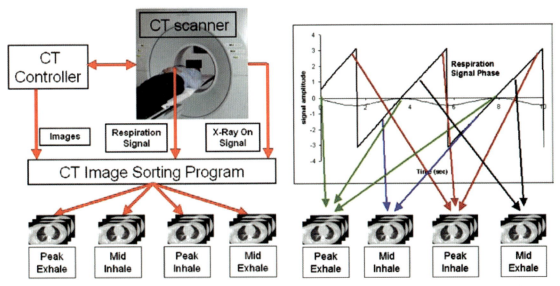

FIGURE 19.16. The 4DCT phase-sorting process: the CT images, breathing tracking signal, and "X-ray ON" signal form the input data stream. The breathing cycle is divided into distinct bins (e.g., peak exhale, mid inhale, peak inhale, and mid exhale). Images are sorted into those image bins depending on the phase of the breathing cycle in which they were acquired.[32] (Vedam SS, Keall PJ, Kini VR, Mostafavi H, Shukla HP and Mohan R Acquiring a four-dimensional computed tomography dataset using an external respiratory signal. *Phys Med Biol*. 2003;48:45–62;with permission of IOP Publishing. All rights reserved.)

Of all the imaging methods that aim to minimize respiration-related motion artifacts, the 4DCT technique is the most comprehensive way to perform such task because it not only reduces motion artifacts but also captures the changing topography of the tumor during the respiratory cycle. This information can be used during treatment planning to optimally delineate treatment volumes and margins under the assumption that the patient will be breathing the same way during treatment as they did during the 4DCT simulation. Irregular breathing (during imaging or treatment) is not desirable and we often use coaching to help the patient breath regularly and reproducible. Coaching can be auditory, where a computerized voice instructs the patient to breath in and out, or visual, where, for example, the patient looks at the superposition of their baseline breathing curve and their real-time breathing curve and tries to match them as they control and pace their breathing.

Ultimately, the goal of simulation is to uniquely and reliably identify in the patient's treatment position anatomy the exact target shape and location that can be reproducibly localized and treated during the daily treatments. 4DCT simulation allows us to segment the target and organ volumes with high specificity resulting in more educated decisions on margin selection but also improved dose calculation during treatment planning.

ACCEPTANCE TESTING AND QUALITY ASSURANCE

When it comes to conventional simulators and CT-simulators, the initial acceptance testing is performed to verify that the unit is operating as specified by the manufacture and to serve as a baseline data pool for future comparisons with periodic quality assurance (QA) testing.

Conventional Simulator

Acceptance testing of a simulator may be divided into two parts: (a) geometric and spatial accuracies verification and (b) performance evaluation of the x-ray generator and the associated imaging system. The first part is similar to the acceptance testing and evaluation of a linac for mechanical performance. Because the simulators are designed to mimic the treatment accelerators, their geometric accuracies should be comparable with those of the accelerators. To minimize differences between the simulator and the accelerator it is desired to use the same table design and accessory holders as those on the treatment machine.

The second part is a performance evaluation of a diagnostic radiographic and fluoroscopic unit.

Several authors have discussed the technical specifications of treatment simulators and the required testing procedures and have presented comprehensive reviews on this subject.[3,4,36-38] The QA for the X-ray generator and the imaging system has been discussed by various groups.[39,40] The most recent recommendations on QA for conventional simulators are coming from American Association of Physicists in Medicine (AAPM) Task Group #40 (Table III in the report).[41] Of course a well-established QA program requires daily and annual testing for simulators, in addition to the monthly testing.

CT-Simulator

Acceptance testing for a CT-simulator requires first, the acceptance testing of the CT scanner as an imaging device to be done, first. This process is described in detail by AAPM Report N. 39.[42] For the purpose of CT-simulation, additional literature needs to be employed to cover the needs of radiotherapy (see, McGee and Das[11]). Due to the complexity of the new technology scanners, the manufacturer's acceptance testing procedure manual provides a great guide to suggested recommendations for testing tolerances for the particular scanner. We recommend that the AAPM Task Group #66 report is followed for all the QA needs of a CT-simulator as it applies to radiotherapy procedures.[13] Table I in Ref. [13] outlines the electromechanical components testing (e.g., lasers, table, gantry, and scan localization). Table II outlines test specifications for image performance evaluation (e.g., CT number vs electron density, image noise, contrast, and spatial resolution). A simplified set of tests are shown in Figure 19.17. Keep in mind that the CT-simulation process QA should be performed along with the treatment planning process QA where information and data are transferred between the CT scanner and the treatment planning computers.

When 4DCT scans are used for simulation, the QA is for the most part the same as that for the CT simulator. In addition to the tests described previously, one could include scans of test phantoms that are placed on a moving platform. Such motorized platforms can be programmed to a user-defined moving cycle that is typically 1D or 2D, which is adequate for QA purposes. Since the physical size of the phantom and any objects embedded inside it are known, a 4DCT scan would test the ability of the scanner and the accompanying software to build the 4D model of the phantom and to reproduce the true dimensions of the imaged objects. Although there is not currently much information on QA for 4DCT, such protocols can easily be developed and incorporated in routine QA programs for CT simulation.

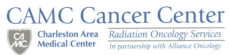

Department of Medical Physics

Date: _____

Physicist: _____

Daily Laser QA LAP Laser Phantom Scan: Horz (x) _____   Vert (y) _____ = 2 mm
                                            (pass / fail)   (pass / fail)

MedTee CT Simulator Laser QA Device centered at lasers:

Longitudinal distance between LAP lasers and Gantry lasers   _____ (500 ± 2 mm)
                                                                           (pass / fail)

        Scanned image checks   (pass / fail)

 + image definition: Right _____   Center _____   Left _____

Vertical centering _____ ± 2 mm   (pass / fail)

Horizontal centering _____ ± 2 mm   (pass / fail)

        Laser Alignment (± 2 mm)   (pass / fail)

LAP side lasers: Alignment   **L** _____   **R** _____

                     Table height   **L** _____   **R** _____   (52 ± 2 mm)

                     Longitudinal tracking **L** _____   **R** _____

                     Vertical tracking   **L** _____   **R** _____

Sagittal LAP laser: Longitudinal tracking _____   Vertical tracking _____

                     Alignment (Displacement at center) _____

Transverse laser: _____

Gantry lasers:

LAP laser motion: X-axis: sagittal laser

Center post _____ (0 ± 2 mm)   Side post _____ (center ± 125 mm ± 1)

Table vertical shift (put coronal lasers @ top of phantom) (25 ± 1 mm) (pass/fail)
Z (coronal sides) _____   A (rt side of pt) _____   B (lt side) _____

Monthly Image Evaluation

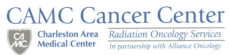

CT # Accuracy:
Use the Monthly QA Worksheet, which will be kept in the CT binder. Open up (preview) a monthly scan of the multi-pin layer of the QA water phantom with various material pins and water visible on the CT computer (or scan it). If you scan it, position it off-center for a more stringent check.

Field Uniformity:
Both the water layer of the head phantom, and the solid body section of the phantom, are scanned daily and checked for uniformity by the CT operator.

Monthly: Check water uniformity in 5 circles on the head phantom water layer scan – one in the center and other in various directions. Circles should be about 1 cm in diameter. If you scanned it, this can be done using the Uniformity Check tool in the Graphics menu on the CT scanner. Average CT# values should be within ± 4 HU of 0.

Examine the image with a narrow window to rule out subtle artifacts (rings, streaks, etc.); repeat scan if necessary.

Do a uniformity check using the solid Body Phantom scan, with the circles away from the pins. The average CT# value in each circle should be 100 ± 15 HU.

Date	H1	H2	H3	H4	H5	H6	B1	B2	B3	B4	B5

Spatial Integrity:
X-dir: On the MedTec phantom scan, check the center-to-center distance of the + (crosses) from the central post to each side post, using the measuring (line) tool.

Rt side = _____ (125 ± 1 mm)   Lt side = _____ (125 ± 1 mm)

Y-dir and X-dir: On the Laser QA phantom scan, check the height ad width of the phantom, using the **IAC** Window/Leveling preset.

Height = _____ (130 ± 1 mm)   Width = _____ (150 ± 1 mm)

Created by: D. Mihailidis, PhD., 6/05/13

FIGURE 19.17. Set of monthly QA tests for CT-simulator. This set of tests is based on AAPM TG-66.[13] (Mutic S, Palta JR, Butker EK, et al. Quality assurance for computed-tomography-simulation process: Report of the AAPM Radiation Therapy Committee Task Group No. 66. *Med Phys.* 2003;30:2762–2792).

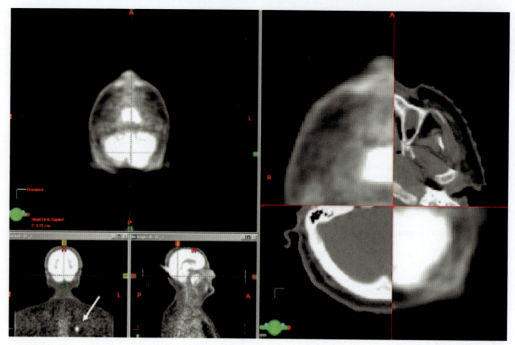

FIGURE 19.18. PET/CT fusion of a patient with nasopharyngeal cancer with an upper left lobe lung nodule (white arrow).

RECENT DEVELOPMENTS IN RADIOTHERAPY SIMULATION

The last decade, PET in combination with CT in hybrid, cross-modality imaging systems (PET/CT) gains more and more importance as a part of the treatment planning procedure in radiotherapy. The fusion of PET with CT adds anatomical information to the physiological information of PET, allowing for improvement in spatial resolution. The high sensitivity and specificity of PET/CT in identifying the areas of tumor involvement in various disease sites[43,44] attracted great interest in integrating functional imaging with PET/CT into the radiotherapy planning process. The aim is to better define and delineate the tumor's extent and its relationship to the surrounding radiosensitive vital structures and to improve the therapeutic index (Fig. 19.18).

MRI is becoming an increasingly important tool in radiation oncology, as it can provide anatomical and functional information regarding the tumor and normal tissues, which may be complementary to information from CT alone. For more than a decade MRI has been successfully used in stereotactic radiosurgery procedures. Thus, MRI has already been integrated into a CT-based RT workflow, using image registration tools. Such tools are already an inherent part of the RT workflow, for multimodality and multiphasic image registration for radiation treatment planning (for MRI, PET, and other imaging) and image guidance at the treatment unit.[45] Further on, with the appearance of the MR-linac technology,[46] MRI-based simulation has been increasingly considered as an integral part of RT planning and workflow.[47,48]

CONCLUSIONS

Treatment simulation is a crucial component of the entire treatment planning process and guarantees successful radiotherapy practice. The advancements of today's technology both in hardware and software allow more accurate patient setup and representation with customization of the treatment plans to the specific patient and site. However, stringent QA procedures are necessary to maintain optimum and safe use of such technologies. The introduction of multimodality imaging for RT introduces the need for deformable image registration early in the RT simulation process, which is a whole exciting topic to investigate.

KEY POINTS

- Treatment planning requires accurate patient data to be acquired through the process of treatment simulation.

- Radiographic, CT, PET/CT, ultrasound, and MRI simulators are essential in modern radiotherapy treatment planning.

- Image fusion between different simulation modalities is necessary for complex modern radiotherapy techniques for mapping out structural or functional anatomy of the targeted areas.

- Important components of CT-simulations and virtual simulation are 3D representation of the patient, DRRs,

image registration and segmentation, and tumor motion management.

- Treatment volume delineation, treatment portal placements, and their directional optimization can be performed as part of the virtual simulation process based on 3D visualization of the patient model.

- Process quality assurance and periodic testing of the radiotherapy simulation equipment should be an integral part of the modern radiotherapy simulation process in order to secure optimal and safe implementation of all aspects of the simulation process.

REVIEW QUESTIONS

1. What is the most common imaging modality used in radiotherapy simulation?
   A. MRI
   B. Planar imaging
   C. Ultrasound
   D. CT E. PET

2. When compared with CT, MRI provides better
   A. spatial resolution
   B. contrast resolution
   C. patient setup
   D. tissue density information
   E. geometrical accuracy

3. When compared with MRI, PET provides better
   A. spatial resolution
   B. patient setup
   C. tissue density information
   D. malignancy differentiation from normal tissue
   E. geometric accuracy

4. During a 4DCT process,
   A. the CT beam is turned on only when the patient's breathing is at a certain window of the respiratory cycle.
   B. a slow CT scan of axial slices is acquired.
   C. multiple scans for each location are obtained and are shorted via retrospective image reconstruction.
   D. a breath-hold technique is used during the image acquisition.

ANSWERS

1. D
2. B
3. D
4. C

REFERENCES

1. Sherouse GW, Bourland JD, Reynolds KL, et al. Virtual simulation in the clinical setting: some practical considerations. *Int J Radiat Oncol Biol Phys.* 1990;19:1059–1065.
2. Sherouse GW. Radiotherapy simulation. In: Khan FM, Potish R, eds. *Treatment Planning in Radiation Oncology.* Baltimore, MD: Williams & Wilkins; 1998:39–53.
3. McCullough EC. Radiotherapy treatment simulators. In: *AAPM Monograph No. 19.* Woodbury, NY: The American Institute of Physics; 1990:491–499.
4. McCullough EC, Earl JD. The selection, acceptance testing, and quality control of radiotherapy treatment simulators. *Radiology.* 1979;131:221–230.
5. Khan FM. *The Physics of Radiation Therapy.* 4th ed. Baltimore, MD: Lippincott Williams & Wilkins;2010.
6. Galvin JM. The CT-simulator and the simulator-CT. In: Smith AR, ed. *Radiation Therapy Physics.* Berlin: Springer-Verlag;1995:19–32.
7. Dahl O, Kardamakis D, Lind B, Rosenwald JC. Current status of conformal radiotherapy. *Acta Oncol.* 1996;35(Suppl. 8):41–57.
8. Rosenwald JC, Gaboriaud G, Pontvert D. Conformal radiotherapy: principles and clarification (in French). *Cancer Radiother.* 1999;3:367–377.
9. Siddon RL. Solution to treatment planning problems using coordinate transformations. *Med Phys.* 1981;8:766–774.

10. Siddon RL. Fast calculation of the exact radiological path for a three-dimensional CT array. *Med Phys.* 1985;12:252–255.

11. Coia LR, Schultheiss TE, Hanks GE, eds. *A Practical Guide to CT Simulation.* Madison, WI: Advanced Medical Publishing;1995.

12. Aird EG, Conway J. CT simulation for radiotherapy treatment planning. *Br J Radiol.* 2002;75:937–949.

13. Mutic S, Palta JR, Butker EK, et al. Quality assurance for computed-tomography-simulation process: Report of the AAPM Radiation Therapy Committee Task Group No. 66. *Med Phys.* 2003;30:2762–2792.

14. Goitein M, Abrams M, Rowell D, et al. Multidimensional treatment planning: II Beam's eye-view, back projection through CT sections. *Int J Radiat Oncol Biol Phys.* 1983;9:789–797.

15. The National Electrical Manufacturers Association (NEMA). *The DICOM Standard.* PS 3.1-2006. http://dicom.nema.org/dicom/2006/06_01pu.pdf.

16. Bosh W. Integrating the management of patient treatment planning and image data. In: Purdy JA, ed. *Categorical Course Syllabus: 3-Dimensional Radiation Therapy Treatment Planning.* Chicago: RSNA;1994:151–160.

17. Ragan D, et al. Semi-automated four-dimensional computed tomography segmentation using deformable models. *Med Phys.* 2005;32:2254–2261.

18. ICRU Report No. 50. Prescribing, recording and reporting photon beam therapy. Bethesda, MD: ICRU;1993.

19. ICRU Report No. 62. Prescribing, recording and reporting photon beam therapy (supplement to ICRU Report 50). Bethesda, MD: ICRU;1999.

20. Rowbottom CG, Oldham M, Webb S. Constrained customization of non-coplanar beam orientations in radiotherapy of brain tumors. *Phys Med Biol.* 1999;44:383–399.

21. Bedford JL, Webb S. Elimination of importance factors for clinically accurate selection of beam orientations, beam weights and wedge angles in conformal radiation therapy. *Med Phys.* 2003;30:1788–1804.

22. Purdy JA, Grant III WH, Palta JR, Butler BE, Perez CA, eds. *3D Conformal and Intensity Modulated Radiation Therapy: Physics and Applications.* Madison, WI: Advanced Medical Publishing, Inc.;2001.

23. Papanikolaou N, et al. Tissue inhomogeneity corrections for megavoltage photon beams. AAPM Task Group Report No. 65, 2004. http://www.aapm.org/pubs/reports/RPT_85.pdf.

24. Van Elmpt W, et al. Dual energy CT in radiotherapy: current applications and future outlook. *Radiother Oncol.* 2017;119:137–144.

25. Möhler C, et al. Methodological accuracy of image-based electron density assessment using dual-energy computed tomography. *Med Phys.* 2017;44:2429–2437.

26. Zhu J, Penfold S. Dosimetric comparison of stopping power calibration with dual-energy CT and single-energy CT in proton therapy treatment planning. *Med Phys.* 2016;43:2845–2854.

27. Jiang S. *Management of Moving Targets in Radiotherapy: Integrating New Technologies into the Clinic: Monte Carlo and Image-Guided Radiation Therapy.* AAPM Monograph No. 32;2006. Madison, WI: Medical Physics Publishing.

28. Mayo JR, Müller NL, Henkelman RM. The double-fissure sign: a motion artifact on thin-section CT scans. *Radiology.* 1987;165:580–581.

29. Ritchie CJ, Hseih J, Gard MF, Godwin JD, Kim Y, Crawford CR. Predictive respiratory gating: a new method to reduce motion artifacts on CT scans. *Radiology.* 1994;190:847–852.

30. Keall PJ, Kini VR, Vedam SS, Mohan R. Potential radiotherapy improvements with respiratory gating. *Australas Phys Eng Sci Med.* 2002;25:1–6.

31. Tarver RD, Conces DJ, Godwin JD. Motion artifacts on CT simulate bronchiectasis. *Am J Roentgenol.* 1998;151:1117–1119.

32. Vedam SS, Keall PJ, Kini VR, Mostafavi H, Shukla HP, Mohan R. Acquiring a four-dimensional computed tomography dataset using an external respiratory signal. *Phys Med Biol.* 2003;48:45–62.

33. Ritchie CJ, Godwin JD, Crawford CR, Stanford W, Anno H, Kim Y. Minimum scan speeds for suppression of motion artifacts in CT. *Radiology.* 1992;185(1):37–42.

34. Kachelriess M, Kalender WA. Electrocardiogram-correlated image reconstruction from sub second spiral computed tomography scans of the heart. *Med Phys.* 1998;25:2417–2431.

35. Wong JW, Sharpe MB, Jaffray DA, Kini VR, Robertson JM, Stromberg JS, Martinez AA. The use of active breathing control (ABC) to reduce margin for breathing motion. *Int J Radiat Oncol Biol Phys.* 1999;44(4):911–919.

36. Connors SG, Battista JJ, Bertin RJ. On technical specifications of radiotherapy simulators. *Med Phys.* 1984;11:341–343.

37. International Electrotechnical Commission. *Functional Performance Characteristics of Radiotherapy Simulators.* Draft Report. Geneva: IEC SubC 62C;1990.

38. Bomford CK, et al. Treatment simulators. *Br J Radiol.* 1989;Suppl. 23:1–49.

39. National Council on Radiation Protection and Measurements. *Quality Assurance for Diagnostic Imaging Equipment.* Report No. 99;1988. Bethesda, MD: National Council on Radiation Protection and Measurements.

40. Boone JM, et al. *Quality Control in Diagnostic Radiology.* AAPM Report No. 74. Report of Task Group #12;2002. Madison, WI: Medical Physics Publishing.

41. Kuthcer GJ, et al. *Comprehensive QA for Radiation Oncology.* AAPM Report No. 46. Report of Task Group #40;1994. College Park, MD: The American Association of Physicists in Medicine.

42. Lin PP-J, et al. *Specification and Acceptance Testing of Computed Tomography Scanners.* AAPM report No. 39. Report of Task Group #2;1993. College Park, MD: The American Association of Physicists in Medicine.

43. Öllers M, et al. The integration of PET/CT scans from different hospitals into radiotherapy treatment planning. *Radiother Oncol.* 2008;87:142–146.

44. Thorwarth D, et al. Physical radiotherapy treatment planning based on functional PET/CT data. *Radiother Oncol.* 2010;6:317–324.

45. Devic S, MRI simulation for radiotherapy treatment planning. *Med Phys.* 2012;39:6701–6711.

46. Liney JP, et al. MRI-linear accelerator radiotherapy systems. *Clin Oncol.* 2018;30:686–691.

47. Schmidt MA, Payne GS. Radiotherapy planning using MRI. *Phys Med Biol.* 2015;60:R323–R361.

48. Tyagi N, et al. Clinical workflow for MR-only simulation and planning in prostate. *Radiat Oncol.* 2017;12:119.

20 Treatment Planning Algorithms: Photon Dose Calculations

John P. Gibbons

INTRODUCTION

Computerized treatment planning systems have been utilized in radiotherapy planning since the 1950s. The first computer algorithm used has been attributed to Tsien[1] who used punch cards to store isodose distributions to allow for the addition of multiple beams. Since that time, advancements in computer speeds and algorithm development have vastly improved our capability to predict photon dose distributions in patients.

In an early attempt to classify computer planning algorithms, the International Commission on Radiation Units and Measurement (ICRU) Report 42[2] divided photon dose calculation methods into two categories: empirical and model-based algorithms. Early empirical algorithms such as Bentley–Milan were developed using clinical beam data measured on a flat water phantom as input. Corrections were then made to incorporate various effects, such as changes in patient external contour, blocking or physical wedges, and so forth. Eventually, patient heterogeneity correction factors were incorporated, but these were applied afterward, that is, after water-based calculations were performed assuming a homogeneous patient geometry. Most of this development occurred prior to the advent of computed tomography (CT), or at least before the incorporation of CT images into the radiotherapy planning process.

However, eventually the commercial utilization of empirical algorithms faded. In the early 1990s, three-dimensional conformal radiation therapy (3D CRT) began to use patient-specific CT-image data in the planning process. Initially, this was limited to virtual simulation. At that time computer-based algorithms that could incorporate the newly available volumetric density information and compute true 3D dose distributions in a reasonable amount of time were not yet available. In order to fully utilize this new information, it was necessary to develop new algorithms that could incorporate variations in individual patient anatomy. As a result, most, if not all, commercial treatment planning systems have moved to model-based photon calculation methods.

In this chapter, we describe three photon calculation models currently in use in radiotherapy clinics. Photon calculation models are an area of continuous development, and it is likely that each commercial vendor's implementation of one or more of these models will differ in many respects. Nevertheless, the intent is to provide a basic understanding of the principles behind each of these algorithms.

REPRESENTATION OF THE PATIENT FOR DOSE PLANNING

Patient representation has evolved dramatically over the past 50 years. Initially, patients were considered as a flat water phantom of a specific source-to-surface distance (SSD) and depth for use in simple dose or monitor unit calculations. Development of external contour tools aided the treatment planner in determining patient-specific dose distributions. Such procedures resulted in the patient being represented as a homogeneous composition (i.e., water) but did allow for the application of surface corrections to the calculation. Patient heterogeneities could be represented in simple ways, such as using internal contours with assigned densities. The electron density to assign to the region could be inferred from CT atlases or, if available, the mean patient-specific CT number within the contoured structure.[3] The problem with this approach was that tissues such as lung and bone are not themselves homogeneous, and their density variations would not be taken into account using this approach.

All modern radiotherapy systems use volumetric imaging data to characterize the patient in a 3D voxel-by-voxel description. The most common imaging dataset used for radiotherapy treatment planning is a treatment-planning CT scan, obtained using a conventional CT simulator. A CT dataset of the treatment region constitutes the most accurate representation of the patient applicable for dose computation, primarily because of the one-to-one relationship between CT number and physical and/or electron density.[3] Dose algorithms that can use the density representation on a point-by-point basis are easier for heterogeneous calculations because contouring of the heterogeneities is typically not required. An exception to this occurs when data are present within the CT scan which will not be present for the treatment. One obvious example is the CT-simulator couch, which is either manually or automatically removed and, in some cases, replaced with a treatment couch by the planning system. Also relevant are temporary contrast agents that can produce a CT number that mimic a higher density material within the body. Usually, the contrast agent is used to aid in the tissue segmentation, and so only the additional step of providing a more realistic CT number in the segmented region is required to correct for the presence of the contrast agent. The spatial reliability of CT scanners is typically within 2%, which leads to dose uncertainties of ~1%.[3]

Other imaging modalities provide information that will aid in the location and delineation of structures, but is of less value in the calculation of dose. For example, the advent of cone-beam CT within the treatment room provides invaluable information regarding patient alignment. However, the scatter contained within the images makes accurate determination of density difficult. Although magnetic resonance imaging (MRI) is often able to provide superior tissue contrast, the information in MRI is not strongly related to electron density. Furthermore, MRI images are more prone to artifacts during image formation, which will degrade the quality of the calculated dose distributions.

In addition to electron density, it is also necessary to determine the tissue composition for more modern calculation algorithms. In convolution/superposition algorithms, fluence attenuation tables are typically computed using mass-attenuation coefficient data, which are somewhat weakly dependent on material. Often these coefficients are determined for each voxel by linearly interpolating between published results of two different materials (e.g., water and bone) based on the density assigned to the voxel. For both Monte Carlo (MC) and Boltzmann transport calculations, a full material assignment must be made to allow for accurate cross-sectional determination of both photon and electron transport throughout the patient volume.

Ideally, the size of the voxels in the treatment planning CT should be close to the dose grid resolution used for calculation. A CT volume set typically consists of 50 to 200 images with a voxel matrix dimension of 512×512 for each image. For a 50-cm field of view, this corresponds to a voxel size of ~1 mm in the transverse direction. The longitudinal voxel size depends on the slice thickness, but is typically from 2 to 5 mm. In many planning systems, the CT slice thickness is chosen as the voxel size of the dose grid. For these systems, it may be appropriate to downsample the CT image set to 256×256. This makes the transverse resolution more closely matched to that of the longitudinal direction, with only a minor degradation in the image. Degrading the resolution further from 256×256 may result in an unacceptable loss of detail.

BASIC RADIATION PHYSICS FOR PHOTON BEAM DOSE CALCULATION

Here, we present an introduction to the important aspects of X-ray production and interaction to understand the capabilities and limitations of model-based photon treatment planning algorithms.

Megavoltage Photon Production

Figure 20.1 displays a cross-sectional view of a linear accelerator treatment head, which consists of a high-density shielding material such as lead, tungsten, or a lead-tungsten alloy. It consists of an X-ray target, flattening filter, ion chamber, and a primary and movable collimator. High-energy electrons are accelerated in the linac's accelerating structure and impinge on the X-ray target.

The production of Bremsstrahlung, or braking radiation, occurs when the high-energy electrons strike a tungsten target located in the head of the accelerator. The size of the focal spot of the electrons on the target is on the order of a few millimeters.[4] This finite size contributes to the penumbra or the blurring of the beam near the edges of the field.

A primary collimator, fabricated from a tungsten alloy, defines the maximum field diameter that can be used for treatment.

At megavoltage energies, Bremsstrahlung is directed primarily in the forward direction. In most conventional C-arm accelerators, to make the beam intensity more uniform, a conical filter positioned in the beam preferentially absorbs the photon fluence along the central axis. The presence of the field-flattening filter alters the energy spectrum, since the beam passing through the thicker central part of the filter has a higher proportion of low-energy photons absorbed by the filter. This may not be necessary for modern treatment deliveries where modulation is used to vary the intensity of the beam. Indeed, many treatment units now have the option of removing the filter for these treatments (e.g., Varian TrueBeam, Palo Alto, CA; Elekta Versa HD, Atlanta, GA), or have removed the flattening filter entirely (e.g., Accuray, Inc. TomoHD, Sunnyvale, CA) when a uniform field is not needed.

Compton Scatter

Photons can inelastically scatter via three main processes: photoelectric absorption, incoherent (Compton) scattering with atomic electrons, and pair production in the nuclear or electron electromagnetic field. In the energy range used for radiation therapy, most interactions are Compton scattering events, which are discussed in more detail here.

Compton-scattered photons may originate in either the accelerator treatment head or the patient (or phantom). Most of the scatter dose generated by the accelerator head is produced within the primary collimator and the field-flattening filter. These scattered photons and electrons are sometimes referred to as "extrafocal radiation" which may be added to the primary photon beam emitted from the source. As the collimator jaws open, more scattered radiation is allowed to leave the treatment head, which results in an increase in the machine output with field size. This effect is known as *collimator scatter*,[5]

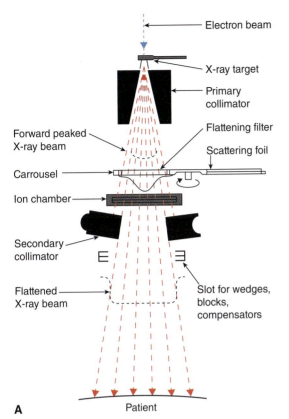
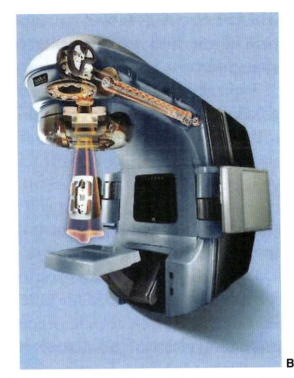

A Patient

B

FIGURE 20.1. Components of the treatment head of a linear accelerator. **A:** A cross-sectional view of the treatment head operating in X-ray therapy mode. **B:** A cut-away diagram of the linac. (Image(s) courtesy of Varian Medical Systems, Inc., Palo Alto, CA. Copyright [2021]. All rights reserved.)

although the collimator jaws themselves contribute little forward scatter. The photons scattered in the primary collimator and field-flattening filter also add to the fluence just outside the geometrical field boundary.

Similar to the accelerator-produced scatter, the phantom scatter primarily occurs in the forward direction and increases with the size of the field. However, for phantom-generated scatter, the penetration characteristics of the beam are also altered. As the field size increases, the phantom scatter causes the beam to be significantly more penetrating with depth. This effect is significant enough that this energy difference must be included in the dose computations.

The behavior of scatter from beam modifiers such as wedges must also be considered within the photon model. When the field size is small, a beam modifier mainly alters the transmission and does not contribute much scatter that arrives at the patient. However, when the field is large, beam modifiers begin to alter the penetration characteristics of the beam, much as the phantom scatter does. This effect is exemplified by the increase in the wedge transmission factor with increasing field size and depth.[6,7]

Electron Transport

Photons are indirectly ionizing radiation. The dose is deposited by charged particles (electrons and positrons)

set in motion from the site of the photon interaction. At megavoltage energies, the range of charged particles can be several centimeters. The charged particles are mainly set in forward motion but are scattered considerably as they slow down and come to rest. Electrons lose energy by two processes: inelastic collisions within the media (primarily with target electrons) and radiative interactions (primarily with target nucleus). Inelastic collisions that ionize the target atom can lead to secondary electrons, known as delta rays. Radiative interactions occur via Bremsstrahlung, which effectively transfers the energy back to a photon. Equations that model these coupled electron–photon interactions are described later on.

The indirect nature of photon dose deposition results in several features in photon dose distributions. Initially, the superficial dose increases or "builds up" from the surface of the patient because of the increased number of charged particles being set in motion. This results in a low skin dose, the magnitude of which is inversely proportional to the path length of the charged particles. The dose builds up to a maximum at a depth, d_{max}, characteristic of the photon beam energy. At a point in the patient with a depth equal to the penetration distance of charged particles, charged particles coming to rest are being replenished by charged particles set in motion, and charged particle equilibrium (CPE) is said to be reached. In this case, the dose at a point is proportional to the energy fluence of photons at the same point. The main criterion for CPE is that the energy fluence of photons must be constant out to the range of electrons set in motion in all directions. This does not occur in general in heterogeneous media, near the beam boundary, or for intensity-modulated beams.

Electrons produced in the head of the accelerator and in air between the accelerator and the patient are called *contamination electrons*. The interaction of these electrons in and just beyond the buildup region contributes significantly to the dose, especially if the field is large.

Perturbation in electron transport can be exaggerated near heterogeneities. For example, the range of electrons is three to five times as long in lung as in water, and so beam boundaries passing through lung have much larger penumbral regions. Bone is the only tissue with an atomic composition significantly different from that of water. This can lead to perturbations in dose of only a few percent,[8] and so perturbations in electron scattering or stopping power are rarely taken into account. Bone can therefore be treated as "high-density water."

SUPERPOSITION/CONVOLUTION ALGORITHM

The most common photon dose calculation in use for radiotherapy planning today is the superposition/convolution algorithm.[8–19] This method incorporates a model-based approach in describing the underlying physics of the interactions, while still being able to calculate dose in a reasonable time.

The convolution/superposition method begins by modeling the indirect nature of dose deposition from photon beams. Primary photon interactions are dealt with separately from the transport of scattered photons and electrons set in motion.

Dose Calculation under Conditions of CPE

To begin, we consider the special case of dose determination under conditions of CPE. In this case, the total energy absorbed by charged particles at position $\mathbf{r}$ is the same as the total energy that escapes due to photon interactions at the same location. Thus, the primary dose D_p and the first-scattered dose from a parallel beam of monoenergetic photons can be computed as[9]

$$D_\mathrm{P}(\mathbf{r}) = (K c(\mathbf{r}))P = \left(\frac{\mu_\mathrm{en}}{\rho}\right)_\mathrm{P} \Psi_\mathrm{P}(\mathbf{r})$$

$$= \left(\frac{\mu_\mathrm{en}}{\rho}\right)_\mathrm{P} \phi_\mathrm{P}(\mathbf{r} = 0) h \nu_\mathrm{P} e^{-\mu r} \quad (20.1)$$

where $\Psi_\mathrm{P}(\mathbf{r})$ and $(K_\mathrm{c}(\mathbf{r}))_\mathrm{P}$ are the *primary* energy fluence and collision kerma, respectively, at point $\mathbf{r}$, $(\mu_\mathrm{en}/\rho)_\mathrm{p}$ is the mass energy absorption coefficient, $\phi_\mathrm{P}(\mathbf{r} = 0)$ is the primary photon fluence at the surface of the phantom, $h\nu_\mathrm{P}$ is the primary photon energy, and μ is the attenuation

coefficient of primary photons. The total dose is the sum of the primary and scatter components

$$D_\mathrm{tot}(\mathbf{r}) = D_\mathrm{P}(\mathbf{r})$$

$$+ \int D_\mathrm{P}(\mathbf{r}')\frac{(\mu_\mathrm{en})_\mathrm{scat}}{(\mu_\mathrm{en})_\mathrm{P}}\frac{(h\nu)_\mathrm{scat}}{(h\nu)_\mathrm{P}}\frac{\mathrm{d}P_\mathrm{scat}(\theta, \mathbf{r}')}{\mathrm{d}V}e^{-\mu_\mathrm{scat}(\mathbf{r}' - \mathbf{r})}\mathrm{d}V$$

$$(20.2)$$

where $\mathrm{d}P_\mathrm{scat}(\theta, \mathbf{r}')/\mathrm{d}V$ is the probability per unit volume of a primary photon being scattered into a solid angle centered about angle θ.

These equations are complicated enough, but they do not take into account any secondary or higher-order photon scatter. They also neglect beam divergence and do not take into account tissue heterogeneities. They are valid only for CPE situations, so that the dose computation is not valid in the buildup region or near the field boundaries, and the scatter dose is perturbed by heterogeneities lying between the scatter site at $\mathbf{r}'$ and the point $\mathbf{r}$, where the total dose is being computed.

Convolution/Superposition Method

Unfortunately, Equation (20.1) is simplistic because it does not take into account the finite range of charged particles. In other words, the energy fluence that was present at the point the charged particles were set in motion upstream should replace the energy fluence in Equation (20.1). We may think of this energy fluence as that originating upstream (i.e., assuming that the charged particles all moved linearly downstream), but in reality, the particles may originate from any location around the calculation point, as long as it is within the particles' range. Thus, rather than a single effective photon interaction site, this expression for dose becomes a convolution integral about $\mathbf{r}$:

$$D(\mathbf{r}) = \int K_\mathrm{c}(\mathbf{r}') A_\mathrm{c}(\mathbf{r} - \mathbf{r}')\mathrm{d}\mathbf{r}' \quad (20.3)$$

where $A_\mathrm{c}(\mathbf{r} - \mathbf{r}')$ describes the contribution of charged particle energy that gets absorbed per unit volume at $\mathbf{r}'$ from interactions at $\mathbf{r}'$ and the integration is over all values of $\mathbf{r}'$ that make up volume $\mathrm{d}\mathbf{r}'$. The charged particle energy absorption kernel has a finite extent because the range of charged particles set in motion is finite.

Equation (20.3) requires knowledge of the energy fluence due to both primary and scattered photons at all points. Time-consuming transport methods, such as the method of discrete ordinates or the MC method, would be needed to compute the scattered component accurately. A simpler solution is to utilize a scatter kernel that includes the scattered photon component along with the contribution from charged particles. The kernel is no longer finite because photon scatter (which has no range) is included. Now, only primary photons are explicitly transported. A convolution equation that separates primary photon transport and a kernel that accounts for the scattered photon and electrons set in motion away from the primary photon interaction site is as follows:

$$D(\mathbf{r}) = \int \frac{\mu}{\rho} \Psi_P(\mathbf{r}')A(\mathbf{r} - \mathbf{r}')d\mathbf{r}'$$

$$= \int T_P(\mathbf{r}')A(\mathbf{r} - \mathbf{r}')d\mathbf{r}' \qquad (20.4)$$

where $\frac{\mu}{\rho}$ is the mass attenuation coefficient, $\Psi_P(\mathbf{r}')$ is the primary energy fluence, and $A(\mathbf{r} - \mathbf{r}')$ includes the contribution of scatter. The product of the mass attenuation coefficient and the primary energy fluence is the primary *term*a (*total energy released per unit mass*) $T_P(\mathbf{r}')$. Terma, first defined by Ahnesjo, Andreo, and Brahme,[20] is analogous to kerma and has the same units as dose.

The convolution kernels can, in principle, be obtained by analytic computation, deconvolution from dose distributions, or even by direct measurement. Most often, the kernels are computed with the MC method by interacting a large number of primary photons at one location and determining from where energy is absorbed, that is, from primary-generated charged particles, charged particles subsequently set in motion from scattered photons, or both.[12,13,20,21] Figure 20.2 illustrates isovalue lines for a 1.25-MeV kernel in water. As is evident from the figure, the kernel is forward directed even at this low energy. As the energy increases, the kernel becomes even more forward peaked.

Modeling Primary Photons Incident on the Phantom

The convolution equation is restricted to describing monoenergetic parallel beams of primary photons interacting with homogeneous phantoms. To model a clinical radiotherapy beam, the contribution for each energy bin of the photon spectrum must be summed. At present, the spectral information is derived from MC simulations benchmarked by measurement. Using the EGS4 MC method, Mohan and Chui[22] first quantified the spectrum of clinical accelerators using the MC method. Since that time, several other authors have performed simulations to calculate photon energy spectrum.[18,23,24]

The spectrum will also vary with off-axis position if a field-flattening filter is used. Figure 20.3 shows that the mean energy of primary radiation (directly from the target) for a Varian 2100C (flattened) 10-MV photon beam decreases off-axis but the extrafocal photons (primary collimator and flattening filter) do not.[18] This off-axis decrease is due to differential hardening of the beam by the field-flattening filter. Since the direct photon component dominates, the model must take into account the change in the energy spectrum across the field.

Collimators and block field outlines are usually modeled with a mathematical *mask function*, which consists of the fraction of the incident fluence transmitted through the modifier. For a collimator, the mask function inside the field is unity, and underneath the collimator it is equal to the primary collimator transmission. For a block, the mask function inside the field is the primary transmission

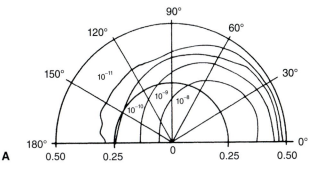

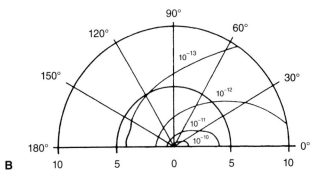

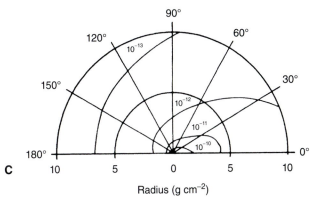

Radius (g cm^{-2})

FIGURE 20.2. Cobalt-60 (more precisely, 1.25-MeV primary photons) kernels for water computed using Monte Carlo simulation (MCS). The isovalue lines are in units of cGy MeV^{-1} photon^{-1}. **A:** The contribution due to electrons set in motion from primary photons (i.e., the primary contribution). **B:** The first scatter contribution. **C:** The sum of the primary and all scatter contributions. (Reprinted from Mackie TR, Bielajew AF, Rogers DW, et al. Generation of photon energy deposition kernels using the EGS4 Monte Carlo code. *Phys Med Biol.* 1988;33:1–2; with permission of IOP Publishing. All rights reserved.)

through the block tray, and underneath the block it is equal to the primary block transmission. The mask function alone would not be able to model the penumbral blurring of the field boundary. This has been modeled by an *aperture function*. The mask function is convolved by a two-dimensional (2D) blurring kernel that represents the finite size of the source. The blurring kernel is usually assumed to be a normal function with a standard deviation equal to the projection of the source spot's width through the collimation system (thereby accounting for magnification of the source at large distances from the collimator system). Finally, the mask function is multiplied by the energy fluence distribution for the largest open field.

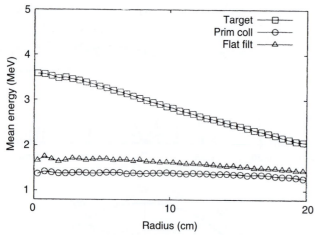

FIGURE 20.3. The photon mean energy distribution in an open 40 × 40-cm field from a 10-MV photon beam target, primary collimator, and field-flattening filter. Values are for in-air photons arriving at the plane of the isocenter. (Reprinted from Liu HH, Mackie TR, McCullough EC. A dual source photon beam model used in convolution/superposition dose calculations for clinical megavoltage x-ray beams. *Med Phys.* 1997;24:1960–1974, with permission.)

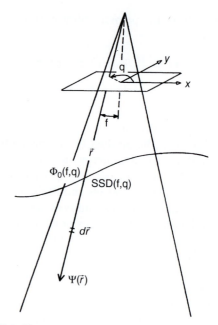

FIGURE 20.4. The ray-tracing of a two-dimensional (2D) energy fluence distribution through the patient to create a three-dimensional (3D) energy fluence distribution in the patient. SSD, source-to-surface distance.

The energy fluence outside the field is greater than that which can be accounted for by collimator transmission of the primary photons generated in the target. It can be modeled by adding short, broad normal distribution to the energy fluence. The source of this component is mainly the extrafocal radiation produced from Compton scattering in the field-flattening filter. The magnitude of the extrafocal radiation source can also be used to account for the variation in the machine-generated output factor, because the scatter outside the field and the increase in machine-generated output are both due to scatter from the accelerator head.[18,25]

Conventional wedges and compensators cannot be accurately modeled with primary attenuation only. These components produce scatter and cause differential hardening of the beam. The hardening of the primary beam can be accounted for according to the material of the wedge and the beam spectrum as a function of radial position. Scatter from the wedge is more difficult to account for. The increased scatter results in the wedge factor increasing by a few percent as a function of field size. This can be adequately modeled by a field size-dependent factor that duplicates the effect. Alternatively, the wedge or compensator can be included as part of the patient representation. This extended phantom has a large heterogeneity in it, namely, the air gap between the device and the patient. This method can predict the variation in the wedge factor as a function of field size.

Ray-Tracing the Incident Energy Fluence Through the Phantom

The incident 2D energy fluence distribution is ray-traced through the patient to create a 3D distribution of energy fluence (Fig. 20.4). The density of the rays followed and the sampling of the rays along their path must be sufficient to represent the attenuation behavior of the phantom. Sufficient sampling density is especially important for head, neck, and breast tangential fields. In general, the sampling density required is higher than the dose resolution desired, so several rays are traversing each calculation voxel.

Terma is computed within the calculation matrix by multiplying the primary fluence by the mass attenuation coefficient. The primary ray attenuation coefficient, weighted to the appropriate beam spectrum, is based on the voxel properties. The energy fluence at a sample point is reduced from the previous sample along the ray. Hardening of the primary energy fluence spectrum with depth and off-axis position is accounted for by changing the attenuation coefficient with position. The speed of the ray-tracing operation can be improved significantly by the use of lookup tables to store precomputed results.

Electron Contamination

The electron contamination of the beam is not accounted for in the conventional convolution method, so an additional independent component must be added to account for this dose. The surface dose from megavoltage photon beams is almost entirely due to the electron contamination component. Studies in which the electron contamination has been removed by magnetically sweeping electrons from the field reveal that the dose from the contaminating electrons resembles an electron beam with a practical range somewhat greater than the depth of the maximum dose. A reasonable agreement with measured depth–dose curves can be obtained by scaling the contamination electron depth–dose curve with the surface dose and adding this component to the convolution-computed dose distribution.

Kernel Spatial Variance and Phantom Heterogeneities

The convolution equation assumes that the kernel is spatially invariant in that the kernel value depends only on the relative geometrical relationship between the interaction and dose deposition sites and not on their absolute position in the phantom. When this is true, the convolution calculation can be done in Fourier space, saving much time. Unfortunately, this is not the case as the kernel varies with position.

The effects of hardening and divergence of the beam are small and can be calculated in a number of ways. A multiplicative correction to the terma in the patient can be used to correct for hardening of the kernel.[17,26] Alternatively, several kernels valid for different depths in the phantom can be used as a basis for interpolation to a specific depth.[17,19] Liu et al. showed that the correction as a function of depth is nearly linear, and not employing any correction results in ~4% discrepancy at 30 cm depth. Tilting the kernel to match the beam divergence results in only a minor improvement in accuracy for the worst-case examples.[19]

Phantom heterogeneities are a more serious problem. Modeling the transport of electrons and scattered photons through a heterogeneous phantom would require a unique kernel at each location. Each kernel would be superimposed on the dose grid and weighted with respect to the primary terma. What is required to make the calculation tractable is to modify a kernel, computed in a homogeneous medium, to be reasonably representative in a heterogeneous situation. If most of the energy between the primary interaction site and the dose deposition site is transported on the direct path between these sites, it is possible to have a relatively simple correction to the convolution equation based on ray-tracing between the interaction and dose deposition sites, and on scaling the path length by density to get the radiologic path length between these sites. The convolution equation modified for radiologic path length is called the superposition equation:

$$D(\mathbf{r}) = \int T_{\mathrm{p}}(\rho_{r'} \cdot \mathbf{r}')\, A(\rho_{r-r'} \cdot (\mathbf{r} - \mathbf{r}'))\, d\mathbf{r}' \quad (20.5)$$

where $\rho_{r-r'} \cdot (\mathbf{r} - \mathbf{r}')$ is the radiologic distance from the dose deposition site to the primary photon interaction site and $\rho_r \cdot \mathbf{r}'$ is the radiologic distance from the source to the photon interaction site.

Woo and Cunningham[15] compared the modified kernel using range scaling for a complex heterogeneous phantom with a kernel computed *de novo* for a particular interaction site inside the phantom. The results shown

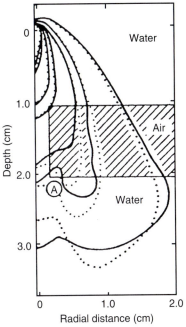

FIGURE 20.5. Comparison of Monte Carlo-generated 6-MeV primary photon kernel in a water phantom containing a ring of air. The dotted line is a kernel modified for the heterogeneous situation using range scaling from the one derived in a homogeneous phantom. The continuous line is a kernel computed expressly for the heterogeneous situation. It is impractical to compute kernels for every possible heterogeneous situation, and there is sufficient similarity to warrant the range scaling approximation. (Reprinted from Woo MK, Cunningham JR. The validity of the density scaling method in primary electron transport for photon and electron beams. *Med Phys.* 1990;17:187–194, with permission.)

in Figure 20.5 indicate that the agreement is not perfect, but the computational trends are clearly in evidence in that isovalue lines contract in high-density regions and expand in low-density regions.

MONTE CARLO

The MC technique of radiation transport consists of using well-established probability distributions governing the individual interactions of electrons and photons to simulate their transport through matter. MC methods are used to perform calculations in all areas of physics and math for any problems that involve a probabilistic nature. Several excellent reviews of MC calculations in radiation therapy exist,[27–31] as well as an American Association of Physicists in Medicine (AAPM) Task Group Report which discusses its clinical implementation.[32]

Although the MC method had been proposed for some time, it was not capable of being fully utilized until the development of the digital computer in the 1940s. Radiation transport was one of the first uses for this methodology at that time, and public codes, such as Monte Carlo N-Particle Transport code (MCNP), began appearing as early as the 1950s. In photon transport calculations, the Electron Transport (ETRAN) code, developed by the

National Bureau of Standards in the 1970s, was based on the condensed history technique (discussed below) first introduced by Berger in 1963. The Electron Gamma Shower (EGS4) code was originally developed at the Stanford Linear Accelerator in the 1980s and is now maintained (as the modified EGSnrc) by the National Research Council of Canada.[33]

Analog Simulations

As pointed out by TG 105, an analog simulation is the random propagation of a particle through the following four steps: (1) determining the distance to the next interaction, (2) transporting the particle to the interaction site, (3) selecting which interaction will take place, and (4) simulating this interaction.[32] The initial step is performed based on the probability that the particle will interact within the medium in question. For example, if the probability of interaction is represented by an attenuation coefficient μ, a random interaction distance r can be determined from a random number ϵ (between 0 and 1) by the following equation[30,32]:

$$r = -\frac{\ln(1-\varepsilon)}{\mu} \qquad (20.6)$$

The second step is relatively straightforward, but knowledge of the mass density (and the corresponding changes in μ) is required for heterogeneous materials. Another random choice will be made for step 3, weighted proportionally to the relative probabilities of interaction choices (e.g., Compton scatter vs. photoelectric absorption vs. pair production). Finally, the results of the interaction must be randomly simulated, including the particles of new energy (if not absorbed) and trajectory.

Condensed Histories

Althoughanalog simulations work well for photon interactions, a practical problem arises for the transport of electrons. The mean free path for electrons in the therapeutic energy range is of the order of 10^{-5} g/cm². This means that a single electron of energy >1 MeV will have more than 10^5 interactions before stopping. To perform an analog simulation of this event is impractical.

The condensed history electron transport technique was first introduced by Berger in 1963. Berger noted that most electron inelastic interactions did not lose a great deal of energy or have a significant directional change. These "soft" interactions could be separated by more significant "catastrophic" events, where the electron had a significant energy loss (e.g., delta ray production, Bremsstrahlung event). The soft interactions could be separately simulated by combining these into single virtual large-effect interactions, while the catastrophic events can be analog simulated as described above.[30] For electrons with energies above an energy threshold, the mean free path for catastrophic interactions is of several orders of magnitude higher.

Although this approach allows for faster computations, the step size choice for the condensed histories has been shown to produce artifacts in the results.[34] However, these issues have led to improved, high-accuracy condensed history methods.[34–36]

Variance Reduction Techniques

Instead of simulating individual events as in an analog simulation, one may employ techniques to improve the MC calculation efficiency in obtaining a particular result. Variance reduction techniques are used to reduce the variance of a given calculation result for a given number of histories. For example, an analog simulation of a Bremsstrahlung event would randomly select an energy and direction (proportional to their respective probabilities) for the resulting photon emission. Alternatively, one could simulate the emission of a large number of photons with lower weights to better mimic the random directional emission of these events. This particular technique is termed Bremsstrahlung splitting[37] and is one of many different techniques which may be employed within a particular MC code. These techniques are important in keeping calculation times practical for most situations. However, care must be taken that the underlying physics is not biased by the results.

MC Radiotherapy Dose Calculations

In principle, it is possible to simulate histories for the entire radiation therapy delivery, that is, from the initial accelerated electron's impact onto the target to the delivery dose. However, this would be a tremendously inefficient process, as few of these histories would make it beyond the accelerator head to the patient. Alternatively, it is possible to transport the particles through the patient-independent structures (e.g., target, primary collimator, ion chamber) and store this information for future use. This information is known as a phase-space file, and it contains information including the position, energy, and direction of the photons and electrons emitted from the accelerator.

Figure 20.6 shows a cross-sectional view of a Varian linac which demonstrates a possible location of a phase-space plane located distal to all the patient-independent components of the accelerator head. Once initially computed, this information may be continually used to calculate the dose to individual patients. It may also be advantageous to create phase-space planes further down the beam path (c.f., phase-space plane 2 in Fig. 20.6), particularly for standard collimator settings and/or beam modifiers. Otherwise, these data can be projected directly onto the patient for dose calculation.

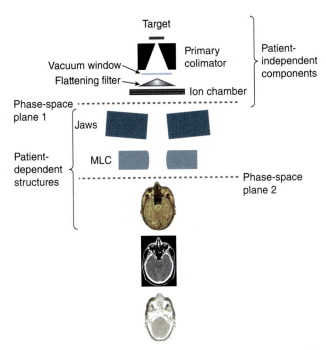

FIGURE 20.6. Illustration of the components of a typical Varian linear accelerator treatment head in photon beam mode. Phase space planes for simulating patient-dependent and patient-independent structures are also represented. (Reprinted from Chetty IJ, Curran B, Cygler JE, et al. Report of the AAPM Task Group No. 105: Issues associated with clinical implementation of Monte Carlo-based photon and electron external beam treatment planning. *Med Phys.* 2007;34:4818–4853, with permission.) MLC.

DISCRETE ORDINATES METHOD

More recently, several authors have reported on a direct numerical solution of the Boltzmann transport equations (BTEs). The approach has been commercialized in the Varian Eclipse Treatment Planning System, under the name Acuros. In particular, this methodology has been proposed as an alternative to MC calculations, in order to produce accurate dose distributions with a substantially reduced calculation time.

Derivation of the Transport Equations

The linear BTE can be derived by assuming particle conservation within a small volume element of phase space.[38–40] We define a quantity called the angular density of electrons, $N_e(\mathbf{r}, \mathbf{\Omega}, E, t)$, which represents the probable number of electrons at location $\mathbf{r}$ and direction $\mathbf{\Omega}$ with energy E at time t per unit volume per unit solid angle per unit energy. $\mathbf{\Omega}$ represents the unit director in the direction of motion, that is, parallel to $\mathbf{v}$. Thus, $N_e(\mathbf{r}, \mathbf{\Omega}, E, t)\, dV\, d\Omega\, dE$ represents the number of electrons at time t in a volume element dV about $\mathbf{r}$, in a narrow beam of solid angle $d\Omega$ about $\mathbf{\Omega}$, and energy range dE about E.

After a time Δt, these electrons have moved to position $\mathbf{r} + \mathbf{v}\,\Delta t$ and have been reduced due to collisions

within the medium by an amount $e^{-\sigma v\Delta t}$. Here σ is the *macroscopic cross section* for electrons and represents $1/\lambda$, where λ is the mean free path. Although not strictly a crosssection, σ is analogous to the photon attenuation coefficient and has units of 1/length. For very short times Δt, the number of electrons from this packet which have reached $\mathbf{r} + \mathbf{v}\Delta t$ is $\approx N_e(1 - \sigma v\Delta t)dV\, d\Omega\, dE$. At the same time scattered electrons from elsewhere in the medium may reach the same position ($\mathbf{r} + \mathbf{v}\,\Delta t$). This quantity may be determined by integrating the angular density over phase space multiplied by the probability for these interactions:

$$N_e^{scatter}(\mathbf{r} + \mathbf{v}\cdot\Delta t, t + \Delta t)$$

$$= \iint N_e(r,t)\left\{\frac{d^2\sigma}{dE\,d\Omega}(\mathbf{\Omega}',E';\mathbf{\Omega},E)\right\}d\Omega\,dE, \quad (20.7)$$

where $\frac{d^2\sigma}{d\Omega\,dE}(\mathbf{\Omega}',E';\mathbf{\Omega},E)$ represents the doubly differential crosssection for electron scatter from energy E' and direction $\mathbf{\Omega}'$ to energy E and direction $\mathbf{\Omega}$.

In addition, any additional sources of electrons produced during time Δt may also reach the position $\mathbf{r} + \mathbf{v}\Delta t$. In this case, the number of additional electrons at $\mathbf{r} + \mathbf{v}\Delta t$ becomes $Q(r, W, E, t)\Delta t$, where $Q(r,\mathbf{\Omega},E,t)$ represents the rate of electron production from other sources. The total number of electrons at position $\mathbf{r} + \mathbf{v}\Delta t$ is now given by the following equation:

$$N_e(\mathbf{r} + \mathbf{v}\Delta t, \mathbf{\Omega}, E, t + \Delta t) = N_e(\mathbf{r}, \mathbf{\Omega}, E, t)(1 - \sigma v\Delta t)$$

$$+ \left\{\iint N_e(\mathbf{r}, \mathbf{\Omega}', E', t)\frac{d^2\sigma}{d\Omega\,dE}(E', \mathbf{\Omega}'; E, \mathbf{\Omega})\right\}\Delta t$$

$$+ Q(\mathbf{r}, \mathbf{\Omega}, E, t)\Delta t \quad (20.8)$$

Dividing the equation by Δt and taking the limit $\Delta t \to 0$, we obtain

$$\lim_{\Delta t\to 0}\left[\frac{N_e(\mathbf{r} + v\Delta t, \mathbf{\Omega}, E, t + \Delta t) - N_e(\mathbf{r}, \mathbf{\Omega}, E, t)}{\Delta t}\right]$$

$$+ \sigma v N_e(\mathbf{r}, \mathbf{\Omega}, E, t)$$

$$= \iint N_e(\mathbf{r}, \mathbf{\Omega}', E', t)\frac{d^2\sigma}{d\Omega\,dE}(E', \mathbf{\Omega}';\ E, \mathbf{\Omega})d\Omega'\,dE'$$

$$+ Q(\mathbf{r}, \mathbf{\Omega}, E, t) \quad (20.9)$$

The limit term represents the total time derivative of N_e for an observer moving with the packet of electrons (i.e., from $\mathbf{r}$ to $\mathbf{r} + v\Delta t$). It may be rewritten to simplify the equation:

$$\lim_{\Delta t\to 0}\left[\frac{N_e(\mathbf{r} + v\Delta t, t + \Delta t) - N_e(\mathbf{r}, t)}{\Delta t}\right]$$

$$= \lim_{\Delta t\to 0}\left[\frac{N_e(\mathbf{r} + v\Delta t, t + \Delta t) - N_e(\mathbf{r}, t + \Delta t)}{\Delta t}\right]$$

$$+ \lim_{\Delta t\to 0}\left[\frac{N_e(\mathbf{r}, t + \Delta t) - N_e(\mathbf{r}, t)}{\Delta t}\right]$$

$$= \mathbf{v}\cdot\nabla N_e(\mathbf{r}, t) + \frac{\partial N_e(\mathbf{r}, t)}{\partial t} \quad (20.10)$$

The first term in Equation (20.10) represents the velocity times the directional derivative of N_e in the direction of Ω. It is known as the *streaming term*, as it represents the difference in the time derivative between the moving and rest frames, the latter of which also includes the effects of electrons moving past **r** without any collisions.

Upon inserting (20.10) into (20.9), the resulting equation becomes

$$\frac{\partial N_e}{\partial t} + \mathbf{v} \cdot \nabla N_e + \sigma v N_e = \iint N_e' \left\{ \frac{d^2\sigma}{dE'd\Omega'} \right\} dE' d\Omega' + Q,$$

(20.11)

where we have removed the arguments for simplicity. This is the basic form of the transport equation, which is often called the Boltzmann equation because of its similarity to the expression derived by Boltzmann involving the kinetic theory of gasses.[39] It is more often written in terms of the angular flux, Ψ_e, where $\Psi_e(\mathbf{r}, \Omega, E, t) = v N_e(\mathbf{r}, \Omega, E, t)$:

$$\frac{1}{v}\frac{\partial \Psi_e}{\partial t} + \Omega \cdot \nabla N_e + \sigma \Psi_e = \iint \Psi_e' \left\{ \frac{d^2\sigma}{dE'd\Omega'} \right\} dE' d\Omega' + Q,$$

(20.12)

Use of the Transport Equations for Photon Beam Calculations

In external beam radiotherapy, the time-independent form of Equation (20.12) is used, since steady state is achieved in a much shorter time than that when the beam is on.[41] Equation (20.12) is an integro-partial-differential equation which can be solved numerically using either stochastic or deterministic methods. Most reports have utilized the latter, employing some form of grid-based numerical method in which phase space is discretized in spatial, angular, and energy coordinates,[40,42,43] although there are some differences in the literature about which techniques are used. Finite difference and finite element methods are used for spatial discretization, and Boman et al. reported using the finiteelement method for all variables.[40] Alternatively, the method of discreteordinates has been employed for angular discretization in the Attila solver,[44,45] and in the subsequent Acuros XB algorithm currently available in the Varian Eclipse treatment planning system (Varian Assoc, Palo Alto, CA). Energy-dependent coupled photon–electron cross-sectional data are available through CEPXS, which uses the multigroup method to discretize the particle energy domain into energy intervals or groups.[46] This class of solvers is commonly known as the discrete ordinates method, although technically the name only refers to the method for numerically discretizing in angle.

Up to now, we have only discussed electron angular density (or angular flux). However, in external beam calculations, collisions involve photons, electrons, and positrons. In principle, Equation (20.12) then becomes a set of coupled equations. For example, excluding positron interactions, we have the following

$$\Omega \cdot \nabla \Psi_\gamma + \sigma_\gamma \Psi_\gamma + \iint \Psi_e' \left\{ \frac{d^2\sigma_{e\gamma}}{dE'd\Omega'} \right\} dE' d\Omega'$$

$$+ \iint \Psi_\gamma' \left\{ \frac{d^2\sigma_{\gamma\gamma}}{dE'd\Omega'} \right\} dE' d\Omega' = Q_\gamma$$

$$\Omega \cdot \nabla \Psi_e + \sigma_e \Psi_e + \iint \Psi_\gamma' \left\{ \frac{d^2\sigma_{\gamma e}}{dE'd\Omega'} \right\} dE' d\Omega'$$

$$+ \iint \Psi_e' \left\{ \frac{d^2\sigma_{ee}}{dE'd\Omega'} \right\} dE' d\Omega' = Q_e$$

(20.13)

where $\frac{d^2\sigma_{12}}{dE'd\Omega'}(\Omega', E', \Omega, E)$ represents the differential crosssection for the creation of particle 2 with energy E, direction Ω, particle 1 of energy E', and direction Ω'.

Acuros XB Implementation of the Linear BTEs

Currently, the only commercial implementation of the linear BTE is the Acuros XB dose calculation algorithm available on the Varian Eclipse treatment planning system. Acuros XB was developed using many of the methods employed with a prototype BTE solver developed at the Los Alamos National Laboratories called Attila, which was co-authored by the founders of Transpire, Inc. (Gig Harbor, WA).[47] Transpire, Inc., established a licensing agreement to commercialize Attila for a broad range of applications. Acuros XB has adapted and optimized the methods within Attila for external photon beam calculations.[48]

Within the Acuros algorithm, both charged pair-production particles are assumed to be electrons, and the contribution of electron-produced Bremsstrahlung within the patient is assumed to be deposited locally.

As already mentioned, energy discretization is performed using a multigroup representation of the crosssection. However, this is difficult for electrons where the inelastic cross-section increases rapidly when energy losses become small. These "soft" interactions would require a very large number of energy bins to accurately describe, which is impractical for an efficient solution. As a result, electron interactions are separated into large and small energy losses, the latter of which are described by a continuous slowing-down (CSD) approximation. In this case, the angular electron fluence is described by the Boltzmann–Fokker–Planck transport equation:

$$\Omega \cdot \nabla \Psi_e + \sigma_e \Psi_e - \frac{\partial S_R}{\partial E} \Psi_e + \iint \Psi_\gamma' \left\{ \frac{d^2\sigma_{\gamma e}}{dE'd\Omega'} \right\} dE' d\Omega'$$

$$+ \iint \Psi_e' \left\{ \frac{d^2\sigma_{ee}}{dE'd\Omega'} \right\} dE' d\Omega' = Q_e$$

(20.14)

In this case σ_{ee} represents larger, "catastrophic" interactions that are represented by standard Boltzmann scattering.[48]

Gifford et al.[44] first performed an evaluation of the prototype solver Attila for radiation therapy dose calculations. Dose calculations performed by Attila were directly compared with those calculated using MC codes MCNPX for a brachytherapy calculation and EGS4 for an

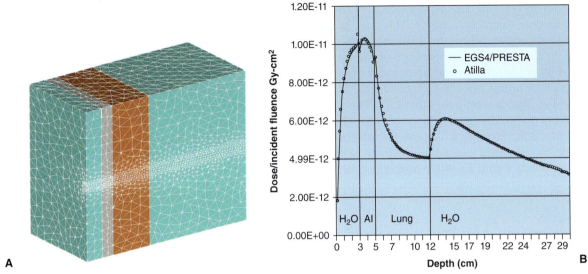

FIGURE 20.7. Comparison of EGS4/PRESTA with Attila for a percent depth–dose calculation in a heterogeneous phantom. (Reprinted from Gifford KA, Horton JL, Wareing TA, et al. Comparison of a finite-element multigroup discrete-ordinates code with Monte Carlo for radiotherapy calculations. *Phys Med Biol*. 2006;51:2253–2265, with permission of IOP Publishing. All rights reserved.)

external photon beam calculation. Differences in doses were compared, along with relative calculation speeds.

The photon dose calculation comparison was made comparing Attila versus EGS4 for an 18-MV photon beam from a Varian 2100 accelerator. A narrow beam geometry was used to highlight any differences in regions of electron disequilibrium. In addition, a heterogeneous multislab phantom was used, which consisted of water, lung, and aluminum. The Attila calculation was divided into 24 and 36 photon and electron energy groups, respectively. A comparison of depth–doses between these two calculations is shown in Figure 20.7. The agreements here were also good, with a root mean square difference of 0.7% of the maximum dose.

Vassiliev et al.[45] extended these comparisons to include external beam calculations of heterogeneous patient geometries. In their work, Attila was compared with EGSnrc MC simulations for a 6-MV photon beam from a Varian 2100 for a prostate and a head and neck case previously treated within their department. For both the BTE and MC calculations, CT datasets were converted into a material map of four materials with fixed densities: air, adipose tissue, soft tissue, and bone. In their comparison, calculations were performed with the same beam geometries as those used clinically, with the exception of beam modulation which was removed for this comparison. Dose calculation differences were investigated along with the resolution of various discretization variables required for accurate Attila calculations.

Figure 20.8 displays the material map for an axial slice through the center of the PTV for the head and neck case.

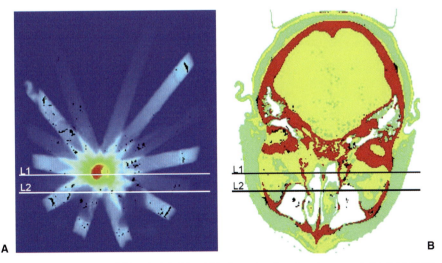

FIGURE 20.8. A: Dose field calculated by Attila for a head-and-neck case on the axial plane through isocenter. Pixels, where the dose difference between Attila and Monte Carlo (EGS) exceeds 3%/3 mm, are shown in black on **A** and **B**. **B:** Material map through the axial plane containing the isocenter for the dose distribution calculated in **A**. (Adapted from Fig. 5 in [25] Safai S, Bortfeld T, Engelsman M. Comparison between the lateral penumbra of a collimated double-scattered beam and uncollimated scanning beam in proton radiotherapy. *Phys Med Biol*. 2008;53:1729–1750.)

Also displayed is the resulting dose distribution performed using the Attila dose calculation engine. The black areas on each image are regions where the difference between the MC and BTE calculations exceeded 5% of the maximum dose. A more quantitative comparison can be seen by looking at a dose profile through the center of the PTV (Line "L1" on Fig. 20.8) and off-axis (Line "L2"). The dose profiles for both the Attila and EGSnrc codes for these lines are displayed in Figure 20.9. The overall agreement between these two methods was good, with over 98% of the calculation points within a ±3%/±3 mm criterion.

Since the release of Acuros XB, there have been a number of planning studies investigating the efficiency and accuracy of the discrete ordinates method. Comparisons are made either with other planning algorithms or with measured results for a variety of treatment sites including lung,[49,50] breast,[51] and nasopharynx.[52] Evaluations of Acuros for calculations within heterogeneous media[53] or for radiosurgery treatments[54] have also been reported. The interested reader is referred to these works for additional information.

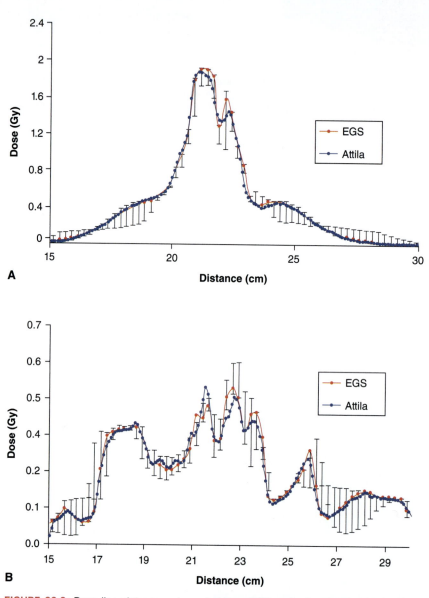

FIGURE 20.9. Dose line plot comparisons between EGSnrc (*red*) and Attila (*blue*) along line L1 **A** and L2 **B** in Figure 20.8. Sharp peaks and dips in the Attila solution correspond to material heterogeneities, which are revolved at the CT image pixel level by Attila. (Reprinted from Vassiliev, Wareing TA, Davis IM, et al. Feasibility of a multigroup deterministic solution method for three-dimensional radiotherapy dose calculations. *Int J Rad Onc Biol Phys.* 2008;72:220–227, with permission.)

KEY POINTS

- Modern radiation therapy planning systems have evolved tremendously over the past few decades. A number of complex model-based photon dose algorithms exist which calculate dose to a 3D representation of the patient. These algorithms have been developed in response to improvements in algorithm development, computing power, and greater availability of volumetric imaging data.

- Today, most commercial photon dose algorithms are a variation of the convolution/superposition method. As algorithm development and computing power improve, the use of MC and discrete-ordinates methods which better incorporate nonequilibrium dosimetry will likely increase.

- A convolution/superposition model should account for the following characteristics:

  - Off-axis energy variations
  - Finite source size

- Extrafocal radiation
- Scatter and attenuation from beam-modifying devices

- MC algorithms track histories of individual photons and electrons that undergo hard ("catastrophic") collisions. Soft electron collisions are dealt with using condensed history methods.

- The discrete ordinates method represents a numerical solution to the coupled Boltzmann transport equations. In this method, the energy, position, and direction of the radiation quanta are discretized for the numerical solution of the integro-differential equations.

- Photon beam optimization presents additional challenges within the planning process. The need to calculate dose rapidly under conditions of changing incident fluence is necessary in a modern radiotherapy clinic.

REVIEW QUESTIONS

1. Which of the following algorithms is/are measurement based?
   A. Bentley–Milan
   B. Convolution/superposition
   C. Monte Carlo
   D. Discrete ordinates

2. Which of the following is/are used to speed up a Monte Carlo dose calculation? Choose all that apply.
   A. Variance reduction technique
   B. Condensed history method
   C. Kernel tilting
   D. Density scaling

3. Which of the following algorithms account for nonequilibrium conditions (e.g., at tissue interfaces)? Choose all that apply.
   A. Bentley–Milan
   B. Convolution/superposition
   C. Monte Carlo
   D. Discrete ordinates

4. For a typical 6-MV beam, an error in CT number of 2% leads to an error in dose of around
   A. 0.1%
   B. 1%
   C. 5%
   D. 10%

5. The inelastic photon scattering processes that must be accounted for include
   A. Rayleigh scattering
   B. Moller scattering
   C. Photoelectric absorption
   D. Bremsstrahlung interactions

6. The convolution dose equation cannot be solved using Fourier analysis primarily because
   A. Scatter kernels are depth dependent
   B. Patient heterogeneities
   C. Beam hardening within the patient
   D. Step-size artifacts

ANSWERS

1. **A**
2. **A and B**
3. **C and D**
4. **B**
5. **C**
6. **B**

REFERENCES

1. Tsien KC. The application of automatic computing machines to radiation treatment planning. *Br J Radiol.* 1955;28(332):432–439.
2. *Use of Computers in External Beam Radiotherapy Procedures with High-Energy Photons and Electrons.* Bethesda, MD:International Commission on Radiation Units and Measurement (ICRU).
3. Sontag MR, Battista JJ, Bronskill MJ, et al. Implications of computed tomography for inhomogeneity corrections in photon beam dose calculations. *Radiology.* 1977;124(1):143–149.
4. Jaffray DA, Battista JJ, Fenster A, et al. X-ray sources of medical linear accelerators: focal and extra-focal radiation. *Med Phys.* 1993;20(5):1417–1427.
5. Khan FM, Gibbons JP. *Khan's the Physics of Radiation Therapy.* 5th ed. Philadelphia, PA: Lippincott, Williams & Wilkins; 2014:624.
6. McCullough EC, Gortney J, Blackwell CR. A depth dependence determination of the wedge transmission factor for 4–10 MV photon beams. *Med Phys.* 1988;15(4):621–623.
7. Palta JR, Daftari I, Suntharalingam N. Field size dependence of wedge factors. *Med Phys.* 1988;15(4):624–626.
8. Sauer OA. Calculation of dose distributions in the vicinity of high-Z interfaces for photon beams. *Med Phys.* 1995;22(10):1685–1690.
9. Mackie TR, Liu HH, McCullough EC. *Treatment Planning Algorithms: Model-Based Photon Dose Calculations in Treatment Planning in Radiation Oncology.* 3rd ed. Philadelphia, PA: Lippincott Williams & Wilkins; 2012:773
10. Battista JJ, Sharpe MB. True three-dimensional dose computations for megavoltage x-ray therapy: a role for the superposition principle. *Australas Phys Eng Sci Med.* 1992;15(4):159–178.
11. Mackie TR, Scrimger JW, Battista JJ. A convolution method of calculating dose for 15-MV x-rays. *Med Phys.* 1985;12(2):188–196.
12. Boyer A, Mok E. A photon dose distribution model employing convolution calculations. *Med Phys.* 1985;12(2):169–177.
13. Mohan R, Chui C, Lidofsky L. Differential pencil beam dose computation model for photons. *Med Phys.* 1986;13(1):64–73.
14. Kubsad SS, Mackie TR, Gehring MA, et al. Monte Carlo and convolution dosimetry for stereotactic radiosurgery. *Int J Radiat Oncol Biol Phys.* 1990;19(4):1027–1035.
15. Woo MK, Cunningham JR. The validity of the density scaling method in primary electron transport for photon and electron beams. *Med Phys.* 1990;17(2):187–194.
16. Metcalfe PE, Hoban PW, Murray DC. Beam hardening of 10 MV radiotherapy x-rays: analysis using a convolution/superposition method. *Phys Med Biol.* 1990;35(11):1533–1549.
17. Papanikolaou N, Mackie TR, Meger-Wells C, et al. Investigation of the convolution method for polyenergetic spectra. *Med Phys.* 1993;20(5):1327–1336.
18. Liu HH, Mackie TR, McCullough EC. A dual source photon beam model used in convolution/superposition dose calculations for clinical megavoltage x-ray beams. *Med Phys.* 1997;24(12):1960–1974.
19. Liu HH, Mackie TR, McCullough EC. Correcting kernel tilting and hardening in convolution/superposition dose calculations for clinical divergent and polychromatic photon beams. *Med Phys.* 1997;24(11):1729–1741.
20. Ahnesjo A, Andreo P, Brahme A. Calculation and application of point spread functions for treatment planning with high energy photon beams. *Acta Oncol.* 1987;26(1):49–56.
21. Mackie TR, Bielajew AF, Rogers DW, et al. Generation of photon energy deposition kernels using the EGS Monte Carlo code. *Phys Med Biol.* 1988;33(1):1–20.
22. Mohan R, Chui C, Lidofsky L. Energy and angular distributions of photons from medical linear accelerators. *Med Phys.* 1985;12(5):592–597.
23. Chaney EL, Cullip TJ, Gabriel TA. A Monte Carlo study of accelerator head scatter. *Med Phys.* 1994;21(9):1383–1390.
24. Lovelock DM, Chui CS, Mohan R. A Monte Carlo model of photon beams used in radiation therapy. *Med Phys.* 1995;22(9):1387–1394.
25. Sharpe MB, Jaffray DA, Battista JJ, et al. Extrafocal radiation: a unified approach to the prediction of beam penumbra and output factors for megavoltage x-ray beams. *Med Phys.* 1995;22(12):2065–2074.

26. Hoban PW, Murray DC, Round WH. Photon beam convolution using polyenergetic energy deposition kernels. *Phys Med Biol.* 1994;39(4):669–685.
27. Rogers DWO, Bielajew AF. Monte Carlo techniques of electron and photon transport for radiation dosimetry. In: Kase K, Bjarngard BE, Attix F, eds. *The Dosimetry of Ionizing Radiation.* New York, NY: Academic Press; 1990:427–539.
28. Mackie TR. Applications of the Monte Carlo Method. In: Kase K, Bjarngard BE, Attix F, eds. *The Dosimetry of Ionizing Radiation.* New York, NY: Academic Press; 1990:541–620.
29. Andreo P. Monte Carlo techniques in medical radiation physics. *Phys Med Biol.* 1991;36(7):861–920.
30. Bielajew AF. The Monte Carlo simulation of radiation transport. In: Curran B, Balter J, Chetty I, eds. *AAPM Monograph No. 32: Integrating New Technologies into the Clinic: Monte Carlo and Image-Guided Radiation Therapy.* Madison, WI: Medical Physics Publishing; 2006:697.
31. Rogers DW. Fifty years of Monte Carlo simulations for medical physics. *Phys Med Biol.* 2006;51(13):R287–R301.
32. Chetty IJ, Curran B, Cygler JE, et al. Report of the AAPM Task Group No. 105: Issues associated with clinical implementation of Monte Carlo-based photon and electron external beam treatment planning. *Med Phys.* 2007;34(12):4818–4853.
33. Kawrakow I. Accurate condensed history Monte Carlo simulation of electron transport. I. EGSnrc, the new EGS4 version. *Med Phys.* 2000;27(3):485–498.
34. Bielajew AF, Rogers DWO, Jenkins TW, et al. *Monte Carlo Transport of Electrons and Photons.* New York, NY: Plenum; 1988:115–137.
35. Kawrakow I, Bielajew AF. On the condensed history technique for electron transport. *Nucl Instrum Methods Phys Res B.* 1998;142:253–280.
36. Seltzer SM. Electron-photon Monte Carlo calculations: The ETRAN code. *Intl J Appl Radiat Isot.* 1991;42:917–941.
37. Kawrakow I, Rogers DW, Walters BR. Large efficiency improvements in BEAMnrc using directional bremsstrahlung splitting. *Med Phys.* 2004;31(10):2883–2898.
38. Case KM, Zweifel PF. *Linear Transport Theory.* Reading, MA: Addison-Wesley; 1967.
39. Bell GI, Glasstone S. *Nuclear Reactor Theory.* New York, NY: Van Nostrand Reinhold Company; 1970:619.
40. Boman E, Tervo J, Vauhkonen M. Modelling the transport of ionizing radiation using the finite element method. *Phys Med Biol.* 2005;50(2):265–280.
41. Borgers C. Complexity of Monte Carlo and deterministic dose-calculation methods. *Phys Med Biol.* 1998;43(3):517–528.
42. Lewis EE, Miller WFJ. *Computational Methods of Neutron Transport.* New York, NY: Wiley; 1984.
43. Dautray R, Lions JL. *Mathematical Analysis and Numerical Methods for Science and Technology.* Berlin: Springer; 1993.
44. Gifford KA, Horton JL, Wareing TA, et al. Comparison of a finite-element multigroup discrete-ordinates code with Monte Carlo for radiotherapy calculations. *Phys Med Biol.* 2006;51(9):2253–2265.
45. Vassiliev ON. Wareing TA, Davis IM, et al. Feasibility of a multigroup deterministic solution method for three-dimensional radiotherapy dose calculations. *Int J Radiat Oncol Biol Phys.* 2008;72(1):220–227.
46. Lorence L, Morel J, Valdez G. Physics guide to CEPXS: a multigroup coupled electron-photon cross section generating code. New Mexico: Sandia National Laboratories: Albuquerque; 1989:110.
47. Wareing TA, McGhee JM, Morel JE, et al., Discontinuous finite element Sn methods on 3-D unstructured grids. *Nucl Sci Eng.* 2001;138:256–268.
48. Eclipse Photon and Electron Algorithms Reference Guide. Varian Medical Systems, Inc., Palo Alto, CA 94304. P1008611-002-B. December 2014.
49. Liu HW, Nugent Z, Clayton R, et al. Clinical impact of using the deterministic patient dose calculation algorithm Acuros XB for lung stereotactic body radiation therapy. *Acta Oncol.* 2014;53(3):324–339.

50. Kroon PS, Hol S, Essers M. Dosimetric accuracy and clinical quality of Acuros XB and AAA dose calculation algorithm for stereotactic and conventional lung volumetric modulated arc therapy plans. *Radiat Oncol.* 2013;8:149.

51. Fogliata A, Nicolini G, Clivio A, et al. On the dosimetric impact of inhomogeneity management in the Acuros XB algorithm for breast treatment. *Radiat Oncol.* 2011;6:103.

52. Kan MW, Leung LH, Yu PK. Dosimetric impact of using the Acuros XB algorithm for intensity modulated radiation therapy and RapidArc planning in nasopharyngeal carcinomas. *Int J Radiat Oncol Biol Phys.* 2013;85(1):e73–e80.

53. Kan MW, Leung LH, So RW, et al. Experimental verification of the Acuros XB and AAA dose calculation adjacent to heterogeneous media for IMRT and RapidArc of nasopharyngeal carcinoma. *Med Phys.* 2013;40(3):031714.

54. Fogliata A, Nicolini G, Clivio A, et al. Accuracy of Acuros XB and AAA dose calculation for small fields with reference to RapidArc(®) stereotactic treatments. *Med Phys.* 2011;38(11):6228–6237.

21 Treatment Planning Algorithms: Brachytherapy

Kenneth J. Weeks

INTRODUCTION

Brachytherapy involves the treatment of cancer using the photon, electron, and positron emissions from radioisotopes. Brachytherapy was developed using naturally occurring radioisotopes such as radium 226. The history, applications, and emission details of radioisotopes are described elsewhere.[1-5] The goal of brachytherapy treatment planning is to determine the number of sources, their individual strengths, and the location of each source relative to the treatment volume, so as to treat a localized volume to a given minimum dose while respecting tolerances of normal tissues. It is important to note that the original brachytherapy clinical applications were developed realizing that brachytherapy demanded three-dimensional (3-D) planning because the sources were distributed in three dimensions. Because of this fact and the absence of computers, these original treatment systems were all inclusive. They were systems with rules for distributing the sources, rules for picking and arranging source strengths, and given the latter, precalculated dose-rate tables for determining the dose to a point. The Manchester, Paris, Stockholm, Memorial, and Quimby systems[1-5] all specified in alternate ways how to do this for interstitial and intracavitary implants. From this history, we can gain knowledge of the range of the radioactive source applications which is important in devising dose calculation algorithms. Thus, we summarize the guidelines, which include the following. When distributing lines of sources, attempt to keep them spaced no closer than 8 mm (smaller volumes) and no farther than 2 cm (larger volumes) apart. The periphery of the treatment volume is generally not much farther than 5 cm from the center of gravity of the source distribution. The very high doses close (less than 5 mm) to the sources are not prescribed or evaluated as to clinical significance. At distances greater than 10 cm from the center of the implant, the dose delivered is low and the precise dose is not considered a treatment objective. Therefore, we conclude that dose calculation algorithms, which are very accurate from 5 mm to 5 cm and generally accurate to 10 cm, are required. The availability of computers and advanced imaging capabilities means precalculated dose tables for predetermined patterns of multiple sources are no longer required. Calculation of the dose distribution for the individual patient's source distribution is possible.

Radioisotopes decay randomly with a time-independent probability.[1,3,5,6] If there are N_0 radioactive atoms at time $t = 0$, then at a later time t, we have $N(t)$ atoms given by

$$N(t) = N_0 e^{-\lambda t} \qquad (21.1)$$

where $\lambda \ (= ln(2)/T_{1/2})$ is the radioisotope's decay constant and $T_{1/2}$ is the half-life (time it takes for half of the isotope to decay). The activity (A) at time t is proportional to the number of radioactive atoms present and is defined by

$$A(t) = \lambda N(t) = A_0 \ e^{-\lambda t} \qquad (21.2)$$

where A_0 is the initial activity. Throughout the following, we will consider the calculation of the dose rate, $\dot{D}$ (in cGy/hour). The total dose D delivered during an implant, which lasts for time t, is obtained from the initial dose rate, $\dot{D}_0$, at the start of the implant from

$$D(t) = \dot{D}_0 (1 - e^{-\lambda t})/\lambda \qquad (21.3)$$

For the case $t \gg T_{1/2}$, for example, a permanent implant, the total dose (D) is simply $D = \dot{D}_0 T_{1/2}/ln(2)$, whereas if $t \ll T_{1/2}$, $D = t\dot{D}_0$. Throughout the following, we will calculate the dose rate at the start of the implant ($\dot{D}_0$). The total dose delivered in time t is then obtained from Equation 21.3.

The isotope emits energy (in the form of photons, electrons, and sometimes positrons) in all directions and that energy is absorbed in the mass (tissue) around the isotope, giving rise to absorbed dose (absorbed energy/mass). The calculation of dose rate depends on the number of radioactive atoms, the types and energies of the emitted particles, the time rate of emission of those particles, and finally, the energy absorption and scattering properties of the surrounding media and the radioactive material itself. In this chapter, we begin with the simplest case of a point source. From there, we will use the point source result to determine the dose rate for an ideal line source and then a clinical cylindrical source. Various parameterized calculation methods are discussed. This leads inevitably to systems that explicitly model the flow of energy from the radioactive sources. These include Monte Carlo and Boltzmann transport theory. These latter techniques owe their existence to the extensive computation power now available. The advantages and disadvantages of these methods are discussed.

CALCULATION OF DOSE RATES AROUND A POINT SOURCE

A point source is the simplest situation to calculate. The first approximation, used in radiation oncology, is to ignore the charged particle emissions and consider only the photons. The significance of this approximation is best understood by reviewing the basic nuclear decay data.[7] Consider the well-known ^{192}Ir which has a half-life of 73.8 days and decays via β decay (95% of the decays) or electron capture (5%). The decay of a single ^{192}Ir nucleus produces on average 2.38 photons (there are 44 possible photon energies ranging from 7.8 to 1,378 keV which can be emitted in a single decay event) and 0.95 β-decay electrons (with the β-decay continuous energy spectrum ranging from 0 to 669 keV). In addition, atomic electrons can be emitted with various discrete energies ranging from 11 to 1,378 keV. In a single decay, the average total energy output from photons is 813 keV (note the average energy per photon is therefore 341 keV from 813 keV/2.38) and the average electron energy output is 216 keV.[7] Therefore, the total average energy output per decay is 1,029 keV. Our decision to ignore the emitted electrons means we are going to ignore around 21% of the total energy output from the point source in our dose-rate calculations. Why is this justified? The reason is that practical commercial sources used for Radiation Oncology will be encapsulated radionuclides and that encapsulation will scatter and slow down the electrons such that most do not leave the source capsule itself and for those that do escape, their range in tissue outside the source is much smaller than 5 mm and thus will not contribute dose at a clinical prescription distance. This encapsulation of the source is essential for the clinical use of most isotopes used in radiation oncology. Historically, in the early days of radiotherapy, in the United States, a clever technique to enclose radon gas in glass capsules was developed. The high energy of the β particles and the light filtration led to unfavorable clinical results.[4] We end this discussion with the observation that there can be a major clinical dose distribution difference between an encapsulated and an insufficiently encapsulated radionuclide.

Consider a sample of radioactive material whose largest dimension is much smaller than 0.1 mm. This will be small enough so that all atoms can be approximately considered as located at a single point. Restricting ourselves to the photon emissions from the point source, we will first think about the dose rate produced in a small volume (dV) of tissue located at a distance (r) from the source. For simplicity, consider the source in vacuum (so no scatter) and that in each decay it emits exactly one photon with energy E. The situation is shown in Figure 21.1. The dose rate in dV must be equal to the product of the following: time rate of emission of the photons, i.e., activity A, the probability of the photon hitting dV (we will abbreviate that as $P(r, dV)$), the probability that the photon of energy E which hits dV actually interacts with

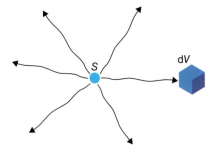

FIGURE 21.1. Point source (S) emission of photons (wavy lines) in vacuum. Direction is random. Only the photon emitted straight at dV can deposit energy in dV and then only if it randomly interacts with the material in dV.

dV as opposed to just passing through ($P(E, dV)$), and the average amount of energy (dE_{abs}) that is absorbed in dV whenever a photon interacts with it, all divided by the mass (m) of dV. The units are energy/mass/time, which is dose rate. Explicitly,

$$\dot{D}(r) = A\, P(r, dV)\, P(E, dV)\, d E_{abs}/m \qquad (21.4)$$

The first question is, what happens to the dose rate in dV if we simply change its distance from r to R (Fig. 21.2)? The two things that do not change, at all, are the activity of the source and the mass of the tissue that we move around. $P(E, dV)$ and dE_{abs} should not change if the angles with which the photons hit the volume are similar, that is, the solid angle subtended by dV is small. So, we are left to focus on the probability of a photon hitting dV. When a nucleus decays and gives off a photon, that photon is emitted isotropically, which means the photon is equally likely to go in any direction. Let the cross-sectional entrance area of the mass m be denoted as da (Fig. 21.2). Of course, the total surface area at a distance r is $4\pi r^2$. So, the probability of a photon emitted in a random direction hitting da after it has traveled a distance r is

$$P(r, dV) = \frac{da}{4\pi r^2} \qquad (21.5)$$

If we move dV to a larger distance R, the probability of hitting da now equals $da/(4\pi R^2)$. Therefore, the probability of hitting da has been reduced by a factor of r^2/R^2

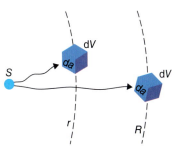

FIGURE 21.2. Point source (S) emission of photon radiation in vacuum. Cross-sectional area (da) of small material volume dV faces the source. dV is moved from radius r to radius R causing a reduced probability of being hit by the photons by the factor r^2/R^2.

in moving from r to R. This suggests that we can try and approximate Equation 21.4 as simply

$$\dot{D}(r) = \frac{cA}{r^2} \qquad (21.6)$$

where we have defined $c = P(E, dV)\, dE_{abs}/m$, and we are hoping that c is constant, under the assumption that the factors in c do not change much as we move the small volume around in vacuum.

In Equation 21.6, it is understood that we should not move the little volume of tissue someplace where it makes no sense to assume that c remains constant. A counterexample best illustrates why it is not true that c is a constant. Suppose that we had moved the volume dV and centered it on $r = 0$, so that it completely surrounded the radioisotope. The factor $P(r, dV)$, where we got r^2 from in the first place, is now $P(r = 0, dV) = 1$, that is, every photon emitted from the radioisotope hits the volume. One can easily see from Equation 21.4 that the dose rate does not become infinite at $r = 0$ (as Equation 21.6 implies); in fact, depending on the photon energy (E) and the size of dV, the dose rate (from the photons emitted) could be extremely small. This example clearly shows that the algorithms we devise to calculate the dose rate have their regions of validity.

Historically, radioisotope emissions were first measured in air. In particular, the concept of exposure[1,3,5,6] (amount of ionization of air per unit mass) was used extensively because charge collection in air-filled cavities are the easiest measurements to make. The process was, first, measurement of exposure rate in air, second, conversion of that exposure rate in air to dose rate to a small amount of tissue in air, and finally, conversion to dose rate to a point in the patient. The result of this process[1,3] led one to define a dose rate to a small amount of water at a distance r surrounded by air as

$$\dot{D}_{air}(r) = \frac{f_{med}\,A\Gamma}{r^2} \qquad (21.7)$$

where the single constant c in Equation 21.6 is split into two constants. Γ is the exposure rate constant[1,3,5] (in units of R cm^2/mCi/h), which represents the conversion of photon energy to ionization of air for the given isotope and f_{med} (in units of cGy/R) is the conversion constant from exposure in air to dose to medium (water) at the average photon energy given off by the radioisotope. Usually, dose to water is calculated since its radiation properties are similar to tissue and measurements were/are made in water. Values of f_{med} (range 0.88–0.97 cGy/R) and Γ (range 1.45–13 R cm^2/mCi/h) for various radioisotopes are summarized in the literature.[1,3,5]

In Equation 21.7, we have the dose rate to water in air, but what we ultimately want is the dose rate in water (i.e., to the patient). Let us look again at a source, radiating photons toward dV but this time in a full water medium. Figure 21.3 shows three examples of photon histories. First, a photon that was going to miss dV (a in Fig. 21.3) is scattered several times, eventually a secondarily scattered

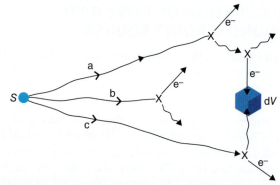

FIGURE 21.3. Point source (S) emission of photon radiation in homogeneous water medium. Wavy lines are photons, straight lines are electrons, and crosses (x) mark photon interaction points. Three photons are followed. Photon a: Compton scatters above dV, the electron produced misses dV, and the Compton photon scatters again (just above dV). The Compton electron after slowing down deposits its remaining energy in dV. Photon b: It was aimed right at dV coming out of S but halfway it was scattered. Both the Compton photon and electron miss dV. Photon c: Compton scatters below dV and the scattered photon heads right for dV and is photoelectrically captured inside dV, its photoelectron (not shown) is absorbed in dV.

electron deposits a fraction of the original energy into dV. Second, a photon (b) which is emitted from the source aimed right at dV interacts on the way there and no part of its energy reaches dV. Finally, a photon (c) which was going to miss dV, interacts and the scattered photon from that interaction is completely absorbed in dV.

One thing we might guess is that inverse square is not going to be valid anymore because how dV absorbs energy is much more complicated. However, we remember that inverse square was not a law anyway, and what we want is an approximation in a restricted region of interest. In any event, we could start by describing the dose rate to a point r in water as

$$\dot{D}(r) = \frac{f_{med}\,A\Gamma}{r^2} e^{-\mu r} + \dot{D}_{scat} \qquad (21.8)$$

In this equation, the major effect of attenuation is represented in the first term where we exponentially attenuate the in-air dose rate of Equation 21.7 with the linear attenuation coefficient (μ) for water for the average energy E emitted by the radionuclide (roughly 0.1 cm^{-1}).[1,3,5] The exponential attenuation factor takes care of one of these effects earlier mentioned (photon [b] in Fig. 21.3), scatter out of the path from the radionuclide to dV. D_{scat} now represents the result of all the various scatter possibilities and is far more complicated. Equation 21.8 has merely organized the calculation into a primary part and a secondary scatter part. Now, we note in Figure 21.3 that the attenuation scattering events [b] reduce the dose rate in dV but the scatter events [a and c] increase the dose rate relative to the (Fig. 21.1) in-vacuum case. Maybe, if we get lucky, these will cancel out. It turns out that scatter and attenuation effects do not cancel out at all distances from the source, but close to the source they almost do and their change with distance farther away can be simply parameterized. Meisberger et al.[8] showed that the measured variation in the dose rate in water as r changed from 1 to 10 cm was such as to establish Equations 21.9 and 21.10 as a good approximation for the dose rate to water

$$\dot{D}(r) = \frac{f_{\text{med}} A\Gamma}{r^2} T(r) \qquad (21.9)$$

$$T(r) = A + Br + Cr^2 + Dr^3 \qquad (21.10)$$

Application of this algorithm (Equation 21.9) has, in the past, been a popular choice in commercial computerized treatment-planning systems. Technically, f_{med} should now be a function of r to account for the lower energy of the scattered photons with greater distance in water[9,10]; however, that detail is usually ignored. Comparing the in-air Equation 21.7 with the in-phantom Equation 21.9, the difference is simply the inclusion of the parameterized factor $T(r)$. $T(r)$, the attenuation and buildup factor, is a polynomial in r (Equation 21.10) which Meisberger et al.[8] used to represent the ratio of the exposure in water to the exposure in air. The free parameters A, B, C, and D are determined by least squares fit to the experimental data for each isotope. One notes[1,3,5,8] that A is close to 1.0 and that B, C, and D are on the order of 10^{-3} or less. Because of this, the value of $T(r)$ is very close to 1.0 for small r. Attenuation and in-scatter are balanced at a distance r_A where $T(r_A) = 1.0$. That in-scatter cancels out the attenuation loss was pointed out by Hale,[11] and is not obvious. For instance, if we consider ^{137}Cs ($E = 662$ keV) that distance is around 3 cm. If we estimate the reduction in dose from attenuation of 3 cm of water (use $\mu = 0.086$ cm^{-1}), we would expect a 23% drop off. Clinically, the fact that a simple dose calculation such as in Equation 21.9 can be used, instead of something as in Equation 21.8, makes calculations easy and has been extremely useful. The mathematical form, Equation 21.10, chosen by Meisberger et al.[8] for $T(r)$ is not a unique parameterization of the attenuation and scatter effects. One could with equal validity use the form proposed by Evans[12]:

$$\dot{D}(r) = \frac{f_{\text{med}} A\Gamma}{r^2} e^{-\mu r} \left[1 + k_a (\mu r)^{kb} \right] \qquad (21.11)$$

Kornelson and Young[13] fit the coefficients k_a and k_b to Monte Carlo results.[14] Venselaar et al.[15] extended the range of the fitted data to 60 cm. Other mathematical expressions[16–18] have been utilized; there is little difference of clinical significance between them or Equations 21.9 and 21.11. The reader should note that Equation 21.9 or 21.11 can be used to quickly calculate verifications of clinical implant plans. If one looks at a dose rate at a point 10 cm from the implant center, all the implanted sources can be considered approximately as a single point source located at the center of gravity of the implant. Add all the activities together and calculate the cGy/hour value expected and compare it to your treatment planning system isodose line. One cannot use this method to determine a small error in the computer plan result, but one can use it to uncover the presence of a major error.

Comparing Equations 21.8 and 21.11, the first term is identical and is the attenuated primary in-air dose rate. Comparing the second terms, one can see that Equation 21.11 assumes that $\dot{D}_{\text{scat}}$ is proportional to the attenuated primary dose rate. This is physically reasonable since scatter comes from the attenuation that occurs in the out-of-path directions, and this should be similar to the in-path attenuation. To the extent that this is not true, we make up for that by letting k_a and k_b be completely free parameters for each different isotope. Fitting the parameters can be done in two ways: one is fitting the free parameters to match measurements in water and the other is fitting[13–15] to match a better calculation such as Monte Carlo. All the parameters (A, B, C, D, and k_i) have no direct physical meaning; they are chosen to allow us to describe the dose rate as accurately as possible. Because of that, it is required to keep track over what range of data the parameters were determined. For example, the best-fit value of D just happens to be negative[1,3,5,8] for ^{192}Ir, ^{198}Au, and ^{137}Cs. Hence, at large distances ($r > 25$ cm), where the r^3 term in Equation 21.10 dominates, $T(r)$ is negative, and therefore, Equation 21.9 predicts a negative dose rate for those isotopes at large distances. This negative dose result arises because we have applied Equation 21.9 outside the range of the fitted parameters and have obtained a nonphysical (wrong) result.

CALCULATION OF DOSE RATES AROUND A LINE SOURCE

In Equation 21.9, we now have an expression for the dose rate in water due to a simple point source. We can now apply this result to calculate the dose rate from different source geometries. The next simplest case is a line (length L) of radioactive material (Fig. 21.4). In the point source case, we had spherical symmetry, which meant that the direction from the source did not change the dose, only the distance (r) did. With a line source, we need to consider direction and distance relative to the center of the line. There is still symmetry remaining, specifically rotational and reflection symmetry, so if we can calculate the dose rate to every point in the shaded region of Figure 21.4, the dose rate anywhere else in the patient volume is determined without calculating. For example, the dose rate at P in Figure 21.4 is the same as at point B (reflection of P with respect to the Y–Z plane), C (reflection of P with respect to the X–Y plane), or D (reflection of B with respect to the X–Y plane). Moreover, any point off the plane ($y \neq 0$) that can be mapped to a point in the plane of Figure 21.4 by a rotation about the z-axis will have the same dose rate as that point in the plane.

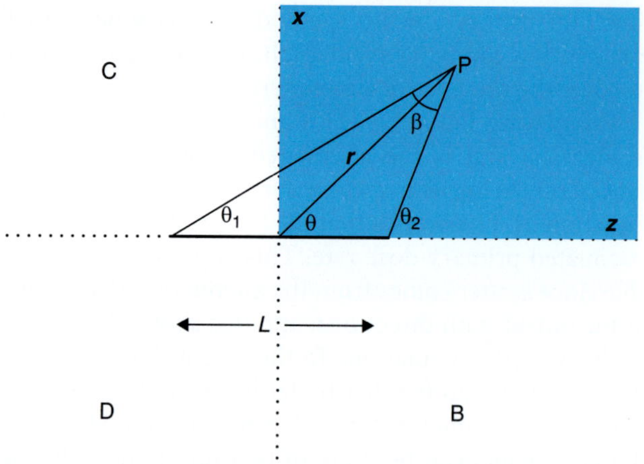

FIGURE 21.4. Line source geometry. Dose-rate calculation to point P depends on distance and direction (r, θ) of P from the source center. The active length (L) defines angles $(\theta_1$ and $\theta_2)$ from the endpoints of the line source to point P. $\beta = \theta_2 - \theta_1$ is the angle from P to the endpoints of the active source. Results need only be calculated for the shaded quadrant, dose to points B, C, and D will be identical to point P by symmetry, likewise for all points in 3-D space obtained by rotation of the source about the z-axis.

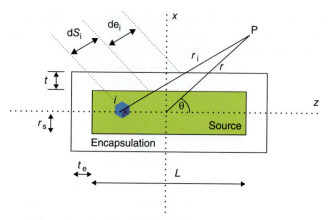

FIGURE 21.5. Cylindrical encapsulated source geometry, thickness of encapsulation is t, radius of source is r_S, and the end cap thickness is t_e. Radioactive material in the source region is subdivided into N tiny regions. Photons from each of the regions are attenuated by their path length through source material and encapsulation. Dose rate at P (located at r, θ from center of source) involves repeated application of point source calculation for all N cubes. For the ith cube, its distance to P is r_i, the path through the source material is d_{Si} and through the encapsulation is d_{ei}.

The solution can be found in an analytic form by defining an activity per unit length (A/L) of source and integrating the point source expression of Equation 21.9 along the line of the source (dl) to obtain the dose rate at any point $P(r, \theta)$ in the plane.[19] The final result for a line source is

$$\dot{D}(r, \theta) = \frac{f_{med}A\Gamma}{L}T(r)\int_{-L/2}^{L/2}\frac{dl}{r'^2} = \frac{f_{med}A\Gamma}{Lr\sin\theta}T(r)\beta \qquad (21.12)$$

where L is the active length of source and $\beta = \theta_2 - \theta_1$ is the angle subtended by the line source when viewed from point P.

CALCULATION OF DOSE RATES AROUND AN ENCAPSULATED CYLINDRICAL SOURCE

Most applications in radiation oncology entail the use of encapsulated (e.g. stainless steel cylinder) sources. Consider a cylindrical source S (radioactive source radius r_S, active length L) and enclose it (Fig. 21.5) inside a cylinder of encapsulation material (radial wall thickness t and end cap thickness t_e). Again, we will consider the active source region to be divided up into many small point sources and determine the contribution from each point source separately using Equation 21.9 and add the results. Clearly the first-order effect of the encapsulation will be to reduce the dose rate by an amount that depends on the path lengths through the encapsulation. As the path length through the encapsulation from every small point source to a given dose point is different, the reduction will be different in different directions. The solution to an encapsulated line source was given by Sievert.[20] He presented the equivalent ($T(r)$ was

ignored in those days) of the following expression for the dose rate at a point P located at planar coordinates r and θ (measured from the radioactive source center, Fig. 21.5):

$$\dot{D}(r, \theta) = \frac{f_{med}A\Gamma}{Lr\sin\theta}T(r)\int_{\theta_1}^{\theta_2}e^{\frac{-\mu_e t}{\cos\gamma}}d\gamma \qquad (21.13)$$

where μ_e is the attenuation coefficient for the radioisotope's photons through the encapsulation material, t is the perpendicular wall thickness of the encapsulation, and θ_1 and θ_2 are the angles from the point P to the ends of the active length of the source (similar to Fig. 21.4). The integral expression in Equation 21.13 is the *Sievert integral*, which can be numerically evaluated with a computer. Young and Batho[21] later provided expressions for an effective wall thickness accounting for source radius. As an aside, Γ would be the unfiltered exposure rate constant in Equation 21.13 because the attenuation of the source's photons by encapsulation is explicitly calculated. The differences between filtered and unfiltered exposure rate constants are discussed in detail elsewhere.[1,3,5,6,22,23]

Equation 21.13 is valid for points (such as P in Fig. 21.5) in the patient where path lengths do not go through the ends of the encapsulated source. The dose rates in the other geometrically distinct regions (through ends of the source capsule) are given elsewhere.[19,20] We can present a single equation for calculation anywhere in the region by numerical integration. We subdivide the source volume into N equal parts. Each little source volume element i contributes independently to the dose rate at P. The dose rate at a point P located at r, θ, from the center of the source is given by adding all N exponentially attenuated point source contributions

$$\dot{D}(r, \theta) = \frac{f_{med}A\Gamma}{N}\sum_{i=1}^{N}\frac{T(r_i)e^{-(\mu_s d_{si}+\mu_e d_{ei})}}{r_i^2} \qquad (21.14)$$

where d_{si} (d_{ei}) (Fig. 21.5) are the individual path length distances through the source (encapsulation) material from tiny source region i to point P. The effect of the attenuation coefficient of the source (μ_s) and its path length (d_{Si}) are included. The numerical integration method in one form or another has been used often in the past.[21,24–28] In Equation 21.14, the coefficients μ are either chosen to give the best fit of Equation 21.14 to experimental measurements or directly measured.

ENCAPSULATION AND THE LOW ENERGY PROBLEM

In our discussion up to now, we have avoided details such as where do we get the activity (A) of a given source, what is the correct way of calculating the exposure rate constant, and how does one calibrate a source and the relationship of the latter procedures to the final step, calculation of dose rate. To get an idea of the ambiguities, consider a hypothetical encapsulated source where a manufacturer makes the encapsulation container from lead and the radioactive material emits a photon of energy 30 keV in half of the nuclear decays and a photon of energy 1 MeV in the other half. If we were to measure the output of this encapsulated source, we would never detect the decays wherein photons of 30 keV are produced because the lead would absorb them. The activity we would infer from measurement would then be less than what it really is because we would only be aware of half the decays. We would be in a dilemma to call that measured activity the activity because the activity is essentially a measure of the actual number of radioactive atoms (Equation 21.2). This extreme example illustrates why there arose a need for "apparent activity." In short, the source manufacturer would tell you the "apparent activity" under the assumption that you would use the same value of Γ that he used to derive his apparent activity. Then, when you multiply A and Γ together, you will get the correct result. Look at Equations 21.9 to 21.14, notice that you need to calculate the value of $A\Gamma$ to obtain the correct dose. You don't need the true activity A and you don't need the theoretical Γ. We emphasize that you have to check that the value of Γ, which the source manufacturer used, matches the value in your treatment planning system in order to use the source manufacturer's apparent activity. As an aside, it is no wonder that the use of mg Ra eq[1,2,3,5] for quantifying activity lasted so long after the abandonment of radium implants because everyone agreed that the value of $\Gamma = 8.25$ (R cm^2/mg Ra eq hour) for radium filtered by 0.5 mm of Pt would be the value you would use for all isotopes.

The second problem (opposite in nature to the first) comes from the details of calibration of the sources. It is easier to measure the emission output of a radioisotope in air than in water. Suppose a low energy photon is given off by the source and it gets out of the capsule or is scattered from the capsule giving rise to a photon even lower in energy and such a photon travels through air and its ionization is measured by the detector. By everything described earlier, for determining the activity, that seems like a good thing (a nucleus decayed and its effect was registered). However, suppose that the photon is so low in energy that it would be absorbed very quickly by the tissue (within an mm or so). Its effect is included in the calibration of the source in air, but clinically, it is of no significance in delivering a dose at a distance in a patient.[29] Therefore, its effects should be excluded.

TWO-DIMENSIONAL DOSE CALCULATION FORMALISM

It should be noted that both these problems were present even from the earliest days of brachytherapy using radium.[1–3] The problems were not a great enough danger to warrant rethinking the dose-rate calculation formalism till low energy sources such as ^{125}I and ^{103}Pd came into clinical use. It has been decided to define a more consistent method. Task Group 43 (TG43) of the American Association of Physicists in Medicine (AAPM) recommended the adoption of a new system[30–34] for calculating the dose rate to water for low energy sources. This system is designed to be consistent from calibration of the source by the accredited calibration laboratories to the final clinical calculation for the patient. The two-dimensional (2-D) dose-rate equation for cylindrically symmetric encapsulated sources in the TG43 formalism[30,34] is given by

$$\dot{D}(r,\theta) = S_K \Lambda \frac{G_X(r,\theta)}{G_X(r_o,\theta_o)} g_X(r) F(r,\theta) \quad X = P \, or \, L \quad (21.15)$$

This dose-rate equation is a 2-D calculation as points in the plane with coordinates r and θ are calculated and all other points in 3-D space are then found by rotation about the z-axis. Equation 21.15 represents two equations, the equation where $X = P$ indicates that you will use a point source geometry factor and the equation where $X = L$ indicates a line source factor is used. All quantities in Equation 21.15 are referenced to a single reference position, $r_o = 1$ cm and $\theta_o = 90°$ (i.e., 1 cm from the source center in a direction perpendicular to the symmetry axis of the source, e.g., 1 cm along the x-axis in Fig. 21.4 or 21.5). The product $S_K \Lambda$ is the dose rate in water at the reference position, r_o and θ_o.

Two new quantities are defined in Equation 21.15. First, the air-kerma strength,[1,30,33] S_K, gives a measure of the absolute amount of radionuclide available. Its source calibration unit U equals cGy cm^2/hour by definition. The air kerma strength is the air kerma rate in vacuum times d^2 (due to photons of energy greater than a cutoff energy, >5 keV, measured with a free air chamber centered at a distance d); d is usually 1 meter. This energy cutoff (5 keV) is chosen so that the calibration effects of low energy photons (which ultimately would not contribute to tissue dose at distances greater than 1 mm from the source) are subtracted from the calibration result. Source manufacturers now provide both the air kerma strength (referenced to the reference position) and the apparent activity (for historical comparison). Typical conversions from air kerma strengths to "apparent activity" for isotopes used clinically are 1.27, 1.29, 2.86, and 4.12 (U/mCi) for ^{125}I, ^{103}Pd, ^{137}Cs, and ^{192}Ir, respectively.

The second new quantity in Equation 21.15 is the radionuclide's dose-rate constant, Λ, (units = μGy/h/U at 1m). The dose-rate constant is the ratio of a reference dose rate $\dot{D}$ (r_o, θ_o) in water to S_K. The dose-rate constant is determined once and for all for each manufacturer's source via Monte Carlo modeling plus experimental measurements usually with thermoluminescent dosimeters (TLDs).[30,31,35–38] There are errors in both methods, so results are averaged to produce a "consensus" value for Λ.[1,5,31,35]

$G(r, \theta)$ is a new symbol for the simple geometry dependence already seen in Equations 21.9 and 21.12, namely, point (P) source and line (L) source.[30,31,39] G accounts for the main effects of distance and direction of source from the point of measurement. TG43 defines G_P and G_L:

$$\text{Point source } G_P\,(r,\theta)\ =\ r^{-2} \qquad (21.16)$$

$$\text{Line source } G_L\,(r,\theta) = \frac{\beta}{L\,r\,\sin\theta},\ \theta \neq 0$$

$$= \frac{1}{z^2 - (L/2)^2},\ \theta = 0 \qquad (21.17)$$

The ratio of $G(r, \theta)$ to the reference value $G(r_o, \theta_o)$ is explicitly indicated in Equation 21.15.

In Equation 21.15, the radial dose function $g(r)$ redefines the traditional attenuation and scatter buildup factor. It accounts for photon attenuation and scatter in water in the radial direction to the source symmetry axis ($\theta_o = 90°$). The radial dose function is essentially $f_{med}(r)T(r)$ renormalized so that $g(r_o) = 1.0$. Since we have long known that the parameters of Equation 21.10 can be fitted accurately, a polynomial expansion is chosen to accurately represent $g(r)$:

$$g_X(r)\ =\ a_0 + a_1 r + a_2 r^2 + a_3 r^3 + a_4 r^4 + a_5 r^5 \quad (21.18)$$

where $X = P$ or L means that one compares their dose-rate data (at varying positions of r with $\theta_o = 90°$) to their calculations using Equation 21.15 and determines the six coefficients a_i in Equation 21.18 using the point or line source formula (Equation 21.16 or 21.17) for the geometry factor. The dose-rate data required to determine the radial dose functions come from Monte Carlo calculations and are verified by measurements. Each radioisotope has its own set of coefficients a_i determined[1,5,30,31,40,41] in this manner.

The anisotropy of the source distribution function $F(r, \theta)$ is introduced to account for differences in the dose rate as a function of angle from the symmetry axis due to the specific geometry of the encapsulation of the radionuclide source. In other words, it takes into account the different path lengths through the source and encapsulation at various angles. If we have information on the dose rate in all directions (such as from Monte Carlo modeling or measured data), then the anisotropy function can be determined[5,30,42–44] from Equation 21.15. The normalization for F is $F(r, \theta_o{=}90°) = 1.0$.

In high-dose-rate afterloader applications using ^{192}Ir (see Chapter 15), there is a single high-activity cylindrical source. Optimization techniques (Chapter 15) are used to vary source dwell times at various positions in fixed implanted catheters. Because you must localize the catheters to plan the patient, you have the orientation of the source symmetry axis in the patient at all possible dwell positions and you can determine the angle θ in Figure 21.4 for any dose point P. Therefore, one uses the 2-D dose calculation ($X = L$) of Equation 21.15. Similarly, ^{125}I seed sources loaded into a fixed geometry eye plaque for ocular melanoma treatment can use the line source form.

There is a practical problem in using Equation 21.15 for cylindrical sources that are not constrained to be in a definitive geometric orientation by the applicator which holds them. Namely, it is not always easy to determine orientation. Consider permanent prostate implants that use ^{125}I seed sources. Computed tomography (CT) scans and/or radiographs cannot provide the necessary resolution to determine the line direction in 3-D space for all the sources (though methods are being developed to do that[45,46]). So, we definitely have line sources but we can't determine each angle θ (from each and every source to each and every point P). Thus, we are forced to use the point source geometry factor. In this event, one can use a better approximation.[31] Although the anisotropy function is a function of r and θ, one can average F over the 4π geometry and F can be approximated by a simple radial function, $\phi_{an}(r)$, called the one-dimensional (1-D) anisotropy function, for example, this is roughly a 5% correction for ^{192}Ir.[5,30,31] Where a 2-D calculation cannot be used for cylindrical sources, the revised TG43 protocol[31] recommends the use of

$$\dot{D}(r,\theta) = S_K \Lambda \, \frac{G_L(r,\theta_o)}{G_L(r_o,\theta_o)} \, g_L(r)\,\phi_{an}(r) \qquad (21.19)$$

Compare Equation 21.19 to Equation 21.15 (with $X = L$) with respect to the geometry function. In Equation 21.19, the line source geometry formula is used but regardless of what the angle θ is on the left side of the equation; we evaluate the right hand side using $\theta = \theta_o = 90°$. The advantage of Equation 21.19 is that it is more accurate for cylindrical sources at distances less than 1 cm than Equation 21.15 with the point source approximation ($X = P$).

It is important to understand the methodology behind the 2-D dose calculation algorithm provided by Equation 21.15. A point or line source approximation for the geometry function is chosen (this choice is determined by practical realities in most cases). Experimental measurements and/or Monte Carlo calculations provide the desired 3-D dose distribution answer. The radial dose-rate function in point source geometry is then determined by choosing the parameters of Equation 21.18 so that multiplying all the factors together at points where $\theta = \theta_0 = 90°$ yields the correct dose rate at those points. Once you have that, you can determine the anisotropy factor, in the same way using the already known 3-D dose distribution. One can either store a table of results[5,30,31] or create a fitting function to reproduce the results. Furhang and Anderson[47] proposed the functional form

$$F(r, \theta) = 1 - (a + b\theta + c\theta^2) \cos(\theta) e^{dr} \quad (21.20)$$

where a, b, c, and d are polynomials in r with a total of 12 free parameters. Sloboda et al.[48] fit those parameters to the results of Monte Carlo calculations. Ling et al.[49] had also used a similar parameterization to fit the dose-rate results for a ^{125}I source.

Finally, let us review the rationale of the change in Equation 21.15. In the old system, calibration in air, calculation in air, and then conversion to dose in medium was the calculation process. The new TG43 system is more akin to external beam calculations. In Equation 21.15, ΛS_K is the cGy/hour calibration in water at a reference position (the analog of linear accelerator calibration at d_{max}). The product of $G(r, \theta_o)$ and $g(r)$ is like a depth dose correction along the x-axis in Figure 21.4 normalized at r_o. Finally, $F(r, \theta)$ is like external beam off-axis ratios. Looked at in this way, the new formalism does not look so foreign.

THREE-DIMENSIONAL DOSE CALCULATIONS: ASYMMETRIC DOSE DISTRIBUTIONS REQUIRED BY APPLICATORS AND SHIELDS

Some treatments involve the use of asymmetric metal applicators to introduce the radioactive sources into the body. In treatment of carcinoma of the uterine cervix,[1,2] some of the applicators have tungsten shields attached, which provide a severe asymmetry in the measured dose-rate distribution. The measurement[27,28,50,51] of dose rate in the presence of these asymmetries shows that the effects are to reduce the dose rate in particular directions (geometric shadow of the shields) by up to 40%. These applicators clearly have an effect on the dose-rate distribution that is different in different directions; hence, the dose-rate algorithm must calculate the dose rate over the entire 3-D grid centered on the source.[25,27,28,52–54] Now because clinical use involves a source loaded into the same applicator with shields every single time, the calculation can be done once for the source/applicator/shield and the result for that dose distribution stored on the computer and used the same way a simple source is used.

Generalization of the TG43 2-D dose calculation formalism, Equation 21.15, to a form suitable for 3-D dose calculation could look something like this.

$$\dot{D}(r, \theta, \varphi) = S_K \Lambda \frac{r_o^2}{r^2} g(r) \, F(r, \theta, \varphi) \quad (21.21)$$

$F(r, \theta, \varphi)$ is extended to explicitly include the angle φ dependence, $0 < \varphi < 2\pi$, and includes all angular variations. F could be described by a function similar to Equation 21.20 with hundreds of free parameters.

At this point, historical review helps us understand that simple equations such as Equation 21.9 or 21.11, among others, arose because the developers needed some simple equation to calculate or check treatments by hand. Today, many parameter fits (such as Equation 21.21 would require) can be done on the computer easily. However, it is also true that characterizing the dose-rate calculation directly using Monte Carlo over a full 3-D volume $20 \times 20 \times 20$ cm^3 and storing such a 3-D matrix would not be a problem either. So one could follow the historical development and precalculate the Monte Carlo result, then fit the parameters of Equation 21.21 to the Monte Carlo, throw away the Monte Carlo result, and use Equation 21.21 with the large number of parameters to calculate the dose distribution. Alternatively, one could just store and use the Monte Carlo results. Therefore, it is unlikely that the description of the results of 3-D dose calculations will follow TG43 in describing the dose rate as a product of several fitted functions whose parameters were found by comparing to Monte Carlo results. Instead, either "consensus" 3-D Monte Carlo-generated dose-rate matrices normalized to the dose at a reference position will be available for use or computers have become so fast that the 3-D Monte Carlo calculations can be generated for an individual patient.

3-D TREATMENT PLANNING WITH 3-D DOSE DISTRIBUTIONS

If we have a precalculated 3-D dose-rate distribution, how do we use it clinically? First, it is necessary to determine the position and orientation of each source's 3-D dose distribution in the patient. Figure 21.6 shows a single source, which is arbitrarily angled in the patient. The patient coordinate system (x, y, z) is defined by a 3-D imaging device such as a CT scanner. The 3-D dose-rate distribution of the source/applicator would have been (pre) calculated in a coordinate system (x', y', z') centered on the source. This is the intrinsic coordinate system of the source/applicator system. If there was cylindrical symmetry about the intrinsic z'-axis, there would be no need to determine in what direction the x' and y' axes are oriented in the CT scan coordinate system, but here we are assuming there is no symmetry whatsoever. $\dot{D}(\vec{r}_P)$ is the calculated dose-rate distribution in its own intrinsic coordinate system $(\vec{r})$ for a unit air kerma strength source. So in Figure 21.6, the dose rate at point P (located at $\vec{r}_P$ in the CT scan) produced by the source (located at $\vec{r}_S$) requires looking up the value for $\dot{D}(\vec{r}_P)$ from the precalculated 3-D matrix. Therefore, we need to determine the vector

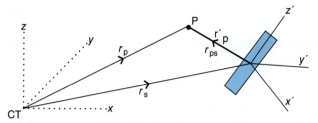

FIGURE 21.6. Relationship between patient coordinate system (as defined by a computed tomography [CT] scan) and the internal dose-rate calculation coordinate system of a precalculated 3-D source, which is rotated relative to the CT system. The center of the source is at r_S (relative to the CT scan). Point P in the patient is located at r_P in the CT scan but at r'_P relative to the internal source coordinate system. r_{PS} and r'_P are physically the same vector, expressed in CT and intrinsic coordinates, respectively.

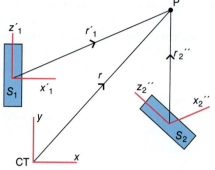

FIGURE 21.7. Superposition approximation. The dose rate at P is found by adding the contribution from source 1 (assuming source 2 is not present) to the contribution from source 2 (assuming source 1 is not present). The internal coordinate system for each source is shown. Only two out of three axes are shown.

(distance and direction) $\vec{r}'_P$. In practice, this requires that we determine which way the x', y', z' axes point in the CT scanner. Now $\vec{r}_{PS}$ the vector from S to P is the same vector as $\vec{r}'_P$ only expressed in the coordinates of the CT scanner. These are shown in Figure 21.6 and related via

$$\vec{r}_P = \vec{r}_S + \vec{r}_{PS} = \vec{r}_S + E(\alpha, \beta, \gamma)\vec{r}'_P \quad (21.22)$$

where $E(\alpha, \beta, \gamma)$ is the rotation matrix[55] for a solid body and α, β, γ are the Euler rotation angles, which rotate the intrinsic coordinate system of the source into correspondence with the CT coordinate system. Our problem is to find the three degrees of rotational freedom, the Euler angles. Finding both ends of the source defines a line in space and decides the z'-axis orientation (equivalent to two degrees of freedom). The last degree of freedom (rotation about that line) is found by identifying a landmark in the CT scan not on the z'-axis. Methods and equations for calculating the Euler angles based on this information have been given for particular 3-D sources/shields/applicators.[56]

Continuing on to the clinical use of multiple sources, in Figure 21.7, the dose at point P from two sources requires that the orientations of both sources be determined. In order to look up the value for $\dot{D}(r'_1)$ and $\dot{D}(r''_2)$, we have to determine r'_1 and r''_2. So the Euler angles for two coordinate systems must be found. For N sources, we use Equation 21.22, and the total dose rate $\dot{D}(\vec{r})$ in the patient's 3-D coordinate system $(\vec{r})$ for N sources is given by

$$\dot{D}(\vec{r}) = \sum_{i=1}^{N} S_{Ki} \dot{D}_i(\vec{r})$$

$$= \sum_{i=1}^{N} S_{Ki} \dot{D}_i [E_i^{-1}(\alpha_i, \beta_i, \gamma_i)(\vec{r} - \vec{rs}_i)] \quad (21.23)$$

where S_{Ki} is the source strength and E_i^{-1} is the inverse of the Euler rotation matrix for the ith source. The Euler angles $(\alpha_i, \beta_i, \gamma_i)$ for each source must be determined. It is the latter task, which is the additional work needed to implement 3-D dose distributions in a clinical real-time setting.[56]

Once a dose-rate calculation algorithm has been implemented, there are two choices in calculating the total 3-D dose-rate distribution in the patient from a multitude of sources. They are (a) dose superposition, that is, addition of individual source/applicator dose distributions independent of the presence of the other sources (Equation 21.23 is dose superposition), or (b) direct dose calculation, that is, using the calculation algorithm with all the sources and applicators accounted for in the calculation. The first is the least computationally taxing because the dose-rate matrices $(\dot{D}_i)$ may be precalculated. The second method is what would be used in real-time clinical Monte Carlo or grid-based Boltzmann solvers (GBBS) applications using CT data.

Commercial treatment-planning systems currently use dose superposition. How important is it to correct for inter-applicator shielding effects and patient inhomogeneities? The answer depends on the number of sources, shields, or applicators and their positions relative to one another. At this time, it is not clear how important these effects are to clinical applications.

In low dose-rate permanent implants of the prostate, one may have up to 100 ^{125}I stainless steel clad sources in a 40 cc volume. Potentially, the overall inhomogeneity effect caused by seed-to-seed attenuations might be severe, especially, since the photon energy is low. Burns and Raeside[57] in a Monte Carlo study of a model two-plane implant showed that the shadowing effect reduces the dose in the interior of the implant, but this reduction was not enough to drop the dose below the reference prescription dose. So, the significance is that very high doses here and there inside the implant region are not really as high as one thought. Meigooni et al.[58] also studied interseed effects for ^{125}I and found through measurements that variations were dependent on direction, but that overall, the dose at the periphery of the implant is reduced by 6%. Chibani et al.[59] used Monte Carlo simulation and found similar results for ^{125}I and ^{103}Pd. Based on these studies, it is not easy to see the need for any correction other than possibly a 5% reduction of the predicted overall dose to the periphery. We emphasize that these studies justify a dose documentation correction, not a 5% increase in dose prescription. The latter is a completely different question which is beyond the scope of this chapter. At the present time, it is unclear[60] whether these corrections are needed in permanent seed implants.

Finally, with respect to patient heterogeneities, this problem is still harder to evaluate since the variations are endless. Das et al.[61] found that the dose beyond bone is most affected and that the perturbations of the dose distribution are too complex to be modeled by simple dose calculation algorithms, so Monte Carlo calculations must be used. Meigooni and Nath[62] used measurements plus Monte Carlo simulation and found in their model that lower energy sources such as ^{125}I and ^{103}Pd have significant changes in dose due to patient heterogeneity whereas ^{192}Ir does not. Calculation methods to produce simple corrections have been proposed by Williamson et al.[63] They used Monte Carlo-generated primary and scatter components and incorporated empiric parameters into a scatter subtraction method to gain the advantages of Monte Carlo computation but with a large saving in computation time. Agreement with full Monte Carlo simulations was within a few percent in most examples considered. Furstoss et al.[64] studied both inter-seed and breast tissue heterogeneity effects for ^{125}I and ^{103}Pd seed permanent breast implants using Monte Carlo simulation. At these low energies, they found that breast tissue can change D90 by 10% relative to the homogeneous water case; inter-seed attenuation is not important.

THREE-DIMENSIONAL DOSE CALCULATIONS: MONTE CARLO AND BOLTZMANN TRANSPORT TECHNIQUES

In this section, we move away from macroscopically parameterized calculations and calculate the dose distribution using microscopically parameterized functions. These calculations can handle all inhomogeneity as straightforwardly as the homogeneous case. The techniques require significant computer power which we now have available. The techniques are feasible for brachytherapy applications because the distances and volumes of interest are small. The method of Monte Carlo[65–68] involves the concepts figuratively expressed in Equation 21.4 at the start of this chapter. Namely, a photon leaves a radioisotope in a random direction and when it hits something, there is a chance of something happening, or not. In Monte Carlo, a photon is randomly created, starts off in a random direction, and each step of the way has a probability (cross section) of photoelectric interaction, Compton interaction, pair production, or coherent scattering. If it splits off an electron at a certain location headed in a certain direction determined by a "roll of the

dice," that electron loses energy as it moves through the medium. The medium is split into small volume regions (e.g., 1-mm cubes), as electrons lose energy in a cube; that energy loss is tallied as being deposited into that cube. So, after the one photon has left and all its scattered photon and electron descendants have ended up as too low in energy to escape any more cubes and all the energy is absorbed, you say that one history has been completed. After that first history, almost every cube volume around the source has zero dose because most cubes were either not geometrically hit by anything or, if hit, no interaction event occurred within them. In order to get useful results, we will have to rerun this "rolling of the dice" process over and over again. The computer is tailor made to handle this task, many billions of times or more to finally get smooth continuous results. We note that Monte Carlo simulation tries to mimic what is happening in the patient. Monte Carlo is sometimes thought[66] of as a simulated measurement process carried out on the computer.

The errors in Monte Carlo are of two types, systematic and statistical. The systematic errors arise from the fact that the scattering cross sections are themselves parameterized approximations to the real atomic scattering. When Monte Carlo is used in Radiation Oncology to predict average macroscopic properties such as dose distributions, these errors are insignificant. The random statistical errors arise because of the need to stop the calculation in some reasonable time, once statistical variation in every important volume element of the patient is rendered insignificant. The details can be misleading. Suppose we use 50 billion histories in a Monte Carlo modeling of an high dose rate (HDR) treatment, this seems like an enormous number. In that case a 10 Ci source can expose the patient for 300 seconds and therefore, the actual treatment involves around 10^{14} photon histories. So, this seemingly huge Monte Carlo computation models 2000 times less decays than the real treatment. Looked at the other way, the 50 billion history Monte Carlo calculation represents what we would expect from a less than one second HDR treatment. In Monte Carlo, the statistical uncertainty in the dose varies in the patient. The uncertainty is larger the farther away from the source distribution which one considers. Near the source distribution, the 50 billion history modeling is acceptable.

Monte Carlo for brachytherapy investigations has a long history starting with Berger's work,[65] which provided analysis and insight into the results of Meisberger et al..[8] The encapsulated radioactive source can be modeled and the relationship between calibration, measurement, and calculation of 3-D distributions determined. An advantage of Monte Carlo is in handling any case regardless of complexity. All that is required is to determine the radionuclide spatial distribution and the positions of the inhomogeneities, subdivide each into regions, subdivide the entire patient region of interest into small regions, and let the Monte Carlo program run until the results stop changing significantly in the region you are concerned with.

This advantage cannot be too highly praised. Consider that the Monte Carlo N-Particle (MCNP)[66] input used for full 3-D calculations of a source/shield/applicator[53] required typing only 100 lines of text to direct the calculation. Meanwhile, experimental measurements of 3-D dose-rate distribution for the same and similar applications[28,50,51] involved machining of positioning devices to allow rotation of applicators with high precision in water tanks. Measurements are made in different orientations, and the results have to be merged together. It is obvious which is easier.

Monte Carlo has been useful even when you are not going to use it explicitly to treat a patient. All the approximations for dose-rate calculation in this chapter involve parameters. If one fits the values of the parameters of your algorithm to best match the results of Monte Carlo simulations,[53] then one obtains a parameterization which one can have more confidence in than from the traditional method of fitting to experimental results.[28] The reasons for this were pointed out by Boyer[69] regarding the limitations of brachytherapy measurement, for example, finite size of detectors, energy response changes of detector with distance, and so on. Monte Carlo does not have these limitations. Monte Carlo does have the limitation or more precisely the requirement that the source emission spectrum[7] must be precisely known and that the exact specifications of source/applicator construction are defined correctly. Because of that, there is still a need for measurement but only to spot check, at a few points, the results for confidence that the earlier mentioned requirements are correct. In summary, one way or another, Monte Carlo simulation is some part of every brachytherapy dose calculation.

Recently a new method[70-72] has been proposed for brachytherapy dose calculation. Suppose we return to our 50 billion history Monte Carlo example and rerun it again on the computer. We would obtain a different (albeit similar) dose distribution result. If we had the time to run the actual 10^{14} histories, get the results, and then rerun that simulation once more and compare, we expect that we would have no significant difference in results between the two calculations. Therefore, there is an expectation that an exact solution exists, i.e., an infinite history solution. To find that solution, we turn to methods for solving the linear Boltzmann transport equation[73] that were developed at Los Alamos National Laboratory.[74,75] The Boltzmann transport equation governs the motion of a particle in a fluid subject to random collisions. It has no analytic solution. To make the problem computationally feasible, the scattering energies and angles are discretized and the equations are solved on a grid of discrete points. The technique is called lattice or GBBS.[76] We can understand this method applied to radiation as having the radioactive source creating the driving flux of photons (see Fig. 21.8). This photon flux flows out, suffers random collisions, and is both modified and creates an electron flux. The solution that GBBS finds is the resulting

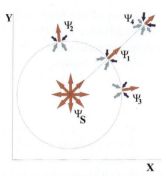

FIGURE 21.8. Point source S of single energy photons, photon flux Ψ_S in homogeneous medium. Resulting identical photon flux Ψ at positions 1–3 and lower energy flux at position 4. Monte Carlo or GBBS can do no better than equal the accuracy of simple parameterized point source dose calculations.

photon and electron final total flux at every grid position throughout the patient. These fluxes are also determined approximately in the Monte Carlo method but far faster in GBBS, 1000s of times faster. Error in GBBS is systematic, not statistical. It is said that the solution is exact.[76] However, the solutions of the differential equations can be affected by the aforementioned discretization approximations. Hence, there is a danger that the solution could be incorrect. As in Monte Carlo, this is a technique wherein more and more computer processing power makes the calculations more and more reliable in shorter times.

In Figure 21.8, we show the photon flux in the homogeneous case, assuming a single energy point source emitter. As one goes away from the source, the intensity of the orange photons drops (line gets shorter), other lower energy photons (shades of blue) appear at different angles. Electron flux is not shown. The assumption with GBBS is that the resulting flux at positions 1–4 can't be random and must be definite and related to each other via the transport equations. Let us compare the use of Equation 21.15 with Monte Carlo and GBBS to illustrate the advantages and disadvantages. In Figure 21.8, if we used Equation 21.15, the dose that we would calculate at equally distant positions 1–3 would be exactly equal and correct. Assuming position 4 is 10 cm away, the dose would be roughly accurate. In contrast, with Monte Carlo the dose would be very close to correct for positions 1–3, but the doses would not be exactly equal because of statistical error. With GBBS, the dose would be exactly equal and correct for positions 1–3. Both Monte Carlo and GBBS would be more accurate for position 4, especially, if it were much greater than 10 cm away. Therefore, for the homogeneous case, really nothing is to be gained over any of the historical methods of dose calculation by using Monte Carlo or GBBS. In Figure 21.9, we show a source distribution S, and dose points in the presence of inhomogeneities, gray is bone, blue is air. If we use Equation 21.15 (assume we can ignore inter-source attenuation effects), the calculated doses at a prescription point such as D_5 or D_1 are very accurate, while the dose at D_2 is fairly accurate (unless position 2 is very close to the bone), the

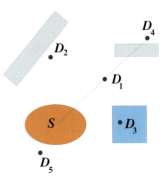

FIGURE 21.9. Source distribution S and dose at five positions in the presence of bone (gray) and air (blue). Only Monte Carlo or GBBS can accurately predict dose at all positions.

dose at D_3 is underestimated and D_4 is overestimated. On the other hand, for Monte Carlo and GBBS, all doses are accurately predicted; moreover, inter-source attenuation effects need not be ignored. There is no question, that if inhomogeneity is be accounted for, the Monte Carlo and GBBS are superior in dose calculation accuracy throughout the patient.

FUTURE DIRECTIONS IN THREE-DIMENSIONAL DOSE-RATE CALCULATION ALGORITHMS

At the present time, commercial treatment-planning systems do not allow precalculated 3-D dose matrices to be used for planning. TG43 formalism is supported for all sources. It is clear that only Monte Carlo and GBBS can handle all difficulties in brachytherapy dose calculation. One reason is that heterogeneities don't hamper the accuracy of these methods. If the Monte Carlo calculation is deciding whether a photon will randomly scatter as it goes through bone or if it is going through water, it is all the same for the computation procedure. A similar statement applies to GBBS. There is not much extra computation power needed for the inter-applicator/patient heterogeneity calculation relative to a homogeneous calculation. Of course, the calculation time plus time for identification and accurate orientation of all sources, and applicators in the CT scan and definition in the Monte Carlo or GBBS calculation framework is still not a real-time clinical reality except in special cases. There are many more considerations[77] with full-scale CT-based Monte Carlo or GBBS. For example, whether it is still appropriate to continue to prescribe dose to water when what you are calculating with Monte Carlo is dose to a specific tissue composition. The question of what is the atomic composition of individual organs, tissues, and what to do about calcifications and artifacts in the CT scans will have to be answered before calculation. Some of these problems will be addressed using increased processing power both for calculations and image analysis. In the future, we expect to be able to take inhomogeneity effects into account, using full clinical Monte Carlo or GBBS calculations.

Recently, BrachyVision (Varian Medical Systems, Palo Alto, CA) has introduced a GBBS option for their HDR treatment planning system. The user generates an optimized plan using Equation 21.15 to calculate dose and thereby determine all dwell times. After completion, they have the option to run a GBBS calculation. This documents the dose distribution in the patient accounting for all inhomogeneities. This calculation takes less than 10 minutes. What the user does with that information is not clear. That the information is now available is noteworthy.

The last paragraph indicates that GBBS has leap-frogged Monte Carlo with respect to individual patient-specific clinical utilization. A problem with commercial implementation of Monte Carlo is when do you stop the calculation, i.e., how many histories? That can be a function of the geometry of the case itself. Since even the homogeneous case takes too long, to design a software system to run more histories than you ever expect to need is not feasible today. The reasons for GBBS success are increased speed and that GBBS provides an "exact" solution. The former is easy to understand, and the latter should be accepted with caution. Since the solution is exact (and hence when it completes, you are finished), then that is a huge advantage. There is one potential problem, namely, what happens to the "exact" solution when you have artifacts in the CT scan, or misinterpretation of the size or density of metal objects or calcifications. Since in GBBS the dose result in all areas of the patient is linked by the differential equations, this could result in the prescription dose result being made inaccurate by other less important regions of the patient being incorrectly specified. This could mean that the "exact" solution is "exactly" wrong. Whether it is possible to be clinically significant wrong is unclear at this time. Having said all that, one has to be excited by this new development as much will be learned from it and in the current GBBS implementation for HDR, Equation 21.15 still determines the actual clinical treatment.

SUMMARY

The history of algorithm development was that extensive use of measurements led to simple calculation algorithms based on a point source. Using numerical integration, these were extended to cylindrical geometries of varying complexity. These developments were then improved by comparison to specialized Monte Carlo studies. The rise in computer power made available more extensive Monte Carlo investigations. These Monte Carlo studies more precisely determined the best parameters of the calculation algorithms to give a better agreement with experiment and later permitted a unification of source calibration and clinical calculation of dose. The ease of these investigations has made extensive 3-D measurement projects a thing of the past. In fact, the GBBS literature bypasses experimental measurements and compares to Monte Carlo for justification. The GBBS will have a greater utilization in clinical practice as it is faster than Monte Carlo and gives definite results. As computer power increases in the future, it is obvious that the power and dominance of these two techniques in providing detailed dose distribution results will increase. It will then seem as if all the simple equations are no longer needed as advanced computer modeling has superseded them. One notes that none of the governing equations for Monte Carlo or GBBS were given in this chapter. There is no need as no one is going to use them to check the dose in a patient. The vast computational labor of these methods is such that only the computer can produce the results. It is then that the historical methods reappear as the only way to check that the computer results can be believed. One is advised to do exactly that.

ACKNOWLEDGMENTS

The author gratefully thanks Vania Arora, M.S., and the late Glenn Glasgow, Ph. D., for useful discussions.

KEY POINTS

- Historical calculations for a source calibrated to specify its activity (use Equation 21.9 or 21.11).

- Modern TG43 calculations for a source calibrated to specify its dose rate in water at a reference position (use Equation 21.15).

- Dose at a point near a cylindrical source should be calculated using a line source approximation.

- Monte Carlo simulation has been essential to accurately determine the basic parameters needed for Equations 21.9, 21.11, or 21.15.

- Increasing computer power will eventually lead to using Monte Carlo and GBBS approaches for individual patient treatment planning.

REVIEW QUESTIONS

1. If the air kerma strength (S_K) doubles and the distance doubles, the dose rate at a given point most nearly
   A. decreases by 50%
   B. doubles
   C. remains the same
   D. decreases by 25%

2. If a 0.5 mCi ^{192}Ir source (Γ = 4.6 Rcm^2/mCi h) is replaced by a 0.5 mCi ^{125}I source (Γ = 1.45 Rcm^2/mCi h), the initial dose rate at 1 cm most nearly
   A. increases by a factor of 2
   B. decreases by a factor of 2
   C. remains the same
   D. decreases by a factor of 3

3. If a S_K = 2.0 U, ^{192}Ir (Λ = 1.12 cGy/hU) source is replaced by a S_K = 2.0 U, Amersham Model 6702 ^{125}I source (Λ = 1.036 cGy/hU), the dose rate at 1 cm most nearly
   A. increases by a factor of 2
   B. decreases by a factor of 2
   C. remains the same
   D. decreases by a factor of 3

4. Consider an ^{192}Ir source and a small detector separated by 3 cm and fixated at the same height in an empty tank. As water is poured into the tank, the ionization signal from the detector is observed in three regions. First region, water level rising to the source-detector height; second region, water level gradually covers the source detector; and third region, water level rising above the source detector. Observation of the signal from the detector as the tank fills would show that the signal in those three regions
   A. remains the same, increases, increases
   B. increases, decreases, increases
   C. increases, stays the same, increases
   D. increases, decreases, decreases

5. Consider an ^{125}I seed source with an air kerma strength of 0.6 U, and use TG43 formalism to calculate the dose rate at r = 2 cm and θ = 30° in Figure 21.4. (Use the line source geometry factor, L = 4 mm, β = 5.8°, $g_L(2)$ = 0.819, Λ = 0.965 cGy/hU, and $F(2,30)$ = 0.842)
   A. 0.02 cGy/h
   B. 0.1 cGy/h
   C. 0.2 cGy/h
   D. 0.4 cGy/h

ANSWERS

1. A From Equation 21.15, the air kerma strength change increases the dose by a factor of 2 and distance change decreases the dose by a factor of 4. Dose drops by a factor of 2.

2. D Exposure rate constant for ^{125}I is more than three times smaller than that for ^{192}Ir.

3. C Dose rate constants for the two isotopes differ by less than 10%.

4. B In the first region, increasing scatter from rising water increases the dose rate; in the second region, as water covers the path from the source to the detector, attenuation decreases the dose rate; and in the third region, increasing scatter from increased water above the source detector increases the dose rate.

5. B Note that when you calculate the line source geometry ratio in Equation 21.15, when $L << r$, the result is very close (in this case, within 1%) to simply using the point source approximation. Far enough away, all source distributions look like point sources.

REFERENCES

1. Gibbons JP. *Khan's The Physics of Radiation Therapy*. 6th ed. Baltimore, MD: Lippincott Williams & Wilkins; 2020.
2. Perez CA, Glasgow GP. Clinical applications of brachytherapy. In: Perez CA, Brady LW, eds. *Principles and Practice of Radiation Oncology*. Philadelphia, PA: JB Lippincott Co; 1987.
3. Johns HE, Cunningham JR. *The Physics of Radiology*. 4th ed. Springfield, IL: Charles C Thomas Publisher; 1983.
4. Pierquin B, Chassagne DJ, Chahbazian CM, et al. *Brachytherapy*. St. Louis, MO: Warren H. Green; 1978.
5. Glasgow GP. Low Dose Rate Brachytherapy. In: Khan F, Gerbi BJ, eds. *Treatment Planning in Radiation Oncology*. 3rd ed. Philadelphia, PA: Lippincott Williams Wilkins; 2012.
6. Attix FA. *Introduction to Radiological Physics and Radiation Dosimetry*. New York: John Wiley & Sons; 1986.
7. Brown E, Firestone RB. In: Shirley VS, ed. *Table of Radioactive Isotopes*. New York: John Wiley & Sons; 1986.
8. Meisberger LL, Keller RJ, Shalek RJ. The effective attenuation in water of the gamma rays of gold 198, iridium 192, cesium 137, radium 226, and cobalt 60. *Radiology*. 1968;90:953–957.
9. Meli JA, Meigooni AS, Nath R. On the choice of phantom material for the dosimetry of 192Ir sources. *Int J Radiat Oncol Biol Phys*. 1988;14:587–594.
10. Dale RG. Some theoretical derivations relating to the tissue dosimetry of brachytherapy nuclides, with particular reference to iodine-125. *Med Phys*. 1983;10:176–183.
11. Hale J. The use of interstitial radium dose-rate tables for other radioactive isotopes. *AJR Am J Roentgenol*. 1958;79:49–53.
12. Evans RD. *The Atomic Nucleus*. New York: McGraw Hill; 1955.
13. Kornelson RO, Young MEJ. Brachytherapy buildup factors. *Br J Radiol*. 1981;54:136–136.
14. Webb S, Fox RA. The dose in water surrounding point isotropic gamma ray emitters. *Br J Radiol*. 1979;52:482–484.
15. Venselaar JL, van der Giessen PH, Dries WJ. Measurement and calculation of the dose at large distances from brachytherapy sources: Cs-137, Ir-192, and Co-60. *Med Phys*. 1996;23:537–543.
16. van Kleffens HJ, Star WM. Application of stereo X-ray photogrammetry (SRM) in the determination of absorbed dose values during intracavitary radiation therapy. *Int J Radiat Oncol Biol Phys*. 1979;5:557–563.
17. Dale RG. A Monte Carlo derivation of parameters for use in the tissue dosimetry of medium and low energy nuclides. *Br J Radiol*. 1982;55:748–757.
18. Park HC, Almond PR. Evaluation of the buildup effect of an 192Ir high dose-rate brachytherapy source. *Med Phys*. 1992;19:1293–1297.
19. Weaver K. Brachytherapy dose calculations: calculational algorithms. In: Thomadsen B, ed. *Categorical Course in Brachytherapy Physics*. Oak Brook, IL: Radiological Society of North America; 1997:41–49.
20. Sievert RM. Die intensitatatverteilung der primaren-strehlung in der nahe medinizinisher radium-praparate. *Acta Radiol*. 1921;1:89–128.
21. Young ME, Batho HF. Dose tables for linear radium sources calculated by an electronic computer. *Br J Radiol*. 1964;37:38–44.
22. Glasgow GP, Dillman LT. Specific γ-ray constant and exposure rate constant of 192Ir. *Med Phys*. 1979;6:49–52.
23. Glasgow GP. Exposure rate constants for filtered 192Ir sources. *Med Phys*. 1981;8:502–503.
24. Diffey BL, Klevenhagen SC. An experimental and calculated dose distribution in water around CDC K-type Cesium-137 sources. *Phys Med Biol*. 1975;20:446–454.
25. van der Laarse R, Meertens H. An algorithm for ovoid shielding of a cervix applicator. In: Cunningham JR, Ragan D, Van Dyk J, eds. *The Proceedings 8th International Conference on the Use of Computers in Radiation Therapy*, Toronto, Canada, July 9–12. Los Angeles, CA: IEEE Computer Society; 1984.
26. Williamson JF. Monte Carlo and analytic calculation of absorbed dose near 137Cs intracavitary sources. *Int J Radiat Oncol Biol Phys*. 1988;15:227–237.
27. Meertens H, van der Laarse R. Screens in ovoids of a Selectron cervix applicator. *Radiother Oncol*. 1985;3:69–80.
28. Weeks KJ, Dennett JC. Dose calculation and measurements for a CT compatible version of the Fletcher applicator. *Int J Radiat Oncol Biol Phys*. 1990;18:1191–1198.
29. Williamson JF. Monte Carlo evaluation of specific dose constants in water for 125I seeds. *Med Phys*. 1988;15:686–694.
30. Nath R, Anderson LL, Luxton G, et al. Dosimetry of interstitial brachytherapy sources: recommendations of the AAPM Radiation Therapy Committee Task Group 43. *Med Phys*. 1995;22:209–234.
31. Rivard MJ, Coursey BM, DeWerd LA, et al. Update of AAPM Task Group No. 43 Report: a revised AAPM protocol for brachytherapy dose calculations. *Med Phys*. 2004;31:633–674.
32. Williamson JF, Butler W, DeWerd LA, et al. Recommendations of the American Association of Physicists in medicine regarding the impact of implementing the 2004 Task Group 43 report on dose specification for 103Pd and 125I interstitial brachytherapy. *Med Phys*. 2005;32:1424–1439.
33. DeWerd LA, Huq MS, Das IJ, et al. Procedures for establishing and maintaining consistent air-kerma strength standards for low-energy, photon-emitting brachytherapy sources: recommendations of the Calibration Laboratory Accreditation Subcommittee of the American Association of Physics in medicine. *Med Phys*. 2004;31:675–681.
34. Rivard MJ, Butler WM, DeWerd LA, et al. Supplement to the 2004 update of AAPM Task Group No. 43 Report. *Med Phys*. 2007;34:2187–2205.

35. Chan GH, Nath R, Williamson JF. On the development of consensus values of reference dosimetry parameters for interstitial brachytherapy sources. *Med Phys.* 2005;31:1040–1045.

36. Karaiskos P, Angelopoulos A, Sakellio L. et al Monte Carlo and TLD dosimetry of an 192Ir high dose-rate brachytherapy source. *Med Phys.* 1998;25:1975–1984.

37. Heintz BH, Wallace RE, Hevezi JM. Comparison of I-125 sources used for permanent interstitial implants. *Med Phys.* 2001;28:671–682.

38. Mainegra E, Capote R, Lopez E. Dose-rate constants for 125I, 103Pd, 192Ir and 169Yb brachytherapy sources: an EGS4 Monte Carlo study. *Phys Med Biol.* 1998;43:1557–1566.

39. Williamson JF. The accuracy of the line and point source approximations in 192Ir Dosimetry. *Int J Radiat Oncol Biol Phys.* 1990;12:409–414.

40. Thomason C, Mackie TR, Lindstrom MJ, et al. The dose distribution surrounding 192Ir and 137Cs seed sources. *Phys Med Biol.* 1991;36:475–493.

41. Mainegra E, Capote R, Lopez E. Radial dose functions for 103Pd, 125I, 169Yb and 192Ir brachytherapy sources: an EGS4 Monte Carlo study. *Phys Med Biol.* 2000;45:703–717.

42. Kirov AS, Williamson JF, Meigooni AS, et al. TLD, diode, and Monte Carlo dosimetry of an 192Ir source for high dose-rate brachytherapy. *Phys Med Biol.* 1995;40:2015–2035.

43. Nath R, Meigooni AS, Muench P, et al. Anisotropy functions for 103Pd, 125I, and 192Ir interstitial brachytherapy sources. *Med Phys.* 1993;20:1465–1473.

44. Capote R, Mainegra E, Lopez E. Anisotropy functions for low energy interstitial brachytherapy sources: an EGS4 Monte Carlo Study. *Phys Med Biol.* 2001;46:135–150.

45. Brunet-Benkhoucha M, Verhaegen F, Lassalle S, et al. Clinical Implementation of a digital tomosynthesis-based seed reconstruction algorithm for intraoperative postimplant dose evaluation in low dose rate prostate brachytherapy. *Med Phys.* 2009;36:5235–5244.

46. Corbett JF, Jezioranski JJ, Crook J, et al. The effect of seed orientation deviations on the quality of 125I prostate implants. *Phys Med Biol.* 2001;46:2785–2800.

47. Furhang EE, Anderson LL. Functional fitting of interstitial brachytherapy dosimetry data recommended by the AAPM Radiation Therapy Committee Task Group 43. *Med Phys.* 1999;26:153–160.

48. Sloboda RS, Menon GV. Experimental determination of the anisotropy function and anisotropy factor for model 6711 I-125 seeds. *Med Phys.* 2000;27:1789–1799.

49. Ling CC, Schell MC, Yorke ED, et al. Two dimensional dose distribution of 125I seeds. *Med Phys.* 1985;12:652–655.

50. Ling CC, Spiro IJ, Kubiatowicz DO, et al. Measurement of dose distribution around Fletcher-Suit-Delclos colpostats using a Therados radiation field analyzer (RFA-3). *Med Phys.* 1984;11:326–330.

51. Mohan R, Ding IY, Martel MK, et al. Measurements of radiation dose distributions for shielded cervical applicators. *Int J Radiat Oncol Biol Phys.* 1985;11:861–868.

52. Williamson JF. Dose calculations about shielded gynecological colpostats. *Int J Radiat Oncol Biol Phys.* 1990;19:167–178.

53. Weeks KJ. Monte Carlo calculations for a new ovoid shield system for carcinoma of the uterine cervix. *Med Phys.* 1998;25:2288–2292.

54. Mohan R, Ding IY, Toraskar J, et al. Computation of radiation dose distributions for shielded cervical applicators. *Int J Radiat Oncol Biol Phys.* 1985;11:823–830.

55. Rose ME. *Elementary Theory of Angular Momentum.* New York: Wiley; 1957.

56. Weeks KJ. Brachytherapy object oriented treatment planning using three dimensional image guidance. In: Thomadsen B, ed. *Categorical Course in Brachytherapy Physics.* Oak Brook, IL: Radiological Society of North America; 1997:79–86.

57. Burns GS, Raeside DE. The accuracy of single-seed dose superposition for I-125 implants. *Med Phys.* 1989;16:627–631.

58. Meigooni AS, Meli JA, Nath R. Interseed effects on dose for I-125 brachytherapy implants. *Med Phys.* 1992;19:385–390.

59. Chibani O, Williamson JF, Todor D. Dosimetric Effect of seed anisotropy and interseed attenuation for 103Pd and 125I prostate implants. *Med Phys.* 2005;32:2557–2566.

60. Yu Y, Anderson LL, Li Z, et al. Permanent prostate seed implant brachytherapy: Report of the American Association of Physicists in Medicine in Medicine Task Group No. 64. *Med Phys.* 1999;26:2054–2076.

61. Das RK, Keleti D, Zhu Y, et al. Validation of Monte Carlo dose calculations near I-125 brachytherapy sources in the presence of bounded tissue heterogeneities. *Int J Radiat Oncol Biol Phys.* 1997;38:843–853.

62. Meigooni AS, Nath R. Tissue inhomogeneity correction for brachytherapy sources in a heterogeneous phantom with cylindrical symmetry. *Med Phys.* 1992;19:401–407.

63. Williamson JF, Li Z, Wong JW. One-dimensional scatter-subtraction method for brachytherapy dose calculation near bounded heterogeneities. *Med Phys.* 1993;20:233–244.

64. Furstoss C, Reniers B, Bertrand MJ, et al. Monte Carlo study of LDR seed dosimetry with an application in a clinical breast implant. *Med Phys.* 2009;36:1848–1858.

65. Berger M. Energy deposition in water by photons from point isotropic sources. MIRD Pamphlet 2. Washington, DC: National Bureau of Standards; 1968.

66. Briesmeister JT. MCNP—A general Monte Carlo N-particle transport code. Version 4a: Los Alamos National Laboratory Report, LA-12625, 1993.

67. Nelson W, Hirayama H, Rogers D. The EGS4 Code System. SLAC Report 265 Stanford University; 1985.

68. Williamson JF. Monte Carlo evaluation of kerma at a point for photon transport problems. *Med Phys.* 1988;14:567–576.

69. Boyer AL. A fundamental accuracy limitation on measurements of brachytherapy sources. *Med Phys.* 1979;6:454–456.

70. Gifford KA, Horton JL, Wareing TA, et al. Comparison of a finite-element multigroup discrete-ordinates code with Monte Carlo for Radiotherapy calculations. *Phys Med Biol.* 2006;51:2253–2265.

71. Daskalov GM, Baker RS, Rogers DW, Williamson JF. Dosimetric modeling of the microselectron high-dose rate 192Ir source by the multigroup discrete ordinates method. *Med Phys.* 2000;27:2307–2319.

72. Zhou C, Inanc F. Integral-transport-based deterministic brachytherapy dose calculations. *Phys Med Biol.* 2003;48:73–93.

73. Lewis EE, Miller WF. *Computational Methods of Neutron Transport.* New York, NY: Wiley; 1984.

74. Alcouffe RE, Baker RS, Brinkley FW, et al. DANTSYS: a diffusion accelerated neutral particle transport code system. LA-12969-M, Los Alamos National Laboratory, Los Alamos, NM; 1995.

75. Wareing TA, McGhee JM, Morel JE. Attila: a three dimensional unstructured tetrahedral mesh discrete-ordinates transport code. *Trans Amer Nucl Soc.* 1996;75:146

76. Vassiliev ON, Wareing TA, McGhee J, et al. Validation of a new grid-based Boltzmann equation solver for dose calculation in radiotherapy with photon beams. *Phys Med Biol.* 2010;55:581–598.

77. Beaulieu L, Carlsson Tedgren A, Carrier JF, Davis SD, Mourtada F, Rivard MJ, Thomson RM, Verhaegen F, Wareing TA, Williamson JF. Report of the Task Group 186 on model-based dose calculation methods in brachytherapy beyond the TG-43 formalism: current status and recommendations for clinical implementation. *Med Phys.* 2012;39:6208–6236.

22 Treatment Planning Algorithms: Electron Beams

Kenneth R. Hogstrom, Garrett M. Pitcher, Robert L. Carver, and John A. Antolak

INTRODUCTION

The evolution of modern electron beam dose algorithms is based on four key technologies: (1) the availability of whole-body CT scanners capable of providing an accurate three dimensional (3D) model of the patient in the late 1970s, (2) the development of electron pencil beam algorithms (PBAs) based on multiple Coulomb scattering (MCS) in the 1980s, (3) the development of fast Monte Carlo (MC) algorithms specific to electron beam therapy in the 1990s, and (4) the geometric growth of computer technology (memory and speed) over the past half century. This chapter focuses on algorithms currently used for electron beam therapy treatment planning. This includes both analytical and MC-based dose algorithms used for treatment planning and algorithms used for electron conformal therapy. Computer algorithms for arc electron therapy and for monitor units are excluded.

Due to lack of these key technologies, dose algorithms, used in treatment planning prior to 1980, were limited to (1) being two dimensional (2D), typically the transverse plane, (2) using a patient skin contour (obtained by manual means) with manually constructed internal heterogeneities (if used at all), (3) computing dose as a depth dose factor times an off-axis factor, and (4) calculating dose considering only the geometry between the source and the point of calculation. These early methods, many reviewed by Sternick,[1] began evolving toward current technology with the use of the age-diffusion equation for modeling off-axis dose by Kawachi[2] and others in the late 1970s.[3] A semiempirical pencil beam model based on age-diffusion equation, as applied by Steben et al.,[4] was available in the Theraplan treatment planning system (Theratronics, Kanata, Ontario) in the late 1970s.

These early dose algorithms had limited accuracy due to their improperly modeling electron MCS. Dose calculations that modeled irregular skin surface and internal heterogeneities were one dimensional (1D), i.e., considered only the anatomy between the virtual source and the point of dose calculation. Because electrons scatter laterally, nearby anatomy can have a significant impact on dose at nearby points and cannot be ignored. With the advent of PBAs based on Fermi–Eyges theory of MCS,[5] algorithms began calculating dose more accurately by considering the anatomy in the plane of calculation, and as computer technology advanced, the same algorithms began calculating dose considering the anatomy in 3D, i.e., 3D dose calculations using 3D heterogeneity corrections started becoming available in the 1990s. Then, as computing technologies further improved, more accurate analytical and MC-based algorithms became available.[6] These algorithms more closely achieved the lower end of the Van Dyk et al.[7] range of suggested criteria of acceptability (± one standard deviation) for accuracy of electron dose calculations in the low-dose gradient/high-dose gradient regions (4%/0.4 cm to 7%/0.5 cm), closely achieving the recommendations (2%/0.2 cm) of ICRU Report No. 42[8] to points of relevance.

To follow, characteristics of these algorithms, i.e., theory of calculation, beam modeling and commissioning requirements, precision (MC algorithms only), documentation of accuracy, and time of calculation are discussed and compared. All electron beam dose algorithms described herein utilize a 3D CT data set to model the patient and compute dose in three dimensions.

The availability of fast, accurate 3D dose algorithms paved the way for the development of electron conformal therapy,[9] which has been available to clinics since 2008 using 3D machined wax and more recently using 3D printed boluses. Treatment sites, design algorithms, and dose accuracy for bolus electron conformal therapy (BECT) will be discussed.

PENCIL BEAM ALGORITHM

Different PBAs have many similarities, but usually a few unique features. This section details the Hogstrom et al.[10] PBA, which has been widely used and has remained in use as late as 2021 for electron dose calculations in the Pinnacle[3] TPS (Philips North America LLC, Cambridge, MA). The dose distribution for an electron beam comprises dose from incident electrons (D_e) and dose from background x-rays (D_x), the latter typically less than a few percent for 6–20 MeV electron beams, i.e.,

$$D_{total}(x,y,z) = D_e(x,y,z) + D_X(x,y,z). \quad (22.1)$$

The electron dose distribution $D_e(x,y,z)$ is calculated using the PBA, and the x-ray dose distribution $D_X(x,y,z)$ is calculated using a simpler broad beam model.

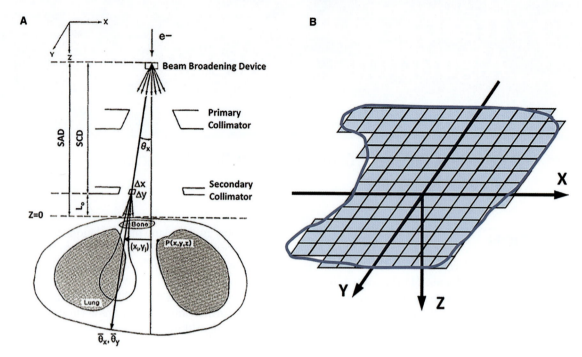

FIGURE 22.1. Pencil Beam Geometry. **(A)** Side view of electron beam and patient geometry for PBA. Beam parameters describe the pencil beam at (x_i, y_j), which contributes dose at each point (x, y, z) in the patient. See text for definition of parameters. From Hogstrom KR, Mills MD, Almond PR. Electron beam dose calculations. *Phys Med Biol.* May 1981;26(3):445–459. doi:10.1088/0031-9155/26/3/008); with permission of IOP Publishing. All rights reserved. **(B)** Irregular field is modeled as the sum of all pencil beams whose centers lie inside it. From Hogstrom KR, Steadham RE. Electron Beam Dose Computation. In: Palta J, Mackie TR, eds. *Teletherapy: Present and Future.* Proceedings of the summar school of the AAPM. Madison, WI: Advanced Medical Publishing;1996:137–174; With permission of Advanced Medical Publishing, Inc [AMP].

Electron Dose Model

A therapeutic electron beam is created from a narrow electron beam exiting an electron accelerator, which is directed toward the patient, typically using one or more bending magnets. That beam is broadened and flattened using a dual scattering foil system or, in prior times, magnetic scanning. The broad beam is collimated by (1) a primary collimator (x-ray jaws), (2) a secondary collimator (applicator) that consists of tiers of collimating bars (trimmers), and (3) a collimating insert located in the final trimmer that creates an irregularly shaped field matched to the patient planning target volume (PTV) (*cf.* Fig. 22.1A). At the plane of the collimating insert, the electron beam is broad and uniform, has a narrow energy distribution, appears to be emitted from a virtual source, and has an approximately Gaussian angular distribution about the mean direction at each point.

For the PBA, the electron beam exiting the collimating insert is modeled as a collection of pencil beams, where a pencil beam is defined as all electrons passing through a small area (Δx by Δy), typically a 0.2 cm square (*cf.* Fig. 22.1B). The electron dose at point $P(x, y, z)$ is the sum of the weighted doses from each pencil beam, i.e.,

$$D_e(x,y,z) = \sum_{i,j\subset\text{aperture}} W(x_i,y_j) \cdot D_{i,j}^{ePB}(x,y,z), \quad (22.2)$$

where $D_{i,j}^{ePB}(x,y,z)$ is the contribution from the (i,j) electron pencil beam centered at (x_i,y_j) to dose at (x,y,z). Each electron pencil beam is characterized initially by

(1) the same energy $(E_{p,0})$, which is the most probable energy of the broad beam energy distribution, (2) a constant planar fluence times an off-axis weighting factor $(\phi_0 \cdot W(x_i,y_j))$, (3) a mean direction at each point that backprojects to a virtual source a distance SAD_{vir} from isocenter, i.e., when projected onto the XZ and YZ planes, and because of small angle scattering, $\bar{\theta}_x \approx \tan(\bar{\theta}_x) = x_i/SAD_{vir}$ and $\bar{\theta}_y \approx \tan(\bar{\theta}_y) = y_j/SAD_{vir}$, respectively, and (4) a root mean square (rms) Gaussian spread or sigma about the mean directions $(\sigma_{\theta_x} = \sigma_{\theta_y})$, which is the same for all pencil beams.

The dose distribution is calculated for each pencil beam incident on a slab phantom, where the depth dependence of the slab phantom equals that in the patient along the central axis of that pencil beam, as illustrated in Figure 22.2. This central-axis approximation, proposed by Perry and Holt[11] and Hogstrom et al.,[10] was necessary to achieve practical calculation times. However, it can result in insufficiently accurate dose calculations for some patient geometries. A pencil beam dose distribution in water, illustrated in Figure 22.3, is characterized by its tear drop shape.[12] The shape of the tear drop changes as beam energy, SSD, and patient anatomy change.

Pencil beam calculations use Fermi–Eyges MCS theory[5] computed for a slab phantom, i.e., one in which the phantom material varies only in the direction of central axis of the beam (z), as illustrated in Figure 22.2. For a pencil beam (Δx by Δy) located at (x_i,y_j), the

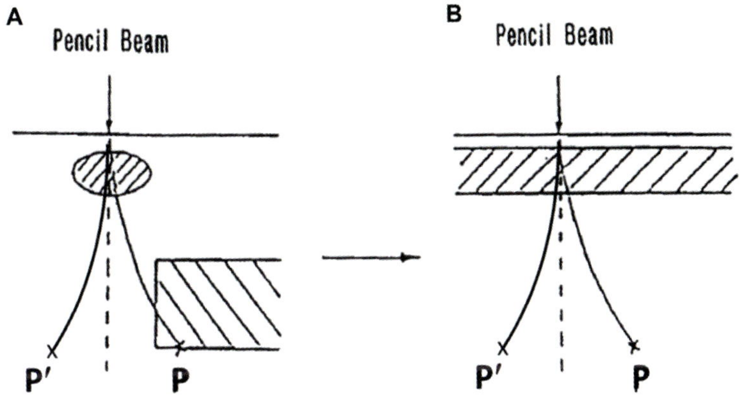

A
Pencil Beam

B
Pencil Beam

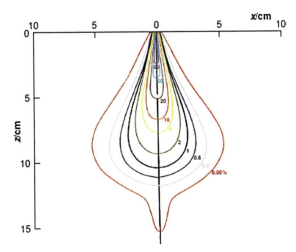

FIGURE 22.2. Central-Axis Approximation. **(A)** Mean paths of electrons from the pencil beam origin on skin surface to points of calculation follow the curved lines, passing through heterogeneities (diagonal fills). **(B)** The anatomy used for calculation of dose from this pencil beam only is a slab phantom matching the anatomy along the central axis of the pencil beam (dashed line). This is a good approximation for point P' but ignores effect of the deeper heterogeneity for point P.

FIGURE 22.3. Pencil beam isodose distribution measured with a narrow electron beam of 22 MeV incident on a water phantom. From Svensson H, Almond P, Brahme A, Dutreix A, Leetz HK. Radiation dosimetry: electron beams with energies between 1 and 50 MeV. 1984. ICRU Report 35.

The first term models the Gaussian off-axis distribution of electrons due to MCS; the second-term models collisional energy loss of the electrons with depth; and the third term corrects for inverse square differences due to distance from the virtual source to the point of calculation (x, y, z), where

- f is the projection factor from the source-to-axis distance (SAD) to the z plane $(1 + z/SAD_{vir})$, a result of beam divergence and all pencil beam coordinates and field dimensions being specified at isocenter;
- $(\sigma_x)_{i,j}$ is the sigma at z of the Gaussian spread in the XZ and YZ planes, i.e., $(\sigma_x)_{i,j} = (\sigma_y)_{i,j}$, according to the Fermi–Eyges theory of MCS for a point beam originating at the center of the (i, j) pencil beam;
- $D_\infty(d_{i,j}^{eff})$ is the dose at depth $d_{i,j}^{eff}$ in water (surface at isocenter) for a field size with side scatter equilibrium on central axis (e.g., ≥12 × 12 cm²); and
- $d_{i,j}^{eff}$ is the depth in water for which electrons have the same energy loss as electrons at position z in the patient along the central axis of the (i, j) pencil beam.

$D_\infty(z)$ is determined using the Fermi–Eyges MCS theory to restore side scatter equilibrium to the measured dose versus depth curve for the reference field size, which typically is the rectangular field size of least area circumscribing the irregularly shaped treatment field, i.e.,

dose contribution to point $P(x, y, z)$ in the patient is given by

$$D_{i,j}^{ePB}(x, y, z) = \iint_{x_i-\frac{\Delta x}{2}, y_j-\frac{\Delta y}{2}}^{x_i+\frac{\Delta x}{2}, y_j+\frac{\Delta y}{2}} dx' dy' \frac{1}{2\pi (\sigma_x)_{i,j}^2}$$

$$\exp\left(-\frac{(x - x')^2 + (y - y')^2}{2\pi (\sigma_x)_{i,j}^2}\right)$$

$$\cdot D_\infty(d_{i,j}^{eff}) \cdot \frac{(SAD_{vir} + d_{i,j}^{eff})^2}{(SAD_{vir} + z)^2}$$

$$= \frac{1}{4}\left\{ erf\left[\frac{(x_i + \frac{\Delta x}{2})f - x}{\sqrt{2}\,(\sigma_x)_{i,j}}\right] - erf\left[\frac{(x_i - \frac{\Delta x}{2})f - x}{\sqrt{2}\,(\sigma_x)_{i,j}}\right]\right\}$$

$$\cdot \left\{ erf\left[\frac{(y_j + \frac{\Delta y}{2})f - y}{\sqrt{2}\,(\sigma_x)_{i,j}}\right] - erf\left[\frac{(y_j - \frac{\Delta y}{2})f - y}{\sqrt{2}\,(\sigma_x)_{i,j}}\right]\right\}$$

$$\cdot D_\infty(d_{i,j}^{eff}) \cdot \frac{(SAD_{vir} + d_{i,j}^{eff})^2}{(SAD_{vir} + z)^2}. \tag{22.3}$$

$$D_\infty(z) = [D_{WX}^{meas}(z) \cdot D_{WY}^{meas}(z)]_{norm}^{1/2}$$

$$\cdot \left[erf\left(\frac{WX \cdot f}{2\sqrt{2}\,\sigma_x^{water}(z)}\right) \cdot erf\left(\frac{WY \cdot f}{2\sqrt{2}\,\sigma_x^{water}(z)}\right)\right]^{-1}, \tag{22.4}$$

where the square root term is the percent central-axis dose versus depth in water for the rectangular field (WX by WY) determined from measured percent central-axis dose versus depth curves in water at isocenter for square fields WX and WY, the erf terms restore side scatter equilibrium for both dimensions of the rectangle, and $\sigma_x^{water}(z)$ is the value in water using Equation 22.5. Using measured central-axis dose versus depth data forces calculated dose to exactly equal measured dose in water, which compensates for the PBA not modeling less important physical interactions such as bremsstrahlung energy loss and delta ray production.

Another important aspect of the PBA is how it determines σ_x, which depends on the initial angular spread of the pencil beam (arising from MCS in the air and secondary scattering foil that lie between the primary scattering foil and the origin of the pencil beam) and MCS in the patient. Hogstrom et al.[10] showed that

$$\sigma_x^2(z) = \sigma_{\theta_x}^2(E) \cdot (L_0 + z)^2 + FMCS \cdot a_2(z), \quad (22.5)$$

where σ_{θ_x} is the initial angular spread for beam energy E, L_0 is the distance from the pencil beam origin to isocenter (cf. Figure 22.1A), and a_2 is the second scattering moment of Fermi–Eyges theory from the patient surface (z_s) to z along the (x_i, y_j) ray line. The latter term, sometimes referred to as the square of the sigma due to scatter in the patient ($\sigma_{x,pat}^2$), is given by

$$a_2(z) = \frac{1}{2}\int_{z_s}^z dz' \left[\frac{T_{pat}(E_{z'}, z')}{T_{water}(E_{z'})}\right] T_{water}(E_{z'})(z - z')^2. \quad (22.6)$$

Because MCS is modeled as a Gaussian, large-angle Molière scattering is not specifically modeled, as done by Lax et al.,[13] resulting in a slight underestimate of penumbral width. This is partially accounted for by FMCS, which is a factor that is adjusted to best fit measured penumbra shape, typically being 1.2–1.4.[6] Calculated values for σ_x^{water} versus depth in water are illustrated for a 13-MeV beam in Figure 22.4. Values for $a_2(z)$, calculated using Equation 22.6, overestimate σ_x at depths greater than $\approx 0.7R_p$, where σ_x peaks due to range straggling. Although this can be modeled by having $\sqrt{a_2(z)}$ fall to 0.0 at R_p,[14] resulting in dashed black line for σ_x in Figure 22.4, Hogstrom et al.[10] found this unnecessary.

In Equation 22.6, $T_{pat}(E_{z'}, z')$ is the linear angular scattering power for the patient tissue and electron energy $E_{z'}$ at z', and $T_{water}(E_{z'})$ is the linear angular scattering power for

water and electron energy $E_{z'}$. $E_{z'} = E_{p,0}\left(1 - \frac{d_{eff}(z')}{R_p}\right)$, where $E_{p,0}$ is the most probable energy of the incident electron beam. $E_{p,0}(MeV) = 0.22 + 1.98R_p$ (cm) $+ 0.0025 R_p^2$ (cm), where R_p, the practical range, is extracted from the measured central-axis dose versus depth curve in water.[12] Similarly, the effective depth is calculated by

$$d_{eff}(z) = \int_{z_s}^z dz' \left[\frac{S_{pat}(E_{z'}, z')}{S_{water}(E_{z'})}\right], \quad (22.7)$$

where $S_{pat}(E_{z'}, z')$ is the linear collisional stopping power for the tissue and electron energy $E_{z'}$ at z', and $S_{water}(E_{z'})$ is the linear collisional stopping power for water and electron energy $E_{z'}$. Both the ratio of linear angular scattering powers and the ratio of linear collisional stopping powers can be assumed independent of energy and correlated to CT number, either directly, as plotted in Figure 22.5, or indirectly by correlating these ratios with density should a CT number to density table be available. Equations 22.6 and 22.7 can be evaluated using the recursion relations of Hogstrom et al.[10] and Hogstrom,[15] which makes the calculation over the entire dose grid more efficient.

Different PBAs have slight differences, e.g., the one developed by Lax et al.[13] used the sum of three Gaussians to model Molière multiple scattering theory, resulting in improved agreement in the penumbra. Hogstrom et al.[10] implemented a unique feature that reduced the error due to the central-axis approximation, significantly improving the calculation of hot and cold spots due to surface irregularities. The feature propagated the broad beam from the beam-defining collimator to the z plane of calculation in the absence of the patient, and then used that relative fluence to weight pencil beams that begin at the patient surface, i.e., the pencil beams were redefined. This improvement was so significant that it led to a subsequent algorithm that redefined pencil beams every 0.5 cm

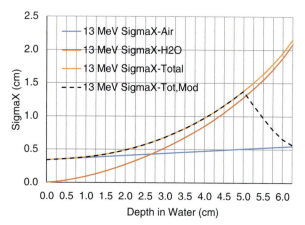

FIGURE 22.4. Comparison of σ_x versus depth in water (yellow line) at 13 MeV. Values are calculated using Equation 22.5 with $L_o = 10$ cm and $FMCS = 1.0$. Note dominance of $\sigma_{air} = \sigma_{\theta_x}(L_o + z)$ (blue line) at shallower depths and $\sigma_{water} = \sqrt{a_2(z)}$ (red line) at deeper depths. Values for $a_2(z)$, calculated using Equation 22.6, overestimate σ_x at depths greater than $\approx 0.7R_p$, where σ_x peaks due to range straggling. Although this can be modeled by having $\sqrt{a_2(z)}$ fall to 0.0 at R_p,[14] resulting in dashed black line for σ_x, Hogstrom et al.[10] found this unnecessary.

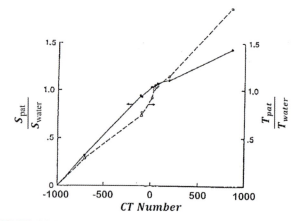

FIGURE 22.5. Electron linear collisional stopping power (S) (solid curve) and linear angular scattering power (T) (dashed curve) relative to that for water at 10 MeV plotted versus CT number (air = −1,000; water = 0 for patient tissues. CT number was computed for 120 kVp x-rays; see reference for data at 140 kVp. From data of Hogstrom KR, Mills MD, Almond PR. Electron beam dose calculations. *Phys Med Biol.* May 1981;26(3):445–459. doi:10.1088/0031-9155/26/3/008; with permission of IOP Publishing. All rights reserved.

throughout the patient, the pencil beam redefinition algorithm (PBRA), discussed in the next section. This feature resulted in the following formula, as reported by Starkschall et al.[16]:

$$D_{ij}(x,y,z) = \quad W_{air}(x_i,y_j) \qquad \text{pencil beam weight}$$

$$\cdot \frac{1}{2}\left\{ erf\left[\frac{\left(x_i + \frac{\Delta x}{2}\right)f - x}{\sqrt{2}\,(a_2)_{i,j}}\right] - erf\left[\frac{\left(x_i - \frac{\Delta x}{2}\right)f - x}{\sqrt{2}\,(a_2)_{i,j}}\right]\right\}$$

x-scatter factor (patient)

$$\cdot \frac{1}{2}\left\{ erf\left[\frac{\left(y_j + \frac{\Delta y}{2}\right)f - y}{\sqrt{2}\,(a_2)_{i,j}}\right] - erf\left[\frac{\left(y_j - \frac{\Delta y}{2}\right)f - y}{\sqrt{2}\,(a_2)_{i,j}}\right]\right\}$$

y-scatter factor (patient)

$$\cdot D_\infty\left(d_{i,j}^{eff}\right) \qquad\qquad \text{depth-dose factor}$$

$$\cdot \frac{\left(SAD_{vir} + d_{i,j}^{eff}\right)^2}{\left(SAD_{vir} + z\right)^2}, \qquad \text{inverse-square factor}$$

$$(22.8)$$

where

$$W_{air}(x_i,y_j) = W(x_i,y_j)$$

$$\cdot \sum_{k=1}^{N}\frac{1}{2}\left\{ erf\left[\frac{\left(x_k + \frac{\Delta x}{2} - x_i\right)f}{\sqrt{2}\,_{air}(z)}\right] - erf\left[\frac{\left(x_k - \frac{\Delta x}{2} - x_i\right)f}{\sqrt{2}\,_{air}(z)}\right]\right\}$$

$$\cdot \sum_{l=1}^{M_k}\frac{1}{2}\left\{ erf\left[\frac{\left(Y_{k,l}^{max}(z) - y_j\right)f}{\sqrt{2}\,_{air}(z)}\right] - erf\left[\frac{\left(Y_{k,l}^{min}(z) - y_j\right)f}{\sqrt{2}\,_{air}(z)}\right]\right\},$$

$$(22.9)$$

where

$Y_{k,l}^{max}$ = maximum y-coordinate of lth strip at x_k (strips comprise irregular field aperture)

$Y_{k,l}^{min}$ = minimum y-coordinate of lth strip at x_k (strips comprise irregular field aperture)

$\sigma_{air}(z) = \sigma_{\theta_x}(E) \cdot (L_o + z)$, the rms spread of pencil-beam propagating (through only air) from the collimator to the z plane of calculation; i.e., Equation 22.5 becomes $(\sigma_x)_{i,j}^2 = (\sigma_{air})^2 + FMCS \cdot (a_2)_{i,j}$

X-Ray Dose Model

The x-ray dose is calculated using the broad beam model of Shiu[17] and Hogstrom et al.,[18] which models inverse square and attenuation, but with the addition of insert attenuation, it makes a 1D heterogeneity correction, resulting in

$$D_X(x,y,z) = D_{X,water}(0,0,d_{eff}) \cdot OAR_{X,water}(x,y,R_p+2)$$

$$\cdot f_{insert}(x,y) \cdot \frac{(SAD + d_{eff})^2}{(SSD + z)^2}, \qquad (22.10)$$

where: $D_{X,water}(0,0,d_{eff})$ is the central-axis x-ray background dose versus depth in water at d_{eff} for the energy

and applicator; $OAR_{X,water}(x,y,R_p+2)$ is the measured off-axis ratio along the x axis times that along the y axis at a depth 2 cm beyond R_p and off-axis position (x,y) projected from z to R_p+2 for the energy and applicator; $f_{insert}(x,y)$ is unity inside the aperture and the insert material's attenuation factor for x-rays beneath the aperture; and the final term is an inverse square correction between the point of calculation and the equivalent point in water whose surface is at the SAD. The central axis term is given by

$$D_{X,water}(0,0,d_{eff}) = D_{water}(0,0,R_p+2)$$

$$\cdot \frac{(SAD + R_p + 2)^2}{(SAD + d_{eff})^2} \cdot exp^{-\lambda(d_{eff}-R_p-2)},$$

$$(22.11)$$

where λ is the linear attenuation coefficient in water that best fits the equation to the measured data for $d_{eff} > R_p + 2$. Equation 22.7 is used to determine d_{eff} along a ray line from the virtual source to (x,y,z).

Beam Data Input and PBA Commissioning

Multiple steps are recommended for algorithm commissioning of electron beams for the radiotherapy machine: (1) inputting parameters that model the electron beam for each beam energy of a machine, (2) inputting measured central-axis dose versus depth and off-axis dose profiles in water, (3) inputting output factors as a function of beam energy, applicator, SSD, and square field size (optional, but recommended if MUs are to be computed), (4) inputting or selecting CT tables for relative scattering power and relative collisional stopping power versus CT number for kVp of x-rays, (5) validation of data input, and (6) establishing a set of tests for future software quality assurance. These steps,[6,15] applicable to most electron dose algorithms, are exemplified for the PBA of Hogstrom et al.[10]

Step 1: Beam parameters for each beam energy:

- Most probable incident electron energy $(E_{p,0})$, determined from the practical range (R_p) of a measured percent dose versus depth curve, according to ICRU Report 35[12]
- Nominal source-to-isocenter distance, typically 100 cm, sometimes used in lieu of SAD_{vir}
- Virtual source-to-isocenter distance (SAD_{vir}), determined from beam profiles at multiple SSDs[19]
- Isocenter to collimating insert distance (L_0)
- Initial projected angular spread of pencil beams at beam-defining collimator $(\sigma_{\theta_x}(E))$, determined from beam profiles at multiple SSDs; these values should closely match those reported by Hogstrom and Steadham[6]

Step 2: Measured relative dose profiles for each beam energy:

- Percent central-axis dose versus depth in water with SSD at isocenter (typically 100 cm SSD) for square field sizes spanning the clinical range, *e.g.*, 2×2, 3×3, 4×4, 6×6, 8×8, 10×10, 15×15, 20×20, and 25×25 cm^2 using the smallest applicator possible

- Off-axis profile at R_{100} or $R_{90}/2$ for each applicator to be used to model off-axis beam nonuniformity (typically within ±3%)
- f_{insert}, λ, and off-axis x-ray profile at $R_p + 2$

<u>Step 3</u>: Dose output factors for each beam energy:

- Output factors (dose per MU) for each applicator and selected field sizes for that applicator (e.g., 2×2, 3×3, 4×4, 6×6, 8×8, 10×10, 15×15, 20×20, and 25×25 cm^2 for the 25×25 applicator) spanning the range of SSDs for clinical use (e.g., 100, 105, 110, 115, and 120 cm), *cf.* Hogstrom et al.[20]

<u>Step 4</u>: CT data tables:

- Tables of relative stopping power and relative scattering power at kVp of x-rays from CT scanner versus CT number (or tables of density versus CT number if TPS code contains fixed tables of relative stopping and scattering powers versus density) for (1) patient tissues, (2) patient tissues with entries to manage bolus, skin, or internal collimating structures, (3) water phantom for beam commissioning verification, and (4) others for any measurement phantoms, *cf.* Hogstrom and Steadham.[6]

<u>Step 5</u>: Quality assurance

- Validate data by computing isodose plots and comparing with plots of measured data in water.

- Validate all dose output values by computing dose in a water phantom and comparing with measured data.
- Establish set of dose calculations using patient CT data set for future QA tests.

Accuracy of the PBA

The accuracy of the PBA is well documented for many clinical situations. PBA calculated dose distributions have been compared with measured dose in water phantoms for incident beams having perpendicular incidence (100 and 110 cm SSD) and angled incidence and for water phantoms having irregular surfaces and containing tissue substitutes for hard bone, lung, and air. Early dose comparisons were made by Hogstrom et al.[10,21] Similar, but more extensive, dose comparisons were made for the Shiu et al.[22] National Cancer Institute (NCI) working group data set for implementation of the Hogstrom PBA by McShan et al.,[23] Cheng et al.,[24] and Hogstrom and Steadham.[6]

Figure 22.6 demonstrates the PBA's accuracy in a water phantom for nominal and extended SSD, for normal and oblique incidence, and for an irregular surface.[21] Figures 22.7, 22.8, and 22.9 illustrate its accuracy in the presence of lung,[6,10] hard bone,[24,25] and air cavities,[6,23] respectively. Overall, results are good, e.g., Cheng et al.[24] reported that pass rates for the 14 test cases (2D dose matrices) of Shiu et al.[22] were 96% for 4% or 0.4 cm distance to agreement (DTA). However, this metric does not reflect small areas for certain geometries where differences can be clinically

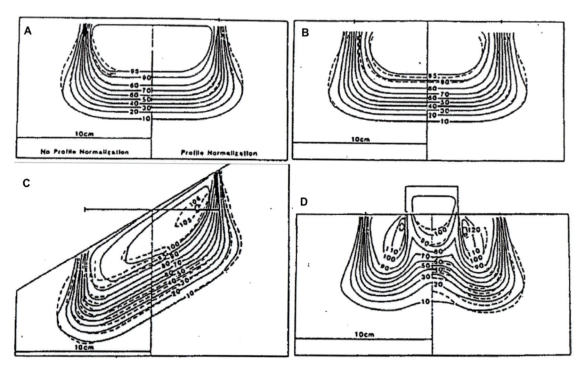

FIGURE 22.6. PBA calculated and measured isoionization curves in water are compared for a 15 MeV 10×10 cm^2 field. **(A)** 100 cm SSD, **(B)** 110 cm SSD, **(C)** 30° from normal incidence, and **(D)** stepped surface. Solid lines are PBA calculation; dashed lines are measurement. From Hogstrom KR, Mills MD, Meyer JA, et al. Dosimetric evaluation of a pencil-beam algorithm for electrons employing a two-dimensional heterogeneity correction. *Int J Radiat Oncol Biol Phys*. Apr 1984;10(4):561–569. doi:10.1016/0360-3016(84)90036-1.

FIGURE 22.7. Comparison of PBA calculated with measured dose in slab lung phantoms. **(A)** Dose versus depth on central axis of 9 MeV 15 × 15 cm² field. From Hogstrom KR, Steadham RE. Electron Beam Dose Computation. In: Palta J, Mackie TR, eds. *Teletherapy: Present and Future*. Proceedings of the summar school of the AAPM. Madison, WI: Advanced Medical Publishing;1996:137–174; With permission of Advanced Medical Publishing, Inc [AMP]. **(B)** Dose normalized to central-axis dose (off-axis response) versus off-axis distance at multiple depths for 17 MeV 10 × 10 cm² field. From Hogstrom KR, Mills MD, Almond PR. Electron beam dose calculations. *Phys Med Biol*. May 1981;26(3): 445–459. doi:10.1088/0031-9155/26/3/008; with permission of IOP Publishing. All rights reserved.

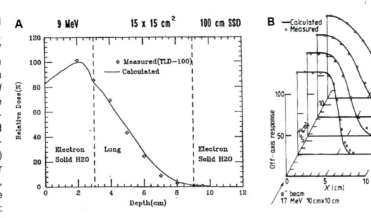

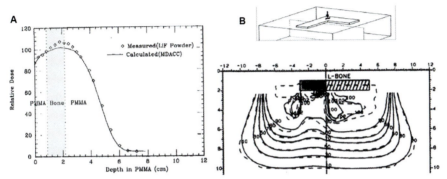

FIGURE 22.8. Comparison of PBA calculated with measured dose in bone phantoms. **(A)** Dose versus depth on central axis of 15 MeV 8 × 8 cm² field with 1.3 cm thick bone slab at 0.9 cm depth. Underestimate of dose (3%) at polymethyl methacrylate (PMMA) bone interface is due to the PBA not modeling backscattered electrons; underestimate of dose (<6%) in and distal to bone is due to the PBA being based on planar fluence rather than fluence. From Shiu AS, Hogstrom KR. Dose in bone and tissue near bone-tissue interface from electron beam. *Int J Radiat Oncol Biol Phys*. Aug 1991;21(3):695–702. doi:10.1016/0360-3016(91)90688-z. **(B)** PBA calculated isodose curves (dashed) compared with measured isodose curves (solid) for a 20 MeV 15 × 15 cm² field with a 1 cm thick L-shaped hard bone substitute at 1 cm depth, which is illustrated. From Cheng A, Harms WB, Sr., Gerber RL, Wong JW, Purdy JA. Systematic verification of a three-dimensional electron beam dose calculation algorithm. *Med Phys*. May 1996;23(5):685–93. doi:10.1118/1.597714.

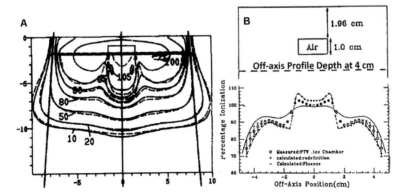

FIGURE 22.9. Comparison of PBA calculated with measured dose in air phantoms. **(A)** PBA calculated isodose curves (solid) and measured isodose curves (dashed) under a 3 cm by 1 cm air column at depth of 1 cm for a 20 MeV 15 × 15 cm² field. From McShan DL, Fraass BA, Ten Haken RK. Dosimetric verification of a 3-D electron pencil beam dose calculation algorithm. *Med Phys*. Jan 1994;21(1):13–23. doi:10.1118/1.597363. **(B)** PBA calculated off-axis dose profile (solid) and measured dose points (circles) under a 2 cm by 1 cm thick air cavity at depth of 2 cm for a 15 MeV 10 × 10 cm² field. Differences as large as 6% are a result of the central-axis approximation of the PBA. From Hogstrom KR, Steadham RE. Electron Beam Dose Computation. In: Palta J, Mackie TR, eds. *Teletherapy: Present and Future*. Proceedings of the summar school of the AAPM. Madison, WI: Advanced Medical Publishing; 1996:137–174; With permission of Advanced Medical Publishing, Inc (AMP).

significant. This is exemplified in Figure 22.10 by comparing results for anthropomorphic phantoms constructed using the central transverse CT plane of patients treated for the retromolar trigone and nose.[21,26] Dose difference histograms showed maximum errors as large as 10% distal to bone and 18% in the septum for the two phantoms, respectively, the latter of particular clinical significance. Also, PBA dose calculations were compared with measurements in phantoms with rehydrated skeletal bones, eye phantoms for treatment of retinoblastoma[27] and inside the spinal column for craniospinal treatment of medulloblastoma.[6,28]

Impact of Central-Axis Approximation

The PBA was a major step forward for electron beam dose calculations because it provided the first electron dose algorithm that (1) modeled the three main physical

effects impacting electron dose calculations—collisional energy loss, MCS, and inverse square effect, (2) was compatible with CT data modeling the patient, (3) was significantly more accurate than previous algorithms, (4) computed quickly, and (5) was openly available to vendors and researchers. Its practicality has been illustrated by its becoming initially available in the RT/Plan software (General Electric, Medical Systems Division, Milwaukee, WI), the first CT-based commercial electron treatment planning system in 1982,[21] and by its still being the electron dose engine for the Pinnacle[3] treatment planning system (Philips North America LLC, Cambridge, MA) in 2021.

Despite being a major advancement and sufficiently accurate for most patient sites, it has clinically significant errors for some sites due to its use of the central-axis approximation. The dose calculation at each point from a single pencil beam assumes a slab phantom geometry

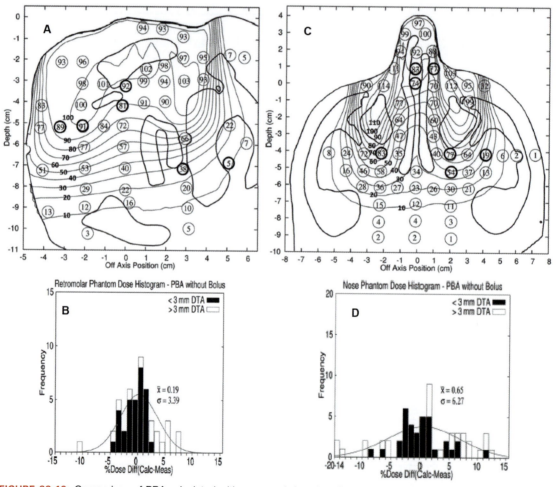

FIGURE 22.10. Comparison of PBA calculated with measured dose in cylindrical anthropomorphic phantoms. **(A)** PBA calculated isodose curves (solid) and measured dose points for retromolar trigone phantom irradiated with a 17 MeV ≈ 8 × 8 cm² field. **(B)** Corresponding dose difference histogram for retromolar trigone phantom dose comparisons. Points having dose difference >5% and DTA >0.3 cm (bold circles) occur distal and lateral to hard bone of mandible and spinal cord. **(C)** PBA calculated isodose curves (solid) and measured dose points for nose phantom irradiated with a 17 MeV ≈ 8 × 8 cm² field. **(D)** Corresponding dose difference histogram for nose phantom dose comparisons. Points having dose difference >5% and DTA >0.3 cm (bold circles) occur in the nasal septum and other tissues distal and lateral to air cavities of the nose and maxillary sinuses. From Carver RL, Hogstrom KR, Chu C, Fields RS, Sprunger CP. Accuracy of pencil-beam redefinition algorithm dose calculations in patient-like cylindrical phantoms for bolus electron conformal therapy. *Med Phys.* Jul 2013;40(7):071720. doi:10.1118/1.4811104.

matching that along the central axis of the pencil beam in the patient (*cf.* Fig. 22.2). This approximation is sufficient so long as the patient anatomy is "slab like," as might be the case for the chest wall. However, it can ignore heterogeneities deep to the patient surface or having long edges near parallel to central axis (*cf.* Fig. 22.2), as might be the case for the external nose and ear or for the spinal column. In such cases, dose inaccuracies can exceed clinically acceptable limits. This limitation was the primary motivation leading to the development of more accurate algorithms such as the PBRA and fast MC algorithms, subsequently described.

PENCIL BEAM REDEFINITION ALGORITHM

The PBRA was so named because it extended the concept of redefining pencil beams at the surface of the patient, a unique feature of the Hogstrom PBA, to continually redefining pencil beams every 0.5 cm in depth. Such redefinition greatly reduced the inaccuracies caused by the central-axis approximation of the PBA. Also different from the PBA, the PBRA computes fluence instead of planar fluence and uses a polyenergetic instead of a monoenergetic energy spectrum. These features result in accuracy better than the PBA and comparable to that of the fast MC algorithms. It offers clinically important advantages of no precision issues, high spatial resolution, fast calculation time that is useful for dose optimization (*e.g.*, BECT), well documented accuracy, and using the same commissioning beam data as the PBA. Presently, a version of the PBRA is used clinically in the p.d bolus design system (.decimal LLC, Sanford, FL).

Theory of Calculation

The PBRA models the same physics as the PBA, continuous energy loss, MCS, and beam divergence, for computing the electron dose component, but differently. It uses the same model for x-ray dose as the PBA. Originally, the PBRA, based on the work of Shiu and Hogstrom,[29] assumed a monoenergetic incident beam; however, this was improved by Boyd et al.[30] by using a polyenergetic incident beam.

In the PBRA, pencil beams are initially defined in the plane of the beam-defining, collimating insert (cutout). Each pencil beam is 0.2 cm square (projected to isocenter), as in the PBA, but the PBRA pencil beams are further partitioned into 1-MeV energy bins. Each pencil beam is characterized by its planar fluence, mean direction using projected angles $\left(\overline{\theta}_x, \overline{\theta}_y\right)$, rms spread about the mean directions $\left(\sigma_{\theta_x}, \sigma_{\theta_y}\right)$, and mean energy $(\overline{E})$. All parameters of the phase space are assumed independent of position in the pencil beam, and all electrons are assumed to have an energy equal to the mean energy of the energy bin.

Initially, the sum of the planar fluences for all energy bins at a single pencil beam location is approximately unity, but weighted for beam nonuniformity. Also, the initial energy distribution is assumed to be independent of the pencil beam location. The mean direction of each pencil beam initially backprojects to the virtual source; however, the rms spread about the mean direction $\left(\sigma_{\theta_x} = \sigma_{\theta_y}\right)$ is independent of position of the pencil beam, but has a 1/E dependence for the different energy bins. The polyenergetic spectrum is extracted from the measured central-axis dose versus depth in water using monoenergetic PBRA-calculated dose versus depth curves. Figure 22.11

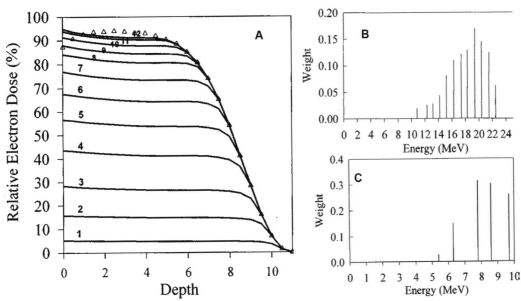

FIGURE 22.11. Initial PBRA energy spectrum. **(A)** PBRA fit (solid lines) to electron component of 20 MeV measured dose versus depth curve in water (Δ). Numbers 1–12 label cummulative sums of differently weighted PBRA calculated, monoenergetic dose versus depth curves. **(B)** Results of 20 MeV fit show magnitude and mean energy in each 1 MeV interval. **(C)** Results of 9 MeV fit show magnitude and mean energy in each 1 MeV interval. From Boyd RA, Hogstrom KR, Rosen II. Effect of using an initial polyenergetic spectrum with the pencil-beam redefinition algorithm for electron-dose calculations in water. *Med Phys.* Nov 1998;25(11):2176–2185. doi:10.1118/1.598414.

Electron Beam

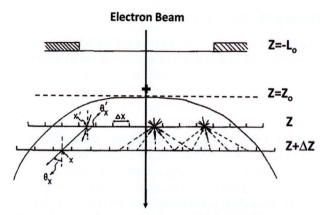

FIGURE 22.12. Illustration of pencil beam redefinition. Electron field defined by cutout at $Z = -L_0$. The electrons are initially transported from the plane of the cutout to the closest plane touching the patient at $Z = Z_0$. Electrons are then sequentially transported from one plane (Z) to the next at $(Z+\Delta Z)$. See text for details. Plus marks isocenter. Modified from Shiu AS, Hogstrom KR. Pencil-beam redefinition algorithm for electron dose distributions. *Med Phys.* Jan–Feb 1991;18(1):7–18. doi:10.1118/1.596697.

Central Axis

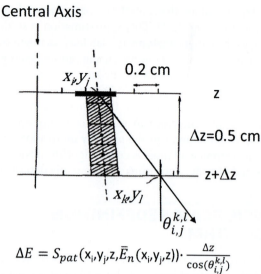

$$\Delta E = S_{pat}(x_i, y_j, z, \bar{E}_n(x_i, y_j, z)) \cdot \frac{\Delta z}{\cos(\theta_{i,j}^{k,l})}$$

FIGURE 22.13. Geometry for transporting planar fluence of pencil beam centered at (x_i, y_j, z) to center of pencil beam at $(x_k, y_l, z + \Delta z)$. This is computed using the mean scattering power in patient along the dashed line through shaded region and by condensing the shaded material to a thin layer (solid black sliver). Energy loss, computed using the mean stopping power in patient along the dashed line through shaded region and the path length connecting the two points, is given by the equation shown. From Shiu AS, Hogstrom KR. Pencil-beam redefinition algorithm for electron dose distributions. *Med Phys.* Jan–Feb 1991;18(1):7–18. doi:10.1118/1.596697.

illustrates initial energy spectra for 9 and 20-MeV beams.[30]

Pencil beams are first transported through air from the secondary collimator (cutout) to the plane intersecting the closest patient point (i.e., non-air voxel) within the radiation beam. There, the pencil beams are redefined, i.e., properties of their phase space are recalculated. Commencing with that plane, the phase space of each pencil beam is transported from z to the next plane at $z + \Delta z$, where the phase space for each pencil beam is recomputed, as illustrated in Figure 22.12. The process from one plane to the next is sequentially repeated until all electrons reach the end of their range.

Each pencil beam at z is transported to the center of each pencil beam at $z + \Delta z$ by condensing the material between the planes into a thin layer at z (*cf.* Fig. 22.13). The PBRA uses the scattering power of that material to determine how much planar fluence each pencil beam at z contributes to the center of each pencil beam at $z + \Delta z$. The energy loss assumes constant collisional energy loss for the patient composition under the pencil beam at z and the path length between the centers of the two pencil beams (*cf.* Fig. 22.13).

Electron dose D^e at the point (x_k, y_l, z) is then computed from the fluence ϕ_m and energy $\bar{E}_m$

$$D^e(x_k, y_l, z) = \sum_{m=1}^{N_e} \phi_m(x_k, y_l, z) \cdot \frac{S}{\rho}(\bar{E}_m) \cdot C(\bar{E}_m), \quad (22.12)$$

where ϕ_m is the electron fluence for the mth energy bin at (x_k, y_l, z), S/ρ is the mass collisional stopping power in water at the mean energy of the bin $\bar{E}_m$, and $C(\bar{E}_m)$ is an energy dependent correction factor that is computed to force the calculated central axis dose versus depth curve in water to best match the measured curve.[30] N_e is the number of 1-MeV energy bins. The fluence is calculated from

electrons of pencil beams at z scattering into the k, l pencil beam at $z + \Delta z$ and falling in the mth energy bin, i.e.,

$$\phi_m(x_k, y_l, z + \Delta z) = \sum_{i=1}^{N_x} \sum_{j=1}^{N_y} \frac{\Delta_m^p(x_k, y_l, x_i, y_j, z + \Delta z)}{\cos(\theta_{i,j}^{k,l})},$$

$$(22.13)$$

where the sum is over the N_x by N_y pencil beams at z, where Δ_m^p is the planar fluence contribution from electrons transported from the pencil beam at (x_i, y_j, z) to the point $(x_k, y_l, z + \Delta z)$ that arrive with an energy in the mth energy bin, and where $\theta_{i,j}^{k,l}$ is the polar angle of the ray from (x_i, y_j, z) to the point $(x_k, y_l, z + \Delta z)$. Details for the calculation of Δ_m^p from the three moments at (x_i, y_j, z) and for the calculation of the new three moments at $(x_k, y_l, z + \Delta z)$ were reported by Shiu and Hogstrom.[29] Electrons are transported according to Gaussian MCS theory, where the linear angular scattering power is extracted from the mean CT number between (x_i, y_j, z) and $(x_i, y_j, z + \Delta z)$, as done in the PBA.

Beam Data Input and PBRA Commissioning

Beam data are the same as that used for the PBA, making the PBRA a plug-in upgrade to the PBA. However, the data are used differently in the calculation. Doses are computed such that 100% equals the "given dose", as in the PBA, so that dose per monitor unit (MU) can be computed using the values entered for dose output as a

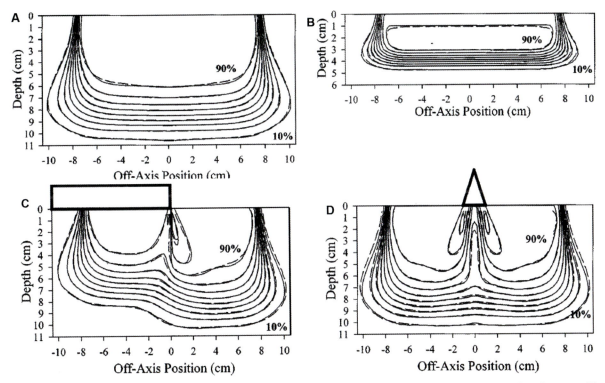

FIGURE 22.14. Comparison of PBRA calculated (solid curves) with measured (dashed curves) dose distributions in water: **(A)** 20 MeV, 100 cm SSD, 15 × 15 cm² field, **(B)** 9 MeV, 100 cm SSD, 15 × 15 cm² field, **(C)** 2-cm stepped surface for 20 MeV, 100 cm SSD, 15 × 15 cm² field, and **(D)** triangular 'nose' surface for 20 MeV, 100 cm SSD, 15 × 15 cm² field. 100% = central axis D_{max} for water phantom only; isodose values every 10%. From Boyd RA, Hogstrom KR, Starkschall G. Electron pencil-beam redefinition algorithm dose calculations in the presence of heterogeneities. *Med Phys.* Oct 2001;28(10):2096–2104. doi:10.1118/1.1406521.

function of SSD, applicator, and square field size for each beam energy. Central-axis dose versus depth in water with SSD at isocenter are stored and assumed independent of applicator, *i.e.*, it is stored for multiple square field sizes at 100 cm SSD. Those curves are used to generate dose versus depth for rectangular fields using the square root method of Hogstrom et al.,[10] from which energy distributions are extracted, as shown in Figure 22.11. The resulting PBRA computed dose versus depth curves do not exactly agree with the measured data for $C(E) = 1$ in equation 22.12; however, a polynomial curve modeling $C(E)$ versus E is determined by a least-squares fit to the measured dose versus depth curve.[30] An off-axis profile at $0.5*R_{90}$ is used to determine the initial beam weighting factors (typically 1.00 ± 0.03) for beam nonuniformity.

The virtual SAD, SAD_{vir}, is the same as that for the PBA, i.e., the initial mean direction of each pencil beam is $\bar{\theta}_{x,0} = \arctan\left(\dfrac{x}{SAD_{vir} - L_0}\right)$ and $\bar{\theta}_{y,0} = \arctan$ $\left(\dfrac{y}{SAD_{vir} - L_0}\right)$. Initially, $\sigma_{\theta_x,0} = \sigma_{\theta_y,0}$, which is independent of pencil beam location. These values, based on those for the PBA, are modified by the mean energy of each energy bin comprising the initial spectrum, *i.e.*, $\sigma_{\theta_x,0}^{PBRA}(\bar{E}_m) = \sigma_{\theta_x}^{PBA} \cdot \left(E_{p,0}/\bar{E}_m\right)$. Lastly, all input data are confirmed by comparing PBRA calculations in water with measured dose distributions and output factors, just as done for the PBA.

Accuracy of the PBRA

The accuracy of the PBRA is well documented. Boyd et al.[31] compared the PBRA calculations with a highly accurate, measured data set[32] for multiple water phantom geometries, i.e., standard and extended SSDs, irregular surfaces, and internal bone and air cavities. The quality of agreement is exemplified for a subset of that data. Figure 22.14 compares PBRA calculated with measured dose in water for 9- and 20-MeV beams incident on a flat surface, and for a 20-MeV beam incident on a stepped surface and a surface simulating a nose. Figure 22.15 compares PBRA calculated with measured dose in water for a 20-MeV beam beneath a bone and air internal heterogeneity. These and other results reported by Boyd et al.[31] showed good agreement, typically more than 97.5% of the dose points in the central region (exclusive of dose fall-off regions) agreeing within 4%.

Accuracy is more relevantly assessed in Figure 22.16 by comparing results for anthropomorphic phantoms constructed using the central transverse CT plane of patients treated for the retromolar trigone and nose.[21,26] These comparisons are for the same measured data set as shown earlier for the PBA, but with significantly better agreement. Dose difference histograms showed all points of comparison to be within 3% or 0.3 cm DTA. Additional comparisons for BECT are discussed in a later section.

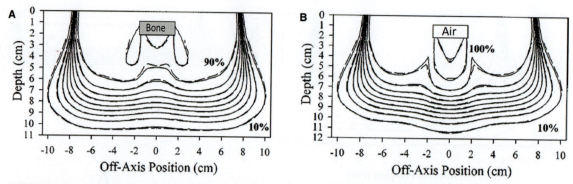

FIGURE 22.15. Comparison of PBRA calculated (solid curves) with measured (dashed curves) dose distributions beneath heterogeneities in water: **(A)** 1 cm thick by 3 cm wide bone material located 1 cm deep in water, 20 MeV, 100 cm SSD, 15×15 cm² field and **(B)** 1 cm thick by 3 cm wide air cavity located 1 cm deep in water, 20 MeV, 100 cm SSD, 15×15 cm² field. From Boyd RA, Hogstrom KR, Starkschall G. Electron pencil-beam redefinition algorithm dose calculations in the presence of heterogeneities. *Med Phys*. Oct 2001;28(10):2096–2104. doi:10.1118/1.1406521.

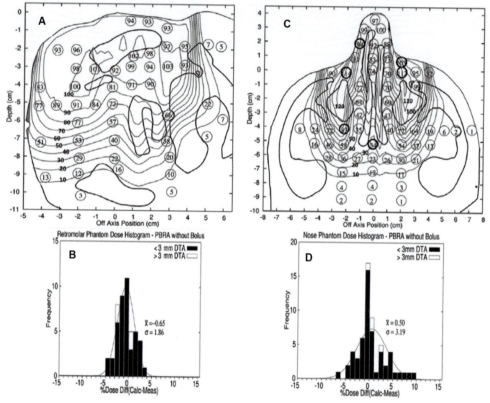

FIGURE 22.16. Comparison of PBRA calculated with measured dose in cylindrical anthropomorphic phantoms. **(A)** PBRA calculated isodose curves (solid) and measured dose points for retromolar trigone phantom irradiated with a 17 MeV ≈8 × 8 cm² field. **(B)** Corresponding dose difference histogram for retromolar trigone phantom dose comparisons. No points have dose difference >5% and DTA >0.3 cm. **(C)** PBRA calculated isodose curves (solid) and measured dose points for nose phantom irradiated with a 17 MeV ≈8 × 8 cm² field. **(D)** Corresponding dose difference histogram for nose phantom dose comparisons. Points having dose difference >5%, but DTA <0.3 cm (bold circles), occur distal to air cavities of the nose and maxillary sinuses and just distal to lateral edge of nose. From Carver RL, Hogstrom KR, Chu C, Fields RS, Sprunger CP. Accuracy of pencil-beam redefinition algorithm dose calculations in patient-like cylindrical phantoms for bolus electron conformal therapy. *Med Phys*. Jul 2013;40(7):071720. doi:10.1118/1.4811104.

Most apropos, Boyd[33] demonstrated PBRA accuracy using patient CT data by comparing PBRA calculated dose with that calculated using EGS4 BEAM and DOSXYZ.[34,35] The EGS4 MC calculations matched the measured data set of Boyd et al.[32] providing confidence

in both measurement and MC calculations. Data for four patient sites—internal mammary chain, ethmoid sinuses, trapezius muscle, and parotid—were compared. Results showed good agreement with dose differences being less than 4% or 0.2 cm DTA for 99%, 97%, 97%, and 96% of the

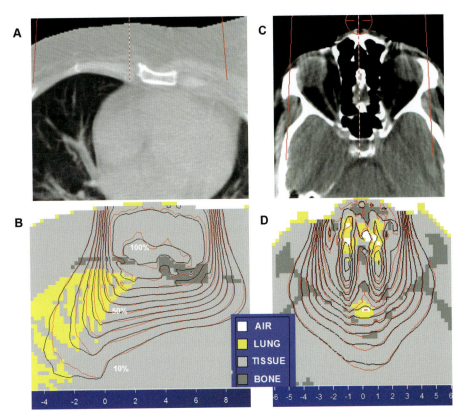

FIGURE 22.17. Comparison of PBRA calculated (black curves) with EGS4 MC calculated (red curves) dose distributions for two patients: **(A)** transverse planar CT image of internal mammary chain patient, **(B)** dose distributions for CT plane above with a 16 MeV, 105 cm SSD beam **(C)** transverse CT planar image of ethmoid sinuses patient **(D)** dose distributions for CT plane above with a 16 MeV, 100 cm SSD beam. Isodose contours every 10% beginning at 10%. From Boyd RA. Pencil-beam redefinition algorithm dose calculations for electron therapy treatment planning. PhD. The University of Texas Graduate School of Biomedical Sciences; 2001.

volume ($D > 5\%$), respectively. Figure 22.17 shows selected planar dose plots for the internal mammary chain and ethmoid sinuses comparisons.

FAST MONTE CARLO ALGORITHMS

MC algorithms have proven accurate and useful for electron beam dose calculations in treatment planning systems. They offer advantages and disadvantages compared to analytical algorithms such as the PBA and PBRA mentioned earlier.

Figure 22.18A shows a measurement of the random tracks of multiple electrons incident on a bubble chamber phantom.[36] Each track is unique because although each electron moves through matter following the same laws of physics, the result of each interaction is random. MC algorithms use pseudo-random numbers (computer-generated numbers uniformly distributed between 0 and 1) to simulate how electron beams interact and contribute dose to a patient on a particle-by-particle basis. For each step, the algorithm computes the electron's next position, direction, and energy using pseudo-random numbers to sample from the probability distributions of those variables, and there are a variety of methods that can be used to do this.[37] Transporting a single electron through its track (history) models multiple interactions (collisional energy loss, MCS, delta ray production, bremsstrahlung energy loss, *etc.*) for many small steps along its path, requiring many random numbers. These simulations can

be very accurate, and Figure 22.18B shows multiple electron tracks (calculated using EGSnrc[38]) that are very consistent with the measured tracks shown in Figure 22.18A. For a more detailed description of the application of the MC method to radiation therapy, the reader is referred to the books by Jenkins et al.[39] and Seco and Verhaegen.[40]

In the MC dose algorithm, the patient (or phantom) is modeled as a 3D array of voxels, each having a specified material (*e.g.*, bone, muscle, fat, or lung) and density, and each track has a unique path through the volume. For each track, the MC algorithm stores the energy $\left(\Delta E_{i,j,k}^{l}\right)$ each particle ($l = 1, N$) deposits in each (i,j,k) voxel it traverses. It then divides the total energy deposited by the mass of the voxel $\left(m_{i,j,k}\right)$ to get total dose deposited, i.e.,

$$D_{i,j,k} = \frac{1}{m_{i,j,k}} \cdot \sum_{l=1}^{N} \Delta E_{i,j,k}^{l}. \qquad (22.14)$$

Note that the PBA, PBRA, and MC algorithms compute average dose to a point, pixel (area), and voxel (volume), respectively. Also, for the PBA and PBRA, dose is the energy per unit mass deposited to the material to which the inputted dose output values are calibrated (e.g., water or muscle); however, for the MC algorithms, dose can be computed to water, muscle, or the material comprising the voxel. Which is selected is important to understand, and users are referred to Kry et al.[41] and their TPS manual for more detail.

Because of the random sampling that is inherent to the MC algorithm, the energy or dose deposited in each voxel varies stochastically (randomly). For example, if the

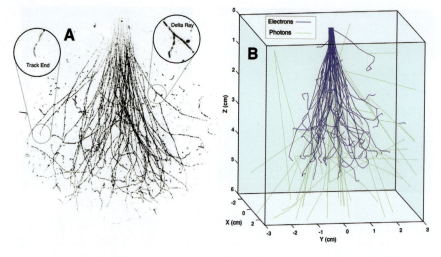

FIGURE 22.18. Random particle tracks, basis of Monte Carlo transport. **(A)** Bubble chamber picture of a 9.3 MeV electron pencil beam in propane (From Harder D, Harigel G, Schultze K. Tracks of fast electrons; pictures of electron and roentgen irradiation of a 35-MeV betatron with a propane-filled bubble chamber. *Strahlentherapie*. May 1961;115:1–21; reproduced with permission of SNCSC.) showing (1) approximately constant energy loss along the track resulting in a relatively constant track width, (2) an approximately constant finite range, (3) a tortuous path caused by multiple Coulomb scattering, and (4) the production of secondary ionizing electrons (delta rays). **(B)** Electron (blue) and photon (green) tracks for a 10 MeV electron pencil beam in water calculated using EGSnrc,[38] showing that detailed Monte Carlo calculations can reproduce realistic electron tracks.

calculation only had 100 tracks and there were 10^6 voxels; then by chance, some voxels would have dose and others none. Hence, there must be an adequate number of tracks to obtain high precision (*e.g.*, 1%). Assuming a 20×20 cm^2 electron field and a voxel dimension of 0.2 cm, the top surface of the calculation volume will have approximately 10^4 voxels within a 20×20 cm^2 field area. The precision of the MC dose calculation is approximately proportional to $(N_v)^{-1/2}$, where N_v is the number of electrons entering the top surface of each voxel. Hence, for a precision of 1%, N_v would have to be approximately 10^4. Over the entire field ($10^2 \times 10^2$ top voxels), there would have to be approximately 10^8 electrons or track histories (10^4/voxel $\times 10^4$ top voxels) computed. This is a large number, so to compute the dose distribution in 100 sec, the track history, which involves many calculations itself, would need to be completed in 10^{-6} sec. Such ability had to be achieved before MC calculations could be practical for the clinic. While the calculation is proceeding, it is possible to estimate the degree of convergence (or uncertainty) in each voxel. Rogers and Mohan[42] suggested that for comparison purposes, a useful measure of the overall uncertainty is the average uncertainty for all voxels with a dose greater than 50% of the maximum dose, and this is the measure of uncertainty used in the RayStation (RaySearch Laboratories AB, Stockholm, Sweden) treatment planning system (TPS) and Eclipse TPS (Varian Medical Systems, Palo Alto, CA), although the latter mistakenly refers to it as accuracy. The XiO TPS (Elekta Instrument AB, Stockholm, Sweden) uses a similar metric, but allows the user to adjust the percentage of maximum dose used in the calculation of the mean uncertainty.

Poor statistics (precision), which arise from the clinical need for short calculation times, result in jagged isodose lines, particularly in areas having low-dose gradient. As illustrated in Figure 22.19, this can be distracting and difficult to interpret for the clinical treatment planner. One solution to improve precision (or statistical noise) is to

increase time of calculation by increasing the number of histories; however, because precision varies as $(N_v)^{-1/2}$, improving the precision by a factor of two requires four times the calculation time. Hence, this might not be practical. Alternatively, statistical noise can be reduced using a smoothing algorithm (*e.g.*, 3D Gaussian); however, it must be done carefully so it does not significantly reduce accuracy,[43] as illustrated in Figure 22.20.

The availability of MC dose calculations for electrons became clinically available around 2000 due to two technological advancements. First was the development of "fast MC" methods, which are found on present TPSs and are further described in later sections. Second was the increased speed of CPUs and the utilization of multiple CPUs (parallel computing).

A full MC calculation requires confidential details of the treatment head configuration in addition to the patient information. Even if the treatment head information was readily available, starting the MC calculation up in the treatment head would be inefficient, since much of the treatment head configuration is invariant from one beam to the next. In general, fast MC algorithms create a source model to describe the electrons emanating from the treatment head, and a separate patient dose calculation using fast MC methods.[44] The two primary fast MC algorithms implemented in commercial TPSs are the Macro Monte Carlo (MMC) algorithm[45] and the Voxel Monte Carlo (VMC) algorithm.[46] The basic implementation of both of these algorithms is described next.

Macro Monte Carlo Algorithm

The MMC algorithm is a fast MC method first reported by Neuenschwander and Born,[45] which is based on the concept of Mackie and Battista[47] of transporting primary electrons in large-scale macroscopic steps through the absorber (patient). Neuenschwander et al.[48] made further improvements, including ability to calculate using CT data.

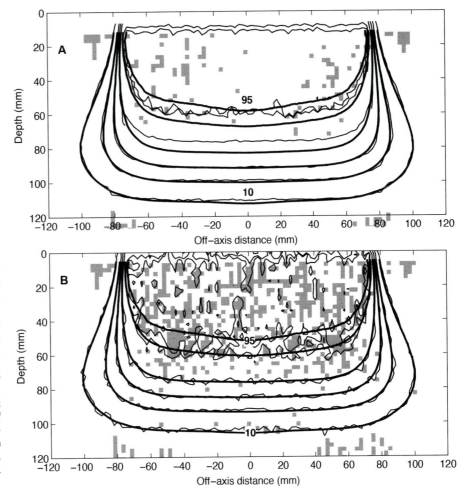

FIGURE 22.19. Comparison of eMC calculated (thin lines) and measured (thick lines) dose for a 20 MeV, 100-cm SSD, 15 × 15 cm² field in water. eMC is calculated with **(A)** 1% and **(B)** 3% statistical precision for (0.25 cm)³ voxels. Isodose curves are 10%, 30%, 50%, 70%, 90%, and 95%. Calculation voxels that violate 3% difference and 0.3 cm distance to agreement (DTA) are shaded gray. From Popple RA, Weinberg R, Antolak JA, et al. Comprehensive evaluation of a commercial macro Monte Carlo electron dose calculation implementation using a standard verification data set. *Med Phys.* Jun 2006;33(6):1540–1551. doi:10.1118/1.2198328.

This algorithm serves as the basis of the electron Monte Carlo (eMC) algorithm currently used in the Eclipse TPS.

The fundamental principle of the MMC is that it precalculates, partitions, and saves the distribution of particles (electrons and photons) exiting a sphere for an electron incident on its polar axis (0°). As illustrated in Figure 22.21A, an electron of initial kinetic energy E_i is incident on a sphere (kugel in German) of radius R, which is composed of a material M (e.g., water, soft tissue, bone, lung) of density ρ. Using EGS4,[34] distributions of electrons exiting spheres have been previously calculated and stored; their distributions are partitioned into final kinetic energy E_f, position as specified by angle of latitude α, and new polar angle θ_f. Azimuthal symmetry is assumed, allowing the azimuthal angle to be randomly selected uniformly during the transport process. This combination of eight parameters requires a large number of one-time precalculations, which are then stored as lookup tables for patient calculations; this is what makes MMC a fast MC algorithm, considerably faster than a MC calculation like EGS4. The MMC algorithm also models secondary electrons (delta rays) and bremsstrahlung x-rays in a simple manner. The difference in the initial and final energy divided by the mass of the sphere computes average dose deposited in the sphere from that electron track.

As discussed earlier, dose is calculated using many electron tracks (or histories) using Equation (22.14). A single history is calculated by stringing together many spheres defining the primary electron track, as illustrated in Figure 22.21B. Each new sphere is oriented such that the electron exiting the previous sphere is incident along the polar axis (i.e., towards the center of the sphere) of the new sphere, and the two spheres intersect at the point where the electron exits the previous sphere. The energy deposited in each sphere is partitioned into voxels intersected by a line segment connecting the entry and exit points of the primary electron in proportion to the product of the line segment through the voxel and the linear stopping power of the voxel.[48] Initially, MMC spheres all had a radius of 0.2 cm; however, for patient calculations Neuenschwander et al.[48] found it beneficial to have adaptive radii (0.05, 0.1, 0.15, 0.2 and 0.3 cm), the smaller values useful where different tissues abut.

Voxel Monte Carlo Algorithm

The Voxel Monte Carlo (VMC) is another useful approach for fast MC calculations in patients. Kawrakow et al.[46] reported the VMC computes approximately 35 times faster than the standard EGS4 MC, making its time of

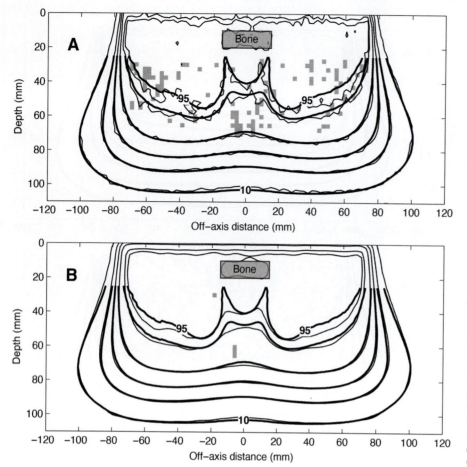

FIGURE 22.20. Comparison of eMC calculated (thin lines) and measured (thick lines) dose for a 20 MeV, 100-cm SSD, 15 × 15 cm² field in water with intervening 1 cm thick by 3 cm wide hard bone material. eMC is calculated with 1% statistical precision for 0.25 cm voxels **(A)** without and **(B)** with smoothing. Isodose lines are 10%, 30%, 50%, 70%, 90%, and 95%. Calculation voxels that violate 3% difference and 0.3 cm distance to agreement (DTA) are shaded gray. Note how the smoothing reduces the fraction of area violating the accuracy standard at the expense of decreasing the magnitude of the "cold spots" inside the edges of the bone. From Popple RA, Weinberg R, Antolak JA, et al. Comprehensive evaluation of a commercial macro Monte Carlo electron dose calculation implementation using a standard verification data set. *Med Phys*. Jun 2006;33(6):1540–1551. doi:10.1118/1.2198328.

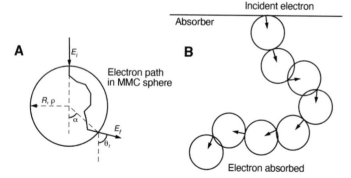

FIGURE 22.21. Principle of MMC. **(A)** For an electron of energy E_i incident on the polar axis of a sphere (kugel) of radius R, density ρ, and material M, the exit energy (E_f), latitude of exit point (α), and polar direction (θ_f) are randomly sampled from precalculated and stored probability distributions. **(B)** String of connected 0.2 cm radius kugels (spheres) specifies a single electron track (history). The exit point and direction of an electron from one kugel specify the location and orientation of the polar axis of the next kugel. The final kugel is when the electron has insufficient energy to exit the kugel. From Neuenschwander H, Born EJ. A macro Monte Carlo method for electron beam dose calculations. *Phys Med Biol*. 1992/01/01 1992;37(1):107–125. doi:10.1088/0031-9155/37/1/007; with permission of IOP Publishing. All rights reserved.

calculation similar to that of the PBAs for 2% precision. However, this was for voxel dimensions of 0.5 cm, which could create inaccuracies near lateral discontinuities in patients. If reduced to the 0.2 cm lateral spatial resolution of the PBA and PBRA, the time of calculation could increase by as much as a factor of six. However, with current computing technology, this presents no known problems. The VMC algorithm (including VMC++ and XVMC) is the basis of the fast MC algorithms currently used in the XiO and RayStation TPSs.

The VMC fast MC algorithm reduces calculation time by a different method than that of the MMC algorithm. Features include (1) approximating MCS with a simpler, Gaussian function, (2) omitting transport of photons from bremsstrahlung in the patient, but modeling its effect on

the electron energy, (3) modeling the x-ray dose from the treatment head (only a few percent of total dose) using a simple model as used by the PBA and PBRA, (4) reducing the total number of steps (increasing distance between interactions) in an electron history, and (5) reusing the same electron history in different patient regions. These modifications are detailed by Kawrakow et al.[46,49]

Commissioning the Fast Monte Carlo Algorithm

Both the MMC and VMC algorithms are designed to speed up the MC calculation inside the voxelized patient geometry and are dependent on an accurate source model to describe the particles incident on the patient. The source model used by the Varian eMC algorithm is based on the work of Janssen et al.,[50] which was improved upon by Fix et al.[51] The former beam model was only applicable to Varian (Palo Alto, CA) linear accelerators, while the latter work generalized the source model so that the eMC algorithm could be applied to linear accelerators from all vendors. As illustrated in Figure 22.22, the beam model includes (1) electron and photons from the primary scattering foils, (2) electrons scattered from the edges of the applicator scrapers, (3) photons that are transmitted though the applicator, and (4) electrons and photons scattering from the jaw faces.

As described by Cygler et al.,[52] the VMC algorithm nominally uses a multi-source model. The source phase space consists of electrons and photons near the scattering foils. The exit phase space, which is the phase space just above the final cutout, is calculated using a dedicated MC code that tracks the source phase space through the collimating geometry. The dedicated code tracks particles that pass through the collimating geometry without interacting with it (the direct component) and those that interact

with it (the indirect component). The indirect component is divided into sub-sources from the various collimating components. The final source is an applicator scatter kernel proposed by Ebert and Hoban[53,54] to account for scattering from the edge of the final electron aperture.

As might be expected, the MMC and VMC source models are similar, as are the data required to commission the source models. While vendor-specific documentation should be consulted for exact details, the measured data usually include data similar to what is documented in the Varian Eclipse Photon and Electron Algorithms Reference Guide,[55] which for each beam energy is:

- Open Field Dose versus Depth Curve: Without an applicator and x-ray jaws open to 40×40 cm^2, dose versus depth on central axis in a water phantom at isocenter (100 cm SSD) is required.
- Applicator Dose versus Depth Curve: For each applicator, dose versus depth on central axis in a water phantom at isocenter (100 cm SSD) is required.
- Dose Output: For each applicator, dose output (cGy/MU) is required.
- Open Field Air Profiles: Without an applicator and x-ray jaws open to 40×40 cm^2, an off-axis scan in air at the location of collimating inserts or cutouts (95 cm source-to-collimator distance, SCD) is required.
- Applicator Air Profiles: For each applicator, with the x-ray jaws at their beam-applicator specific settings, but without the applicator in place, in-plane and cross-plane off-axis scans in air at the location of collimating inserts or cutouts (95 cm SCD) are optional.

In the Eclipse TPS, the measured data are entered by the user into the beam configuration module, and the source model is calculated by the user. For the VMC algorithm, the user measures the data required for the source model, and the vendor prepares and installs the model for the user.[52,56,57] Similar to any other dose calculation algorithm, the user must then validate the accuracy of the source model and dose algorithm together.

Impact of Precision, Voxel Size, and Data Smoothing

The precision of MMC calculations is dependent on the voxel dimension and the number of particle histories, as discussed earlier. Precision of each voxel is computed by subdividing a dose calculation into segments (number of particles) and then computing the standard deviation of the mean for the dose to each voxel. The user specifies the desired precision, e.g., 1%–5%, and this impacts the agreement between measured and calculated dose at each point in the patient, i.e., the respective isodose curves. Figure 22.19 compares the dose distribution measured in water for a 20 MeV beam with the MMC calculation for 1% and 3% specified precision, and there are two noticeable results.[43] First, the MMC dose lines for 3% precision are highly erratic (noisy), particularly for doses greater than

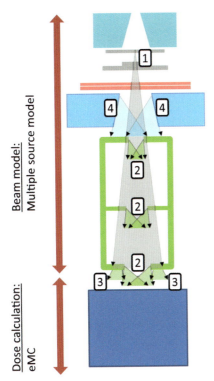

FIGURE 22.22. Schematic overview of the generalized eMC. The upper part shows the different parts of the radiotherapy accelerator treatment head: primary collimator, first scattering foil, second scattering foil, monitor chamber, secondary collimator jaws, and applicator (top to bottom) and the sources of the beam model: (1) the main electron source and the main photon source; (2) edge source of electrons; (3) transmission source of photons; and (4) line source of electrons and photons. The bottom blue box illustrates a water phantom. From Fix MK, Cygler J, Frei D, et al. Generalized eMC implementation for Monte Carlo dose calculation of electron beams from different machine types. *Phys Med Biol.* May 7 2013;58(9):2841–2859. doi:10.1088/0031-9155/58/9/2841; with permission of IOP Publishing. All rights reserved.

80% (low-dose gradient regions). This can be annoying to radiation oncologists and the treatment planning staff, and it makes coverage of the PTV, typically by the 90% dose line, difficult to assess. Second, the statistical noise makes dose readings more inaccurate, causing a greater number of voxels failing dose agreement criteria (e.g., 3% or 0.3 cm DTA).

Statistical noise can be reduced by applying Gaussian smoothing to the dose matrix; however, too much smoothing can come at the expense of blurring sharp dose gradients. Figure 22.20 illustrates this by comparing no smoothing with 3D medium smoothing (convolution with a Gaussian of standard deviation equal to the 0.25 cm grid spacing) for a 20 MeV dose distribution under a bone heterogeneity.

Voxel spacing also impacts the dose calculation. Results of 0.1–0.5 cm spacing showed that too coarse of a spacing led to increased dose calculation error due to how the MMC managed discontinuities in the anatomy like the skin surface or bone-muscle interface. On the other hand, too fine of a spacing significantly increased time of calculation, e.g., from approximately 19 min to 334 min at 20 MeV. Popple et al.[43] stated that the grid spacing should be chosen to be sufficiently small to minimize errors due to uncertainty in the surface position and to appropriately model heterogeneities. They suggested a rule of thumb of approximately $0.1R_{80-20}$, which for 6 and 20 MeV beams is 0.1 and 0.25 cm, respectively.

Popple et al.[43] showed that precision, voxel size, and smoothing of an MMC calculation can significantly impact accuracy, precision, time of calculation, and hence, the utility of the dose calculation. Using current computer hardware and a statistical precision of 1%, calculation times of a few minutes are easily achievable; hence, 1% or better precision is recommended with or without the application of smoothing. It is recommended that selecting the parameters for MMC calculations for the site of interest be well understood and properly used by the treatment planner.

Accuracy of the MMC

The MMC dose calculation can be highly accurate if the algorithm parameters are appropriately selected. Popple et al.[43] demonstrated the accuracy of MMC dose calculations by comparing results of its implementation into Eclipse with the standard data set of Boyd et al.[32] discussed earlier. The quality of agreement is exemplified for a subset of that data, in Figure 22.23 for irregular surfaces of a water phantom at 9 and 20 MeV, and in Figure 22.24 for a 20 MeV beam with internal bone and air heterogeneities. The MMC (eMC) agreed within 3% or 0.3 cm DTA for 99.5% of all dose measurements, when computed using 1% precision (mistakenly called accuracy), 0.1 cm (0.25 cm) grid spacing, and 3D medium smoothing for

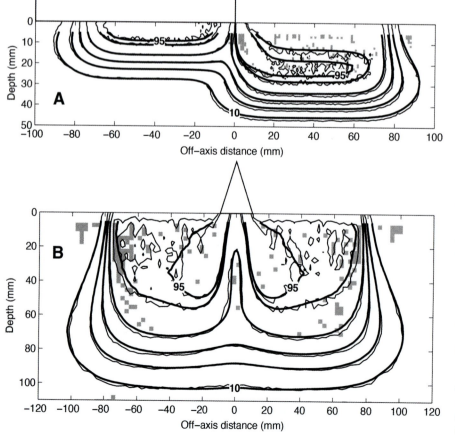

FIGURE 22.23. Comparison of eMC calculated (thin curves) with measured (thick curves) dose distributions in water with irregular surfaces: **(A)** 2-cm stepped surface for 9 MeV, 100 cm SSD, 15 × 15 cm² field. **(B)** Triangular 'nose' surface for 20 MeV, 100 cm SSD, 15 × 15 cm² field. eMC calculation had 1% statistical precision, 0.1 (9MeV) and 0.25 (20 MeV) cm grid spacing, no smoothing. 100% = central axis D_{max} for water phantom only; isodose values are 10%, 30%, 50%, 70%, 90%, and 95%. From Popple RA, Weinberg R, Antolak JA, et al. Comprehensive evaluation of a commercial macro Monte Carlo electron dose calculation implementation using a standard verification data set. *Med Phys.* Jun 2006;33(6):1540–1551. doi:10.1118/1.2198328.

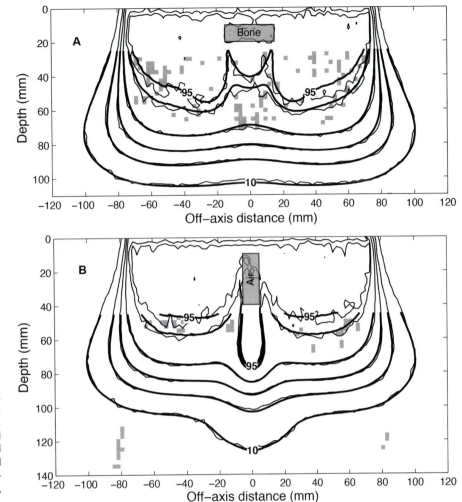

FIGURE 22.24. Comparison of eMC calculated (thin curves) with measured (thick curves) dose distributions beneath heterogeneities in water: **(A)** 1 cm thick by 3 cm wide bone material located 1 cm deep in water, 20 MeV, 100 cm SSD, 15 × 15 cm² field. From Popple RA, Weinberg R, Antolak JA, et al. Comprehensive evaluation of a commercial macro Monte Carlo electron dose calculation implementation using a standard verification data set. *Med Phys.* Jun 2006;33(6):1540–1551. doi:10.1118/1.2198328. **(B)** 3 cm thick by 1 cm wide air cavity located 1 cm deep in water, 20 MeV, 100 cm SSD, 15 × 15 cm² field. eMC calculations had 1% statistical precision, 0.25 cm grid spacing, no smoothing. 100% = central axis D_{max} for water phantom only; isodose values are 10%, 30%, 50%, 70%, 90%, and 95%.

the 9 (20) MeV data in the Boyd et al.[32] data set. Zhang et al.[58] compared eMC calculations with measured profiles under a half-field lung slab for 12 and 16 MeV beams, and results agreed well for all measured profiles. Zhang et al.[58] reported "generally speaking" the eMC to be accurate to within 3% or 0.2 cm DTA.

Accuracy has been further assessed by comparing results for cylindrical anthropomorphic phantoms constructed using the central transverse CT plane of patients treated for the retromolar trigone and nose.[21,26] These comparisons are for the same measured data set as shown earlier for the PBA and PBRA without bolus. Additionally, dose calculated by the PBA, PBRA, and eMC algorithms for BECT in the same phantoms and compared with measured data were reported by Carver et al.[26,59] and will be shown in the subsequent section on BECT.

Accuracy of the VMC

The accuracy of VMC, evaluated by Kawrakow et al.[46] for select geometries with air, lung, and aluminum

heterogeneities, demonstrated a high degree of agreement with respect to EGS4 MC calculations. Fippel et al.[60] compared absolute dose calculations with the measured NCI Electron Working Group data set,[22] which consisted of 28 different geometries simulating electron patient heterogeneities and geometries. VMC calculations were done using 0.5 cm voxels with sufficient histories for 0.7% precision. A subset of these comparisons is provided in Figure 22.25, which for 20 MeV shows comparisons for a water phantom and under a bone heterogeneity mimicking the mandible, and for 9 MeV shows comparisons for an irregular triangular "nose" surface. Good agreement was found between VMC calculation and measured data, for most cases within 3% in low-dose gradient regions and 0.3 cm DTA in high-dose regions. Validation of recent implementations of VMC has been done by Vandervoort et al.[56] for the XiO TPS and Huang et al.[57] for the RayStation TPS; both results showed considerably improved accuracy as compared to the Hogstrom PBA and acceptable accuracy for clinical use.

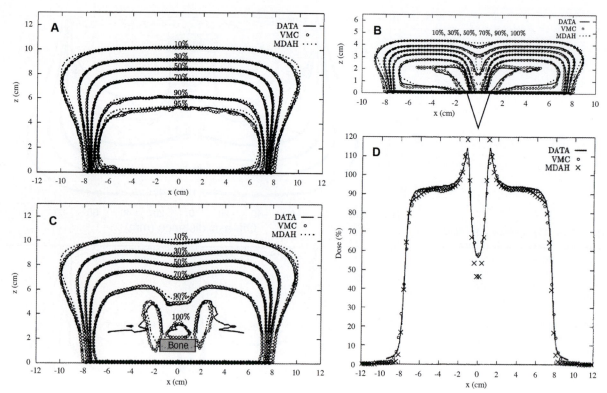

FIGURE 22.25. Comparison of VMC calculated (open circles) with measured (dotted curves) for select data from NCI Electron Collaborative Working Group data set.[22] **(A)** 20 MeV, 100 cm SSD, 15 × 15 cm² field in water. **(B)** 9 MeV, 100 cm SSD, 15 × 15 cm² field with irregular triangular "nose" surface, **(C)** 20 MeV, 100 cm SSD, 15 × 15 cm² field in water with 1 cm thick by 3 cm wide bone material located 1 cm deep in water. **(D)** Off-axis profile at depth z = 1.0 cm in water, distal to irregular triangular "nose" surface above, 9 MeV, 100 cm SSD, 15 × 15 cm² field; MDAH points show PBA[10] calculation for comparison. 100% = central axis D_{max} for water phantom. From Fippel M, Kawrakow I, Friedrich K. Electron beam dose calculations with the VMC algorithm and the verification data of the NCI working group. *Phys Med Biol*. Mar 1997;42(3):501–520. doi:10.1088/0031-9155/42/3/005; with permission of IOP Publishing. All rights reserved.

BOLUS ELECTRON CONFORMAL THERAPY ALGORITHMS

Modulated electron therapy utilizes multiple strategies for achieving electron conformal therapy[9], and one of these, BECT, is presently clinically available. BECT development can be attributed to the availability of accurate dose algorithms (PBRA and fast MC), computerized numerical control (CNC) milling machines for wax boluses,[61,62] 3D printing of boluses using polylactic acid (PLA),[63] and the development of computer algorithms that design bolus for BECT. BECT has been used for multiple clinical sites, e.g., scalp, ear, parotid, buccal mucosa, eye, nose, postmastectomy chest wall, paraspinal muscles, and extremities.[62–70] Fig. 22.26 illustrates use

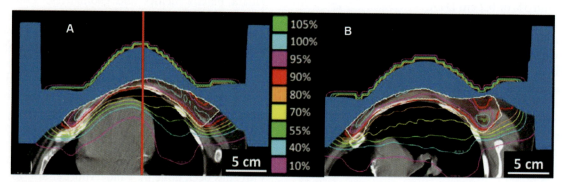

FIGURE 22.26. Postmastectomy dose plan for chest wall using 16 MeV BECT. **(A)** Transverse plane through center of heart demonstrates heart sparing. **(B)** Transverse plane through upper lung demonstrates lung sparing. Modest intensity modulation reduced hot spots in PTV (white contour) near field edges. From Wang SL. Benefits of continuously spaced energies and scanned beams for electron bolus conformal therapy for left-side post-mastectomy chest wall. Louisiana State University and Agricultural and Mechanical College; 2020.

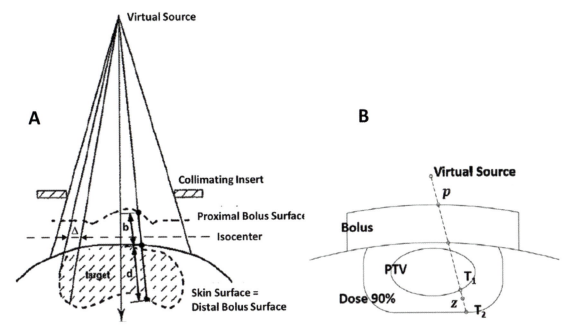

FIGURE 22.27. Electron bolus is designed with a variable thickness b along ray lines from the virtual source through a grid of points at isocenter to the distal surface of the planning target volume (PTV). The bolus is shaped to conform the therapeutic isodose surface (e.g., 90%) to the distal PTV surface. **(A)** Using the Low et al.[71] creation "based on physical thickness" operator, the bolus is created such that $b + d = R_{90}$ for ray lines located a margin Δ inside the outer edge of the PTV, and the bolus height is extended outside the electron field. Modified from Low DA, Starkschall G, Bujnowski SW, et al. Electron bolus design for radiotherapy treatment planning: bolus design algorithms. *Med Phys*. Jan–Feb 1992;19(1):115–124. doi:10.1118/1.596885. **(B)** Contrastingly, Su et al.[63] create the bolus shape by first computing dose without a bolus, then creating bolus thicknesses along ray lines whose radiological thickness equals that in the patient between points (T_1, T_2). From Su S, Moran K, Robar JL. Design and production of 3D printed bolus for electron radiation therapy. *J Appl Clin Med Phys*. Jul 8 2014;15(4):4831. doi:10.1120/jacmp.v15i4.4831. Both methods subsequently modify the created bolus using a sequence of operators that modify bolus thickness to shape the 90% dose contour and smooth its proximal surface to reduce dose heterogeneity in the PTV.

of BECT for the postmastectomy chest wall. Because of the MCS of the electrons, boluses abut the patient skin surface and require complex design algorithms.

Bolus Design Algorithms

These algorithms design a bolus such that the therapeutic isodose surface (e.g., 90% of given dose) conforms to and circumscribes the PTV, providing maximum sparing of distal normal tissues. The bolus is specified by its thicknesses along ray lines from the virtual source, as illustrated in Figure 22.27. Because of MCS, the bolus is best located abutting the patient surface. Also, thickness along each ray line impacts the coverage of the 90% dose along nearby ray lines, making this a complex optimization problem (*cf*. Fig. 22.28).

Low et al.[71] first developed a forward planning algorithm that is comprised of a sequence of operators (creation, modification, and extension) that design the upstream bolus shape. The creation operator creates the

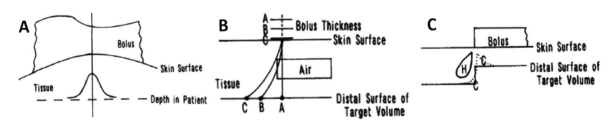

FIGURE 22.28. Challenges in bolus design due to MCS. **(A)** Due an approximately Gaussian spread, electrons from a single pencil beam impact the dose in the nearby lateral volume. **(B)** As the electrons from a single pencil beam travel to nearby points (A, B, C), their mean paths differ, resulting in the impossible need of different bolus thicknesses. **(C)** If a bolus is designed without consideration of MCS, the bolus reflects the shape of the distal surface of the PTV, which can create hot and cold spots. From Low DA, Starkschall G, Bujnowski SW, et al. Electron bolus design for radiotherapy treatment planning: bolus design algorithms. *Med Phys*. Jan–Feb 1992;19(1):115–124. doi:10.1118/1.596885.

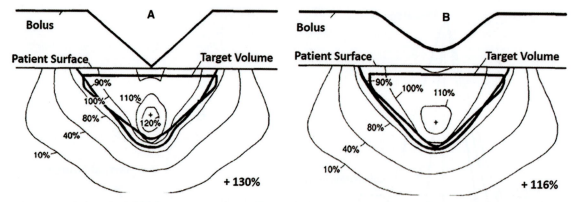

FIGURE 22.29. Example of effect of smoothing modification operator. **(A)** Initial bolus design comparing 90% isodose surface with target volume (home plate shape). The V-shaped bolus creates a hot spot (130%) and the 90% isodose surface overshoots the underlying target volume. **(B)** Applying Gaussian smoothing to the top surface of the bolus improves conformity of the 90% isodose surface to the PTV and reduces the hot spot (116%). From Low DA, Starkschall G, Bujnowski SW, et al. Electron bolus design for radiotherapy treatment planning: bolus design algorithms. *Med Phys.* Jan–Feb 1992;19(1):115–124. doi:10.1118/1.596885.

initial shape by setting the water equivalent bolus thickness (b) plus the physical distance from the skin surface to the distal PTV surface (d) equal to the therapeutic range, e.g., R_{90} along each ray line (*cf.* Fig. 22.27). Modification operators fine tune the bolus surface by smoothing the surface, shifting the surface by different amounts along each ray line, or shifting the surface by the same amount for all ray lines (*cf.* Fig. 22.29). The creation and modification operators only impact bolus design a specified distance (Δ) inside the PTV's outer edge, and the extension operator extends the bolus laterally to just outside the penumbra of the field. Other operators control the bolus shape outside the radiation field, minimizing its size and weight. A useful operator sequence for a specific site can be a good sequence to start planning for a similar, future patient.

Many of the Low et al.[71] operators and an additional marching operator are used in the p.d bolus design software (.decimal LLC, Sanford, FL). The p.d system uses the PBRA to calculate dose during the design process, and upon completion of design it transfers its shape to the cancer center's treatment planning system for dose calculation for the patient chart. The difference between that final dose calculation and that used to design the bolus could be clinically significant if the center is using a TPS with an electron beam dose algorithm not as accurate as the PBRA, such as the PBA.

More recently, Su et al.[63] developed a similar algorithm for bolus design. A major difference in their algorithm (basis of software by Adaptiiv, Halifax, NS, Canada) is that at each stage during the design process it transfers the bolus shape to the TPS for dose calculation, then returns those results to the design algorithm for modifications. Also, its creation operator creates a bolus by computing the radiological path length between the distal PTV surface and the 90% dose surface computed without the bolus in place along each ray line (*cf.* Fig. 22.27B). Subsequent modification and extension operations are similar, to those of Low et al.[71] Either algorithm should design a clinically suitable bolus.

Accuracy of Dose Algorithms for BECT

As the treatment plan becomes more conformal, the accuracy of the dose calculation becomes more important. The accuracy of the PBA, PBRA, and eMC has been investigated by Carver et al.[26,59] for BECT using cylindrical phantoms having transverse cross sections based on the CT scans of a retromolar trigone patient and a nose patient. Isodose plots of the calculated dose distributions are each compared to a set of measured point doses in Figures 22.30 and 22.31 for the retromolar trigone and nose phantoms, respectively. Also shown are the dose difference histograms.

The accuracies of these algorithms are best summarized by the standard deviation (sigma) of the dose difference plots. For the retromolar trigone phantom, in order from most to least accurate, sigmas for the PBRA, eMC, and PBA were 1.78%, 2.55% and 3.27%, respectively. For the nose phantom, sigmas for the PBRA, eMC, and PBA were 1.52%, 3.30%, and 6.01%, respectively. The eMC results were for 1% precision, 0.2 cm grid spacing, and no smoothing. For the nose phantom, adding smoothing worsened accuracy, and using maximum histories (to improve precision) did not improve accuracy.[59]

Future Potential for Intensity Modulated Bolus Electron Conformal Therapy (IM-BECT)

Kudchadker et al.[65] showed that dose heterogeneity created by an irregular bolus surface due to MCS and variance in SSD can be significantly reduced by using intensity modulation with BECT, called IM-BECT. In such case, BECT planning is followed by an intensity modulation operator, which subsequently requires slight modification of the bolus design due to a small, but significant, interdependence between range modulation (bolus) and intensity modulation, as exemplified in Figure 22.32.

IM-BECT gained interest following the development of a passive radiotherapy intensity modulator for electrons

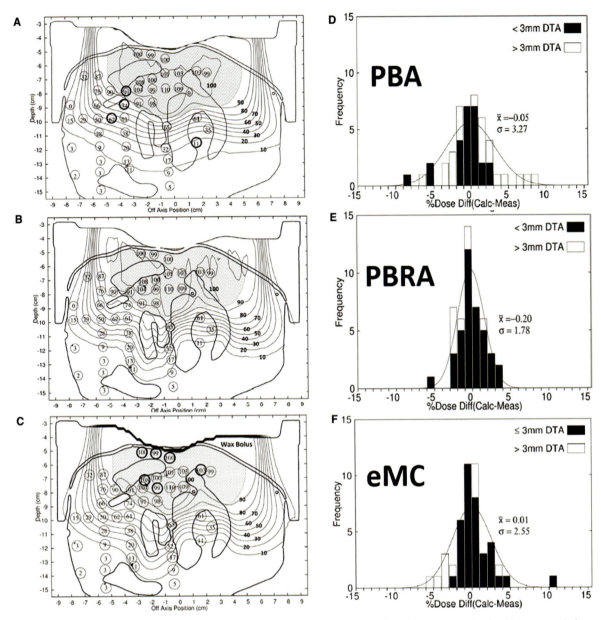

FIGURE 22.30. Comparison of calculated dose distribution (100% = given dose in water phantom) with measured dose points for a BECT plan in a retromolar trigone phantom for **(A)** PBA, **(B)** PBRA, and **(C)** eMC (1% precision, no smoothing, 0.2 cm grid) calculated dose. PTV is shaded gray; bolus is closed outline resting on patient surface. Points having a dose difference >3% and distance to agreement (DTA) >3 mm are indicated by bold circles. **(D)**, **(E)**, and **(F)** show the corresponding dose difference histograms. Portions of histogram shaded black show points within 0.3 cm DTA. Solid curves show Gaussian plots with same mean and standard deviation as data. From Carver RL, Hogstrom KR, Chu C, et al. Accuracy of pencil-beam redefinition algorithm dose calculations in patient-like cylindrical phantoms for bolus electron conformal therapy. *Med Phys.* Jul 2013;40(7):071720. doi:10.1118/1.4811104; Carver RL, Sprunger CP, Hogstrom KR, et al. Evaluation of the Eclipse eMC algorithm for bolus electron conformal therapy using a standard verification dataset. *J Appl Clin Med Phys.* May 8 2016;17(3): 52–60. doi:10.1120/jacmp.v17i3.5885.

(PRIME) device.[72,73] The PRIME device is a set of tungsten pins of varying diameter placed in a hexagonal array located inside the field-defining aperture (cutout). IM-BECT planning and delivery process using PRIME has been demonstrated by Hilliard et al.[74]

IM-BECT is planned by adding an intensity modulation operator to the current BECT forward planning algorithm. The resulting intensity distribution must then be segmented into a hexagonal grid of tungsten island blocks of varying diameters, using an algorithm developed by Chambers;[74,75] optimal pin separation depends on the range of intensity modulation, beam energy, and SSD.[76] Because current treatment planning systems do not manage intensity modulation for electron beams, this feature along with BECT planning tools will have to be added to future electron beam TPSs to support clinical use of IM-BECT.

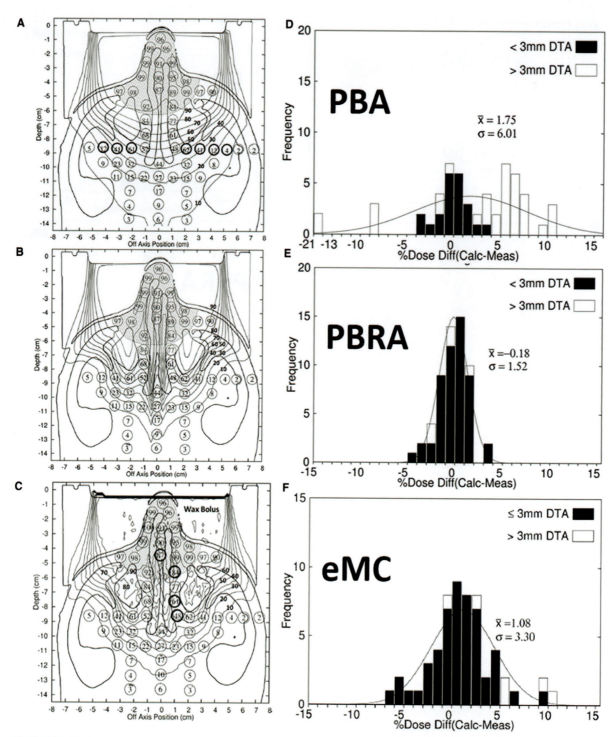

FIGURE 22.31. Comparison of calculated dose distribution (100% = given dose in water phantom) with measured dose points for a BECT plan in a nose phantom for **(A)** PBA, **(B)** PBRA, and **(C)** eMC (1% precision, no smoothing, 0.2 cm grid) calculated dose. PTV is shaded gray; bolus is closed outline resting on patient surface. Points having a dose difference >3% and distance to agreement (DTA) >3 mm are indicated by bold circles. **(D)**, **(E)**, and **(F)** show the corresponding dose difference histograms. Portions of histogram shaded black show points within 0.3 cm DTA. Solid curves show Gaussian plots with same mean and standard deviation as data. From Carver RL, Hogstrom KR, Chu C, et al. Accuracy of pencil-beam redefinition algorithm dose calculations in patient-like cylindrical phantoms for bolus electron conformal therapy. *Med Phys.* Jul 2013;40(7):071720. doi:10.1118/1.4811104; Carver RL, Sprunger CP, Hogstrom KR, et al. Evaluation of the Eclipse eMC algorithm for bolus electron conformal therapy using a standard verification dataset. *J Appl Clin Med Phys.* May 8 2016;17(3):52–60. doi:10.1120/jacmp.v17i3.5885.

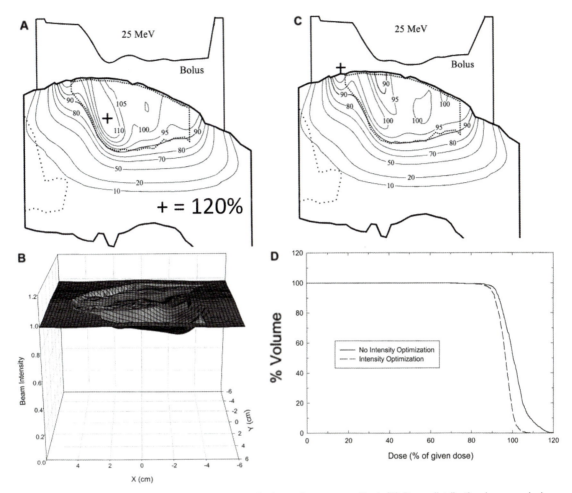

FIGURE 22.32. IM-BECT versus BECT dose plan for buccal mucosa patient. **(A)** Dose distribution in coronal plane for BECT plan shows 90% dose surface conforming to distal PTV (dotted structure) and hot spot of 120%. **(B)** Intensity modulation (80%–100%) is applied to BECT plan (-X is superior). **(C)** Bolus shape is modified in IM-BECT dose plan to restore 90% dose surface conforming to distal PTV. **(D)** Comparison of dose-volume histograms, DVHs for PTV show IM-BECT dose plan has less dose spread with D_{90-10} being reduced from 15% to 9%. From Kudchadker RJ, Hogstrom KR, Garden AS, McNeese MD, Boyd RA, Antolak JA. Electron conformal radiotherapy using bolus and intensity modulation. *Int J Radiat Oncol Biol Phys*. 2002;53(4):1023–1037. doi:10.1016/S0360-3016(02)02811-0.

KEY POINTS

- The <u>pencil beam algorithm (PBA)</u> models irregular fields as a collection of small pencil beams (≈0.2-cm square pixels), and the electron dose at each point in the patient is the sum of dose contribution from each pencil beam.

- Each pencil beam's dose distribution models (1) collisional energy loss along its central axis, (2) lateral spread using Fermi–Eyges multiple Coulomb scattering (MCS) theory, and (3) beam divergence. Using measured central axis dose versus depth in water as input accounts for other physical processes not specifically modeled.

- The PBA can accurately calculate patient dose distributions for irregular field shape, variable SSD (i.e., air gap), oblique incidence, irregular patient surface, and internal patient heterogeneities using CT data. Unique to the Hogstrom PBA, it accurately models the effect

- of irregular patient surface on the dose distribution by redefining pencil beams at the patient surface.

- PBA dose distributions can become unacceptably accurate distal to internal heterogeneities that are deep to the surface or have edges long and parallel to the beam. This is due to its central axis approximation, which assumes a slab phantom geometry for each pencil beam's dose calculation.

- The <u>pencil beam redefinition algorithm (PBRA)</u> differs from the PBA in that it (1) redefines pencil beams every 0.5 cm in depth along central axis, greatly reducing inaccuracies due to the central-axis approximation, (2) partitions pencil beams into 1-MeV energy bins, (3) uses an incident polyenergetic spectrum, and (4) computes dose using fluence, not planar fluence.

● Benefits of the PBRA are (1) its accuracy compares well with that of MC calculations, (2) its commissioning requires the same input data as the PBA, (3) its dose never fluctuates due to stochastic (precision) processes, and (4) its speed makes it useful for optimizing dose distributions, e.g., its use for BECT.

● MC algorithms compute dose by accumulating energy in voxels from multiple electron histories (tracks). Fast Monte Carlo algorithms make approximations that reduce the calculation time for individual tracks.

● The macro Monte Carlo (MMC) algorithm constructs tracks by stringing together many spheres (kugels). The MMC is fast because for spheres of differing radius, tissue type, and density and for an electron of kinetic energy E_i incident along its polar axis, the distribution of exiting electrons partitioned into final kinetic energy, exit latitude, and polar angle is precalculated using EGS4.

● The voxel Monte Carlo (VMC) algorithm reduces calculation time by (1) approximating multiple Coulomb scattering using a Gaussian function, (2) omitting transport of bremsstrahlung photons, (3) modeling x-ray dose from the treatment head using an analytical model, (4) increasing the distance between interactions along an electron track, and (5) reusing the same electron history in different patient regions.

● The number of histories, voxel size, and smoothing of a fast MC calculation should be carefully selected to meet the clinical need for accuracy, precision, and time of a patient dose calculation.

● The commissioning process for the PBA, PBRA, MMC, and VMC and each's accuracy for calculating patient dose is well understood and documented. The PBRA, MMC, and VMC are approximately equally accurate and suitable for all patient dose calculations. The PBA is less accurate, but suitable for patient dose calculation except for some patients having tissue heterogeneities that are deep to the surface or have long edges parallel to central axis.

● Bolus electron conformal therapy (BECT), which reduces dose to distal normal tissue by conforming the dose distribution to the distal PTV surface, requires greater dose calculation accuracy, as provided by the PBRA, MMC, and VMC. Optimization of bolus shape is achieved by application of multiple operators, requiring multiple dose calculations, which benefits from faster algorithms such as the PBRA or fast MC algorithms with multiple processors.

❓ REVIEW QUESTIONS

1. The Hogstrom pencil beam algorithm is least accurate:
   A. In the penumbral region at extended treatment distances
   B. In the penumbral region for irregularly shaped fields
   C. Distal to irregular patient surfaces such as the ear or nose
   D. Distal to air cavities long and parallel to central axis (e.g., those abutting nasal septum)
   E. Distal to lung along central axis of oblique beams irradiating the chest wall

2. Which of the following is not an attribute of the PBA?
   A. Uses Fermi–Eyges MCS theory to determine the Gaussian off-axis dose distribution for each pencil beam at depth
   B. Uses Klein–Nishina theory to determine the off-axis dose distribution of background x-ray beam component
   C. Uses inputted measured central-axis dose versus depth to account for unmodeled physics
   D. Uses tables of relative linear collisional stopping power and relative linear scattering power versus CT number for the kVp used to acquire patient CT scans

3. The feature of the PBRA that most improves accuracy as compared to the PBA is
   A. Redefining pencil beams every 0.5 cm in depth
   B. Computing dose using fluence rather than planar fluence
   C. Modeling the incident beam as polyenergetic rather than monoenergetic
   D. Forcing agreement of calculation with measured central axis dose versus depth in water

4. The PBRA uses measured central-axis dose versus depth in determining all but the following:
   A. Incident polyenergetic spectrum
   B. Energy dependent correction factor forcing calculated to best match inputted, measured central-axis dose versus depth in water
   C. Lateral spread of electrons in a pixel at depth Z to other pixels at depth $Z+\Delta Z$
   D. Background x-ray dose distribution

5. The VMC algorithm is a fast MC algorithm that reduces calculation time by using the following schemes with the exception of
   A. Approximating multiple Coulomb scattering with a simpler, Gaussian function

B. Omitting transport of photons from bremsstrahlung energy loss in the patient

C. Decreasing the distance between interactions in an electron history

D. Reusing the same electron history in different patient regions

6. The MMC algorithm is a fast MC algorithm that reduces calculation time by precalculating, partitioning, and storing the distribution of electrons exiting a sphere of specified radius, material, and density for an electron of initial kinetic energy E_i incident on its polar axis. Resulting distributions are partitioned into all of the following physical quantities for the exiting electron except for

A. Kinetic energy

B. Position as specified by angle of latitude

C. Position as specified by azimuthal angle

D. Direction as specified by polar angle

7. Which of the following does not impact statistical noise (precision) of MC calculated dose?

A. Voxel size

B. Beam energy

C. Number of histories

D. Data smoothing

8. Smoothing of MC calculated dose results in all but which of the following?

A. Increased dose accuracy in high-dose gradient regions

B. Decreased time of calculation for equal precision

C. Blurring of dose in high-dose gradient regions

D. Smoothing kinks in isodose curves in low-dose gradient regions

9. BECT algorithms select and design a bolus shape of varying thickness using a forward planning process. Which of the following best describes such algorithms?

A. Creation operator only; followed by single dose calculation

B. Dose calculation followed by single modification operator; followed by second dose calculation

C. Creation operator followed by modification operators; dose calculation after each operator

D. Creation operator followed by modification operators; dose calculation after final operator only

10. BECT requires accurate dose algorithms. Which of the current electron beam dose algorithms is least accurate and potentially insufficiently accurate for some BECT patient treatments? Which of the current electron beam algorithms has been demonstrated most accurate for BECT in a nose phantom?

A. PBRA, MMC

B. MMC, PBRA

C. PBA, MMC

D. PBA, PBRA

ANSWERS

1. **D**
2. **B**
3. **A**
4. **C**
5. **C**
6. **C**
7. **B**
8. **A**
9. **C**
10. **D**

REFERENCES

1. Sternick E. Algorithms for computerized treatment planning. In: Orton CG, Bagne F, eds. *Practical aspects of electron beam treatment planning*. American Institute of Physics; 1978;2:52.

2. Kawachi K. Calculation of electron dose distribution for radiotherapy treatment planning. *Phys Med Biol*. Jul 1975;20(4):571–577. doi:10.1088/0031-9155/20/4/004.

3. Andreo P. Broad beam approaches to dose computation and their limitations. In: Nahum AE, ed. *The Computation of dose distributions in electron beam radiotherapy*. Umeå University; 1985:128–150.

4. Steben JD, Ayyangar K, Suntharalingam N. Betatron electron beam characterisation for dosimetry calculations. Research Support, U.S. Gov't, P.H.S. *Phys Med Biol*. Mar 1979;24(2):299–309. doi:10.1088/0031-9155/24/2/006.

5. Eyges L. Multiple scattering with energy loss. *Phys Rev*. 1948;74:1534–1535.

6. Hogstrom KR, Steadham RE. Electron Beam Dose Computation. In: Palta J, Mackie TR, eds. *Teletherapy: Present and Future*. Madison, WI: Advanced Medical Publishing; 1996:137–174.

7. Van Dyk J, Barnett RB, Cygler JE, Shragge PC. Commissioning and quality assurance of treatment planning computers. *Int J Radiat Oncol Biol Phys*. May 20 1993;26(2):261–273. doi:10.1016/0360-3016(93)90206-b.

8. Möller TR, Rosenow U, Bentley RE, et al. *ICRU Report 42: Use of computers in external beam radiotherapy procedures with high-energy photons and electrons*. 1987:70. ICRU report. 42.

9. Hogstrom KR, Antolak JA, Kudchadker RJ, Ma CM, Leavitt DD. Modulated Electron Therapy. In: Palta JR, Mackie TR, eds. *Intensity-Modulated Radiation Therapy:The State of the Art*. Madison, WI: Medical Physics Publishing; 2003:749–786.

10. Hogstrom KR, Mills MD, Almond PR. Electron beam dose calculations. *Phys Med Biol*. May 1981;26(3):445–59. doi:10.1088/0031-9155/26/3/008.

11. Perry DJ, Holt JG. A model for calculating the effects of small inhomogeneities on electron beam dose distributions. *Med Phys*. May-Jun 1980;7(3):207–215. doi:10.1118/1.594687.

12. Svensson H, Almond P, Brahme A, Dutreix A, Leetz HK. *Radiation dosimetry: electron beams with energies between 1 and 50 MeV*. 1984. ICRU Report 35.

13. Lax I, Brahme A, Andreo P. Electron beam dose planning using Gaussian beams. Improved radial dose profiles. *Acta Radiol Suppl*. 1983;364(1):49–59.

14. Werner BL, Khan FM, Deibel FC. A model for calculating electron beam scattering in treatment planning. *Med Phys*. Mar-Apr 1982;9(2):180–7. doi:10.1118/1.595157.

15. Hogstrom KR. Evaluation of electron pencil beam dose calculation. In: Kereiakes JG, Elson HR, Born CG, eds. *Radiation Oncology Physics (Medical Physics Monograph No 15)*. American Institute of Physics; 1987:532–557.

16. Starkschall G, Shiu AS, Bujnowski SW, Wang LL, Low DA, Hogstrom KR. Effect of dimensionality of heterogeneity corrections on the implementation of a three-dimensional electron pencil-beam algorithm. *Phys Med Biol*. Feb 1991;36(2):207–227. doi:10.1088/0031-9155/36/2/006.

17. Shiu AS. *Three-dimensional electron beam dose calculations*. Houston, TX: The University of Texas Graduate School of Biomedical Sciences; 1988.

18. Hogstrom KR, Kurup RG, Shiu AS, Starkschall G. A two-dimensional pencil-beam algorithm for calculation of arc electron dose distributions. *Phys Med Biol*. Mar 1989;34(3):315–341. doi:10.1088/0031-9155/34/3/005.

19. Meyer JA, Palta JR, Hogstrom KR. Demonstration of relatively new electron dosimetry measurement techniques on the Mevatron 80. *Med Phys*. Sep-Oct 1984;11(5):670–677. doi:10.1118/1.595550.

20. Hogstrom KR, Steadham RE, Wong PF, Shiu AS. Monitor Unit Calculations for Electron Beams. In: Gibbons JP, ed. *Monitor Unit Calculations for External Photon and Electron Beams*. Advanced Medical Publishing, Inc.; 2000:113–125.

21. Hogstrom KR, Mills MD, Meyer JA, et al. Dosimetric evaluation of a pencil-beam algorithm for electrons employing a two-dimensional heterogeneity correction. *Int J Radiat Oncol Biol Phys*. Apr 1984;10(4):561–569. doi:10.1016/0360-3016(84)90036-1.

22. Shiu AS, Tung S, Hogstrom KR, et al. Verification data for electron beam dose algorithms. *Med Phys*. May-Jun 1992;19(3):623–636. doi:10.1118/1.596808.

23. McShan DL, Fraass BA, Ten Haken RK. Dosimetric verification of a 3-D electron pencil beam dose calculation algorithm. *Med Phys*. Jan 1994;21(1):13–23. doi:10.1118/1.597363.

24. Cheng A, Harms WB, Sr., Gerber RL, Wong JW, Purdy JA. Systematic verification of a three-dimensional electron beam dose calculation algorithm. *Med Phys*. May 1996;23(5):685–693. doi:10.1118/1.597714.

25. Shiu AS, Hogstrom KR. Dose in bone and tissue near bone-tissue interface from electron beam. *Int J Radiat Oncol Biol Phys*. Aug 1991;21(3):695–702. doi:10.1016/0360-3016(91)90688-z.

26. Carver RL, Hogstrom KR, Chu C, Fields RS, Sprunger CP. Accuracy of pencil-beam redefinition algorithm dose calculations in patient-like cylindrical phantoms for bolus electron conformal therapy. *Med Phys*. Jul 2013;40(7):071720. doi:10.1118/1.4811104.

27. Kirsner SM, Hogstrom KR, Kurup RG, Moyers MF. Dosimetric evaluation in heterogeneous tissue of anterior electron beam irradiation for treatment of retinoblastoma. *Med Phys*. Sep-Oct 1987;14(5):772–779. doi:10.1118/1.596002.

28. Dominiak GS. *Dose in spinal cord following electron irradiation*. Houston, TX: The University of Texas Graduate School of Biomedical Sciences; 1991.

29. Shiu AS, Hogstrom KR. Pencil-beam redefinition algorithm for electron dose distributions. *Med Phys*. Jan-Feb 1991;18(1):7–18. doi:10.1118/1.596697.

30. Boyd RA, Hogstrom KR, Rosen II. Effect of using an initial polyenergetic spectrum with the pencil-beam redefinition algorithm for electron-dose calculations in water. *Med Phys*. Nov 1998;25(11):2176–2185. doi:10.1118/1.598414.

31. Boyd RA, Hogstrom KR, Starkschall G. Electron pencil-beam redefinition algorithm dose calculations in the presence of heterogeneities. *Med Phys*. Oct 2001;28(10):2096–2104. doi:10.1118/1.1406521.

32. Boyd RA, Hogstrom KR, Antolak JA, Shiu AS. A measured data set for evaluating electron-beam dose algorithms. refereed paper/manuscript. *Med Phys*. Jun 2001;28(6):950–958. doi:10.1118/1.1374245.

33. Boyd RA. *Pencil-beam redefinition algorithm dose calculations for electron therapy treatment planning*. PhD. Houston, TX: The University of Texas Graduate School of Biomedical Sciences; 2001.

34. Nelson WR, Hirayama H, Rogers DWO. *The EGS4 code system*. 1985. SLAC Report 265.

35. Rogers DW, Faddegon BA, Ding GX, Ma CM, We J, Mackie TR. BEAM: a Monte Carlo code to simulate radiotherapy treatment units. *Med Phys*. May 1995;22(5):503–524. doi:10.1118/1.597552.

36. Harder D, Harigel JG, Schultze K. [Tracks of fast electrons; pictures of electron and roentgen irradiation of a 35-MeV betatron with a propane-filled bubble chamber]. *Strahlentherapie*. May 1961;115:1–21.

37. Haghighat A. *Monte Carlo methods for particle transport*. Boca Raton, FL: CRC Press; 2016.

38. Kawrakow I, Mainegra-Hing E, Rogers DWO, Tessier F, Walters BRB. *The EGSnrc Code System: Monte Carlo simulation of electron and photon transport*. 2017. PIRS-701. http://nrc-cnrc.github.io/EGSnrc/doc/pirs701-egsnrc.pdf.

39. Jenkins TM, Nelson WR, Rindi A. *Monte Carlo transport of electrons and photons*. Ettore Majorana international science series Physical sciences. New York, NY: Plenum Press; 1988:638.

40. Seco J, Verhaegen F. *Monte Carlo techniques in radiation therapy*. Imaging in medical diagnosis and therapy. Boca Raton, FL: CRC Press/Taylor; 2013:318.

41. Kry SF, Feygelman V, Balter P, et al. AAPM Task Group 329: Reference dose specification for dose calculations: Dose-to-water or dose-to-muscle? *Med Phys*. Mar 2020;47(3):e52–e64. doi:10.1002/mp.13995.

42. Rogers DWO, Mohan R. Questions for comparison of clinical Monte Carlo codes. In: Schlegel W, Bortfeld T, eds. *The Use of Computers in Radiation Therapy*. Springer-Verlag; 2000:120–122.

43. Popple RA, Weinberg R, Antolak JA, et al. Comprehensive evaluation of a commercial MMC electron dose calculation implementation using a standard verification data set. *Med Phys*. Jun 2006;33(6):1540–1551. doi:10.1118/1.2198328.

44. Jabbari K. Review of fast monte carlo codes for dose calculation in radiation therapy treatment planning. *J Med Signals Sens*. Jan 2011;1(1):73–86.

45. Neuenschwander H, Born EJ. A MMC method for electron beam dose calculations. *Phys Med Biol*. Jan 01 1992;37(1):107–125. doi:10.1088/0031-9155/37/1/007.

46. Kawrakow I, Fippel M, Friedrich K. 3D electron dose calculation using a Voxel based Monte Carlo algorithm (VMC). *Med Phys*. Apr 1996;23(4):445–457. doi:10.1118/1.597673.

47. Mackie TR, Battista JJ. A macroscopic Monte Carlo method for electron beam dose calculations: a proposal. In: *Proc. 8th Conf. on Use of Computers in Radiation Therapy (Toronto, 1984)*. Silver Spring, MD: IEEE Computer Society Press; 1984:123–127.

48. Neuenschwander H, Mackie TR, Reckwerdt PJ. MMC--a high-performance Monte Carlo code for electron beam treatment planning. *Phys Med Biol*. Apr 1995;40(4):543–574. doi:10.1088/0031-9155/40/4/005.

49. Kawrakow I. Improved modeling of multiple scattering in the Voxel Monte Carlo model. *Med Phys*. Apr 1997;24(4):505–517. doi:10.1118/1.597933.

50. Janssen JJ, Korevaar EW, van Battum LJ, Storchi PR, Huizenga H. A model to determine the initial phase space of a clinical electron beam from measured beam data. *Phys Med Biol*. Feb 2001; 46(2):269–286. doi:10.1088/0031-9155/46/2/301.

51. Fix MK, Cygler J, Frei D, et al. Generalized eMC implementation for Monte Carlo dose calculation of electron beams from different machine types. *Phys Med Biol*. May 7 2013;58(9):2841–2859. doi:10.1088/0031-9155/58/9/2841.

52. Cygler JE, Daskalov GM, Chan GH, Ding GX. Evaluation of the first commercial Monte Carlo dose calculation engine for electron

beam treatment planning. *Med Phys.* Jan 2004;31(1):142–153. doi:10.1118/1.1633105.

53. Ebert MA, Hoban PW. A Monte Carlo investigation of electron-beam applicator scatter. *Med Phys.* Sep 1995;22(9):1431–1435. doi:10.1118/1.597414.

54. Ebert MA, Hoban PW. A model for electron-beam applicator scatter. *Med Phys.* Sep 1995;22(9):1419–1429. doi:10.1118/1.597415.

55. Systems VM. *Eclipse Photon and Electron Algorithms 15.5 Reference Guide.* Varian Medical Systems; 2017:332–332.

56. Vandervoort EJ, Tchistiakova E, La Russa DJ, Cygler JE. Evaluation of a new commercial Monte Carlo dose calculation algorithm for electron beams. *Med Phys.* Feb 2014;41(2):021711. doi:10.1118/1.4853375.

57. Huang JY, Dunkerley D, Smilowitz JB. Evaluation of a commercial Monte Carlo dose calculation algorithm for electron treatment planning. *J Appl Clin Med Phys.* Jun 2019;20(6):184–193. doi: 10.1002/acm2.12622.

58. Zhang A, Wen N, Nurushev T, Burmeister J, Chetty IJ. Comprehensive evaluation and clinical implementation of commercially available Monte Carlo dose calculation algorithm. *J Appl Clin Med Phys.* Mar 4 2013;14(2):4062. doi:10.1120/jacmp.v14i2.4062.

59. Carver RL, Sprunger CP, Hogstrom KR, Popple RA, Antolak JA. Evaluation of the Eclipse eMC algorithm for bolus electron conformal therapy using a standard verification dataset. *J Appl Clin Med Phys.* May 8 2016;17(3):52–60. doi:10.1120/jacmp.v17i3.5885.

60. Fippel M, Kawrakow I, Friedrich K. Electron beam dose calculations with the VMC algorithm and the verification data of the NCI working group. *Phys Med Biol.* Mar 1997;42(3):501–520. doi:10.1088/0031-9155/42/3/005.

61. Low DA, Hogstrom KR. Determination of the relative linear collision stopping power and linear scattering power of electron bolus material. *Phys Med Biol.* Jun 1994;39(6):1063–1068. doi:10.1088/0031-9155/39/6/012.

62. Low DA, Starkschall G, Sherman NE, Bujnowski SW, Ewton JR, Hogstrom KR. Computer-aided design and fabrication of an electron bolus for treatment of the paraspinal muscles. *Int J Radiat Oncol Biol Phys.* 1995;33(5):1127–1138.

63. Su S, Moran K, Robar JL. Design and production of 3D printed bolus for electron radiation therapy. *J Appl Clin Med Phys.* Jul 8 2014;15(4):4831. doi:10.1120/jacmp.v15i4.4831.

64. Perkins GH, McNeese MD, Antolak JA, Buchholz TA, Strom EA, Hogstrom KR. A custom three-dimensional electron bolus technique for optimization of postmastectomy irradiation. *Int J Radiat Oncol Biol Phys.* 2001/11/15/ 2001;51(4):1142–1151. doi:10.1016/S0360-3016(01)01744-8.

65. Kudchadker RJ, Hogstrom KR, Garden AS, McNeese MD, Boyd RA, Antolak JA. Electron conformal radiotherapy using bolus and intensity modulation. *Int J Radiat Oncol Biol Phys.* 2002/07/15/ 2002;53(4):1023–1037. doi:10.1016/S0360-3016(02)02811-0.

66. Kudchadker RJ, Antolak JA, Morrison WH, Wong PF, Hogstrom KR. Utilization of custom electron bolus in head and neck radiotherapy. refereed paper/manuscript. *J Appl Clin Med Phys.* Autumn 2003;4(4):321–333. doi:10.1120/1.1621494.

67. Zeidan OA, Chauhan BD, Estabrook WW, Willoughby TR, Manon RR, Meeks SL. Image-guided bolus electron conformal therapy - a case study. *J Appl Clin Med Phys.* Oct 7 2010;12(1):3311. doi:10.1120/jacmp.v12i1.3311.

68. Kim MM, Kudchadker RJ, Kanke JE, Zhang S, Perkins GH. Bolus electron conformal therapy for the treatment of recurrent inflammatory breast cancer: a case report. *Med Dosim.* Summer 2012;37(2):208–213. doi:10.1016/j.meddos.2011.07.004.

69. Opp D, Forster K, Li W, Zhang G, Harris EE. Evaluation of bolus electron conformal therapy compared with conventional techniques for the treatment of left chest wall postmastectomy in patients with breast cancer. *Med Dosim.* Winter 2013;38(4): 448–453. doi:10.1016/j.meddos.2013.08.002.

70. Wang SL. *Benefits of continuously spaced energies and scanned beams for electron bolus conformal therapy for left-side post-mastectomy chest wall.* Baton Rouge, LA: Louisiana State University and Agricultural and Mechanical College; 2020.

71. Low DA, Starkschall G, Bujnowski SW, Wang LL, Hogstrom KR. Electron bolus design for radiotherapy treatment planning: bolus design algorithms. *Med Phys.* Jan-Feb 1992;19(1):115–124. doi:10.1118/1.596885.

72. Hogstrom KR, Carver RL, Chambers EL, Erhart K. Introduction to passive electron intensity modulation. *J Appl Clin Med Phys.* Nov 2017;18(6):10–19. doi:10.1002/acm2.12163.

73. Hogstrom KR, Carver RL, inventors; PRIME. USA patent 10,751,549. patent application 16/039,251. August 25, 2020.

74. Hilliard EN, Carver RL, Chambers EL, Kavanaugh J, Erhart K, Hogstrom KR. Planning and delivery of intensity modulated bolus electron conformal therapy. *J Appl Clin Med Phys.* 2021; In press.

75. Chambers EL. *Design of a passive intensity modulation device for bolus electron conformal therapy.* Baton Rouge, LA: Louisiana State University and Agricultural and Mechanical College; 2016.

76. Chambers EL, Carver RL, Hogstrom KR. Useful island block geometries of a passive intensity modulator used for intensity-modulated bolus electron conformal therapy. *J Appl Clin Med Phys.* Dec 2020;21(12):131–145. doi:10.1002/acm2.13079.

Hanne M. Kooy, Benjamin M. Clasie, and Nicolas Depauw

INTRODUCTION

A clinical dose computation algorithm must satisfy requirements such as clinical accuracy in the patient, computational performance, representations of patient devices and delivery equipment, and specification of the treatment field in terms of equipment input parameters. A dose algorithm has been invariably imbedded within a larger treatment planning system (TPS) whose requirements and behavior often affect the dose algorithm. Current clinical emphasis on the patient workflow and advanced delivery technologies such as adaptive radiotherapy require different dose algorithm implementations and deployments depending on the context. For example, a treatment planner needs highly interactive dose computation and optimization in a patient to allow rapid evaluation of a clinical treatment plan. A quality assurance physicist, on the other hand, needs an accurate dose algorithm whose requirements could be simplified considering that Quality Assurance (QA) measurements are typically done in simple homogeneous phantoms.

Phenomenological models and Monte Carlo are the two methods to compute dose in patient. The first relies on pencil-beam models that decompose the field in narrow (in the isocentric plane) beamlets. Each pencil beam is transported through the patient by considering the physics interactions along the pencil-beam axis. A pencil-beam model typically models the external patient devices as changes in the pencil-beam parameters. A Monte Carlo uses a large number (10^6) of individual particles, each of which is traced through the patient. The particle trace is fragmented at particle interaction points and geometry boundaries and particle physics parameters are adjusted along each fragment. Pencil-beam models are being replaced by Monte Carlo models given the comparable computational performance afforded by (for example) Graphics Processing Unit (GPU) hardware.

Modern calculation algorithms and Monte Carlo should yield dose representations appropriate for calculation optimization functions. Such a representation maintains the dose response of a particular dose-delivery device control element (a multi-leaf collimator settings or a proton scanning spot). This requires a significant indexing overhead for such calculations compared to traditional bulk dose calculations.

For rapid dose calculation inside an optimization loop it is necessary to index fractional dose per control element. For protons, the dose to a point i is the sum over the product of the spot j charge Q_j and the unit-charge spot dose evolution D_{ij} to each point i in the patient

$$D_i = \Sigma j Q_j D_{ij} \qquad (23.1)$$

The proton D_{ij} matrices are sparse but, for protons, very large (O(10,000–100,000 MB)). Other scalar quantities such as LET (the mean rate of energy loss of a particle per unit length of its track) can similarly be computed (see below). The matrices allow an optimization algorithm, deep inside the inner loops, to rapidly obtain the dose given new optimized parameters.

This chapter describes the physical processes of proton transport, phenomenological and Monte Carlo models, implementation detail (primarily through analytical forms) and results for these models.

PHYSICS OF PROTON TRANSPORT IN MEDIUM

Interactions

The physics of proton interactions for clinical energies, that is, between 50 and 350 MeV, is well understood. The publication "Passive Beam Spreading in Proton Radiation Therapy" by Bernard Gottschalk[7] is an in-depth elaboration of this physics.

Protons lose energy in medium through interactions with orbital electrons, scatter through electromagnetic Coulomb interactions with the nuclear electric field, and have inelastic interactions with the nucleus. Proton–electron interactions produce delta electrons that deposit dose in proximity to the proton geometric track. The mass of the proton is about 2,000 times that of the electron and hence the collision is analogous to a blue whale moving at near-relativistic speed toward you: the proton scatters minimally. Proton–nucleus Coulomb interactions result in small angular deviations in the proton direction and produce a Gaussian diffusion profile in a narrow parallel beam of protons. The Gaussian form is a consequence of the large number of scattering events, which, as described by the central limit theorem, approximate to a continuous Gaussian function.

Protons have inelastic interactions with the nucleus and produce secondary protons, neutrons and α particles. The secondary protons contribute up to 10% of the dose within a proton depth dose.[3] The long-range effect of secondary neutron production is of specific concern. These neutrons deposit dose to healthy tissues throughout the patient, far from the target region, and impact on the shielding requirements of a proton therapy facility. The neutron contribution to the dose distribution is only considered implicitly through their contribution in the physics parameters such as a depth-dose distribution. The effect of heavier secondaries can be ignored for dose calculation purposes.

Stopping Power

The proton energy is reduced in electromagnetic interactions that transfer energy to electrons in the medium. The proton stopping power S to the medium is the rate of energy loss per unit length and defined in combination with the local material density ρ (g/cm^3)

$$\frac{S}{\rho} = -\frac{1}{\rho}\frac{dE}{dx}(\text{MeV cm}^2/\text{g}) \qquad (23.2)$$

The mass stopping power in Equation 23.2 is a function of the proton energy E and increases significantly near the end of the proton track. The proton mass stopping power can be calculated using the Bethe-Bloch equation[1]

or from tables.[13,15] The rapid increase in energy loss per unit length, combined with minimal proton scatter, leads to the characteristic Bragg peak of the proton depth-dose distribution (see Fig. 23.1 for individual Bragg peaks that comprise a spread-out Bragg peak [SOBP]). A Bragg peak is a characteristic feature of all charged particles but disappears for electrons due to their large scattering angle. The track "tangles-up" and the Bragg peak averages out over all the entwined tracks. Thus, a monoenergetic electron depth-dose distribution has a broad and flat high-dose region followed by the Bragg-like distal falloff.

The proton mass stopping power is analogous to the photon mass attenuation. Protons can be used, like X-rays, for tomography and measure the mass attenuation power for a patient directly.[4] Such an image measures the energy loss, a function of the integrated stopping power, along a particular proton ray instead of an attenuation loss, a function of the integrated electron density, along an X-ray. The reconstructed tomographic image is thus a stopping power distribution. There is considerable interest in this technology to improve range precision (estimated at 2%–3%[22]) with volumetric imaging at very low doses.[29]

Relative Biological Effectiveness

Clinically, the proton physical dose (in Gy) is scaled by a relative biological effectiveness (RBE) factor of 1.1 to yield the proton biological dose with units of Gy (RBE).[14] Thus,

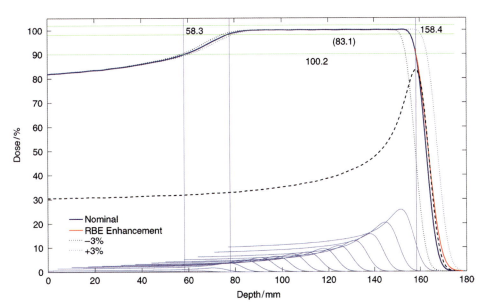

FIGURE 23.1. An SOBP depth-dose distribution with its constituent pristine Bragg peak depth-dose distributions scaled relative to their contribution. The deepest pristine peak is at 160 mm, which results in a lower SOBP range of 158.4 mm because of the other peak contributions. The 90–90 modulation width is 100.2 mm while the 90–98 is 83.1 mm. The range uncertainties create a band of uncertainty both distally and proximally (see dashed distal fall-offs). The effect is most pronounced at the distal fall-off and the error must be considered to ensure that the target coverage is respected. The 80% depth, R80, of a pristine peak correlates accurately with the proton energy in MeV. The clinical historical range is in reference to the 90% depth, which also depends on the energy spread. The difference in practice is on the order of 1 mm. Care should be practiced especially considering calibration and reference conditions.

a photon fraction prescription of 1.8 Gy (which has an RBE of 1 as Co60 dose quantifies clinical empirical knowledge) is delivered with a proton fraction of 1.8 Gy (RBE), which corresponds to 1.64 Gy physical proton dose. The latter is the value measured in a radiation detector.

Proton RBE is assumed 1.1 irrespective of organ, LET or dose prescription or clinical end-point. A constant RBE of 1.1 was chosen as a minimum value to ensure proton target doses equal or greater compared to photon target doses. This implies, however, that organs at risk could receive more compared to an equivalent photon dose of great concern (see Gottschalk[10]).

Dose-averaged LET_D is a predictor for variable biological response. Monte Carlo allows for a direct computation of LET_D using Equation 23.3 (see also Bertolet et al.[2]). (We use a 1 MeV cutoff in our computations.)

$$LET_D = \frac{\int D(L)\,L\,dL}{\int D(L)\,dL} \tag{23.3}$$

where $D(L)$ is the dose deposited by the track energy loss L.

An indirect Monte Carlo calculation can use a phenomological model such as described by Wilkins and Oelfke[31] (Equation 23.4).

$$LET_D(z) = \frac{\langle S^2 \rangle_z}{\langle S \rangle_z} \tag{23.4}$$

where $\langle S^2 \rangle$ and $\langle S \rangle$ are weighted values over the residual range spectrum at z.

The LET_D can be tabulated as a function of radiological depth and energy and used algorithmically in a non-Monte Carlo calculation (see Fig. 23.2).

An RBE optimization objective function $F(D, {}^{\alpha}/_{\beta}, L)$ used in an optimization for the proton spot charges Q_j given a set of constraints has as arguments dose D, organ-specific ${}^{\alpha}/_{\beta}$ ratios, and dose-averaged LET L. The dose in a voxel is $d_i = \Sigma_j Q_j D_{ij}$ (Equation 23.1) and dose-averaged LET in a voxel is $L_i = (\Sigma_j D_{ij} L_{ij})/d_i$, where L_{ij} is parallel to D_{ij} in Equation 23.1 and provides the LET at voxel i from protons originating in spot j and uses these quantities to compute the RBE (see Unkelbach et al.[30] for an example of LET optimization and McNamara et al.[19] for RBE calculation).

Water-Equivalent Depth and proton range, R

The water-equivalent thickness, τ_{wet} [g/cm^2], of a proton track in medium is the thickness in water that produces the same proton energy at the track end-point location in the medium. It is calculated from the mass stopping power ratio, S_W^V, defined as the ratio of the stopping power of protons in the medium V over that in water W. In practice S_W^V is known for the materials such as polyethylene used in range-compensators but generally derived from CT (Computed Tomography) Hounsfield numbers (see Schneider et al.[28]). The proton water-equivalent thickness is[21]

$$\tau_{wet} = \tau_m \frac{\rho_v S_v}{\rho_w S_w} \tag{23.5}$$

where ρ is the density. The mass stopping power ratio is almost independent of therapeutic proton energies for biological materials.[12] If this ratio is unity the radiological pathlength and water equivalent thickness are mathematically equivalent.

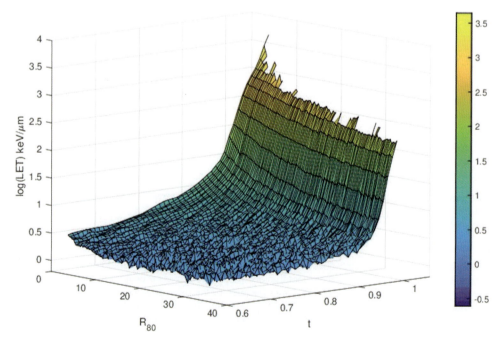

FIGURE 23.2. The LET_D is computed with TOPAS as a function of range R_{80} and range-normalized depth $t = d/R_{80}$. The surface (note the $\log(LET_D)$!) is parameterized for ready LET_D lookup in a voxel given the radiological depth τ. This yields the required LET_{ij} matrix in analogy to the D_{ij} to rapidly compute dose for optimization.

In treatment planning, however, the differences between ρ_{rpl} and ρ_{wet} can be clinically significant and limited by the uncertainties in local material properties.

The mean proton range R is the average water-equivalent depth at which protons stop in the medium. This is a very close approximation to the range in the continuous slowing down approximation, R_{CSDA}, and the depth at distal 80% of maximum dose, R_{80} of a pristine proton Bragg peak (see Fig. 8.1). The pristine peak R_{80} is independent of proton energy spread and directly relates to proton energy. Definitions of range are often used interchangeably in proton therapy.

Dose to Medium

The dose to a volume element, of thickness t along, and area A, perpendicular to the proton direction, is given by the energy lost in the volume-let (voxel) divided by its mass

$$D \equiv \frac{\text{Energy}}{\text{Mass}}\left[\frac{J}{kg}\right] = \frac{\frac{dE}{dx}tN}{\rho At} = \Phi\frac{S}{\rho}[\text{Gy}] \quad (23.6)$$

where $\Phi = N/_A$ is the proton fluence in $[\text{cm}^{-2}]$. Dose for a fluence of 10^9 (1 gigaproton) per cm^2 of 100 MeV protons in water where $S/\rho = 7.3 \text{ MeV.cm}^2/g$ is (Equation 23.6)

$$D = \frac{10^9}{\text{cm}^2}\frac{7.3\,\text{MeVcm}^2}{10^{-3}\,\text{kg}}\frac{0.162\,10^{-12}\text{J}}{\text{MeV}} = 1.17[\text{Gy}]$$

$$(23.7)$$

at the entrance of the water (where the proton energy is 100 MeV) and where we used the factor 10^{-3} to convert from g to kg and the conversion factor $0.1602\,10^{-12}$ J/MeV. Equation 23.7 shows that the number of protons to deliver a clinical dose is on the order of gigaprotons, a number less than 10^{-15} of the number of protons in a gram of water! A convenient rule of thumb is that 1 Gp delivers about 1 cGy to a 1 liter volume.

The mass stopping power quantifies energy loss from electromagnetic interactions but excludes energy deposited from secondary particles. In computational practice, a measured depth-dose can be a substitute for the mass stopping power even in Monte Carlo calculations (see below).

A CT volume of the patient provides electron density in a precise geometry. The conversion from electron density to relative (to water) stopping power is empirical and based on an average for particular organs over all patients.[28] The conversion has inherent uncertainties due to (1) the non-specificity for a particular patient, and (2) the lack of knowledge of precise stopping powers for particular organs. A 3% uncertainty in the relative stopping power in patient (see Fig. 23.1) is assumed, which directly translates to range uncertainty. Dose uncertainty thus can range from 0% to 100% depending on the dose gradients.

Depth-Dose Distributions

A dose algorithm may use axial, integrated over the lateral dimension, depth-dose distributions in water for

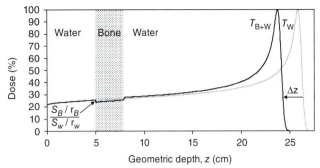

FIGURE 23.3. T_W is the depth-dose distribution in a homogenous water phantom and T_{W+B} is the depth-dose distribution in a water phantom with bone at 5 cm depth. The relative mass stopping power, $S_B/\rho_B/S_W/\rho_W$, of bone to water gives the ratio of the dose deposited in bone to water in the shaded region. Bone has larger relative stopping power compared to water and for 2.9 cm geometric thickness of bone with 1.72 relative stopping power the Δz is -2.1 cm by Equation 23.8.

all available proton energies. Dose distributions in the patient are calculated from the dose in water using the local density and relative stopping power derived from CT data. In the presence of heterogeneities, the broad-field depth-dose distribution in the medium, $T_m(E,\tau_{wet})$ $[\text{Gy.mm}^2/\text{gigaproton}]$, is obtained from that in water by (following from Equation 23.6)

$$T_m^\infty(E, \tau_{wet}) = T_w^\infty(E, z\rho_w)\frac{S_m/\rho_m}{S_w/\rho_w}$$

where E is the incident proton energy, z is the geometric depth in cm and the superscript ∞ indicates that broad beam depth-dose distributions are at infinite source to axis distance (SAD). The effect of inhomogeneities is twofold. First, the physical depth of the Bragg peak is shifted relative to a water phantom based on the water equivalent depth in the patient. The shift for material M with geometric thickness z_m and water equivalent thickness $\tau_{wet,m}$ is

$$\Delta z = z_m - \frac{\tau_{wet,m}}{\rho_w}$$

Second, the dose in the heterogeneity is scaled by the ratio of relative mass stopping powers. This ratio is close to 1 and typically ignored in dose algorithm implementations. These effects are illustrated in Figure 23.3.

Proton Lateral Spread

The numerous multiple elastic scattering events produce, for an initial parallel and infinitesimally narrow beam of protons, a Gaussian lateral distribution profile. The characteristic spread of this Gaussian profile in the Bragg peak region is about 2% of the range (in cm). Thus, a proton beam of 20 cm penetration range in water has a spread of 4 mm in the Bragg peak region. In comparison, an electron beam has a spread of about 20% of its range (Fig. 23.5).

Molière investigated proton scattering in the Coulomb field of the nucleus and multiple scattering as a consequence of numerous interactions.[20] In practice, the Highland approximation,[8] or analytical variants, are used to compute the lateral beam spread in matter. For dose calculations in thick, heterogeneous matter, the volume is divided into N homogeneous slabs that represent the material along the particle track. The standard deviation of the Gaussian spread σ_p at radiological depth L due to the i-th slab is

$$\sigma_{p,i} = \left[1 + \frac{1}{9}\log_{10}\left(\frac{L_i - L_{i-1}}{L_{R,i}}\right)\right]$$
$$\left[\int_{L_{i-1}}^{L_i}\left(\frac{14.1\,\text{MeV}}{pv}\frac{L - L'}{\rho_i}\right)^2\frac{1}{L_{R,i}}dL'\right]^{1/2} \text{[cm]} \quad (23.8)$$

where pv is the product of the proton momentum and speed (in MeV), L_R is the radiation length (in g/cm^2) and the i-th slab extends from radiological depth L_{i-1} to L_i. The total Gaussian spread, σ_p, is the quadrature sum of the individual Gaussian spreads from each slab

$$\sigma_p = \left[\sum_{i=1}^{N}\sigma_{p,i}^2\right]^{1/2} \text{[cm]} \quad (23.9)$$

Solving Equation 23.9 is not practical. With two clinically acceptable simplifications—the radiation length L in the patient equals the radiation length of water (36.1 g/cm^2) and the density ρ equals the density of water (1 g/cm^3)—the Gaussian spread

$$\sigma_p = \left[1 + \frac{1}{9}\log_{10}\left(\frac{L}{L_{R,\text{water}}}\right)\right]$$
$$\left[\int_0^L\left(\frac{14.1\,\text{MeV}}{pv}\frac{L - L'}{\rho_{\text{water}}}\right)^2\frac{1}{L_{R,\text{water}}}dL'\right]^{1/2} \text{[cm]} \quad (23.10)$$

is only a function of the radiological depth L in the media. Consider protons with 100 MeV energy incident on a homogeneous water phantom, then σ_p at the maximum water-equivalent depth is 0.179 mm. If the same beam passes through 1 g/cm of compact bone (L_R = 16.6 g/cm^2 and ρ = 1.85 g/cm^3) followed by water then σ_p at the maximum water-equivalent depth is 0.169 mm, an acceptable difference compared to the homogeneous phantom. One should in general give special attention to treatment plans that have materials with properties significantly different than water.

Treatment planning algorithms use tables or parameterizations of σ_p in water to improve the computation time. Numerical solutions of Equation 23.10 are described in Hong et al.[12] and Lee et al.[18] Figure 23.6 shows a similar calculation in water where the momentum and velocity of protons at radiological depth, L, and range, R, are calculated through range-energy tables from J Janni.[15]

Nuclear Interactions

The proton interaction with a nucleus was originally ignored due to its complex scatter profile, secondary protons, and lack of models. Scattered proton fields, in the absence of absolute dose calculation models, relied on manual field calibrations to correct for any effect on the total dose. The proton–nucleus dosimetric effect is dubbed the "halo" effect and is described in Gottschalk et al.[9] and parameterized in Gaussian form (with a halo spread σ_H) in Clasie et al.[3] The proton–nucleus interaction causes a nuclear build-up effect at the entrance dose and has a maximum build-up at about half the range.

The biological and dosimetric effect of these nuclear interactions can only be quantified through Monte Carlo.[23] Algorithmically, the range (energy) and depth-dependent effect can be parameterized as a reduction in the depth dose where the form below parameterizes the fraction of the total depth dose due to these nuclear interactions.

$$\alpha\left(t = \frac{d}{R}, R\right) = 1, \alpha_0(R) + \alpha_1(R)t + \alpha_2(R)t^2 \quad (23.11)$$

The α_i factors in turn are parameterized as

$$\alpha_i(R) = b0,i + b1,iR + b2,iR2 \quad (23.12)$$

where the b values are in Table 23.1.

We consider the algorithmic compensation of the disequilibrium of a single pencil beam placed within a set of pencil-beam spots analogous to secondary scatter build-up in photon fields. We use the Clarkson sector summation algorithm over the N triangles created by boundary polygon point pairs (x_i, x_{i+1}) and the position x_s of a spot. We use an Gaussian form for the halo disequilibrium $H(r) = 1 - \exp(-r^2/2\sigma_H^2)$. The equivalent radius satisfies the equality

$$H(r_{eq}) = \sum_{i=1,N} S_i\frac{\theta_i}{2\pi}H(r_i)$$

where r_i is the average distance from the spot position x_s to the triangle boundary points, $S_i = \pm 1$ considers convexity and concavity of the boundary and θ_i is the triangle angle at the spot position. The corrected depth dose is

$$D_H(d, r_{eq}, R) = D(d, R)\left[\alpha\left(\frac{d}{R}, R\right) + \left(1 - \alpha\left(\frac{d}{R}, R\right)\right)\right.$$
$$\left. H(r_{eq})\right] \quad (23.13)$$

The depth-dose correction is used in the analytical forms and the Monte Carlo below by correcting T_w^∞ (see Fig. 23.4).

TABLE 23.1	Fit Parameters to Obtain the Coefficients a_i to Compute the Depth-dependent Halo Fraction $\alpha(d/R, R)$		
	a_0	a_1	a_2
$b_{0,i}$	1.002	2.128e-03	−2.549e-03
$b_{1,i}$	−5.900e-04	−2.044e-02	2.125e-02
$b_{2,i}$	0	3.178e-04	−3.788e-04

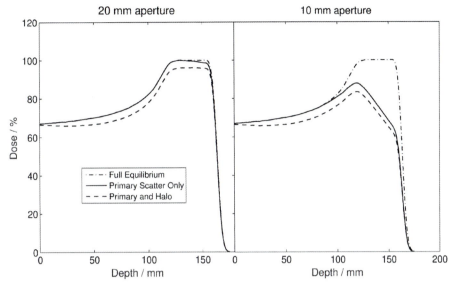

FIGURE 23.4. The effect of primary and secondary (halo) disequilibrium on an SOBP field passing through a 20 and 10 mm aperture (s_H = 30 mm³).

MODELS OF DOSE DEPOSITION

Gaussian Proton Pencil-Beam Model

The Gaussian form of charged particle spread in medium was first used in an electron pencil-beam algorithm by Hogstrom et al.[11] Gaussian functions have the convenient properties of well-behaved integration and summation to describe the field profile and lateral penumbrae. In a pencil-beam model, the radiation field is subdivided into narrow pencil-beam subfields. The central axis of the pencilbeam is traced through the medium and only density variations along the axis are considered. The density lateral to the pencil-beam axis is considered equal the on-axis density and the calculation is thus insensitive to heterogeneity variations comparable to the width of the pencilbeam at depth. The Gaussian description for electron beams works well in homogeneous medium but less so in heterogeneous media as a consequence of the large scattering angle of electrons. The Gaussian model improves in accuracy and performance when the spread is small as is the case for proton beams.

Hong et al.[12] describe a Gaussian pencil-beam model by a general delivery device. Such a device contains beam scatterers, an aperture, a rangecompensator or shifter, an air-gap between the range-compensator and the patient, and the patient itself (Fig. 23.8). A physical narrow pencilbeam of protons can be mathematically modeled even in the presence of heterogeneities while retaining good resolution. For example, an infinitesimal pencilbeam of 15 cm range still has better than 4 mm resolution at depth. The model applies equally to pencil-beam scanning (PBS) devices (Fig. 23.5). The dose D to a point (x,y,z) from a pencil-beam field is

$$D(x, y, z) = \sum_i \Psi_i \frac{T_w^\infty(R_i, \tau_{wet})}{2\pi\, \sigma_T(\tau_{wet})^2}$$

$$\exp\left(-\frac{(x - x_i)^2 - (y - y_i)^2}{2\, \sigma_T(z)^2}\right) \qquad (23.14)$$

where the sum is overall pencilbeam i (each of range R_i) whose central axis at a depth (at the coordinate z) is at (x_i, y_i), Ψ_i is the "intensity" of the pencilbeam, σ_T is the total spread of the pencilbeam at z, and $T_w^\infty(R_i, \tau_{wet})$ are broad-field depth-dose distributions in water with infinite SAD. $T_w^\infty(R_i, \tau_{wet})$ can be measured in broad fields or for a single spot/pencil using a sufficiently broad chamber ($\phi > 12$ cm). Measurements are best used to validate Monte Carlo and use Monte Carlo generated depth doses at high resolution[3] (Fig. 23.6).

Equation 23.14 is a general description of protons diffusion through medium as a function of depth. Its form is used for describing a scattered proton field, where a proton beam is passively scattered in the lateral dimension and modulated in depth, and a PBS field, where a narrow beam of proton pencils are scanned magnetically in the lateral dimension and modulated in depth. The PBS context overloads the term *pencilbeam* and we distinguish between the mathematical pencilbeams of the algorithm and the physical pencilbeams delivered to the beams. The first have a small area to allow representative sampling of the patient geometry; the latter have a large area (on the order of 3–20 mm (1σ!). In our implementation, for example, we transport a large number of mathematical pencilbeams and subsequently convolve the physical pencilbeams over that transport space (Equation 23.18).

Scattered fields and PBS fields differ in the use of inverse square. In scattered fields, the source of the field is also the source of the depth-dose divergence.

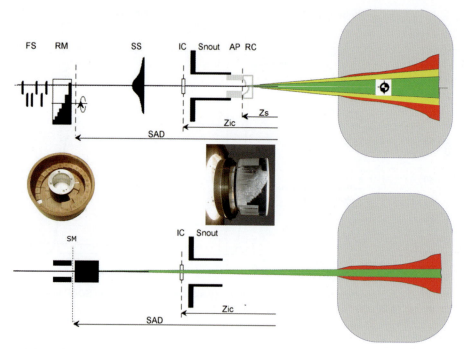

FIGURE 23.5. A double scattering (DS) system (top) and pencil-beam scanning (PBS) system (bottom) are shown. The DS requires mechanical systems (FS and SS) to scatter the proton laterally to a uniform field and to modulate (RM) the energy in depth. The ionization chamber (IC) measures the dose in the central region of the field. A DS field always requires an aperture, to create a sharp penumbra, and range-compensator, to minimize distal dose. A PBS uses SM to move the beam over the lateral dimension and uses the beamline switching mode to change energy. The IC now covers the extent (plus margin) of the scanning area. PBS may obviate the need for apertures and compensators but are not excluded per se. The in-patient dose is characterized by sharp penumbrae for both DS and PBS (red). DS, however has an increase in in-field sharpness due to the range-compensator scatter (yellow). A DS field has no dose modulation control inside the field. Dose modulation control for a PBS field is a function of the spot size and in-patient scatter.

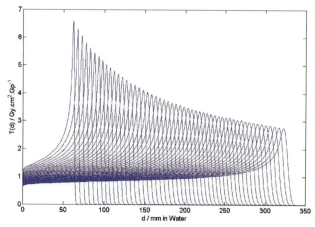

FIGURE 23.6. High-resolution (depth and dose) pristine peaks in absolute units obtained from Monte Carlo calibrated against water measurements. The peaks report dose per gigaproton, which is an equipment independent unit as Monitor Unit, is not a standard definition in proton radiotherapy.

Thus T_w^∞ is replaced by $I^2 T_w^\infty$ where I^2 is the inverse correction. In PBS[26] the pencil-beam geometry emanates from the origin(s) of the magnet center(s) and the pencil-beam depth dose is given by Equation 23.8.

One computational burden in a pencil-beam ray-trace algorithm implementation is the association of dose to points surrounding the ray (see Fig. 23.7). One has to search an area perpendicular to the Z-axis at depth z of radius $\geq 3\sigma(z)$ as this, for a Gaussian distribution, contains 99% of the laterally distributed profile. Efficient algorithms use sorting and indexing algorithms.[17] A general, and fast, implementation relies on indexing and sorting the dose points in the beam coordinate system, in the isocentric plane and along the axis of the beam or ray.

Scattered Field Implementation

A scattered proton field is similar to an electron scattered field. The scattered field is characterized by a virtual source, with a spread σ_S from which the protons appear to emanate and diverge. The source position and size can be determined by measuring the field width and the penumbral width of an aperture as a function of distance from the aperture. The field width projects back to the source position while the penumbral width is given by the back-projection of the measured penumbra through the aperture, where the penumbra is 0, to that position (as described, for example, in[11]). The resultant "virtual" source size of the proton beam is large with σ_S between 5 and 10 cm as a consequence of the proton scatter in the scattering system (see Fig. 23.8). This large source size can only be mitigated by placing an

FIGURE 23.7. A patient (curved contour) is irradiated by a set of spots S of optical spread σ_o, charge G_S and range R_S emanating for a source (possibly with dual source positions). The spot beam's eye view (BEV) shows the location of a mathematical pencilbeam k of extent A_k. The spot S contributes a number of protons to spot k per Equation 23.18, where $\Delta_{S,k}$ are the extents of A_k in S. The in-patient transport by the set of mathematical unit-charge pencilbeams k starts at the entrance to the patient. At the depth $\rightarrow x = (x,y,z)$, at τ_{wet}, the pencil has a spread σ_p and contributes a dose-fraction given by Equation 23.18. Transformations between coordinate systems are required but implicit here and in Equation 23.18.

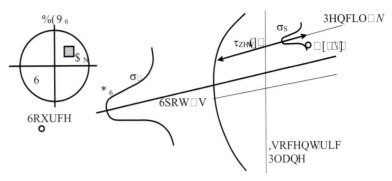

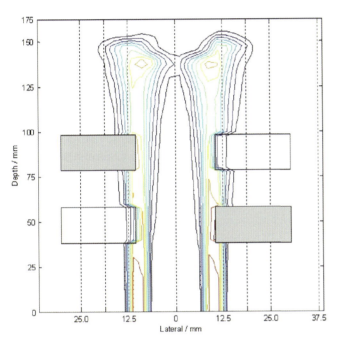

FIGURE 23.8. Passage of two broad pencilbeams through a geometry with discrete heterogeneities. The Monte Carlo models the differential penetration, straggling, and lateral spread.

aperture as close to the patient as possible (as is the practice for electron aperture) and to move the source position as far as possible from the patient (the SAD at the Harvard Cyclotron Laboratory was 600 cm). The latter is one reason for the size of proton gantries; the other being the magnetic rigidity necessary to bend the proton beam toward the patient.

The effective source size (the projection of the source to $Z = 0$ through a pinhole at the aperture) is

$$\sigma_{s,eff} = \sigma_s \frac{SAD - Z_A}{Z_A} \qquad (23.15)$$

which for a typical beamline, with an SAD of 300 cm and an aperture distance Z_A to patient of 10 cm, reduces the source size by a factor of $(300-10)/10 = 29$ and the contribution of the virtual source is reduced to $\sigma = 3$ mm or less.

The proton beam passes through the aperture and subsequently through the range-compensator, which shifts the proton range over the field area such that the distal surface of the field is placed beyond, and conformed to, the distal target volume surface (with respect to the beam

axis). Passage through the range-compensator introduces local compensator thickness dependent scatter with a penumbral spread in the patient at depth z given by

$$\sigma_R = \theta_0(t(x,y))(z - Z_R) \qquad (23.16)$$

where $\theta_0(t)$ is the scattering angle produced by the protons passing through the local thickness t at (x, y) of the range-compensator (see Figure A2 in[12]).

The protons scatter in the patient quantified by a third spread factor, σ_p. The derivation of σ_p is computed, for example, from the generalized Highland formula (Equation 23.8). The total spread of the pencil beam is the quadratic sum of the three spread factors in Equations 23.8, 23.15, and 23.16 (Fig. 23.8).

The complete algorithm divides the scattered field extent circumscribed by the aperture into many small pencilbeams, typically spaced in a rectangular grid of 2 mm resolution. This high resolution ensures that heterogeneities within the patient are sufficiently sampled in the lateral extent. Each pencil beam axis is traced through the CT volume from the virtual source through a grid point and through the CT. The calculation points (x, y, z) are transformed to the beam coordinate system and are sorted in z (Figure 23.7). The ray trace evaluates the water-equivalent depth for the point whose z is first in this sorted list and whose $\sqrt{(x - x')^2 + (y - y')^2} < 3\sigma_T$, that is, those points close enough to the pencil-beam axis to receive sufficient dose. For those points, the evaluation of Equation 23.14 yields the dose to those points. The ray trace continues and repeats the procedure for the next point z in the list.

Scattered Proton Field Superposition

Scattered fields use superposition of individual pristine peak doses to create SOBP distribution in depth. The lateral profile is flat or near-flat depending on the upstream scattering system.[7] The SOBP is the summation of the dose distribution of the peak dose distributions $D_{P,i}$ in patient

$$SOBP(z) = \sum_{i=1}^{N} W_i D_{P,i}(z) \qquad (23.17)$$

where W_i is the (relative) contribution of each peak dose distribution (see Fig. 23.1).

The superposition of Bragg peaks is achieved by mechanically inserting range-shifting material in the monoenergetic proton beam with the insertion time proportional (times the current if not constant) to the required contribution of a peak to the SOBP. The common method is to use a rotating wheel with increasing step thicknesses and where the angular extent of the step is proportional to the weight. A rotating wheel can produce SOBPs of varying modulation by turning the beam off before a full rotation has been completed (ref). The use of a stepped rotation wheel and the large proton source size results in a softening of the proximal plateau, which can be considered by convolving the source size over the wheel segment and adjusting W_i.

The modulation width is the distance between the distal and proximal 90%. This definition, however, leads to modulation values larger than the range value for some fields and is hard to measure in the shallow entrance dose region. In our practice we specify the modulation width between the distal 90% and the proximal 98% (see Fig. 23.1).

Absolute dose calculations for SOBP models have not been implemented and output calculations rely on empirical models (see Kooy et al.[16]). The large number of mechanical components in a scattering nozzle make a description very difficult. This complexity increases the burden on the physicist to establish a practical quality assurance protocol for output calibrations (see Engelsman et al.[5]).

Pencil-Beam Scanning Field Implementation

PBS fields comprise numerous (O(1000)) physical narrow proton beams, spots, whose lateral position is controlled by scanning magnets (SM) and whose penetration depth is set by energy. Spots are (because energy switching is "slow") grouped in constant energy layers. Spot protons are nearly monoenergetic with an energy spread dE/E on the order of 0.5% or less.

One could use the physical pencilbeam directly as a representation for the Gaussian form in Equation 23.14. Such an implementation is insensitive to patient heterogeneities given the large spot size of physical pencilbeams of (σ) 3–15 mm in the isocentric plane) at the entrance as a consequence of the beam transport system and scatter in air and windows. Thus a dose algorithm of Equation 23.14 is unable to discern inhomogeneities smaller than that spread. Schaffner et al.[27] describe various techniques of modeling dose distributions near lateral heterogeneities. Other solutions are Monte Carlo or a higher-resolution decomposition as described below (see Fig. 23.8).

The physical pencil-beam field of spots S is convolved over constituent narrow mathematical pencilbeams k with initial spread $\sigma_p = 0$ (including spread due to inserted shifters) to retain sufficient resolution of the proton transport inside the patient (see Fig. 23.7)

$$D\left(\vec{x}\right) = \sum_S G_S$$
$$\times \sum_k \int \frac{1}{2\pi\sigma_o^2(R_S, z)} \exp\left(-\frac{\Delta_{S,k}^2}{2\sigma_o^2(R_S, z)}\right) dA_k$$
$$\times \frac{T_w^\infty(R_S, \tau_{\text{wet}})}{2\pi\sigma_p^2(R_S, \tau_{\text{wet}})} \exp\left(-\frac{\Delta_k^2\left(\vec{x}\right)}{2\sigma_p^2(R_S, \tau_{\text{wet}})}\right) \quad (23.18)$$

where the first term is the number of protons G_S (in units of billions, or giga, protons Gp) in the spot S with optical lateral spread σ_o and the second term is the apportionment of these G_S protons over the set k given the distance $\Delta_{S,k}$ between the spot axis and pencil beam k. The set k in is high resolution (O(1 mm)) necessary to compute the dose in patient in the presence of heterogeneities. Equation 23.18 models the diffusion of the number of protons, in the patient given the scatter spread in the patient due to multiple Coulomb scattering. The spot lateral spread in Equation 23.18 is determined by the scatter in air, magnetic steering, and focusing properties of the PBS system (see Fig. 23.8) and is a function of the spot range R_S and position z along the pencil-beam spot axis. The parameter $\Delta_{S,K}$ denotes the location of the computational pencil-beam area A_K with respect to the spot coordinate system. The final term follows Pedroni et al.,[24] where T (in units of Gy.cm^2.Gp^{-1}) is the absolute measured depth dose per gigaproton (see Fig. 23.9) integrated over an infinite plane at water-equivalent depth. σ_p is the pencilbeam spread at τ_{wet} caused by multiple Coulomb scatter in patient (see Hong et al.[12]), and Δ_k is the displacement from the calculation point to the k pencil-beam axis. In our implementation, we first transport all pencilbeams k and "re-use" a pencilbeam k in case of overlap between two spots (see also Fippel et al.[6] for a decomposition of spots in to sub-beams).

A Monte Carlo for Proton Transport in Patient

Monte Carlo methods improve on dose calculations in heterogeneous medium. We describe a minimal Monte Carlo algorithm for proton dose calculation which correctly models primary scatter in heterogeneous medium and derives dose deposited per proton track from measured depth-dose data. The latter avoids the typical arbitrary calibration of physics parameters in fundamental Monte Carlo's such as GEANT4 to achieve clinical correspondence, and it maintains a direct traceability between Monte Carlo and clinical practice for dose reporting.

Figure 23.9 [Left] shows the geometry of the particle transport at the voxel level and the use of the pristine depth dose to compute energy loss. A particle, of initial energy E_0 at the patient surface, enters a voxel (volume V, density ρ) with certain input parameters: current energy E_i, relative position (x_i, y_i, z_i) and direction cosines (u_i, v_i, w_i) in the voxel, and initial energy E_0 (energy at the entrance of the phantom/patient). A cord length L is computed from the path elements to and from the center of the voxel. The mean radial Coulomb scattering angle in the voxel is computed per Gottschalk[8] in a "differential Molière—dM" model (Equation 23.19) and applied in the center of the voxel:

$$\langle\theta^2\rangle = \int_0^L T_{dM} dx \approx T_{dM} L \quad (23.19)$$

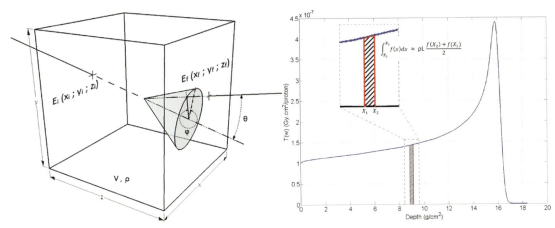

FIGURE 23.9. [Left] Voxel geometry for a proton entering and exiting the voxel. The proton is scattered in the center of the voxel at an angle given by Equation 23.19 and only the azimuthal angle is given by a random variable. [Right] Derivation of energy loss in a voxel from the area under the curve between the entrance and exit depths.

where

$$T_{dM} = f_{dM}(E_i, E_0)\left(\frac{E_s}{E_i}\right)^2 \frac{1}{X_s}$$

and

$$f_{dM} = 0.5244 + 0.1975\log_{10}\left(1 - \left(\frac{E_i}{E_0}\right)^2\right)$$

$$+ 0.2320\log_{10}\left(\frac{E_i}{\mathrm{MeV}}\right) - 0.0098\log_{10}$$

$$\left(\frac{E_i}{\mathrm{MeV}}\right)\log_{10}\left(1 - \left(\frac{E_i}{E_0}\right)^2\right)$$

θ is the average radial scattering angle, E_i and E_0 are entry and exit energies, x the distance already traveled by the particle along its track in cm, $E_s = 15.0$ MeV, and $X_s = 46.88$ cm.

The mean energy loss ΔE is given by a trapezoidal approximation of the integral under the pristine Bragg peak curve at the voxel entrance and exit energies (Fig. 23.9 [Right]). The local dose deposited ΔD is computed from Equation 23.6.

The Monte Carlo models devices as slabs with optional holes to represent apertures and range-shifters. Transport through these slabs is along fixed length step L_C and at each step the scattering angle is given by Equation 23.19 and the energy loss by the step length and material density. This part of the transport is simple polygonal math and extremely fast.

The Monte Carlo models heterogeneity features at the scale of the feature and correctly models lateral spread and range-straggling (see Fig. 23.8). Figure 8.10 compares dose distributions obtained with our TPS astroid™ (.decimal Sanford, FL), this Monte Carlo (GMC) and TOPAS.[25] The dose distributions are qualitatively equivalent. The astroid and GMC dose calculations report dose as dose to water while TOPAS reports dose to medium. Astroid and GMC are closest in their prediction of target doses while GMC and TOPAS are closest in their prediction for other structures. Such expected differences need to be properly aligned with clinical expectations based on long-standing dose prescription reporting and conventions and correlated

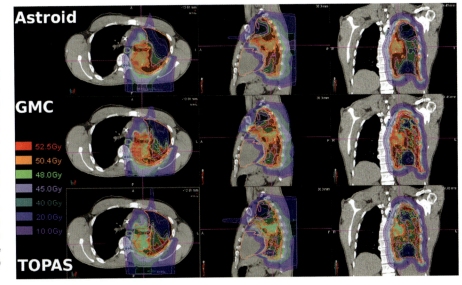

FIGURE 23.10. Dose on orthogonal sections for a lung calculation. The computations represent a pencil-beam algorithm (astroid), this Monte Carlo (GMC) and the TOPAS (GEANT4) Monte Carlo. The pencil-beam algorithm produces a smooth distribution and (by design) has full target coverage. GMC and TOPAS show more nuanced detail because of accurate tracking in heterogeneities and indicate deviations from target coverage. Quantitative clinical consequences between practice-based dosimetry (astroid) and more accurate physical calculations (Monte Carlo) must be carefully considered.

empirically with clinical outcomes. Astroid and GMC directly report dose per equipment Gp through the use of equipment calibrated depth doses (see Fig. 23.6). TOPAS requires a calibration from equipment protons to internal protons because its internal dose per proton depends on numerous modeled physics processes not traceable to equipment.

The Monte Carlo is implemented on a GPU and achieves a metric of 510^7 cm/s. That is, for a proton range of 10 cm, 510^6 protons per second are transported.

REFERENCES

1. Amsler C, Doser M. et al. Review of particle physics. *Phys Lett.* 2008;B667:1–6.
2. Bertolet A, Baratto-Roldán A, Barbieri S, Baiocco G, Carabe A, CortØs-Giraldo MA. Dose-averaged LET calculation for proton track segments using microdosimetric Monte Carlo simulations. *Med. Phys.* 2019;46(9):4184–4192.
3. Clasie B, Depauw N, et al. Golden beam data for proton pencil-beam scanning. *Phys Med Biol.* 2012;57:1147–1158.
4. Cormack AM, Koehler AM. Quantitative proton tomography: preliminary experiments. *Phys Med Biol.* 1976;21:560–569.
5. Engelsman M, Lu HM, Herrup D, Bussiere MR, Kooy HM. Commissioning a passive scattering proton therapy nozzle for accurate SOBP delivery. *Med Phys.* 2009;36:2172–2180.
6. Fippel M, Soukup M. A Monte Carlo dose calculation algorithm for proton therapy. *Med Phys.* 2004;31:2263–2273.
7. Gottschalk B. Passive beam spreading in proton radiation therapy. http:huhepl.harvard.edu/gottschalk/
8. Gottschalk B. On the scattering power of radiotherapy protons. *Med Phys.* 2010;37:352–367.
9. Gottschalk B, Cascio EW, Daartz J, Wagner MS. On the nuclear halo of a proton pencil beam stopping in water. *Phys Med Biol.* 2015;60:5627–5654.
10. Haas-Kogan D, Indelicato D et al. National Cancer Institute workshop on proton therapy for children: considerations regarding brainstem injury. *Int J Radiat Oncol Biol Phys.* 2018;101(1):152–168.
11. Hogstrom KR, Mills MD, Almond PR. Electron beam dose calculations. *Phys Med Biol.* 1981;26:445–459.
12. Hong L, Goitein M, Bucciolini M, Comiskey R, Gottschalk B, Rosenthal S, Serago C, Urie M. A pencil beam algorithm for proton dose calculations. *Phys Med Biol.* 1996;41:1305–1330.
13. Stopping Powers and Ranges for Protons and Alpha Particles (ICRU Report 49). *J ICRU.* 1993;25(2):1993.
14. Prescribing, Recording, and Reporting Proton-Beam Therapy (ICRU Report 78). *J ICRU.* 2007;7(2).
15. Janni J. Proton range-energy tables, 1 keV–10 GeV atomic data and nuclear data tables, 27. *Numbers.* 1982:147–339.
16. Kooy HM, Schaefer M, Rosenthal S, Bortfeld T. Monitor unit calculations for range modulated spread-out Bragg peak fields. *Phys Med Biol.* 2003;48:2797–2808.
17. Kooy HM, Rashid H. A three-dimensional non-coplanar electron pencil beam algorithm. *Phys MedBiol.* 1989;34:229–243.
18. Lee M, Nahum A, Webb S. An empirical method to build up a model of proton dose distribution for a radiotherapy treatment-planning package *Phys Med Biol.* 1993;38:989–998.
19. McNamara AL, Schuemann J, Paganetti H. *Phys. Med Biol.* 2015;60:8399–8416.
20. Moliere G. Theorie der Streuung schneller geladener Teilchen II Mehrfach und Vielfachstreuung, Z. Naturforsch. B 1948;3A:78–97.
21. Zhang R, Newhauser WD. Calculation of water equivalent thickness of materials of arbitrary density, elemental composition and thickness in proton beam irradiation. *Phys Med Biol.* 2009;54:1383–1395.
22. Paganetti H. Range uncertainties in proton therapy and the role of Monte Carlo simulations. *Phys Med Biol.* 2012;57:R99–R117.
23. Paganetti H. Nuclear interactions in proton therapy: dose and relative biological effect distributions originating from primary and secondary particles. *Phys Med Biol.* 2002;47:747–764.
24. Pedroni E, Scheib S, Bohringer T, Coray A, Grossmann M, Lin S, Lomax A. Experimental characterization and physical modelling of the dose distribution of scanned proton pencil beams. *Phys Med Biol.* 2005;50:541–561.
25. Perl J, Shin J, Schuemann J, Faddegon B, Paganetti H. TOPAS: an innovative proton Monte Carlo platform for research and clinical applications. *Med Phys.* 2012;39:6818–6837.
26. Safai S, Bortfeld T, Engelsman M. Comparison between the lateral penumbra of a collimated double-scattered beam and uncollimated scanning beam in proton radiotherapy. *Phys Med Biol.* 2008;53:1729–1750.
27. Schaffner B, Pedroni E, Lomax A. Dose calculation models for proton treatment planning using a dynamic beam delivery system: and attempt to include density heterogeneity effects in the analytical dose calculation. *Phys Med Biol.* 1999;44:27–41.
28. Schneider U, Pedroni E. A Lomax The calibration of CT Hounsfield units for radiotherapy treatment planning. *Phys Med Biol.* 1996;41:111–124.
29. Schneider U, Pemler P, Besserer J, Pedroni E, Lomax A, KaserHotz B. Patient specification optimization of the relation between CT-Hounsfield units and proton stopping power with proton radiography. *Med Phys.* 2005;32:195–199.
30. Unkelbach J, Botas P, Giantsoudi D, et al. Reoptimization of intensity modulated proton therapy plans based on linear energy transfer. *Int J Radiation Oncol Biol Phys.* 2016;96:1097–1106.
31. Wilkens J, Oelfke U. A phenomenological model for the relative biological effectiveness in therapeutic proton beams. *Phys Med Biol.* 2004;49:2811–2825.

24 Commissioning and Quality Assurance

Francisco J. Reynoso and James A. Kavanaugh

INTRODUCTION

Modern radiation therapy requires increasingly sophisticated technologies to accurately deliver high doses of radiation to very specific anatomic targets. The successful administration of a patient's radiation treatment is the final step of a complex process that includes the acquisition of patient volumetric data, target and normal tissue delineation, development of treatment plan, verification of the plan integrity, and finally treatment delivery. Errors at any step in the process can cause deviations between the radiation therapy plan and the intended prescription, with such deviations having the potential to produce markedly inferior clinical outcomes compared with those whose treatment was initially protocol compliant.[1] On rare occasions, these deviations can have catastrophic consequences to the patient's health.[2,3] To ensure accuracy of the prescription and the fulfillment of treatment intent, a rigorous *quality assurance* (QA) program is required at all stages of the radiation treatment process. The purpose of a QA program is to provide systematic evaluations and necessary corrective actions to maintain the quality and safety of a radiation therapy program. These evaluations, or *quality controls* (QC), measure a specific quality metric, compare it to an existing standard baseline, and adjust the metric to conform to the baseline as necessary. The baselines used within a QA program are typically defined during the initial *commissioning* process.[4] Commissioning is the preparation of new device, technique, or procedure for clinical use.

The continued development of modern tools to aid in the generation of radiation treatment plans has made the treatment planning system (TPS) process one of the most complex in the entire radiation oncology workflow. Tools to assist in automated optimization,[5] beam intensity modulation,[6] the use of a variety of imaging modalities,[7] and the inclusion of biological parameters[8] to calculate tumor control probabilities (TCP) and normal tissue complication probabilities (NTCP) are now considered standard in most TPSs. More recently, developments in auto-segmentation contouring algorithms,[9] automated/ knowledge-based planning (KBP) techniques,[10] adaptive radiation therapy (ART),[11] and advanced dose calculation algorithms, such as Monte Carlo simulations,[12] have further compounded this complexity. The extent of this complexity has resulted in treatment planning and dose calculation being related to almost one-third of reported accidental exposures in radiation therapy.[13]

The continually expanding complexity of the modern TPS has made the commissioning process one of the most challenging and error-prone steps in modern radiation therapy.[14–16] Historically, measurements and modeling of the basic radiation data set needed to accurately commission a TPS have been the responsibility of the local medical physicist. Despite comprehensive guidance documents,[17–21] the variation in skill level and experience of local physicists has produced drastic variations in the accuracy of the calculated dose distributions across institutions utilizing the same linear accelerator (LINAC) technology.[22] In the early years of LINAC manufacturing, each machine possessed unique characteristics that made it imperative to carefully characterize each LINAC separately, with reference data provided as a guide for data comparison. Modern LINACs are manufactured to tight specifications with highly reproducible dose characteristics for machines of the same model and energy,[23] and manufacturer-provided reference data is now routinely used for TPS beam modeling with beam-matched machines sharing the same model.[22,24–26] To minimize errors in TPS beam modeling, many modern LINACs come with prepackaged beam data that users have limited ability to modify. For linear accelerators that require manual TPS modeling, the vendor-supplied standardized reference data set minimizes the variation in TPS commissioning and modeling process. When using a standard reference data set, local verification measurements are still required to ensure they match the dose delivery data. Utilizing a vendor-supplied reference data set has an added benefit of reducing the time needed for commissioning, allowing a facility to start operations sooner and minimize the loss in revenue. While utilization of standard reference data has historically been controversial, it has become much more common in recent years and is widely used throughout the field.[26–28] However, care must be taken to ensure an accurate match between standard reference data and local LINACs for small field dosimetry, particularly when used for SBRT and SRT/SRS where the reference data set may not be appropriate.[29] It is imperative that the limitations of any vendor-supplied reference data set are well understood prior to clinical use.

The overall need for QA in radiation therapy is well defined.[30] As mentioned previously, comprehensive reports on treatment planning QA have been developed by the International Atomic Energy Agency (IAEA)[20,21] with a comprehensive commissioning and QA practice guideline recently developed by the American Association of Physicist in Medicine (AAPM).[17] This chapter addresses issues related to the use of treatment planning computers in the context of acceptance testing, commissioning, and routine clinical application. Although the emphasis is on commissioning and QC, there is also some discussion on QA of the total treatment planning process. The intent of this chapter is to be as generic as possible so that it applies to both conventional and more sophisticated radiation treatment techniques; however, because of page limitations, details for specialized techniques are confined to references where indicated.

TREATMENT PLANNING PROCESS

In its broader sense, treatment planning includes all the steps from therapeutic decision making to target volume and normal tissue delineation, selection of treatment technique, determination of the direction of radiation beams, simulation, fabrication of ancillary devices and treatment aids, monitor units (MU) calculations, treatment verification, and finally, first treatment. In its narrower sense, treatment planning includes the outlining of target and critical volumes[31]; the determination of the number, directions, and modality/energy of radiation beams; and the corresponding MU calculations. In this narrower definition, treatment planning involves the use of image information and the computer to perform the appropriate virtual simulation and dose calculations. The QA considered in this chapter primarily addresses the use of the TPS to generate appropriate beam arrangements and dose calculations. The following specific issues are associated with that part of the QA process.

Patient Data

The accuracy and integrity of patient imaging data comprise the foundation of the treatment planning and delivery process. The primary data set typically consists of a simulation computed tomography (CT) scan, with additional information obtained from magnetic resonance imaging (MRI) and positron emission tomography (PET) imaging. Image registration techniques (rigid and deformable) are used to accurately overlay the patient's anatomy from these various secondary imaging modalities so each can be fully used during contour delineation.[7] It is important that the data be transferred accurately to the TPS, with the simulation CT correctly displaying the spatial and radiographic composition of the patient while in the intended treatment position. This includes ensuring volume integrity, slice thickness, scan resolution, and patient orientation. Additionally, conversion of digitized data, such as the conversion of CT numbers to electron densities via electron and physical density tables, must be verified within the TPS.

Display of Patient and Beam-Related Information

Once the data have been transferred to the TPS, the treatment planner can manipulate the information, look at the data on various slices or in 3D, and allow the system to perform reconstructions of images. The radiation oncologist and treatment planner are able to outline target volumes and critical organs-at-risk (OAR) on the appropriate slices.[31] Standardization of contour names and colors should be implemented for an entire institution to minimize errors associated with variance in the names and interpretations of structures within the 3D and DVH displays. The correctness of the display of patient data is important not only for target/OAR delineation but also for the treatment planner to accurately design the placement and optimization of radiation beams.[32] Beam placement is often performed by entering parameters such as field size, collimator rotation, couch angles, and gantry direction, including rotation angles for arc therapy. At this stage, various options can be used for the definition of the field shape. In each case, the beam edges can be displayed either on a beam's-eye-view (BEV) perspective or as perspectives of the beam edges intersecting any specified plane. Associated with the beam edge display, information demonstrating gantry angle, collimator angle, beam energy, collimator size, multileaf collimator (MLC) motion, arc motion, and wedge orientation should also be displayed on the screen. Efficiency gains and variability reduction can be achieved using standard clinical templates that replicate most of the treatment planning parameters for patients with similar planning modalities and objectives.

Dose Calculation and Display

Once the beam geometry has been determined, the dose distribution can be calculated and displayed. Displays vary from simple colored isodose lines to color washes to individual point doses. The accuracy of the geometric correctness of isodose lines on the display is very difficult to assess, although very specific phantom geometries, whereby one can assess the position of a specific isodose line, can help with this process. Doses calculated at individual points can be correlated to the isodose lines as well as measured data. Additionally, the corresponding DVH displayed should similarly be verified. Finally, the integrity of the displayed composite dose plans should be verified by comparing doses calculated at individual points in the individual subplans. Similar to ROI naming and color templates, the visible displayed dose levels should be standardized across all treatment modalities within each institution to minimize errors produced by interpretation differences in the displayed data.[33]

DEVELOPMENT AND IMPLEMENTATION OF TREATMENT PLANNING ALGORITHMS

The clinical implementation of treatment planning programs involves a number of steps. Some are under the control of the user, and some are not user controlled because they depend on software developed by others. The typical clinical implementation of treatment planning programs usually takes the following steps.

Development of Calculation Algorithms

Dose calculation algorithms are based on the physics of radiation interactions within a tissue. Because of the complexity of the physics of these types of interactions, the algorithms usually involve simplifications, allowing the calculations to be completed fast enough to be useful to the treatment planner. These simplifications result in approximations to the complicated physics, and therefore the algorithms have inherent uncertainties and generally work well only over a limited range of conditions. Usually, the more complex algorithms not only handle the physics in more detail but also require longer calculation times. The extreme example of this is Monte Carlo calculations, which can take up to several hours, depending on the mode of treatment, the complexity of the plan, and calculation resolution settings.[34,35] To be practical, a clinical algorithm should generate dose distributions nearly in real time but usually in seconds. The details of the algorithm implemented on a given commercial TPS are not in the control of the user.

Development of the Computer Programs Implementing the Algorithms

Once the developer of a TPS has determined the nature of the algorithm, the algorithm must be coded into software. This software must include appropriate input–output routines, image display and manipulation routines, options that allow the user to define the treatment technique, and plan optimization and evaluation routines. The development of the software is not under the control of the user. It is the responsibility of the developer of the software to ensure that the algorithms are properly coded.

It is important for the user to have some knowledge of the nature of the dose calculation algorithms to help understand their capabilities and limitations. Furthermore, a basic knowledge will also help the user diagnose specific TPS problems and can be of some help in developing an appropriate QA process. A detailed description of different dose calculation algorithms can be found in the preceding chapters. A detailed report on external beam tissue inhomogeneity corrections for photon beams has been produced by AAPM Task Group 65.[36] For brachytherapy, an interesting review of the evolution of treatment planning has been provided by Rivard et al.[37]

Determination of the Radiation Database Required by the Algorithms

All algorithms, even sophisticated Monte Carlo procedures, require a basic radiation data set as input. As discussed earlier in this chapter, the data used to create a basic radiation data set originate from two possible sources. Traditionally, the data are independently measured for each energy on each therapy machine in every radiation therapy department. The quality and accuracy of such data depend on the individuals commissioning the TPS. Alternatively, one can commission the TPS using a reference data set supplied by the system manufacturer and validate the supplied data against a subset of beam measurements from the local radiation therapy machines.

Such data are always determined over a limited range of conditions. Thus, calculations that extend beyond the range of the original measurements may be subject to question, depending on the extrapolation procedures used by the calculation algorithms. Furthermore, measured data have their own inherent uncertainties and depend on the type and size of detectors used and the care taken by the clinical physicist.[18] Appropriate detectors and their intended use within the commissioning process are extensively described in AAPM Medical Physics Practice Guideline 5.a.[17] The accuracy of the measured data also depends on the stability of the radiation therapy machine and its ability to yield the same kind of radiation characteristics from day to day.

The input data required by TPSs at minimum are relative, in the form of dose ratios, with the denominator being the dose under some reference condition. Any TPS capable of calculating MU or treatment times also requires absolute information in the form of MUs per gray or grays per minute. These are all part of the input data set required by the TPS.

Modern Computational Demands

Over the past two decades, the utilization of multiple imaging modalities and the ever-increasing computational demands of more sophisticated algorithms have necessitated changes in the TPS hardware and storage capabilities. Modern fluence optimization and dose calculations require significantly more computational power, resulting in a migration from local desktop PCs to large local and cloud-based server farms.[38] Storing the vast amount of on-treatment and historical treatment planning data often requires utilizing picture archiving and communications systems (PACS). While the installation of these systems is often completed by industry experts, it is typically the responsibility of the local physics or information technology (IT) staff to provide management for routine data backup/restoration, software/hardware issues, and future upgrades. While larger institutions may have the necessary resources to fully support all components of a modern local server-based TPS, the increased hardware/software components may be beyond the means and expertise available for smaller clinics.

The ubiquity of modern high-speed fiber-optic communications now allows clinics to outsource the dose computation, data archiving, and other TPS functionalities to professionally managed server farms. Cloud computing allows radiation oncology clinics to install modern TPS functions without extensively investing in hardware or specialized staff. Implementing cloud computing provides several other advantages, including easy sharing of plan data, standardization of TPS parameters between institutions with matched machines, and scalable computation power, which can dramatically decrease the computational time. Several determents of cloud computing systems include increased complexity for data transfer between the local user and the storage/computation facility, which can increase the possibility of extended downtime whenever connectivity problems arise. Additionally, bandwidth issues and data security/privacy can be of increased concern and require extensive testing prior to implementation. QA for cloud-based TPS is another topic that may require special attention due to the increased capacity/frequency of vendors to supply system updates. Automated computational tools need to be developed and implemented in order to handle this increased frequently and the reliance on vendor-provided data.

Clinical Application

Finally, the clinical use of the TPS requires patient-specific information in the form of patient contours, usually generated with the aid of CT, PET, and/or MRI. Appropriate parameters must be entered to determine the treatment configuration. Dose calculations are usually performed for each beam independently, with the summed doses displayed on a monitor. This clinical application of treatment planning depends entirely on the user and their knowledge of the capabilities and limitations of the TPS. Admittedly, the newer inverse planning optimization routines[5] used for Intensity-Modulated Radiation Therapy (IMRT) are automated and leave little in the control of the user other than entering the dose-volume constraints as required by the objective function for the optimization.

TREATMENT PLANNING SYSTEM COMMISSIONING AND QUALITY ASSURANCE

Terminology Associated with Quality Assurance

Four major topics that are associated with the installation of any major piece of apparatus are *specifications, acceptance testing, commissioning,* and *QC*. In the context of TPS, the distinction between some of these terms is not entirely clear, and therefore they warrant special discussion.

System Specifications

In the context of treatment planning computers, specifications define the detailed functionality criteria of how the TPS will be utilized within the clinical workflow. Until relatively recently, there have been numerous commercial and home-grown TPSs, with each offering unique functionality. This broad selection made it extremely important for an end user to carefully match system specifications to their current/future clinical workflow. Currently, there are only a few commercially available systems, each offering a standard range of functions that facilitate all applications used within most clinical workflows. Manufacturers of these modern TPSs provide specifications that define the capabilities of their equipment. For TPSs, the specifications tend to include necessary hardware, system administration software, networking software, and dose planning software. Software specifications include detailed descriptions of what the software is capable of doing and how accurate the dose calculations can be made. Networking software specifications should detail the ability for the TPS to be fully integrated with the electronic medical record, information management, and record and verify software systems.

Acceptance Testing

Upon the installation of any new device, the user should assess the device to ensure that it behaves according to its vendor-defined specifications. For a TPS, this takes at least two forms: assessment of the hardware and the software. The latter can also be divided into several components, including assessment of the integrity of the operating system, dose calculations, image transfer, and image display. Acceptance testing is typically conducted with the vendor's installation engineers, who must show the accuracy of the dose calculation algorithm under specific circumstances is within pre-agreed standards. The acceptance testing should be carried out on the system after it has been installed in the clinic but before it is used clinically. A detailed test procedure and results from the acceptance testing should be carefully documented, along with any variation from the defined procedures, and kept as long as the TPS is used in the department. Successful completion of acceptance testing represents the final stage of the installation contract.

Commissioning

Commissioning is the process of putting the system into active clinical service. A commissioned TPS is deemed ready for clinical service after passing several milestones. Equipment is installed and tested, problems are identified and corrected, and the prospective users are extensively trained. A commissioned TPS is one whose specifications, systems, and staff have successfully completed a thorough QA process. Commissioning should include dosimetric as well as non-dosimetric testing. Dosimetric testing includes the production of a basic radiation database, which is entered into the TPS, after which the user tests the system over a range of clinically relevant conditions.

Quality evaluations of the programs' outputs are then made. Such a process cannot test all the system's pathways or subroutines; however, it does provide the user with a level of confidence over a wide variety of often-used treatment conditions. In addition, it helps the user understand the degree of uncertainty associated with these specific calculations. Non-dosimetric testing includes but is not limited to image geometry, CT-density table information, contouring accuracy, beam information and display, as well as isodose and DVH display. Finally, during commissioning the user produces a baseline of performance standards to be utilized for future QC.[4]

Quality Control

Quality is often equated with a general sense of goodness, but a more precise definition is necessary in Radiation Oncology. Quality can be defined as characteristics that meet the medical needs of the patient free from errors and mistakes. As indicated earlier, QA and QC are closely related and are meant to maintain a high level of quality. QA is the total process required to ensure that a certain level of quality is maintained for a defined product or service. QC consists of systematic actions necessary to ensure that the product or process performs according to specification. QC contains three components: (1) the measurement of the performance, (2) the comparison of this performance with existing baselines or specifications defined during commissioning, and (3) the appropriate actions necessary to keep or regain agreement with the baseline.

In the context of the TPS, QA and QC require the definition of a series of specifications that determine quality. Acceptance tests ensure that the system meets these basic requirements as defined by the specifications. Commissioning ensures the TPS is ready for clinical use and provides a series of baselines that can be used for ongoing QC in order to ensure that the system is maintaining the required standards. Ongoing QC must be performed at predefined intervals to confirm that there have been no changes in the basic radiation and machine parameter data files, in the input–output hardware, in the CT, MRI, or other imaging-related software or hardware, or with the transfer of data between clinical systems. Each of these four sections will be described in detail throughout the remainder of the chapter.

System Specifications

Sources of Uncertainties

Specifications take various forms. One form is simply a statement of whether the TPS is capable of doing a particular function or not. Another form is a quantitative definition of performance, for example, calculation speed, number of images it can hold, machine limitations, and so on. A third form is a statement of dose calculation accuracy. In order to assess the accuracy of a TPS and define realistic accuracy specifications, it is necessary to understand the sources of uncertainties.

The determination of uncertainties in dose calculations is complex because dose calculation algorithms depend on input information, which is usually generated by measurement. Thus, the uncertainty in the calculation output depends on the uncertainties associated with the measurements as well as the limitations of the calculation algorithms. This is true even with manufacturer-provided reference data as it also originates from measurements and includes typically measurement-based uncertainties, specifically at the extreme conditions, such as small field sizes. Measured data can be of various types, including relative doses in water phantoms, absolute dose calibrations for MU calculations, patient anatomy using imaging techniques or contouring devices, electron and physical density measurements, as well as physical characterization of compensators, bolus, and other treatment devices.

Suggested Tolerances

Criteria of acceptability for dose calculations have been described by various authors, including AAPM Task Group 53 and IAEA TRS-430.[39–41] More recently, AAPM MPPG 5.a provided updated discussions on criteria of acceptability and tolerances generally considered achievable for modern TPSs.[17] All tolerance values vary depending on the region of calculation. Greater accuracy can be achieved on the central ray in a homogeneous phantom than in the penumbra region at the beam edge. Generally, the five regions depicted in Figure 24.1 can be considered: (1) normalization point, (2) regions of low-dose gradients in the central axis (CAX) portion of the beam, (3) regions of large-dose gradients such as those occurring in the penumbra or in the fall-off region for electron beams, (4) regions of low-dose gradients in low-dose areas such as those occurring out of field or under large shielded areas, and (5) doses in the buildup or build-down regions at the entrance and exit surfaces of the patient. Criteria of acceptability are generally quoted as a percent of the reference dose except in regions of high-dose gradients, where a spatial agreement in millimeters is a better descriptor, since the dose uncertainties in such regions can be very large. The AAPM Medical Physics Practice Guideline 5.a provides a set of criteria of acceptability for TPS validation tests.[21] These include criteria for percentage depth doses (PDDs) and profiles used for TPS beam modeling and composite criteria to be applied in patient plans. A summary of these criteria is provided in Table 24.1.

For brachytherapy calculations, uncertainty estimates are more difficult to determine because of the very short treatment distances and the corresponding large-dose gradients. Furthermore, brachytherapy calculations usually include absolute dose estimates, which require a detailed understanding of absolute source output specifications. AAPM TG-138 suggests that when all uncertainties are combined, the two standard deviations (or two sigma uncertainty, $k = 2$ in the report) of dose rates

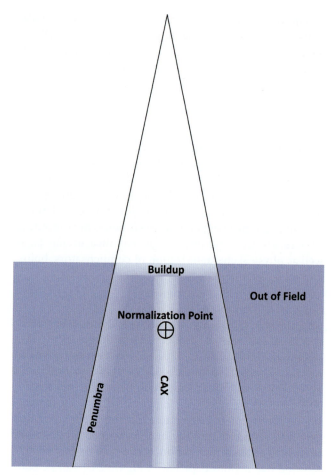

FIGURE 24.1. TPS accuracy and tolerance values can vary depending on the region of calculation and limitations of dose calculation algorithms and beam modeling. Greater accuracy can be achieved on the central ray in a homogeneous phantom than in the penumbra region at the beam edge.

TABLE 24.1	Criteria of Acceptability for Photon and Electron Dose Calculations
Descriptor	**Criterion**
Photon beams	
Homogeneous calculations (no shields)	
Reference dose conditions/Normalization Point	0.5%
High-dose region, low-dose gradient	2%
Large-dose gradients (>30%/cm)	3 mm
Small-dose gradients, low-dose region (<7% or normalization dose)*	3%
Inhomogeneity calculations	
Central ray (slab geometry, electron equilibrium)	3%
Composite, anthropomorphic phantom	
Off axis, contour, inhomogeneities, shields, electronic equilibrium, attenuators	
High-dose region, low-dose gradient**	5%
Large-dose gradient (>30%/cm)	3 mm
Small-dose gradient, low-dose region (<7% normalization dose)	3%
Electron beams	
Homogeneous calculations (no shields)	
Reference dose conditions/Normalization Point	0.5%
Central ray data (excluding buildup region)	3%/3 mm
High-dose region, low-dose gradient	3%
Large-dose gradients (>30%/cm)	3 mm
Small-dose gradients, low-dose region (<7% of normalization dose)*	4%
Inhomogeneity calculations	
Central ray (slab geometry, electron equilibrium)	7%
Composite, anthropomorphic phantom	
Off axis, contour, inhomogeneities, shields, electronic equilibrium, attenuators	
High-dose region, low-dose gradient	7%
Large-dose gradient (>30%/cm)	5 mm
Small-dose gradient, low-dose region (<7% normalization dose)	3%

Relative to local dose, unless otherwise specified.
*Percentage relative to maximum field dose
**Limit applicable for combination of several factors, listed earlier.

used in treatment planning are approximately 9% and 7% for low-energy and high-energy photon-emitting brachytherapy sources, respectively.[42] These stated uncertainties are for a single location, 1 cm from the source along the transverse plane. It should be noted that the one standard deviations (or one sigma uncertainty, $k = 1$ in the report) are less than 5% for both low-energy and high-energy sources. These findings keep in agreement with the suggested criteria of acceptability for brachytherapy calculations with a confidence interval of one standard deviation given in Table 24.2.

Acceptance Testing

The system specifications determine the acceptance tests that have to be performed. As a first step upon completion of the installation of a new system, the user should determine that all the components have been delivered and are consistent with the specifications. This includes a review of each component of the hardware. With rapidly changing technologies, manufacturers often switch one piece of

hardware with an updated version or with a device from another manufacturer. It is up to the user to ensure that the new hardware equals or surpasses the specifications set out in the purchase document.

The next step is to ensure that each component of the hardware functions at a simple level, that is, assess the monitor, mouse, printer, scanner, storage media, network connection, and other hardware items. A check that all the relevant manuals and schematics have been delivered is also important. The next level of hardware testing is to use the diagnostic programs provided with the system to ensure that all the hardware components assessed by the

TABLE 24.2 Sample Criteria of Acceptability for Brachytherapy Calculations

Descriptor	Criterion[a]
Single point source	
Distances of 0.5 to 5 cm	5%
Single line source	
Points along lines normal to the central 80% of the active length, distances of 0.5 to 5 cm	5%
Source end effects are difficult to quantify; therefore, no specification is given.	

[a]Percent of local dose.

diagnostic routines are functioning properly. This provides both a test of the system and a baseline for the user to understand any changes that may be observed in the follow-up QA tests.

The next step is to run the system software and to ensure that each component of the software listed in the specifications is actually installed and functional. This includes third-party software (commercial software purchased by the vendor and included in the TPS), in addition to the treatment planning software.

The TPS software acceptance can be very complex, primarily because the testing of the software requires input data specific to the therapy machines to allow direct comparisons of calculations with measurements. A practical approach is to test the system's input–output hardware to ensure that the system is capable of providing the options as defined in the specifications and then to assess the accuracy of the calculations as part of the commissioning process. In the signing of the acceptance document, the purchaser should indicate that the software acceptance will be completed as part of the commissioning process.

It should be noted that acceptance testing for IMRT requires a special emphasis on the system's capability of handling the penumbra region of small radiation fields as well as the leakage radiation outside the field. Small differences between measured and calculated doses in these regions can yield relatively large-dose differences when many of these small fields are summed together. Due to the difficulty of small field dosimetric measurements, extreme care should be taken to ensure the input data accurately represent the radiation delivery system.

A major component of potential error relates to maintaining the spatial integrity of imaging data sets during input–output with the TPS. Analysis of the spatial integrity during input–output should include validating the consistency of size, shape, distance, and orientation of the data set, and the uncertainty should be <1 mm. All contours, target volumes, normal tissue structures, CT images, beam outlines, ancillary devices such as wedges and blocks, and isodose lines should be accurate and consistent between screen display and hard-copy output. Scales, distance calipers, and any other measurement routines should be assessed for both function and accuracy. This includes autocontouring, automatic contour expansion for target volume margins, density assessments, automatic field shaping, and other features used by the planning software.

A more comprehensive process for acceptance testing has been proposed by the IAEA.[20] The consultant group for the IAEA proposed that vendors should perform a series of "type" tests for their system, the results of which should be provided by the vendor to the user as part of the purchase documentation.[20] Type tests refer to those tests that are to be done by the manufacturer, normally at the factory, to establish compliance with specified criteria. The type tests proposed by the IAEA are based on an intercomparison of photon dose calculation data.[43] Once the TPS is installed at the user's site, a select subset of tests should be performed to demonstrate consistency with the vendor's type tests. The vendors should update the type test results, if necessary, whenever software changes or upgrades are made, and again these should be documented and provided to all purchasers of that software. At the time of software updates by the user, another select subset of tests can be made to ensure consistency of results between the vendor's calculations in the factory and the user's calculations in the clinic.

Commissioning

As discussed in the introduction, there is still some ongoing debate on the utilization of a vendor-provided standard reference data set for commissioning a TPS. Supporters of the historical customized method of using institution-specific beam data contend that manufacturing and installation variations between linear accelerators require unique beam models developed from the beam data produced by extensive commissioning measurements.[18] In this approach, it is the responsibility of the physicist, guided by numerous formalized documents, to correctly commission the TPS and develop ongoing QA processes.[40,18] Proponents of using the vendor-provided data set contend that variations between machines from the same vendor/series are minimal and reference several studies indicating measurement and modeling errors during TPS commissioning and QA produce more extensive dose calculation inaccuracies.[26–28] Furthermore, prepackaged TPSs modeled on extensively validated vendor supplied reference beam data have the potential to drastically reduce gross systematic errors and standardize delivery quality across the entire radiation oncology industry. Several vendors of both generalized and specialized commercial TPSs install units using manufactured measured the vendor-provided data set.[44–46] Validation of the vendor-provided data set to the measurements made on the local linear accelerator is still needed to ensure an accurate match between the planned and delivered dose. There are several beam configuration parameters that are not specified in prepackaged data sets and must be carefully determined and validated against published data.[22] Regardless of which set of beam data is used during TPS commissioning, the same general measurement and comparison methodology should be followed, including comprehensive end-to-end testing for the entire treatment planning and delivery process. The commissioning process should also incorporate the development of treatment planning procedures, training for staff, and designating expert users who will be responsible for the continually TPS QA program. The remainder of this section provides examples and highlights of tests that should be conducted during TPS commissioning.

Photon Beams

The clinical implementation of the TPS can be divided into several components. These include entry of basic radiation data, entry of machine-specific parameters, entry of data related to ancillary treatment devices, verification of the accuracy of electron and physical density tables, and the validation of data transfer between all systems in the clinical workflow. Each of these components involves data entry and subsequent software validation. For each component, it is important for the user to understand the capabilities and limitations of the TPS and all software systems that are involved in the clinical workflow.

For beam model commissioning that is based on unique local beam data, the data entry for each algorithm requires a manufacturer-specific format from the beam data collection software or manually generated data set. The beam data collection software and dose calculation algorithms evolve with time, and the formatting requirement may change with it. As such, it is important that the adequacy of beam data formatting is verified to be compatible with the TPS and dose calculation algorithm being commissioned

Basic radiation data can be entered in various forms, including tissue–air ratios, tissue–phantom ratios, tissue–maximum ratios, PDD, and cross-beam profiles. Cross-beam profiles may also have to be measured under a variety of conditions, including profiles for the machine collimators, shielding blocks, wedges, and multileaf collimators. The quality and accuracy of the measured basic radiation data should be evaluated prior to implementation in the TPS. A standard set of procedures for acquiring radiation beam data, along with examples of commonly identified errors, are provided by the AAPM.[18] Limitations of physical measurements, specifically for small fields, high gradients such as the penumbra and buildup regions, and peripheral dose regions should be carefully evaluated. In all situations, it is imperative that the user ensures the accuracy of the entered data by looking at the numerical values on the screen or by plotting out the data and comparing directly with what has been entered. An independent verification of the beam data using either Monte Carlo–generated data or manufacturer-provided standard data should be considered.

In cases where manufacturer-provided standard data form the basis of the beam model commissioning, thorough validation measurements should be taken on the LINAC and validated against the data being used. Any discrepancies should be evaluated, and if necessary, modifications can be made to the delivery system in order to ensure each beam matches the data provided. It is important to understand the limitations of the data being used and if necessary to supplement the data with local beam data based on the types of treatment to be delivered on the machine (e.g. appropriate small field beam data for SRS or SBRT treatments).

The types of tests that should be used to assess the quality of the algorithms are summarized through working group reports as seen in references.[17,40,41] Table 24.3 provides a summary of the relevant parameters and variables that should be included in the testing process. The following section outlines a list of examples of photon commissioning tests and the kinds of issues that should be considered when assessing the calculation capabilities of the TPS.

Examples of Photon Commissioning Tests

The type of photon beam commissioning tests, possible methods of evaluation, and some additional issues to consider are provided for non-IMRT photon beam commissioning. These examples do not represent extensive commissioning testing and primarily serve to illustrate possible methods for completing the commissioning process. Figure 24.2 illustrates an example of simple CAX PDD data for a 10 cm × 10 cm 6 MV photon beam. A comparison is made between the calculated data (circles) and the measured data (*solid line*) using a 1D gamma index analysis criteria of 1% dose difference and 1 mm distance-to-agreement, where a gamma index value less than 1.0 indicates the calculated TPS data is within the assessment criteria. It is clear that beyond the buildup depth (15 mm), the differences are minimal but in the buildup region the differences can be quite large. This is a reasonable difference, given the difficulty of measuring dose close to the phantom surface, and highlights the importance of understanding the limitations of the TPS and measured data being used for comparison. Figure 24.3 shows a difference comparison for cross-beam profiles for a 4.0 cm × 4.0 cm 6 MV photon beam with a 45° wedge. A similar 1D gamma index analysis using 1%/1 mm criteria shows the largest differences in the penumbra region or in areas of steep change within the wedged field. This is also another reasonable expectation, given the volume averaging effects in steep regions of beam profiles.

The accurate modeling of dosimetric characteristics for MLCs has increased importance in modern radiation therapy as they not only shape most treatment fields but also generate modulated dose distributions through the summation of numerous subfields. Thus, the uncertainty in the MLC model is compounded in IMRT and volumetric modulated arc therapy (VMAT) plans, often resulting

TABLE 24.3 Initial Dose Calculation Tests: Variables to Consider

Photon beam point calculations

TAR, TPR, PDD, PSF for square fields
TAR, TPR, PDD, PSF for rectangular fields
TAR, TPR, PDD, PSF for complex fields
Inverse square law, distance corrections
Attenuation, tray, wedge, compensator factors
Output or collimator scatter factors

Photon beam dose profiles or distributions

Square fields, normal incidence
Rectangular fields normal incidence
Effects of SAD or SSD
Wedged fields
Contour corrections
Bars or blocks
Multileaf collimators
Asymmetrical fields
Multiple beams
Arcs and rotations
Off-axis calculations
Collimator rotation and/or rotation of plane of calculation
Inhomogeneity corrections
Compensators
Anthropomorphic phantom tests

Electron beam point doses, distributions, or profiles

Square fields PDD and dose profiles
Extended distances
Rectangular fields, normal incidence
Contour corrections
Inhomogeneity corrections
Output factors
Effects of shields and irregular field shapes
Anthropomorphic phantom tests

Brachytherapy calculations

Entered data
Exposure or air kerma rate constants
Parameters for tissue attenuation and scatter
Half-life and decay calculation
Source wall information
Activity
Anisotropy
Dose calculations
Single and multiple source distributions
Line source calculations
Rotation and translation of plane of calculation
Source trajectories for special applicators
Use of orthogonal and/or stereotactic films
Automatic source identification schemes
Source display routines
Automated optimization, evaluation routines

PDD, percentage depth dose; PSF, peak scatter factor; SAD, source-to-axis distance; SSD, source-to-surface distance; TAR, tissue–air ratio; TPR, tissue–phantom ratio.

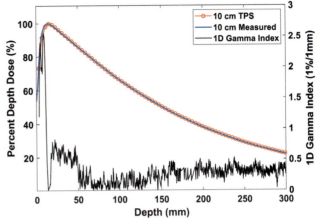

FIGURE 24.2. Central ray percentage depth doses (PDD) for an energy of 6MV and a field of size of 10 cm × 10 cm. The data points entered into the treatment planning system are shown as solid lines, and the calculated data are shown by the circles. The 1D gamma index uses criteria of 1% dose difference and 1 mm distance-to-agreement.

TPS, treatment planning system.

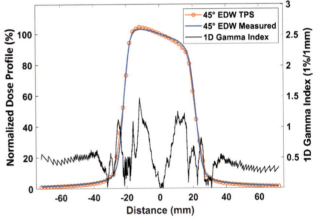

FIGURE 24.3. Calculated and measured normalized dose profiles under an enhanced dynamic wedge with an angle of 45°. Profiles are shown for the 4 cm × 4 cm at 2.5 cm depth. The measured data points entered into the treatment planning system are shown as solid lines, and the calculated data are shown by the circles. The 1D gamma index uses criteria of 1% dose difference and 1 mm distance-to-agreement.

TPS, treatment planning system.

in larger total dosimetric uncertainty in the aggregate delivered plan. Figure 24.4 shows measured and calculated cross-beam dose profiles at 2.5 cm depth for a round 9 cm MLC delineated field with two 5 mm MLCs covering the central portion of the beam to produce a central beam block. A 1D gamma index analysis using 1%/1 mm criteria shows the largest differences under the blocked region. This type of analysis demonstrates the limitations of the TPS to accurately model intraleaf and interleaf leakage with a single parameter. The dosimetric leaf gap (DLG) characterizes the dose through the minimum physical leaf gap between opposing pairs of leaves to incorporate the rounded leaf end into the MLC model

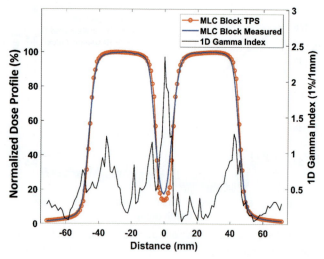

FIGURE 24.4. Comparison of measured and calculated cross-beam profiles under a central MLC block covering the center of a 9 cm circular MLC delineated field. 1D gamma index analysis using a 1% dose difference and 1 mm distance to agreement shows the largest differences occur under the centrally shielded region of the multileaf collimator.

MLC, multi-leaf collimator; TPS, treatment planning system.

in the TPS. Figure 24.5 shows a profile across a closed pair of 5 mm MLCs demonstrating the dose through the closed region as well as the transmission under the MLCs. The TPS can be tuned to accurately match the dose at the gap and under the leaf but may fail to accurately calculate the dose across the rounded leaf end. These differences may be due to the TPS's inability to characterize the complex characteristics of MLCs (i.e. rounded leaf end,

tongue and groove, drive screw cavity), with a few fixed parameters like the DLG and MLC transmission values, and failure to handle electron contamination under the leaves or shields. This is a physics problem that occurs in older algorithms but has been improved in most new commercial treatment planning programs.[47,48] Differences could also be originating from the limitations of physical measurements within these regions.

Intensity-Modulated Radiation Therapy

There are some unique aspects to commissioning IMRT compared to 3D conformal radiation therapy (CRT). IMRT uses automated inverse planning routines, which use iterative algorithms to yield acceptable plans based on specified dose-volume constraints. The resulting dose distribution can have steep gradients between the target and the organs at risk, and the commissioning tests need to reflect this added consideration. Because IMRT could involve the summation of very many small fields, multiple field edges, dynamic delivery, and multiple arc delivery, it is extremely important to ensure that the modeling of the penumbra and the low-dose region outside the beam is handled accurately. As previously discussed, the accurate calculation of the leakage radiation through the body, side, and end of the leaves, especially those with curved ends, is very important to yield an accurate penumbra.[49,50] Because of these small field considerations, International Commission on Radiation Units and Measurements (ICRU) Report 83[51] and AAPM MPPG 5.a[17] indicate a criteria of acceptability of 2% in the low-gradient high-dose target region and 3% in low-dose regions. More importantly, planar dose verification using gamma analysis with a criteria of 2% dose difference and 2 mm distance may uncover correctable problems with IMRT commissioning that may be hidden with the more common 3%/3 mm criteria.[17]

It should also be noted that the delivered dose distribution is dependent on the leaf sequencing algorithm that is used to convert the TPS-derived intensity maps to a deliverable set of MLC sequences. The results are dependent on leaf width, leaf-travel distance, speed, and acceleration, interdigitization of leaves, gantry speed and acceleration, DLG, and maximum field size. Using smaller MLC steps and a larger number of intensity levels can result in many segments with small field sizes again compounding the need for accuracy in MLC positioning and penumbra modeling. Furthermore, there may be accelerator constraints on the delivery of many segments, each with a small number of MUs.

Because of the difficulty in measuring doses in small fields and potential accelerator constraints, the ICRU Report 83[51] suggests that the use of end-to-end testing is integral to the beam commissioning process. End-to-end testing validates the entire treatment planning process, including data collection, beam modeling, treatment planning and delivery, data transfer from the TPS to the record-and-verify system, and QA of the delivered

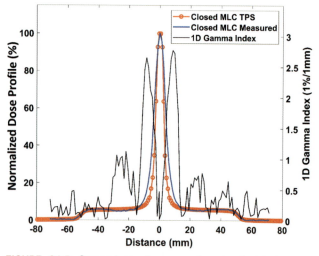

FIGURE 24.5. Comparison of measured and calculated cross-beam profiles across a closed, rounded leaf MLC pair. 1D gamma index analysis using a 1% dose difference and 1 mm distance to agreement shows the largest differences occur as the dose falls across the rounded leaf end. This shows the limitation of modeling the complex shape of modern MLCs with a few fixed a parameters.
MLC, multi-leaf collimator; TPS, treatment planning system.

absorbed dose. A typical end-to-end test involves scanning a QA phantom, creating an IMRT plan on the image data set, measuring the delivered dose within the phantom, and comparing the measurements to the calculated dose distribution.[19] The AAPM Task Group 119 provides an end-to-end testing suite for IMRT planning.[19]

Automated Treatment Planning System Validation

The wide range of clinical beams and dose calculation algorithms of increasing complexity, from simple convolution-superposition algorithms towards more complex algorithms that rely on Monte Carlo simulations, place a heavy burden on clinical physicists to validate and commission the TPS properly. The ever-increasing use of cloud-based TPS also suggests a future where TPS version upgrades will be much more common, given the relative ease of implementation, further imposing additional commissioning frequency and requirements. It is important that TPS commissioning remains comprehensive enough so that the limitations are well understood and a high level of confidence exists in the accuracy of the dose calculation and treatment planning algorithms of the future. To this end, automated TPS commissioning should play an important role to complete all the necessary commissioning testing. Manufacturers now develop application programming interfaces (API), allowing for the direct scripted manipulation of the TPS in order to generate commissioning testing plans, analyze results, and programmatically detect undesired changes to the database.

Automated and Knowledge-based Planning

Automated and KBP techniques have recently been developed to improve both treatment planning efficiency and plan quality.[52–54] Automated techniques replace repetitive steps of the manual workflow typically completed by a planner by automatically applying predefined site-specific parameters (structure names, beam angles, weighted optimization objectives) to a new patient data set. These predefined parameters provide a standardized basis to begin the optimization process and help minimize the variations introduced by planner. KBP is an additional method that aims to reduce the variation in IMRT plan quality and improve efficiency by providing achievable, patient-specific optimization objectives derived from a model trained with a cohort of previously treated site-specific plans.[55,56] This database of existing treatment plans is used to create a dose prediction model that correlates patient-specific anatomic relationships (contours) with prior dose distributions and can be applied to future patients being treated to a similar anatomic site. Recent research for automated, knowledge-based contour validation has also shown promise.[57]

Commissioning automated treatment planning software requires a thorough understanding of how the program takes input data and creates treatment plans. Ideally, predefined planning parameters, as discussed earlier, are evaluated to ensure they correlate to an institution's treatment planning practice. To ensure acceptable quality is achieved, plans generated using the automated software should be evaluated at specific dosimetric endpoints against manually generated plans for several patients across all treatment sites for which the software will be clinically used. If acceptable plan quality is not achieved, the predefined planning parameters should be adjusted until the necessary quality is met.

Additional considerations are necessary when commissioning KBP software, as discussed in AAPM Task Group 308.[10] Users have the option to commission their own local KBP model or to utilize existing global models created by another institution. KBP models are intrinsically dependent on the anatomic relationships (contours), clinical trade-offs, and dosimetric endpoints of the initial IMRT plans selected to train the model. Global models are sometimes provided by the vendor with a detailed description of the parameters associated with these dependencies, and each should be carefully compared to the clinical practice before being considered for implementation. When creating a local model, the quality and diversity of the plans included should reflect the intended scope for which the model will be clinically applied. Both local and global models should be extensively validated against an independent validation cohort of manually created clinical plans to ensure the model will meet or exceed expected target and OAR dosimetric goals.[10] If plans created with the model are not consistently comparable or superior to manually created plans, the model should not be selected for use within the clinical workflow.

Image Registration

The utilization of multi-modality imaging in the definition of anatomic OARs and targets has become increasingly common in the modern radiation therapy clinical workflow.[58,59] While CT imaging still remains the primary modality for radiation treatment planning, it is often inadequate when attempting to accurately delineate the tumor.[60] Tumors located in the central nervous system, abdomen, pelvis, breast, or head and neck may require MRI/ultrasounds to provide high contrast between soft tissues.[61] Other sites in the thorax, abdomen, pelvis, and head and neck benefit from metabolic information provided from PET and single-photon emission computerized tomography (SPECT) imaging.[7,62,63] Additionally, specialized CT scans (4DCT) may be necessary to assist in the management of tumor motion in the thorax or abdomen.[64] In order for the physician to accurately and efficiently use the information provided by all imaging modalities, it is necessary for all imaging data sets to be geometrically associated via a process called image registration.

Image registration creates a vector transformation that maps specific anatomic structures in the secondary imaging data set to the corresponding anatomic structures in the primary imaging data set (typically the planning CT). This transformation may be a rigid (consisting of a global shift/rotation) or deformable (incorporating relative local modifications of the secondary data set). Once the image data sets are registered, it is possible to map information such as soft tissue contrast, metabolic uptake, tissue boundaries, or previously delivered dose from the secondary data sets onto the primary CT data set. This combination of information from various imaging modalities is known as image fusion. Many modern TPSs have developed integrated image registration and fusion software. Due to their role in delineating radiation targets and healthy tissue, the accuracy and reliability of the registration and fusion software necessitates a thorough commissioning process.

The process of validating image registration and fusion software is relatively new. To thoroughly evaluate the accuracy and uncertainties of any registration software, it is necessary to quantitatively compare the generated coordinate system changes to known true changes within baseline image data sets. These tests should be completed across all imaging modalities using virtual geometric and anatomic phantoms and include both rigid and deformable registration techniques.[65] Virtual phantoms allow for predetermined changes to an imaging set against which registration algorithms can be evaluated.[52] AAPM Task Group 132 describes a series of virtual phantoms and related tests to be used during commissioning and proposes making this standard set of virtual phantoms available via download in order to standardize the commission process.[7] Additional end-to-end tests using physical phantoms, such as those supplied by the Imaging and Radiation Oncology Core (IROC) in Houston, should also be conducted. A series of typical clinical images should also be evaluated qualitatively, and an ongoing patient-specific QA process should be developed to efficiently evaluate image registration within the treatment planning workflow.

Auto-Segmentation

Clinical auto-segmentation algorithms significantly improve the efficiency of the contouring process but can produce contours with small to moderate errors.[66,67] Commissioning tests for auto-segmentation algorithms should identify the frequency and magnitude of consistently occurring deviations from the clinically accepted manual contours for each structure, and all treatment planning staff should be familiar with these deviations. Continuing patient-specific contour QA should be incorporated into the clinical treatment planning workflow.

Adaptive Radiation Therapy

ART seeks to account for the dosimetric impact of daily anatomical variations that occur during treatment to ensure the initial planned dose distribution matches the final delivered dose distribution. Online ART requires the rapid implementation of many of the typical treatment planning steps, including image acquisition, image registration, anatomic contouring, dose optimization, daily/cumulative plan evaluation, and patient-specific QA.[11]

While each of the hardware and software components for the ART process may have been independently commissioned in the normal TPS, their specific application in the ART workflow should be evaluated.[68] In order to minimize the time needed for online ART, many of the planning steps are automated. The accuracy and functionality of any automated tools, such as DVH evaluation scripts, cumulative dose analysis, and OAR/target assessment, should be validated for all treatment sites. Finally, due to the time sensitivity of online ART, each member of the staff should be extensively trained in each of their roles. End-to-end tests of both the system and workflow should be conducted with the staff to ensure the online ART can be accurately and efficiently completed under the necessary time constraints.[68] A thorough evaluation of the integrated ART workflow using modern process improvement tools has been shown useful in identifying potential sources of error and should be conducted for each unique ART workflow during the commissioning process.[69]

Electron Beams

Good examples of specific tests for electron beams can be found in recent working group reports.[40,41] Tests of specific concern to electrons relate to changes in source-to-skin distance (SSD), output factor calculations, oblique beam incidence, and variations in output for shaped fields. Additional tests to validate the accuracy of the calculated dose in heterogeneous medium, such as bone, fat, and lung, should also be conducted.

Brachytherapy

Verification of brachytherapy dose calculation should be approached similarly to the external beam tests. In this situation, however, it becomes much more difficult to compare measurements with calculations because of the difficulty in performing measurements over the short distances involved in brachytherapy. The user may have to resort to comparing calculations with previously published source data. Relevant information can be found in various reports.[40,41,70,71] One unique test for brachytherapy is the assessment of anisotropy calculations if these are provided by the system. A recent report by Rivard et al.[72] provides enhancements to commissioning techniques and QA of brachytherapy TPS that use model-based dose calculation algorithms. Additional information regarding model-based dose calculation algorithms has been included in a recent AAPM Task Group 186.[73] As previously noted, a recent joint AAPM-ESTRO Working Group addressed the uncertainty in dose calculation accuracy for brachytherapy TPSs.[42]

Proton Therapy

Commissioning proton beam models within a TPS is often accomplished through a combination of simulated Monte Carlo data and measured beam data.[74] Requirements for specific commissioning tests depend on the type of proton system (dual passive scatter vs. active spot scanning), and examples of each have been described thoroughly.[75–78] For dual passive scattering systems, validation will typically include measuring longitudinal fluence, virtual source position, effective source position, source size, Bragg peaks, and lateral beam profiles. Active spot scanning may require validation of spot size, in-air lateral profiles, and integral depth dose data. During commissioning, the lateral and range uncertainties associated with the accuracy of the model for the full range of treatment conditions should be carefully evaluated and accounted for within the clinical treatment planning process.[79,80] Consideration needs to be given to accurately correlate proton stopping power ratios to CT numbers within a patient, and difference between phantom stopping powers and patient tissue stopping power should be evaluated.[81]

Commissioning of Other Components

Modern TPSs contain many other commissioning aspects than those related to dose calculations. Examples of other types of issues that must be considered and verified are shown in Table 24.4. The ability of the TPS to accurately handle tissue heterogeneities when calculating dose is of particular importance and validation requires the use of a specialized phantom.[21] Other non-dosimetric parameters, such as image transfer and contouring validation, can also be evaluated using specialized phantoms specifically to address some commissioning and QA issues.[21,82]

Special Techniques

Special and individualized techniques require their own unique evaluation. Examples of special techniques that require additional workup and commissioning are summarized in Table 24.5. In addition, there are now a number of new technologies that have specialized TPS specifically made for that technology. Examples include helical tomotherapy,[44] robotic radiation therapy,[83] onboard MRI-guided radiation therapy,[45] online ART systems[84] and multiple cobalt source, small field radiation therapy, used mostly for neurological sites.[46]

Quality Assurance and Quality Control

QC of a product or process involves three steps: (1) the measurement of the performance, (2) the comparison of the performance with a given standard, and (3) the actions necessary to keep or regain the standard. The commissioning process of the TPS provides the standard for comparison. Once the TPS is fully commissioned, a QA program should be implemented to ensure the system is able to remain within the standards determined during commissioning. However, the problems associated with maintaining consistency and quality within a TPS are quite different from the problems associated with QA of a CT simulator or accelerator, which has electrical and mechanical components that can wear and change with time.

Closely associated with QA is *risk management*. Risk management consists of four components: (1) identifying

TABLE 24.4	Commissioning of Other Components

Image-related issues
Image acquisition
Image transfer
Conversion of CT numbers to electron densities
MRI distortions
Automatic contouring routines
Effects of autocontouring routines with incomplete image sets
Effects of unequally spaced slices
Partial volume effects due to slice thickness
Image artifacts
Image registration
Image reconstructions
Image enhancement tools

Anatomical structures
Contour determination and entry
3D reconstruction of contours
3D surface displays
Bolus generation
Beam display in 3D
Irregular field display
Multileaf collimator display
Wedge display
Display of isodose lines and surfaces
Labeling of relevant parameters and dimensions
Coordinate determination and display
Beam's eye view
Room views
Source display for brachytherapy

Miscellaneous issues
Digitally reconstructed radiographs
Dose-volume histograms
Tumor control and normal tissue complication probabilities
Isocenter moves
Data transfer to therapy machine

the possible sources of risk of failure or malfunction, (2) analyzing the frequency of incidents of failure or malfunction, (3) taking corrective action to minimize such failure, and (4) monitoring the outcome of such changes. Thus, to develop an appropriate QA program for treatment planning computers, an assessment of the likelihood of failure helps focus on the issues of concern. IAEA TRS-430[14] provides a good summary of reported errors associated with radiation treatment planning. For the "accidents" (major clinically significant errors) associated with TPSs, they determined that the key contributory factors include the following:

1. A lack of understanding of the TPS
2. A lack of appropriate commissioning (no comprehensive tests)
3. A lack of independent calculation checks

TABLE 24.5	Techniques Requiring Special Workup
Beam junctions for both photons and electrons	
Electron arcs	
Stereotactic radiation therapy	
Stereotactic brachytherapy	
High-dose rate brachytherapy	
Low-dose rate brachytherapy	
Bolus Electron Conformal Therapy	
Automatic optimization routines	
Total body irradiation	
Total skin irradiation	
Intraoperative radiation therapy	
Dynamic wedges	

The major issues related to treatment planning errors were summarized by four key words: (1) education, (2) verification, (3) documentation, and (4) communication.

The development of a thorough QA program is a compromise between cost and benefit. An appropriate program has specific QC to identify and mitigate high probability and high impact errors without being excessively burdensome on a facility's resources. However, as new technology is implemented in the clinic, it can be challenging to identify the appropriate QC tests that provide the necessary balance. A careful evaluation of a new process should be conducted before determining changes and additions to any QA program.

AAPM Task Group 100[85] is attempting to deal with the issue of ever-increasing QA activity as new and more complex technologies evolve. The central idea of TG-100 is to transition from traditional device-centered QA to a more comprehensive risk-based, process-centered approach. To implement a process-centered QA program, the task group describes three techniques that have been historically used in engineering circles: process tree mapping, failure mode and effects analysis (FMEA), and fault tree analysis (FTA). Process tree mapping is a visual illustration of all the relationships of each step for a specific process. It tracks the physical and temporal flow of each step, from start to finish, and is useful in easily identifying and tracking weaknesses and error migration. FMEA is a prospective approach to QA. When used in conjunction with a process tree map, it assesses the potential risks (failure modes), likelihood of errors, and impact of such errors for each step defined within the process. For each step, there may be many potential failure modes, and each one may have several potential causes and outcomes. For each potential cause of failure, values are assigned in three categories: O, the probability that a specific cause will result in a failure mode; D, the probability that the failure mode

resulting from the specific cause will go undetected; and S, the severity of the effects resulting from a specific failure mode should it go undetected throughout treatment. Convention uses numbers between 1 and 10. Category O ranges from 1 (unlikely failure, <1 in 10^4) to 10 (highly likely, >5% of the time). Category D ranges from 1 (undetected only <0.01% of the time) to 10 (undetected >20% of the time). Category S ranges from 1 (no appreciable danger) to 10 (catastrophic if persisting through treatment). The product of these three indices forms the risk probability number (RPN = $O \times S \times D$). A complete FMEA applied to an entire process helps develop an FTA, which is a visualization of all errors at each step and associated root causes for each error. By applying an FTA, it is possible to determine appropriate QC measures that can be implemented at the necessary steps to accurately mitigate identified root causes of failure. The prospective approach described by TG-100 provides guidelines to determine an efficient application of resources within a QA program that accurately minimizes all major sources of error. Examples of FMEA analyses have been published for the external beam radiation therapy process[86] and dynamic MLC tracking systems.[87]

A necessary element in developing a prospective QA program is the inclusion of an electronic incident event reporting system.[88,89] A department-level reporting system provides a platform for all employees to voluntarily and anonymously report events, the severity of which ranges from minor miscommunication to near-miss to severe treatment error. Submitted events can be analyzed, and previously unidentified patterns can be systematically addressed prior to the occurrence of serious errors.[89] Several major groups have recently begun development of national/international reporting systems (ASTRO's RO-ILS and IAEA's SAFRON), which will provide the possibility of shared learning across all participating institutions.

Program and System Documentation and Training

At the most basic level of QA, the user must be aware of what the computer programs are doing when any specific option is requested. Even if the programs are perfectly accurate, any error in data entry results in an error in the output. Thus, the user must have adequate information in terms of manuals and online help to aid in the commissioning and operational process of the TPS. The types of documentation that should be available are listed in Table A1–1 of AAPM TG53.[40]

A significant amount of documentation occurs during the commissioning process and encompasses all systems and software that were tested. Appropriate documentation should include detailed descriptions of all tests run, origin of data used in the TPS, and baselines for the QA program. Documentation detailing the treatment planning procedures should also be developed during the commissioning process, and all appropriate staff should be provided training to fulfill their roles.

User Training

Closely associated with proper manuals and information is user training. The user must be clearly aware of normalization procedures, dose calculation algorithms, image display and reconstruction procedures, and program calculation capabilities and limitations. This training can be carried out at three levels at least: (1) vendor training courses, (2) in-house staff training, and (3) special training courses set up by user groups or third-party software vendors.

TPS training has traditionally been formatted for dosimetrists and physicists, and often only limited training is available to physicians. Physicians should be able to effectively operate the simple tools of any planning system (setting beams parameters, defining field sizes, contour tools). Beyond the basic functionality, in order to accurately evaluate a treatment plan, physicians need to be aware of inaccuracies and limitations of the planning system. This includes the inherent inaccuracies of the dose calculation algorithms (CAX, buildup region, penumbra, heterogeneities) and clinical situations in which these inaccuracies are commonly a factor. Additionally, physicians should be aware of the capabilities and limitations of IMRT optimization algorithms to achieve organ/target specific dosimetric planning goals and the common clinical trade-offs. Finally, physicians should be able to evaluate the quality of image registration/fusion and understand the processes of rigid and deformable image registration.

Reproducibility Tests

A normally functioning TPS is unlikely to generate small changes in output. TPS system hardware malfunctions are likely to be obvious. A more probable issue of concern is inadvertent access by treatment planners to the basic radiation or machine data files. This can result in changes to accuracy of calculations without the user being aware that changes have taken place.

For inadvertent software or hardware changes, a binary comparison of all the software and data files can test whether any changes have occurred. If changes are found, the details of the changes must be assessed, and a partial system recommissioning may have to be implemented. Alternatively, as described in the IAEA report,[21] a select subset of the vendor type tests should be performed to demonstrate consistency with previous results.

From a risk management perspective, other possible sources of error include intended or unintended changes in software or data files. These can occur within the TPS or in the systems associated with data generation, such as CT scanners and water phantom systems. Software upgrades in these external systems can result in changes to the data entered into the TPS.

To aid in the assessment of any software changes, a series of reproducibility tests of the dose calculation algorithms, the image display algorithms, and the plan evaluation tools should be undertaken on a regular basis. Examples of such reproducibility tests can be found in the reports from the AAPM[40] and the IAEA.[41] Users should develop their own tests based on their particular TPS and what components of the hardware, software, and data files have any likelihood of being changed.

Patient-Specific Tests

Since no system of computer programs is error-free, nor are users of such programs perfect, routine inspection of each treatment plan is a requirement for proper QA. Calculation of the external beam dose usually consists of two components: (1) calculation of a relative dose distribution and (2) calculation of the machine output in terms of MUs. Both of these components require a check by a participant independent of the first calculation. For relative dose distributions, secondary checks, either conducted manually or with a third-party software, can be performed by choosing a specific point, usually on the central ray, and calculating a dose estimate for each of the beams using simplified tables to generate the results. These checks should agree to within about 2% to 3% of the computer-calculated values in regions of uniform dose delivery and relatively simple inhomogeneity corrections.[90] More complicated plans have to be evaluated on an individual basis to assess the trends of the numerical values. Similarly, the machine setting calculation should be checked independently of the first calculation.

With the advent of more complex segmented or dynamic conformal therapy and IMRT, such manual checks become very difficult if not impossible. In these situations, the absolute dose is determined as part of the planning process, with the MUs being defined for each component of the treatment. QC checks must be developed for each individual technique. AAPM Task Group 218 describes recommendation for the prioritization of patient-specific QA delivery methods as follows[91]:

- Measurement of the true composite dose in phantom using treatment delivery method
- Measurement of the individual field-by-field fluence, perpendicular to the field CAX
- All measurements analyzed in absolute dose mode with global normalization

For brachytherapy, manual single-point calculations are more difficult, and therefore a check can be performed with one of the conventional systems of dosage calculations, such as the Manchester system. This approach can be used to make crude checks to an accuracy of about 10%. Again, assessing trends is crucial in evaluating the quality of the calculation.

In vitro and in vivo Dosimetry Checks

As a final check of the quality of the overall treatment planning process, it is useful to perform measurements using special-purpose or anthropomorphic phantoms (in vitro dosimetry) or to perform measurements on or in the patient while in treatment position (in vivo dosimetry). In vitro dosimetry is an important component of the implementation of any new treatment technique or clinical procedure. Generally, it is performed with thermoluminescent dosimetry

(TLD) in a phantom containing human-like tissue densities and composition, such as an anthropomorphic phantom. More recently, optically stimulated luminescence (OSL) is being used in place of TLD.[92] Diodes and metal-oxide semiconductor field-effect transistor (MOSFET)[93] dosimetry systems are now readily available and provide instant read-out capability. This type of dosimetry ensures that the basic procedures associated with a new treatment technique are in agreement within a predetermined range of accuracy. A report by Dunscombe et al.[94] gives a good overview of the use of an anthropomorphic phantom to evaluate the quality of treatment planning computer systems. While providing a good indication of the accuracy of the dose delivery process near the center of the target volume, differences between measurements and calculations away from the central region were difficult to interpret as to whether the calculations were off, the measurements were off, or the beam placement was inaccurate. Thus, in vitro dosimetry must be established in such a manner that differences between measurements and calculations can be readily interpreted.

Similar concerns of interpretation also apply to in vivo dosimetry.[95] There is a tendency by radiation oncologists to request in vivo measurements to give them an assurance that the dose delivery process is accurate, especially in regions where there is concern about critical structures such as the eyes, gonads, or a fetus. Sometimes, these regions are close to the edge of the radiation beams. Under such circumstances, small changes in beam alignment can generate large changes in measured dose, leaving ambiguity in the interpretation of the results. These interpretation difficulties should be clearly explained to the radiation oncologist requesting the measurements. Better comparisons of calculations and measurements can be made in regions where doses are not changing as rapidly—either on the entrance or exit surfaces or, if possible, by placing dosimeters in body cavities such as the mouth, trachea, esophagus, vagina, uterus, or rectum. In vivo dosimetry is a recommended check under some treatment conditions and it may provide an opportunity to mitigate treatment errors,[96] but it should not replace pre-treatment in vitro phantom measurements for more complex treatment techniques, such as IMRT. AAPM Task Group 158 has been charged with assessing the current status of in vivo dosimetry for non-target, out-of-field exposures and to formulate recommendations for methods to improve measurements and calculations for doses outside the treatment volume.[97]

Quality Audits

It is always useful to review the QA activities of individual institutions. Recent years have seen the public reporting of various errors or "accidents" in radiation therapy. While such errors can have a devastating effect on individual patients, the actual error rate in radiation therapy is very low. However, it is the responsibility of members of the radiation therapy team to ensure that proper procedures are in place to minimize such errors. As a first approach, an institutional self-auditing process is beneficial. This is best done in the context of a QA committee that should exist in every radiation therapy department. External audits have proven to be extremely beneficial for finding inadvertent deviations from acceptable practice. The IROC in Houston, Texas, has done this for years for institutions participating in clinical trials involved with the Radiation Therapy Oncology Group (RTOG).[98,14] Dosimetry intercomparisons are also useful especially in the development of new techniques such as IMRT and provide a means to standardized the quality of radiation treatment facilities.[14,99]

The IAEA has developed an external audit process, which involves a review of the total treatment process.[100] They do this through the use of a quality assurance team in radiation oncology (QUATRO), which consists of a radiation oncologist, medical physicist, radiation therapist, and sometimes a specialist in radiation protection. A similar external quality audit has been incorporated into the American Society of Radiation Oncologist (ASTRO) Apex and American College of Radiology (ACR) radiation therapy accreditation process.[101] Dosimetric comparisons and external audits provide a substantial benefit to improve the overall quality of radiation therapy across all facilities.

Quality Assurance Administration

An important component of any QA program is its effective organization and administration. Any QA program should be carried out according to a predetermined schedule and ongoing records of the activities and the results should be maintained. Proper administration requires that one person, usually a qualified medical physicist, be responsible for the QA program. Although this individual does not necessarily have to carry out all the tests and their evaluations, they must ensure that there is written documentation on the QA process, that the tests are carried out according to their specified frequency, and that appropriate actions are taken as needed.

As TPSs become networked into clusters with various planning and target volume delineation stations, servers, and peripheral devices, system management becomes an integral component of the entire QA of the TPS. This management includes maintaining an adequate check on system security and limiting user access not only to the system but also to specific software and data file modifications. It is important that the radiation data files not be inadvertently changed and that patient confidentiality be fully maintained.

To avoid the possibility of any undesired loss of information, a regular schedule for system backup is essential.[40] This may include daily backups of the most recent patient additions and changes, weekly backups of all patient information, and monthly backups of the entire TPS. Backups are also warranted immediately after any major changes to the software of the system.

In addition to standard backups, it may also be desirable to archive specific patient information, especially if patients are to be grouped for study purposes. In some cases, patient data may have to be forwarded to clinical trial groups such as the RTOG, which accepts such information through the internet. However, patient data must also be archived in case the patient comes back for retreatment.

Proper QA of the modern 3D TPS is a time-consuming process. Adequate staff resources must be allocated to ensure that the QA is completed in an appropriate manner.

SUMMARY

QA programs for radiation therapy machines, especially with the clinical implementation of high-energy accelerators have been well defined for many years. Formalized (CT) simulator QA is a more recent phenomenon.[82] While redundant checks for MU and time calculations have also been standard practice, the formalization of a QA program for treatment planning computers occurred more recently. This is partly due to the tremendous variation in TPSs and their algorithms and partly to the complexity of treatment planning QA, since it involves multiple facets and is inherently centered on the entire process and not specific equipment. Because of these complexities, it is clear that a comprehensive program depends on institutional procedures, the type of planning system in use, and the entire treatment planning workflow.

Treatment planning errors can be minimized with a good QA program. As indicated earlier in this chapter, the major issues that relate to treatment planning errors can be summarized by four keywords: (1) education, (2) verification, (3) documentation, and (4) communication.[41] Education is required not only at the technical and professional level in terms of the use of the TPS but also at the organizational level with respect to institutional policies and procedures. A very important component of education relates to understanding the software capabilities and limitations. Secondary dose verification of TPS-produced plans are also important as many reported errors involved a lack of an appropriate independent secondary check of the treatment plan or dose calculation. Clear documentation is required both of each patient's individual treatment plan and of departmental policies and procedures. Finally, communication among staff members is essential for all aspects of treatment, since various individuals at various professional levels are involved in the treatment process. Poor communication was a key factor in a number of the errors reported that relate to treatment planning.

A carefully executed program of treatment planning computer commissioning and ongoing QA assessment provides users with confidence that their work is being carried out accurately. Furthermore, it gives the user a clear understanding of the TPS's capabilities and limitations. Finally, the quality of the delivered radiation dose to the patient depends on the quality of all the steps in the treatment planning process, including patient imaging, simulation, target volume delineation, treatment planning, treatment verification, and quality factors associated with dose delivery and related to the radiation therapy machine. Thus, it is imperative that the medical physicist, as well as all other staff associated with the radiation therapy process, be actively involved in the QA process at all stages. This provides both full awareness of the capabilities and limitations of each step of the process and a mechanism for decision-making about any corrective action deemed to be necessary.

ACKNOWLEDGMENTS

Contributions of Dr. Jacob Van Dyk to previous editions of this chapter are still prevalent throughout the content in current edition, as his expertise in treatment planning system commissioning and quality assurance is unparalleled.

KEY POINTS

- Key contributing factors for major treatment planning system (TPS) accidents typically involve at least one of the following:
  - Lack of understanding of the TPS
  - Lack of appropriate commissioning
  - Lack of independent calculation checks

- A rigorous quality assurance (QA) program for TPS is necessary to ensure an accurate delivery of the treatment intent. Such a QA program consists of the following components:
  - *System specifications*: definitions of the capabilities of the software and the accuracy of the dose calculations.

- *Acceptance testing*: assessment of the hardware and software to ensure the accuracy of all system specifications.
- *Commissioning*: acquisition of all data needed to bring the system into clinical service.
  - Radiation beam data can be acquired onsite for each individual radiation producing device or be a validated universal set of vendor-provided reference data.
  - Baselines of performance standards used for quality controls are determined during commissioning.
- *Quality controls*: systematic actions to ensure specific performance standards are maintained.

- The uncertainty of the calculated dose depends on the accuracy of the beam data used during commissioning and the limitations of the calculation algorithms.
  - For external photon beam calculations in a homogenous phantom, this uncertainty is typically smallest on the central axis and largest in the buildup region.
  - Criteria of acceptability should be based on what is realistically achievable and include statements of confidence.

- Commissioning of a TPS typically requires basic radiation data which may include tissue–air ratios, tissue–phantom ratios, percentage depth doses, cross-beam profiles, and output factors.

- Additional measurements are needed for any ancillary devices such as wedges, blocks, and MLCs.

- End-to-end validation of the TPS and treatment workflow should be conducted for each unique treatment modality. End-to-end tests typically include the following:
  - Acquiring a CT simulation of a QA phantom
  - Creating a treatment plan on the image data set
  - Validating the calculated dose to the measured dose
  - Modern TPSs include new functionalities such as image registration, auto-segmentation, automated planning/knowledge-based planning, and adaptive radiation therapy. While specific commissioning and quality assurance tasks differ for each functionality, end-to-end tests and validations against the existing manual workflow should be included prior to clinical implementation.

- Quality assurance for the total radiation therapy planning process incorporates all steps from the initial simulation to the treatment delivery. Quality controls need to be developed for each aspect of the treatment planning workflow. Several tools that can aid in developing a strong QA program include the following:
  - An FMEA analysis provides the framework to identify key steps in the treatment planning workflow at which implementing quality controls will provide the greatest utility.
  - Reproducibility tests of the dose calculation, image display, and plan evaluation tools are useful quality controls that easily determine no significant changes have occurred to the planning system hardware/software.
  - In vivo and in vitro patient-specific checks provide a useful final validation of the dose distribution and can identify gross errors that may result in harm to the patient.
  - Quality audits of treatment planning process, either conducted internally or by an external third party, can identify weaknesses prior to implementing a new planning system, treatment modality, or treatment technique. Such quality audits can incorporate end-to-end tests to validate the entire treatment planning workflow.
  - A proper training program for all staff should be developed or re-evaluated during the commissioning process. Annual credentialing should be considered to ensure everyone is up-to-date on any new changes that may have been implemented.

❓ REVIEW QUESTIONS

1. Dose calculations for an enface photon beam in a homogenous phantom exhibit the highest absolute uncertainty in which region?
   A. Central axis after a depth of maximum dose
   B. Lateral penumbra
   C. Build up
   D. Out of field

2. When upgrading a TPS, it is important to complete the following tests except
   A. End-to-end tests
   B. In-phantom patient-specific dose measurements
   C. Third-party linear accelerator output audits
   D. Reproducibility tests of basic dose calculations

3. Implementation of effective quality controls with the treatment planning process is aided by a prospective quantitative technique that assesses potential risks, likelihood of errors, and impact of such errors. This technique is known as
   A. Process Tree Mapping
   B. Fault Tree Analysis
   C. Risk Management
   D. Failure Modes and Effects Analysis

4. The advantages of using standardized reference beam data sets when commissioning a treatment planning system include all of the following except
   A. All standardized reference beam data sets properly account for small field dosimetry.

B. Reference data sets allow for much of the TPS commissioning process to be "prepackaged" and minimize the chance of gross systematic errors arising from the input of incorrect data.

C. Reference data sets standardize the delivery quality of all linear accelerators from a specific vendor.

D. Reference data sets eliminate the possibility of poor quality commissioning measurements being used for the basic radiation data needed to define beam models.

ANSWERS

1. **C** Uncertainties in the dose calculation are dependent on the accuracy of the measured data used to create the beam model and the inherent accuracy of the dose calculation algorithm. Both exhibit the lowest uncertainty on the central axis. Measurements in the buildup region are inherently challenging, and vary greatly with detectors typically available to physicist acquiring the basic radiation data. In addition, many dose calculation algorithms do not handle the physics of electron contamination very well.

2. **C** End-to-end tests, patient-specific QA, and reproducibility tests all validate either the integrity of the dose calculation algorithms or the planning workflow. As a TPS system upgrade does not impact the linear accelerator output and reproducibility tests will confirm minimal changes to the basic beam data, third-party output audits are unnecessary.

3. **D** While process tree mapping and fault tree analysis can be useful in determining effective quality controls, FMEA provides the quantitative framework to examine the balance between risks, probability of occurrence, and impact.

4. **A** Vendor-provided reference data sets are intended to standardize the delivery of basic radiation data used during commissioning; thus, it does not account for small local variations that may exist between linear accelerators. Validation measurements of the basic radiation data should be conducted and compared to the reference data set to determine if any differences exist.

REFERENCES

1. Peters LJ, O'Sullivan B, Giralt J, Fitzgerald TJ, Trotti A, Bernier J, Bourhis J, Yuen K, Fisher R, Rischin D. Critical impact of radiotherapy protocol compliance and quality in the treatment of advanced head and neck cancer: results from TROG 02.02. *J Clin Oncol.* 2010;28(18):2996–3001.

2. Bogdanich W. The Radiation Boom. As technology surges, radiation safeguards lag. *New York Times*, January 27th, 2010: A1, New York edition.

3. Bogdanich W. The Radiation Boom. Radiation offers new cures, and ways to do harm. *New York Times*, January 24th, 2010:A1, New York edition.

4. Klein EE, Hanley J, Bayouth J, et al. Task Group 142 report: quality assurance of medical accelerators. *Med Phys.* 2009;36(9): 4197–4212.

5. Wu Q, Xing L, Ezzell G, et al. Inverse treatment planning. In: Van Dyk J, ed. *The Modern Technology of Radiation Oncology: A Compendium for Medical Physicists and Radiation Oncologists.* Volume 2. Madison, WI: Medical Physics Publishing, 2005:131–183.

6. Xia P, Verhey LJ. Intensity-modulated radiation therapy. In: Van Dyk J, ed. *The Modern Technology of Radiation Oncology: A Compendium for Medical Physicists and Radiation Oncologists.* Volume 2. Madison, WI: Medical Physics Publishing; 2005:221–258.

7. Brock KK, Mutic S, McNutt TR, et al. Use of image registration and fusion algorithms and techniques in radiotherapy: report of the AAPM Radiation Therapy Committee Task Group No. 132. *Med Phys.* 2017;44(7):e43–e76.

8. Li XA, Alber M, Deasy JO, et al. The use and QA of biologically related models for treatment planning: Short report of the TG-166 of the therapy physics committee of the AAPM. *Med Phys.* 2012;39(3):1386–1409.

9. Hatt M, Lee JA, Schmidtlein CR, et al. Classification and evaluation strategies of auto-segmentation approaches for PET: Report of AAPM task group No. 211. *Med Phys.* 2017:44(6). e1–e42.

10. Moore KL, Olsen LA, Kavanaugh JA, et al. Clinical Implementation of Data-driven Quality Control and Automated Treatment Planning: Report of the TG-308 of the Therapy Physics Committee of the AAPM.

11. Wu QJ, Li T, Wu Q, Yin FF. Adaptive radiation therapy: technical components and clinical applications. *Cancer J.* 2011;17(3): 182–189.

12. Ma CM, Chetty IJ, Deng J, et al. Beam modeling and beam model commissioning for Monte Carlo dose calculation-based radiation therapy treatment planning: report of AAPM Task Group 157. *Med Phys.* 202;47(1):e1–e18.

13. Annals of the ICRP. ICRP publication 86. Prevention of Accidental Exposures to Patients Undergoing Radiation Therapy. Editor Valentin, J. The International Commission on Radiological Protection. 2001

14. Gershkevitsh E, Pesznyak C, Petrovic B, et al. Dosimetric inter-institution comparison in European radiotherapy centres: results of IAEA supported treatment planning system audit. *Acta Oncol.* 2014;53;628–636.

15. Glenn MC, Peterson CB, Howell RM, Followill DS, Pollard-Larkin JM, Kry SF. Sensitivity of IROC phantom performance to radiotherapy treatment planning system beam modeling parameters based on community-driven data. *Med Phys.* 2020;47(10):5250–5259.

16. Kerns JR, Stingo F, Followill DS, Howell RB, Melancom A, Kry SF. Treatment planning system calculation errors are present in most Imaging and Radiation Oncology Core-Houston phantom failures. *IJROBP.* 2017;98(5):1197–1203.

17. Smilowitz JB, Das IJ, Feygelman V, Fraass BA, Kry SF, Marshall IR, Mihailidis DN, Ouhib Z, Ritter T, Snyder MG, Fairobent L. AAPM Medical Physics Practice Guideline 5.a.: commissioning and QA of treatment planning dose calculations – megavoltage photon and electron beams. *J Appl Clin Med Phys.* 2015;16(5):14–34.

18. Das IJ, Cheng CW, Watts RJ, Ahnesjö A, Gibbons J, Li XA, Lowenstein J, Mitra RK, Simon WE, Zhu TC. Accelerator beam data commissioning equipment and procedures: report of the TG-106 of the Therapy Physics Committee of the AAPM. *Med Phys.* 2008;35(9):4186–4215.

19. Ezzell GA, Burmeister JW, Dogan N, et al. IMRT commissioning: multiple institution planning and dosimetry comparisons, a report from AAPM Task Group 119. *Med Phys.* 2009;36(11):5359–5373.

20. International Atomic Energy Agency. IAEA-TECDOC-1540. Specification and acceptance testing of radiotherapy treatment planning systems. Vienna, Austria: International Atomic Energy Agency, 2007.

21. International Atomic Energy Agency. IAEA-TECDOC-1583: commissioning of radiotherapy treatment planning systems: testing for typical external beam treatment techniques. Vienna, Austria: International Atomic Energy Agency, 2008.

22. Glenn MC, Peterson CB, Followill DS, Howell RM, Pollard-Larkin JM, Kry SF. Reference dataset of users' photon beam modeling parameters for the Eclipse, Pinnacle, and RayStation treatment planning systems. *Med Phys.* 2020;47:282–288. doi:10.1002/mp.13892

23. Watts RJ. Comparative measurements on a series of accelerators by the same vendor. *Med Phys.* 1999;26(12):2581–2585.

24. Sjöström D, Bjelkengren U, Ottosson W, Behrens CF. A beam-matching concept for medical linear accelerators. *Acta Oncologica.* 2009;48(2):192–200.

25. Chang Z, Wu Q, Adamson J, et al. Commissioning and dosimetric characteristics of TrueBeam system: composite data of three TrueBeam machines. *Med Phys.* 2012;39(11):6981–7018.

26. Glide-Hurst C, Bellon M, Foster R, et al. Commissioning of the Varian TrueBeam linear accelerator: a multi-institutional study. *Med Phys.* 2013;40(3):031719.

27. Beyer GP. Commissioning measurements for photon beam data on three TrueBeam linear accelerators, and comparison with Trilogy and Clinac 2100 linear accelerators. *J Appl Clin Med Phys.* 2013;14:273–288. doi:10.1120/jacmp.v14i1.4077

28. Tanaka Y, Mizuno H, Akino Y, Isono M, Masai N, Yamamoto T. Do the representative beam data for TrueBeam™ linear accelerators represent average data? *J Appl Clin Med Phys.* 2019;20(2):51–62. doi:10.1002/acm2.12518

29. Irmen P, Reft C, Fitzherbert C, Solin L, Hand C. Verification of representative data for output factors of SRS cones utilizing IAEA TRS 483 recommendations. *Phys Med Biol.* 2019 Nov 4;64(21):215011. doi:10.1088/1361-6560/ab47dd

30. Williamson JF, Thomadsen BR, eds. Quality assurance for radiation therapy: the challenges of advanced technologies symposium. *Int J Radiat Oncol Biol Phys.* 2008;72(Suppl 1):S1–S214.

31. International Commission on Radiation Units and Measurements. ICRU Report 62. Prescribing, recording, and reporting photon beam therapy (Supplement to ICRU Report 50). ICRU 1999. Bethesda, MD.

32. Bevins, MB, Flynn, MJ, Silosky, MS, et al. Display Quality Assurance. The Report of AAPM Task Group 270. 2019. https://doi.org/10.37206/183

33. Mayo CS, Moran JM, Bosch W, et al. Standardization Nomenclatures in Radiation Oncology. The Report of AAPM Task Group 263. 2018. https://doi.org/10.37206/171

34. Siebers JV, Keall PJ, Kawrakow I. Monte Carlo dose calculations for external beam radiation therapy. In: Van Dyk J, ed. *The Modern Technology of Radiation Oncology: A Compendium for Medical Physicists and Radiation Oncologists.* Volume 2. Madison, WI: Medical Physics Publishing; 2005:91–130.

35. Chetty IJ, Curran B, Cygler JE, et al. Report of the AAPM Task Group No. 105: issues associated with clinical implementation of Monte Carlo-based photon and electron external beam treatment planning. *Med Phys.* 2007;34:4818–4853.

36. Papanikolaou N, Battista JJ, Boyer AL, et al. Tissue inhomogeneity corrections for megavoltage photon beams. Report by Task Group 65 of the Radiation Therapy Committee of the American Association of Physicists in Medicine. AAPM Report 85. Madison, WI: Medical Physics Publishing; 2004.

37. Rivard MJ, Venselaar JL, Beaulieu L. The evolution of brachytherapy treatment planning. *Med Phys.* 2009;36:2136–2153.

38. Moore KL, Kagadis GC, McNutt TR, Moiseenko V, Mutic S. Vision 20/20: automation and advanced computing in clinical radiation oncology. *Med Phys.* 2014;41(1):010901.

39. Venselaar J, Welleweerd H, Mijnheer B. Tolerances for the accuracy of photon beam dose calculations of treatment planning systems. *Radiother Oncol.* 2001;60:191–201.

40. Fraass B, Doppke K, Hunt M, et al. American Association of Physicists in Medicine Radiation Therapy Committee Task Group 53: quality assurance for clinical radiotherapy treatment planning. *Med Phys.* 1998;25:1773–1829.

41. Van Dyk J, Rosenwald J-C, Fraass B, et al. Commissioning and quality assurance of computerized planning systems for radiation treatment of cancer. IAEA TRS-430. Vienna: International Atomic Energy Agency; 2004.

42. DeWerd LA, Ibbott GS, Meigooni AS, et al. A dosimetric uncertainty analysis for photon-emitting brachytherapy sources: report of AAPM Task Group No. 138 and GEC-ESTRO. *Med Phys.* 2011;38:782–801.

43. Venselaar J, Welleweerd H. Application of a test package in an intercomparison of the photon dose calculation performance of treatment planning systems used in a clinical setting. *Radiother Oncol.* 2001;60:203–213.

44. Mackie TR. History of tomotherapy. *Phys Med Biol.* 2006;51: R427–R453.

45. Mutic S, Dempsey JF. The ViewRay system: magnetic resonance-guided and controlled radiotherapy. *Semin Radiat Oncol.* 2014; 24:196–199.

46. Wowra B, Muacevic A, Jess-Hempen A, et al. Safety and efficacy of outpatient gamma knife radiosurgery for multiple cerebral metastases. *Expert Rev Neurother.* 2004;4:673–679.

47. Zhu TC, Palta JR. Electron contamination in 8 and 18 MV photon beams. *Med Phys.* 1998;25:12–19.

48. Bedford JL, Childs PJ, Nordmark H, et al. Commissioning and quality assurance of the Pinnacle(3) radiotherapy treatment planning system for external beam photons. *Br J Radiol.* 2003;76: 163–176.

49. Cadman P, McNutt T, Bzdusek K. Validation of physics improvements for IMRT with a commercial treatment-planning system. *J Appl Clin Med Phys.* 2005:6:74–86.

50. Cadman P, Bassalow R, Sidhu NP, et al. Dosimetric considerations for validation of a sequential IMRT process with a commercial treatment planning system. *Phys Med Biol.* 2002;47:3001–3010.

51. International Commission on Radiation Units and Measurements. ICRU Report 83: Prescribing, Recording, and Reporting Photon-Beam Intensity-Modulated Radiation Therapy (IMRT). Bethesda, MD: International Commission on Radiation Units and Measurements; 2010.

52. Craft DL, Hong TS, Shih HA, et al. Improved planning time and plan quality through multicriteria optimization for intensity-modulated radiotherapy. *Int J Radiat Oncol Biol Phys.* 2012;82(1):e83–e90.

53. Voet PWJ, Maarten DLP, Breedveld S, et al. Toward fully automated multicriterial plan generation: a prospective clinical study. *Int J Radiat Oncol Biol Phys.* 2012;85(3):866–872.

54. Moore KL, Brame RS, Low DA, et al. Experience-based quality control of clinical intensity-modulated radiotherapy planning. *Int J Radiat Oncol Biol Phys.* 2011;81(2):545–551.

55. Good D, Lo J, Lee WR, et al. A knowledge-based approach to improving and homogenizing intensity modulated radiation therapy planning quality among treatment centers: an example application to prostate cancer planning. *Int J Radiat Oncol Biol Phys.* 2013;87(1):176–181.

56. Appenzoller LM, Michalski JM, Thorstad WL, et al. Predicting dose-volume histograms for organs-at-risk in IMRT planning. *Med Phys.* 2012;39(12):7446–7461.

57. Altman MB, Kavanaugh JA, Green OL, et al. Addressing the issues limiting rapid contour evaluation to facilitate On-line Adaptive Radiation Therapy (OL-ART) with MR-IGRT. *Int J Radiat Oncol Biol Phys.* 2014;90(1):S860.

58. Caldwell C, Mah K. Imaging for radiation therapy planning. In: Van Dyk J, ed. *The Modern Technology of Radiation Oncology: A Compendium for Medical Physicists and Radiation Oncologists.* Volume 2. Madison, WI: Medical Physics Publishing; 2005:31–89. (#5 in current version).

59. Kessler ML. Image registration and data fusion in radiation therapy. *Br J Radiol.* 2006;70:S99–S108.

60. Njeh CF. Tumor delineation: The weakest link in the search for accuracy in radiotherapy. *J Med Phys.* 2008;33(4):136–140. doi:10.4103/0971-6203.44472

61. Khoo VS, Joon DL. New developments in MRI for target volume delineation in radiotherapy. *Br J Radiol.* 2006;79:S2–S15.

62. Price PM, Green MM. Positron emission tomography imaging approaches for external beam radiation therapies: current status and future developments. *Br J Radiol.* 2011;84:S19–S34.

63. Macmanus M, Nestle U, Rosenweig KE, et al. Use of PET and PET/CT for Radiation Therapy Planning: IAEA expert report 2006–2007. *Radiother Oncol.* 2008;91:85–94.

64. Li G, Citrin D, Camphausen K, et al. Advances in 4D medical imaging and 4D radiation therapy. *Technol Cancer Res Treat.* 2008;7:67–81

65. Brock KK. Deformable Registration Accuracy Consortium. Results of a multi-institution deformable registration accuracy study (MIDRAS). *Int J Radiat Oncol Biol Phys.* 2010;76(2):583–596.

66. Teguh DN, Levendag PC, Voet PWJ, et al. Clinical validation of atlas-based auto-segmentation of multiple target volumes and normal tissue (swallowing/maticiation) structures in the head and neck. *Int J Radiat Oncol Biol Phys.* 2011;81(4):950–957.

67. Gambacorta MA, Valentini C, Dinapoli N, et al. Clinical validation of atlas-based auto-segmentation of pelvic volumes and normal tissue in rectal tumors using auto-segmentation computed system. *Acta Oncol.* 2013;52:1676–1681.

68. Glide-Hurst CK, Lee P, Yock AD. Adaptive radiation therapy (ART) strategies and technical considerations: A state of the ART review from NRG Oncology. *Int J Radiat Oncol Biol Phys.* 2020. https://doi.org/10.1016/j.ijrobp.2020.10.021

69. Noel CE, Santanam L, Parikh PJ, Mutic S. Process-based quality management for clinical implementation of adaptive radiotherapy. *Med Phys.* 2014;41(8), Article 081717.

70. Rivard MJ, Coursey BM, DeWerd LA, et al. Update of AAPM Task Group No. 43 Report: a revised AAPM protocol for brachytherapy dose calculations. *Med Phys.* 2004;31(3):633–674.

71. Perez-Calatayud J, Ballester F, Das RK, et al. Report of the High Energy Brachytherapy Source Dosimetry (HEBD) Working Group: Dose Calculation for Photon-Emitting Brachytherapy Sources with Average Energy Higher than 50 keV: Full Report of the AAPM and ESTRO. College Park, MD: AAPM; 2012.

72. Rivard MJ, Beaulieu L, Mourtada F. Enhancements to commissioning techniques and quality assurance of brachytherapy treatment planning systems that use model-based dose calculation algorithms. *Med Phys.* 2010;37:2645–2658.

73. Beaulieu L, Tedgren AC, Carrier JF, et al. Report of the Task Group 186 on model-based dose calculation methods in brachytherapy beyond the TG-43 formalism: Current status and recommendations for clinical implementation. *Med Phys.* 2012;39(10):6208–6236.

74. Paganetti H, Jiang H, Lee SY, Kooy HM. Accurate Monte Carlo simulations for nozzle design, commissioning and quality assurance for a proton radiation therapy facility. *Med Phys.* 2004;31:2107–2118.

75. Zhu XR, Poenisch F, Sawakurchi GO, et al. Commissioning dose computation models for spot scanning proton beams in water for a commercially available treatment planning system. *Med Phys.* 2013;40(4):041723.

76. Slopsema RL, Lin L, Flampouri S, Yeung D, et al. Development of a golden beam data set for the commissioning of a proton double-scatter system in a pencil-beam dose calculation algorithm. *Med Phys.* 2014;41(9):091710.

77. Paganetti H. *Proton Therapy Physics, Series in Medical Physics and Biomedical Engineering.* Boca Raton, FL: CRC Press; 2012

78. International Commission on Radiation Units and Measurements. ICRU Report 78: Prescribing, Recording, and Reporting Proton-Beam Therapy. Bethesda, MD: International Commission on Radiation Units and Measurements; 2007.

79. Park PC, Zhu XR, Lee AK, et al. A beam-specific planning target volume (PTV) design for proton therapy to account for setup and range uncertainties. *Int J Radiat Oncol Biol Phys.* 2012;82(2):e329–e336.

80. Paganetti H. Range Uncertainties in proton therapy and the role of Monte Carlo simulations. *Phys Med Biol.* 2012;57:R99–R117.

81. Paganetti H. Dose to water versus dose to medium in proton beam therapy. *Phys Med Biol.* 2009;54(14):4399–4421.

82. Mutic S, Palta JR, Butker EK, et al. Quality assurance for computed-tomography simulators and the computed-tomography-simulation process: report of the AAPM Radiation Therapy Committee Task Group No. 66. *Med Phys.* 2003;30:2762–2792.

83. Calcerrada Diaz-Santos N, Blasco Amaro JA, Cardiel GA, et al. The safety and efficacy of robotic image-guided radiosurgery system treatment for intra- and extracranial lesions: a systematic review of the literature. *Radiother Oncol.* 2008;89:245–253.

84. Hu Y, Byrne M, Archibald-Heeren B, et al. Validation of the pre-configured Varian Ethos Acuros XB Beam Model for treatment planning dose calculations: a dosimetric study. *J Appl Med Phys.* 2020. doi:10.1002/acm2.13056

85. Huq MS, Fraass BA, Dunscombe PB. The report of Task Group 100 of the AAPM: application of risk analysis methods to radiation therapy quality management. *Med Phys.* 2016;43(7):4209–4262.

86. Ford EC, Smith K, Terezakis S, Croog V, et al. A streamlined failure mode and effects analysis. *Med Phys.* 2014;41(6):061709.

87. Sawant A, Dieterich S, Svatos M, et al. Failure mode and effects analysis-based quality assurance for dynamic MLC tracking systems. *Med Phys.* 2010;37:6466–6479.

88. Ford EC, Fong de Los Santos L, Pawlicki T, et al. Consensus recommendations for incident learning database structures in radiation oncology. *Med Phys.* 2012;39:7272–7290.

89. Terezakis SA, Harris KM, Ford EC, et al. An evaluation of departmental radiation oncology incident reports: anticipating a national reporting system. *Int J Radiat Oncol Biol Phys.* 2013;85:919–923.

90. Stern RL, Heaton R, Fraser MW, et al. Verification of monitor unit calculations for non-IMRT clinical radiotherapy: report of AAPM Task Group 114. *Med Phys.* 2011;38(1):504–530.

91. Miften M, Olch A, Mihailidis D, et al. Tolerance limits and methodologies for IMRT measurement-based verification QA: recommendations of AAPM Task Group No. 218. *Med Phys.* 2018;45(4):e53–e83.

92. Yukihara EG, McKeever SW. Optically stimulated luminescence (OSL) dosimetry in medicine. *Phys Med Biol.* 2008;53:R351–R379.

93. Jornet N, Carrasco P, Jurado D, et al. Comparison study of MOS-FET detectors and diodes for entrance in vivo dosimetry in 18 MV x-ray beams. *Med Phys.* 2004;31:2534–2542.

94. Dunscombe P, McGhee P, Lederer E. Anthropomorphic phantom measurements for the validation of a treatment planning system. *Phys Med Biol.* 1996;41:399–411.

95. Van Dam J, Marinello G. Methods for in vivo dosimetry in external radiotherapy. Brussels, Belgium: ESTRO; 2006.

96. World Health Organization (WHO). Radiotherapy risk profile: technical manual. Geneva: World Health Organization; 2008.

97. Kry SF, Bednarz B, Howell RM, et al. AAPM Task Group 158: Measurements and calculations of doses outside the treatment volume from external beam radiation therapy. *Med Phys.* 2017;44(10):e391–e429.

98. Ibbott G, Ma CM, Rogers DW, et al. Anniversary paper: fifty years of AAPM involvement in radiation dosimetry. *Med Phys.* 2008;35:1418–1427.

99. Schiefer H, Fogliata A, Nicolini G, et al. The Swiss IMRT dosimetry intercomparison using a thorax phantom. *Med Phys.* 2010;37:4424–4431.

100. International Atomic Energy Agency. Comprehensive audits of radiotherapy practices: a tool for quality improvement, quality assurance team for radiation oncology (QUATRO). Vienna, Austria: International Atomic Energy Agency, 2007.

101. Zietman A, Palta J, Steinberg M, et al., 2019. *Safety Is No Accident, A Framework for Quality Radiation Oncology Care.* ASTRO.

25 Intensity-Modulated Radiation Therapy: Photons

Jan Unkelbach

INTRODUCTION

The Rationale for IMRT: Concave Target Volumes

The development of intensity-modulated radiation therapy (IMRT) was preceded by two important technologic developments: computed tomography (CT) and multileaf collimators (MLCs). Before the widespread availability of CT scanners, radiotherapy planning was based on two-dimensional X-ray images. In these images, the projection of the target volume could be delineated, which led to the design of two-dimensional treatment fields. With the development of CT imaging, a three-dimensional model of the patient became available. The target volume, as well as organs at risk, could be delineated in three dimensions and their spatial relation became known. This led to the development of three-dimensional conformal radiotherapy. Conforming the radiation dose to the target volume required improved ways of collimating the radiation field. The solution to this problem was the MLC. Three-dimensional conformal radiotherapy is still the standard for many treatment sites today. However, conforming the dose distribution to the tumor is limited to round or convex shapes of the target volume. In three-dimensional conformal radiotherapy, the tumor is treated with one radiation field from each incident beam direction, where the shape of the radiation field is the projection of the target volume in beam's eye view. The incident fluence is homogeneous over the field. This makes it impossible to carve out concavities in the target volume. The problem is illustrated in Figure 25.1, which shows a patient treated for a spinal metastasis. The target volume shown in red includes the entire vertebral body, which surrounds the spinal cord. An emerging treatment paradigm for such cases consists in delivering a single fraction dose of 18 to 24 Gy to the target volume. This treatment approach requires that the dose to the spinal cord is limited to approximately 10 Gy. With three-dimensional conformal radiotherapy, it is impossible to spare the spinal cord. As a first approach, the projection of the spinal cord in beam's eye view could be removed from the treatment field, and the area to the right and to the left be treated as two separate fields. However, this strategy would yield an inhomogeneous dose distribution to the target volume and would underdose the target volume near the spinal cord. More specifically, in order to deliver the prescribed dose to the target, the fluence at the edge of the spinal cord has to be increased. Anders Brahme had studied this phenomenon for a stylized geometry in his 1982 paper.[1] The work can be considered as one of the first papers illustrating the need for inhomogeneous fluence distributions across the treatment field when treating concave target volumes. This eventually led to the development of *IMRT*.

Typical Applications of IMRT

The treatment of spinal metastasis using stereotactic body radiotherapy (SBRT) is a recent application of IMRT. However, over the past years, IMRT has become the standard of care for a variety of treatment sites. Two of the established applications are prostate cancer and head-and-neck tumors, which are illustrated in Figures 25.2 and 25.3. The prostate lies in the midsagittal plane between the bladder and the rectum. In radiotherapy of prostate cancer, the target volume contains the entire prostate gland. The main dose-limiting normal tissue is the anterior rectal wall. In many patients, the lateral lobes of the prostate partially wrap around the rectum, as illustrated in Figure 25.2. Only millimeters separate the prostate gland from the radiosensitive lining of the rectal wall. Historically, the prescription dose was therefore limited by rectal toxicity as the anterior rectal wall received the full prescription dose. Today, in the era of IMRT, a commonly used prescription dose is 79 Gy using standard fractionation, which is among the highest prescriptions throughout radiotherapy. This necessitates that the high-dose region carves out the concavity formed by the rectum, which became possible with IMRT. The improved conformity further allows for SBRT treatments delivering 35–40 Gy in 5 fractions to the prostate, and even single fraction treatments are being explored.[2]

Tumors in the head-and-neck region represent a third example in which IMRT has replaced three-dimensional conformal techniques for the most part. This includes tumors arising in the oral cavity, the nasopharynx, and the oropharynx. These tumors are often inoperable and

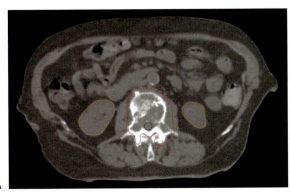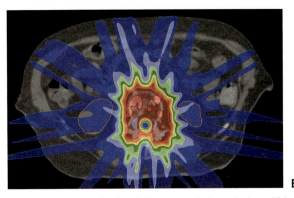

A   B

FIGURE 25.1. **A:** Geometry of a spinal metastasis treated with IMRT. The target volume (*red*) entirely surrounds the spinal cord (*dark green*), which is to be spared. Additional organs at risk are the kidneys (*orange*). **B:** IMRT provides the means to spare the spinal cord while delivering a high dose to the target volume, as shown in the dose distribution.

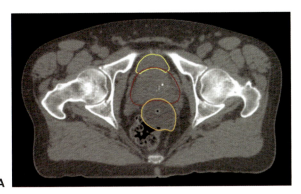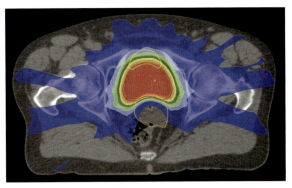

A   B

FIGURE 25.2. **A:** Prostate cancer represents a typical application of IMRT. The prostate (*red*) abuts the rectum (*orange*) and the bladder (*yellow*). **B:** IMRT has the ability to conform the high dose to the prostate while carving out the concavity formed by the rectum.

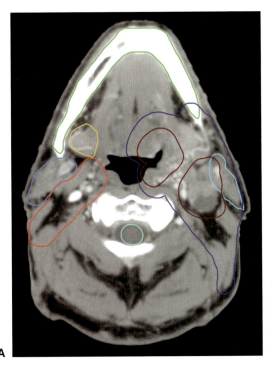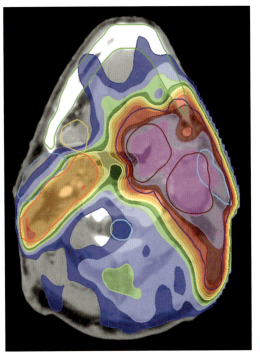

A   B

FIGURE 25.3. **A:** A head-and-neck cancer patient treated with IMRT. The target consists of multiple volumes prescribed to different doses: GTV (*brown*), high-risk clinical target volume (CTV) (*purple*), and low-risk nodal CTV (*red*). Radiosensitive structures, including the parotid glands (*blue*), the submandibular glands (*yellow*), and the spinal cord (*light blue*), are near the target volume. **B:** IMRT allows for conformal dose distribution to complex-shaped target volumes.

are close to a variety of radiosensitive structures. These include the saliva secreting glands, such as the parotid glands, as well as structures related to swallowing, such as the pharyngeal constrictor muscles. Thus, radiotherapy to cancers of the head and neck is associated with acute and long-term side effects that seriously impact quality of life, including xerostomia and dysphagia. IMRT allows for sparing of the parotid glands and carefully distributing dose in normal tissues. Furthermore, IMRT allows for complex dose prescriptions that are standard of care today. Nowadays, treatment protocols often use three dose levels, in which 70 Gy is delivered to the gross tumor volume (GTV) containing the primary tumor and macroscopic lymph node metastases, 60 Gy to high-risk clinical target volumes (CTV), and 54 Gy to low-risk nodal levels. This type of dose painting approach would be very difficult to mimic using forward planning techniques and three-dimensional conformal radiotherapy.

These examples illustrate problems in oncology in which the technical development of IMRT had profound impact on the way patients were treated. In the case of prostate cancer, the widespread availability of IMRT causes a shift from radical prostatectomy toward radiotherapy as the mainstay of therapy. In the case of spinal metastasis, IMRT offers the option of high single fraction doses with the intent of local control, where the role of radiotherapy was limited to palliative treatments before.

Scope and Organization of This Chapter

This chapter focuses on the concepts of IMRT, the treatment planning process, and the mathematical methods used. It discusses steps in the planning process and the user interface between treatment planner and planning software, and it provides an understanding of the algorithms used behind the scenes by modern treatment planning systems (TPS). For a review of the history of IMRT, the reader is referred to the paper by Bortfeld[3] and references therein. For a comprehensive review of IMRT including the physics and technology aspects, we recommend the book by Webb.[4] The remainder of this chapter is organized as follows:

- The section IMRT—Concepts and Planning Process introduces the main concepts in IMRT and illustrates the planning process step by step using a head-and-neck cancer example.
- The section Fluence Map Optimization discusses fluence map optimization (FMO) in more detail, which represents the most important concept in IMRT planning. In that context, the formulation of IMRT treatment planning as a mathematical optimization problem is discussed.
- The section Leaf Sequencing describes the leaf sequencing problem, that is, the method to deliver intensity-modulated radiation fields using MLCs.

The aforementioned sections reflect the historical development of IMRT, and thereby the functionality and algorithmic foundation of the first-generation IMRT planning systems. In recent years, TPS have evolved to more advanced planning algorithms and support more complex delivery techniques. To that end, the remaining sections describe more recent developments in IMRT planning.

- The section Direct Aperture Optimization describes methods for direct aperture optimization (DAO), which aims to overcome problems of the traditional two-step approach of FMO plus leaf sequencing.
- The section Arc Therapy describes treatment planning for volumetric-modulated arc therapy (VMAT), that is, a delivery technique where the gantry continuously rotates around the patient while radiation is delivered.
- The section Automated Planning and Multi-criteria Optimization provides an introduction to approaches aiming at automating most of the treatment plan optimization process. This includes methods to utilize data bases of previously delivered treatment plans for designing objective functions. In addition, methods to deal with inherent tradeoffs between conflicting planning goals are introduced. This includes prioritized optimization as well as interactive Pareto-surface navigation techniques.
- The section Specialized Topics in Treatment Planning considers current areas of research and development in IMRT including noncoplanar arc therapy, robust optimization for handling uncertainty and motion, and treatment plan optimization for multi-modality radiotherapy combining photons with electrons or protons.

IMRT—CONCEPTS AND PLANNING PROCESS

This section demonstrates the concepts of IMRT planning step by step for an example case. We consider the head-and-neck cancer patient shown in Figure 25.3, which represents a typical application of IMRT. The target consists of multiple volumes, the GTV, the high-risk CTV, and the elective nodal CTV, which are prescribed to different dose levels. In addition, several radiosensitive structures are located in proximity of the tumor. This includes the saliva-producing parotid glands, the spinal cord, the pharyngeal constrictor muscles, and the larynx.

The Fluence Map

IMRT refers to radiotherapy delivery methods for which the fluence distribution in the plane perpendicular to the incident beam direction is modulated. To that end, the radiation beam is divided into small beam segments, which are in principle deliverable by an MLC, as further described in the Leaf Sequencing section. The lateral fluence distribution of the beam is thereby discretized into small elements, which are commonly referred to as *beamlets* or *bixels*. Modern MLCs typically have a leaf width of 5 mm. Thus, the fluence distribution is represented by the intensities of 5 × 5 mm beamlets. The discrete representation of the fluence is commonly referred to as the *fluence map*. In IMRT planning, the goal is to find the fluence maps of all incident beam directions that yield the best possible dose distribution in the patient. This problem is referred to as FMO and is the topic of this section and the following one.

The definition of the fluence map is illustrated in Figure 25.4. Similar to three-dimensional conformal therapy, this starts with the definition of the isocenter. For IMRT planning, we subsequently determine the set of all beamlets that are potentially helpful in finding the most desirable treatment plan. Loosely speaking, this corresponds to all beamlets that contribute a significant dose to the target volume. A common method for initializing the fluence map consists in including all beamlets for which the central axis of the corresponding beam segment intersects the target volume.

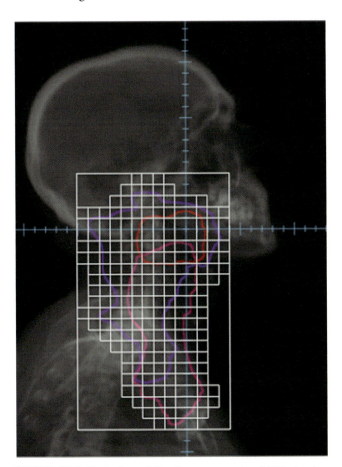

FIGURE 25.4. Illustration of the fluence map for IMRT planning for a head-and-neck cancer patient. The figure shows the digitally reconstructed radiograph (DRR) for one of the incident beam directions. The contours show the projections of the three target volumes in beam's eye view. The fluence map consists of all beamlets that cover the projection of the target volume.

The Dose-Deposition Matrix

The quality of a treatment plan is primarily judged based on the dose distribution in the patient. Thus, we would like to determine the fluence maps of the incident beams as to best approximate a desired dose distribution. To that end, we have to relate the incident fluence to the dose distribution in the patient. The *dose-deposition matrix* concept, which is frequently used in IMRT planning, provides this link.

For dose calculation, the patient is discretized into small volume elements referred to as voxels. A dose calculation algorithm is used to calculate the dose distribution of every beamlet in the fluence map in the patient. Let us denote the dose that beamlet j contributes to voxel i in the patient as D_{ij}, and let us denote the intensity of beamlet j as x_j. The total dose d_i delivered to voxel i is then simply given by the superposition of all beamlet contributions:

$$d_i = \sum_j D_{ji} x_j \qquad (25.1)$$

Here, the matrix of dose contributions D_{ij} of beamlets j to voxels i is referred to as the *dose-deposition matrix*. In practice, the fluence is commonly quantified in monitor units (MU). In this case, the natural unit of the dose-influence matrix is Gy/MU, such that the resulting dose distribution in the patient is obtained in Gy. The dose-deposition matrix concept is convenient since it allows for a separation of the mathematical optimization of beamlet intensities x_j from the dose calculation algorithm. In IMRT planning, the dose-deposition matrix is often calculated up front and held in memory. Subsequently, the dose distribution is obtained by a simple matrix multiplication $d = Dx$.

Formulation of IMRT Planning as an Optimization Problem

In order to determine the optimal fluence map for every incident beam direction, we have to specify the desired dose distribution. In other words, we have to characterize what a *good* treatment plan is. In the example case in Figure 25.3, treatment planning aims at different goals including the following:

1. A prescribed dose d^{pres} should be delivered to all parts of the target volume. In this case, the target volume consists of multiple parts. The GTV is often prescribed to 70 Gy; the surrounding CTV at high risk of microscopic tumor invasion is prescribed to an intermediate dose of 60 Gy; and more distant elective lymph node levels that may contain occult metastases but with lower probability are prescribed to 54 Gy. The elective lymph node targets essentially consist of normal tissue such that treatment planning aims at a homogeneous dose in the target, avoiding both under- and overdosing.

2. The dose distribution should conform to the target volume. Outside the target volume, a steep dose falloff is desired, and unnecessary dose to all healthy tissues should be avoided.
3. The dose delivered to the parotid glands is to be minimized to avoid or reduce side effects such as xerostomia (mouth dryness).
4. The dose to the spinal cord has to be limited. The maximum dose delivered to any part of the spinal cord has to stay below a maximum tolerance dose d_s^{max}.

For IMRT planning, these goals have to be translated into mathematical terms. This is done by defining functions, which represent measures for how good a treatment plan is, and whether it is acceptable at all. In this context, we distinguish objectives and constraints:

Constraints are conditions that are to be satisfied in any case. Every treatment plan that does not satisfy the constraint would be unacceptable.

Objectives are functions that measure the quality of a treatment plan. They may represent measures to quantify how close a treatment plan is to the ideal or desired treatment plan.

In the example provided earlier, the first three goals can be formulated as objectives; the fourth goal of enforcing a strict maximum on the spinal cord dose represents a constraint. The goal of delivering a homogeneous dose to the target volume can be formulated via a quadratic objective function:

$$f_T(d) = \frac{1}{N_T}\sum_{i=1}^{N_T}(d_i - d_i^{pres})^2$$

Ideally, every voxel that belongs to the target volume receives the prescribed dose d^{pres}, which corresponds to a value of zero for the function f_T. Otherwise, f_T yields the averaged quadratic deviation from the prescribed dose. The larger the objective value is, the more the dose deviates from the prescription dose, corresponding to a worse treatment plan.

Similarly, the goal of minimizing the dose to the parotid glands can be formulated as an objective function. For example, we can define the objective f_P as

$$f_P(d) = \frac{1}{N_p}\sum_{i=1}^{N_p}d_i$$

which aims at minimizing the mean dose to the parotid glands. The goal of conforming the dose distribution to the target volume can, for example, be described via a piecewise quadratic penalty function

$$f_H(d) = \frac{1}{N_H}\sum_{i=1}^{N_H}(d_i - d_i^{max})_+^2$$

where the + operator is defined through $(d_i - d_i^{max})_+ = d_i - d_i^{max}$ if $d_i \geq d_i^{max}$, and zero otherwise. Thus d_i^{max} is a maximum dose that is accepted in voxel i; dose values

exceeding d_i^{max} are penalized quadratically. Clearly, in normal tissue voxels directly adjacent to the target volume, high doses are unavoidable, whereas at large distance from the target volume, treatment planning should aim at avoiding unnecessary dose. Therefore, d_i^{max} can be chosen based on the distance of voxel i to the target volume. For example, d_i^{max} is set equal to the prescribed dose in voxels directly adjacent to the target volume and to half the prescription at 1 cm distance.

Finally, we would like to ensure that the dose in all voxels that belong to the spinal cord does not exceed a maximum tolerance dose d_s^{max}. If we do not accept any treatment plan that exceeds the maximum dose, this can be implemented as a constraint, not an objective. In this case we can formulate the constraint as

$$d_i \leq d_s^{max} \quad \text{for all } i \in S$$

where S is the set of all voxels belonging to the spinal cord.

Treatment planning simultaneously aims at minimizing the aforementioned objective functions; that is, ideally we would like each tumor voxel to receive the prescribed dose while no dose is delivered to the normal tissues. It is clear that the objectives associated with different structures are inherently conflicting. Thus, the treatment planner will have to weigh these conflicting objectives relative to each other and accept a compromise. The traditional approach in IMRT planning consists in manually assigning importance weights w to each objective, using a high weight for the most important objective, and a smaller weight for less important goals. The best treatment plan is then defined as the one that minimizes the weighted sum of objectives.

$$w_T f_T(d) + w_P f_P(d) + w_H f_H(d)$$

IMRT planning uses mathematical optimization algorithms in order to determine the fluence map x, corresponding to the dose distribution $d = Dx$, which minimizes the weighted sum of objectives, subject to all constraints on the dose distribution, and under the condition that all beamlet weights have to be positive. We will further discuss optimization algorithms in the section Fluence Map Optimization. First, we look at the result of such an optimization for a specific choice of optimization parameters.

Solution to the IMRT Problem: The Optimal Treatment Plan

Figure 25.5 illustrates an IMRT treatment plan using 11 incident beam directions. It shows the dose distribution overlaid on a coronal slice of the patient's CT. Also shown are the 11 beams together with the effective fluence that is incident from each direction. One of the radiation fields is illustrated in more detail in Figure 25.6, in which the

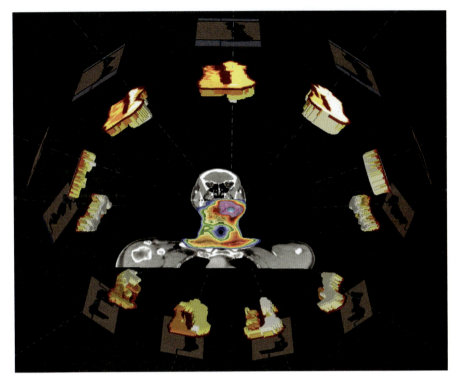

FIGURE 25.5. Illustration of an IMRT plan for the head-and-neck cancer patient generated in the RayStation planning system, version 4.0. The dose distribution is shown on a coronal slice of the patient's CT scan. The *blue circle* indicates the isocenter. The 11 beam directions are displayed with their respective fluence. *Red color* indicates a low fluence, white a high fluence.

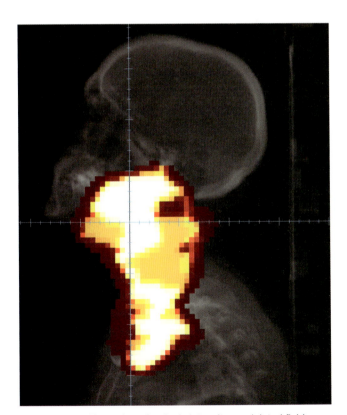

FIGURE 25.6. Illustration of a single intensity-modulated field overlaid on the DRR. The figure shows the effective fluence that is incident on the patient surface for the final treatment plan. This includes modification of the optimized fluence map through leaf sequencing (see Leaf Sequencing section) and refinement of MLC leaf positions (see Direct Aperture Optimization section). The latter also applies to Figure 25.5.

fluence is overlaid on the digitally reconstructed radiograph (DRR). The figure illustrates the modulation of the intensity over the radiation field.

The resulting dose distribution of the IMRT plan is shown in Figure 25.7. The middle panel shows the cumulative dose distribution of all beams. IMRT allows for dose distributions that conform to complex-shaped, concave target volumes. A single IMRT plan allows for different dose levels in high- and low-risk lymph node targets, as well as a simultaneous integrated boost (SIB) to the GTV. The peripheral images in Figure 25.7 show the dose contributions of 6 of the 11 incident beams.

Controlling Tradeoffs

Different objectives in IMRT planning are inherently conflicting. Clearly, there is a tradeoff between delivering dose to the tumor and reducing dose to healthy tissues. In the example described earlier, the target volume is directly adjacent to the parotid glands. Sparing the parotid glands from radiation will lead to a dose reduction in the adjacent part of the target volume. Ensuring coverage of the target will in turn lead to higher doses to the parotid glands. In addition, there are tradeoffs between different normal tissues. In order to deliver the prescribed dose to the target volume, some dose to the normal tissues is unavoidable. However, using intensity modulation and enough beam directions, the dose distribution in the normal tissue can be shaped according to the physician's preference.

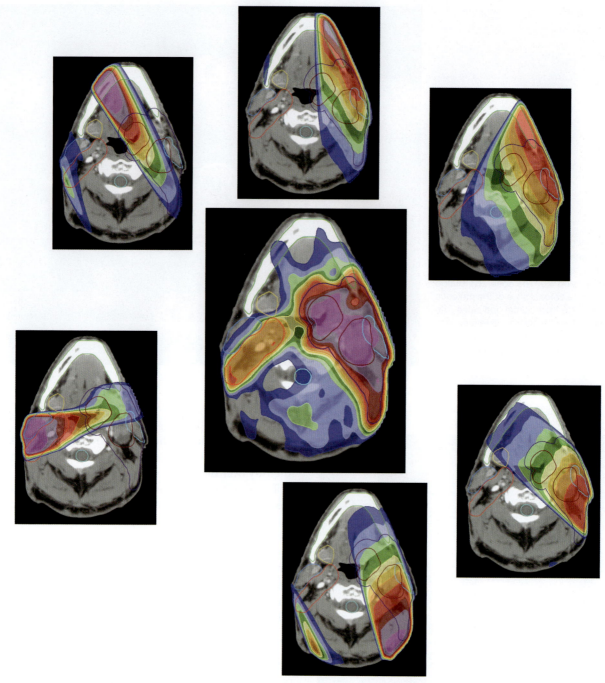

FIGURE 25.7. IMRT dose distribution for the head-and-neck case example, demonstrating the ability of IMRT to conform the dose distribution to complex target volumes (middle panel). Also shown are the dose contributions of 6 (out of 11) beam directions (surrounding images).

In most TPS that are in use today, treatment planners control the tradeoffs between different planning goals manually by manipulating the relative weights w of objective functions. This can lead to a time-consuming trial-and-error process. Different approaches have been suggested to improve the interaction of the treatment planner with the TPS, including interactive Pareto-surface navigation methods, which are discussed in the section Automated Planning and Multi-criteria Optimization.

Delivery of Intensity-Modulated Fields

In order to deliver an intensity-modulated field, the fluence map is decomposed into a number of smaller radiation fields that can be delivered using an MLC. This process is called sequencing and is described in more detail in the Leaf Sequencing section. As an outlook to subsequent sections, Figure 25.8 illustrates how the fluence shown in Figure 25.6 is delivered as a sequence of three MLC openings.

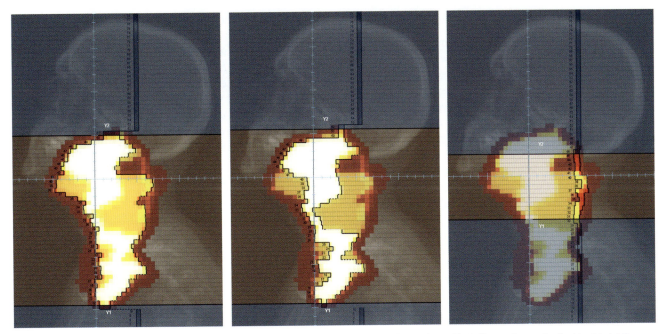

FIGURE 25.8. Delivery of an intensity-modulated field through a sequence of MLC openings. Each figure shows the incident total fluence overlaid on the DRR, together with the leaf positions of the multileaf collimator that define the field opening. Also shown are the positions of the Y-jaws that reduce transmission through closed MLC leaves (*blue*).

FLUENCE MAP OPTIMIZATION[1]

The previous section illustrated the main concepts in IMRT planning for an example case. In this section we take a more formal look at IMRT planning as a mathematical optimization problem. We first discuss some of the frequently used objective and constraint functions, in particular the handling of dose–volume effects. The subsequent section briefly outlines the use of outcome models in IMRT planning and their limitations. Finally, the section Optimization Algorithms introduces basic mathematical optimization algorithms to solve IMRT planning problems.

In mathematical terms, a general FMO problem can be formulated as the following mathematical optimization problem:

$$\begin{aligned} \text{minimize} \quad & f(d) \\ \text{subject to} \quad & g_s(d) \leq c_s \\ & d_i = \sum_j D_{ij} x_j \\ & x_j \geq 0 \end{aligned}$$

Treatment planning involves balancing different clinical objectives. Therefore, the objective function f is a weighted sum of individual objectives:

$$f(d) = \sum_n w_n f_n(d)$$

Here, w_n are positive weighting factors, which are used to control the relative importance of different terms in the composite objective function.

The objective function that may be the most commonly used in current TPS is a piecewise quadratic penalty function:

$$f_n(d) = \frac{1}{N_n} \sum_{i=1}^{N_n} (d_i - d_i^{max})_+^2 \quad \text{or}$$

$$f_n(d) = \frac{1}{N_n} \sum_{i=1}^{N_n} \left(d_i^{min} - d_i\right)_+^2 \qquad (25.2)$$

Here, d^{max} is a maximum tolerance dose for an organ, which is usually specified by the treatment planner through the graphical user interface in the TPS. Similarly, for target volumes d^{min} is a minimum dose that is to be delivered to the target volume.

The functions $g_s(d)$ correspond to hard constraints on the dose distribution. Common constraints are maximum dose values in organs at risk and minimum doses in target volumes. In this case, c_s is the maximum dose in a structure, s is an index over all voxels in the structure, and $g_s(d)$ is simply the dose in voxel s. In the subsection Dose–Volume effects, additional commonly used objectives and constraints are discussed.

---

[1]*This section was in parts adapted from the book chapter Boyer A, Unkelbach J. Intensity-modulated radiation therapy planning. In: Brahme A, ed. Comprehensive Biomedical Physics, Vol 9, Chapter 17, Elsevier; 2014.*

Dose–Volume Effects

An organ at risk will typically receive an inhomogeneous dose distribution. The question arises whether it is better to irradiate a small part of the organ to a large dose while sparing the remaining parts to a large extent; or whether it is better to spread out the dose and avoid large doses in all parts of the organ. In that context, one distinguishes parallel organs and serial organs. For organs with a serial structure, the function of the whole organ will fail if one part of the organ is damaged. One prominent example for a serial organ is the spinal cord. For serial organs, it is therefore crucial to limit the maximum dose delivered to the organ, rather than the mean dose. For a parallel organ, the function of the organ as a whole is preserved even if a part of the organ is damaged. The lungs are an example of a parallel organ. The dependence of a clinical outcome on the irradiated volume of an organ is commonly referred to as a *volume effect* or *dose–volume effect*. For IMRT planning, clinical knowledge on dose–volume effects are to be translated into appropriate objective functions. Today, mainly two types of objective/constraint functions are being applied: dose–volume histogram (DVH) constraints and the concept of equivalent uniform dose (EUD).

Equivalent Uniform Dose

One approach to quantifying dose–volume effects consists of using generalized mean values of the dose distribution:

$$EUD(d) = \left[\frac{1}{N}\sum_{i=1}^{N}(d_i)^\alpha\right]^{1/\alpha}$$

where the exponent α is larger than 1 for organs at risk (OARs). For the special case $\alpha = 1$, $EUD(d)$ is equivalent to the mean dose in the organ. In the limit of large α values, the value of $EUD(d)$ approaches the maximum dose in the organ. Thus, parallel organs are described via a small value of α close to 1, whereas serial organs are described via large values of α (approximately 10). The generalized mean value is commonly referred to as EUD. The generalized mean value can also be applied to target volumes by using negative exponents. For a large negative value of α, the EUD approaches the minimum dose in the target volume. In practice, exponents in the range of $\alpha = -10 \ldots -20$ are considered. The EUD can be used as both an objective function and a constraint function.

DVH Objectives and Constraints

The clinical evaluation of treatment plans often uses the DVH. A typical evaluation criterion for the target volume is as follows: at least 95% of the target volume should receive a dose equal to or higher than the prescription dose. Similarly, a criterion for an OAR could be as follows: at most 20% of the organ should receive more than 30 Gy. From an optimization perspective, it is not straightforward to handle DVH constraints in a rigorous way. In practice, DVH constraints are therefore handled approximately using a quadratic penalty function. We consider the

example that no more than 20% of an organ should receive a dose higher than d^{max}. Given an initial dose distribution, one can identify the fraction of voxels that exceed the dose level d^{max}. If this fraction is smaller than 20%, the DVH constraint is fulfilled. Otherwise, a quadratic penalty function is introduced that aims at reducing the dose to those voxels that exceed d^{max} by the least amount. For example, if 30% of the organ receives a higher dose, the 20% of voxels receiving the highest dose are ignored. For the remaining 10% of overdosed voxels a quadratic penalty term as in Equation 25.2 is added to the objective function.

The Use of Clinical Outcome Models in IMRT Optimization

Since the beginning of the IMRT era, the question regarding the adequate objective function has persisted. Intuitively, we would like to translate the notion of "maximizing the tumor control probability (TCP)" while "minimizing the normal tissue complication probability (NTCP)" more directly into mathematical terms.

One of the most common methods for relating treatment outcome to the dose distribution is logistic regression. As an example, we consider NTCP models; however, the same methodology can be applied to TCP models. The severity of a radiation side effect is clinically assessed in discrete stages. Typically, one is interested in avoiding severe complications. For example, in the treatment of lung cancer, treatment planning may aim at minimizing the probability for radiation pneumonitis of grade 2 or higher. This converts the observed clinical outcome into a binary outcome label. NTCP modeling can thus be considered as a classification problem, which aims at estimating the probability of a complication, given features of the dose distribution. Standard statistical classification methods, such as logistic regression, can be applied to this problem. In logistic regression, the NTCP model is as given by:

$$NTCP(d) = \frac{1}{1 + \exp(-f(d,q))}$$

Here, f is a function of the dose distribution d and the model parameters q. The central problem in statistical analysis and modeling of patient outcome consist in determining the function f, that is, selecting features of the dose distribution that are correlated with outcome. One of the most commonly used representations of f is given by:

$$NTCP(d) = \frac{1}{1 + \exp\left[\gamma(TD_{50} - EUD(d))\right]}$$

In this case, f is a linear function of a single feature of the dose distribution, namely the EUD. For $EUD(d) = TD_{50}$, the value of NTCP evaluates to 0.5, that is, TD_{50} corresponds to the effective dose that leads to a complication probability of 50%. The parameter γ determines the slope of the dose-response relation. The NTCP model has three parameters (TD_{50}, γ, and the EUD exponent α), which can be fitted to outcome data, for example, through maximum likelihood methods. This NTCP model is equivalent to the Lyman–Kutcher–Burman (LKB) model, except that the LKB model traditionally uses a different functional form of the sigmoid.

Although phenomenological outcome models play an increasing role in treatment plan evaluation, their capabilities from a treatment plan optimization perspective have remained limited so far. One reason for that is the uncertainty in outcome models. A second reason is that currently used models are not more powerful than dose-based objective functions. The NTCP model discussed here represents an increasing function of the EUD, that is, independent of the parameters TD_{50} and γ, higher EUD always leads to higher NTCP. As a consequence, the dose distribution that minimizes EUD is the same as the dose distribution that minimizes NTCP. Hence, from an IMRT optimization perspective, minimizing EUD and NTCP is equivalent.[5]

Optimization Algorithms

Our goal in this section is to provide the reader with an understanding of the most basic optimization algorithms, which do not require advanced knowledge of optimization theory. We start with a geometric visualization of the IMRT optimization problem. Subsequent, the gradient descent algorithm is described, which is in principle sufficient to optimize fluence maps. Afterward, extensions of gradient descent methods toward quasi-Newton algorithms are outlined. Certainly, the field of IMRT optimization has advanced significantly, and more sophisticated algorithms for constrained optimization are being applied in modern TPS. These algorithms require knowledge of optimization theory, which is beyond the scope of this chapter. The interested reader is referred to the optimization literature.[6,7] Ehrgott et al.[8] provide a review of radiotherapy planning from a mathematical optimization perspective.

Visualization of The Fluence Map Optimization Problem

Due to the large number of beamlets (optimization variables), it is not possible to visualize the objective and constraint functions for a full IMRT planning problem. Nevertheless, it is helpful to understand its structure. To that end, we consider a simplified version of an IMRT planning problem in which only two beamlets and four voxels are considered. We consider the following dose-deposition matrix:

$$D = \begin{pmatrix} 1.3 & 0.7 & 0.1 & 1.0 \\ 0.7 & 1.3 & 0.5 & 0.3 \end{pmatrix}$$

where the first two columns correspond to the tumor voxels, and columns 3 and 4 correspond to OAR voxels. We further assume that we aim to deliver a dose of 2 to both of the tumor voxels, and we impose maximum dose constraints on OAR voxels 3 and 4 of 0.8 and 1.0, respectively.

The goal of delivering the prescribed dose to the tumor voxels is expressed via a quadratic objective function. The optimization problem for this illustrative example can be formulated as follows:

$$\text{minimize} \quad \frac{1}{2}\sum_{i=1}^{2}(d_i - 2)^2$$

$$\text{subject to} \quad d_3 \leq 0.8$$

$$d_4 \leq 1.0$$

$$d_i = \sum_{j=1}^{2}D_{ij}x_j$$

$$x_j \geq 0$$

Since we have only two optimization variables, the objective and constraint functions can be visualized explicitly (see Fig. 25.9). The objective function is illustrated via isolines. Since we consider a quadratic objective function, it represents a two-dimensional parabola. The minimum of the objective function is located at beamlet

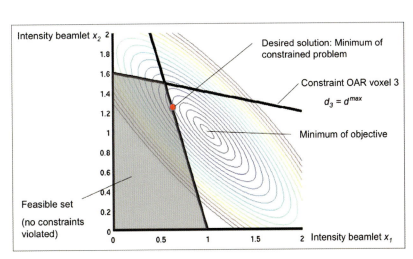

FIGURE 25.9. Visualization of the IMRT optimization problem for two beamlets. The quadratic objective function is shown via isolines; the linear maximum dose constraints of OAR voxels are shown as thick *black lines* (with permission reproduced from (69)).

intensities $x_1 = 1$ and $x_2 = 1$. At this point, both tumor voxels receive the prescribed dose and the objective function is zero.

We now consider the constraints on the OAR voxels. Since the dose in each voxel is a linear function of the beamlet intensities, the constraints represent hyperplanes in beamlet intensity space, that is, lines in two dimensions. In Figure 25.9 we show the lines where the constraints $d_3 = 0.8$ and $d_4 = 1.0$ are met exactly. For all beamlet intensity beyond these lines, the maximum dose to an OAR voxel is exceeded. All beamlet intensity combinations below the lines form the *feasible region*. Thus, the optimal solution to the IMRT planning problem is given by the point within the feasible region that has the smallest value of the objective function. In this example, the optimal solution is given by $x_1 = 0.7$ and $x_2 = 1.2$ and is indicated by the red dot in Figure 25.9. By multiplying this solution with the dose-deposition matrix, we obtain the corresponding optimal dose distribution.

In this case, the constraint for OAR voxel 3 is binding, that is, the OAR voxel receives the maximum dose we allow for. We further note that the minimum of the objective function is outside of the feasible region, which means that, in order to fulfill the maximum OAR dose constraint, we have to accept a compromise regarding target dose homogeneity.

Approximate Handling of Constraints via Penalty Functions

In IMRT planning, maximum dose constraints in OARs are often approximated via penalty functions. More specifically, we can consider the composite objective function where a quadratic penalty function, multiplied with a weight w, is added to the original objective for target dose homogeneity:

$$f(d) = \frac{1}{2}\sum_{i=1}^{2}(d_i - 2)^2 + w\left[(d_3 - 0.8)_+^2 + (d_4 - 1.0)_+^2\right]$$

Adding the penalty function does not change the objective function within the feasible region; only the objective function values outside of the feasible region are increased. This is shown in Figure 25.10 for penalty weights of $w = 5$ and $w = 20$. While w is increased, the unconstrained minimum of the function f moves closer to the optimal solution of the constrained problem.

The Basic Gradient Descent Method

In this section we introduce the most generic optimization algorithm, which can in principle be used to generate an IMRT treatment plan. To that end, we assume that we want to minimize an objective function f, subject to the constraint that all beamlet intensities are positive. We do not consider additional constraints g on the dose distribution, that is, all treatment goals are included in the objective function.

The gradient of the objective function is the vector of partial derivatives of f with respect to the beamlet intensities x_j:

$$\nabla f = \begin{bmatrix} \dfrac{\partial f}{\partial x_1} \\ \vdots \\ \dfrac{\partial f}{\partial x_j} \end{bmatrix}$$

The gradient vector is oriented perpendicular to the isolines of the objective function; it points in the direction of maximum slope in the objective function landscape. Thus, taking a small step into the direction of the negative gradient yields a fluence map x that corresponds to a lower value of the objective function, that is, an improved plan. This gives rise to the most basic nonlinear optimization algorithm: In each iteration k, the current fluence map x^k is updated according to the following:

$$x^{k+1} = x^k - \alpha \nabla f(x^k)$$

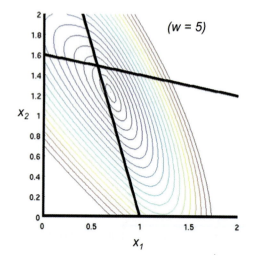
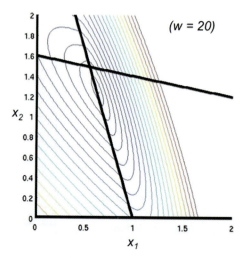

FIGURE 25.10. Visualization of the composite objective function containing quadratic penalty functions to approximate maximum dose constraints. For increasing weights w for the penalty function, the minimum of the composite objective function moves closer to the optimal solution of the constrained problem (with permission reproduced from (69)).

where α is a step size parameter, which has to be sufficiently small in order for the algorithm to converge.

Gradient Calculation. The gradient of the objective function with respect to the beamlet intensities can be calculated by using the chain rule in multiple dimensions: Given that the objective is a function of the dose distribution, we have

$$\frac{\partial f}{\partial x_j} = \sum_{i=1}^{N} \frac{\partial f}{\partial d_i} \frac{\partial d_i}{\partial x_j}$$

The partial derivative of the voxel dose d_i with respect to the beamlet weight x_j is simply given by the corresponding element of the dose-deposition matrix:

$$\frac{\partial d_i}{\partial x_j} = D_{ij}$$

The partial derivative of the objective function with respect to dose in voxel i describes by how much the objective function changes by varying the dose in voxel i. For the quadratic objective function

$$f(d) = \frac{1}{N} \sum_{i=1}^{N} (d_i - d^{pres})^2$$

the components of the gradient vector are given by

$$\frac{\partial f}{\partial x_j} = \frac{1}{N} \sum_{i=1}^{N} 2(d_i - d^{pres}) D_{ij}$$

which has an intuitive interpretation. The total change in the objective function value due to changing the intensity of beamlet j is obtained by summing over the contributions of all voxels. The contribution of a voxel is given by the dose error $(d_i - d^{press})$ multiplied by the influence D_{ij} of beamlet j onto the voxel i. If the dose d_i exceeds the prescribed dose, the voxel's contribution is positive; voxels that are underdosed yield a negative contribution to the gradient component. If the gradient component is negative after summing over the contributions of all voxels, the impact of the underdosed voxels dominates. A step in the direction of the negative gradient corresponds to increasing the beamlet weight x_j, thus reducing the extent of underdosing.

Handling the Nonnegativity Constraint. So far, only the objective function f was considered, not taking into account the nonnegativity constraint on the beamlet intensities. Applying the gradient descent algorithm without accounting for the nonnegativity constraint leads to negative intensities for some of the beamlets, which is not meaningful. Different extensions of the gradient descent algorithm exist in order to ensure positive beamlet weights.

One method consists in simply setting all negative beamlet intensities to zero after each gradient step. Formally, this corresponds to a projection algorithm for handling bound constraints. An alternative approach is based on a variable transformation. In this case, a new optimization variable is introduced for every beamlet, which is defined as the square root of the intensity. Thus, the beamlet intensity, given by the squared value of the variable, is always positive, while the optimization variable can take any value. This way, the constrained optimization problem is converted into a fully unconstrained problem.

Improvements to Gradient Descent
The generic gradient descent algorithm shows slow convergence in practical IMRT optimization problems. Improvements to the generic gradient descent algorithm can be made mainly in three aspects:

1. Selecting an appropriate step size using line search algorithms.
2. Improving the descent direction by including second-derivative information.
3. Improving the handling of constraints using more advanced algorithms for constrained optimization.

For the first and third aspects, the reader is referred to the advanced optimization literature. The second aspect is outlined in the following section.

Including Second Derivatives. The generic gradient descent algorithm considers the first derivative of the objective function at the current fluence map x. This can be interpreted as finding a hyperplane that is tangential to the objective function at x. The convergence properties of iterative optimization algorithms can be improved by including second derivative (i.e., curvature) information. This can be interpreted as finding a quadratic function that is tangential to the objective function at x. The iterative optimization algorithm, known as the *Newton method*, then performs a step to the minimum of the quadratic approximation.

To formalize this concept, we consider a second-order Taylor expansion of the objective function f at the fluence map x:

$$\tilde{f}(x + \Delta x) = f(x) + \sum_{j} \frac{\partial f}{\partial x_j} \Delta x_j + \sum_{j,k} \frac{\partial^2 f}{\partial x_j \partial x_k} \Delta x_j \Delta x_k$$

By defining the Hessian H as the matrix of second derivatives, this can be written as

$$\tilde{f}(x + \Delta x) = f(x) + \nabla f(x) \Delta x + \Delta x^T H(x) \Delta x$$

The idea of the Newton method consists in taking a step Δx such that we reach the minimum of the quadratic approximation. For the special case that the original objective function f is a quadratic function, the approximation is exact, and thus the Newton method finds the optimal solution in a single step. Generally, f will not be a purely quadratic function. However, it is assumed that Newton steps will approach the optimum in fewer iterations than steps along the gradient direction.

To calculate the Newton step Δx^*, we set the gradient of $\tilde{f}$ with respect to Δx to zero, which yields the condition

$$\nabla f(x) + H(x)\Delta x^* = 0$$

Thus, the Newton step is given by

$$\Delta x^* = -H(x)^{-1}\, \nabla f(x)$$

This leads to a modified iterative optimization algorithm in which the beamlet intensities are updated according to

$$x^{k+1} = x^k - \alpha H\left(x^k\right)^{-1} \nabla f\left(x^k\right)$$

We can further note that the Newton method has a natural step size $\alpha = 1$. In practical IMRT optimization, the pure Newton method is not applied. A naïve computation of the Newton step involves the calculation of the Hessian matrix at point x, inverting the Hessian matrix, and multiplying the inverse Hessian $H(x^k)^{-1}$ with the gradient vector. In IMRT optimization, the size of the Hessian matrix is given by the number of beamlets squared. Therefore, the explicit calculation and inversion of the Hessian are often computationally expensive. Thus, IMRT optimization often employs so-called quasi-Newton methods, which rely on an approximation of the Newton step. One of the most popular methods is the limited memory L-BFGS quasi-Newton algorithm. In this algorithm, the descent direction $H(x^k)^{-1}\nabla f(x^k)$ is approximated based on the fluence maps and gradients evaluated during the previous iterations of the algorithm, which avoids a costly matrix inversion. A comprehensive description of the L-BFGS algorithm can be found in the textbook by Nocedal and Wright.[6]

Convexity

Many objective functions commonly applied in IMRT planning are convex. This is in particular the case for the piecewise quadratic objective, linear objectives, and the generalized EUD for exponents $|\alpha| > 1$. The convexity property of objective and constraint functions has important implications for the optimization of fluence maps. An optimization problem defined through a convex objective function f and convex constraint functions g_s has a unique global minimum, that is, there are no local minima, which are not the global minimum. Thus, gradient descent–based optimization algorithms do reliably find the optimal fluence map. The only nonconvex objectives commonly applied in practice are DVH criteria. However, practical experience suggests that the nonconvexity of DVH criteria does not cause severe local minima-related issues in IMRT planning.

LEAF SEQUENCING

In this section, we discuss ways to deliver intensity-modulated radiation fields. The section is focused on IMRT delivery using conventional Linacs equipped with an MLC. This represents, by far, the most widely used IMRT technique, although it is not the only possible form of IMRT. Historically, IMRT delivery with compensators has been performed in many centers. In that technique, an intensity-modulated field is created using an absorber placed in the beam path in the Linac head. The absorber causes an exponential attenuation of the fluence. By varying the thickness of the absorber across the beam profile, the desired intensity-modulated field can be created. Compensators had to be custom made for every patient and every field, and were typically cast in lead. This required a machine shop connected to the radiotherapy department. Nowadays, the use of computer-controlled MLCs, which eliminates the need for patient-specific hardware, has replaced compensator-based IMRT delivery.

Beam Shaping and Multi-leaf Collimators

This section briefly introduces MLCs. We focus on the main aspects of MLCs that are relevant for IMRT planning and delivery as described in the remainder of this chapter. For details on the mechanical and technical aspects, the reader is referred to the literature.[4] Figure 25.11 illustrates the main components used to collimate the radiation beam: the jaws and the MLC. The MLC is the primary collimation device that defines the shape of the beam. It consists of thin sheets of tungsten, which are moved in and out of the beam using computer-controlled electric motors. Each leaf has a considerable height (measured in beam direction) of approximately 5 to 10 cm in order to keep the transmission of radiation through closed leaves low. In contrast, each leaf is only a few mm thick to yield a projected beamlet size of 5 mm or 10 mm at the isocenter. The jaws represent rectangular field collimators upstream of the MLC. Figure 25.12 illustrates the use of the MLC for

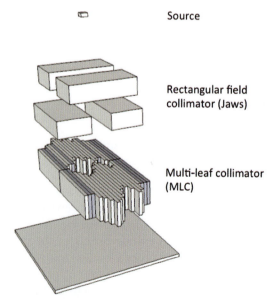

FIGURE 25.11. Illustration of beam collimation for IMRT delivery using multileaf collimators and jaws.

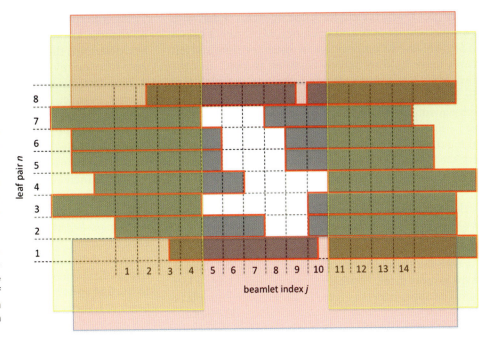

FIGURE 25.12. Illustration of beam collimation in beam's eye view using an MLC and jaws. The MLC leaves (*gray bars*) are used primarily for beam shaping. The jaws (*red and yellow blocks*) are typically placed in a post-processing step to irradiate the smallest rectangular field that covers the MLC aperture. The jaws reduce transmission through closed MLC leaves. In addition, for MLCs that require a finite gap between the left and right leaf tip, closed leaf pairs can be hidden behind the jaws, as illustrated in rows 1 and 8.

beam collimation in beam's eye view. A variety of terms are used to refer to a radiation field produced by an MLC. In this chapter, we use the term *aperture*; other common terms are *segment* or *MLC opening*.

Depending on the MLC model, there are a number of constraints on leaf motion and leaf positioning. This limits the set of apertures that can be delivered by an MLC. With the latest generation of MLCs, some of these restrictions are eliminated, but especially for older models some of the following restrictions may apply:

- Interdigitation: For some MLCs it is not possible for neighboring leaf pairs to cross, that is, the tip of the left leaf cannot move past the tip of a neighboring right leaf. The leaf configuration of leaf pairs 7 and 8 in Figure 25.12 would be prohibited. The interdigitation constraint has been eliminated for most modern MLCs.
- Maximum overtravel: Most linear accelerators have a 40 × 40 cm field of view at the isocenter. However, for some MLCs it is not possible for the left leaf to travel all the way to the right side of the field of view. The maximum distance that the leaf tip can travel beyond the isocenter projection is called the maximum overtravel. The constraint implies that the MLC cannot deliver small apertures far away from the isocenter.

- Minimum leaf gap: For some MLCs a leaf pair cannot fully close; that is, a minimum gap between the right and left leaf tips has to remain.
- Maximum leaf speed: In addition to restrictions on leaf positioning, MLCs have dynamic constraints. Leaves cannot move faster than a maximum speed; typical values are 3 cm/s or 6 cm/s.

Aperture Decomposition of Fluence Maps

It is intuitively clear that the superposition of multiple distinct radiation fields formed by an MLC may yield an intensity-modulated field. This is schematically illustrated in Figure 25.13.

In IMRT planning, the inverse problem needs to be solved, that is, given an optimized fluence map, we have to determine a set of apertures that closely reproduces the fluence map. This is called the *leaf sequencing* problem. We assume for now that the fluence map is discretized into evenly spaced fluence levels. A closer look at Figure 25.13 demonstrates that the leaf sequencing problem does not have a unique solution; that is, a given fluence map can be decomposed into a set of apertures in many different ways. We consider MLC rows 3 and 4 in

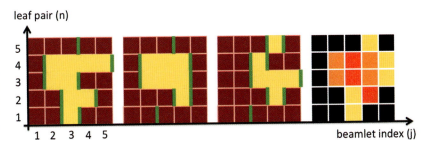

FIGURE 25.13. Schematic illustration of the decomposition of a fluence map (right panel) into apertures. The positions of MLC leaf ends are indicated by the *green bars*. It is assumed that each aperture delivers one unit of fluence; the colors *yellow, orange,* and *red* indicate one, two, and three units of fluence, respectively.

Figure 25.13, which yield the same fluence, created with a distinct sequence of leaf openings. MLC row 3 uses a *sliding window* decomposition, in which the right and left leaves move unidirectionally from left to right. In contrast, MLC row 4 uses a *close-in* technique, in which case the first aperture corresponds to the largest field opening. Subsequent apertures shrink the field and deliver additional fluence at the beamlets that have higher intensity. In Figure 25.13 and throughout this section, we assume that the fluence over an open field is homogeneous, which is applicable to Linacs with flattening filter. Although not discussed here, leaf sequencing methods can be extended to flattening filter free (FFF) delivery of IMRT, which has the advantage of higher dose rates.

Sliding Window Sequencing

We consider the sliding window decomposition of fluence maps in more detail.[9] To that end, we consider a single leaf pair. The upper panel in Figure 25.14 shows an example of one row of a fluence map for a single leaf pair. The bottom panel shows the sliding window type aperture decomposition. In the example, both leaves move unidirectionally from left to right.

It is intuitive that the gradients in the fluence map, that is, changes in the intensity between neighboring beamlets, determine the leaf positions. In the example, the fluence increases by 4 units between beamlet 1 and beamlet 2. This determines that, during the delivery of 4 units of fluence, beamlet 1 has to be blocked by the left leaf while beamlet 2 is exposed. Likewise, the fluence decreases by 1 unit between beamlets 2 and 3, which determines that during the delivery of 1 unit of fluence, beamlet 3 has to be blocked by the right leaf while beamlet 2 is exposed. We call an increase in the fluence from one beamlet to the next higher numbered beamlet a positive gradient, and a decrease a negative gradient. It is clear that the *sum of positive gradients* (SPG) equals the sum of negative gradients. In sliding window sequencing, the positive gradients uniquely determine the left leaf positions, while the negative gradients uniquely determine the right leaf positions. In the first aperture, the left leaf is positioned to the left of beamlet 1, the right leaf is positioned where the first negative gradient occurs, which is between beamlet 2 and 3. For the second aperture, the left leaf stays in the same position while the right leaf moves to the next negative gradient position, which is between beamlets 3 and 4.

It is intuitive that an irregularly shaped fluence map with several peaks and valleys requires more apertures to deliver than smooth fluence maps. It can be shown that the minimum total number of MU to deliver a fluence map is given by the SPG. Sliding window sequencing is therefore optimal regarding the total number of MU since it always reproduces a fluence map with the shortest possible beam-on time.

Sequencing as an Optimization Problem

As illustrated in Figure 25.13, the leaf sequencing problem does not have a unique solution. The degeneracy of the problem provides some freedom that can be exploited, that is, the sequencing step can aim at determining apertures that have desirable features. Criteria for good aperture sets are as follows:

- The total number of MU to be delivered is small, which corresponds to the total beam-on time.
- The total number of apertures is small.
- Leaf travel is minimized; that is, the MLC leaves move as little as possible
- Apertures should have regular shapes and very small apertures are avoided.
- The fluence map is reproduced exactly or as closely as possible without prior discretization.
- All MLC constraints are satisfied.

The sliding window sequencing method is optimal regarding the total number of MU. However, other sequencing methods can potentially reduce the total number of apertures needed. To that end, the sequencing problem can be formulated as an optimization problem. While the FMO problem is a continuous optimization problem for which gradient-based optimization

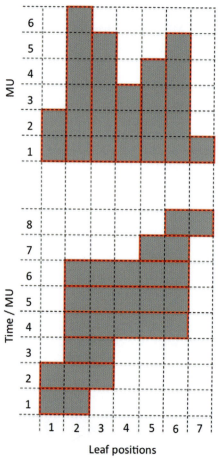

FIGURE 25.14. Illustration of sliding window sequencing. The upper panel shows the fluence map (*vertical bars*) corresponding to a single leaf pair. The bottom panel shows the set of apertures (*horizontal bars*) to realize the fluence map.

methods are applied, the sequencing problem is discrete and requires different optimization techniques. The interested reader is referred to the literature. For example, the work by Engel[10] describes a sequencing algorithm that yields the minimum number of MU and simultaneously approximately minimizes the number of apertures.

Step-and-Shoot Delivery Versus Dynamic Delivery

In IMRT, two types of delivery are distinguished: step-and-shoot delivery and dynamic delivery. In step-and-shoot IMRT, the fluence map is sequenced into a set of apertures as described earlier. Each aperture is irradiated individually, that is, the MLC leaves move to the desired position, and the beam is turned on to deliver the specified number of MU. Subsequently, the beam is turned off while the MLC leaves are moved to shape the next aperture. In dynamic delivery, the MLC leaves move while the treatment beam is on. In this case, the sequencing task consists in determining the trajectories of MLC leaves, that is, the leaf positions as a function of time.

Dynamic delivery is frequently associated with a sliding window type delivery, because this gives rise to a constructive method to determine the leaf trajectories.[11] To that end, we consider a generalization of the sliding window aperture decomposition in Figure 25.14. Figure 25.15 schematically illustrates continuous trajectories of the left and right leaf in one MLC row. The horizontal axis shows the position of the leaf end, while the vertical axis shows the time when the leaf end traverses a given position. At every beamlet position in the MLC row, the effective fluence of the beamlet is given by the exposure time. Initially, both leaves are positioned on the left side and the right leaf covers the beamlet. At time t_1, the right leaf end traverses the beamlet and opens the radiation field at that position. At a later time point t_2 the left leaf traverses the beamlet and closes the radiation field. The fluence of the beamlet is proportional to the time interval $t_2 - t_1$ during which the beamlet is exposed. Thus, the distance of right and left leaf on the vertical axis determines the corresponding fluence profile (green line in the bottom panel).

In practice, the MLC leaves cannot move arbitrarily fast and have to respect a maximum leaf speed. In Figure 25.15, the maximum leaf speed constraint corresponds to a minimum slope of the leaf trajectory. To allow a leaf to move a certain distance on the horizontal axis, a minimum amount of time has to pass. This is indicated by the black dashed line in the upper panel.

Dynamic delivery is frequently associated with sliding window type delivery and used synonymously by some people. However, dynamic delivery is not per se tied to sliding window trajectories. In principle, other sequencing methods that allow for bidirectional leaf motion could be developed and used. In fact, delivery of VMAT can be considered as dynamic delivery with bidirectional leaf motion.

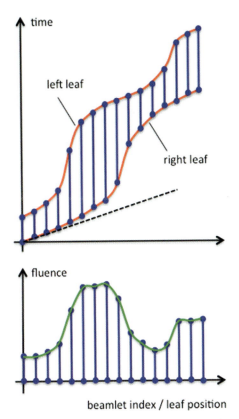

FIGURE 25.15. Illustration of dynamic IMRT delivery using a sliding window technique. The *red lines* in the upper panel show the positions of the left and right leaf as a function of time. The *green line* in the bottom panel shows the corresponding fluence profile.

DIRECT APERTURE OPTIMIZATION

Historically, IMRT planning was developed as the two-step approach of FMO plus sequencing. However, there are a number of disadvantages related to the two-step approach. For example, in step-and-shoot IMRT, a large number of apertures may be required to faithfully reproduce a fluence map. Other problems relate to dose calculation accuracy during the FMO step. In order to cope with the limitations of the two-step approach, DAO methods were developed and integrated into commercial TPS. In this section, we first summarize some of the limitations of the two-step approach. Subsequently, approaches to DAO are discussed, which directly determine the shapes and intensities of apertures.

Limitations of the FMO + Sequencing Approach

Limitations of the two-step approach can broadly be categorized into three types:

1. The fluence map is not accurately reproduced by the set of apertures. This is primarily a problem in step-and-shoot IMRT if the total number of apertures is kept small.

2. In step-and-shoot IMRT, the leaf ends are positioned at the boundary between two beamlets after the sequencing step. The dose distribution may be improved by positioning the leaves at intermediate positions.

3. Even if the leaf sequencing step reproduces the fluence map exactly, there will still be a discrepancy between the FMO dose distribution used during plan optimization and the dose that is actually delivered by the set of apertures.

While the first two limitations are quite apparent, the third aspect is more complex. There are multiple reasons for dose discrepancy. Some are inherent to the dose-deposition matrix concept, which does not take into account higher-order effects on the incident fluence that the MLC causes. Others are related to compromises being made between accuracy and computational performance in the FMO stage.

Dose calculation accuracy: The calculation of the dose-deposition matrix often uses a simplified dose calculation algorithm to speed up the computation. For example, the dose-deposition matrix may be based on a pencil beam algorithm, while the final dose distribution of the apertures may be calculated with a convolution–superposition algorithm. In addition, the dose-deposition matrix may not store small scatter dose contributions far away from the central axis of the beamlet in order to reduce memory requirements. This leads to dose discrepancy between the sequenced FMO solution and the final dose distribution. This issue is not an inherent limitation of the two-step approach, and using accurate dose calculation methods for computing the dose-deposition matrix could mitigate the problem. However, in practice fast treatment plan optimization is desired, which requires compromises.

Tongue-and-groove effect: Other dose calculation problems are inherent to the dose-deposition matrix concept. For mechanical reasons, two neighboring MLC leaves cannot be arbitrarily close to each other. However, a small gap between MLC leaves would lead to radiation leaking through. In order to avoid such inter-leaf leakage, many MLCs adopt a tongue-and-groove design, which is schematically illustrated in Figure 25.16. Let us consider an aperture consisting of two neighboring beamlets in adjacent leaf pairs. The dose-deposition matrix concept used in FMO assumes linearity. This means, if both beamlets are combined to a single aperture, the resulting dose distribution is predicted to be the same compared to the situation in which both beamlets are delivered individually as separate apertures. However, for MLCs with tongue-and-groove design, this is not true. The regions where both leaves overlap are now blocked as soon as one of the

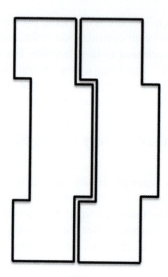

FIGURE 25.16. Illustration of MLC leaves with tongue-and-groove design.

two leaves is closed. This leads to an underdosage of the region of the beamlet boundary if both beamlets are delivered as separate apertures.

Leaf transmission: During the FMO step, the fluence of beamlets may be zero if the beamlet is not beneficial for the treatment plan. Also, the sequencing method typically assumes that the fluence for closed leaves is zero. In reality this is only approximately true as there is some transmission of radiation through closed MLC leaves. The effect is mitigated by the jaws and is small when considering a single aperture. However, the leaf transmission effect can add up for treatment plans consisting of a large number of small apertures.

Mitigation of dose discrepancies: There are approaches to mitigate the effects that lead to discrepancies between the dose distributions at the FMO stage and after sequencing. One approach consists in adding regularization terms to the FMO problem to favor smooth fluence maps that require fewer apertures to deliver. In this context, the L_1-norm regularization term is of particular interest, which has edge-preserving properties and favors piecewise constant fluence maps.[12,13] Furthermore, enhancements to the sequencing algorithm have been devised, which, for example, aim to reduce tongue-and-groove effects.[14]

Direct Aperture Optimization for Step-and-Shoot IMRT

In light of the aforementioned limitations of the two-step approach of FMO plus sequencing, it appears desirable to directly optimize the shapes and intensities of apertures based on the dosimetric objective function $f(d)$. As a modification of the FMO problem, the DAO problem can be stated as follows:

Determine the intensities and shapes of K apertures that minimize the objective function f(d) subject to the constraints $g_s(d) \leq c_s$. Optimizing shapes of the apertures refers to optimizing the positions of all MLC leaves.

In order to appreciate the inherent difficulties in DAO, we recall the favorable properties of the FMO problem. For FMO, the optimization variables are the beamlet intensities, while the objective is a function of the dose distribution. Given the dose-deposition matrix elements as fixed parameters, the dose distribution is a linear function of the beamlet intensities. A small change in the intensity of one beamlet leads to a small linear change in the dose to a voxel. Thus, the objective function can be written explicitly as a function of the optimization variable. In addition, if the objective is a convex function of dose, the overall optimization problem is convex, and gradient-based algorithms converge to the global optimum.

The DAO problem does not have this favorable property. The dose distribution is a more complex and nonconvex function of the optimization variables (the MLC leaf positions), which cannot easily be stated in closed form. If we consider the dose in a voxel as a function of the position of an MLC leaf, the dependence is given by a smoothed step function. While both leaves are fully open, the leaf pair contributes its maximum dose to the voxel. While one leaf moves to close the field, the leaf pair's dose contribution goes to zero. However, for most parts, a change in the leaf position has little impact on the dose to a particular voxel. Only in a small region that corresponds to the projection of the voxel onto the MLC plane, a small change in the leaf position yields a steep change in the voxel's dose.

In addition, there is a combinatorial aspect to the DAO problem. An IMRT plan typically consists of 7 to 11 beam directions. Some beams contribute more dose than others, and not all beam directions require the same amount of intensity modulation. Therefore, the best distribution of a limited number of apertures over the incident beam angles is not clear a priori. Assigning the same number of apertures to every beam may not yield the best treatment plan.

All approaches to DAO have to cope with these intrinsic difficulties. DAO approaches can broadly be categorized into three types:

1. Stochastic search methods
2. Aperture generation methods
3. Gradient-based leaf position optimization

Stochastic Search Methods

Stochastic search methods for DAO include simulated annealing[15] and genetic algorithms.[16,17] These approaches typically start with a geometry-based initialization of aperture shapes, that is, apertures that conform to the target volume, possibly excluding projections of the OARs. Subsequently, random perturbations of leaf positions are generated, and dose distribution d and objective function $f(d)$ are evaluated. If the treatment plan improves, the modification of the aperture set is accepted; otherwise, it is rejected with some probability. Stochastic search methods have a number of advantages. First, random perturbations of leaf positions can be restricted such that all MLC constraints are fulfilled. In addition, these methods can in principle escape from local optima of the objective function. Simulated annealing–based DAO had been commercialized by PROWESS in the Panther TPS for step-and-shoot IMRT. Furthermore, the method has been adapted to VMAT (section Arc Therapy) and is used in the RapidArc module in the Eclipse TPS marketed by Varian.

Aperture Generation Methods

The second class of methods refers to techniques that iteratively generate new apertures that are added to a treatment plan. Such an approach has been suggested by Romeijn et al.[18] and Carlsson.[19] Here, we illustrate the main idea behind the approach. We assume that the current treatment plan consists of $n - 1$ apertures, and we are interested in generating the nth aperture that yields a large improvement to the current treatment plan. To that end, we consider the partial derivative $\partial f / \partial x_j$ of the objective function f with respect to the intensity of a beamlet j. If the derivative is negative, adding the beamlet with a small positive intensity reduces the objective function, that is, improves the treatment plan. Furthermore, if $\left| \partial f / \partial x_j \right|$ is large, the beamlet promises a large improvement to the treatment plan. Therefore, a plausible approach to identifying a valuable new aperture consists in finding a deliverable aperture that contains many beamlets j for which $\partial f / \partial x_j < 0$ and $\left| \partial f / \partial x_j \right|$ is large. Romeijn et al.[18] describe an efficient algorithm to identify the aperture A for which

$$\sum_{j \in A} \frac{\partial f}{\partial x_j}$$

is minimized. The aperture is added to the treatment plan, and the intensities of all n apertures are optimized. The problem of optimizing the aperture intensities is formally identical to the FMO problem and can be solved using the algorithms described in the section Fluence Map Optimization. The dose distribution of an aperture A_k in the patient is obtained by summing the dose-deposition matrix elements over the beamlets contained in the aperture,

$$D_i^k = \sum_{j \in A_k} D_{ij}$$

and the dose distribution is simply given by summing the contributions of all apertures,

$$d_i = \sum_k D_i^k y_k$$

where y_k is the intensity of aperture k. The iterative generation of new apertures can be stopped once a maximum number of apertures is reached or the plan quality is sufficiently high.

Local Leaf Position Optimization[2]

In the remainder of this section, we describe the third approach of gradient-based leaf position optimization in more detail. The reason is that this approach is implemented in several of the widely used commercial TPS, including Pinnacle (Philips),[20] RayStation (Raysearch Laboratories), and Monaco (Elekta).

In this approach to DAO, we assume that we are given an initial set of apertures. This set of apertures can, for example, be obtained by sequencing a fluence map solution, or from the aperture generation method discussed earlier. Due to the nonconvex nature of the problem, the initial set of apertures should represent a good starting point for leaf position refinement, that is, ideally forms a decent treatment plan already. The set of K apertures, indexed by k, is characterized by the following:

- aperture intensities y_k
- leaf positions for the left and right leaf edges: L_{kn} and R_{kn} where n is the index of the MLC leaf pair

The goal of gradient-based leaf refinement is to optimize the objective function $f(d)$ with respect to the leaf positions and aperture weights. In particular, we allow the leaf positions to change continuously, that is, the leaf edge does not have to be positioned at a beamlet boundary.

Approximate Dose Calculation

We first formulate the dose distribution as a function of the optimization variables, that is, leaf positions and aperture intensities. The dose in voxel i is given by the sum of the contributions of the individual apertures, weighted with their intensity y_k. Furthermore, the dose contribution of each aperture is given by the contributions ψ_{kn}^i of each MLC leaf pair:

$$d_i = \sum_k \sum_n y_k \psi_{kn}^i(L_{kn}, R_{kn})$$

To proceed, we have to further characterize the function $\psi_{kn}^i(L_{kn}, R_{kn})$. For that purpose, we consider a particular MLC row n in aperture k. We first imagine that the left leaf is located at the left-most position at the edge of the field, and we consider the dose contribution of the MLC row as a function of the right leaf position, which we denote by the function $\phi_{kn}^i(R_{kn})$. Let us further assume that the voxel i is within the beam's eye view of the MLC row such that the MLC row contributes a significant dose

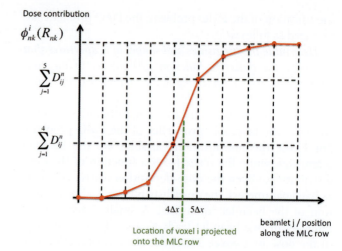

FIGURE 25.17. Illustration of the function $\phi_{kn}^j(R_{kn})$, representing the dose contribution of an MLC row to a voxel as a function of the right leaf position. The function is known at discrete positions where the right leaf is positioned at a beamlet boundary, and the dose contribution can be expressed as a sum of dose-deposition matrix elements. In between, the dose contribution is interpolated linearly (with permission reproduced from (69)).

to voxel i. We know that the function $\phi_{kn}^i(R_{kn})$ has the shape of a smooth step function: If the right leaf is located at the left-most position, the MLC row is closed and the dose contribution is zero. While the right leaf is moving to the right, the dose contribution increases monotonically. This is illustrated in Figure 25.17.

We now consider the dose-deposition matrix representation of the dose to further characterize the function $\phi_{kn}^i(R_{kn})$. We note that we know the function $\phi_{kn}^i(R_{kn})$ at discrete points, namely when the right leaf is positioned at the edge of a beamlet. Let Δx denote the size of a beamlet, and let j denote the beamlet index in leaf motion direction. At position $j\Delta x$, the dose contribution is simply given by the sum over the exposed beamlets, that is,

$$\phi_{kn}^i(R_{kn} = j_{kn}\Delta x) = \sum_{j=1}^{j_{kn}} D_{ij}^n$$

where we introduce the dose-deposition matrix notation D_{ij}^n to denote the dose contribution of beamlet j in MLC row n to voxel i. For a continuous leaf position in between, we consider a linear interpolation (see Fig. 25.17). This corresponds to the assumption that the dose distribution of a beamlet that is half exposed is given by the beamlet dose distribution with half the intensity. This approximation will break down for large beamlet size Δx; however, for practical beamlet sizes of 5 mm, the approximation yields adequate results. Using the function ϕ_{kn}^i, we can express the dose contribution of an MLC row as

$$\psi_{kn}^i(L_{kn}, R_{kn}) = \phi_{kn}^i(R_{kn}) - \phi_{kn}^i(L_{kn}).$$

[2]*This section was in parts adapted from the book chapter Boyer A, Unkelbach J. Intensity-modulated radiation therapy planning. In: Brahme A, ed. Comprehensive Biomedical Physics, Vol 9, Chapter 17, Elsevier; 2014.*

The first term represents the beamlets that are exposed by the right leaf; the second term subtracts the beamlets that are blocked by the left leaf.

Optimizing Leaf Positions

To optimize leaf positions and aperture intensities, we can utilize gradient descent–based algorithms for nonlinear optimization. To apply the generic gradient descent algorithm described in the section Fluence Map Optimization, we have to evaluate the gradient of the objective function with respect to leaf positions and aperture intensities.

This can be achieved with the help of the function ϕ. Let us consider the derivative with respect to one of the right leaves, R_{kn}:

$$\frac{\partial f}{\partial R_{kn}} = \sum_{i=1}^{N} \frac{\partial f}{\partial d_i} \frac{\partial d_i}{\partial R_{kn}} = \sum_{i=1}^{N} \frac{\partial f}{\partial d_i} y_k \frac{\partial \phi_{kn}^i(R_{kn})}{\partial R_{kn}}$$

The calculation of the partial derivatives $\partial f / \partial d_i$ is identical to the case of FMO. Using the linear approximation illustrated in Figure 25.17, the derivative of the dose contribution function $\phi_{kn}^i(R_{kn})$ only depends on the beamlet where the leaf edge is currently located. If we further assume that the leaf position is measured in units of beamlets (i.e., moving a leaf by the width of one beamlet corresponds to a distance of 1), the derivative of $\phi_{kn}^i(R_{kn})$ is simply given by

$$\frac{\partial \phi_{kn}^i(R_{kn})}{\partial R_{kn}} = D_{ij_{kn}}^n$$

where j_{kn} is the index of the beamlet where the leaf edge is located. The derivative of the voxel dose with respect to the aperture intensity is simply given by the dose contribution of the aperture for unit intensity:

$$\frac{\partial d_i}{\partial y_k} = \sum_n \Psi_{kn}^i(L_{kn}, R_{kn})$$

Evaluating the dose gradient of the objective function with respect to the optimization variables provides the prerequisites for the use of a gradient-based nonlinear optimization algorithm. In contrast to FMO, DAO considers two types of optimization variables simultaneously, that is, leaf positions and aperture intensities. Therefore, the use of second derivatives in the optimization algorithm is important. In particular, the quasi-Newton methods like L-BFGS can be used. Variations of gradient-based leaf position optimization are described by De Gersem et al.[21] and Cassioli and Unkelbach.[22]

DAO provides the opportunity to account for restrictions of the MLC directly. These can be integrated into the optimization problem in the form of bound constraints and linear constraints. In addition, DAO provides better ways of mitigating dose calculation inaccuracies compared to FMO. For example, at an intermediate stage of gradient-based leaf position optimization, the dose distributions of the current aperture set can be calculated using a convolution–superposition algorithm. In subsequent iterations, changes can be approximated by a pencil beam–based dose-deposition matrix. If leaf position changes remain small, the error in the dose distribution is minor.

ARC THERAPY

In IMRT, the patient is irradiated from discrete beam directions. Typically, between 7 and 11 beam directions are used. While the gantry moves from one angle to the next, the treatment beam is off. *Arc therapy* refers to a radiotherapy delivery mode in which the treatment beam is continuously on while the gantry rotates around the patient. Conformal arc therapy has long been used as a delivery mode for conformal therapy, especially for small spherical lesions that do not require intensity modulation. In conformal arc therapy, the treatment field is fixed during gantry rotation or conforms to the projection of the target volume. VMAT refers to an extension of IMRT to a rotational treatment mode, delivered at conventional Linacs equipped with an MLC. The treatment field does not necessarily conform to the target at every angle. Instead, an effectively intensity-modulated field is delivered over an arc sector.

The motivation for VMAT has been twofold: First, the patient is irradiated from all gantry angles rather than a relatively small number of discrete angles. This bears the potential for better and more conformal treatment plans. Second, VMAT bears the potential for shorter treatment times because the treatment beam is continuously on. The idea of delivering intensity-modulated fields through arc therapy was suggested by Yu as early as 1995.[23] However, clinical implementation of VMAT was delayed in part due to TPS lacking support for this technique. In 2008, Varian introduced the RapidArc planning module in the Eclipse planning system and provided a commercial VMAT solution. Around the same time, Philips Medical Systems provided the SmartArc module in the Pinnacle planning system to support VMAT. Today, most treatment systems including Monaco (Elekta) and RayStation (Raysearch Laboratories) support VMAT planning.

Before the clinical adaptation of VMAT, specialized hardware to deliver intensity-modulated fields in a rotational mode was developed. The device has been proposed by Mackie[24] and was commercialized as *Tomotherapy*, resulting in the first patient treatment in 2002. The design of Tomotherapy machines resembles a serial CT scanner in which the X-ray tube is replaced by a Linac that produces a therapeutic megavoltage treatment beam. The radiation source continuously rotates while the patient is shifted through the device. The patient is irradiated slice by slice using a fan beam, whose intensity is modulated using a customized binary MLC. From a treatment planning perspective, Tomotherapy can build on the FMO concepts described in the

Fluence Map Optimization section. The leaf sequencing problem is simple compared to MLCs at conventional Linacs. In this section, we therefore focus on VMAT, which poses new challenges for treatment planning. For further details on Tomotherapy, we refer the interested reader to the review by Mackie[25] and references therein. A more extended review of treatment plan optimization approaches to VMAT is provided by Unkelbach.[26] For further information on the clinical implementation of VMAT, we suggest the review by Yu.[27]

The VMAT Treatment Planning Problem

VMAT can be thought of as a dynamic MLC technique to deliver IMRT, with the modification that the gantry does not stand still at discrete angles but continuously rotates while radiation is delivered. The dose distribution delivered by a VMAT plan is determined through three types of variables:

1. The MLC leaf trajectories, that is, the positions of the left leaves L_n and the right leaves R_n as a function of time;
2. The gantry angle $\varphi(t)$ as a function of time;
3. The dose rate $\delta(t)$ as a function of time.

In principle, the jaws, collimator, and treatment couch also could move. However, here we assume that the collimator and couch are at fixed angles and that the jaws can be positioned in a post-processing step with minor impact on the treatment plan. For dose calculation, a VMAT arc is discretized into small arc sectors. For example, a 360° arc is divided into 180 arc sectors of 2° length. For treatment planning, a dose-deposition matrix can be calculated at the center of each arc sector.

Given the trajectories for leaves, gantry, and dose rate, a VMAT plan delivers an effective fluence x_{nj}^{φ} at any gantry angle φ. The relation between effective fluence and leaf trajectories is illustrated in Figure 25.18 for a single leaf pair n. Let us for simplicity assume that the dose rate is constant over the arc sector φ. Then the effective fluence x_{nj}^{φ} is determined by the time that beamlet j is exposed by the MLC leaves. In Figure 25.18, the red-colored area enclosed by the leaf trajectories and the beamlet boundaries corresponds to the effective exposure time. This method to relate leaf positions to fluence involves the common approximation made in Figure 25.17: If at time t, a beamlet is partially exposed by the MLC leaves, the time point's contribution to the beamlet's effective fluence is proportional to the exposed fraction of the beamlet. The dose distribution is obtained by multiplying the effective fluence with the dose-deposition matrix at each arc sector.

VMAT planning aims at determining efficient trajectories that lead to high plan quality, that is, VMAT plans that only take a short amount of time to deliver. Thereby, the trajectories have to satisfy a number of machine constraints. In particular, the MLC leaves have to satisfy the

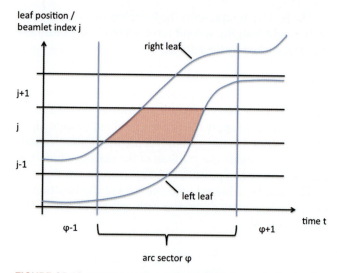

FIGURE 25.18. Relation between leaf trajectories and effective fluence in VMAT delivery. The *red area* corresponds to the exposure time of the beamlet in arc sector φ and is proportional to the beamlet's effective fluence.

maximum leaf speed constraint. In addition, the gantry speed is limited to one full rotation per minute. Limitations on the dose rate are highly machine dependent. Some Linacs allow for continuously varying dose rates, while others allow for discrete values only. All machines have a maximum dose rate.

DICOM Specification of a VMAT Plan

VMAT planning approaches differ in the way that the leaf trajectories are parameterized. The most common representation is driven by the Digital Imaging and Communications in Medicine (DICOM) specification of a treatment plan, which is used to communicate the plan between the TPS and the treatment machine control system. Using DICOM standard, the treatment plan is defined via a sequence of control points. Each control point is defined through a set of leaf positions, a gantry angle, and the total number of MU that is delivered up to that control point. Thereby, the DICOM specification gives rise to formulating VMAT planning as a DAO problem. For example, a prostate patient may be treated with a single 360° arc, which is divided into 90 arc sectors of 4° length. For VMAT planning, one control point (i.e., one aperture) is assigned to the center of each arc sector. Subsequently, the DAO methods discussed in the Direct Aperture Optimization section can be applied for plan optimization.

The DAO algorithm will return the aperture shapes and aperture intensities for each control point along the arc. It is apparent that a given aperture intensity y_{φ}, which corresponds to the number of MU delivered over the arc sector, depends on the gantry speed s_{φ}, the dose rate δ_{φ}, and the length of the arc sector Δ_{φ} and is given by

$$y_{\varphi} = \frac{\Delta_{\varphi}\,\delta_{\varphi}}{s_{\varphi}}$$

Large aperture intensities can be realized by a large dose rate or a slow gantry speed. Since the motivation for VMAT treatments is in part the reduction in treatment time, the machine controller should select the largest possible gantry speed.

In principle, a DAO algorithm applied to VMAT planning yields a deliverable plan if the gantry speed can vary between the maximum and very small values. However, without modifications, the resulting treatment plan may be inefficient regarding delivery time. As an example, we assume that we want to deliver a 360° arc in 90 seconds at constant gantry speed. Then, the gantry sweeps over each 4° arc sector in 1 second. If the maximum leaf speed of the MLC is 3 cm/s, the MLC leaves can only move by 3 cm between two neighboring control points. Otherwise, the gantry speed has to be reduced, leading to longer delivery times. Hence, VMAT planning typically aims at limiting the leaf travel between adjacent control points—in the interest of treatment time and also dose calculation accuracy. For gradient-based leaf position optimization methods, constraints on leaf travel correspond to linear constraints on the leaf positions.

Illustration of a VMAT Plan

Figure 25.19 illustrates a VMAT plan for a patient with prostate cancer treated with a single 360° arc, delivered by moving the gantry counter-clockwise from 180 to −180°. The arc is evenly divided into 90 arc sectors that are assigned one aperture each. The circle around the patient indicates the coplanar incident beam directions. The yellow bars depict the number of MU that is delivered over each arc sector. In the foreground, one of the apertures along the arc is shown.

Approaches to VMAT Plan Optimization

The VMAT implementations in commercial systems heavily build on the concepts that were previously developed for IMRT planning. Bzdusek et al.[28] suggest a three-step approach to VMAT, using all three concepts of IMRT planning.

1. In the first step, FMO is performed at discrete, equi-spaced beam angles. In practice, 15 to 20 beam angles are used.
2. In the second step, the resulting fluence maps are converted into apertures that are distributed over the corresponding arc sector. Assuming 15 beam angles are considered in the FMO step, leading to 24° arc sectors, each fluence map can be segmented into six apertures, which results in one control point every 4°. The *arc sequencing* step should aim for neighboring apertures that are similar to limit leaf travel. For that reason, most arc sequencing methods use a sliding window type decomposition, which leads to a natural ordering of the apertures.
3. In the third step, DAO methods are applied to refine the leaf positions and aperture intensities. Assuming that the first two steps yield a good starting point, local gradient-based DAO methods can be used in the third step.

Such a three-step approach is implemented in several commercial systems including the SmartArc module in Pinnacle (Philips Medical Systems), the RayArc module in RayStation (Raysearch Laboratories), and in Monaco (Elekta). Planning systems differ in the exact implementation of each step and not all details are disclosed.

The work by Otto[29] is the basis for the RapidArc module in the Eclipse planning system (Varian). This approach primarily depends on DAO using simulated annealing as described by Shepard et al.,[15] and uses a geometry-based initialization of aperture shapes. Other VMAT optimization approaches proposed in the literature are based on sliding window delivery of a fluence map over an arc sector.[30–32] An overview of VMAT planning approaches can be found in the review by Unkelbach et al.[26]

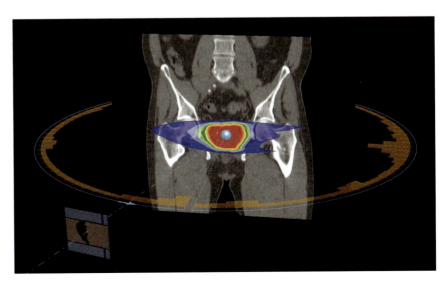

FIGURE 25.19. Illustration of a VMAT plan for a prostate cancer patient generated in RayStation 4.0. The treatment plan consists of a single 360° arc divided into 90 sectors. The dose distribution is shown on a coronal slice of the patient's CT.

AUTOMATED PLANNING AND MULTICRITERIA OPTIMIZATION

IMRT treatment planning is based on mathematical optimization, as explained earlier. To that end, clinical goals have to be formulated mathematically in terms of objective functions. In addition, IMRT treatment planning has to find a tradeoff between inherently conflicting clinical goals. The traditional planning approach consists in manually varying the different parameters in the objective function (relative objective weights w_n, maximum doses d^{max} and minimum doses d^{min}, and dose–volume parameters). This may lead to a time-consuming trial-and-error process. To address this, methods referred to as *Multi-criteria planning* and *Knowledge-based* planning are being developed to automate the planning process or make the interaction of treatment planner and planning software more efficient. A review of automated planning methods is provided by Hussein (33) and Moore (34).

Knowledge-Based Treatment Planning

Treatment planning should aim for an IMRT plan that minimizes dose to normal tissues for a given prescription dose delivered to the tumor, e.g. 60 Gy. In principle, this could be represented by setting d^{max} to zero in a quadratic penalty function. However, this would be far from achievable, and thus the obtained dose distribution would strongly depend on the weight w for this objective and would usually not represent the desired tradeoff. Setting d^{max} to 50 Gy would be closer to being achievable, but there would be no incentive to reduce dose below 50 Gy even if this was physically possible. One of the approaches to automate treatment planning consists of estimating the lowest physically achievable dose distribution in the normal tissue and defining objective functions based on that.

Simple examples are conformity objectives. In a normal tissue voxel adjacent to the planning target volume (PTV), the dose will be similar to a dose d^{pres} prescribed to the tumor. In a voxel at 1 cm distance from the PTV, it may be possible to achieve a dose that is only half the prescribed tumor dose. A quadratic penalty function of the form

$$f_R(d) = \frac{1}{N_R}\sum_{i=1}^{N_R}\left(d_i - d^{pres}\left(1 - \frac{z_i}{2}\right)\right)_+^2$$

may be applied to all normal tissue voxel in a 1 cm rim R around the PTV, where z_i is the Euclidean distance of voxel i from the PTV contour. Such objectives are available in several TPS with user-defined parameters for the steepness of the desired dose falloff.

A further step toward knowledge-based planning is to estimate the achievable steepness of the dose falloff from a database of previously delivered treatment plans. For example, for the treatment of brain metastases, one can determine the average dose in voxels that have a

certain distance from the PTV contour, which is then used as d^{max} in a quadratic penalty function for the corresponding normal tissue voxels surrounding the PTV. The achievable dose falloff also depends on the size of the brain metastasis. Small targets will allow for a steeper falloff than large targets. Therefore, one could introduce the size of the PTV as an additional parameter and train a simple regression model that predicts the dose in a normal tissue voxel depending on the distance from the PTV and the size of the PTV. This represents the basic idea of knowledge-based treatment planning in the sense of using a database of previously delivered plans for the construction of objective and constraint functions for treatment planning for a new patient.

Unlike single brain metastases, most target volumes are not spherical. For more complex-shaped targets, the dose to a voxel will not only depend on the distance but also where the voxel is located with respect to the PTV and OARs. Given a CT scan of a patient plus the contours for the target volumes, one would like to know the best achievable dose in each voxel. This problem can be approached with a variety of machine learning algorithms such as convolutional neural networks.[35,36] Similar to predicting achievable doses in individual voxels, one may also predict achievable dose–volume parameters for entire structures. For example, for head-and-neck cancer patients, one may develop regression models that predict the mean dose to the parotid gland based on several features such as the volume of the parotid gland and the volume overlap with the PTV.

Prioritized Optimization

In the previous subsection, methods to define objectives that reflect achievable goals were discussed. One of the main additional difficulties in treatment planning amounts to the handling of tradeoffs between conflicting goals. One approach to address this problem is referred to as *prioritized optimization* or *lexicographic ordering*.[37–40] It is motivated by the assumption that the clinical goals can be ranked according to their priority. For example, in the prostate cancer example shown in Figure 25.2, the main planning goal may be to deliver the prescribed dose to the target volume. The second planning goal is the sparing of the anterior rectal wall. Additional objectives are related to bladder dose and conformity but are considered lower priority.

A prioritized optimization scheme performs a sequence of IMRT optimizations. In the first step, we obtain the treatment plan that yields the best possible plan only considering the highest-ranked objective. In the prostate example, we may minimize a quadratic objective function for the target volume:

$$\text{minimize} \quad \frac{1}{N_T}\sum_{i=1}^{N_T}(d_i - d^{pres})^2$$
$$\text{subject to} \quad g_s(d) \leq c_s$$

where $g_s(d) \le c_s$ represents the hard constraints on the dose distribution. This yields an optimal value f_T^* for the quadratic objective function for the target volume. In the second step, the target objective is turned into a constraint, while minimizing the objective with the second-highest priority, which could be the EUD in the rectal wall:

$$\text{minimize} \quad \left[\frac{1}{N_R}\sum_{i=1}^{N_R}(d_i)^\alpha\right]^{\frac{1}{\alpha}}$$

$$\text{subject to} \quad g_s(d) \le c_s$$

$$\frac{1}{N_T}\sum_{i=1}^{N_T}(d_i - d^{pres})^2 \le f_T^* + \varepsilon$$

In this formulation, the EUD in the rectal wall is minimized, subject to the constraint that the target dose homogeneity deteriorates by at most ε compared to the optimally achievable value f_T^*. Solving this optimization problem yields the optimal rectal wall EUD f_R^* that is achievable under the given constraints. In the third step, the objective function for dose conformity can be minimized as the only objective, subject to the constraints that the target and rectum objectives only deteriorate by a small ε from their optimal values f_T^* and f_R^*.

Pareto-Optimality

Prioritized optimization schemes rely on a ranking of the objectives and make the assumption that higher ranked objectives are not compromised to improve lower ranked objectives. This is a potential drawback in situations where a large improvement in one objective can be achieved by only a minor degradation of a higher ranked objective, or if the ranking is unclear a priori.

For simplicity, we consider only two objectives later, for example, target dose homogeneity and rectal wall EUD in a prostate case. By varying the tolerance level ε in the prioritized optimization scheme, one can generate a sequence of treatment plans as illustrated in Figure 25.20. The plans obtained in this manner define the set of *Pareto-optimal* treatment plans that form the *Pareto surface*. A treatment plan is Pareto-optimal if it is not possible to improve the plan in one objective without worsening at least one other objective.

Interactive Pareto-Surface Navigation Methods

For radiotherapy planning, we are interested in choosing a treatment plan from the Pareto surface. However, it may depend on the patient's or physician's preference which treatment plan to pick. Especially for difficult cases such as the head-and-neck cancer example in Figure 25.3, the physician or treatment planner may want to explore the tradeoffs between different planning goals. Both tasks are straightforward in a two-dimensional tradeoff, as illustrated in Figure 25.20. In this case, the Pareto surface can be approximated with a few treatment plans that are evenly spaced on the one-dimensional Pareto surface in the clinically relevant range. The treatment planner can then choose one of these precomputed treatment plans. However, IMRT planning typically involves tradeoffs between more than two objectives (say, 5 to 10). It is apparent that in higher dimensions, the approximation of the Pareto surface is more challenging due to the curse of dimensionality. In addition, exploring the tradeoff space is nontrivial. The development of a treatment planning framework has to address two problems:

1. Developing methods to efficiently represent the Pareto surface with a small number of Pareto-optimal treatment plans, which are called database plans. One method to achieve this is the so-called Sandwich method described by Craft et al.[41]
2. Providing a graphical user interface and the underlying mathematical methods that allow the treatment planner to interactively explore and visualize the tradeoffs between conflicting planning goals.

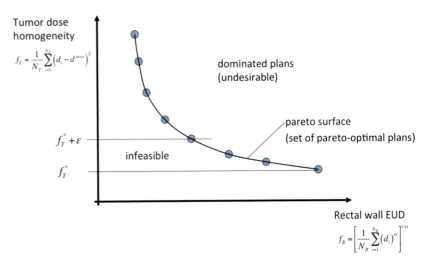

FIGURE 25.20. Schematic illustration of the Pareto surface for the tradeoff between target dose homogeneity and rectal wall EUD. All treatment plans below the Pareto surface are impossible to achieve; treatment plans above the Pareto surface are undesirable because they can be improved in one objective without worsening the second objective. Points on the Pareto surface can be generated using the constrained method, that is, by minimizing the rectal wall EUD, subject to different target homogeneity constraints (with permission reproduced from (69)).

One goal of Pareto-surface navigation methods is to allow for a continuous exploration of treatment plans. To that end, not only the discrete database plans are considered but also linear combinations of plans. We assume that a treatment plan is defined through the fluence map x. Given two treatment plans with fluence maps x^1 and x^2, we can form a convex combination of the two treatment plans by considering the averaged fluence map

$$x = qx^1 + (1 - q)x^2$$

which is obtained by averaging the beamlet intensities beamlet-by-beamlet, using a mixing parameter $q \in [0,1]$. If x^1 and x^2 are Pareto-optimal treatment plans, the convex combination of two plans is expected to be also a "good" treatment plan (although not strictly Pareto-optimal).

In a TPS, the planner has to be provided with tools to navigate in the space of convex combinations of database plans. In a practical scenario, the planner may have evaluated a current treatment plan, and would like to improve the treatment plan regarding one particular objective, say the rectum dose. The TPS has to provide a user interface to express this request. Figure 25.21 shows the Pareto-surface navigation interface in the RayStation TPS (version 4.0), distributed by RaySearch Laboratories. Each objective is associated with a slider. By moving the slider, the user can request an improvement of the treatment plan with respect to the chosen objective. In the background, the TPS translates the slider movement into a new convex combination of database plans.

Here, continuous navigation is facilitated by considering convex combination of fluence maps. It is not straightforward to extend such pareto-surface navigation methods to DAO and VMAT algorithms. The reason is, there is no natural way to average the set of apertures of two distinct treatment plans. However, multi-criteria extensions have been suggested, for example, in the context of aperture generation methods for DAO[42] as well as sliding window delivery of IMRT and VMAT.[43]

SPECIALIZED TOPICS IN TREATMENT PLANNING

Beam Angle Optimization and 4π Radiotherapy

Beam angle optimization for IMRT

IMRT planning primarily refers to determining the fluence maps of incident beam directions and their delivery with MLCs. In this context, it is assumed that the incident beam directions are given. In practice, treatment planners often use a template of standardized beam directions for a given treatment site. For example, for prostate treatments a set of nine evenly spaced coplanar beam directions may be used. For treatment sites that exhibit relatively little geometric variation across patients, such templates often provide satisfying plan quality. However, treatment planning studies suggest that some treatment sites, for example intracranial lesions, may benefit from individualized noncoplanar beam directions. Despite this benefit, current TPS have very limited support for automated selection of optimized beam directions. Typically, the treatment planner selects beam angles manually based on experience and the patient's geometry.

Approaches to automated *beam angle optimization* (BAO) in the literature can broadly be categorized into two types:

- Beam angle selection and FMO are considered jointly, which means the quality of a treatment plan is judged by an objective function $f(d)$ as used for FMO. The goal of BAO is then to simultaneously select a set of beam angles and their associated fluence maps such that the objective function f is minimized.
- Beam angle selection is separated from the FMO problem. In the first step, beam angles are selected based on simplified measures to score the quality of a beam direction. This is done mostly based on geometric features. In the second step, FMO is performed for the fixed set of beam angles.

Approaches in the first category are typically formulated as a combinatorial optimization problem. In that

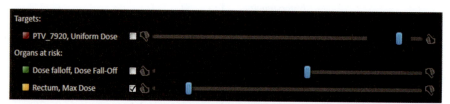

FIGURE 25.21. Graphical user interface for multi-criteria IMRT planning in the RayStation treatment planning system (version 4.0). Each objective is associated with a slider. The user can drag sliders to improve the treatment plan regarding the corresponding objective. The user request is translated into a new convex combination of database plans, and the corresponding DVH and the dose distribution are displayed. By locking sliders (visible as the check boxes to the left of each slider) the user has additional control over the navigation process. For example, by locking the slider for target dose homogeneity, the user can request that the navigation is restricted to treatment plans for which the target homogeneity is no worse than indicated by the current slider position.

setting, BAO aims to select a small subset of n beams from a larger pool of N candidate beam directions. This yields a very large number of possible beam ensembles given by the binomial coefficient. No computationally efficient algorithms exist to determine the optimal beam ensemble, and it is in part this combinatorial nature of BAO that has prevented a practical implementation in commercial TPS. Most approaches to combined FMO and beam angle selection amount to solving a large number of FMO problems for different beam ensembles. This includes stochastic search methods like simulated annealing[44] as well as integer programming methods.[45] For a review of BAO from a methodology perspective, we suggest the paper by Ehrgott et al.[8] BAO research suffers from the lack of shared patient data sets. Works that compare different BAO algorithms on a common patient data set using the same objective functions are scarce. The work by Bangert et al.[46] is an exception and compares three stochastic search methods and an iterative beam selection heuristic, observing similar performance of the investigated methods.

Trajectory Optimization for Noncoplanar Arc Therapy

In current practice, most VMAT treatments are based on one or multiple coplanar arcs selected by the treatment planner. However, similar to adding optimized noncoplanar beam angles in IMRT, some treatment sites may benefit from using noncoplanar arcs. One can distinguish two approaches to noncoplanar arc therapy.

1. A treatment plan consists of one or more arcs. For each arc, the couch is at a fixed position while the gantry rotates; however, couch angles differ between arcs. The problem then consists of selecting the couch angles as well as the gantry start and end positions for each arc. This type of treatment can be delivered clinically with current treatment machines.
2. Both the gantry and the couch rotate while radiation is delivered. In this case, the goal is to determine the sequence of gantry-couch angle pairs, which determine the trajectory of the incident beam direction. This more complex version of noncoplanar arc therapy is within the technical ability of current treatment machines but is not available in treatment mode. This method is sometimes referred to as 4π radiotherapy, where 4π alludes to the solid angle of a complete sphere around the isocenter.

The first version is similar to the BAO problem in IMRT except that the problem amounts to selecting a small set of arcs from a large pool of candidate arcs rather than selecting beams from a pool of candidate beams. Therefore, similar combinatorial optimization algorithms may be applied. Most algorithms that have been suggested for the second version can be thought of as having three components.[47-50]

1. First, a set of beneficial beam angles is determined. This component may apply any of the BAO algorithms previously developed for IMRT.

2. Second, beneficial beam angles that should be visited along the gantry-couch trajectory are connected in an efficient way in order to limit treatment time to an acceptable duration. This is similar to the well-studied traveling salesman problem.
3. The first and second components together determine the trajectories of gantry and couch. In the third step, any of the previously described VMAT algorithms can be applied to determine the MLC leaf positions along the trajectory of control points with given couch and gantry angles.

Integrating Uncertainty and Organ Motion in IMRT Planning

Setup uncertainties and organ motion in radiotherapy are traditionally handled via a safety margin approach. The clinical target volume (CTV) is expanded by a margin to form the PTV. Radiotherapy planning aims at delivering the prescribed dose to the PTV. As long as the CTV stays within the PTV, it can be assumed that the CTV receives the prescribed dose despite variations of the CTV location. IMRT planning is formulated as a mathematical optimization problem, which provides the possibility of incorporating a model of patient motion directly into the IMRT treatment planning problem, leading to so-called robust or probabilistic planning methods. In this case, the manual definition of the PTV becomes obsolete and, in some cases, better sparing of normal tissues can be achieved. An extensive review of robust radiotherapy planning is provided by Unkelbach.[51] Some of the key ideas are outlined in the following section.

Accounting for Respiratory Motion

As an example, we consider the handling of respiratory motion in the lung. Tumors located close to the diaphragm that are not attached to the chest wall may move approximately 2 cm in superior–inferior direction between exhale and inhale. Nowadays, the magnitude of motion can be assessed using four-dimensional CT, which provides snapshots of the patient geometry at 10 phases during the respiratory cycle. Traditionally, motion is accounted for using the internal target volume (ITV) concept. The ITV represents the union of the target volume defined on each individual phase. Treatment planning aims at delivering the prescribed dose to the entire ITV to ensure that the target volume receives the prescribed dose in any phase of the breathing cycle.

The dose delivered to the surrounding lung tissue can be reduced via a nonuniform dose distribution within the ITV. Rather than irradiating the ITV homogeneously with the prescription dose, the dose can be higher in regions that are covered by the tumor most of the time. Thereby, the dose can be reduced in regions that are occupied by lung tissue most of the time, and only rarely by the tumor. The dose inhomogeneities are to be designed such that the tumor eventually receives the prescribed dose while accumulating dose contributions from different phases in the respiratory cycle. IMRT optimization provides the means to formalize this idea.

We assume that a four-dimensional CT provides a CT image for each respiratory phase s. Typically, the exhale phase is used as a reference phase, which is used to define OAR voxels and tumor voxels. IMRT planning can be based on the cumulative dose that a voxel accumulates over the breathing cycle, which can be approximated as

$$d_i = \sum_s p_s d_i^s = \sum_s \left[p_s \sum_j x_j D_{ij}^s \right] = \sum_j x_j \left[\sum_s p_s D_{ij}^s \right]$$

Here, d_i^s is the dose received by voxel i in phase s, D_{ij}^s is the dose-deposition matrix in phase s, and p_s is the relative amount of time that the patient spends in phase s. The calculation of the dose-deposition matrices in phase s represents a substantial practical difficulty. D_{ij}^s represents the dose that the anatomical voxel i defined on the reference phase receives from beamlet j in another phase s. Its calculation requires not only a dose calculation on phase s but also a deformable registration of the dose distribution to the reference phase.

In the respiratory motion case, as described so far, the motion is assumed to be predictable in the sense that the cumulative dose distribution can be calculated. Although this involves practical challenges, it does not require conceptual changes in terms of the optimization method used. IMRT planning can be performed by minimizing the objective function f evaluated for the cumulative dose:

$$\text{minimize } f\left(\sum_s p_s d^s \right)$$

Handling Uncertainties

The presence of uncertainty is different from the case of predictable motion. For example, a systematic setup error implies that the dose distribution delivered to the patient is not predictable and is inherently uncertain. This requires conceptual changes regarding the formulation of the treatment planning problem.

To illustrate the handling of uncertainty, we consider systematic setup errors. As an example, we can consider six patient shifts of ±3 mm in anterior–posterior, superior–inferior, and left–right direction. For each patient shift, a separate dose-deposition matrix D_{ij}^s can be calculated, leading to different dose distributions d^s (where s is now an index for the error scenario). Since we consider a systematic error, only one of the dose distributions d_i^s can be realized, not an average. Generally, the goal is to obtain a treatment plan that is good or acceptable for any error scenario that is accounted for. There are mainly two approaches to translate this notion into mathematical terms: the *probabilistic approach* and the *worst-case approach*.

In the probabilistic approach, a probability p_s is assigned to each scenario s. For example, a higher probability can be given to the nominal scenario (i.e., no setup error occurs), and a lower probability is assigned to setup error scenarios. IMRT treatment plan optimization is performed by minimizing the expected value of the objective function f:

$$\text{minimize } \sum_s p_s f(d^s)$$

In words, the composite objective function is a weighted sum of objectives evaluated for each error scenario, where a higher weight may be given to likely scenarios, and a lower weight to less likely scenarios. While the probabilistic approach can be seen as optimizing the average plan quality, the worst-case approach aims at finding the treatment plan that is as good as possible for the worst error scenario that is accounted for. Formally, this can be formulated as

$$\text{minimize } \max_s f(d^s)$$

Methods to incorporate motion and uncertainty in IMRT planning have been investigated in the literature (see[51] for a review). For example, Bohoslavsky et al.[52] consider random and systematic setup errors for prostate treatments. Trofimov et al.[53] consider respiratory motion for lung tumors based on a four-dimensional CT. Heath et al.[54] extend this work to include uncertainties in the breathing trajectory through robust optimization techniques. While many robust optimization techniques have initially been investigated for IMRT, they have subsequently been applied to intensity-modulated proton therapy (IMPT) to handle range and setup uncertainties. In IMPT, the PTV concept is fundamentally limited[55] and cannot generally ensure robust treatment plans. The need for methods to incorporate uncertainty directly into IMPT planning has led to implementations of robust planning in the main commercial IMPT planning systems. However, RayStation (Raysearch Laboratories) is currently the only commercial planning system that also supports robust optimization for photons. This is in part because robust planning methods for IMRT reproduce PTV-like treatment plans in many situations. In contrast to IMPT, the benefit of robust planning over PTV margins is therefore more difficult to demonstrate for IMRT.

Treatment Planning for Multi-Modality Treatments

Most radiotherapy treatments are delivered using photons as the only radiation modality. However, in some situations, the combination of different types of radiation may be beneficial. This is illustrated here for photon–electron and photon–proton combinations, and the corresponding treatment planning methodology is outlined.

Combined Electron–Photon Treatments

Electrons have the advantage of a finite range, which may allow for normal tissue dose reduction distal to the target volume compared to photons. However, electrons have also significant disadvantages. First, the penetration depth of electrons is limited to a few cm for clinically available energies. Therefore, electrons can reach only superficial parts of the target volume. Second, lateral scattering of electrons leads to a broad beam penumbra and thereby suboptimal conformity of dose distributions (chapters 22 and 31). Consequently, there is a role for combined photon–electron treatments that best exploit the distinct advantages of both modalities.

In current practice, electron fields are typically delivered with add-on collimators. Hence, electron fields are forward-planned and not optimized by algorithms. However, it is possible to optimize IMRT or VMAT treatments, taking into account the dose distribution d^e delivered by electron fields. For example, to optimize the photon fluence maps x^y of IMRT fields, that deliver the residual dose to reach the prescription d^{pres}, the objective function can be minimized as follows:

$$f_T(x^y) = \frac{1}{N_T}\sum_{i=1}^{N_T}\left(d_i^e + \sum_j D_{ij}x_j^y - d_i^{pres}\right)^2$$

It has also been suggested to deliver electron fields of different energies with the MLC, which allows for intensity-modulated electron fields. To that end, electron fluence maps can be created with associated electron beamlet intensities x_k^e and a corresponding electron dose-influence matrix D_{ik}^e. In contrast to the photon fields that are typically delivered with the same energy, there is a separate electron fluence map for each available electron energy. Subsequently, electron and photon beamlet intensities x_k^e and x_j^y can be simultaneously optimized by minimizing the objective function evaluated for the cumulative dose of electrons and photons combined.[56–61]

$$\underset{x_j^y, x_k^e}{\text{minimize}}\ f\left(\sum_j D_{ij}^y x_j^y + \sum_k D_{ik}^e x_k^e\right)$$

In principle, this yields the optimal combination of electron and photon dose contributions. To obtain a deliverable treatment plan, one may apply an MLC leaf sequencing algorithm to obtain electron apertures for all energies. If this step is approximate to keep the number of electron apertures small, the resulting dose degradation can be compensated for by reoptimizing the photon fields using DAO or VMAT algorithms, taking the total dose delivered by electrons as given. Current treatment machines and planning systems do not support this optimized form of combined photon–electron therapy, arguably leading to an underutilization of electrons. However, current linacs are already capable of delivering photon MLC collimated electron beams in a research mode.[62,63]

Combined Proton–Photon Treatments

The concept of simultaneous optimization of electron and photon fluence maps can equally be applied to combinations of protons and photons, or even the combination of all three modalities.[64] A proton beamlet corresponds to a proton pencil beam characterized by its lateral position in the fluence map and its energy, which is conceptually similar to electrons except that proton beamlets are delivered with pencil beam scanning rather than an MLC (chapters 23 and 32).

Unlike electrons, protons cannot be delivered at the same machine and in the same treatment room as photons. In addition, protons are superior to photons in many situations—in contrast to electron–photon combinations

where there are complementary advantages of both modalities. Consequently, the value of jointly optimizing the combination of protons and photons for their cumulative dose distribution is not immediately apparent.

Fabiano et al.[65] described a future concept of proton therapy without gantry, which may potentially allow for a more widespread and less costly implementation of proton therapy in existing bunkers. The idea is to install a fixed proton beamline within a conventional treatment room containing a Linac for photon therapy and a treatment couch. Thereby, protons and photons may be delivered in the same fraction in the same treatment position. The rationale for combining protons and photons in this way is as follows. With only a fixed horizontal proton beamline and treatment in lying position, single-modality proton treatments may be suboptimal since proton beams are limited to a coronal plane. Thus, a photon contribution may improve conformity of the dose distribution compared to protons only. By delivering most of the dose with protons, integral dose to normal tissues can be reduced compared to photons only. This idea is illustrated in Figure 25.22 for a head-and-neck cancer patient.

Another way of combining protons and photons is to deliver a subset of n_p fractions with IMPT and the remaining n_y fractions with IMRT. However, this requires that fractionation effects are considered. For example, splitting the combined proton–photon treatment plan in Figure 25.22 into proton fractions and photon fractions would represent a substantial deviation from the current clinical paradigm of treating head-and-neck cancer with fractionated radiotherapy—because parts of the target volume would receive high doses in one fraction and low doses in others. The issue can be addressed by introducing an additional objective to enforce that both protons and photons individually deliver homogeneous doses to the target volume.[66] However, this limits the benefit of combining the two modalities.

One approach to account for fractionation effects in treatment planning consists in simultaneous optimization of IMRT fluence maps x_j^y and IMPT pencil beam intensities x_k^p based on their cumulative biologically effective dose (BED)[67,68]:

$$\underset{x_j^y, x_k^p}{\text{minimize}}\ f\left(n_\gamma\left(d_i^\gamma + \frac{(d_i^\gamma)^2}{\alpha/\beta}\right) + n_p\left(d_i^p + \frac{(d_i^p)^2}{\alpha/\beta}\right)\right)$$

$$d_i^\gamma = \sum_j D_{ij}^\gamma x_j^\gamma, \quad d_i^p = \sum_k D_{ik}^p x_k^p$$

Potential applications of this approach are described in[67,68] for patients in whom a part of the target volume is eligible for hypofractionation while other parts overlay dose-limiting OARs. In this case, IMRT and IMPT fractions may have to deliver similar doses per fraction to volumes where target and OARs overlap in order to protect the OARs through fractionation. However, in parts of the target volume that are eligible for hypofractionation, protons can deliver an overproportionate dose, which reduces the photon dose bath.

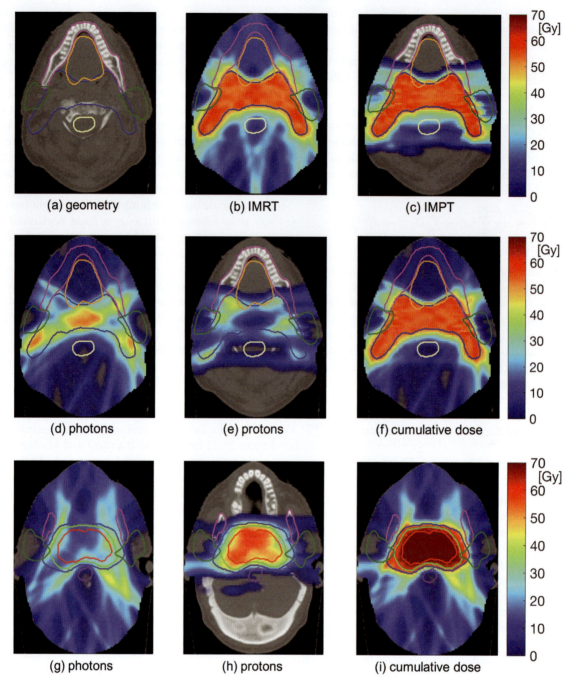

FIGURE 25.22. Illustration of a combined proton–photon treatment for a head-and-neck cancer patient on two axial slices. The treatment uses four horizontal IMPT beams with different couch angles and 19 coplanar IMRT beams. Due to the horizontal beam arrangement, protons alone yield suboptimal spar30ing of the parotid glands (green contour) (c), while photons alone feature a dose bath, e.g. in the oral cavity (orange contour) (b). The optimal combination uses both modalities. The majority of the dose to the target volume (blue contour) is delivered with protons (g–i). However, photons are used to improve conformity of the dose distribution and reduce dose to the parotid glands (d-f).

KEY POINTS

- Intensity-modulated treatment techniques are needed when treating concave target volume such as head-and-neck tumors, prostate cancer, or spinal metastasis
- IMRT planning is formulated as a mathematical optimization problem, where objective and constraint functions are defined to characterize the desired dose distribution. Optimization algorithms are used to determine the optimal incident radiation fields to come as close as possible to the desired dose distribution.
- Traditionally, IMRT planning was based on a two-step approach. First, the fluence map optimization problem (FMO) was solved to determine the optimal incident fluence. Second, leaf sequencing was applied to decompose the fluence map into a sequence of MLC apertures.
- Nowadays, most commercial treatment planning systems support DAO, where mathematical algorithms are used to directly optimize MLC leaf positions and aperture intensities.
- VMAT is an intensity-modulated technique where radiation is delivered while the gantry rotates. Planning algorithms for VMAT are based on the three modules, FMO, leaf sequencing, and DAO and combine these in different ways.
- Automated planning techniques aim to improve the IMRT planning workflow, which is often a time-consuming trial-and-error process. Knowledge-based planning techniques use a database of treatment plans to automatically define objective functions; Multi-criteria planning techniques aim to improve the handling of tradeoffs between conflicting planning objectives.
- Many further improvements to IMRT planning are being developed. This includes BAO, noncoplanar arc therapy, robust optimization for incorporating uncertainty and motion, and multi-modality treatments combining photons with electrons or protons.

REVIEW QUESTIONS

1. How is a VMAT plan communicated between the treatment planning system (TPS) and the Linac?
   A. The TPS determines the optimal MLC leaf positions as a function of time as well as the gantry speed and dose rate.
   B. The TPS generates a sequence of control points defined through leaf positions, gantry angle, and cumulative MU.
   C. The TPS optimizes incident fluence maps and the Linac control system converts these into MLC apertures.

2. What are the advantages of the sliding window leaf sequencing method?
   A. The conversion of a fluence map into a sliding window leaf trajectory can be performed analytically without the need for time-consuming optimization.
   B. Sliding window sequencing yields the smallest number of apertures.
   C. Sliding window sequencing yields the smallest total number of MU.

3. Which statement about DAO is appropriate?
   A. DAO is an important component of many VMAT planning algorithms.

   B. DAO has been developed for step-and-shoot IMRT and is therefore not applicable to dynamic delivery techniques such as VMAT.
   C. DAO eliminates the need for mathematical optimization methods in IMRT planning and hence makes IMRT planning faster and better.
   D. DAO can in part overcome the problem of dose degradation that may occur in the leaf sequencing step following FMO.
   E. The DAO problem can be solved much more reliably compared to the traditional FMO approach and therefore leads to better treatment plans.

4. What is the motivation for multi-criteria optimization (MCO)?
   A. MCO potentially provides better treatment plans because the traditional planning approach does not yield Pareto-optimal plans.
   B. Allowing the treatment planner to assess tradeoffs is one of the main motivations for MCO.
   C. In MCO, BAO or VMAT planning can more easily be integrated compared to the traditional planning approach.
   D. MCO is a way to overcome the cumbersome tweaking of objective weights, which can be time-consuming in traditional planning.

ANSWERS

1. B VMAT plans are communicated via DICOM standard, that is, via a sequence of control points. Gantry speed, dose rate, and MLC leaf trajectories are determined by the machine controller based on the sequence of apertures generated by the TPS.
2. A and C It is the main disadvantage of sliding window sequencing that it may generate a large number of small apertures.
3. A and D DAO addresses the shortcomings of the traditional fluence map plus sequencing IMRT planning approach. Although DAO was originally developed for step and shoot IMRT, it is widely used in VMAT algorithms, in parts due to the DICOM specification of a VMAT plan as a sequence of apertures.
4. B and D The main motivation for MCO is to provide methods for an efficient and interactive exploration of tradeoffs between planning goals. This may in turn translate into improved treatment plans. It is a common misconception that the traditional planning method of assigning importance weights does not yield Pareto-optimal plans. In fact, the same optimization methods are used in MCO, except that importance weights are determined by an algorithm rather than manually. Incorporating DAO or VMAT into an MCO framework is difficult and subject to ongoing research.

REFERENCES

1. Brahme A, Roos JE, Lax I. Solution of an integral equation encountered in radiation therapy. *Phys Med Biol.* 1982;27:1221–1229.
2. Zilli T. et al., ONE SHOT-single shot radiotherapy for localized prostate cancer: study protocol of a single arm, multicenter phase I/II trial. *Radiat Oncol.* 2018;13(1):166. doi:10.1186/s13014-018-1112-0
3. Bortfeld T. IMRT: a review and preview. *Phys Med Biol.* 2006;51(13):R363–R379.
4. Webb S. *Intensity-modulated Radiation Therapy.* Boca Raton, FL: CRC Press; 2001.
5. Romeijn HE, Dempsey JF, Li JG. A unifying framework for multi-criteria fluence map optimization models. *Phys Med Biol.* 2004;49(10):1991–2013.
6. Nocedal J, Wright SJ. *Numerical Optimization.* 2nd ed. New York: Springer; 2006.
7. Bertsekas DP. *Nonlinear Programming.* 2nd ed. Belmont, MA: Athena Scientific; 1999.
8. Ehrgott M, Güler C, Hamacher HW, et al. Mathematical optimization in intensity-modulated radiation therapy. *Ann Oper Res.* 2010;175:309–365.
9. Bortfeld TR, Kahler DL, Waldron TJ, et al. X-ray field compensation with multileaf collimators. *Int J Radiat Oncol Biol Phys.* 1994;28(3):723–730.
10. Engel K. A new algorithm for optimal multileaf collimator field segmentation. *Discrete Appl Math.* 2005;152(1):35–51.
11. Stein J, Bortfeld T, Dorschel B, et al. Dynamic x-ray compensation for conformal radiotherapy by means of multileaf collimation. *Radiother Oncol.* 1994;32:163–173.
12. Li R, Xing L. Bridging the gap between IMRT and VMAT: Dense angularly sampled and sparse intensity modulated radiation therapy. *Med Phys.* 2011;38(9):4912–4919.
13. Kim H, Li R, Lee R, et al. Dose optimization with first-order total-variation minimization for dense angularly sampled and sparse intensity modulated radiation therapy (DASSIM-RT). *Med Phys.* 2012;39(7):4316–4327.
14. Kamath S, Sahni S, Palta J, et al. Optimal leaf sequencing with elimination of tongue-and-groove underdosage. *Phys Med Biol.* 2004;49(3):N7–N19.
15. Shepard DM, Earl MA, Li XA, et al. Direct aperture optimization: a turnkey solution for step-and-shoot IMRT. *Med Phys.* 2002;29(6):1007–1018.
16. Li Y, Yao J, Yao D. Genetic algorithm based deliverable segments optimization for static intensity-modulated radiotherapy. *Phys Med Biol.* 2003;48:3353–3374.
17. Cotrutz C, Xing L. Segment-based dose optimization using a genetic algorithm *Phys Med Biol.* 2003;48:2987–2998.
18. Romeijn HE, Ahuja RK, Dempsey JF, et al. A column generation approach to radiation therapy treatment planning using aperture modulation. *SIAM J Optim.* 2005;15:838–862.
19. Carlsson F. Combining segment generation with direct step-and-shoot optimization in intensity-modulated radiation therapy. *Med Phys.* 2008;35:3828–3838.
20. Hardemark A, Liander H, Rehbinder H, et al. *Direct machine parameter optimization* with RayMachine in Pinnacle. RaySearch Laboratories White Paper; 2003.
21. De Gersem W, Claus F, De Wagter C, et al. Leaf position optimization for step-and-shoot IMRT. *Int J Radiat Oncol Biol Phys.* 2001;51:1371–1388.
22. Cassioli A, Unkelbach J. Aperture shape optimization for IMRT treatment planning. *Phys Med Biol.* 2013;58(2):301–318.
23. Yu CX. Intensity-modulated arc therapy with dynamic multileaf collimation: an alternative to tomotherapy. *Phys Med Biol.* 1995;40(9):1435–1449.
24. Mackie TR, Holmes T, Swerdloff S, et al. Tomotherapy: a new concept for the delivery of conformal radiotherapy. *Med Phys.* 1993;20:1709–1719.
25. Mackie TR. History of tomotherapy. *Phys Med Biol.* 2006;51:R427–R453.
26. Unkelbach J, Bortfeld T, Craft D, et al. Optimization approaches to volumetric modulated arc therapy planning. *Med Phys.* 2015;42(3):1367–1377.
27. Yu CX, Tang G. Intensity-modulated arc therapy: principles, technologies and clinical implementation. *Phys Med Biol.* 2011;56(5):R31–R54.
28. Bzdusek K. Friberger H, Eriksson K, et al. Development and evaluation of an efficient approach to volumetric arc therapy planning. *Med Phys.* 2009;36:2328–2239.
29. Otto K Volumetric modulated arc therapy: IMRT in a single gantry arc. *Med Phys.* 2008;35:310–317.
30. Craft D, McQuaid D, Wala J, et al. Multicriteria VMAT optimization. *Med Phys.* 2012;39:686–696.
31. Papp D, Unkelbach J. Direct leaf trajectory optimization for volumetric modulated arc therapy planning with sliding window delivery. *Med Phys.* 2014;41(1):011701.
32. Wang C, Luan S, Tang G, et al. Arc-modulated radiation therapy (AMRT): a single-arc form of intensity-modulated arc therapy. *Phys Med Biol.* 2008;53(22):6291–6303.

33. Hussein M, Heijmen BJM, Verellen D, et al. Automation in intensity modulated radiotherapy treatment planning—a review of recent innovations. *BJR*. 2018;91 (1092):20180270. doi: 10.1259/bjr.20180270.

34. Moore KL. Automated Radiotherapy Treatment Planning. *Semin Radiat Oncol*. 2019;29(3):209–218. doi: 10.1016/j.semradonc.2019.02.003.

35. Fan J, Wang J, Chen Z, et al. Automatic treatment planning based on three-dimensional dose distribution predicted from deep learning technique. *Med Phys*. 2019;46(1):370–381. doi: 10.1002/mp.13271.

36. Nguyen D, et al. 3D radiotherapy dose prediction on head and neck cancer patients with a hierarchically densely connected U-net deep learning architecture. *Phys Med Biol*. 2019;64(6):065020. doi: 10.1088/1361-6560/ab039b.

37. Wilkens JJ, Alaly JR, Zakarian K, et al. IMRT treatment planning based on prioritizing prescription goals. *Phys Med Biol*. 2007;52:1675–1692.

38. Jee KW, McShan DL, Fraass BA. Lexicographic ordering: intuitive multicriteria optimization for IMRT. *Phys Med Biol*. 2007;52 1845–1861.

39. Breedveld S, Storchi PRM, Voet PWJ, et al. iCycle: Integrated, multicriterial beam angle, and profile optimization for generation of coplanar and noncoplanar IMRT plans. *Med Phys*. 2012;39(2):951–963. doi: 10.1118/1.3676689.

40. Heijmen B, et al. Fully automated, multi-criterial planning for Volumetric Modulated Arc Therapy - An international multi-center validation for prostate cancer. *Radiother Oncol*. 2018;128(2):343–348. doi: 10.1016/j.radonc.2018.06.023.

41. Craft D, Halabi TF, Shih HA, et al. Approximating convex Pareto surfaces in multiobjective radiotherapy planning. *Med Phys*. 2006;33(9):3399–3407.

42. Salari E, Unkelbach J. A column-generation-based method for multi-criteria direct aperture optimization. *Physics in medicine and biology*. 2013;58(3):621–39. doi: 10.1088/0031-9155/58/3/621.

43. Craft D, Papp D, Unkelbach J. Plan averaging for multicriteria navigation of sliding window IMRT and VMAT. *Medical physics*. 2014;41(2):021709. doi: 10.1118/1.4859295.

44. Stein J, Mohan R, Wang XH. Number and orientations of beams in intensity-modulated radiation treatments. *Med Phys*. 1997;24(2):149–160.

45. Lee EK, Fox T, Crocker I. Integer programming applied to intensity-modulated radiation treatment planning. *Annals of Operations Research*. 2003;119:165–181.

46. Bangert M, Ziegenhein P, Oelfke U. Comparison of beam angle selection strategies for intracranial IMRT. *Med Phys*. 2013;40:011716.

47. Papp D, Bortfeld T, Unkelbach J. A modular approach to intensity-modulated arc therapy optimization with noncoplanar trajectories. *Physics in medicine and biology*. 2015;60(13):5179–98. doi: 10.1088/0031-9155/60/13/5179.

48. Fix MK, et al. Part 1: Optimization and evaluation of dynamic trajectory radiotherapy. *Medical physics*. 2018;45(9):4201–4212. doi: 10.1002/mp.13086.

49. Smyth G, Bamber JC, Evans PM, et al. Trajectory optimization for dynamic couch rotation during volumetric modulated arc radiotherapy. *Phys Med Biol*. 2013;58(22):8163–8177. doi: 10.1088/0031-9155/58/22/8163.

50. Lyu Q, Yu VY, Ruan D, et al. A novel optimization framework for VMAT with dynamic gantry couch rotation. *Phys Med Biol*. 2018;63(12):125013. doi: 10.1088/1361-6560/aac704.

51. Unkelbach J, et al. Robust radiotherapy planning. *Physics in Medicine & Biology*. 2018;63(22):22TR02.

52. Bohoslavsky R, Witte MG, Janssen TM, et al. Probabilistic objective functions for margin-less IMRT planning. *Phys Med Biol*. 2013;58(11):3563–3580.

53. Trofimov A, Rietzel E, Lu HM. Temporo-spatial IMRT optimization: concepts, implementation and initial results. *Phys Med Biol*. 2005;50(12):2779–2798.

54. Heath E, Unkelbach J, Oelfke U. Incorporating uncertainties in respiratory motion into 4D treatment plan optimization. *Med Phys*. 2009;36:3059–3071.

55. Unkelbach J, Bortfeld T, Martin B, et al. Reducing the sensitivity of IMPT treatment plans to setup errors and range uncertainties via probabilistic treatment planning. *Med Phys*. 2009;36(1):149–163.

56. Mueller S, et al. Part 2: Dynamic mixed beam radiotherapy (DYMBER): Photon dynamic trajectories combined with modulated electron beams. *Medical physics*. 2018;45(9):4213–4226. doi: 10.1002/mp.13085.

57. Palma BA, et al. Combined modulated electron and photon beams planned by a Monte-Carlo-based optimization procedure for accelerated partial breast irradiation. *Physics in medicine and biology*. 2012; 57(5):1191–202. doi: 10.1088/0031-9155/57/5/1191.

58. Miguez C, et al. Clinical implementation of combined modulated electron and photon beams with conventional MLC for accelerated partial breast irradiation. *Radiother Oncol*. 2017;124(1):124–129. doi: 10.1016/j.radonc.2017.06.011.

59. Xiong W, et al. Optimization of combined electron and photon beams for breast cancer. *Physics in medicine and biology*. 2004;49(10):1973–89. doi: 10.1088/0031-9155/49/10/010.

60. Renaud MA, Serban M, Seuntjens J. On mixed electron-photon radiation therapy optimization using the column generation approach. *Medical physics*. 2017;44(8):4287–4298. doi: 10.1002/mp.12338.

61. Mueller S, et al. Simultaneous optimization of photons and electrons for mixed beam radiotherapy. *Physics in medicine and biology*. 2017;62(14):5840–5860. doi: 10.1088/1361-6560/aa70c5.

62. Lloyd SAM, Gagne IM, Bazalova-Carter M, et al. Validation of Varian TrueBeam electron phase-spaces for Monte Carlo simulation of MLC-shaped fields. *Medical physics*. 2016;43(6):2894–2903. doi: 10.1118/1.4949000.

63. Mueller S, et al. Electron beam collimation with a photon MLC for standard electron treatments. *Physics in medicine and biology*. 2018;63(2):025017. doi: 10.1088/1361-6560/aa9fb6.

64. Kueng R, et al. TriB-RT: simultaneous optimization of photon, electron and proton beams. *Phys Med Biol*. 2020;66(4):045006. doi: 10.1088/1361-6560/ab936f.

65. Fabiano S, Balermpas P, Guckenberger M, et al. Combined proton–photon treatments – A new approach to proton therapy without a gantry. *Radiotherapy and Oncology*. 2020;145:81–87.

66. Gao H. Hybrid proton-photon inverse optimization with uniformity-regularized proton and photon target dose. *Phys Med Biol*. 2019;64(10):105003. doi: 10.1088/1361-6560/ab18c7.

67. Unkelbach J, Bangert M, De Amorim Bernstein K, et al. Optimization of combined proton-photon treatments. *Radiother Oncol*. 2018:128(1):133–138. doi: 10.1016/j.radonc.2017.12.031.

68. Fabiano S, Bangert M, Guckenberger M, et al. Accounting for Range Uncertainties in the Optimization of Combined Proton-Photon Treatments Via Stochastic Optimization. *Int J Radiat Oncol Biol Phys*. 2020;108(3):792–801. doi: 10.1016/j.ijrobp.2020.04.029.

69. Boyer A, Unkelbach J. Intensity-modulated radiation therapy planning. In: Brahme A, ed. *ComprehensiveBiomedical Physics*. Vol 9, Chapter 17. Amsterdam, NL: Elsevier; 2014.

26 Patient and Organ Movement

Paul J. Keall and James M. Balter

INTRODUCTION

The driving tenet of external-beam radiotherapy is the precise delivery of focal radiation doses to the target so that an effective dose can be delivered while limiting concomitant normal tissue irradiation and related toxicity risk. Technical advancements, such as intensity-modulated radiation therapy (IMRT), volumetric-modulated arc therapy (VMAT), and image-guided radiotherapy (IGRT), have provided significant gains in specifying means to provide such dose distributions. Accurate delivery, so that intended and actual doses agree, is a more complicated matter.

The problems of patient positioning and motion have been studied extensively. Although there are currently areas that need further exploration, it is possible to consider the magnitude of various uncertainties in dose delivery due to variation of patient position and organ movement and to discuss rational strategies for dealing with these uncertainties in the context of precision radiotherapy.

DESCRIPTION OF THE PROBLEM OF GEOMETRIC VARIATION

International Commission on Radiation Units and Measurements (ICRU) has addressed the relative problem of geometric variations. In reports 50[1], 62[2], and 83[3], concepts are evolved to attempt to standardize means of reporting doses. Some of the concepts presented in these reports have served as the basis for numerous investigations over the past few years and have been adopted as standards for clinical trials. A brief discussion of the key concepts as they apply to geometric variation follows.

The key structures that are delineated are the gross tumor volume (GTV) and organs at risk (OARs). The "GTV" is generally defined as the "visible" target, that is, that can be delineated from imaging or related information. The OARs are tissue structures that are dose-limiting due to risk of radiation-induced toxicity.

The next volume of interest is the clinical target volume (CTV). This target volume ideally expands about the GTV to include a reasonable expectation of the true target extent on a (static) patient model. The CTV expansion includes a reasonable expectation of the extent of disease below the sensitive range of the imaging modality.

The planning target volume (PTV) adds a margin to the CTV to account for organ motion or setup error. Margins, allowing for positioning, motion, and anatomical changes, may also be required for the OAR to arrive at the planning organ-at-risk volume (PRV). A margin provides a buffer in the delineation of tissues to account for uncertainties.[3] These structures are used for the treatment planning process.

When the patient is imaged to define the CTV and critical structures, the position is sampled. In general, this sample occurs once, specifically during the computed tomography (CT) scan for treatment planning. To obtain this sample, the patient is immobilized and positioned with typical reference marks placed on the skin and/or immobilization device at the principal axes of the CT scanner for verification of position and orientation. The sample of the patient serves as the model for treatment planning, and all subsequent targeting and density modeling are based on the information obtained during this session. With the advent of broadly available in-room imaging modalities, such as cone beam CT[4–7] and the emerging integrated Magnetic Resonance Imaging (MRI)-radiotherapy systems,[8–10] adaptive strategies which can account for inter and potentially infraction anatomic changes are emerging.

Multiple samples of patient position will form a distribution. If we set the position at the initial (treatment planning) CT scan as the "true" patient position, then a reasonable method of describing this distribution of subsequent positioning is by the translation necessary to make the patient position match that of the treatment planning CT scan. Conventionally, the average coordinate of this distribution is considered as the "systematic" error, in that it is the effective transformation that persists throughout the samples (multiple CT scans in the example given earlier or multiple patient positions over a course of treatment). The spread of sampled positions about this average coordinate represents the random setup variation. It is important to note that the average coordinate may never be sampled. An excellent overview of margins in radiotherapy is given by van Herk.[11]

MINIMIZING THE IMPACT OF SETUP VARIATIONS ON TREATMENT

Obviously, these setup variations require margins to create the PTV to ensure proper coverage of the CTV. Reducing the margins yields a smaller volume of tissue irradiated to high doses and can potentially reduce the toxicity to normal tissues. As such, significant efforts have been made to minimize the range of variations and their resulting impact on treatment.

POSITIONING SYSTEMS

A significant variety of equipment is in use to aid in repeat setup of patients. This equipment attempts to address a dual role: immobilization and localization. These dual roles are not necessarily compatible to any given piece of technology.

IMMOBILIZATION

Quite simply, the process of immobilization involves limiting or eliminating movement for the time period of imaging or treatment. The primary objective is to limit target movement, although critical normal tissue movement also needs to be considered. There is a large amount of literature on immobilization; however, as the technology is evolving, it is important to consider a number of key aspects in deciding on a technology and strategy for use of an immobilization system.

The advantage of a given immobilization method may be compromised by the complexity of use. If an immobilization system has many degrees of freedom, improper configuration of the device may lead to systematic errors in patient position or shape at treatment. Examples of complex systems are multiuse boards for fixation, in which the angles and positions of arm supports, angle of the upper thorax, shape of neck support, and other components are adjustable. These devices are very cost effective and can be used effectively, but special care must be taken to properly verify the patient configuration, including notation of all configuration parameters and documented photographs of proper setup.

Some systems (e.g., alpha cradle and vacuum loc) form directly to the person's shape. This can be beneficial in positioning, but it is important to separate comfort from immobilization. Formed immobilization that extends to distal regions from the target has been shown to be beneficial in reproducing positions.[12] However, studies have shown that simple or no immobilization, when used well, can be as effective as more complex systems.[13] Therefore, the training, use, protocols, documentation, and in-house expertise are as important as the systems themselves, and there is no substitute for qualified expert staff.

LOCALIZATION TECHNOLOGY

A wealth of technology has been applied to localization in radiation therapy. At present, the most prevalent technology includes in-room lasers, gantry-mounted kilovoltage X-ray imaging systems, and electronic portal imaging devices (EPIDs), though in-room localization is a very fast-changing field.

In-room diagnostic radiography is, in fact, a very old concept. Film-based radiographic systems have existed on linear accelerators for over 30 years.[14] Room-based digital systems have been used for radiographic[15–18] and fluoroscopic[19] procedures.

A number of different localization technologies have been used to treat radiotherapy patients. These include dedicated systems such as the real-time tracking radiotherapy system,[20] tomotherapy,[21] CyberKnife,[22] and Vero[23] linear accelerators. A number of additional localization methods have been developed based on markers, including Calypso,[24] Navotek,[25] and Raypilot.[26] Emerging localization technologies include ultrasound[27] integrated MRI-radiotherapy systems[10,28–30] and kilovoltage intrafraction monitoring (KIM).[31,32] Given the reduction in the cost of camera-based surface imaging for recreational (typically gaming) applications, surface imaging[33] is anticipated to grow rapidly in use to assist with both setup reproducibility and intratreatment patient monitoring.

STRATEGIES FOR POSITION CORRECTION

Online Correction

Generally, online position correction refers to the processes of measuring and correcting setup error at the start of each treatment fraction. This is the area in which the vast majority of technical developments have focused recently. The process of online correction includes three steps: measurement, decision, and adjustment. A fourth step (verification) may also be used.

Measurement systems include data collection and analysis. Data can be from imaging (e.g., radiographs, CT scan images, ultrasound, and video) or other markers (e.g., electromagnetic and external fiducial). Analysis is the comparison of reference image or position information to that gathered at treatment.

Decision is the process of choosing to act or not on information from measurements. It is valuable to consider that the measurement systems, as well as correction technology, are not perfect, and therefore the errors in these systems may increase errors in certain circumstances. The use of thresholds for corrections allows a trade-off between the cost (frequency of adjustment) and benefit (actual reduction of errors). Figure 26.1 shows the cost versus threshold for setup adjustment in prostate patients. Of course, the definition of cost in setup adjustment is important here.

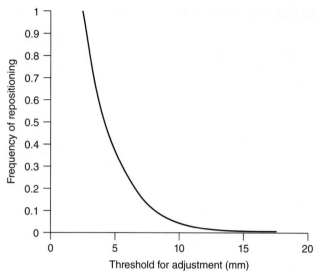

FIGURE 26.1. Cost (frequency of adjustment) versus threshold for online setup adjustment (based on 6-mm σ for pelvic patients).

If integrated, for example, real-time adaptation, the cost of correction is very low. If the setup adjustment involves a manual procedure, including treatment pause, reimaging, position shift, and verification, then the time is long and the cost is high. Automation can substantially reduce the cost of radiotherapy. Figure 26.2 shows the impact of positioning strategy on margins under assumptions of systematic error versus none.

Offline Correction

One of the earlier forms of position correction was offline correction. Studies of the dosimetric impact of setup error[34–37] demonstrate that systematic error has the largest

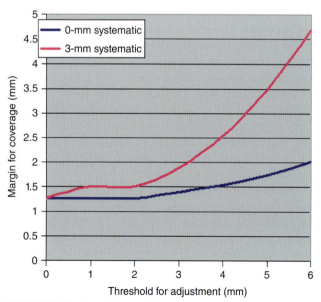

FIGURE 26.2. Benefit (margin) versus threshold for adjustment (4-mm σ setup, 1.5-mm σ measurement uncertainty, and 1.0-mm σ setup correction uncertainty).

impact on margin needed to adequately dose a target and that the geometric expansion to account for random error is generally small (less than one standard deviation). Given this observation, it can be seen that, as long as random errors are not exceedingly large, the most significant patient benefit comes from strategies that rapidly reduce the magnitude of systematic setup variation.

A number of strategies have been used to minimize systematic error. Two strategies are the shrinking action level (SAL) and no action level (NAL) methods.[38–40] In the SAL protocol, setup is verified daily for the first few fractions, and adjustments are made with tolerances that reduce in magnitude as the fractions progress. This strategy has shown promising results.

The NAL protocol has also been used. In this method, images from setup are acquired for n (typically 3 to 5) fractions. These images are analyzed offline (thereby minimizing the delay needed to analyze and act on images at the treatment unit), and the best prediction of the systematic error (typically the average position of the fractions analyzed) is corrected before the next fraction is treated. This protocol has been tested and shown to dramatically reduce systematic errors.

ADAPTIVE RADIOTHERAPY STRATEGIES

Adaptive strategies for position adjustment were first proposed by Yan et al.[41] The adaptive process extends the concept of offline and online strategies. Essentially, the patient position variability is assumed to follow a population model before patient-specific measurements. As information about that patient's variation is acquired (e.g., through multiple CT scans or daily portal images), the model of variation is refined, and predictions from this refined model can be used to adjust position and margins. The frequency of further measurement can be similarly adjusted as increased confidence in the patient variation is gained, and similarly increased frequency of measurement can be reinstated if, for example, an unexpected outlying measurement occurs during the treatment course. Such strategies form a basis for plan modification, which is a topic of active research and development in radiation therapy.

ORGAN MOVEMENT

Internal organ movement is a further, sometimes significant, factor in dose-limiting geometric uncertainty. The most studied forms of organ movement have been prostate movement and breathing-induced movement in (primarily) the thorax and abdomen. Langen and Jones have published an excellent review of the magnitude of organ movement, as studied by several investigators[42] With the availability of real-time localization systems, rich datasets of tumor position are now available.[24,43,44]

Prostate position variability is a combination of pelvic setup variation (mentioned earlier) with internal movement of the prostate within the pelvis.[45–54] The primary factors affecting prostate movement are rectal and bladder filling, with differential influence of these forces in prone versus supine patients. The vast majority of prostate patients are positioned supine, both for patient comfort and owing to observed improvements in setup variation of the pelvis. Prone positioning has been reported advantageous due to a separation of the rectal wall from the prostate, although both setup variation and (breathing-related) internal movement have been observed to increase in these patients.

Internal movement of the prostate has generally been observed in the anterior–posterior (AP) and cranial-caudal (CC) directions. Furthermore, a significant component of this movement has been correlated to rotations of the prostate about the left–right (LR) axis, with a pivot at or near the prostatic apex[7] (Fig. 26.3). The magnitude of this movement (of the prostate relative to the pelvic bones) is typically 1 cm or less in the AP and CC directions, and 5 mm in the LR direction.

Although most prostate movement studies have examined interfractional position changes (i.e., on the order of days), some measurements have been made of

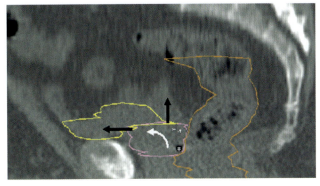

FIGURE 26.3. Graphic representation of the dominant modes of prostate movement (bladder—*yellow*, rectum—*brown*, prostate—*pink*, intraprostatic implanted markers—*white stars*). The major translation axes (*black arrows*) about the left–right and anterior–posterior axes have also been significantly attributed as rotation about the left–right axis (*white arrow*).

intrafractional movement. Breathing has been shown to impact prostate movement, most notably during deep breathing and in prone patients.[55,56] Peristalsis, gas in the rectum, and bladder filling have a more significant influence on prostate position and potentially short-term movement. The complexity of prostate motion is shown in Figure 26.4. In most cases, there is little motion, but

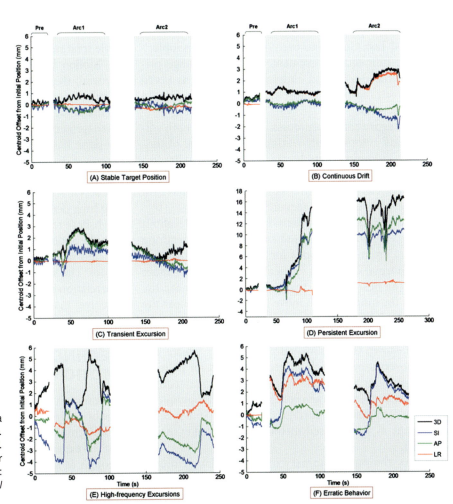

FIGURE 26.4. Prostate motion exhibits a variety of different motion characteristics. From Ng JA, Booth JT, Poulsen PR, et al. Kilovoltage intrafraction monitoring for prostate intensity modulated arc therapy: first clinical results. *Int J Radiat Oncol Biol Phys.* 2012;84(5):e655–e661.

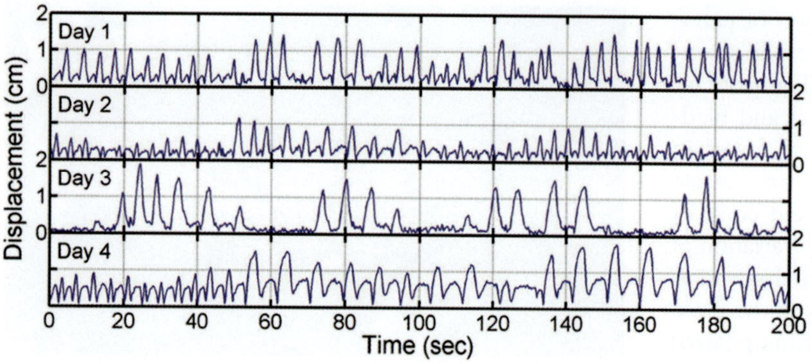

FIGURE 26.5. Calypso-measured lung tumor motion traces over 4 consecutive days. Note the large changes within and between fractions. From Shah AP, Kupelian PA, Waghorn BJ, et al. Real-time tumor tracking in the lung using an electromagnetic tracking system. *Int J Radiat Oncol Biol Phys.* 2013;86(3):477–483.

motion of over 15 mm can be observed with a variety of motion types.

Prostate movement has been addressed by attempts at reducing motion by diet, as well as immobilization through a rectal balloon. Most common attempts at managing prostate movement, however, have focused on localization. Radiographic localization and tracking of implanted markers, studied by several investigators, are routine practices, with initial localization (before subsequent movement) accuracy of better than 2 mm. Ultrasound and in-room CT scan have also been used for prostate localization before treatment.

Vast efforts have recently been focused on the problem of breathing-related movement in radiation therapy. An AAPM Task Group has been dedicated to this topic.[57] Breathing influences movement and shape change primarily in the thorax and abdomen, although, as noted earlier, breathing-related movements can also be seen in pelvic structures.

Breathing is a complex process. It is controlled both voluntarily and automatically. Various combinations of thoracic and abdominal muscles (including the diaphragm) can be used to control breathing, and therefore the shape of a patient can vary for the same estimated "phase" of breathing when evaluated sequentially.

A few general observations have been made about breathing in population studies. A typical breathing cycle lasts around 4 seconds for lung cancer patients.[58] During normal breathing, patients tend to spend more time to (or near) exhale than inhale. Tumors near the apices of the lungs tend to move less than those near the diaphragm. Although these general observations represent a reasonable population summary, numerous studies have shown that individual patients may violate any of the observations just described. The need for patient-specific motion assessment has been demonstrated.[59,60] The advent of four-dimensional (4D) CT techniques[61] provides data that help further elucidate patient-specific movement. A widely used method now in radiotherapy is 4D CT.

A very thorough summary of the ventilatory movement patterns of intrathoracic tumors was published by Seppenwoolde.[43] In addition to the observations

described earlier, this study further showed the influence of heartbeat on some tumors, especially those near the mediastinum. An observation of complex, elliptical movement ("hysteresis") was also noted in this study and observed by several other investigators. This elliptical movement can be attributed to the complex elastic properties of lung tissue, coupled with the different interactions of muscles and force between the inhale and exhale portions of the breathing cycle. Lung tumor motion induced by respiration changes with time. The daily variation of lung tumor motion traces over 4 consecutive treatment days is shown in Figure 26.5. A large variation in motion within and between fractions is observed, which challenges the ability to determine suitable treatment margins.

Motion has been studied in breast cancer as well. In general, the breast and chest wall move <1 cm within a single treatment fraction. Such small movements may not demand significant intrafraction intervention for motion management. Larger interfraction variation of chest wall position has been seen in portal imaging studies. Of note, however, is the potentially significant advantage of deep-inspiration breathhold,[62–67] not only for immobilizing the chest wall temporarily but also, more importantly, for reducing lung density and separating the heart from the medial high-dose region.

The abdomen has demonstrated significant breathing-related movement with typical amplitudes of 1.5 cm or more. The superior region of the liver moves with strong correlation to the diaphragm, while more caudal regions of the liver may move differentially due to deformation.[68–71]

TECHNOLOGY TO MANAGE ORGAN MOTION

A number of technologies have been introduced to manage breathing movement. The most common method currently employed involves using larger margins to account for the expected inter- and intrafraction motion variation, though as shown in Figure 26.5, this motion is variable and difficult to estimate. Another system involves gating (turning on and off) the treatment beam. The feedback

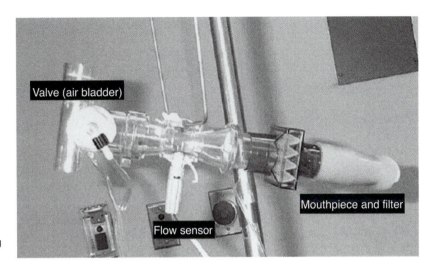

FIGURE 26.6. Components of an active breathing control (ABC) system.

for gating has generally been from the monitoring of an externally placed reflective marker on the patient's abdomen, although fluoroscopic tracking systems have also been used with tolerance windows for gating.[72] Gating involves a trade-off of residual motion versus efficiency. The narrower the acceptance range for motion, the less frequently the beam is on. The most significant concern with external gating is the relationship between the external marker position and the tumor location. While targets near the skin surface (e.g., breast) may have significant correlation with external references, other targets, especially those in the thorax, have been shown to vary in location at the same phase (as estimated from external motion) over multiple breathing cycles.[73–76]

Another commonly used technology is active breathing control (ABC) (Fig. 26.6). First introduced by Wong,[77] this concept involves using a system that monitors breathing and occludes breath at a given phase of the breathing cycle and/or volume of air relative to exhalation. Various studies have shown excellent short-term reproducibility of target position in the thorax and abdomen using this technology.[15,78–82] Decreased accuracy in long-term reproducibility suggests the advantage of image-guided localization at the start of a treatment fraction, in combination with ABC-aided ventilatory immobilization.

More complex technology for managing breathing movement involves tracking. In this process, an estimate of the target's trajectory is used to adjust the couch, linear accelerator orientation, or field aperture. The available systems to perform real-time adaptation, along with the year they were first implemented clinically, are shown in Figure 26.7. Of the four systems shown, the most widely available are the multileaf collimator (MLC) and couch. The MLC is the lightest and as each leaf can be controlled

Robotic linac head
CyberKnife
Synchrony, Accuray
Clinical 2004

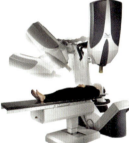

Gimbaled linac
Vero/Mitsubishi
Clinical 2011

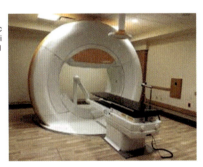

MLC adaptation
Clinical 2013
Smallest
Lightest
6 DoF
Deformation

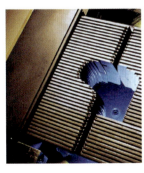

Robotic couch
Clinical ?

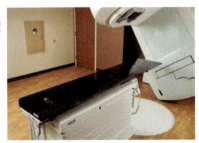

FIGURE 26.7. The four systems investigated to realign the radiation beam and tumor due to intrafraction motion.

individually, higher order corrections such as rotation[83] and deformation[84] can be performed.

Some breathing management systems rely on the relationship of a surrogate to estimate tumor position at any given time or patient state. Various surrogates have been employed, including implanted fiducial markers, external fiducials (usually tracked in real time by video systems), external surface monitoring, and lung volume and airflow. The relationship between surrogate state/position and tumor position may be variable, and the influence of this variability on geometric accuracy of target position prediction should determine the extent of additional verification needed or residual error expected. Two commercial systems, the CyberKnife and Vero, currently employ a hybrid approach to tracking, in which implanted radiopaque fiducials are periodically localized using biplanar radiographs, and their position is used to update a correlation with the constantly monitored external surface of the patient.

SUMMARY

The influence of geometric variations in radiation therapy increases in significance with the conformality of the planned treatment. Our understanding of motion and its effects is growing. Interventions to better reduce these movement-related uncertainties are evolving rapidly. A fundamental understanding of the limitations of any given monitoring or tracking system, coupled with the impact of uncertainty in target position on dose, will yield efficient strategies for implementing technology to limit the impact of patient and organ movement on treatment outcome.

KEY POINTS

- Organ structure nomenclature has been standardized by the ICRU in reports 50, 62, and 83. The visible GTV may be expanded into a CTV to include microscopic disease, and further expanded into a PTV, to account for organ motion or setup error. Similarly, the OARs may be expanded to planning organs at risk (PRVs) to account for patient position and organ motion.

- Patient positioning systems are designed to immobilize the patient and/or improve the localization of the treatment site. Immobilization devices should limit target movement but not so complex that systematic setup errors could be introduced. A number of in-room localization technologies have been introduced in the past few years to assist with setup reproducibility and intrafractional target monitoring.

- Patient positioning corrections can be made online or offline. Online corrections include measurement, decision as to whether to shift, adjustment, and in some cases verification. Offline corrections are important in minimizing systematic errors, which have a significant impact on the margin necessary for adequate treatments. Adaptive strategies can serve to modify the aforementioned corrections, based on the variations observed with individual patients.

- Organ motion within the patient represents another source of positional uncertainty. Several site-specific studies of interfractional organ motion have been performed, many of which have focused on the prostate gland. Intrafractional organ motion may also be significant, especially for diseases within the lung, which has motivated the development of a number of techniques to manage treatment of this site.

REVIEW QUESTIONS

1. Which of the following nomenclature did ICRU 50 first introduce?
   - **A.** Gross treatment volume (GTV)
   - **B.** Off-axis ratios (OARs)
   - **C.** Clinical target volume (CTV)
   - **D.** Normal tissue complication probability (NTCP)

2. Which of the following is/are used to immobilize patients?
   - **A.** Alpha cradle and/or vacuum loc
   - **B.** Calypso
   - **C.** Electronic portal imaging systems
   - **D.** ABC systems

3. Which two strategies are adopted to perform offline corrections to minimize systematic error?
   A. Inter- and intrafractional motion management
   B. Adaptive and nonadaptive margin adjustments
   C. System gating and/or tracking
   D. Shrinking action level and no action level

4. What is typically the magnitude of the interfractional movement of the prostate relative to the pelvic bones?
   A. 1 cm or less in the anterior–posterior direction
   B. 1 to 2 cm in the cranial–caudal direction
   C. 5 mm or less in the left–right direction
   D. <5 mm in any direction

5. The following technologies was/were developed to help manage breathing movement:
   A. Ultrasound
   B. In-room CT
   C. Treatment beam gating
   D. Tracking using multileaf collimator

ANSWERS

1. C
2. A
3. D
4. A and C
5. C and D

REFERENCES

1. International Commission on Radiation Units and Measurements. Prescribing, recording and reporting photon beam therapy. ICRU Report 50. 1993.
2. International Commission on Radiation Units and Measurements. Prescribing, recording and reporting photon beam therapy (Supplement to ICRU Report 50). ICRU Report 62. 1999.
3. International Commission on Radiation Units and Measurements. Prescribing, recording, and reporting photon-beam intensity-modulated radiation therapy (IMRT). ICRU Report 83. 2010.
4. Jaffray DA, Siewerdsen JH, Wong JW, et al. Flat-panel cone-beam computed tomography for image-guided radiation therapy. Int J Radiat Oncol Biol Phys. 2002;53(5):1337–1349.
5. Cho PS, Johnson RH, Griffin TW. Cone-beam CT for radiotherapy applications. Phys Med Biol. 1995;40(11):1863–1883.
6. Pouliot J, Bani-Hashemi A, Chen J, et al. Low-dose megavoltage cone-beam CT for radiation therapy. Int J Radiat Oncol Biol Phys. 2005;61(2):552–560.
7. Smitsmans MH, de Bois J, Sonke JJ, et al. Automatic prostate localization on cone-beam CT scans for high precision image-guided radiotherapy. Int J Radiat Oncol Biol Phys. 2005;63(4):975–984.
8. Fallone BG. The rotating biplanar linac–magnetic resonance imaging system. Semin Radiat Oncol. 2014;24:200–202.
9. Lagendijk JJ, Raaymakers BW, van Vulpen M. The magnetic resonance imaging–linac system. Semin Radiat Oncol. 2014;24:207–209.
10. Mutic S, Dempsey JF. The ViewRay system: magnetic resonance-guided and controlled radiotherapy. Semin Radiat Oncol. 2014;24:196–199.
11. Van Herk M. Errors and margins in radiotherapy. Semin Radiat Oncol. 2004;14:52–64.
12. Bentel GC, Marks LB, Sherouse GW, et al. The effectiveness of immobilization during prostate irradiation. Int J Radiat Oncol Biol Phys. 1995;31(1):143–148.
13. Song PY, Washington M, Vaida F, et al. A comparison of four patient immobilization devices in the treatment of prostate cancer patients with three dimensional conformal radiotherapy. Int J Radiat Oncol Biol Phys. 1996;34(1):213–219.
14. Biggs PJ, Goitein M, Russell MD. A diagnostic X ray field verification device for a 10 MV linear accelerator. Int J Radiat Oncol Biol Phys. 1985;11(3):635–643.
15. Balter JM, Brock KK, Litzenberg DW, et al. Daily targeting of intrahepatic tumors for radiotherapy. Int J Radiat Oncol Biol Phys. 2002;52(1):266–271.
16. Litzenberg D, Dawson LA, Sandler H, et al. Daily prostate targeting using implanted radiopaque markers. Int J Radiat Oncol Biol Phys. 2002;52(3):699–703.
17. Schewe JE, Lam KL, Balter JM, et al. A room-based diagnostic imaging system for measurement of patient setup. Med Phys. 1998;25(12):2385–2387.
18. Murphy MJ. An automatic six-degree-of-freedom image registration algorithm for image-guided frameless stereotaxic radiosurgery. Med Phys. 1997;24(6):857–866.
19. Shirato H, Shimizu S, Kitamura K, et al. Four-dimensional treatment planning and fluoroscopic real-time tumor tracking radiotherapy for moving tumor. Int J Radiat Oncol Biol Phys. 2000;48(2):435–442.
20. Shimizu S, Shirato H, Kitamura K, et al. Use of an implanted marker and real-time tracking of the marker for the positioning of prostate and bladder cancers. Int J Radiat Oncol Biol Phys. 2000;48(5):1591–1597.
21. Mackie TR, Holmes T, Swerdloff S, et al. Tomotherapy: a new concept for the delivery of dynamic conformal radiotherapy. Med Phys. 1993;20(6):1709–1719.
22. King CR, Brooks JD, Gill H, et al. Stereotactic body radiotherapy for localized prostate cancer: interim results of a prospective phase II clinical trial. Int J Radiat Oncol Biol Phys. 2009;73(4):1043–1048.
23. Kamino Y, Takayama K, Kokubo M, et al. Development of a four-dimensional image-guided radiotherapy system with a gimbaled X-ray head. Int J Radiat Oncol Biol Phys. 2006;66(1):271–278.
24. Kupelian P, Willoughby T, Mahadevan A, et al. Multi-institutional clinical experience with the Calypso System in localization and continuous, real-time monitoring of the prostate gland during external radiotherapy. Int J Rad Onc Biol Phys. 2007;67(4):1088–1098.
25. de Kruijf WJ, Verstraete J, Neustadter D, et al. Patient positioning based on a radioactive tracer implanted in patients with localized prostate cancer: a performance and safety evaluation. Int J Radiat Oncol Biol Phys. 2013;85(2):555–560.
26. Castellanos E, Ericsson MH, Sorcini B, et al. RayPilot – Electromagnetic real-time positioning in radiotherapy of prostate cancer – Initial clinical results. Radiother Oncol. 2012;103, Supplement 1(0):S433.
27. Ballhausen H, Li M, Hegemann NS, et al. Intra-fraction motion of the prostate is a random walk. Phys Med Biol. 2015;60(2):549–563.
28. Fallone B. Murray B, Rathee S, et al. First MR images obtained during megavoltage photon irradiation from a prototype integrated linac-MR system. Med Phys. 2009;36(6):2084–2088.
29. Raaymakers BW, Lagendijk JJ, Overweg J, et al. Integrating a 1.5 T MRI scanner with a 6 MV accelerator: proof of concept. Phys Med Biol. 2009;54(12):N229–N237.

30. Keall PJ, Barton M, Crozier S, et al. The Australian magnetic resonance imaging–linac program. *Semin Radiat Oncol.* 2014;24:203–206.

31. Poulsen PR, Cho B, Langen K, et al. Three-dimensional prostate position estimation with a single x-ray imager utilizing the spatial probability density. *Phys Med Biol.* 2008;53(16):4331–4353.

32. Keall PJ, Aun Ng J, O'Brien R, et al. The first clinical treatment with kilovoltage intrafraction monitoring (KIM): a real-time image guidance method. *Med Phys.* 2015;42(1):354–358.

33. Bert C, Metheany KG, Doppke K, et al. A phantom evaluation of a stereo-vision surface imaging system for radiotherapy patient setup. *Med Phys.* 2005;32(9):2753–2762.

34. Bel A, van Herk M, Lebesque JV. Target margins for random geometrical treatment uncertainties in conformal radiotherapy. *Med Phys.* 1996;23(9):1537–1545.

35. Remeijer P, Rasch C, Lebesque JV, et al. Margins for translational and rotational uncertainties: a probability-based approach. *Int J Radiat Oncol Biol Phys.* 2002;53(2):464–474.

36. van Herk M, Remeijer P, Lebesque JV. Inclusion of geometric uncertainties in treatment plan evaluation. *Int J Radiat Oncol Biol Phys.* 2002;52(5):1407–1422.

37. Balter JM, Brock KK, Lam KL, et al. Evaluating the influence of setup uncertainties on treatment planning for focal liver tumors. *Int J Radiat Oncol Biol Phys.* 2005;63(2):610–614.

38. de Boer HC, van Sörnsen de Koste JR, Creutzberg CL, et al. Electronic portal image assisted reduction of systematic set-up errors in head and neck irradiation. *Radiother Oncol.* 2001;61(3):299–308.

39. de Boer HC, Heijmen BJ. A protocol for the reduction of systematic patient setup errors with minimal portal imaging workload. *Int J Radiat Oncol Biol Phys.* 2001;50(5):1350–1365.

40. van Lin EN, Nijenhuis E, Huizenga H, et al. Effectiveness of couch height–based patient set-up and an off-line correction protocol in prostate cancer radiotherapy. *Int J Radiat Oncol Biol Phys.* 2001;50(2):569–577.

41. Yan D, Vicini F, Wong J, et al. Adaptive radiation therapy. *Phys Med Biol.* 1997;42(1):123–132.

42. Langen KM, Jones DT. Organ motion and its management. *Int J Radiat Oncol Biol Phys.* 2001;50(1):265–278.

43. Seppenwoolde Y, Shirato H, Kitamura K, et al. Precise and real-time measurement of 3D tumor motion in lung due to breathing and heartbeat, measured during radiotherapy. *Int J Radiat Oncol Biol Phys.* 2002;53(4):822–834.

44. Suh Y, Dieterich S, Cho B, et al. An analysis of thoracic and abdominal tumour motion for stereotactic body radiotherapy patients. *Phys Med Biol.* 2008;53(13):3623–3640.

45. Balter JM, Sandler HM, Lam K, et al. Measurement of prostate movement over the course of routine radiotherapy using implanted markers. *Int J Radiat Oncol Biol Phys.* 1995;31(1):113–118.

46. Beard CJ, Kijewski P, Bussière M, et al. Analysis of prostate and seminal vesicle motion: implications for treatment planning. *Int J Radiat Oncol Biol Phys.* 1996;34(2):451–458.

47. Booth JT, Zavgorodni SF. Set-up error & organ motion uncertainty: a Review. *Australas Phys Eng Sci Med.* 1999;22(2):29–47.

48. Crook JM, Raymond Y, Salhani D, et al. Prostate motion during standard radiotherapy as assessed by fiducial markers. *Radiother Oncol.* 1995;37(1):35–42.

49. Dawson LA, Mah K, Franssen E, et al. Target position variability throughout prostate radiotherapy. *Int J Radiat Oncol Biol Phys.* 1998;42(5):1155–1161.

50. Melian E, Mageras GS, Fuks Z, et al. Variation in prostate position quantitation and implications for three-dimensional conformal treatment planning. *Int J Radiat Oncol Biol Phys.* 1997;38(1):73–81.

51. Padhani AR, Khoo VS, Suckling J, et al. Evaluating the effect of rectal distension and rectal movement on prostate gland position using cine MRI. *Int J Radiat Oncol Biol Phys.* 1999;44(3):525–533.

52. Roeske JC, Forman JD, Mesina CF, et al. Evaluation of changes in the size and location of the prostate, seminal vesicles, bladder, and rectum during a course of external beam radiation therapy. *Int J Radiat Oncol Biol Phys.* 1995;33(5):1321–1329.

53. van Herk M, Bruce A, Kroes AP, et al. Quantification of organ motion during conformal radiotherapy of the prostate by three dimensional image registration. *Int J Radiat Oncol Biol Phys.* 1995;33(5):1311–1320.

54. Zimmermann FB, Molls M. Influence of organ and patient movements on the target volume in radiotherapy of prostatic carcinoma. *Strahlenther Onkol.* 1997;173(3):172–173.

55. Dawson LA, Litzenberg DW, Brock KK, et al. A comparison of ventilatory prostate movement in four treatment positions. *Int J Radiat Oncol Biol Phys.* 2000;48(2):319–323.

56. Malone S, Crook JM, Kendal WS. Respiratory-induced prostate motion: quantification and characterization. *Int J Radiat Oncol Biol Phys.* 2000;48(1):105–109.

57. Keall PJ, Mageras GS, Balter JM, et al. The management of respiratory motion in radiation oncology report of AAPM Task Group 76. *Med Phys.* 2006;33(10):3874–3900.

58. George R, Vedam SS, Chung TD, et al. The application of the sinusoidal model to lung cancer patient respiratory motion. *Med Phys.* 2005;32(9):2850–2861.

59. Allen AM, Siracuse KM, Hayman JA, et al. Evaluation of the influence of breathing on the movement and modeling of lung tumors. *Int J Radiat Oncol Biol Phys.* 2004;58(4):1251–1257.

60. Stevens CW, Munden RF, Forster KM, et al. Respiratory-driven lung tumor motion is independent of tumor size, tumor location, and pulmonary function. *Int J Radiat Oncol Biol Phys.* 2001;51(1):62–68.

61. Rietzel E, Pan T, Chen GT. Four-dimensional computed tomography: image formation and clinical protocol. *Med Phys.* 2005;32(4):874–889.

62. Barnes EA, Murray BR, Robinson DM, et al. Dosimetric evaluation of lung tumor immobilization using breath hold at deep inspiration. *Int J Radiat Oncol Biol Phys.* 2001. 50(4):1091–1098.

63. Chen MH, Cash EP, Danias PG, et al. Respiratory maneuvers decrease irradiated cardiac volume in patients with left-sided breast cancer. *J Cardiovasc Magn Reson.* 2002;4(2):265–271.

64. Hanley J, Debois MM, Mah D, et al. Deep inspiration breath-hold technique for lung tumors: the potential value of target immobilization and reduced lung density in dose escalation. *Int J Radiat Oncol Biol Phys.* 1999;45(3):603–611.

65. Rosenzweig KE, Hanley J, Mah D, et al. The deep inspiration breath-hold technique in the treatment of inoperable non–small-cell lung cancer. *Int J Radiat Oncol Biol Phys.* 2000;48(1):81–87.

66. Sixel KE, Aznar MC, Ung YC. Deep inspiration breath hold to reduce irradiated heart volume in breast cancer patients. *Int J Radiat Oncol Biol Phys.* 2001. 49(1):199–204.

67. Stromberg JS, Sharpe MB, Kim LH, et al. Active breathing control (ABC) for Hodgkin's disease: reduction in normal tissue irradiation with deep inspiration and implications for treatment. *Int J Radiat Oncol Biol Phys.* 2000;48(3):797–806.

68. Brock KK, Hollister SJ, Dawson LA, et al. Technical note: creating a four-dimensional model of the liver using finite element analysis. *Med Phys.* 2002;29(7):1403–1405.

69. Brock KM, Balter JM, Dawson LA, et al. Automated generation of a four-dimensional model of the liver using warping and mutual information. *Med Phys.* 2003;30(6):1128–1133.

70. Brock KK, Sharpe MB, Dawson LA, et al. Accuracy of finite element model-based multi-organ deformable image registration. *Med Phys.* 2005;32(6):1647–1659.

71. Brock KK, McShan DL, Ten Haken RK, et al. Inclusion of organ deformation in dose calculations. *Med Phys.* 2003;30(3):290–295.

72. Shirato H, Shimizu S, Kunieda T, et al. Physical aspects of a real-time tumor-tracking system for gated radiotherapy. *Int J Radiat Oncol Biol Phys.* 2000;48(4):1187–1195.

73. Berbeco RI, Nishioka S, Shirato H, et al. Residual motion of lung tumours in gated radiotherapy with external respiratory surrogates. *Phys Med Biol.* 2005;50(16):3655–3667.

74. Jin JY, Yin FF. Time delay measurement for linac based treatment delivery in synchronized respiratory gating radiotherapy. *Med Phys.* 2005;32(5):1293–1296.

75. Ozhasoglu C, Murphy MJ. Issues in respiratory motion compensation during external-beam radiotherapy. *Int J Radiat Oncol Biol Phys.* 2002;52(5):1389–1399.

76. Vedam SS, Keall PJ, Kini VR, et al. Determining parameters for respiration-gated radiotherapy. *Med Phys.* 2001;28(10):2139–2146.

77. Wong JW, Sharpe MB, Jaffray DA, et al. The use of active breathing control (ABC) to reduce margin for breathing motion. *Int J Radiat Oncol Biol Phys.* 1999;44(4):911–919.

78. Cheung PC, Sixel KE, Tirona R, et al. Reproducibility of lung tumor position and reduction of lung mass within the planning target volume using active breathing control (ABC). *Int J Radiat Oncol Biol Phys.* 2003;57(5):1437–1442.

79. Dawson LA, Brock KK, Kazanjian S, et al. The reproducibility of organ position using active breathing control (ABC) during liver radiotherapy. *Int J Radiat Oncol Biol Phys.* 2001;51(5):1410–1421.

80. Dawson LA. Eccles C, Bissonnette JP, et al. Accuracy of daily image guidance for hypofractionated liver radiotherapy with active breathing control. *Int J Radiat Oncol Biol Phys.* 2005;62(4):1247–1252.

81. Remouchamps VM, Letts N, Vicini FA, et al. Initial clinical experience with moderate deep-inspiration breath hold using an active breathing control device in the treatment of patients with left-sided breast cancer using external beam radiation therapy. *Int J Radiat Oncol Biol Phys.* 2003;56(3):704–715.

82. Sarrut D, Boldea V, Ayadi M, et al. Nonrigid registration method to assess reproducibility of breath-holding with ABC in lung cancer. *Int J Radiat Oncol Biol Phys.* 2005;61(2):594–607.

83. Wu J, Ruan D, Cho B, et al. Electromagnetic detection and real-time DMLC adaptation to target rotation during radiotherapy. *Int J Radiat Oncol Biol Phys.* 2012;82(3):e545–e553.

84. Ge Y, O'Brien RT, Shieh CC, et al. Toward the development of intrafraction tumor deformation tracking using a dynamic multi-leaf collimator. *Med Phys.* 2014;41(6):061703.

27 Linac Radiosurgery: System Requirements, Procedures, and Testing

Frank J. Bova, William A. Friedman, and Jonathan G. Li

The goal of teletherapy planning has always been to concentrate a radiation dose over the target tissues while minimizing dose to all normal tissues. It did not take long for clinicians to realize that a very strong tool for such dose optimization was the use of multiple beams with separate entrance and exit pathways, beams that only intersected over the targeted tissues. This simple and effective geometric principle has been leveraged in megavoltage teletherapy throughout the body.

The number of unique beam paths is often limited by the size of the target volume, the anatomic target location and the geometry of the teletherapy equipment. For a vast majority of targets a full 360degrees of access around the cephalo-caudal axis is available for unique beam entrance-exit pathways. Due to patient geometry and the design of most teletherapy units, available beam trajectories along the remaining two anatomic axes are limited. However, these geometric and anatomic constraints are greatly reduced for most intracranial targets. For these targets a full hemisphere, 2 pi radians, of potential entrance space can be accessed. This broadened geometric space allows for a larger number of unique beam pathways to be leveraged for the purpose of dose concentration. The increase in the number of beams results in a dose distribution with gradients over the entire surface of the target volume that are significantly steeper than can be obtained elsewhere in the body.

Lars Leksell realized that the spreading of entrance doses across a hemisphere would produce dose distributions with sufficient concentration as to allow for a safe and effective single fraction therapy to be administered. A significant body of literature now exists that supports the safety and efficacy of radiosurgery in treating malignant and benign tissues. This chapter will discuss the dose characteristics, that is, target conformality and dose gradients, that are responsible for these published clinical results. It will also examine the required end to end accuracy that these distributions demand to avoid underdosing target tissues or overdosing normal structures. While plan optimization parameters will be discussed, the algorithms used to optimize the dose distributions will not. This is simply because, while the criteria for spatial dose requirements have been relatively constant, the development of these algorithms continues to be very fluid, leaving any detailed discussion dated prior to publication.

Over the past four decades, the practice of radiosurgery has undergone a broadening in the underlying algorithms used for localization, planning, and treatment delivery. These changes have come about for both linear accelerator and GammaKnife-based treatments. For linear accelerator-based systems treatment delivery, new approaches leveraging multileaf collimation have aimed at decreasing the overall time required to deliver the optimized dose plan. Immobilization and localization approaches aimed at replacing neurosurgical-specific equipment, such as stereotactic headframes, with methods familiar in radiation oncology, such as thermoplastic immobilization and orthogonal and conebeam-based treatment alignment procedures, have continued to gain acceptance. For GammaKnife treatments, dynamic intra-treatment movement of the patient has been introduced as well as conebeam verification. There are no hard-and-fast rules as to when some of these new techniques will provide a clinical advantage or when they will require increased precision of the delivery system. The number of targets and their size and location, both absolute and relative, the prescribed dose, and pathology all place requirements on planning and delivery. As these new techniques are applied to an ever-increasing array of clinical targets, the radiosurgeon must ensure that each new innovation maintains the accuracy and precision responsible for radiosurgery's established clinical results.

Chapters on radiosurgery traditionally begin by exploring the background of Radiosurgery followed by a discussion of the special parameters that are considered responsible for the clinical success of this treatment paradigm. We often forget that these treatments were not derived from a perfectly understood set of interactions. The relationship between effective doses and complications are reported observations from carefully controlled clinical trials. While underlying principles are understood, the accurate prediction of clinical effect based on first principles remains beyond our understanding. It must also be remembered that a radiosurgery practice consists of not only treatments for malignant disease but for significant number of benign targets. The radiosurgeon needs to be particularly careful not to accept that therapeutic equivalence based on short-term results, a few months or a year, will be representative of the results of safety and efficacy when measured in decades.

HISTORIC DEVELOPMENT OF RADIOSURGICAL PRINCIPLES

In the mid-20th century, the advent of cobalt teletherapy units and, subsequently, linear accelerators helped radiation therapy play an increasingly important role in cancer treatment. During this time, external beam radiation therapy relied heavily upon the fact that normal cells are better than cancer cells at repairing sub-lethal radiation damage. Typically, a course of therapy would be divided into small fractions, each delivering a sub-lethal dose of radiation to a specified target volume. In the time between therapeutic fractions, the normal tissues would recover more quickly than the cancerous cells, and by the end of a course of treatment, the targeted cancer cells would have amassed significantly more radiation damage (see Fig. 27.1).

Reliance upon this delivery technique was necessary for two reasons. First, in the mid-20th century, neither computed tomography (CT) nor magnetic resonance imaging (MRI) was yet available, limiting the clinician's ability to map out and plan three-dimensional (3D) target volumes for conformal radiation planning. Second, it is not unusual for the relative ratio of normal tissue cells to cancer cells to vary considerably through the volume requiring treatment. Some regions of a target volume may have a high concentration of tumor cells, while other regions only contain microscopic levels of disease. To accommodate for this variation of target cell concentration it was necessary to develop a therapeutic tool that resulted in more cancer cell death relative to normal tissue cell death for a given course of therapy. Dose fractionation provided such a tool.

Radiosurgery, defined as a single fraction, stereotactically targeted, radiation therapy, proposed a paradigm shift in the art of radiation delivery. This new approach would not attempt to leverage differential repair of sublethal cell damage, but instead deliver a highly concentrated dose of radiation to the targeted volume. The very steep dose gradient would be the mechanism for protecting normal tissues. The result of this paradigm change would allow an unprecedented escalation in dose, allowing for safe and effective single fraction radiation delivery.

The term "radiosurgery" was initially conceived by a Swedish neurosurgeon, Lars Leksell.[1,2] Leksell's first attempt at a delivery scheme was to provide such a concentrated radiation dose by attaching an X-ray tube onto an arc-centered stereotactic frame system. This placed the X-ray source to be moved along two orthogonal arcs (see Fig. 27.2). When used for routine neurosurgical procedures, the arc-centered stereotactic frame was fitted with a probe holder. The probe holder could then be moved along either arc while maintaining a trajectory that pointed to the center of the arcing planes. Mounting an X-ray tube in place of the probe holder provided a method of delivering a radiation beam that would also remain focused at the center of the arcing planes. The center of the arcing planes would be translated to coincide with the center of the target volume. This provided a means for delivering multiple non-coplanar beams, each with a separate entrance and exit pathway, that all intersected over the target. The two arcs provided the ability to deliver beams from an entire hemisphere, 2 pi radians. While Leksell had developed a technique for producing focused, concentrated, dose distributions, his ability to define the target volume was based upon state of the art orthogonal X-rays, which, as will be discussed later, is insufficient to define irregular 3D structures.

In the 1950s, while teletherapy was still in its infancy, a transition from radiation delivery with orthovoltage X-ray tubes and teleradium systems to cobalt-based units was underway. Leksell was familiar with the state-of-the-art teletherapy radium devices. Due to limited specific

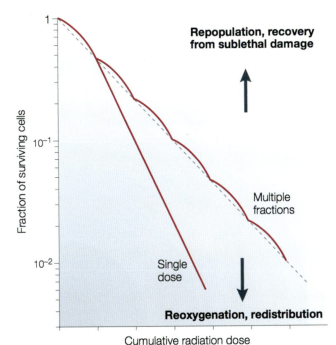

FIGURE 27.1. Figure shows the effects of a single dose therapy vs. that of a fractionated therapy. After each fraction cells repair sublethal damage before the next fraction is administered.

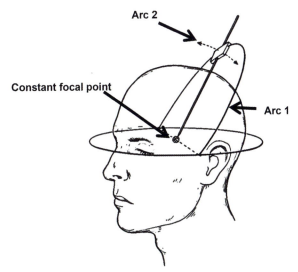

FIGURE 27.2. The two bicentered arc geometry with the focal point shown at the center of two arcs. The user can move a probe or x-ray tube along each of the arcs maintaining a trajectory that will always go through the focal point.

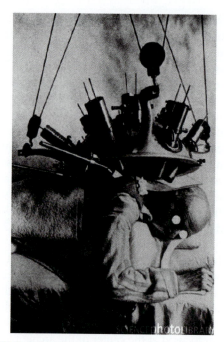

FIGURE 27.3. Tele-radium device for increasing doserate over a target volume. Multiple sources are focused at a distance providing unique entry and exit pathways while only overlapping at the target volume.

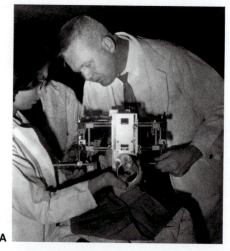

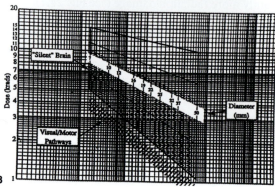

FIGURE 27.4. A: Kjellberg, proton therapy procedure. **B:** Adaption of the Kjellberg's proton therapy data relating volume to complication demonstrating that as the treatment volume increases the safe dose must decrease to remain below the 1% probability of radiation necrosis.

activity, and the resultant self-shielding, a single tele-radium source had a very low output, that is, dose rate at a distance. This resulted in very long treatment times. Novel approaches to address the low-dose rate issue were developed. One such approach was a device that could simultaneously focus multiple radium sources at a specific target [3] (see Fig. 27.3). The set of tele-radium beams were focused on a specific depth, that is, converging at a point in space and then diverging as they left the target volume. This geometric focusing technique is very similar to the approach Leksell first used in his arc-mounted orthovoltage X-ray tube design and later in his 179 Cobalt-60 source GammaKnife design.[4,5] Leksell's contribution to radiosurgery also included the coupling of a multifocused radiation-beam delivery system to a stereotactic reference system. This coupling enabled the highly focused dose of radiation to be delivered to a defined target volume, a development that preceded isocentric teletherapy designs.

Prior to Leksell's development of the GammaKnife unit, Leksell and Kjellberg, in separate efforts, had adapted fixed-port proton beam units for stereotactic radiosurgical applications (see Fig. 27.4). These pioneering systems treated significant numbers of patients and provided early data on appropriate doses for malignant and benign targets. The proton units used by Leksell and Kjellberg were both initially constructed for physics experiments and then retrofitted for patient application and were not readily available to the therapeutic community at large. This limited the widespread application of this new technique. Leksell's subsequent development of the self-contained Cobalt-60 based teletherapy unit, GammaKnife, provided

the first commercial unit to offer dose distributions that rivaled the dose concentration and dose gradient of particle-beam therapy (see Fig. 27.5).

The GammaKnife's concentration of dose simply relied upon the geometric convergence of a fixed array of Co-60 sources. With a half-life over 300 times shorter than Ra-226, Co-60 allowed for the fabrication of small

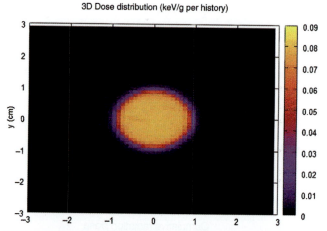

FIGURE 27.5. GammaKnife with dose distribution for an 18 mm helmet. The distribution and gradient is relatively symmetric about the vertical axis of the displayed dose distribution.

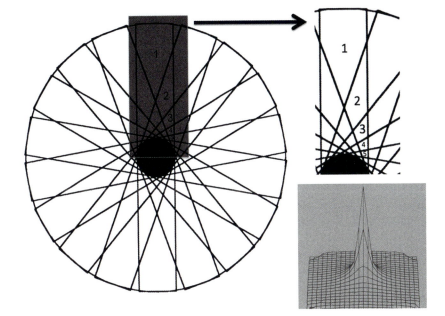

FIGURE 27.6. The intersection of multiple trajectories on a target point showing the pattern of interesting and diverging pathways. As can be seen from the blowup in the upper right, the number of interesting beams (1 through 5 are indicated) provides a steep geometric defined dose gradient. The lower right diagram shows the resultant doseintensity profile of 36 beams each 1 cm in diameter.

pencil-beam sources with high-dose outputs. A large number of these pencil-beam sources could be packed into a focused array. The design spread these pencil Co-60 sources over approximately a hemisphere and ensured all sources were accurately focused to the same point in space, that is, to a 0.3 mm tolerance. Each source produced a circular dose distribution. At the point of convergence, the resultant 3D dose profile was spherical. The convergence and divergence of the beams caused the dose at the edges of the dose sphere to quickly decrease (see Fig. 27.6). Leksell's intention was to use this new device for functional neurosurgical procedures. For malignant and benign targets, the only tools available were plain film X-rays. The tools readily available today, CT and MR imaging, would not be available for several decades. However, the principles of radiosurgery were established and were being applied to targets that could be defined through orthogonal X-ray imaging.

Techniques for CT-based stereotactic frame localization developed in the 1980s and the MR-CT image fusion techniques of the 1990s began to provide a solution to the problems of 3D target definition.[8] Combining these imaging techniques with a new dose computation algorithm allowed for a paradigm shift in the treatment of intracranial targets. For the first time, the ability to deliver a high dose of radiation that conformed to a 3D target shape and provided an exceedingly steep dose gradient along the entire target-to-normal tissue interface would become widely available to clinicians.

Over the past two decades, radiosurgery has gone from a novel treatment approach, limited to a few academic centers, to a treatment modality available in most communities. Systems capable of delivering these precise conformal doses with steep gradients have been developed on multiple platforms. Joining the isotope-based GammaKnife device are a multitude of linear accelerator-based systems. These include traditional gantry-based Linac approaches, robotic arm-mounted systems,[6,7] and gimbal-mounted approaches. These first two approaches can provide intracranial and extracranial radiosurgical treatments. While each of these delivery platforms presents unique challenges, the underlying principles for targeting and the desired characteristics of the prescribed dose distributions remain the same.

PRIMARY OBJECTIVES OF RADIOSURGICAL LOCALIZATION, PLANNING, AND TREATMENT

The combination of stereotactic localization and the ability to produce a highly focused dose distribution with exceedingly high gradients provided a radical change from the existing fractionated treatment paradigm. This new imaging/treatment technique could successfully address intracranial targets in a single-fraction therapy, eliminating the dependence upon the rate of radiation repair in normal tissue cells versus cancerous cells. This paved the way for clinicians to think of radiation as a tool of target elimination similar to a surgical procedure but in an outpatient setting.

Radiosurgery allowed ionizing radiation to be applied to targets previously resistant to fractionated therapy. Dose distributions developed with an ever-evolving set of tools for high conformality and with steep dose gradients provided new optimization parameters that were effectively leveraged against both benign and malignant targets. Radiosurgery treatment of arteriovenous malformations (AVMs) is an example of a successful application of a single fraction radiation therapy when relying on the differential repair of target to normal tissue did not provide a sufficient therapeutic advantage.

It is difficult to separate the effects of conformality and gradient on the success of radiosurgery treatments. The GammaKnife allowed for the treatment of spherical and irregular targets with a planning/delivery tool commonly referred to as "sphere packing." An array of collimators provides a means for the creation of spherical distributions of varying diameters. For round targets, a sphere can be simply fitted to the target volume. For nonspherical targets, the sphere packing technique fits the largest possible sphere inside the target, removes the volume covered by that sphere, and repeats the process as many times as necessary until the entire target volume is treated. The result is an alignment of the entire target-normal tissue surface with the dose-sphere's steep gradient.

While eliminating normal tissue from the prescription volume is generally accepted as a necessary parameter for a safe and effective therapy, a high-dose gradient has not been universally recognized as an equally important parameter.[10] When radiosurgery gradients are examined, special attention is paid to the portion of the distribution where the delivered dose decreases from the prescribed target dose to one-half the target dose.[9,11-13] As the target volume increases, the volume of normal tissue contained in this "target to half target" dose volume rapidly expands. Therapies for both malignant and benign disease have shown limitations on the safe maximum target volume of a single fraction dose. It is widely accepted that the dose that can be safely delivered decreases as the target volume, as well as the volume of this rim of normal tissue, increases. It is the expansion of the normal tissue volume receiving the "target to one half the target dose" that is

responsible for the dose-volume limit placed on radiosurgery treatments.

The importance of gradient can be appreciated by examining the volume enclosed in the high-dose gradient, the shell defined by the edge of the prescribed isodose volume to the volume receiving one-half the prescription dose. The first evidence of a volume-limiting normal tissue threshold was the safe-dose threshold versus target size published for particle beams (see Fig. 27.4B).[9] This curve demonstrates the relationship between complications and increasing target volume. Many other reports have provided clinical evidence demonstrating the correlation between increasing volumes and radiosurgery complications. Several reports have associated an increase in complications with the increase in the volume receiving 12 Gy. As can be seen in Figure 27.7, the high-dose shell exposing normal tissue exponentially increases in volume as the target linearly increases. The lower curve in Figure 27.7 demonstrates the increase in this shell's volume if the steep dose gradient, defined as the average distance between the prescribed isodose surface and the isodose surface of one-half the prescribed dose, is maintained at 3 mm. The upper curve is the volume of this shell if the gradient is allowed to degrade from 3 mm to 6 mm. The net effect of the lower dose gradient is that the limiting dose-volume is reached at smaller target volumes. For example, assume that it is safe to expose a rim of normal tissue, 2.0 cc in volume, to a gradient that is decreasing from 20 Gy to 10 Gy. If a plan has a high dose gradient, 3 mm, as described above, this volume will not be reached until target of ~4 cc (2.0 cm average diameter) is treated. However, if the high-dose gradient is allowed

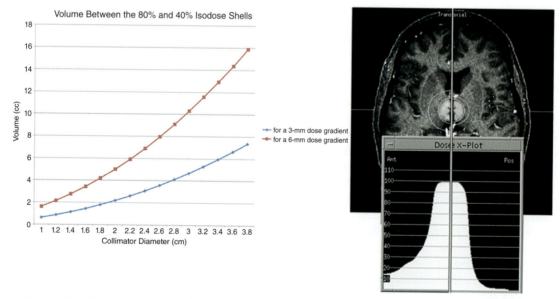

Dose distribution on the right has a gradient of 3 mm and the dose distribution on the left has a gradient of 6 mm.

FIGURE 27.7. Volume of steep dose shell for 3 and 6 mm gradients. Figure on the left demonstrates the increase in volume of the encompassed by the 80% to 40% isodose shells for a 3 mm gradient and a 6 mm gradient. The figure on the right shows the effect of this change on a metastatic target.

to degrade to 6 mm, then the 2.0 cc rim of normal tissue volume is reached when a target of only 0.9 cc (1.2 cm average diameter) is treated. Paying careful attention to the high-dose gradient is critical to the delivery of a safe and effective therapy.

Early radiosurgery literature was based on particle-beam treatments. For these treatments, the Bragg peak provided a delivery tool that allowed for both high conformality and little exit dose. The absence of an exit dose provides for a smaller integral dose to be delivered. Due to the necessary broadening of the proton's Bragg peak, the proximal, upstream dose is approximately equal to the prescription dose. When this upstream dose is coupled with the smaller number of beams used in a routine proton plan, the percent of clinical cases where protons can outperform photons is small.

The high degree of conformality coupled with the steep dose gradients places a very high requirement on the spatial accuracy of target localization. With a CTV equal to the PTV and with doses decreasing at rates of 15% to 30% over a single millimeter, accuracy of delivery measured in millimeters can no longer be considered sufficient. Each portion of the imaging-planning-treatment process must be optimized, and all possible tolerances examined to ensure that target tissues are accurately aligned with a reference which is then accurately aligned to the dose delivery platform. The radiosurgery team must be diligent, ensuring that the accumulation of tolerances do not result in the misalignment of the prescribed dose distribution to the target or the misalignment of complex radiation modulation during treatment delivery.

The literature that established the long-term efficacy and safety of intracranial radiosurgery, using both GammaKnife and Linac, has several treatment techniques in common. A vast majority of the large clinical studies are based on dose optimization and delivery through the use of sphere packing, the first clinical application of intensity modulation. The second is that in order to create the spherical dose distribution, the target, or a portion of the target, was placed at the center of the teletherapy system's isocenter. The third is the alignment of the patient through the use of a rigid stereotactic head-ring system.[15] Placing the treatment's focus at the isocenter eliminated all but a few of the delivery machine's mechanical parameters. Under these conditions, a few degrees of rotational error in the collimator and gantry continue to produce a spherical dose distribution. As long as the center of the sphere is aligned with the targeted tissues the rotation of a spherical distribution has little effect on the delivered dose. However, if multiple targets are treated simultaneously, coupled with image-based alignment of the patient's anatomy through treatment unit-based imaging, that is, cone-beam CT, these parameters can affect both the accuracy of beam placement as well as the distribution's resultant dose gradient.[16,17] Take for example the treatment of

two targets 8 cm apart. Instead of treating each target separately at isocenter, assume that the first target is set at the unit's isocenter and the other is targeted off-axis. Also assume 1-degree resolution in the teletherapy unit's readouts and 1 mm in image-based patient alignment accuracy. With 1-degree resolution an error of half a degree in each rotation is undetectable. This undetectable error can result in more than a millimeter in delivery error for the second target. It can also degrade the dose gradient and result in dose errors at the target-normal tissue interface of 20% or more. It is therefore recommended that before such "efficient" approaches are applied, the individual clinical situation is carefully evaluated and the potential and consequence for such inadvertent errors are considered.

IMAGING: BI-PLANAR IMAGE-BASED TARGET DEFINITION

To provide a highly conformal treatment with steep dose gradients, the system must be able to provide a spatially accurate description of the tissues to be targeted. While suffering from a lack of true 3D target descriptions, fiducial-based plain film systems can provide the position of a point within a stereotactic reference frame to within a few tenths of a millimeter (see Fig. 27.8). The overly defined fiducial system and solution, as described by Siddon and Barth,[14] not only provides high-precision spatial accuracy but also removes the previously required orthogonal geometry. As late as the 1980s and early 1990s, images used to define intracranial targets, such as AVMs, were obtained on plain X-ray films. These systems utilized flat-imaging planes that in turn provided the clinician with spatially undistorted projections. The temporal resolution was limited to the speed at which film changers could shuffle film in and out of cassettes, approximately two images per view per second. As X-ray film gave way to higher-speed image intensifiers, these un-warped projections were lost. The image intensifier's distortions were not only complex in any single orientation but could vary nonlinearly with the orientation of the image intensifier. With the adoption of solid-state detectors, these projections are again able to be presented without spatial distortion.

Simple orthogonal image sets are not capable of providing 3D descriptions of such vascular targets. Figure 27.9 shows a series of objects for which the orthogonal projections do not provide the information required for true 3D reconstructions. While such views have been used for decades to reconstruct implanted radiation sources, the vascular images differ in that unique points in each projection cannot be matched. Although these solid-state imaging systems provide clinicians with the perception of the 3D nature of the vasculature, these systems have not been formatted and mapped to a stereotactic reference system.

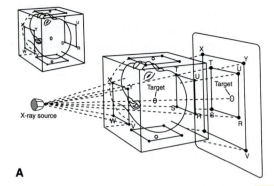

A

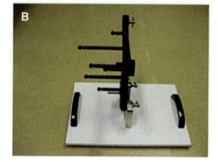

B

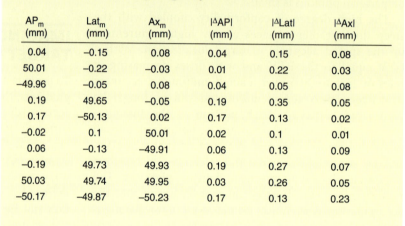

C

Coordinates of Test Points Determined from Angiographic Films

AP_m (mm)	Lat_m (mm)	Ax_m (mm)	$|\Delta AP|$ (mm)	$|\Delta Lat|$ (mm)	$|\Delta Ax|$ (mm)
0.04	−0.15	0.08	0.04	0.15	0.08
50.01	−0.22	−0.03	0.01	0.22	0.03
−49.96	−0.05	0.08	0.04	0.05	0.08
0.19	49.65	−0.05	0.19	0.35	0.05
0.17	−50.13	0.02	0.17	0.13	0.02
−0.02	0.1	50.01	0.02	0.1	0.01
0.06	−0.13	−49.91	0.06	0.13	0.09
−0.19	49.73	49.93	0.19	0.27	0.07
50.03	49.74	49.95	0.03	0.26	0.05
−50.17	−49.87	−50.23	0.17	0.13	0.23

FIGURE 27.8. Showing stereotactic system for plane films and target localization data. Figure in upper left is from Siddon's description of the mathematic solution. Lower left shows the variable phantom that allows for targets to be set throughout the entire stereotactic volume. Table on the right shows the data from 9 experiments that examine the results along individual axis and in combinations.

While angiography remains the gold standard for detection of most vascular targets, due to the above limitations, computed tomography angiography (CTA) and magnetic resonance angiography (MRA) have become the stereotactic targeting modalities of choice. This has resulted in many commercial stereotactic systems abandoning radiographic fiducial frames. Newly introduced imaging platforms capable of rapid rotation during angiographic image acquisition and conebeam reconstructions, cone beam CT angiogram (CBCT-A), compete with MRA and CTA as viable stereotactic imaging modalities.[23] Fusing the CBCT-A dataset to a CTA or MRA can allow the images from this high sensitivity exam to be incorporated into the identification of vascular targets.

IMAGING CT

The first significant advance in the ability to define a true 3D intracranial target volume relative to a rigid reference system was the CT fiducial rod system[15,18]

(see Fig. 27.10). The addition of the CT fiducial reference to a stereotactic frame provided a means by which target tissues could be accurately and precisely mapped to a stereotactic reference platform.[19] The stereotactic frame provided a method of analyzing each CT slice by mapping CT pixels to stereotactic based voxels.[15,20–22] By analyzing the rods on each image, a framework for image-by-image quality control can be incorporated directly into the image processing pathway. Such fiducial systems removed the need for strict adherence of scanner-dependent alignments, such as gantry to table alignment as well as patient-scanner alignment. All data necessary for mapping of every image pixel to the reference frame's coordinate system is incorporated into each slice.

Not all scanner-patient alignments are controllable or easily observed during the scanning process. As CT tables are made more radio-translucent, they begin to lose rigidity. If a patient's longitudinal movement is tilted 0.5 degrees relative to the CT gantry, an error of 2.6 mm in the superior-inferior axis across a 300 mm diameter

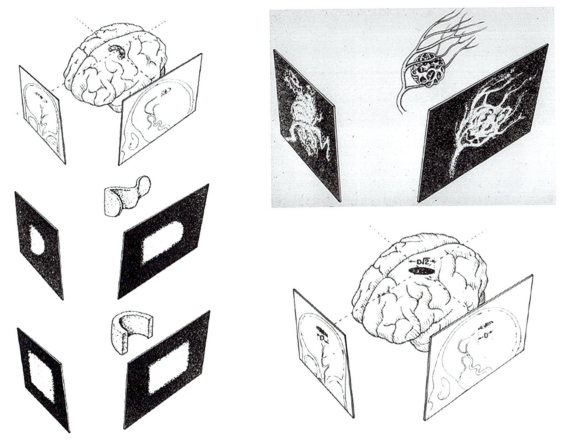

FIGURE 27.9. Series of objects for which a 2D projection are inadequate for an accurate 3D description.

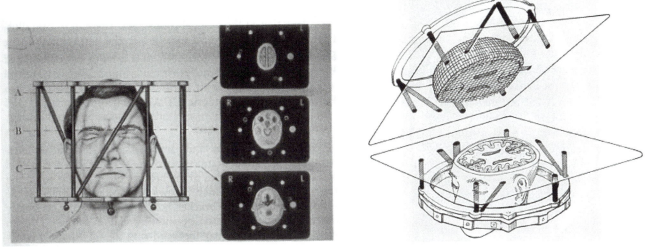

FIGURE 27.10. A fiducial cage is shown with three transaxial plains. Each image intersects all 9 fiducial rods. The right-most figure shows the fiducial cage attached to a headring with the stereotactic grid mapped onto the upper projection.

scan will result. If the stereotactic mapping algorithm is not capable of detecting these misalignments, errors of several millimeters can quickly accumulate. Some systems have approached stereotactic mapping by simply analyzing a single axial slice and then assuming all subsequent slices to be perfectly parallel. This procedure can result in millimeters of error as more anterior and posterior targets are localized. It is difficult to guarantee that small misalignments are detected for an individual scan without a rigid fiducial reference system. It is therefore critical for the stereotactic imaging system to be rigorously tested for accurate identification and correction of these potential imaging anomalies.

It is advisable to incorporate detection of misalignment into radiosurgical image-processing algorithms. For example, as the patient is extended through CT gantry the

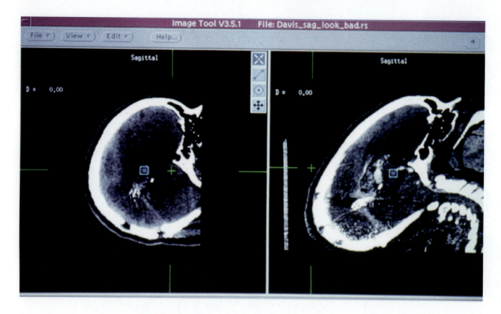

FIGURE 27.11. Image of effects of severe CT gantry tilt (30 degrees).

table can exhibit a downward deflection. While a severe gantry tilt (shown in Fig. 27.11) can be readily identified at the time of image acquisition, small tilts may be more difficult to detect by visual inspection of the data set. Such an analysis can be done with a high degree of certainty when a fiducial array is used. When, however, such systems are not present, as is the case in many mask-based procedures, these subtle errors become difficult to detect and correct. One potential solution is to place a known rigid object in the imaged volume.[24-26] Figure 27.12 shows a CT scan for a mask-based system. Prior to treatment, an algorithm is executed that analyses the reconstructed geometry of the sphere array and provides an estimate of the error in the volumetric dataset. The fiducial system can be placed in the mask system's base frame or as a temporary set of markers that is fitted to the outside of the mask frame. If sub-millimeter precision is to be maintained, the solutions to these potential problems must be incorporated into the stereotactic image processing-planning-treatment algorithms.

The ability to perform a local test of stereotactic localization requires assessment of computed stereotactic coordinates relative to a known standard. It is important not only for the center of the stereotactic coordinates to be tested, but also the points distributed throughout the defined stereotactic volume. As with the above example, a small tilt may correctly calculate the center of the defined stereotactic space. However, as the stereotactic mapping moves away from the center of the imaged volume, the errors are magnified.

A simple test object has been developed initially for frame-based quality assurance.[27] This object contains spherical targets spaced throughout the frame's defined stereotactic volume, allowing for a series of tests to be performed that verifies the correct computation of these known stereotactic coordinates under varying patient-scanner alignments. Misalignments that can be

individually tested or tested in combination are: (1) gantry tilt, (2) patient frame tilt, and (3) patient frame rotation. Such a distributed target test object can also assist in evaluating the accumulation of errors for single isocenter treatment of multiple targets.

Figure 27.13 shows two types of phantoms: a fixed absolute phantom and a variable phantom. Each phantom can be attached to a fixture that allows for the attachment of a CT localizer as well as to a fixture that allows the system to be mounted onto the treatment unit. Such phantoms provide a methodology for examining the alignment of the stereotactic process, beginning with imaging, moving through planning and culminating in treatment delivery. The fixed phantom has six targets at known stereotactic positions. Figure 27.14 shows the results of a series of tests. In these tests the phantom was first aligned as precisely as possible to the CT scanner. Then patient tilts, spins as well as gantry tilts were introduced. The CT scans were then processed by a stereotactic localization program by first locating the fiducial rods in each CT image. The algorithm then processed each image, mapping the voxels to the stereotactic ring's reference coordinate system. The results of this test show that the center of each of the known targets was correctly mapped to within one pixel, demonstrating the system's ability to correct for misalignments that occur during routine scanning. Figure 27.15 shows the absolute phantom being used with an optical alignment system, also referred to as a motion capture (MOCAP) system. If a ring-based system and known fiducial device is not available, then a hidden phantom test can be utilized. The hidden target test can provide a test of the entire imaging-planning-treatment delivery process. If an error is detected in the end-to-end test then more testing of the sub systems can be conducted. The common availability of 3D printers makes the manufacture of special phantoms for such testing within the reach of every

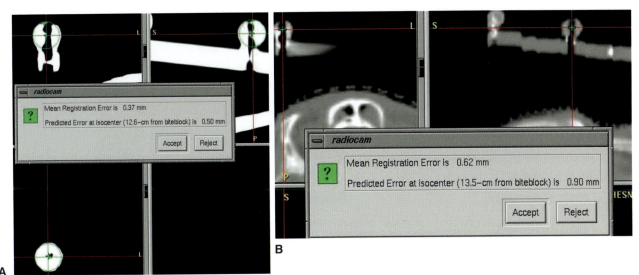

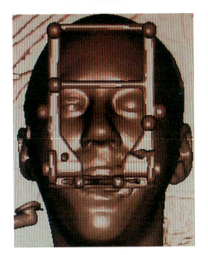
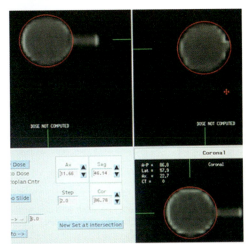
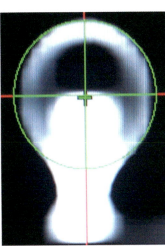

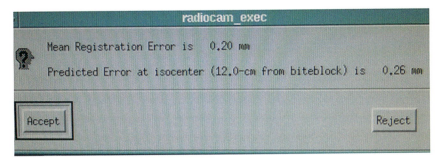

FIGURE 27.12. Optical target system with a known geometry can be used to detect CT scan error or patient inter-scan movement. **A:** Image on the left shows an acceptable scan with the reconstructing of the known fiducial system predicting errors less than a pixel in dimension at 10 cm from the array and **B:** a failed test with the errors predicting approximately two pixel error at 10 cm from the array.

clinic. Figure 27.16 shows a skull printed in a 3D printer within which hidden targets can be placed. This allows the full effect of a mask-based teletherapy with image-based alignment treatment delivery system to be tested on a realistic anatomic model to better replicate the real-world situation.

One important factor in calculating stereotactic coordinates is the ability to account for errors inherent in the pixilation of fiducial systems. With a routine CT image matrix of 512×512 pixels and a scan diameter of approximately 350 mm to encompass a stereotactic fiducial reference system, the in-plane pixels have dimensions of 0.67 mm $\times$ 0.67 mm. A fiducial rod of 4 mm in diameter that is randomly aligned in the field of view can demonstrate significant sampling errors. Using prior knowledge that the rod is straight and that the multislice assembly of rod images must therefore fit a straight line, many of the errors introduced by the relatively large pixel dimension can be corrected. For the optical system shown in Figure 27.12, the knowledge that the passive fiducials are round is routinely used in most motion capture (MOCAP) (what is MOCAP?) systems.

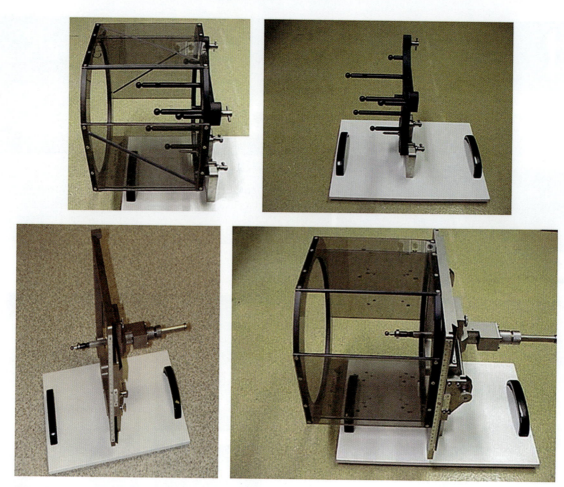

FIGURE 27.13. lower images show variable Winston-Lutz phantom and angiographic with and without fiducial system, upper image pair show fixed six target absolute phantom with CT with and without localizer attached.

Scan Descriptor	Calculated Coordinates			Absolute Coordinates			Error			Vector Error	Average Vector Error
	AP	Lat	Axial	AP	Lat	Axial	AP	Lat	Axial		
Ring no Tilt no Spin	24.90	−43.80	50.00	25.00	−43.30	50.00	0.10	0.50	0.00	0.51	0.57
	−50.20	−0.50	29.60	−50.00	0.00	30.00	0.20	0.50	0.40	0.67	
	24.80	43.10	9.50	25.00	43.30	10.00	0.20	0.20	0.50	0.57	
	−100.10	−0.40	−10.40	−100.00	0.00	−10.00	0.10	0.40	0.40	0.57	
	49.80	86.20	−30.50	50.00	86.60	−30.00	0.20	0.40	0.50	0.67	
	49.80	−86.90	−50.20	50.00	−86.60	−50.00	0.20	0.30	0.20	0.41	
Ring Tilt 3 deg	25.00	−43.70	49.80	25 00	−43.30	50.00	0 00	0.40	0.20	0.45	0.56
	−50.40	−0.40	29.80	−50.00	0.00	30.00	0.40	0.40	0.20	0.60	
	24.80	42.80	9.40	25.00	43.30	10.00	0.20	0.50	0.60	0.81	
	−100.40	−0.30	−10.30	−100.00	0.00	−10.00	0.40	0.30	0.30	0.58	
	49.90	86.30	−30.50	50 00	86.60	−30.00	0.10	0.30	0.50	0.59	
	50.00	−86.90	−50.20	50.00	−86.60	−50.00	0.00	0.30	0.20	0.36	
Ring Spin 3 deg	25.30	−43.30	50.10	25.00	−43.30	50.00	−0.30	0.00	−0.10	0.32	0.49
	−49.70	−0.10	29.90	−50.00	0.00	30 00	−0 30	0.10	0.10	0.33	
	25.10	43.30	9.80	25.00	43.30	10.00	−0.10	0.00	0.20	0.22	
	−99.30	0.20	−10.00	−100.00	0.00	−10.00	−0.70	−0.20	0.00	0.73	
	50.20	86.10	−30.30	50 00	86.60	−30.00	−0.20	0.50	0.30	0.62	
	50.20	−86.00	−49.70	50.00	−86.60	−50.00	−0.20	−0.60	−0.30	0.70	
Ring Tilt 3 deg Spin 3 deg	25.30	−43.50	49.80	25 00	−43.30	50.00	−0.30	0.20	0.20	0.41	0.49
	−49.60	−0.10	29.80	−50.00	0.00	30.00	−0.40	0.10	0.20	0.46	
	25.20	43.10	9.70	25 00	43.30	10.00	−0.20	0.20	0.30	0.41	
	−99.40	0.10	−10.10	−100.00	0.00	−10.00	−0.60	−0.10	0.10	0.62	
	50.00	86.20	−30.20	50.00	86.60	−30.00	0.00	0.40	0.20	0.45	
	50.00	−86.00	−50.00	50.00	−86.60	−50.00	0.00	−0.60	0.00	0.60	

Absolute phantom, scan diameter 350 mm 512 · 512 matrix, pixel size 0.67 · 0.67 mm.

FIGURE 27.14. Table shows the results of scanning the absolute phantom (see Figure 27.13) with CT localization. Separate runs for phantom spin, tilt, and combination spin and tilt and gantry tilt are shown.

Delivery Testing

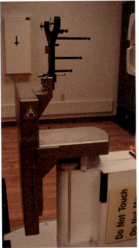

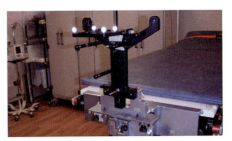

Optical Table Mount

Accuracy Winston–Lutz test for each target

FIGURE 27.15. Absolute phantom and optical positioning system used for end-to-end testing, from image acquisition through delivery.

Floorstand

Example of a 1.0-mm WL test error

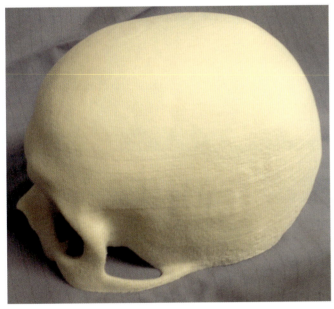

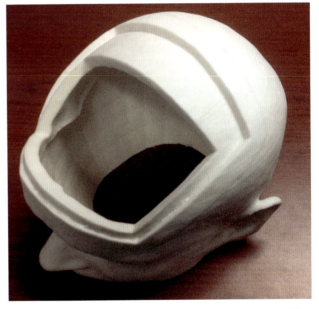

FIGURE 27.16. Two skulls reproduced using a 3D printer. The use of such devices allows the user to reproduce anatomic structures providing a means of testing image-based time-of-treatment positioning system.

MR IMAGING

Over the past three decades, MRI has become the dominant imaging modality for soft-tissue target definition. A host of sequences have been developed that assist in the differentiation between normal tissues and target tissues. Most systems rely heavily upon MRI to provide the target-to-normal tissue contrast necessary for targeting definition. While the superior contrast of MR scanning for most solid targets is critical for planning, MRI has limitations in providing pristine spatial uniformity. The perturbations in the magnetic fields introduced by the patient result in susceptibility errors that warp the MR image. These errors are most dominant at the interface of changes in soft tissue and bone and again at the interface of tissue and air and in the vicinity of any materials that introduce magnetic perturbations.[28] A second set of errors in direct fiducial-based MR stereotactic imaging are introduced by the positioning of the fiducial systems at the outer most diameter of the image, an area where magnetic fields are least uniform. A third issue that arises when direct MR stereotactaxis is attempted is that the size of the fiducial system and the stereotactic ring system often do not fit into head coils that have been optimized to provide the best tissue contrast and image uniformity.

Many systems have adopted MR-CT image-registration techniques, also referred to as "image fusion techniques." These approaches allow the best MR images to be obtained, often requiring head coils that cannot accommodate a stereotactic localizer. Image fusion techniques register these images with the spatially more accurate, but often lower contrast, CT dataset. The fused datasets provide the best of both systems while compensating for each individual imaging system's limitations. Figure 27.17 shows a typical MR-CT dataset aligned. The structures identified on both scanning systems provide images of common tissue boundaries, thereby allowing clinicians to judge the acceptability of the fusion-alignment process. By evaluating the fused images at the level of the ventricles and the sulci the clinician can observe any changes in intracranial alignment that may have taken place between images taken day or days before the procedure and the CT scan on the day of the procedure.

One other advantage of nonstereotactic MR scanning is that the imaging of the target tissues can be obtained hours or days before the radiosurgical procedure is to be carried out. For procedures where stereotactic rings are used, this allows for complete preplanning of the procedure prior to the day of treatment.

As mentioned previously, the resolution of each dataset affects the end accuracy of the procedure. CT scanners are usually set to reconstruct with 512×512 in-plane matrix size and a square in-plane pixel dimension of 0.67 mm. It is important to ensure that the in-plane dimensions of the MR images are comparable. The same is true for the thickness of the slices used for each exam. Figure 27.18 shows a 3D reconstruction of a test object using different slice thickness. While thicker slices often provide improved signal to noise ratios, this improvement

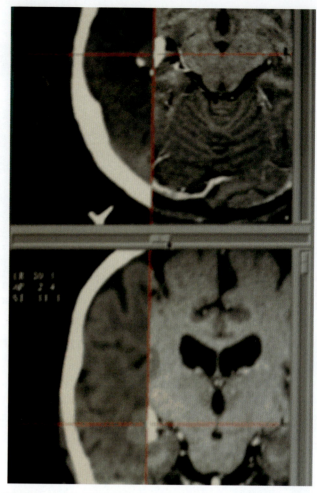

FIGURE 27.17. Right image demonstrating successful CT-MR image fusion. Image alignment is inspected in all three anatomic planes. Left image demonstrating alignment at target location.

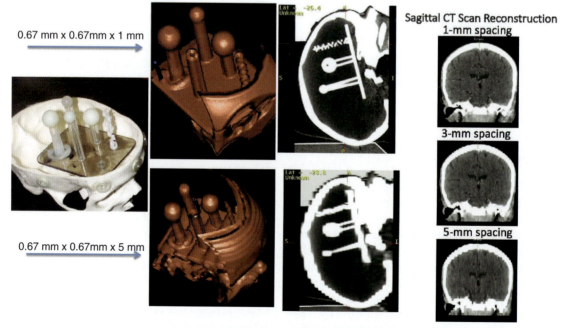

FIGURE 27.18. (From left to right) A test phantom, 3D reconstructions form CT scans using contiguous slice thicknesses of 1 and 5 mm and reformatted sagittal planes from CT contiguous slice thicknesses of 1, 3, and 5 mm showing respective decreasing axial spatial resolution.

comes at the cost of spatial resolution. With high conformality and steep dose gradients, the CT and MR slice thickness should not exceed 1 mm.

DOSE PLANNING

As previously mentioned, the criteria of conformality and gradient have been the primary focus for plan optimization. The first radiosurgical dose planning was the creation of a spherical dose distribution. As 3D target definition became available, planning was extended to "packing" the target volume with spherical distributions, Figure 27.19. While these multispherical plans contain overlaps of spherical distributions within the target volume, such hotspots have not been associated with increased complications. In GammaKnife procedures it is not unusual for these hot spots to be anywhere from 120% to 200% of the prescribed target dose, or stated another way, for the prescribed dose to be 80% to 50% of the distribution's maximum dose. These same sphere-packing techniques were adopted by early linear accelerator radiosurgery systems. Due to the near-uniform sensitivity of intracranial tissues, a uniformly steep gradient is most times considered optimal. A notable exception is for targets near the optic processes, which are considered more sensitive for both single and fractionated treatments. In these cases, gradients can be altered to produce a steeper

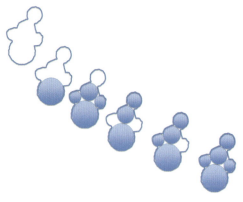

FIGURE 27.19. A hypothetical target being progressively covered, starting in the upper left and progressing to the lower right, by varying diameter spherical dose projections.

gradient in the direction of the chiasm. For example, gradient alteration is often used in the optimization of treatments involving pituitary targets. In the case of the pituitary, the optic chiasm lies just superior to the target volume. Producing a steeper dose gradient in the superior direction, at the sacrifice of a less steep lateral gradient, is often considered beneficial, Figure 27.20.

Many systems that approach dose planning from other perspectives have been introduced. Dynamic conformal planning and various forms of inverse planning have been applied to radiosurgical treatment. Dynamic conformal

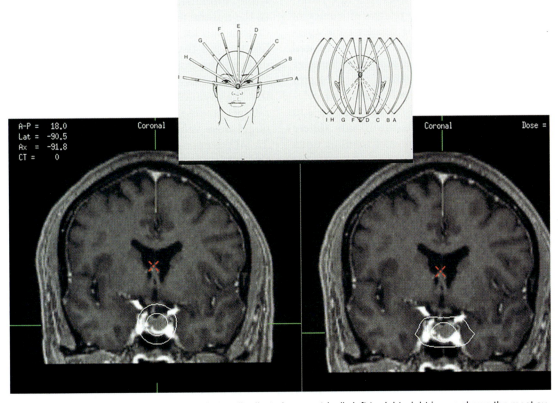

FIGURE 27.20. Left image shows arcing planes distributed symmetrically left to right, right image shows the most superior beams eliminated increasing the dose gradient in the superior-inferior direction, decreasing the dose to the optic chiasm, while decreasing the gradient in the lateral direction.

planning, a technique that uses multiple non-coplanar arcs and beam's eye collimation, has difficulty providing a high degree of conformality when addressing very small, irregular targets.[29,30] The issue of conformality is better addressed by inverse planning and intensity-modulated radiotherapy (IMRT). Dose gradients can be steepened when dealing with specified adjacent critical tissues. However, optimizing the dose gradient over 4pi provides a challenge for IMRT and must be carefully evaluated. The gradient over the entire surface of the target volume is particularly critical in most intracranial radiosurgery. As intensity modulation algorithms have matured more non-coplanar beams have been leveraged resulting in steeper gradient over 4pi. However, as with the above discussion of teletherapy unit tolerances, moving from a single target volume treatment to multiple targets treated with a single isocenter, the same concerns surface when dealing with dose gradients. Careful evaluation of the gradients for targets distant from the isocenter must be carefully evaluated.

While sphere packing and the spectrum of intensity modulation algorithms are often seen as competing technologies, they are in fact one and the same. Early publications proposing intensity modulation as a potential approach to dose optimization actually suggested packing the target volume with spheres of differing intensities (Fig. 27.21).[31] To appreciate the similarities of these approaches, one needs to examine the relative output of the circular cones used to create the spheres. Figure 27.22 shows the output for a set of 6-MV radiosurgical cones. As can be seen, the relative efficiency of monitor unit to dose decreases for smaller cone apertures. Let's assume that the target volume to be treated can be covered by two spheres, one 24 mm in diameter and one 10 mm in diameter. The output of the 24 mm collimator is .94 and the 10 mm collimator is .84, relative to that of the reference 10 x 10 cm field. If one is to deliver 15 Gy to the target volume, the 10 mm sphere would require 1.12 times the number of monitor units

as the 24 mm collimator (0.94/0.84 = 1.12). This is easily achieved if the spherical dose distributions are delivered one at a time, as they are in a sphere-packing approach or if the dose to different portions of the target volume can be modulated. However, if they are to be treated on one beam, as with conformal arc therapy, then there are four options: (1) under dose the 10 mm spherical volume, (2) overdose the 24 mm spherical volume, (3) increase the 10 mm sphere to sacrifice conformality for increased output, or (4) temporally modulate the beam to compensate for the output factors. Figure 27.23 shows a dose distribution for treating an acoustic neuroma where the degree of modulation where each of the spherical dose distributions is provided. This modulation can be provided through modulating the dose to each sphere. It can also be modulated by adjusting the fluence of an intensity modulated set of beams. The only criterion for the latter approach is that the beam plan utilizes a significant number of non-coplanar beams. While beam modulation can compensate for the effects seen in Figure 27.22, it cannot replace the multiple non-coplanar beam geometric effect that produces the overall steep 4 pi gradient.

PRESCRIPTION ISODOSE

As previously mentioned, the goals of radiosurgery are to eliminate all of the tissue within the target volume while minimizing the dose to all normal tissues, that is, the normal tissue volume. Figure 27.24 shows a dose distribution for a metastatic lesion using a conical collimator and five 100-degree non-coplanar arcs. Cross plots of the dose along the lateral axis are shown in Figures 27.24A–D. The first plot in Figure 27.24 A shows that the distance required for the dose to decrease from a target isodose shell of 95% of max to 47.5%, half the target dose value, is 5.7 mm. Figures 27.24B through 27.24D denote the distance required if the 90%, 80%, and 70% isodose shells are selected as the target isodose. As can be seen, the minimum distance between target and half-target dose of 3.8 mm coincides with selecting the 80% isodose shell as the prescription isodose shell. This selection results in the lowest integral dose over the high-dose volume to normal tissue.[32] Looking at the dose distributions one observes that this selects a prescription point just past the high-dose shoulder of the dose profile, beyond the 90% shoulder. This dose profile holds true for distributions with significant non-coplanar beam sets, whether they are plan optimized using a sphere packing approach or a temporal intensity modulation algorithm.

If sphere-packing is employed, and more than one isocenter is combined for coverage of an irregular target volume, small hot spots are often present within the target volume. When normalizing to the maximum dose this hot spot can shift the optimized prescription

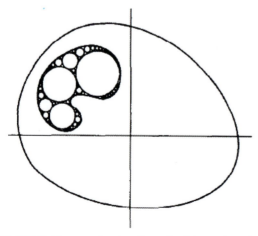

FIGURE 27.21. Diagram showing the potential creation of an intensity-modulated plan by packing the target volume with spheres.

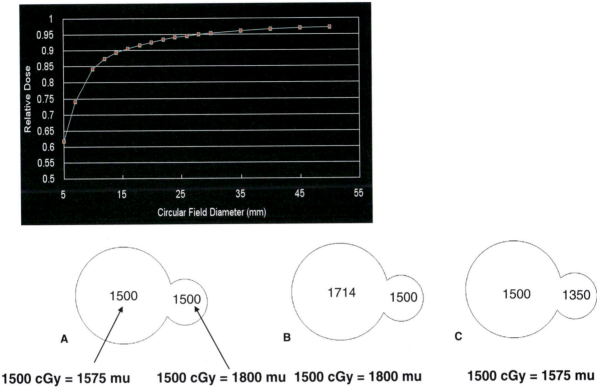

FIGURE 27.22. Relative output of spherical collimators with three potential scenarios of covering a target volume. **A:** Covering the volume with two different spheres allowing for the required monitor units of each segment to be separately calculated. **B** and **C:** the under- and overdose resulting from treating the entire target with one conformal field allowing for only one monitor unit setting to be selected.

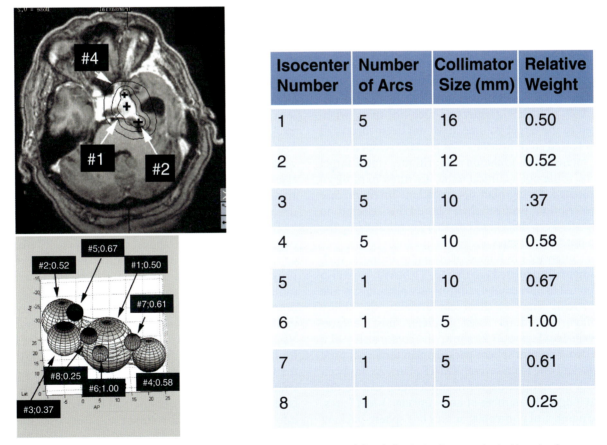

Isocenter Number	Number of Arcs	Collimator Size (mm)	Relative Weight
1	5	16	0.50
2	5	12	0.52
3	5	10	.37
4	5	10	0.58
5	1	10	0.67
6	1	5	1.00
7	1	5	0.61
8	1	5	0.25

FIGURE 27.23. Modulating sphere intensities to provide an intensity modulated plan to treat a nonspherical target volume.

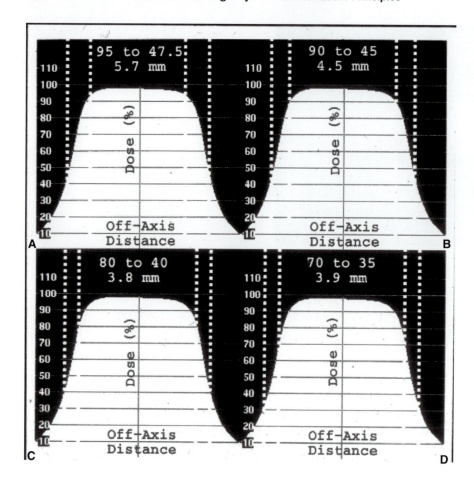

FIGURE 27.24. Dose cross plot of a single isocenter, multiple non-coplanar arcing plan. The effect of selecting the prescription isodose 95%,90%, 80%, 70% of maximum dose, demonstrating the dose falls most rapidly to one half the dose when the 80% of maximum dose shell is selected. This provides maximum normal tissue sparing for near target doses.

shell down to a lower value. Although tools are available to help dampen the extent of these hotspots, prescription isodose shells of 70% through 50% are commonly encountered. As previously mentioned, the target volume is void of normal tissue, and such hot spots, when confined to the target volume, have not been correlated with increased complications. For plans developed using other intensity modulation algorithms, intra-target hotspots, while not a clinical issue, are often minimized or eliminated during plan optimization. In either case the prescription isodose shell should be selected to leverage the steep dose gradient, thereby minimizing the dose to nontarget tissues.

Other intensity modulated planning techniques, such as volumetric modulated arc therapy (VMAT), have also been applied to intracranial radiosurgery planning. While these systems show excellent conformality, the ability to maintain exceedingly tight gradients must be carefully evaluated. Figure 27.25 shows the conformality of a simple two-isocenter sphere-packing plan for an acoustic neuroma and one from several VMAT plans. As has been observed, the optimal degree of modulation can be difficult to judge. The number of non-coplanar VMAT arcs, like the number of non-coplanar arcs in a sphere-packing plan, has been shown to affect the overall 4 pi dose gradient.[16,35] While both plans provide excellent conformality,

conformal VMAT plans can, if not carefully optimized, produce a less steep dose gradient for small and midsize targets, thereby increasing the volume of tissue exposed to near target dose levels. For larger targets, 2.4 to 3.0 cm average diameters, the ability of circular field sphere packing to rapidly converge and then diverge becomes less effective due to the increased distance from isocenter required for overlapping beam trajectories to diverge. For these larger target volumes intensity modulation begins to outperform sphere packing, especially in the arena of dose gradient.

Because of the rapid development in treatment planning algorithms, the above comparisons in planning approaches are in a constant state of flux. However, the primary objectives of the planning process remain the same: a high degree of conformality with exceedingly steep dose gradients. Many groups have suggested both conformality and gradient as critical planning parameters.[30,33,34] Wagner introduced a Conformality Gradient Index (CGI) for both conformality (CGIc) and gradient (CGIg).[30] For the Gradient Score (CGIg), the formulation converts the volume of the prescription isodose and the volume of the isodose that encompasses one-half the treatment isodose into effective spherical volumes and then uses the radii of these effective spheres to compute an average effective radius. Assigning a score of 100 to an average radius of

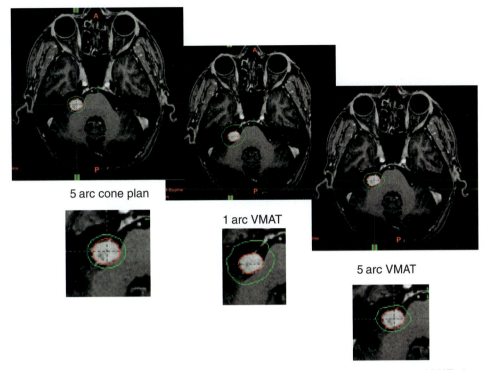

5 arc cone plan

1 arc VMAT

5 arc VMAT

FIGURE 27.25. Plans for a simple acoustic two-isocenter plan for sphere packing and VMAT plan. Also a more complex plan showing favorable VMAT planning.

3 mm, from prescription to one-half the prescription isodose, the score is calculated as

$$CGIc = 100 \left(\frac{Target\ volume}{Perscription\ isodose\ volume} \right)$$
$$= (PITV)^{-1} \times 100$$
$$UFIg = 100 - \left\{ 100 \cdot \left[\left(R_{Eff,\ 50\%Rx} - R_{Eff,\ Rx} \right) - 0.3\ cm \right] \right\}$$
$$R_{eff} = \sqrt[3]{\frac{3V}{4\pi}}$$
$$CGI = (CGIc + CGIg)/2.$$

where PITV is the ratio of Prescription isodose volume to the target volume. Other conformality indexes have also been defined by the ICRU 62[38] as the ratio of the prescription isodose volume to that of the planning target volume (PTV).

$$CI_{ICRU} = \frac{V_{Rx}}{V_{PTV}}$$

Another suggested conformality index utilizes the volume of the prescription isodose that encompasses 95% of the PTV divided by the PTV. In yet another conformality index formulation, suggested by Paddick, the volume of the treatment isodose that does not include target volume is not counted in the denominator[33] to ensure that the planning volume counted overlaps with the target volume.

$$CI_{Inv-Paddick} = \frac{V_{Rx} \times V_{PTV}}{V_{Rx \cap PTV}^2}$$

The goal of radiosurgery is to mimic a surgical resection. The coverage of the PTV is set equal to the imaging target volume. The goal of the planning process is to ensure that the full imaged target is covered. Because of the steep dose gradient, the omission of any portion of the target volume is analogous to a subtotal surgical resection. It is therefore common for the prescribed plan to encompass the entire imaged target volume. The sensitivity of the intracranial tissues requires that safe and effective treatments result in conformality indexes between 1.0 and 2.0. With average target volumes on the order of 4 cc to 5 cc, these plans result in less than 1 cc of normal tissue being exposed to the prescription dose. The steep dose gradient also minimizes the exposure of normal tissue adjacent to the target volume. Some typical treatment plans with conformality indexes and dose gradients are shown in Figure 27.26.

TREATMENT MARGIN, PTV VS. CTV

Historically, for both benign as well as malignant targets, the prescription isodose has been set to coincide with the enhancing volume. This sets the clinical target volume (CTV) or imaging target volume equal to the PTV. As with the discussion of gradient, increasing target volume ultimately results in the lowering of the safely administrable, although less effective, dose. With sub-millimeter localization and treatment delivery accuracy, nearly all centennial studies establishing safety and effectiveness have adopted setting the PTV equal to the CTV.[36,37]

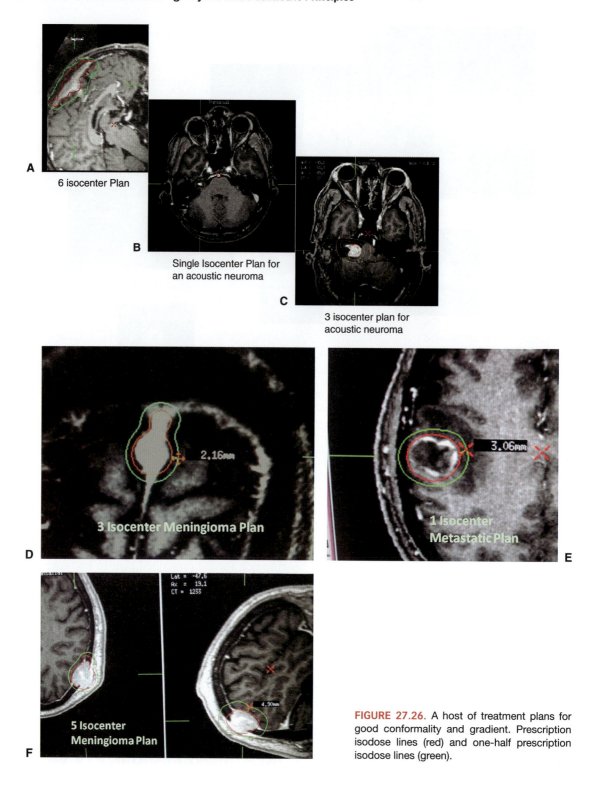

6 isocenter Plan

Single Isocenter Plan for
an acoustic neuroma

3 isocenter plan for
acoustic neuroma

3 Isocenter Meningioma Plan

1 Isocenter
Metastatic Plan

5 Isocenter
Meningioma Plan

FIGURE 27.26. A host of treatment plans for good conformality and gradient. Prescription isodose lines (red) and one-half prescription isodose lines (green).

TREATMENT DELIVERY

The previously discussed imaging and highly conformal planning requirements with steep dose gradients require a highly accurate delivery system. This necessitates that stereotactic targets be aligned with delivery systems, and that delivery systems be able to deliver multiple non-coplanar beams while maintaining accurate alignment.

With the need for non-coplanar beam for optimization, the delivery often requires multiple patient table angles as well as multiple gantry positions or arcs. These treatment parameters result in the need to maintain a high accuracy alignment of the target volume to the treatment device for tens of minutes. Studies have shown that for the more common mask-based immobilization systems movement over such times can be challenging.

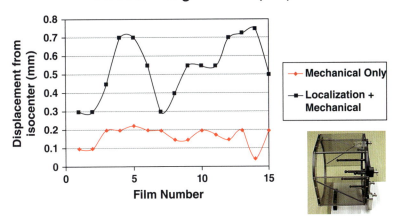

Hidden Targets Test (CT)

FIGURE 27.27. Left—Data shows the results of a hidden target test. Targets are CT imaged, planned, and Winston-Lutz films are taken and analyzed for total vector error. Right—experiment setup for Floorstand and optical guidance systems.

System with average delivery error of 0.2 mm has an overall error dominated by the image localization accuracy.

Early GammaKnife units provided the gold standard for stereotactic delivery. The design of the rigid source alignment with the system's stereotactic reference provided a stereotactic target to isocenter alignment of 0.3 mm.[39] Early linear accelerator systems had trouble maintaining such critical alignments.[40,41] Winston and Lutz introduced a system that allowed for the evaluation of stereotactic target alignment to the delivery system.[42] This design provided a means by which non-coplanar delivery accuracy could be measured. In 1988, Friedman and Bova introduced a system to correct the linear accelerator's gantry and patient support "wobble".[11] Redesigned linear accelerators, capable of maintaining sub-millimeter delivery alignments, were introduced in the mid-1990s. For such systems, the Winston-Lutz delivery testing procedure remains the standard for certifying accuracy in delivery.

The phantoms shown in Figure 27.13 can be used with the Winston-Lutz test to provide end-to-end system testing. After evaluation of the CT mapping program, the computer stereotactic coordinates can be used to "treat" the phantom. This provides a process by which the entire image-planning-treatment chain can be evaluated. Figure 27.27 shows the results of such a test. Again, as with previous evaluations, it is critical that targets throughout stereotactic space be evaluated. Testing only at the center of the defined stereotactic volume can mask errors in both image mapping and treatment delivery.

The beams used in radiosurgery treatment are often significantly smaller than those used in routine radiation therapy. The complement of beams usually does not exceed 40 mm and usually includes beams as small as 4 mm to 5 mm. The measurement of these small beams poses special problems and requires very small detectors.[43] If routine "Farmer-style" chambers are employed for such small beams, then significant errors in both beam profiles and output factors can be made (see Fig. 27.28). Figure 27.29 shows beam profiles using numerous high spatial resolution/small cross-section detectors Figure 27.30 shows first how a set of small beams behaves

Effect of Detector Dimension on Penumbra Measurements

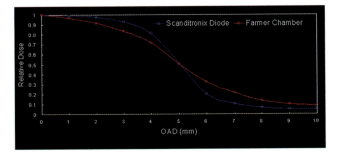

Finite dimensions of larger detectors cause rounding or smoothing of profile

FIGURE 27.28. Beam profiles using small diode detector and larger ion chamber demonstrating the errors possible when detectors of large size are used on small radiosurgical beams.

Radiosurgery OAR Detectors (AAPM TG 42)

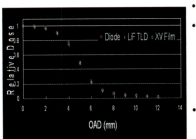

- Film is best.
- Diodes, plastic scintillators, TLDs, and ion chambers are all acceptable.
- Detector dimensions must be <2 mm.

FIGURE 27.29. Beam profile of a 10 mm circular beam data taken with three high spatial resolution detectors. (American Association of Physicist in Medicine Task Group 42 [AAPM TG 42].)

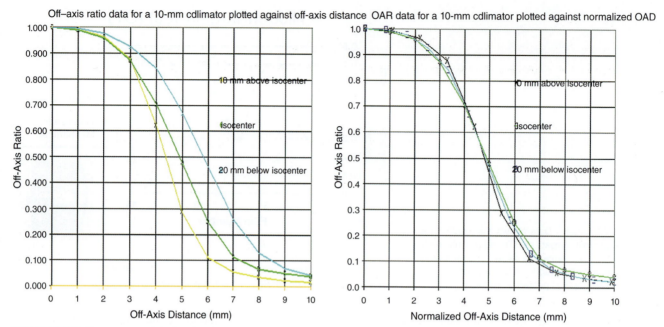

FIGURE 27.30. Beam cross-plots for absolute distance from central axis and again as percentage of off-axis-distance that can be used to check for effects of detector size.

when plotted against off-axis distance and again how they agree when normalized to the beam's diameter. Such cross tests should be carried out to ensure that detector sizes are not affecting measurement results. Figure 27.31 shows the output factors for a set of circular beams as well as a set of small square fields. Again, cross-checking using multiple detectors is critical in ensuring that errors can be identified when these exceedingly small beams are measured.

Recently single isocenter treatments of multiple targets have placed more demands on small beam dosimetry. It is becoming common to treat sub-centimeter targets that are five to eight centimeters from the central axis. Dosimetry for these small off axis beams must be carefully validated to ensure that an accumulation of small errors do not result in significant dose delivery errors.

Services such as those provided by calibration and quality assurance labs are critical in the commissioning of each radiosurgery system to ensure that all such parameters

have been correctly measured and correctly incorporated into the system's treatment planning and delivery system services. The ability to localize, plan, and treat a test phantom and to have an independent laboratory verify the end result in both accuracy and prescribed dose is critical. Utilizing such services should be part of each new installation's calibration and certification procedure.

SYSTEM CRITERIA

While it is difficult to define absolute accuracy or precision in stereotactic imaging or treatment delivery, it is possible to examine and provide perspective on the effect of misalignments and errors. Figure 27.32 shows the addition of treatment errors to imaging errors and how these added errors can quickly dominate the overall system accuracy. Accuracy and precision can be affected by

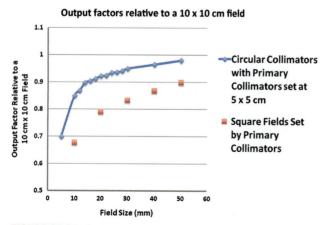

FIGURE 27.31. Output factors for cones and small square fields.

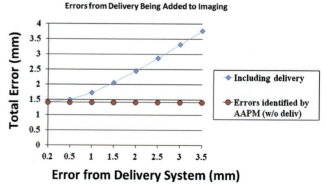

FIGURE 27.32. Demonstrating the effects of treatment errors when delivery error is added to imaging errors (AAPM report 42).

(1) incorrect mapping of stereotactic coordinates during image analysis, (2) planning that does not provide sufficient conformality or gradient, and (3) delivery systems that do not maintain sufficient rigidity and precision during non-coplanar beam delivery. The first two effects have been discussed previously. The third can be simulated in the radiosurgery planning system.

During treatment planning, a simulated radiation source is maneuvered to deliver beams from various directions. The mathematic model is designed to point at a specific stereotactic coordinate without error. This specific error is referred to as the teletherapy unit's isocentric accuracy. This accuracy is determined by different design and manufacturing parameters that vary with each type of delivery system. In every case, the first critical alignment is the system's ability to place a specific stereotactic coordinate at the unit's nominal isocenter or reference point. In the case of the GammaKnife, the unit's delivery accuracy is determined by how accurately the collimators are aligned within the treatment head. For a linear accelerator delivery system, it is the system's ability to accurately rotate the gantry and patient support unit about this isocenter. For robotic systems, it is the robot's ability to maintain alignment of the beam to a point in space. And for tomographic units, it is the combination of the isocentric rotation of the source and the system's ability to accurately translate the patient through the gantry.

To help understand how isocentric accuracy can affect dose delivery, one can simulate isocentric inaccuracy in the planning system. The resultant dose distributions can then be compared to those derived from perfectly aligned simulations. For an arcing linear accelerator delivery system, dividing the arc into several segments and allowing each segment to aim at a different stereotactic coordinate can accomplish this simulation. Such a simulation was conducted with the gantry and patient support rotation maintaining a plus or minus 1 mm isocenter accuracy along each orthogonal axis. For a typical mid-size target of 18 mm diameter, the effects of this degree of inaccuracy result in a shrinking of the 80% prescription isodose shell's volume by 15% and a decrease in the sharpness of the isodose fall off from 80% to 40% isodose shells by 33%. While it is difficult to translate these effects into treatment failures or treatment complications, it does demonstrate the striking effect of small errors in isocentric accuracy on the delivery of the prescribed dose as well as the maintenance of the steep dose gradient.

THE TREATMENT PROCEDURE

Unlike routine fractionated radiation delivery, radiosurgery requires more of a surgical mindset. With a single-fraction therapy, all QA and checking must be completed prior to the initiation of the first and only treatment. This places special demands on the radiation oncology department's teletherapy delivery team, who are more aligned with an incremental treatment technique.

To assist in the procedure, many departments have adopted a rigid checklist to help ensure that each critical step is performed and verified by more than one member of the clinical team. For a ring-based stereotactic radiosurgery surgery (SRS) procedure, this checklist would begin when the clinical team meets the patient and continue until the treatment is complete and the ring is removed. The procedure would include:

- A "time out": Prior to ring placement, a "time out" is used to ensure that the team is focused on the correct radiosurgical target for that individual patient. Figure 27.33 shows a typical "time out" checklist with the accompanying MR image showing the radiosurgical target.
- Specific written orders to accompany the patient to CT scanning
- A signoff by the treatment team on the quality of image fusion
- A signoff by the treatment team on the final plan
- The development of a treatment checklist that includes
  - A check of the plan's transfer to the treatment system's record and verify system
  - The pretreatment QA ensuring that
    - The correct patient and prescription have been transferred
    - The unit's accuracy is verified prior to each treatment
    - A step-by-step procedure to ensure that every step is documented and verified, including
      - Verification of the stereotactic coordinates
      - The cone and/or the collimator settings
      - The monitor unit setting for each treatment segment

An example checklist, automatically generated by the treatment planning system, is shown in Figure 27.34. The use of such a checklist is usually accompanied by a minimum of one double-check and often with a third "blind check" to ensure that each parameter is properly set prior to the initiation of each treatment segment.

It is also critical to provide an atmosphere that allows the treatment team to concentrate on delivery and not be distracted by phone calls, scheduling questions or any other unrelated tasks. While an awareness of the distraction of cell phones during tasks such as driving a motor vehicle are being realized, similar distractions during complex procedures, such as radiation delivery, are often not appreciated. Forwarding the phones at the treatment unit's console and inside the treatment vault, prohibiting the use of cell phones, texting, and voice, throughout the procedure and minimizing any discussions that distract the treatment team from the delivery process should be enacted. Providing the proper environment as well as a thoroughly planned procedure and post-procedure reviews are critically important to the reduction of human errors and the identification of general system failures.

Procedure Checklist

Instructions for Staff: Place Initials in the appropriate box indicating complete or enter NA

Step: Process Verification	Radiation Oncology Nurse LPN or RN Complete	Attending Physician Immediately Before any Radioactive Procedure
A. Patient identification: Name and at least one other ☐MRN ☐SSN ☐DOB		
B. Procedure verified with consent for treatment		
C. Procedure verified with history and physical or progress note		
D. Verified availability of materials or treatment unit		
E. "Time Out." The treatment team, led by the attending physician, actively participating in verbal notification of: ☐ Patient name ☐ Patient MRN ☐ Procedure ☐ Procedure site		

Signature signifies verification of patient ID, intent, correct procedure site

FIGURE 27.33. Checklist for time-out prior to initiation of the radiosurgical procedure.

```
        STEREOTACTIC RADIOSURGERY TREATMENT CHECKLIST

    Date :

    Patient Name: Gator, Al E.

    Prescribed dose: 1750.0  energy: 6MV Trilogy

    Prescription Percent Line: 70.0 % of Maximum Dose
    ----------------------------------------------------------
           Setup and Validation Procedure

    ____ Collimator rotation set to 0 degrees.

    ____ Field size set to 5 × 5 cm with collimator symmetric.

    ____ Patient on table in position, table, collimator, and
         jaw movements disabled.

    ____ Collision avoidance enabled

    ____ Patient wristband ID checked prior to treatment

    ____ Patient verified again patient signed picture

    ____ Prescription validated in Record and Verify System against
         Physician signed prescription

    ____ Set Winston-Lutz variable phantom to first Isocenter values

    Isert collimator and carryout the following test film shots:
          Gantry     PSU
    ____   270         0
    ____    0          0
    ____    0         270
    ____    90         0

    ____ Visual approval of test film

    ____ Second Dosimetry Check compared to Physician signed treatment plan.
    ----------------------------------------------------------

    ____  1.  Verify First isocenter coordinates:
                   A-P = -19.3
                       Lat = -29.5
                       Axl = -39.3
    ____  2.  Install 18nm collimator.

    ____  3.  Set patient table to 20 degrees.

    ____  4.  Treat  : Start angle = 120
                       End angle  = 30
                       Mon units  = 567

    ____  5.  Set patient table to 55 degrees.

    ____  6.  Treat  : Start angle = 120
                       End angle  = 30
                       Mon units  = 630
```

```
    ------------------------------------------------------------
    ____  7.  Set patient table to 340 degrees.

    ____  8.  Treat  : Start angle = 240
                       End angle  = 330
                       Mon units  = 704
    ------------------------------------------------------------
    ____  9.  Set patient table to 305 degrees.

    ____ 10.  Treat  : Start angle = 240
                       End angle  = 330
                       Mon units  = 744
    ------------------------------------------------------------
    ____ 11.  Set patient table to 270 degrees.

    ____ 10.  Treat  : Start angle = 240
                       End angle  = 330
                       Mon units  = 718
    ------------------------------------------------------------
    ____ 13.  Set Coordinates to A-P = -14.9
                                Lat = -42.7
                                Axl = -41.2

    ____ 14.  Install 10nm collimator.

    ____ 15.  Set patient table to 20 degrees.

    ____ 16.  Treat  : Start angle = 120
                       End angle  = 30
                       Mon units  = 315
    ------------------------------------------------------------
    ____ 17.  Set patient table to 55 degrees.

    ____ 18.  Treat  : Start angle = 120
                       End angle  = 30
                       Mon units  = 348
    ------------------------------------------------------------
    ____ 19.  Set patient table to 340 degrees.

    ____ 20.  Treat  : Start angle = 240
                       End angle  = 330
                       Mon units  = 449
    ------------------------------------------------------------
    ____ 21.  Set patient table to 305 degrees.

    ____ 22.  Treat  : Start angle = 240
                       End angle  = 330
                       Mon units  = 461
    ------------------------------------------------------------
    ____ 21.  Set patient table to 270 degrees.

    ____ 22.  Treat  : Start angle = 240
                       End angle  = 330
                       Mon units  = 418
    ------------------------------------------------------------
    END OF TREATMENT PROCEDURE
```

FIGURE 27.34. Checklist for SRS procedures automatically produced by treatment planning system.

KEY POINTS

- Radiosurgery does not depend upon the differential sensitivity between health and diseased tissue.

- Radiosurgery requires extremely high conformality.

- Radiosurgery requires very steep dose gradients over the entire 4 pi of the target's surface.

- The radiosurgery process is perhaps the most demanding radiation treatment process and requires redundancy throughout the process.

- From imaging through planning and delivery it is essential to provide end-to-end testing of all components and processes.

- Radiosurgery requires 3D targeting. Two-dimensional targeting can lead to either over- or under-coverage of target structures.

- Prescription isodose is chosen to provide the maximum gradient at the target to normal tissue interface.

REVIEW QUESTIONS

1. Which of the following imaging techniques is not recommended for defining the 3D shape of a vascular intracranial target?
   A. Computed tomographic angiography
   B. MRA
   C. Cone-beam angiography
   D. Orthogonal angiography

2. Which of the following is usually part of a radiosurgery quality assurance testing procedure?
   A. CT slice–thickness assessment
   B. MR uniformity assessment
   C. Hidden target testing
   D. Field flatness assessment

3. Which of the following factors limit the application of dynamic conformal dose optimization?
   A. The size of multileaf collimators
   B. The rapid change in output factor for small field sizes
   C. The isocentric accuracy of teletherapy units
   D. The nonlinearity of film dosimetry

4. Which of the following radiation detectors are not used in small field measurements?
   A. Parallel plate buildup detectors
   B. Diamond detectors
   C. Diode detectors
   D. Radiochromic film

5. Why do most radiosurgery treatment units utilize either Co-60 or 6 MV as opposed to 18-MV photons?
   A. 18 MV has lower penetration
   B. 18 MV has a greater penumbra
   C. 18 MV has a steeper dose fall-off at the edge of the field
   D. 18-MV beams are more polychromatic

ANSWERS

1. D   Figure 27.9 demonstrates a few potential shape errors when a three-dimensional object is projected onto two orthogonal planes. Simple orthogonal planar images are incapable of providing 3D descriptions of vascular targets. See the discussion in the "Imaging: Bi-Planar Image-Based Target Definition" section.

2. C   Figures 27.13 and 27.14 show the results from a hidden target test. It is important for the targets be disbursed through the volume that can potentially contain clinical targets. A hidden target test can provide verification of the entire imaging-planning-treatment delivery process. See the discussion in the "Imaging: CT" section.

3. B   Figure 27.22 demonstrates the rapid decrease in dose relative to fluence as the size of the radiation field decreases. With many targets having small irregularities, it is common for regions of the beam's eye view to have areas less than 5 millimeters in diameter. This figure demonstrates the inability of such fields to provide a uniform dose.

Dynamic conformal planning has difficulty when treating small, irregularly shaped targets. See the discussion in the "Dose Planning" section, and reference 29 (Wagner TH et al.).

4. A   The small field required for radiosurgery targets require very small radiation detectors. Larger detectors can exhibit partial volume effects. The reference Rice 43 was the first to examine this potential pitfall for radiosurgery size fields. Measurement of small, radiosurgical beams requires very small detectors. The dimensions for parallel plate chambers are too large (i.e., >2 mm) for these beams. See Reference 37, AAPM Task Group 42 Report (Schell et al.)

5. B   Figure 27.7 demonstrates the effect of dose gradient on the volume of normal tissue that receives a potentially therapeutic dose. The reference of Wagner et al.[30] demonstrates the need for both conformality and gradient to maximize the therapeutic effect while minimizing complications. For small fields, the off-axis profiles are influenced by the lack of lateral electronic equilibrium present in higher energy beams.

REFERENCES

1. Leksell L. The stereotaxic method and radiosurgery of the brain. *Acta Chir Scand.* 1951;102:316–319.
2. Leksell L. Cerebral radiosurgery. I. Gammathalamotomy in two cases of intractable pain. *Acta Chir Scan.* 1968;134:585–589.
3. Mould R. *Mould's medical anecdotes omnibus edition.* CRC Press;1966.
4. Lunsford LD, Flickinger J, Lindner G, et al. Stereotactic radiosurgery of the brain using the first United States 201 cobalt-60 source gamma knife. *Neurosurgery.* 1989;24(2):151–159.
5. Mehta M. The physical, biologic, and clinical basis of radiosurgery. *Curr Probl Cancer.* 1995;19(5):270–328.
6. Rahimian J, Chen L, Rao A, et al. Geometrical accuracy of the Novalis stereotactic radiosurgery system for trigeminal neuralgia. *J Neurosurg.* 2004;101(Suppl 3):352–355.
7. Chang J, Yenice K, Narayana A, et al. Accuracy and feasibility of conebeam computed tomography for stereotactic radiosurgery setup. *Med Phys.* 2007;34:2077–2084.
8. Wu A, Lindner G, Maitz AH, et al. Physics of gamma knife approach on convergent beams in stereotactic radiosurgery. *Int J Radiat Oncol Biol Phys.* 1990;18:941–949.
9. Kjellberg R, Hanamura T, Davis KR, et al. Bragg-Peak proton-beam therapy for arteriovenous malformations of the brain. *N Engl J Med.* 1983;309:269–274.
10. Chin L, MA L, DiBiase S. Radiation necrosis following gamma knife surgery: a case-controlled comparison of treatment parameters and long-term clinical follow up. *J Neurosurg.* 2001;899–904.
11. Friedman WA, Bova FJ. The University of Florida radiosurgery system. *Surg Neurol.* 1989;32(5):334–343.
12. Liu R, Wagner TH, Buatti JM, et al. Geometrically based optimization for extracranial radiosurgery. *Phys Med Biol.* 2004;49(6):987–996.
13. Pike GB, Podgorsak EB, Peters TM, et al. Three-dimensional iso-dose distributions in stereotactic radiosurgery. *Stereotact Funct Neurosurg.* 1990;54(55):519–524.
14. Siddon RL, Barth NH. Stereotaxic localization of intracranial targets. *Int J Radiat Oncol Biol Phys.* 1987;13(8):1241–1246.
15. Heilbrun M, Roberts T, Apuzzo M. Preliminary experience with Brown-Roberts-Wells (BRW) computerized tomography stereotaxic guidance system. *J Neurosurg.* 1983;59:217–222.
16. Audet C, Poffenbarger B, Chang P, et al. Evaluation of volumetric modulated arc therapy for cranial radiosurgery using multiple non-coplanar arcs. *Med Phys.* 2011;38(11):5863–5872.
17. Shirashi S, Tan J, Olsen LA. Knowledge-based prediction of plan quality metrics in intracranial stereotactic radiosurgery. *Med Phys.* 2015;42(3):908–917.
18. Leksell L. Stereotactic radiosurgery. *J Neurol Neurosurg Psychiatry.* 1983;46(9):797–803.
19. Leksell L. *Stereotaxis and radiosurgery: An operative system.* Thomas; 1971.
20. Verellen D, Linthout N, Bel A, et al. Assessment of the uncertainties in dose delivery of a commercial system for linac-based stereotactic radiosurgery. *Int J Radiat Oncol Biol Phys.* 1999;44:421–433.
21. Roberts T, Brown R. Technical and clinical aspects of CT-directed stereotaxis. *Appl Neurophysiol.* 1980;43:170–171.
22. Saw CB, Ayyangar K, Suntharalingam N. Coordinate transformations and calculation of the angular and depth parameters for a stereotactic system. *Med Phys.* 1987;14(6):1042–1044.
23. Lightstone A, Benedict S, Bova F, et al. American Association of Physicists in Medicine Radiation Therapy Committee. Intracranial stereotactic positioning systems: Report of the American Association of Physicists in Medicine Radiation Therapy Committee Task Group no. 68. *Med Phys.* 2005;32:2380–2398.
24. Meeks SL, Bova FJ, Wagner TH, et al. Image localization for frameless stereotactic radiotherapy. *Int J Radiat Oncol Biol Phys.* 2000;46:1291–1299.
25. Meeks S, Bova F, Friedman W, et al. IRLED-based patient localization for linac radiosurgery. *Int J Radiat Oncol Biol Phys.* 1998;41:433–439.
26. Ryken T, Meeks S, Pennington E, et al. Initial clinical experience with frameless stereotactic radiosurgery: analysis of accuracy and feasibility. *Int J Radiat Oncol Biol Phys.* 2001;51:1152–1158.
27. Phillips MH, Singer K, Miller E, et al. Commissioning an image-guided localization system for radiotherapy. *Int J Radiat Oncol Biol Phys.* 2000;48(1):267–276.
28. Li L, Leigh J. Quantifying arbitrary magnetic susceptibility distributions with MR. *Magn Reson Med.* 2004;51(5):1077–1082.
29. Wagner TH, Yi T, Meeks SL, et al. A geometrically based method for automated radiosurgery planning. *Int J Radiat Oncol Biol Phys.* 2000;48(5):1599–1611.
30. Wagner TH, Bova FJ, Friedman WA, et al. A simple and reliable index for scoring rival stereotactic radiosurgery plans. *J Radiat Oncol Biol Phys.* 2003;57(4):1141–1149.
31. Barth NH. An inverse problem in radiation oncology. *Int J Radiation Oncology Biol Phys.* 1990;18:425–431.
32. Schell MC, Smith V, Larson DA, et al. Evaluation of radiosurgery techniques with cumulative dose volume histograms in linac-based stereotactic external beam irradiation. *Int J Radiat Oncol Biol Phys.* 1991;20(6):1325–1330.
33. Paddick A. A simple scoring ratio to index the conformity of radiosurgical treatment plans. Technical note. *J Neurosurg.* 2000;93(Suppl 3):219–222.
34. Bolsi A, Fogliata A, Cozzi L. Radiotherapy of small intracranial tumours with different advanced techniques using photon and proton beams: A treatment planning study. *Radiother Oncol.* 2003;68:1–14.
35. Tan J, Olsen L, Moore K. Knowledge-based prediction of plan quality metrics in intracranial stereotactic radiosurgery. *Med Phys.* 2015;42(2):908–917.
36. Ma L, Sahgal A, Larson DA, et al. Impact of millimeter-level margins on peripheral normal brain sparing for gamma knife radiosurgery. *Int J Radiat Oncol Biol Phys.* 2014;89:206–213.
37. Schell M, Bova F, Larson D, et al. *"TG-42 Report on stereotactic external beam irradiation. AAPM Report No. 54." Stereotactic Radiosurgery.* American Association of Physicists in Medicine. College Park: AAPM; 1995.
38. ICRU, 6. *ICRU Report 62. Prescribing, recording, and reporting photon beam therapy.* International Commission on Radiation Units and Measurements. Bethesda, MD: ICRU;1999.
39. Lindquist C. Gamma knife radiosurgery. *Semin Radiat Oncol.* 1995;5(3):197–202.
40. Betti OO, Galmarini D, Derechinsky V. Radiosurgery with a linear accelerator: methodological aspects. *Stereotact Funct Neurosurg.* 1999;57(1–2):87–98.
41. Colombo F, Benedetti A, Pozza F. Stereotactic radiosurgery utilizing a linear accelerator. *Appl Neurophysiol.* 1985;48(1–6):133–145.
42. Lutz W, Winston KR, Maleki N. A system for stereotactic radiosurgery with a linear accelerator. *Int J Radiat Oncol Biol Phys.* 1988;14(2):373–381.
43. Rice RK, Hansen JL, Svensson GK, et al. Measurements of dose distributions in small beams of 6 MV X-rays. *Phys Med Biol.* 1987;32(9):1087–1099.

28 Stereotactic Ablative Radiotherapy

Mu-Han Lin, Andrew Godley, and Robert D. Timmerman

INTRODUCTION

Stereotactic ablative radiotherapy (SAbR), also known as stereotactic body radiation therapy (SBRT), which delivers punishing potent radiotherapy dose to achieve tumor control, has been established over the past few decades as a highly effective local therapy for a wide variety of tumor sites and indications. SAbR requires accurate targeting, effective immobilization, and tumor motion management to deliver an ablative dose to tumors in a few fractions (typically less than 5), while sparing surrounding normal tissues via a steep dose gradient outside the target. SAbR can be performed on a variety of radiation delivery platforms provided the required mechanical accuracy can be achieved and the system has the appropriate image guidance for the disease sites that will be treated. The latter feature is deemed "geometric avoidance" and constitutes a powerful example of targeted therapy in oncology. SAbR has become the standard of care for certain patient populations, including common indications such as inoperable early stage lung cancer, inoperable liver metastases, inoperable primary liver cancer, lung metastases, breast cancer, and prostate cancer. SAbR is a larger and more diverse extension of cranial stereotactic radiosurgery (SRS) and has many of the same characteristics, including a heterogeneous dose inside the tumor, sharp dose gradients outside the tumor, highly effective patient immobilization, and the use of many beams. Since the first publications outside the brain for spine by Hamilton[1] and the seminal publications of Lax and Blomgren et al.[2,3] describing extracranial stereotactic irradiation using a linear accelerator in the mid-1990s, thousands of publications related to SAbR have appeared on PubMed searches, indicating the intense interest in and rapid adoption of this evolving therapy. While the early SAbR treatments made use of an external stereotactic coordinate system, which was usually embedded in a body frame similar to intracranial SRS, the advancement and improvement of in-room imaging has made the need for a stereotactic coordinate system less common (Fig. 28.1).

Similar to surgical resection, SAbR has blossomed into a well-established therapy for localized gross disease and is considered standard of care for some disease subsites, thanks to impressive local control results. SAbR is being investigated as a potential therapy in an increasing number of disease sites and patient populations. Techniques to optimize this therapy are still being explored. This chapter guides the reader through many aspects of SAbR conduct, including patient simulation, quality assurance, and treatment planning. Recent clinical results for a variety of disease sites will be briefly summarized.

RATIONALE AND GOALS

Historically, radiation therapy has been fractionated because spreading out a large dose over many treatments is better tolerated by normal tissue by allowing time for damaged cells to repair. Until recently, fractionation of radiation therapy was the only way to give tumoricidal doses to deep-seated tumors with the available technology. The disadvantage of fractionation is that tumor cells also can repair and repopulate over a protracted course of therapy. The underlying reason for the success of SAbR is still the subject of much debate. Postulations of a "new biology" have taken root whereas others have made the case for increased cell kill using the fractionation era modeling, for example, due to an increased biological equivalent dose (BED).[4-7] Beyond direct tumor cell effects, the hypothesis is that devascularization, which is greater with SAbR, leads to indirect cell death. Furthermore, it has been shown that extensive tumor cell death can lead to an immune response which may promote further cell death.[8] While the linear-quadratic (LQ) model is clearly ill-suited for the ablative dose range, modifications to the LQ model have been proposed and occasionally demonstrate utility for both SAbR-range ablative and hypo-fractionated treatment regimens.[9] But in the end, it is the clinical results that best support the use of SAbR.

The initiation of an antitumor immune response as a result of focal irradiation is particularly exciting, increasing the role SAbR could play in therapy for patients with widespread metastatic disease. Certainly systemic therapy has struggled to eradicate gross deposits of cancer providing a strong rationale for ablative local therapy. There are mostly isolated reports of an abscopal effect

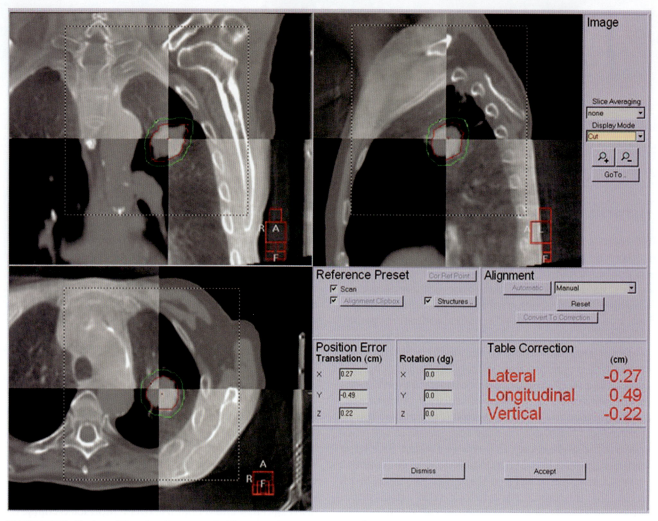

FIGURE 28.1. Fusion of the planning computed tomography scan to a cone beam computed tomography scan acquired on the treatment machine allows for accurate repositioning of lung targets.

in patients with metastatic melanoma treated with local radiotherapy.[10,11] In a recent case reported in the New England Journal of Medicine, a patient was treated to a para-spinous lesion to 28.5 Gy in 3 fractions while tumors in the hilum and the spleen were not treated with radiation. The patient also received ipilimumab, a monoclonal antibody. The untreated tumors underwent a partial response 3 months after radiotherapy and the response was durable out to 9 months post-radiation. The combination of SAbR and immunotherapy may prove to be a novel application of this highly focused form of radiation therapy and this application will certainly be studied extensively in the coming years.

SAbR has been made possible by technological advances such as 3D treatment planning, tumor motion assessment and visualization, highly accurate dose calculation algorithms, and in-room image guidance. The goal of delivering an ablative dose to non-cranial lesions while sparing nearby normal tissues was not possible previously. Due to the technological advances and impressive clinical results, SAbR has rapidly become an important tool for clinicians and patients in their fight against cancer.

SIMULATION

The SAbR process starts with patient simulation, which includes several key elements that will determine the success of the course of therapy. Those elements include patient (target) immobilization, motion management, and accurate patient imaging. The first aspect of the patient simulation that must be optimized is patient immobilization. Patients must be immobilized in an effort to minimize voluntary motion. But the method used must be comfortable and reproducible to also minimize involuntary motion. Various methods of immobilization have been shown to be effective. Body frames,[12,13] vacuum fixation,[14] and alpha-cradles[15] have all been used successfully for patient immobilization during SAbR. The main goal of patient immobilization is to ensure that the patient is in a reproducible "state" at the simulation and subsequently, in the same state at each treatment. Patient immobilization aids typically consist of a custom-formed cushion that molds closely to the patient surface (Fig. 28.2).

In most cases, the arms are positioned over the patient's head and must also be supported by a custom-formed

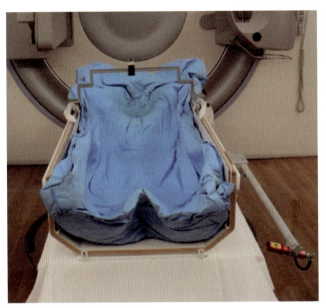

FIGURE 28.2. The vacuum cushion and the stereotactic body frame used for SBRT patient immobilization at UT Southwestern.

cushion. If possible, the patient should be supported on three sides to increase surface contact, with a molded cushion formed beneath and along the sides of the patient. Increased surface contact distributes the patient's weight and relieves pressure points that would otherwise confound set-up accuracy. Poor design of patient immobilization aids can cause the patient discomfort and it may be difficult for them to remain still for the long treatment times that accompany SAbR. In the end, effective immobilization can allow smaller planning target volume (PTV) margins at the time of planning, thus reducing the amount of normal tissue receiving a high dose.

At the time of simulation, the target motion must be assessed for patients receiving treatment to the lung or abdomen. For tumors in these locations, motion due to respiration can be as large as several centimeters and must be minimized or accounted for. Motion assessment can be in the form of fluoroscopy, 4 dimensional computed tomography (4DCT) or cine magnetic resonance imaging (MRI). Motion assessment provides the clinician with information about how the tumor moves (period, amplitude, direction, regularity) and should guide the use of motion management. The goal of the motion management should be to reduce the motion envelop around the GTV to ideally no more than 5 mm larger than the gross tumor volume (GTV) itself in any one direction. As with patient immobilization, there are several strategies available for motion management, including abdominal compression,[12,14] breath hold,[16,17] gating,[18] and tumor tracking.[19,20] Abdominal compression is the simplest method for motion management, utilizing a compression plate or belt to encourage chest wall breathing. Unlike more routine diaphragmatic breathing, chest wall breathing results in more limited intra-thoracic and intra-abdominal target motion. Chest wall breathing utilizes

the accessory muscles of respiration (e.g., intercostal and scalene) to provide lung inflationary force.[22] At UT Southwestern, tumor motion is assessed via fluoroscopy or mini 4DCT encompassing the tumor area before the regular planning computed tomography (CT) to determine if compression is necessary. Our current threshold for using compression is tumor motion more than 1 cm in the superior–inferior direction. A potential disadvantage of compression, patient discomfort, can be alleviated by proper coaching. If compression is to be used, the patient must be both simulated and treated with the compression applied.

Breathhold has been used successfully for limiting respiratory motion. Patients take a deep breath and hold it ideally assisted with a device that reliably measures a stable tidal volume and prevents expiration for a short period of time. Patients receive training at the time of simulation. The patient is treated only during the time they are holding their breath and the breathholds typically last for 15 to 30 seconds, depending on the patient's tolerance. Patients with poor lung function are not good candidates for breathhold techniques because they are unable to hold their breath for a significant length of time. In addition, breathhold significantly increases the overall length of treatment potentially reducing set-up accuracy.

Another method for motion management is to gate the delivery of the radiation so that the beam is delivered only during specific parts of the patient's respiratory cycle. Gating thresholds are determined during treatment planning and the beam is only on when the tumor is inside the gating limits. The tumor motion is typically accessed via its external surrogate. A recent advancement of MRI guided linac offers direct tumor motion assessment via real time cine MR images during the treatment.[23,24] The gating can be performed manually or can be interfaced with the accelerator, allowing automated gating. As with breathhold, the major disadvantage of beam gating is that it has a low duty cycle and increases treatment times. Another concern is the validity of the correlation between tumor and surrogate motion.

The final method for motion management, tumor tracking, is technically more challenging and is not currently a widely used technique.[25] Currently available tracking methods correlate the internal tumor motion and external surrogate motion[25–27] and adapt treatment delivery in real time. It has advantages over the other techniques in that it is not uncomfortable for the patient and does not require the beam to turn off during delivery. Currently available tracking methods track either an external tumor surrogate or markers implanted in or near the tumor to create a motion model of tumor position over time. The accuracy of this model is critical to the success of the method.

Accurate patient imaging is a great enabler for SAbR treatment planning and treatments. Considering the small fields, sharp dose gradients, and high doses characteristic of SAbR, the geometric and density information acquired with the simulation CT must be accurate. Scan length should be sufficient to include any potential organs at risk and the entrance point of all non-coplanar beams. Importantly, external contours extending 15 to 20 cm above and below the center of all targets should be acquired to insure accurate modeling of both entry and exit of all beams used for treatment. For accurate contouring of small lesions, CT slice thickness less than 3 mm is recommended. 4DCT is recommended for imaging moving tumors and organs in order to account for residual motion despite motion management techniques. 4D scans can be reconstructed into minimum, maximum, and average intensity projection data sets. The maximum intensity projections (MIP) reconstruction is useful for contouring the internal target volume (ITV) for targets within low-density lung because it provides the motion envelope for the tumor. The 0% and 50% phase reconstructions represent the limits of respiration and can be used to help determine the craniocaudal limits of the ITV. These images are particularly useful if tumor abuts denser normal tissue that would be consolidated on the MIP. The minimum intensity projections (MinIP) reconstruction can be used when contouring the ITV for liver tumors because those lesions are often less dense than the surrounding liver. Since actual treatments are long compared to the planning scan acquisition time, the average data set is used for dose calculation and as the reference for the conebeam CT (CBCT) localizations at the time of treatment.

Additional imaging modalities may be required to accurately delineate the tumor for certain disease sites. For example, tumors in the liver and spine will be easier to contour on MRI than on CT and MRI allows the spinal cord itself to be contoured, as opposed to the entire spinal canal. Additional imaging that will be fused with the treatment planning CT should be acquired in treatment position to allow for more accurate fusion and contouring. Positron emission tomography (PET) is currently used less often during treatment planning for SAbR due to motion artifacts that obscure the tumor size and location, but is frequently used for evaluation of post-therapy response. Any registration between a secondary image set and the planning CT must be evaluated for accuracy before contouring begins.

TREATMENT PLANNING AND DOSIMETRY

One of the most important steps in treatment planning is contouring of targets and critical structures. In general, any internal critical structure that is within 10 cm of the target should be contoured to help obtain accurate dose to these structures from the planning system. The PTV is determined based on the motion management used for treatment and the intra- and interfractional setup uncertainties as illustrated in Figure 28.3. The ITV accounts for the residual motion. The PTV expands on the ITV to account for daily setup, contouring and tumor changes.

An example of lung case contouring at UT Southwestern Medical Center follows:

1. ITV: Contoured by the physician using the MIP (or MinIP for liver tumors), 0%, and 50% (when requested). Represents the envelope of motion of the GTV. Isocenter is placed in the geometric center of the ITV for planning.
2. PTV: 5 mm expansion around ITV in all dimensions.
3. Proximal bronchial tree: The most inferior 2 cm of the distal trachea as well as the bilateral proximal airways.
4. Proximal trachea: Contoured beginning 2 cm above the carina and extends 10 cm superior to the PTV.
5. Spinal cord: Contoured based on the bony limits of the spinal canal and extends at least 10 cm above and below the PTV.
6. Esophagus: Contoured at least 10 cm superior and inferior to the PTV.
7. Heart: Contoured along with pericardial sac. The superior aspect begins at the aorta-pulmonary window and extends inferiorly to the apex.
8. Total lung: Contoured to include both lungs subtracting out the ITV.
9. PTV + 2 cm: PTV expanded by 2 cm in all dimensions (uniform expansion)
10. Body: Contoured as the patient's body at least 10 cm superior and inferior to the PTV.
11. Body–PTV + 2 cm: The PTV + 2 cm will be subtracted from the outer contour (body) and is used to

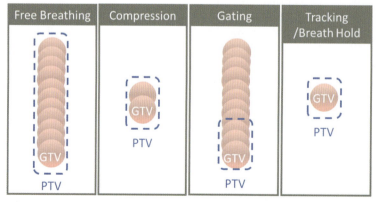

FIGURE 28.3. PTVs for various motion management methods including free breathing, compression, gating, tracking, and breath hold.

evaluate dose fall-off 2 cm in every dimension of the PTV ($D_{2\,cm}$).

12. Brachial plexus: Contoured from the spinal nerves exiting from C5 to T2. This contour extends along the subclavian and axillary vessels to the level of the second rib.

13. Skin ring: Contoured to evaluate the skin dose and is a 0.5 cm ring inside body.

14. Ribs: Contoured as all ribs in close proximity to PTV.

The goal of SAbR planning is to achieve highly conformal high dose volume to the PTV, a very compact intermediate dose region, and rapid isotropic dose fall-off outside the target volume, which can be achieved by using many non-coplanar non-overlapping beams.[28] There are several delivery techniques that can be used in SAbR treatment planning and the choice of technique often depends on an individual patient's tumor location and magnitude of motion, but the most reliable method for SABR is 3D conformal. The use of intensity modulated radiation therapy (IMRT) or volumetric modulated arc therapy (VMAT) for SAbR is typically reserved for tumors that exhibit limited motion and when intensity modulation is necessary for concave targets or critical structure sparing, such as spine lesions and prostate lesions. Static fields (3D and IMRT) and arc (3D conformal arc and VMAT) techniques both offer conformal high dose volume. Dose contribution from many, typically non-coplanar beams is the key to achieve isotropic high and intermediate rapid dose fall-off outside the tumor volume, which is crucial to avoid toxicity. More isotropic rather than polarized fall-off may also better kill potential invisible microscopic

tentacles around the tumor and improve the tumor control. Unfortunately, with current linac configurations, non-coplanar arcs are collision-prone and have less flexibility to utilize the non-coplanar angle in the 4π solid angle space compared to the static beam arrangements. Therefore, arcs are more suitable for the lesions with anatomy boundary or tumor barrier in the superior and inferior directions, such as prostate and spine, preventing microscopic spread in these directions. The static fields offer more flexibility in non-coplanar beam arrangement for SBRT planning. The drawback, longer treatment time for multiple couch rotations, is often well worth the cost.

The 3D conformal beam arrangement for right and left-sided lung lesions are shown in Figure 28.4 and the gantry and couch angles for right and left lung SAbR treatments are found in Table 28.1. The non-coplanar beams are conventionally manually selected, which can be tedious and collision-prone. Dong et al. proposed automatic beam orientation optimization to select the optimal beam arrangement from 1,162 non-coplanar isocentric beams throughout the entire 4π solid angle space to improve the dose conformality and dose fall-off.[29,30]

The intermediate dose is the most challenging aspect of SAbR treatment planning and achieving this compactness separates a good plan from a bad plan because the intermediate dose is responsible for most normal tissue toxicity. radiation therapy oncology group (RTOG) 0236 specified a maximum dose at 2 cm outside the PTV($D_{2\,cm}$) and a ratio of the 50% isodose volume to the PTV volume ($R_{50\%}$) and on average 10 beams were required to meet these compactness constraints.[31] There was no relationship found

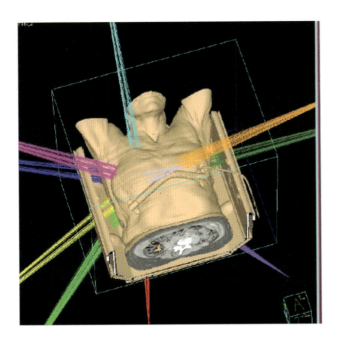

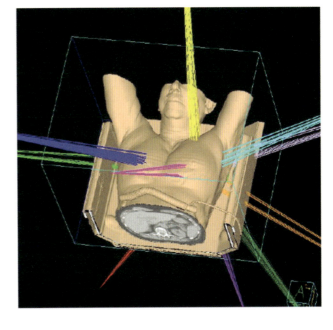

Right Sided Angles   Left Sided Angles

FIGURE 28.4. Reconstructed simulation computed tomography of a lung patient showing the use of non-coplanar beams for left side and right side lesions.

TABLE 28.1 Stereotactic Body Radiation Therapy Couch and Gantry Angles for Right- and Left-Sided Lung Lesions			
Right lung		**Left lung**	
Couch angle	Gantry angle	Couch angle	Gantry angle
0	180	0	210
10	220	0	270
345	270	15	315
15	270	90	30
0	315	90	330
90	30	0	50
90	330	15	90
345	45	345	90
0	90	350	160
0	150	0	180

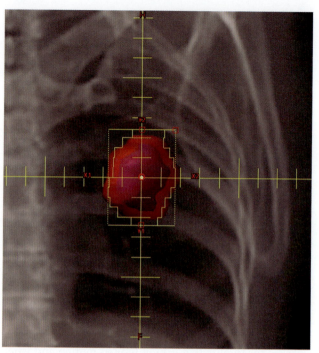

FIGURE 28.5. Beams eye view for a lung stereotactic body radiation therapy 3D conformal multileaf collimator aperture. The aperture is 2 mm smaller than the PTV in the radial direction and 2 mm larger in the superior–inferior directions.

between PTV size and number of beams needed. Due to the large number of beams, SAbR dose distributions are also characterized by a large low-dose region. However, given that nearly all radiation dose response effects follow a sigmoid relationship, large low-dose exposure below the threshold for toxicity is a reasonable tradeoff for limiting high and intermediate dose.

In addition to the number and arrangement of the beams, the beam apertures can be made smaller than the PTV to reduce the volume of normal tissue treated. At our institution, the Multileaf collimator (MLC) aperture is 2 mm smaller in the radial direction and 2 mm larger in the superior–inferior directions, as shown in Figure 28.5.

The dose distribution within the PTV will be highly heterogeneous and the edges of the PTV will likely be underdosed if "negative margins" are used. To cover 95% of the PTV with the prescription isodose line, the plan will be normalized to the 60% to 90% (usually around 80%) isodose line, resulting in a large hot spot in the tumor. The planner must balance the need for a conformal dose distribution with the mechanical limitations of the radiation delivery equipment and treatment delivery efficiency. Beam weighting is chosen to be ideally even between beams so that dose fall-off is isotropic unless an adjacent organ at risk makes isotropic fall-off undesirable.

Figure 28.6 shows the dose distributions of 3D conformal, coplanar VMAT, and non-coplanar VMAT plans for a lung SBRT case. The 3D plan features a conformal distribution in the high and the intermediate dose volumes, as well as a sharp dose fall-off from 90% to 50% isodose curves. While the coplanar VMAT plan offers a fairly conformal high dose volume, the dose contribution from the numerous coplanar beams polarizes the intermediate dose laterally and broadens dose fall-off. Non-coplanar setting

can be used to replicate the intermediate dose distribution in the 3D plan. However, with the nature of beam modulation increasing scatter from adjacent fields/aperture, the dose distribution of non-coplanar VMAT is not as compact as non-coplanar 3D plan. As shown by the 75% and 50% isodose curves, the non-coplanar VMAT improves the intermediate dose conformality. But, the 75% isodose curve is not as compact as the one in the 3D plan. The R50 and the $D_{2\,cm}$ are able to flag this intermediate dose difference. The R50 is a quantitative measure of 50% isodose volume, but, it does not consider the spatial dose distribution while the $D_{2\,cm}$ can pick up the dose spill of the intermediate dose volume and compensate R50 evaluation. In our example, the 3D plan resulted in the best R50 and $D_{2\,cm}$ and the two VMAT plans resulted in identical R50, but, the $D_{2\,cm}$ implies the intermediate dose conformality is better in the non-coplanar VMAT. As a summary, 3D is the preferred technique for SBRT while IMRT/VMAT can be considered when the target is in proximity to organ at risk (OAR) and can't meet the planning goal with 3D.

Beam energies used for lung SAbR plans are typically 6 MV and no higher than 10 MV for beams that must traverse more than 10 cm of tissue. Lower energy beams have a sharper penumbra, which is especially important in the low-density lung and for the small fields used for SAbR due to the lateral electron disequilibrium.[32] Higher energy beams can be used for targets in the liver, prostate, and spine, where tumors and the surrounding tissues are of similar density. Flattening filter free (FFF) beams have been shown to decrease treatment times with the efficiency improvements most significant for larger doses per

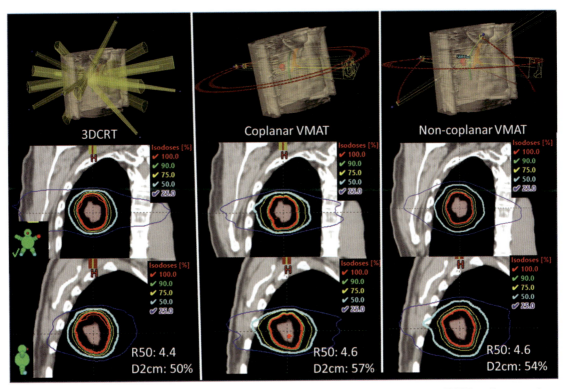

FIGURE 28.6. Dose distribution comparison among non-coplanar 3D conformal, coplanar VMAT, and non-coplanar VMAT for a lung stereotactic ablative radiotherapy case. All three techniques result in clinically acceptable plan quality, however, 3D conformal technique features the sharpest dose fall-off and most conformal intermediate dose bath.

fraction, such as those delivered with SAbR.[33–36] By removing the flattening filter, there is much less attenuation of the beam between the target and the patient and dose rates as high as 2,400 cGy per minute at d_{max} can be achieved. These beams are also more peaked and softer (lower average beam energy) than their flattened counterparts.

When planning lung SAbR, accurate heterogeneity corrections in the planning system become extremely important. An analysis of patients treated on RTOG 0236, which required homogenous calculations, found that the true delivered dose was approximately 10% lower than the homogeneous dose.[31] Task Group 101 from the American Association of Physicists in Medicine (AAPM) recommends against using pencil beam algorithms for lung SAbR planning because of the over-prediction of the dose in low-density tissues.[37] More sophisticated heterogeneity corrections, such as superposition/convolution algorithms (analytical anisotropic algorithm and collapsed cone convolution), principle based algorithms (e.g., Acuros XB), and Monte Carlo method should be used for SBRT dose calculation to properly handle the heterogeneity.[38–40]

Plan evaluation is a critical component of SAbR planning and all contours should be reviewed by the radiation oncologist to ensure that the contours are accurate and that dose being reported to critical structures as well as the PTVs meet expectations. Chapter 2 contains updated normal tissue constraints for 1-, 3-, and 5-fraction SAbR regimens used at University of Texas Southwestern (UTSW). The spinal cord and brachial plexus constraints take priority and are met, even if it requires the tumor to be underdosed. Occasionally, the brachial plexus constraint can be exceeded if informed consent is given by the patient. As mentioned previously, 95% of the PTV should be covered by the prescription dose and 99% of the PTV should be covered by 90% of the prescribed dose. Hot spots should ideally be inside the PTV, but any volume receiving 105% of the prescription dose should be no larger than 15% of the PTV volume. Guidelines for the use of $D_{2\,cm}$ and $R_{50\%}$, which are used to evaluate the compactness of the intermediate dose, can be found in the RTOG guidelines (www.rtog.org). The conformality of the prescription dose can be determined by calculating the ratio of the volume covered by the prescription dose to the volume of the PTV. Ideally, this ratio will be close to 1.

The critical volume dose is also an important tool in plan evaluation for parallel tissues, such as the liver and lung. The critical volume represents the volume of an organ that must be spared from toxic dose in order to maintain organ function. Here, toxic dose is beyond the threshold of the tissue's sigmoid dose response curve (effect as a function of dose). For lung, this threshold dose is around 20 Gy for conventional fractionation and around 12 to 13 Gy for 5 fractions (Chapter 2). In these tissues, the amount of tissue damaged or the severity of the damage is not as important as the remaining functional volume. Evaluating a parallel structure to determine if the critical volume is respected is illustrated in Figure 28.7. By definition, critical volume max dose is an absolute volume

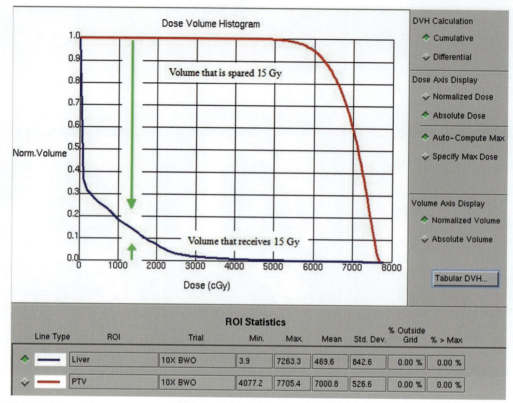

FIGURE 28.7. DVH showing the concept of the critical volume maximum, which is the volume of an organ that must be spared to avoid dysfunction.

COMMISSIONING AND QUALITY ASSURANCE

of an organ that is spared a specific dose in order to avoid an endpoint effect.[41] Dose–volume constraints for parallel organs can be found in Chapter 2.

COMMISSIONING AND QUALITY ASSURANCE

The safe and accurate delivery of SAbR would not be possible without the technology that has been developed over the last several decades. The quality assurance activities of the medical physicist ensure that this advanced technology is functioning properly and is instrumental in ensuring the success of a SAbR program. Initially, the physicist will be responsible for commissioning new equipment that will be used for SAbR, such as immobilization devices, planning systems and linear accelerators. If existing equipment will be used, the medical physicist should evaluate its suitability for use in SAbR. AAPM Task Group 142 provides test tolerances for linacs that will be used for SAbR.[42] As expected, mechanical tolerances for these linacs are stricter than those that will be used for conventional treatments. Planning systems must be commissioned to accurately calculate dose distributions and monitor units for small fields in heterogeneous tissues. Errors made in commissioning of small fields, in particular measuring output factors, have led to serious overdoses.[43,44] Guidance for small field measurements

is provided in AAPM Task Group 101[37] and an average set of small field output factors has been published by the Imaging and Radiation Oncology Core (IROC), formerly the Radiological Physics Center, for several linac models.[45,46] Institutions can compare their measurements to the radiological physics center (RPC) dataset to ensure that there are no major errors in their data. End to end tests using anthropomorphic phantoms, such as those available from the IROC quality assurance centers (Fig. 28.8) for institutions participating in clinical trials, can provide an independent evaluation of the entire SAbR process, including the simulation, treatment planning, image guidance, and delivery. Resulting uncertainties can be used to set the PTV expansions needed to cover targets reliably. End to end testing should be performed before commencing a SAbR program, annually, and after any change to the process to reduce systematic errors and deviations from the normal processes.

Pretreatment quality assurance (QA) is an important component of the treatment process, which aids the physicist to identify any issues associated with the plan design, dose calculation or delivery system. Typically delivered dose is measured in a phantom or reconstructed from the MLC positions recorded during the QA delivery. The use of small fields in SAbR techniques requires high spatial resolution devices for their measurement. The tolerance and action levels of the pretreatment QA should be determined based on the measurement uncertainties of

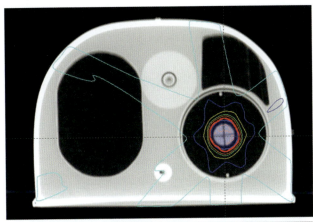

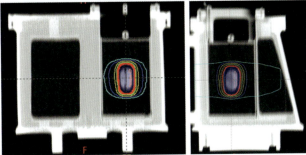

FIGURE 28.8. Lung phantom for the end to end test of stereotactic ablative radiotherapy credentialing process provided by Imaging and Radiation Oncology Core.

the device and the measurement workflow. AAPM task group 218 provides the comprehensive review and recommendation of various measurement devices, dose analysis methods and tolerance limits that can be utilized to establish the pretreatment QA process.[47] These practices should be applied to measure 3D conformal SAbR plans pretreatment as well.

The physicist will also be responsible for developing the patient-specific checks to ensure that the entire process is performed as planned. Items in the SAbR process that should be part of the patient specific checks include verification that normal tissue constraints are met, that the treatment planning and patient positioning parameters have been independently verified, the correct patient is treated, and that the correct dose has been delivered.

AAPM published a comprehensive practice guideline on the medical physics support for the linac-based SRS–SBRT and summarized the medical physicist's role and responsibility from staff training to commissioning, clinical practice, and periodic QA.[48] Guidelines for implementing a safe and high-quality SAbR program can be found in the white paper[49] endorsed by the American Society for Radiation Oncology, AAPM, the American Society of Radiologic Technologists, and the American Association of Medical Dosimetrists. This white paper also includes recommendations on personnel, training and technology requirements and provides example checklists and forms that can be amended for use according to the individual institution's needs.

LUNG CANCER

More than 25% of all cancer deaths every year can be attributed to lung cancer, making it the leading cause of cancer related death in the United States.[50] Lung was one of the first sites treated using SAbR[2] and it continues to be the site most frequently treated with this technique.[51] Clinical use of lung SAbR has increased in the last several years, with more than half of surveyed radiation oncologists reporting that they began using SAbR after 2008.[51] The most common reported fractionation scheme was 18 to 20 Gy × 3 (43%), likely due to the success of RTOG 0236, which showed a 3-year primary tumor control rate of 98% and overall survival (OS) of 56%[52] in medically inoperable patients with early stage non-small cell lung cancer (NSCLC). The long-term results from the trial found rates for 5 year primary tumor control and OS to be 93% and 40%, respectively.[53,54] Excess late toxicities have not been observed, dispelling fears of such late toxicities with hypofractionation. Results from RTOG 0236 and similar results from other countries have cemented SAbR as the standard of care for medically inoperable early stage NSCLC.

Optimal regimens for centrally located tumors continue to be an area of active investigation (Fig. 28.9). RTOG 0813, a phase I/II trial to determine the maximal tolerated dose for central lung tumors in a 5-fraction regimen recently closed after meeting the accrual goal. Efficacy of SAbR for controlling centrally located tumors has been shown to be nearly equivalent to control of peripheral tumors,[55–57] demonstrating that SAbR is indicated for these tumors when appropriate fractionation schemes are used.

For patients who are medically operable and treated with 54 Gy in 3 fractions, RTOG 0618 found that 2-year progression-free survival and OS were 65.4% and 84.4%, respectively.[58] Only four patients on the trial experienced treatment related grade 3 adverse events while no patients had grade 4 to 5 toxicity. A multi-center, multi-national phase III trial comparing this RTOG 0618 regimen to standard surgery for high-risk operable patients has enrolled >150 patients by this writing. Likewise, a 400+ Veterans Administration phase III trial (VALOR) in the US comparing surgery to SAbR is enrolling well for average-risk operable patients. These trials will be crucial for finding the proper place of SAbR for a wide spectrum of patients with this deadly disease.

In addition to stage I patients, use of SAbR is being expanded to other patient populations who historically did not receive radiation therapy or received no therapy at all. Results from a phase II trial investigating SAbR and erlotinib for patients with metastatic (stage IV) NSCLC who progressed after chemotherapy were recently published.[59] Patients with fewer than six metastatic extracranial lesions were treated to all sites of disease with SAbR to a modest tumor debulking equivalent dose. With median follow-up of 16.8 months, progression-free survival was

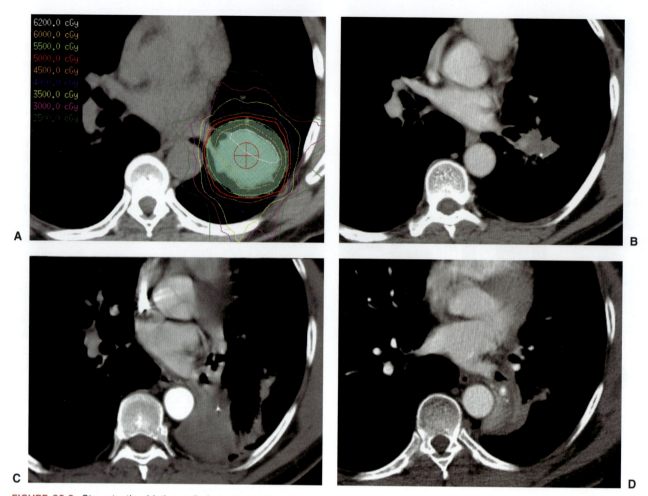

FIGURE 28.9. Stereotactic ablative radiotherapy of a central lung tumor treated on protocol. Panel A shows the isodose plan. While follow-up scans are shown at 3 months, 6 months, and 1 year in panels B–D, respectively. There was an excellent initial response with eventual collapse of the downstream lung.

14.7 months and OS was 20.4 months, both superior to patients historically treated with systemic therapy alone. The pattern of failure also changed, from predominantly existing sites to new sites. This data along with a similar randomized phase II trial from MD Anderson[60] form the basis for a large ongoing phase III trial sponsored by the NRG (LU001) adding SAbR to standard of care systemic therapy for patients with newly diagnosed metastatic lung cancer that will complete enrollment soon.

LIVER METASTASES

Approximately 150,000 Americans are diagnosed with colorectal cancer annually, making it the third most common cancer diagnosed.[61] Approximately one-third of these patients die from the disease, with liver metastases a leading cause of death.[62,63] The liver receives nutrient rich blood from the digestive system (stomach, intestines, spleen, and pancreas) via the portal vein, making it a common site for trafficking and growth of metastases from gastrointestinal cancers. Other primary cancers including lung, breast, and melanoma also frequently metastasize to the liver. Surgery is the treatment of choice because it offers the most established chance of long-term survival. However, despite advances in surgical techniques, only 10% to 25% of patients have metastases that are considered resectable due to existing liver disease, number and size of the lesions, liver damage from chemotherapy, and location of the metastases within the liver as well as coexisting patient medical comorbidities.[64,65] As a result, there is great interest in minimally invasive ablation technologies to include radiofrequency ablation (RFA), cryosurgery, and laser-induced thermotherapy.[66–72] However, these treatments are all invasive, efficacy rates are dubious, and patients are frequently not eligible for these procedures for various reasons. RFA, a commonly used ablation method, is limited in efficacy by tumor size as well as vascular heat sink effects common in larger tumors.[73] Cryosurgery can cause significant morbidity and has a high local recurrence rate.[74] No studies have shown that any one of these therapies has clear advantages over the others.

Historically, the use of whole or large volume liver radiation therapy has been limited due to the risk of radiation-induced liver disease (RILD), a variably defined condition marked by ascites, rapid weight gain, elevated liver enzyme levels, and anicteric hepatomegaly. Histologically, RILD appears as a form of veno-occlusive disease (VOD)[75,76] with venous congestion of the central portion of the liver lobules. RILD can lead to liver failure. The whole liver tolerance of 30 to 35 Gy is insufficient to achieve reasonable tumor control. In contrast to conventional radiotherapy, SAbR has allowed radiation oncologists to focally target lesions and deliver high doses of radiation very accurately to the tumor while sparing the healthy tissue around it. SAbR provides certain advantages relative to thermal ablations technologies, chief among them the non-invasive nature of the treatment as well as the lack of a heat-sink problem. Several groups have published studies using SAbR for tumors in the liver.[77–85] Overall, SAbR has shown to provide excellent local control for patients with liver metastases with little toxicity including no meaningful observation of RILD. As such, RILD appears more a manifestation of large volume liver irradiation than used for SAbR. However, patients with larger tumors or treated with lower doses have been shown to have worse local control and survival,[79,86,87] particularly for colorectal metastatic histology.

Although prior studies established dose limits for irradiation of the entire liver, dose–volume limits for partial liver irradiation are less well established. Schefter and colleagues from the University of Colorado and Indiana University performed a prospective dose escalation trial where the maximum tolerated dose (MTD) was not found even for the high dose ranges investigated.[88] Patients treated in this study had tumor diameters less than 6 cm and at least 700 mL of normal liver (the presumed critical volume) was restricted to receiving a total dose less than 15 Gy (the presumed tolerated threshold dose). Total dose was escalated to 60 Gy in 3 fractions without any RILD or grade ≥3 dose limiting toxicities. The median gross tumor volume (GTV) was 18 cc and the median planning target volume (PTV) was 41 cc. Phase II results of this trial using the 20 Gy × 3 dose regimen have been encouraging; actuarial local control 2 years after SAbR was 92% and for lesions less than 3 cm in diameter, it was 100%.[84] At UT Southwestern, we have conducted two dose-escalation SAbR liver studies, one using 3 to 5 fractions[85] and another using a single fraction.[89] The multi-fraction trial found that 60 Gy can be safely delivered in 5 fractions as long as normal liver constraints were met and local control rates at 12 and 24 months were both 100%, respectively (Fig. 28.10). The single-fraction study found 40 Gy in a single fraction to be a tolerable dose and at 2.5 years median follow-up, no patients had experienced local progression and 69% of the imaging-evaluable tumors had undergone a complete response. In general, it's been determined that

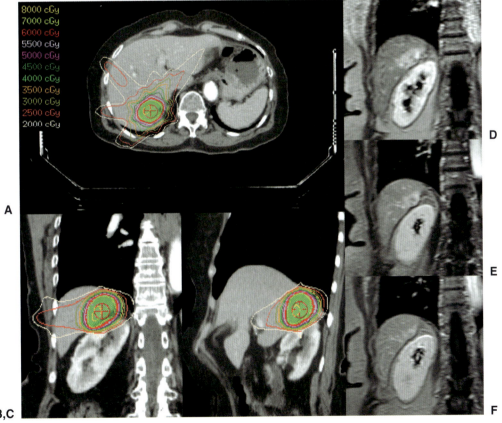

FIGURE 28.10. Axial, coronal, and sagittal isodoses from liver stereotactic ablative radiotherapy treated to 60 Gy are shown in panels A–C, respectively. Panels D–F show 3-month, 6-month, and 1-year follow-up.

local control increases with increased dose, particularly for larger tumors and larger tumors can be treated so long as the critical volume is respected.

Patients with tumors at or near the hilum of the liver (central liver zone) and thus near major vessels, such as the portal vein and hepatic artery as well as large-caliber bile ducts, are ineligible not only for invasive treatments, but are also often excluded from treatment with thermal ablation and single-fraction SAbR courses, including our own phase I single-fraction trial. The tissue at the liver hilum likely has a lower tolerance to ablative radiation doses, similar to that seen in SAbR treatment of central lung tumors.[90] Biliary sclerosis and jaundice requiring stenting have been seen in patients treated with SAbR to the central zone of the liver. A better understanding of the central zone tolerance to ablative radiation doses will be important in order to make this treatment option available for patients with tumors in the central zone of the liver.

HEPATOCELLULAR CARCINOMA

Experience with SAbR for hepatocellular carcinoma (HCC) is certainly more limited than that for liver metastases due to the underlying liver disease that accompanies HCC. Patients with HCC often are not eligible for curative treatments due to disease stage or poor liver function.[91] With an already diseased liver and loss of hepatic reserve, the critical volume spared with SAbR for treatment tolerance must be appropriately adjusted (more liver spared than for a healthy liver). Despite this, SAbR is emerging as a potential definitive therapy or as a bridge to transplant. Researchers from Indiana University published their experience for Child–Turcotte–Pugh (CTP) Class A and B patients treated with median of 44 Gy in 3 fractions and 40 Gy in 5 fractions, respectively.[92] Their median follow-up was 27 months and the 2 year local control, progression-free survival and OS were 90%, 48%, and 67%, respectively. The reported 2 year local control was better than that from a previously reported study,[93] likely due to the larger tumor volumes treated in the earlier study. All ≥grade 3 toxicity was hematologic, but 7 of 36 patients with CTP Class A progressed to CTP Class B and 5 of 24 patients with CTP Class B progressed to CTP Class C. The authors found that pretreatment CTP Class and development of toxicity were related. Another study treated patients with more advanced liver disease to a median dose of 34.4 Gy in 6 fractions.[94] Median survival was 7.9 months and OS at 1 year was 32.3%. During follow-up, no patients experienced progression of irradiated HCC and there were no grade III or higher acute toxicities. In general, studies for SAbR as a definitive treatment for HCC have found that tumor size and liver function should be carefully considered before treating these patients. Hypofractionation is also being explored as a bridge to liver transplants. Radiotherapy can be used

to downsize or stabilize tumors prior to liver transplant. A 10-fraction regimen delivering 50 Gy was found to be very effective with 12 patients receiving liver transplant or resection following irradiation and were alive at a median follow-up of 19.6 months.[95] SAbR appears to be a suitable option to bridge patients scheduled for liver transplant, which shows similar response rates but very modest toxicity profiles as compared to other local treatment options.

SPINE

The spine is a frequent site of metastases from primary cancers of the prostate, lung, breast, and kidney. Spine metastases can cause pain and lead to fractures and spinal cord compression. Historically, spinal metastases have been treated with 30 Gy in 10 fractions for palliation and this dose regimen has provided good pain relief. However, higher dose are needed to provide durable pain and tumor control. There are a variety of fractionation schemes being used including single and multifraction regimens. Figure 28.11 illustrates a spine SAbR plan prescribing 20 Gy in 1 fraction. A recently published study of a 3-fraction regimen with total doses ranging from 27 to 30 Gy found significant reduction in patient reported pain at 6 months post-SAbR, progression-free survival was 80.5% at 1 year and 72.4% at 2 years.[96] A study of spine SAbR for renal cell metastases to a median dose of 24 Gy in 2 fractions found 1-year OS and local control rates of 64% and 83% with oligometastatic disease status a positive prognosticator for OS. The phase II portion of RTOG 0631 demonstrated that spine SAbR/SRS was feasible, safe and could be performed at a high level by a cooperative group.[97] The phase III portion of the trial compared 3 month pain relief and quality of life for patients treated with single fraction 16 to 18 Gy SAbR versus patients treated conventionally with 8 Gy in a single fraction and has yet to be published.

Spine SAbR is being used increasingly in the reirradiation setting for patients who progress through conventional palliative courses,[98] but the optimal dose and fractionation scheme for the reirradiation has been confounded by a poor understanding of the spinal cord tolerance and its ability to repair previous radiation damage. Sahgal et al. analyzed myelopathies that occurred after reirradiation with SAbR and provided guidelines for presumed tolerant SAbR following conventional treatment for spinal metastases. Pre-clinical studies in a large animal model have shown that reirradiation 1 year after a conventional course of radiation therapy had the same ED_{50} for paralysis as those that received single-fraction therapy alone.[99] While animal data may not be directly applicable for human spinal cord tolerance, it can be useful in guiding the development of clinical trials. The most common toxicities following spine SAbR are myelopathy[100] and iatrogenic vertebral compression fracture (VCF)[101,102] and

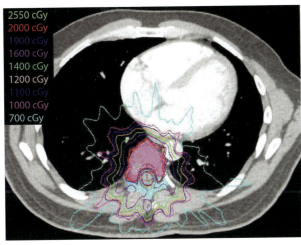 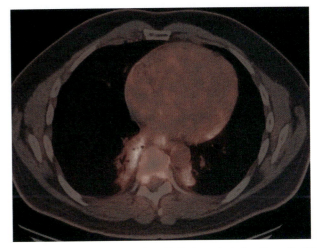

2550 cGy
2000 cGy
1900 cGy
1600 cGy
1400 cGy
1200 cGy
1100 cGy
1000 cGy
700 cGy

A

B

FIGURE 28.11. Panel A shows a stereotactic ablative radiotherapy isodose plan of a patient treated to 20 Gy in a single fraction with IMRT used to create a sharp dose gradient toward the spinal cord. Panel B shows follow-up at 6 weeks with radiation pneumonitis corresponding to the 10 Gy line.

both are associated with higher doses while probability of VCF is also correlated with preexisting tumor-related VCF.[102,103]

PROSTATE

Prostate cancer accounts for 21% of new cancer cases diagnosed in men in the United States and is the second leading cause of cancer-related death in men.[50,104] Prostate cancer is often diagnosed early due to effective screening programs. Prostate cancer is conventionally treated to 79.2 Gy in 40+ fractions with IMRT and image guidance, with the bladder, urethra, erectile tissues and rectum serving as the most important organs at risk. Other options for early stage prostate cancer include watchful waiting, surgery, and brachytherapy. While all options have excellent survival in low-risk disease (Gleason < 7, prostate specific antigen [PSA] < 10), cancer death rates increase with intermediate- and high-risk patients.

SAbR is an attractive option for these patients because it can be delivered in fewer fractions, is non-invasive and has been shown to be more cost-effective than a protracted course of conventional IMRT, provided that outcomes and quality of life are similar,[105] though longer follow-up and more mature data are needed to determine if that is the case. A recent analysis of Medicare beneficiaries treated with SAbR for prostate cancer found more frequent genitourinary (GU) toxicity for patients treated with SAbR when compared to IMRT.[106] However, their retrospective analysis was confounded by a lack of information on grade of toxicity experienced, differences in baseline function, SAbR dose, or treatment technique. In contrast, a multi-institutional report on quality of life after prostate SAbR found that at 3-year median follow-up SAbR is well tolerated and that after a decline shortly following completion of therapy, urinary and gastrointestinal (GI) quality of life returns to baseline and remains

high long term.[107] These patients received a median dose of 36.25 Gy in 4 or 5 fractions. The same group retrospectively reported the clinical outcomes of nearly 1,100 patients treated at eight centers between 2003 and 2011.[108] They reported that with median follow-up of 36 months, 40 patients experienced PSA failure. Their reported 5-year biochemical relapse free survival for Gleason score ≤6, 7, and ≥8 were 95%, 83%, and 78%, respectively and 93% for all patients. Updated follow-up from a multi-institutional phase I/II trial reported excellent PSA control of 99% at median follow-up of 42 months for all patients (phase I and II) and 54 months for patients treated on the 50 Gy arm in the phase I study.[109] To reduce incidental dose to the rectum and rectal toxicity, anatomic modulating devices have been developed to distance the anterior rectum from the prostate. Such a strategy using an injectable rectal spacer has been investigated and implemented for the prostate SAbR. Figure 28.12 shows an example plan for a prostate SAbR patient with rectal spacer. The spacer created about 1 cm extra space allowing the dose to cool down from 100% to 50% of the prescribed dose and effectively reduced the GI and GU toxicity.[110]

PANCREAS

Prognosis for patients diagnosed with pancreatic cancer is extremely poor as it remains the fourth leading cause of cancer-related death in the United States and together with lung cancer, has seen the least improvement in survival over the last three decades.[50] Five-year survival remains below 10%. Surgery is the only potentially curable treatment but unfortunately, very few patients present with resectable disease. Several recently published studies have found that SAbR for locally advanced pancreatic cancer is promising. Potential advantages of SAbR for pancreatic cancer include shorter treatment courses, better local control and earlier start of chemotherapy.

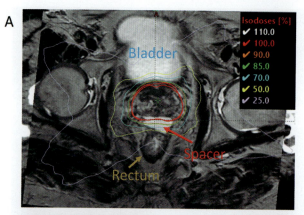

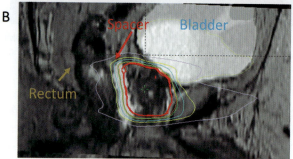

FIGURE 28.12. Representative treatment plan for prostate stereotactic ablative radiotherapy patients treated spacer at the UT Southwestern. The spacer created addition space between the prostate and the rectum and allowed dose to cool off from the prescription dose to a more tolerable dose to the rectum.

In as single institution study, patients were treated with 3 fractions of 8, 10, or 12 Gy, depending on the proximity of the tumor to organs at risk, which was followed 1 month later with 6 months of weekly gemcitabine.[111] With median follow-up of 24 months, local control was 78% and median OS was 14.3 months. Eight percent of patients experienced acute grade 3 toxicities and two patients experienced late toxicity. A multi-institutional trial examined a single fraction of 25 Gy preceded by three cycles of gemcitabine and followed by three to five cycles.[112] All 20 enrolled patients completed SAbR and received a median of five cycles of systemic therapy. No grade 3 or greater nonhematologic acute toxicities were seen and one late Grade 3 toxicity occurred. Median survival was 11.8 months and 1- and 2-year survival was 50% and 20%, respectively.

A single institution retrospective review of locally advanced and borderline resectable patients treated with three cycles of gemcitabine-based chemotherapy followed by SAbR was recently published.[113] SAbR was delivered in 5 consecutive daily fractions to a median dose of 25 to 30 Gy to the GTV and a simultaneous integrated boost of 35 to 50 Gy to the region of vessel abutment/encasement. For the borderline resectable patients, 77.2% underwent an exploratory laparotomy and 56.1% underwent resection, with 96.9% of those resected having negative margins. Two of the locally advanced patients underwent surgical exploration but neither was found to be resectable.

Median OS and 1-year progression-free survival for borderline resectable patients was 16.4 months and 42.8% and for locally advanced patients was 15 months and 41%, respectively. Patients who were resected had significantly better median OS and median progression-free survival compared to all patients who remained unresectable. No acute grade 3 or greater toxicities occurred but four patients experienced late grade 3 adverse events. The effect of SAbR on local control was clearly demonstrated in that 37% of patients had distant failure only, indicating the need for improved systemic therapies for pancreatic cancer. Another multi-institutional phase II trial using a 33 Gy in 5-fraction regimen found 1- and 2-year OS rates of 59% and 18% with low toxicity.[114] Short-term and long-term gastrointestinal toxicity limited the dose escalation of pancreas SAbR. Strategies including increasing the number of fractions in the SAbR, allowing for ablative hotspots to be placed in the hypoxic core in the tumor, prioritizing gastrointestinal tract dose sparing in planning have been recommended to improving the tumor control. Recent advancement of magnetic resonance-guided adaptive radiation therapy (RT) adapting the treatment plan based on daily motion and deformation of the tumor and OAR opens up opportunity to reduce margin and potentially improve the therapeutic ratio.[115]

METASTASES

Patients with metastases are often treated with systemic therapy in an effort to improve survival and quality of life. Systemic therapy is necessary to reach all sites of known metastases and to treat microscopic disease that is assumed to be present. However, certain patients with limited metastatic disease can have excellent long-term outcomes with surgical resection, even without systemic treatment[116] leading many to believe that similar results could be achieved with ablative radiotherapy. Long-term follow-up of a prospective study treating patients with five or fewer metastases from any primary site found 6-year OS and freedom from distant metastasis rates of 20% and 21%, respectively, and approximately one-third of patients survived more than 4 years.[117] Doses were determined by the adjacent organs at risk, with a preferred schedule of 50 Gy in 10 fractions. Patients with metastatic breast cancer experienced significantly better outcomes than those who had metastases from non-breast cancer and non-breast cancer tumor burden was significant for worse OS and local control.

A dose escalation study from the University of Chicago reported 1- and 2-year survival rates of 81.5% and 56.7%, respectively for patients receiving SAbR to one to five metastatic sites.[118] They began with 24 Gy in 3 fractions and escalated 2 Gy per fraction to a total of 60 Gy. They found that patients tolerated this treatment regimen and 27% of patients developed no new metastatic lesions during the reported median follow-up of 20.9 months for all patients and 31.3 months for living patients. A retrospective review of 14 patients with 74 lung metastases from soft-tissue sarcomas treated with SAbR reported excellent 3 year local control of 82% with a preferred treatment scheme of 50 Gy in 5 fractions.[119] The median number of lesions treated per patient was four and the median GTV was 5.1 cc. Excluding a single patient treated with 30 Gy in 3 fractions, the local control rate was 97%. Multiple retrospective series and a prospective trial have shown local control rates >85% at 1 to 2 years for metastatic lesions from renal cell

carcinoma (RCC) and median OS rates of 12 to 51.[120,121] Our institution also demonstrated that SAbR is an effective treatment for patients with oligometastatic RCC. With a median follow-up of 30 months, the 1- and 2-year OS after SAbR were 93.1% and 84.8%, respectively.[122] Dose received by 99% of the target volume was the strongest dosimetric predictor for local control rate.[123] These results are promising, but determining which patients will benefit the most from local ablative therapies is still challenging and better systemic treatments are needed.

KEY POINTS

- SAbR requires optimal patient immobilization, motion management, and accurate targeting to deliver an ablative dose to tumors while sparing surrounding normal tissues.

- The biology of SAbR is not well-understood, but the excellent local tumor control is believed to be a result of vascular damage and abscopal effects are likely a result of an antitumor immune response to massive cancer cell death in the irradiated tumor.

- A successful SAbR program requires careful commissioning and a comprehensive quality assurance program developed by the medical physicist.

- SAbR dose distributions are characterized by a highly conformal but heterogeneous high dose volume, a compact intermediate dose volume and a large low-dose volume.

- Treatment plans should be scrutinized carefully to ensure that the attending physician's goals are being met for organs at risk and targets.

- SAbR is the standard therapy for early stage inoperable lung and liver cancer and lung and liver metastases.

- SAbR is being studied under clinical trials for prostate and pancreatic cancers and for metastatic disease.

QUESTION AND ANSWER

1. According to the RTOG 0236 guidelines, which parameters determine the quality of the dose distribution for a lung SAbR treatment plan?
   A. The mean lung dose
   B. the mean heart dose
   C. $R_{50\%}$ and $D_{2\,cm}$
   D. Tumor BED.

2. Lung tumor motion assessment provides all of the following information except for
   A. Tumor motion amplitude
   B. Tumor size
   C. Tumor motion period
   D. Tumor motion regularity

3. The concept of the critical volume of an organ that must be spared to prevent dysfunction would apply to which pair of organs?
   A. Lung and liver
   B. Lung and spinal cord
   C. Lung and esophagus
   D. Liver and spinal cord

4. In low-density tissues such as the lung, simplistic treatment planning heterogeneity corrections such as the pencil beam algorithm
   A. Under predict the actual delivered dose
   B. Calculate the correct delivered dose
   C. Over-predict the delivered dose
   D. Are recommended by the AAPM Task Group 101

5. Which one of the following treatments is established as standard of care?
   A. SAbR for primary esophageal squamous cancer
   B. SAbR for unresectable mesothelioma.
   C. SAbR for a primary 1 cm lung bronchioalveolar cancer in a healthy Asian woman
   D. SAbR for a primary 2 cm lung adenocarcinoma in a patient with severe emphysema

ANSWERS

1. C
2. B
3. A
4. C
5. D

REFERENCES

1. Hamilton AJ, et al. Preliminary clinical experience with linear accelerator-based spinal stereotactic radiosurgery. *Neurosurgery*. 1995;36(2):311–319.
2. Blomgren H, et al. Stereotactic high dose fraction radiation therapy of extracranial tumors using an accelerator: clinical experience of the first thirty-one patients. *Acta Oncol*. 1995;34(6):861–70.
3. Lax I, et al. Stereotactic radiotherapy of malignancies in the abdomen: methodological aspects. *Acta Oncol*. 1994;33(6):677–83.
4. Brown JM, Carlson DJ, Brenner DJ. The tumor radiobiology of SRS and SBRT: are more than the 5 Rs involved? *Int J Radiat Oncol Biol Phys*. 2014;88(2):254–262.
5. Brown JM, Carlson DJ, Brenner DJ. Dose escalation, not "new biology," can account for the efficacy of stereotactic body radiation therapy with non-small cell lung cancer. In reply to Rao et al. *Int J Radiat Oncol Biol Phys*. 2014;89(3):693–694.
6. Rao SS, et al. Dose escalation, not "new biology," can account for the efficacy of stereotactic body radiation therapy with non-small cell lung cancer. In regard to Brown et al. *Int J Radiat Oncol Biol Phys*. 2014;89(3):692–693.
7. Song CW, et al. Radiobiological basis of SBRT and SRS. *Int J Clin Oncol*. 2014;19(4):570–578.
8. Finkelstein SE, et al. The confluence of stereotactic ablative radiotherapy and tumor immunology. *Clin Dev Immunol*. 2011;2011:439752.
9. Park C, et al. Universal survival curve and single fraction equivalent dose: useful tools in understanding potency of ablative radiotherapy. *Int J Radiat Oncol Biol Phys*. 2008;70(3):847–8452.
10. Postow MA, et al. Immunologic correlates of the abscopal effect in a patient with melanoma. *N Engl J Med*. 2012;366(10):925–931.
11. Stamell EF, et al. The abscopal effect associated with a systemic anti-melanoma immune response. *Int J Radiat Oncol Biol Phys*. 2013;85(2):293–295.
12. Foster R, et al. Localization accuracy and immobilization effectiveness of a stereotactic body frame for a variety of treatment sites. *Int J Radiat Oncol Biol Phys*. 2013;87(5):911–916.
13. Negoro Y, et al. The effectiveness of an immobilization device in conformal radiotherapy for lung tumor: reduction of respiratory tumor movement and evaluation of the daily setup accuracy. *Int J Radiat Oncol Biol Phys*. 2001;50(4):889–898.
14. Han K, et al. A comparison of two immobilization systems for stereotactic body radiation therapy of lung tumors. *Radiother Oncol*. 2010;95(1):103–108.
15. Shah C, et al. Intrafraction variation of mean tumor position during image-guided hypofractionated stereotactic body radiotherapy for lung cancer. *Int J Radiat Oncol Biol Phys*. 2012;82(5):1636–1641.
16. Boda-Heggemann J, et al. Clinical outcome of hypofractionated breath-hold image-guided SABR of primary lung tumors and lung metastases. *Radiat Oncol*. 2014;9:10.
17. Eccles C, et al. Reproducibility of liver position using active breathing coordinator for liver cancer radiotherapy. *Int J Radiat Oncol Biol Phys*. 2006;64(3):751–759.
18. Berbeco RI, et al. Residual motion of lung tumours in gated radiotherapy with external respiratory surrogates. *Phys Med Biol*. 2005;50(16):3655–3667.
19. Falk M, et al. Motion management during IMAT treatment of mobile lung tumors: a comparison of MLC tracking and gated delivery. *Med Phys*. 2014;41(10):101707.
20. Depuydt T, et al. Geometric accuracy of a novel gimbals based radiation therapy tumor tracking system. *Radiother Oncol*. 2011;98(3):365–3672.
21. Hoogeman M, et al. Clinical accuracy of the respiratory tumor tracking system of the cyberknife: assessment by analysis of log files. *Int J Radiat Oncol Biol Phys*. 2009;74(1):297–303.
22. Heinzerling JH, et al. Four-dimensional computed tomography scan analysis of tumor and organ motion at varying levels of abdominal compression during stereotactic treatment of lung and liver. *Int J Radiat Oncol Biol Phys*. 2008;70(5):1571–1578.
23. Menten MJ, Wetscherek A, Fast MF. MRI-guided lung SBRT: present and future developments. *Phys Med*. 2017;44:139–149.
24. Alongi F, et al. 1.5 T MR-guided and daily adapted SBRT for prostate cancer: feasibility, preliminary clinical tolerability, quality of life and patient-reported outcomes during treatment. *Radiat Oncol*. 2020;15(1):69.
25. Keall PJ, et al. The first clinical implementation of electromagnetic transponder-guided MLC tracking. *Med Phys*. 2014;41(2):020702.
26. Kurosu K, et al. Dosimetric and clinical effects of interfraction and intrafraction correlation errors during marker-based real-time tumor tracking for liver SBRT. *J Radiat Res*. 2018;59(2):164–172.
27. Sothmann T, et al. Real time tracking in liver SBRT: comparison of CyberKnife and Vero by planning structure-based gamma-evaluation and dose-area-histograms. *Phys Med Biol*. 2016;61(4):1677–1691.
28. Papiez L, et al. Extracranial stereotactic radioablation: physical principles. *Acta Oncol*. 2003;42(8):882–894.
29. Dong P, et al. 4pi non-coplanar liver SBRT: a novel delivery technique. *Int J Radiat Oncol Biol Phys*. 2013;85(5):1360–1366.
30. Woods K, et al. Viability of non-coplanar VMAT for liver SBRT as compared to coplanar VMAT and beam orientation optimized 4pi IMRT. *Adv Radiat Oncol*. 2016;1(1):67–75.
31. Xiao Y, et al. Dosimetric evaluation of heterogeneity corrections for RTOG 0236: stereotactic body radiotherapy of inoperable stage I-II non-small-cell lung cancer. *Int J Radiat Oncol Biol Phys*. 2009;73(4):1235–1242.
32. Disher B, et al. An in-depth Monte Carlo study of lateral electron disequilibrium for small fields in ultra-low density lung: implications for modern radiation therapy. *Phys Med Biol*. 2012;57(6):1543–1559.
33. Lang S, et al. Clinical application of flattening filter free beams for extracranial stereotactic radiotherapy. *Radiother Oncol*. 2013;106(2):255–259.
34. Ong CL, et al. Fast arc delivery for stereotactic body radiotherapy of vertebral and lung tumors. *Int J Radiat Oncol Biol Phys*. 2012;83(1):e137–e143.
35. Prendergast BM, et al. Flattening filter-free linac improves treatment delivery efficiency in stereotactic body radiation therapy. *J Appl Clin Med Phys*. 2013;14(3):4126.
36. Thomas EM, et al. Effects of flattening filter-free and volumetric-modulated arc therapy delivery on treatment efficiency. *J Appl Clin Med Phys*. 2013;14(6):4328.
37. Benedict SH, et al. Stereotactic body radiation therapy: the report of AAPM Task Group 101. *Med Phys*. 2010;37(8):4078–4101.
38. Aarup LR, et al. The effect of different lung densities on the accuracy of various radiotherapy dose calculation methods: implications for tumour coverage. *Radiother Oncol*. 2009;91(3):405–414.
39. Chen H, et al. Stereotactic, single-dose irradiation of lung tumors: a comparison of absolute dose and dose distribution between pencil beam and Monte Carlo algorithms based on actual patient CT scans. *Int J Radiat Oncol Biol Phys*. 2010;78(3):955–963.
40. Tsuruta Y, et al. Dosimetric comparison of Acuros XB, AAA, and XVMC in stereotactic body radiotherapy for lung cancer. *Med Phys*. 2014;41(8):081715.
41. Ritter TA, et al. Application of critical volume-dose constraints for stereotactic body radiation therapy in NRG radiation therapy trials. *Int J Radiat Oncol Biol Phys*. 2017;98(1):34–36.
42. Klein EE, et al. Task Group 142 report: quality assurance of medical accelerators. *Med Phys*. 2009;36(9):4197–4212.
43. Borius PY, et al. Dosimetric stereotactic radiosurgical accident: study of 33 patients treated for brain metastases. *Neurochirurgie*. 2010;56(5):368–373.
44. Derreumaux S, et al. Lessons from recent accidents in radiation therapy in France. *Radiat Prot Dosimetry*. 2008;131(1):130–135.
45. Followill DS, Kry S. Response to Thomsen et al.: comments on "The Radiological Physics Center's standard dataset for small field size output factors." *J Appl Clin Med Phys*. 2014;15(2):4841.
46. Followill DS, et al. The Radiological Physics Center's standard dataset for small field size output factors. *J Appl Clin Med Phys*. 2012;13(5):3962.
47. Miften M, et al. Tolerance limits and methodologies for IMRT measurement-based verification QA: recommendations of AAPM Task Group No. 218. *Med Phys*. 2018;45(4):e53–e83.

48. Halvorsen PH, et al. AAPM-RSS medical physics practice guideline 9.a. for SRS-SBRT. *J Appl Clin Med Phys.* 2017;18(5):10–21.

49. Solberg TD, et al. Quality and safety considerations in stereotactic radiosurgery and stereotactic body radiation therapy: executive summary. *Pract Radiat Oncol.* 2012;2(1):2–9.

50. Siegel RL, Miller KD, Jemal A. Cancer statistics, 2020. *CA Cancer J Clin.* 2020;70(1):7–30.

51. Pan H, et al. Clinical practice patterns of lung stereotactic body radiation therapy in the United States: a secondary analysis. *Am J Clin Oncol.* 2013;36(3):269–272.

52. Timmerman R, et al. Stereotactic body radiation therapy for inoperable early stage lung cancer. *JAMA.* 2010;303(11):1070–1076.

53. Timmerman RD, et al. Long-term results of stereotactic body radiation therapy in medically inoperable stage I non-small cell lung cancer. *JAMA Oncol.* 2018;4(9):1287–1288.

54. Videtic GM, et al. A randomized phase 2 study comparing 2 stereotactic body radiation therapy schedules for medically inoperable patients with stage I peripheral non-small cell lung cancer: NRG oncology RTOG 0915 (NCCTG N0927). *Int J Radiat Oncol Biol Phys.* 2015;93(4):757–764.

55. Senthi S, et al. Outcomes of stereotactic ablative radiotherapy for central lung tumours: a systematic review. *Radiother Oncol.* 2013;106(3):276–282.

56. Rowe BP, et al. Stereotactic body radiotherapy for central lung tumors. *J Thorac Oncol.* 2012;7(9):1394–1399.

57. Arnett ALH, et al. Long-term clinical outcomes and safety profile of SBRT for centrally located NSCLC. *Adv Radiat Oncol.* 2019;4(2):422–428.

58. Timmerman RD, et al. RTOG 0618: stereotactic body radiation therapy (SBRT) to treat operable early-stage lung cancer patients. *ASCO Meeting Abstracts.* 2013;31(15_suppl):7523.

59. Iyengar P, et al. Phase II trial of stereotactic body radiation therapy combined with erlotinib for patients with limited but progressive metastatic non-small-cell lung cancer. *J Clin Oncol.* 2014;32(34):3824–3830.

60. Gomez DR, et al. Local consolidative therapy versus maintenance therapy or observation for patients with oligometastatic non-small-cell lung cancer without progression after first-line systemic therapy: a multicentre, randomised, controlled, phase 2 study. *Lancet Oncol.* 2016;17(12):1672–1682.

61. Siegel RL, et al. Colorectal cancer statistics, 2020. *CA Cancer J Clin.* 2020;70(3):145–164.

62. Ercolani G, et al. Liver resection for multiple colorectal metastases: influence of parenchymal involvement and total tumor volume, vs number or location, on long-term survival. *Arch Surg.* 2002;137(10):1187–1192.

63. Welch JP, Donaldson GA. The clinical correlation of an autopsy study of recurrent colorectal cancer. *Ann Surg.* 1979;189(4):496–502.

64. Adam R, et al. Rescue surgery for unresectable colorectal liver metastases downstaged by chemotherapy: a model to predict long-term survival. *Ann Surg.* 2004;240(4):644–657; discussion 657–658.

65. Fusai G, Davidson BR. Management of colorectal liver metastases. *Colorectal Dis.* 2003;5(1):2–23.

66. de Baere T, et al. Radiofrequency ablation of 100 hepatic metastases with a mean follow-up of more than 1 year. *AJR Am J Roentgenol.* 2000;175(6):1619–1625.

67. Kerr DJ, et al. Intrahepatic arterial versus intravenous fluorouracil and folinic acid for colorectal cancer liver metastases: a multicentre randomised trial. *Lancet.* 2003;361(9355):368–373.

68. Solbiati L, et al. Percutaneous radio-frequency ablation of hepatic metastases from colorectal cancer: long-term results in 117 patients. *Radiology.* 2001;221(1):159–166.

69. Sotsky TK, Ravikumar TS. Cryotherapy in the treatment of liver metastases from colorectal cancer. *Semin Oncol.* 2002;29(2):183–191.

70. Tandan VR, Harmantas A, Gallinger S. Long-term survival after hepatic cryosurgery versus surgical resection for metastatic colorectal carcinoma: a critical review of the literature. *Can J Surg.* 1997;40(3):175–181.

71. Vogl TJ, et al. Malignant liver tumors treated with MR imaging-guided laser-induced thermotherapy: technique and prospective results. *Radiology.* 1995;196(1):257–265.

72. Vogl TJ, et al. Malignant liver tumors treated with MR imaging-guided laser-induced thermotherapy: experience with complications in 899 patients (2,520 lesions). *Radiology.* 2002;225(2):367–377.

73. Haas RJ, Wicherts DA, Adam R. Oncosurgical strategies for unresectable liver metastases. In Vauthey J-N, Hoff PM, Audisio RA, Poston GJ, editors. *Liver Metastases*; Springer. 2009:1–13.

74. Blazer DG, Anaya DA, Abdalla EK. Destructive therapies for colorectal cancer metastases. In *Liver Metastases*; 2009:1–11.

75. Reed GB, Jr., Cox AJ, Jr. The human liver after radiation injury: a form of veno-occlusive disease. *Am J Pathol.* 1966;48(4):597–611.

76. Yannam GR, et al. A nonhuman primate model of human radiation-induced venocclusive liver disease and hepatocyte injury. *Int J Radiat Oncol Biol Phys.* 2014;88(2):404–411.

77. Herfarth KK, et al. Stereotactic single-dose radiation therapy of liver tumors: results of a phase I/II trial. *J Clin Oncol.* 2001;19(1):164–170.

78. Hoyer M, et al. Phase II study on stereotactic body radiotherapy of colorectal metastases. *Acta Oncol.* 2006;45(7):823–830.

79. Lee MT, et al. Phase I study of individualized stereotactic body radiotherapy of liver metastases. *J Clin Oncol.* 2009:JCO.2008.20.0600.

80. Mendez Romero A, et al. Stereotactic body radiation therapy for primary and metastatic liver tumors: a single institution phase I–II study. *Acta Oncol.* 2006;45(7):831–837.

81. Milano MT, et al. A prospective pilot study of curative-intent stereotactic body radiation therapy in patients with 5 or fewer oligometastatic lesions. *Cancer.* 2008;112(3):650–658.

82. Zhang Y, et al. Hypofractionated stereotactic body radiotherapy for primary and secondary liver tumors. *Int J Radiat Oncol Biol Phys.* 2008;72(Supplement 1):S247–S248.

83. Katz AW, et al. Hypofractionated stereotactic body radiation therapy (SBRT) for limited hepatic metastases. *Int J Radiat Oncol Biol Phys.* 2007;67(3):793–798.

84. Rusthoven KE, et al. Multi-institutional phase I/II trial of stereotactic body radiation therapy for liver metastases. *J Clin Oncol.* 2009;27(10):1572–1578.

85. Rule W, et al. Phase I dose-escalation study of stereotactic body radiotherapy in patients with hepatic metastases. *Ann Surg Oncol.* 2011;18(4):1081–1087.

86. Milano MT, et al. Descriptive analysis of oligometastatic lesions treated with curative-intent stereotactic body radiotherapy. *Int J Radiat Oncol Biol Phys.* 2008;72(5):1516–1522.

87. McCammon R, et al. Observation of a dose-control relationship for lung and liver tumors after stereotactic body radiation therapy. *Int J Radiat Oncol Biol Phys.* 2009;73(1):112–118.

88. Schefter TE, et al. A phase I trial of stereotactic body radiation therapy (SBRT) for liver metastases. *Int J Radiat Oncol Biol Phys.* 2005;62(5):1371–1378.

89. Meyer JJ, et al. A phase I dose-escalation trial of single-fraction stereotactic radiation therapy for liver metastases. *Ann Surg Oncol.* 2016;23(1):218–224.

90. Timmerman R, et al. Excessive toxicity when treating central tumors in a phase II study of stereotactic body radiation therapy for medically inoperable early-stage lung cancer. *J Clin Oncol.* 2006;24(30):4833–4839.

91. Bruix J, Sherman M, American Association for the Study of Liver Diseases. Practice guidelines committee, management of hepatocellular carcinoma. *Hepatology.* 2005;42(5):1208–1236.

92. Andolino DL, et al. Stereotactic body radiotherapy for primary hepatocellular carcinoma. *Int J Radiat Oncol Biol Phys.* 2011;81(4):e447–e453.

93. Tse RV, et al. Phase I study of individualized stereotactic body radiotherapy for hepatocellular carcinoma and intrahepatic cholangiocarcinoma. *J Clin Oncol.* 2008;26(4):657–664.

94. Culleton S, et al. Outcomes following definitive stereotactic body radiotherapy for patients with Child-Pugh B or C hepatocellular carcinoma. *Radiother Oncol.* 2014;111(3):412–417.

95. Katz AW, et al. Stereotactic hypofractionated radiation therapy as a bridge to transplantation for hepatocellular carcinoma: clinical outcome and pathologic correlation. *Int J Radiat Oncol Biol Phys.* 2012;83(3):895–900.

96. Wang XS, et al. Stereotactic body radiation therapy for management of spinal metastases in patients without spinal cord compression: a phase 1-2 trial. *Lancet Oncol.* 2012;13(4):395–402.

97. Ryu S, et al. RTOG 0631 phase 2/3 study of image guided stereotactic radiosurgery for localized (1–3) spine metastases: phase 2 results. *Pract Radiat Oncol.* 2014;4(2):76–81.

98. Sahgal A, et al. Stereotactic body radiotherapy is effective salvage therapy for patients with prior radiation of spinal metastases. *Int J Radiat Oncol Biol Phys.* 2009;74(3):723–731.

99. Medin PM, et al. Spinal cord tolerance to reirradiation with single-fraction radiosurgery: a swine model. *Int J Radiat Oncol Biol Phys.* 2012;83(3):1031–1037.

100. Sahgal A, et al. Probabilities of radiation myelopathy specific to stereotactic body radiation therapy to guide safe practice. *Int J Radiat Oncol Biol Phys.* 2013;85(2):341–347.

101. Cunha MV, et al. Vertebral compression fracture (VCF) after spine stereotactic body radiation therapy (SBRT): analysis of predictive factors. *Int J Radiat Oncol Biol Phys.* 2012;84(3):e343–e349.

102. Thibault I, et al. Spine stereotactic body radiotherapy for renal cell cancer spinal metastases: analysis of outcomes and risk of vertebral compression fracture. *J Neurosurg Spine.* 2014;21(5):711–718.

103. Sahgal A, et al. Vertebral compression fracture after spine stereotactic body radiotherapy: a multi-institutional analysis with a focus on radiation dose and the spinal instability neoplastic score. *J Clin Oncol.* 2013;31(27):3426–3431.

104. Siegel R, et al. Cancer statistics, 2014. *CA Cancer J Clin.* 2014;64(1):9–29.

105. Hodges JC, et al. Cost-effectiveness analysis of SBRT versus IMRT: an emerging initial radiation treatment option for organ-confined prostate cancer. *Am J Manag Care.* 2012;18(5):e186–e193.

106. Yu JB, et al. Stereotactic body radiation therapy versus intensity-modulated radiation therapy for prostate cancer: comparison of toxicity. *J Clin Oncol.* 2014;32(12):1195–201.

107. King CR, et al. Health-related quality of life after stereotactic body radiation therapy for localized prostate cancer: results from a multi-institutional consortium of prospective trials. *Int J Radiat Oncol Biol Phys.* 2013;87(5):939–945.

108. King CR, et al. Stereotactic body radiotherapy for localized prostate cancer: pooled analysis from a multi-institutional consortium of prospective phase II trials. *Radiother Oncol.* 2013;109(2):217–221.

109. Kim DW, et al. Stereotactic body radiation therapy for prostate cancer: review of experience of a multicenter phase I/II dose-escalation study. *Front Oncol.* 2014;4:319.

110. Chen L, et al. Safety and outcome of stereotactic body radiation therapy (SBRT) with rectal hydrogel spacer for prostate cancer. *J Clin Oncol.* 2020;38(6_suppl):76–76.

111. Mahadevan A, et al. Stereotactic body radiotherapy and gemcitabine for locally advanced pancreatic cancer. *Int J Radiat Oncol Biol Phys.* 2010;78(3):735–742.

112. Schellenberg D, et al. Single-fraction stereotactic body radiation therapy and sequential gemcitabine for the treatment of locally advanced pancreatic cancer. *Int J Radiat Oncol Biol Phys.* 2011;81(1):181–188.

113. Chuong MD, et al. Stereotactic body radiation therapy for locally advanced and borderline resectable pancreatic cancer is effective and well tolerated. *Int J Radiat Oncol Biol Phys.* 2013;86(3):516–522.

114. Herman JM, et al. Phase 2 multi-institutional trial evaluating gemcitabine and stereotactic body radiotherapy for patients with locally advanced unresectable pancreatic adenocarcinoma. *Cancer.* 2015;121(7):1128–1137.

115. Reyngold M, Parikh P, Crane CH. Ablative radiation therapy for locally advanced pancreatic cancer: techniques and results. *Radiat Oncol.* 2019;14(1):95.

116. Ollila DW, Caudle AS. Surgical management of distant metastases. *Surg Oncol Clin N Am.* 2006;15(2):385–398.

117. Milano MT, et al. Oligometastases treated with stereotactic body radiotherapy: long-term follow-up of prospective study. *Int J Radiat Oncol Biol Phys.* 2012;83(3):878–886.

118. Salama JK, et al. Stereotactic body radiotherapy for multisite extracranial oligometastases: final report of a dose escalation trial in patients with 1 to 5 sites of metastatic disease. *Cancer.* 2012;118(11):2962–2970.

119. Dhakal S, et al. Stereotactic body radiotherapy for pulmonary metastases from soft-tissue sarcomas: excellent local lesion control and improved patient survival. *Int J Radiat Oncol Biol Phys.* 2012;82(2):940–945.

120. Svedman C, et al. A prospective Phase II trial of using extracranial stereotactic radiotherapy in primary and metastatic renal cell carcinoma. *Acta Oncol.* 2006;45(7):870–875.

121. Kothari G, et al. Outcomes of stereotactic radiotherapy for cranial and extracranial metastatic renal cell carcinoma: a systematic review. *Acta Oncol.* 2015;54(2):148–157.

122. Zhang Y, et al. Stereotactic Ablative Radiation Therapy (SAbR) used to defer systemic therapy in oligometastatic renal cell cancer. *Int J Radiat Oncol Biol Phys.* 2019;105(2):367–375.

123. Wang CJ, et al. Safety and efficacy of stereotactic ablative radiation therapy for renal cell carcinoma extracranial metastases. *Int J Radiat Oncol Biol Phys.* 2017;98(1):91–100.

29 Low Dose–Rate Brachytherapy

Yun Yang and Mark J. Rivard

INTRODUCTION

Brachytherapy is a form of radiation therapy in which the source of radiation is placed close to or within the patient. The origin of the word *brachytherapy* is from the ancient Greek word βραχύς or *brachys*, which means *short distance* as relating to the proximity of the radiation source to the patient. As a co-discoverer of radium with Marie Curie (née Skłodowska) in 1898, Pierre Curie suggested to a fellow Frenchmen, Henri-Alexandre Danlos, to use the radioactive material for therapeutic purposes. With the assistance of the physicist Paul Bloch, Dr. Danlos proceeded to treat a patient with tuberculosis—this was the first brachytherapy treatment.[1] This form of treatment would be termed radium therapy until Forssell associated the term *brachyradium*,[2] and later simplified it as brachytherapy with the availability of other radiation sources. Prolific historian and practicing radiation oncologist Aronowitz has researched much of the early history of brachytherapy; the interested reader should examine these readily available summaries.[3-16]

Clinical applications of brachytherapy may be applied with the radiation source on the patient's skin surface, sometimes referred to as plesiotherapy in historical documents (think of the plesiosaurus dinosaur that lived on the water surface). Other means of treatment delivery can place the source within a naturally occurring cavity within the patient (i.e., intracavitary brachytherapy), into a naturally occurring channel or lumen such as the esophagus (i.e., intraluminal brachytherapy), into a blood vessel (i.e., intravascular or endovascular brachytherapy), percutaneously into the tumor volume via a needle (i.e., interstitial brachytherapy), and within the tumor volume via an open surgical procedure (i.e., intraoperative brachytherapy). All these delivery methods require (semi)invasive placement techniques and contrast with teletherapy, nowadays commonly referred to as external-beam radiotherapy (EBRT), where the radiation source is positioned relatively far from the patient.

Brachytherapy may be further portioned in terms of the means of delivery. The first treatments were delivered with needle-tipped ^{226}Ra sources directly inserted into the lesion. This is now referred to as manual loading. Soon thereafter, ^{222}Rn sources were developed to provide sources with higher specific activity, that is, Ci/g, and allow implantation with thinner perforations. After physicians and surgeons exhibited toxicities such as blackened digits and subsequent amputations due to high radiation exposures for manually inserting the sources, an alternate method of implantation was developed, now referred to as manual afterloading. Here, the lesion was implanted with needles during surgery, and the sources were implanted afterward. This approach allowed careful needle positioning without rush, especially important at the academic centers where brachytherapy was most active at the time. Further, radiation exposure to hospital personnel was minimized since patients located in recovery rooms were not emitting radiation—sources were inserted into the needles after surgical recovery. A further advancement was implemented with remote afterloading, where the placement of the radiation source within the patient was done through electromechanical means instead of manually, with negligible radiation exposure to hospital personnel.

All these delivery methods can utilize low dose–rate (LDR) brachytherapy sources, which are classified to administer radiation at a dose rate of 0.4–2 Gy/h (i.e., 0.67–3.33 cGy/minute). High dose–rate (HDR) sources are classified to administer radiation at a dose rate exceeding 12 Gy/h (i.e., 20 cGy/minute). This categorization of dose rate was established in Report 38[17] by the International Commission on Radiation Units and Measurements (ICRU). ICRU 38 categorization also includes medium dose–rate sources that administer radiation at a dose rate of 2–12 Gy/h (i.e., 3.33–20 cGy/minute), or pulsed dose–rate brachytherapy (using HDR sources positioned within the target for a short time, but as an in-patient procedure with the treatment course extending over a few days), but these intermediary approaches have all but stopped and are used now only in a handful of clinics in the United States. Nevertheless, LDR brachytherapy has key advantages over HDR brachytherapy such as greatly diminished upfront and ongoing costs, improved radiobiology, and direct placement when concurrent to surgery.

A key issue with the clinical delivery of brachytherapy is patient safety and implant quality.[18] The European

Society for Radiotherapy & Oncology (ESTRO) Booklet 8 established quality standards for brachytherapy equipment and quality assurances practices,[19] but did not offer much guidance on the quality measures governing the practice of clinical brachytherapy. This topic is covered in greater detail within societal reports such as the TG-56[20] and the TG-64[21] reports by the American Association of Physicists in Medicine (AAPM), and also the book by Thomadsen[22] dedicated to the subject of achieving quality in brachytherapy.

LDR BRACHYTHERAPY SOURCES

So what is a brachytherapy source? Brachytherapy sources differ from other internally placed sources of radiation used in medicine (e.g., nuclear medicine) in that the radiation source does not chemically interact with the patient. Brachytherapy sources will often have a single or double layer of encapsulation to contain a radionuclide, whereas nuclear medicine has a radionuclide bound to a chemical that will preferentially locate within the body after being injected. This difference even applies to ^{90}Y microspheres for selective internal radiation therapy,[23] where the radionuclide is contained within a resin or glass matrix,[24] approximately 30 μm in diameter, and injected for permanently lodging within the micro vessels of an organ such as a lobe of the liver. Radionuclides used in nuclear medicine will typically clear the body based on a biological half-life related to fluid flow and metabolism.

The radiation source for brachytherapy may also be generated electrically, such as through an internally or externally positioned X-ray tube.[25-27] However, these radiation sources are designed to deliver a therapeutic dose within a matter of minutes and are categorized as HDR brachytherapy sources.

This leaves the most popular type of brachytherapy source, which is a radionuclide contained within an inert encapsulation for permanent or temporary implantation within a patient. LDR sources in use today contain radionuclides that emit radiation described as low-energy radiation, typically photons with mean energy <50 keV.[28] The decision to use low-energy radiation helps both the patient (to make the dose distribution more conformal with local dose deposition) and the hospital personnel (to readily permit shielding and radiological protection). Some radiological properties of common low-energy photon-emitting brachytherapy sources are included in Table 29.1. These three radionuclides decay via electron capture, in which a proton-rich nucleus absorbs an electron from an inner atomic shell, subsequently transforming a proton into a neutron. When the atom relaxes to its ground state, energy is released as photons. This can occur through X-rays generated by electrons from outer atomic shells filling the void of the inner shell and sometimes also with nuclear relaxation (as is the case for ^{103}Pd and ^{125}I) with gamma-ray emission from the excited nucleus. These X-ray and γ-ray photons have discrete energies and intensities for a given radionuclide disintegration. Auger electrons may also be emitted by the excited atom, but these low-energy particles are blocked from exiting the brachytherapy source due to the encapsulation.

Some examples of low-energy LDR brachytherapy sources are included in Figure 29.1 with images adapted

TABLE 29.1 Some radiological properties of low-energy, photon-emitting brachytherapy sources. X-ray transitions are listed after the elemental symbols for the daughter nuclides. The lower-probability X-ray transitions (i.e., <10 keV) and Auger electrons are not listed

^{125}I (half-life = 59.41 days)		^{103}Pd (half-life = 16.991 days)		^{131}Cs (half-life = 9.689 days)	
Photon energy (keV)	Photons/ disintegration	Photon energy (keV)	Photons/ disintegration	Photon energy (keV)	Photons/ disintegration
27.202 Te K$_{\alpha2}$	0.406	20.073 Rh K$_{\alpha2}$	0.224	29.461 Xe K$_{\alpha2}$	0.211
27.472 Te K$_{\alpha1}$	0.757	20.216 Rh K$_{\alpha1}$	0.423	29.782 Xe K$_{\alpha1}$	0.389
30.945 Te K$_{\beta3}$	0.0683	22.700 Rh K$_{\beta3}$	0.0352	33.562 Xe K$_{\beta3}$	0.0364
30.996 Te K$_{\beta1}$	0.132	22.724 Rh K$_{\beta1}$	0.0681	33.624 Xe K$_{\beta1}$	0.0702
31.698 Te K$_{\beta2}$	0.0381	23.173 Rh K$_{\beta2}$	0.0163	34.419 Xe K$_{\beta2}$	0.0213
35.4925 γ	0.0668	39.748 γ	0.000683		
		62.41 γ	0.0000104		
		294.98 γ	0.000028		
		357.45 γ	0.000221		
		497.080 γ	0.0000396		
28.4 keV mean	1.47 total	20.7 keV mean	0.77 total	30.4 keV mean	0.73 total

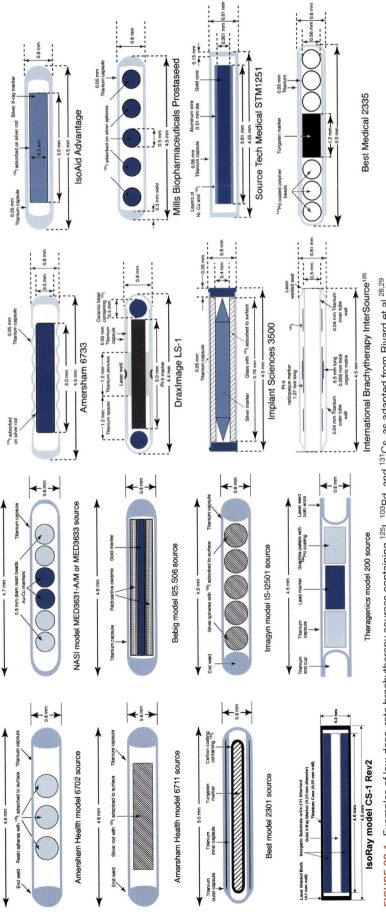

FIGURE 29.1. Examples of low dose–rate brachytherapy sources containing ^{125}I, ^{103}Pd, and ^{131}Cs, as adapted from Rivard et al.[28,29]

from Rivard et al.[28,29] These images of ^{125}I, ^{103}Pd, and ^{131}Cs seeds depict the various designs that have been developed to provide source localization with imaging from X-ray computed tomography (CT) scans, as well as to facilitate some novel features such as localization with ultrasound imaging, thinner diameters to minimize tissue trauma following interstitial implantation, and flexibility of the encapsulation.

LDR brachytherapy sources have been used, and may still be in use in some clinics, which contain other radionuclides that emit high-energy photons. These sources contained ^{198}Au, ^{137}Cs, or ^{192}Ir. However, their use in LDR brachytherapy sources has greatly diminished over the past decade due to limited availability from manufacturers and excellent clinical results using low-energy brachytherapy sources, which greatly restrict the radiation exposure to the patient. Further, high-energy, photon-emitting brachytherapy sources may have higher doses in contact with their encapsulation than low-energy sources due to electrons escaping.[30]

DOSIMETRY

The following section describes the current means in which dose distributions are determined in the vicinity of LDR brachytherapy sources and how these dose distributions are integrated into clinical treatment planning systems (TPSs). Historical dosimetry systems[31-34] that came to light before the advent of computerized treatment planning are available to the interested reader for gaining insight on general principles that still apply today. Currently, dose specification to water is the standard for which brachytherapy prescriptions are generally based. This is due to historical reasons, as the earliest brachytherapy sources (i.e., ^{226}Ra, ^{222}Rn, ^{60}Co, and ^{192}Ir) were high-energy photon emitters and the radiological equivalence of water and soft tissue was within about 1% of unity due to similarities in the mass-attenuation coefficients (i.e., μ/ρ, governing attenuation in medium) and mass-energy absorption coefficients (i.e., μ_{en}/ρ, governing dose deposition).[35] For the low-energy photon-emitting LDR sources, differences between water and soft tissue for μ/ρ and μ_{en}/ρ can exceed a couple percent such as for ^{103}Pd,[36] causing differences between prescribed and administered dose by over 10% in some instances.

However, a key point to note is that current prescriptions are generally based on trial-and-error with years of historical data.[37,38] The doses prescribed as standard-of-care are based on the assumption of the water equivalence of human tissue.[39] One cannot simply update the medium for dose calculation without also coordinating a thoughtful change in the prescription paradigm to correct for the radiological differences between water and soft tissue—often a 3D phenomenon and not simply a scalar value.

Given the prevalence of computerized TPSs, the current worldwide standard method is the AAPM TG-43 formalism, based on the seminal report from 1995,[40] the most cited publication in the scientific journal *Medical Physics*.[41] This approach sets water as the reference medium, with a fixed-dose calculation formulism, and parameters within the formulism that are specific to each brachytherapy source model. The TG-43 formalism is based upon prior approaches that also parameterized source-specific terms.[42-47] For clinical dose calculations to occur, the dose distribution must first be determined in the vicinity of a given brachytherapy source model. From the measured or calculated dose distributions, brachytherapy dosimetry parameters are obtained. The TG-43 formulism relies on widespread adoption of dosimetry parameters for a given source model, resulting in consistent dose calculation for all that utilize accepted dosimetry parameters. The AAPM establishes consensus data on brachytherapy dosimetry parameters as they are invested in the safe and uniform implementation of clinical brachytherapy.

But how are radiation dose distributions around brachytherapy sources determined in the first place? These are often performed by dosimetry investigators, who use measurement techniques or computational methods to derive the dose distribution around a given model for a single brachytherapy source. The dose gradients are smoother in EBRT than with brachytherapy, where changes in dose exceeding a factor of two can occur within 1 mm.[48] In EBRT, there also is an established infrastructure of measurement devices and measurement protocols for evaluating the dose distribution under reference conditions from a linear accelerator;[49] brachytherapy dosimetry requires larger detector corrections than for EBRT,[50] where the photon energy is usually a factor of 100 or more higher than that measured in brachytherapy dosimetry. Prescriptions in brachytherapy are sometimes at a distance of 5 mm from the source, where a positioning uncertainty of just 0.5 mm can result in a change in dose at that location of 20%. Issues on the methods of measuring brachytherapy dose distributions are discussed in detail by Williamson and Rivard.[51,52]

The practice of measuring radiation doses in EBRT radiation fields is also supported due to the electrical nature of radiation generation and the beam tailoring devices that can alter the dose delivered to the patient. In brachytherapy, the radiation is almost always generated via radionuclide decay, which is a predictable process that lends itself to determination through strict computational methods.[53,54] Due to the low-energy photons prevalent in LDR brachytherapy, assumptions of charged particle equilibrium and the approximation of absorbed dose equivalence to collisional kerma can simplify the calculations while introducing minimal errors.

Monte Carlo (MC) methods for radiation transport calculations are a crucial component for brachytherapy dosimetry evaluations performed recently and expected for the foreseeable future. MC methods have been used for over four decades for this purpose.[55,56] A thorough description of the process is described by Williamson and by Thomadsen et al.[57,58] Briefly, the dose distribution around a given model for a single brachytherapy source is determined. From this dose distribution and attributes describing the spatial distribution of the radionuclide, the brachytherapy dosimetry parameters for that particular source model are determined. These brachytherapy dosimetry parameters are then entered into a brachytherapy TPS and used for all subsequent clinical applications so that there is uniformity in the dosimetry of patient treatments with that source model.

In practice, one of the following two equations[28,29,59,60] is used for clinical dose calculations:

$$\dot{D}(r) = S_K \cdot \Lambda \cdot \left(\frac{r_0}{r}\right)^2 \cdot g_P(r) \cdot \phi_{an}(r) \quad (29.1)$$

$$\dot{D}(r,\theta) = S_K \cdot \Lambda \cdot \frac{G_L(r,\theta)}{G_L(r_0,\theta_0)} \cdot g_L(r) \cdot F(r,\theta) \quad (29.2)$$

where the dose rate at any location is simply the product of a few brachytherapy dosimetry parameters. If the source orientation is unknown, then Eq. 29.1 is used. This 1D dose calculation formalism is the most popular means of determining dose distributions for LDR brachytherapy sources, which results in a spherically symmetric dose distribution.

For the 2D dose calculation formalism, the source is assumed to be designed cylindrically symmetric with a resultant cylindrically symmetric dose distribution. Almost always the source is assumed to be designed with further symmetry about the transverse plane bisecting the source length. Dose rate is determined as a function of radial distance r from the source center to the point of interest and the polar angle θ as measured from the source long axis. The polar coordinate system of the TG-43 formalism is depicted in Figure 29.2. Note that the relevant length for dose calculations is the radioactivity extent and not the length of the encapsulation. The reference position is at a distance of $r_0=1$ cm and a polar angle $\theta_0=90°$.

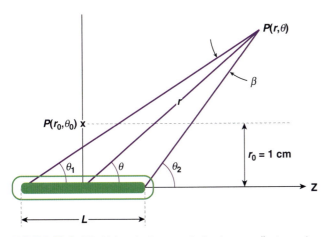

FIGURE 29.2. TG-43 brachytherapy dosimetry coordinate system for dose calculations, adapted from Rivard et al.[28]

The source strength is specified in terms of air-kerma strength, S_K. It has units of "U," where 1 U = 1 μGy·m²/h = 1 cGy·cm²/h. For a given source model, this is the only dosimetry parameter specific to the source inventory within the clinic. Source strength is reported by the source manufacturer and measured in the clinic. This is discussed in greater detail in the next section.

The dose–rate constant Λ is specific to a given source model and is the ratio of the dose rate at the reference position, $\dot{D}(r_0,\theta_0)$, to the source strength. The units of Λ are cGy/h/U. Low-energy LDR brachytherapy sources have Λ values near equal to unity, with Λ approximately equal to 0.68 cGy/h/U for [103]Pd sources, 0.93 cGy/h/U for ^{125}I sources, and 1.06 cGy/h/U for [131]Cs sources.[61]

The geometry function is the most important dosimetry parameter toward approximating the dose rate distribution using the TG-43 dose calculation formalism. It can account for a factor of 10,000 gradient in the dose distribution between near and far positions from the source, that is, positions 0.1–10 cm from the source. Use of the geometry function (and typically coarse evaluation matrices) obscures the fact that doses exceeding 10,000 Gy may occur at the surface of LDR brachytherapy seeds following clinical implantation. For the 1D dose calculation formalism, a simple inverse-square relationship is used to approximate the dose falloff. A complementary term r_0 is in the numerator to balance the units of $1/r^2$. For the 2D dose calculation formalism, the spatial distribution of the radionuclide is approximated as a line segment that typically covers the physical extent of the radioactivity within the encapsulation. The active length (or effective length for sources containing multiple pellets of radioactivity) is used for derivation of the 2D geometry function, $G_L(r,\theta)$. The geometry function takes the following form based on the polar angle:

$$G_L(r,\theta) = \begin{cases} \frac{1}{(r^2 - L^2/4)} & \text{if } \theta=0° \\ \frac{\beta}{Lr\sin\theta} & \text{if } \theta\neq0° \end{cases}$$

The term β is the angle (in radians) subtended by the ends of the radioactive part of the source and the point of interest. When the point of interest is more than three times the distance from the center of the source than the active length, any differences between the 1D and 2D dose calculation formalism results amount to less than 5%.[59] For sources with an active length of about 0.3 cm, this occurs at a distance of about 1 cm.

The radial dose function, $g(r)$, is the dosimetry parameter used to obtain the dose rate in water at positions on the source transverse plane beyond the trend expected by correcting dose rate at the reference position by the geometry function. For instance, if the medium were not water but a more attenuating material, the radial dose function would falloff more steeply than in water due to increased radiation attenuation. While the radiological properties associated with this dosimetry parameter are radiation attenuation and scatter, it is used simply to permit replication of the dose rate distribution on the transverse plane beyond any corrections provided by the geometry function.

In the original (1995) TG-43 report,[20] a single radial dose function g(r) was introduced to account for the deviation from the geometry function on the transverse plane. However, since there are differences between the 1D and 2D geometry functions, there should consequently be different radial dose functions for each formalism to reproduce the original dose rate distribution. These radial dose functions, $g_P(r)$ and $g_L(r)$, were introduced in the 2004 report update (TG-43U1) by Rivard et al.[59] Because there may be 1D or 2D geometry functions used based on knowledge of source orientation, it is imperative that the correct radial dose function, either $g_P(r)$ or $g_L(r)$ respectively, be used to properly replicate the original dose rate distribution. Especially at locations near the source, the use of a radial dose function for the wrong formalism can cause errors in dose by more than a factor of two.

The last term to account for dose anisotropy may be thought of as "everything else" to address what is not accounted for by the combination of the geometry function and the radial dose function to reproduce dose rates away from the transverse plane. This concept is explained elsewhere in greater detail.[62] Like the geometry function and radial dose function, the anisotropy function can be for either the 1D or 2D formalism. For the case of the 1D formalism, the 1D anisotropy function, $\phi_{an}(r)$, is the ratio of the solid-angle weighted dose rate, averaged over the entire 4π steradian space, divided by the dose rate at that same distance r on the transverse plane. Due to anisotropy of dose as a function of polar angle at large distances from low-energy LDR brachytherapy sources (primarily due to photon attenuation by the encapsulation), values for $\phi_{an}(r)$ are typically slightly less than unity. However, the dose rate is higher at locations close to the source off the transverse plane for a given r value due to the nonspherical geometry of the source. Consequently, volume averaging of dose over the entire 4π steradian space at these close distances tends to produce values for $\phi_{an}(r)$ are typically greater than unity. In fact, the volume averaging will include locations within the source for positions closer than half the encapsulation length. Care must be made by dosimetry investigators to exclude these locations for $\phi_{an}(r)$ derivation.

The 2D anisotropy function, $F(r, \theta)$ is slightly more complicated in that it is the ratio of the dose rate at any location off the transverse plane to the dose at the same r on the transverse plane, after accounting for the geometry function. Consequently, the perturbing effect on the dose distribution by the spatial distribution of radioactivity will alter calculations of $\phi_{an}(r)$ but not $F(r, \theta)$. In the end, if properly derived, this difference does not matter as the use of the appropriate geometry function and radial dose function in combination with the anisotropy function will reproduce the original dose distribution.

Once all the dosimetry parameters are available for a given model of a brachytherapy source, the AAPM, in concert with other professional societies such as the ESTRO, will review the literature to evaluate candidate datasets and then establish consensus brachytherapy dosimetry parameters based on robust and unbiased methods.[28] These data will then become available to clinical users through publication in AAPM reports, posting on the Brachytherapy Source Registry as managed jointly by the AAPM and the Imaging and Radiation Oncology Core Houston Quality Assurance Center (IROC Houston, formerly the Radiological Physics Center), through web-based resources under development, or through inclusion in vendor-provided software by TPS manufacturers. It is always the responsibility of the clinical medical physicist to evaluate any data used for clinical applications and to document this evaluation methodically. Implementation of new dosimetry parameters can have a profound influence on the resultant dose distribution that the patient would receive.[63-65]

SOURCE CALIBRATIONS

Source strength is typically the only dosimetric quantity of a brachytherapy source that is measured by a clinical medical physicist. In the United States, these assays of source strength should be traceable to the National Institute of Standards and Technology (NIST), the US primary standard dosimetry laboratory. The practice for making calibrations of clinical instruments traceable to the NIST standard is covered in depth in the AAPM reports by DeWerd et al.[66] and by Butler et al.[67]

The report by the Calibration Laboratory Accreditation subcommittee of the AAPM set practice standards for LDR brachytherapy source manufacturers and dosimetry investigators.[65] Source manufacturers are to establish internal standards for source calibrations as used for providing calibration certificates to customers. These calibrations are to be traceable to NIST on an ongoing basis. Further, measurements of the dose–rate constant (as performed by brachytherapy source dosimetry investigators) are taken from a subset of the sources used to establish the calibration standard at NIST. In this way, the seeds used in patients and the dosimetry parameters used in clinical applications are both connected through NIST-traceable calibrations. This process has extended the dosimetric prerequisites[68] necessary for sources to satisfy the AAPM criteria for placement on the Brachytherapy Source Registry.

The report by the Low Energy Brachytherapy Source Calibration Working Group of the AAPM set standards for clinical medical physicists on the practice standards for assaying brachytherapy sources.[66] Specific to brachytherapy source strength measurements, these practice standards supersede those of the AAPM TG-56 report.[20] The responsibility for such calibrations was clearly identified as being that of the clinical medical physicist. This clarified ambiguity where some source manufacturers offered calibrations from third-party services where seeds were placed in strands or prepared with spacers into needle assemblies. Clinical medical physicists are required to assay sources preceding clinical use because of the lack of NIST-traceability sometimes and the increased uncertainties associated with using third-party calibration services. The report outlined standards for the number of sources to be assayed, the permissible tolerances between measurements performed by the clinical medical physicist and the source manufacturer calibration certificate, and actions to be taken by the end-user medical physicist based on the level of agreement between the two values of the brachytherapy source strength. Interestingly, the tolerances in this report can be extended to account for statistical variations in the reported source strength for a batch of seeds, where the number of sources to be assayed in a given batch can be derived based on the desired level of agreement with the manufacturer calibration certificate.[69–72] However, this statistical approach was deemed too complicated for setting widespread use and clinical practice standards.

For the low-energy photon-emitting radionuclides included in Table 29.1, the LDR brachytherapy seeds should have a primary calibration standard established by NIST. This calibration standard is made through measurements performed using the NIST wide-angle free-air chamber (WAFAC) as described by Seltzer et al.,[73] which has been extended beyond ^{125}I and [103]Pd to include [131]Cs seeds. A schematic diagram of the NIST WAFAC device is given in Figure 29.3, where it is indicated that the source rotates during measurements, radiation is filtered

through an aluminum foil, and the chamber can collapse in length to remove measurement artifacts. As there are photons emitted by brachytherapy sources with energies less than 5 keV, such as characteristic X-rays from the frequently used titanium encapsulation, the measurement of source strength includes corrections to remove these low-energy photons that do not significantly contribute to absorbed dose in tissue, yet significantly contribute to source strength measurements.[74,75]

The source strength is measured in air at a distance of 30 cm from the source with an 8 cm diameter tungsten aperture that collimates the photons before reaching the ionization chamber. This collimation results in a high signal due to the sampling angle (explaining use of the words "wide-angle" in the WAFAC designation), which spans $\pm 7.6°$ from the seed transverse plane (i.e., 82.4°–97.6°). Corrections to the reported source strength (in terms of air-kerma rate in vacuum) are made for radiation attenuation by the aluminum filter, attenuation in air, radiation scatter, and several other effects. All these corrections total to approximately 5% for ^{125}I, 11% for [103]Pd, and 4% for [131]Cs sources.

It is important to recognize the robust processes in place for establishing traceable calibrations of brachytherapy sources, requirements of manufacturers to have their products included on the Brachytherapy Source Registry, and the standards of the clinical practices developed for clinical medical physicists. An example of how the dose delivered to a patient may vary based on nonrobust calibration methods is given in Figure 29.4, adopted from Williamson et al.,[63] where undesirable dose variations of up to 17% occurred.

There are still some clinics in the United States that use the antiquated unit of apparent activity (A_{app}) for specifying brachytherapy source strength.[76] Another antiquated unit of source strength is the source equivalence to milligrams of radium (i.e., mg Ra eq). These units of source strength are not traceable to NIST and must not be used for clinical applications. As a requirement for transportation paperwork to ship sources to and from the manufacturer to the clinic, the contained source strength in units of MBq or mCi is specified. However, the clinical medical physicist *should not* use this information for the derivation of dose in the patient, this is the role of S_K with units of U. Confusion by clinical medical physicists on this issue has resulted in numerous medical errors in brachytherapy, for example, with some patients receiving 27% higher dose than intended for treatment with ^{125}I seeds.[63,77] While the radiation oncologist will be familiar with concepts like standards of care, he or she will likely not be familiar with concepts like calibration traceability, and it is the responsibility of the clinical medical physicist to convey the importance of following the long-standing recommendations of the AAPM[78] for only using S_K with units of U for brachytherapy source when ordering sources, independently measuring their source strength, and using this in clinical treatment plans.

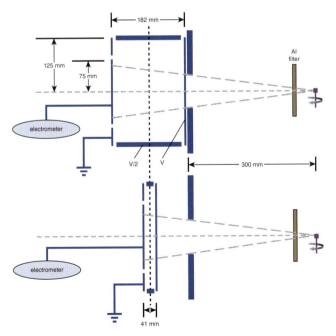

FIGURE 29.3. Schematic depiction of the wide-angle free-air chamber (WAFAC) at the National Institute of Standards and Technology, as adapted from Rivard et al.[28]

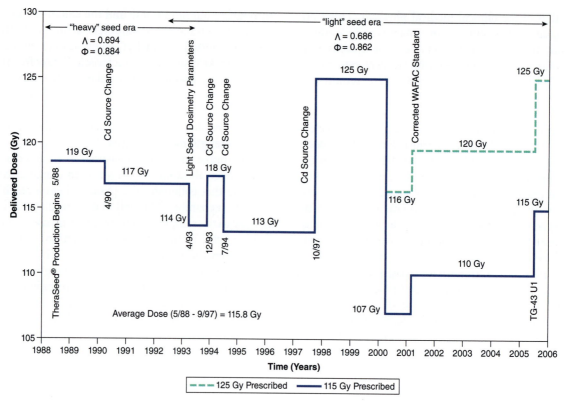

FIGURE 29.4. Variations in the delivered dose as a function of time when prescribing either 125 or 115 Gy with the model 200 [103]Pd source using the 1D dose calculation formalism in Eq. 29.1, as adapted from Williamson et al.[63] The solid line indicates a prescribed dose of 115 Gy, which initially delivered a dose of 119 Gy in May of 1988. Through changes in the [109]Cd calibration source at Theragenics, Corp. (Buford, GA), the delivered dose varied from 113 to 125 Gy preceding the establishment of the National Institute of Standards and Technology (NIST) Wide-Angle Free-Air Chamber (WAFAC) calibration standard. After implementation of this calibration standard and correction for a detector response anomaly, a prescribed dose of 115 Gy corresponded to a delivered dose of 115 Gy through use of the AAPM TG-43U1 brachytherapy dosimetry parameters. For those physicians that changed their prescription dose from 115 to 125 Gy in the year 2000, as indicated by the dashed line, the delivered dose ranged from 116 to 125 Gy at present.

TREATMENT PLANNING

The treatment planning process for brachytherapy has advanced considerably over the past decade. Modern brachytherapy treatment planning relies on computer-based approaches for dose calculation.[58,79,80] Optimization of source strength is not typically used for LDR brachytherapy, where it is most helpful for HDR brachytherapy using ^{192}Ir sources when a single source traverses the implant with varying dwell times. Even with modern computational tools and technological advances such as the ability to perform intraoperative brachytherapy treatment planning without a preimplant plan, all participants in the process must recognize that a poorly executed brachytherapy implant cannot be salvaged afterward.

Use of film or other 2D means of identifying the spatial relationship between the brachytherapy sources and the patient is discouraged given the widespread availability of CT scanners used in the clinic primarily for EBRT treatment planning.[81,82] Image-based, 3D treatment planning for brachytherapy will produce a more realistic representation of the implant conditions.[83,84] 3D imaging is now used for both identifying the structures within the patient as well as guiding the prescription in a volumetric manner instead of simply prescribing dose to an arbitrary point.[85,86] While CT remains the gold standard in general for brachytherapy imaging, use of magnetic resonance imaging (MRI) is becoming more prevalent due to its ability to discern soft issues better than ~100 kV X-rays.[87–90] Ultrasound (US) also has a strong role for source delivery and postimplant treatment planning in permanent prostate implants given its nonionization nature and ability to discern soft tissue. However, probe placement during transrectal US imaging displaces the anatomy and produces differences in implanted dose distributions and related plan evaluation metrics. It is now standard of practice to perform image fusion of CT with any pertinent and available dataset(s), for example, MRI or positron emission tomography (PET).

There are many dosimetric uncertainties associated with clinical brachytherapy. The joint AAPM+ESTRO report TG-138 estimated the total dose calculation uncertainty ($k=1$) to be about 4.4% for a single ^{125}I source.[91] The propagation of uncertainties from source measurement to utilization in the brachytherapy TPS is given in Table 29.2.

Propagation of best practice uncertainties and a standard uncertainty of k=1 (unless stated otherwise with a coverage factor of 2) for derivation of dose at 1 cm on the transverse plane for an LDR ^{125}I brachytherapy source.[90] The measured source strength S_K is added in quadrature with the Monte Carlo–derived brachytherapy dosimetry parameters and the uncertainties associated with treatment planning system (TPS) interpolation uncertainties, yielding a total dose calculation uncertainty of 4.4%. The expanded uncertainty (k=2) is simply double the standard uncertainty and differs slightly from 8.8% due to rounding of the preceding values.

TABLE 29.2

Uncertainty component	Relative propagated uncertainty (%)
S_K measurement by the clinical medical physicist	1.3
Measured dose	3.6
Monte Carlo dose estimate	1.7
TPS interpolation uncertainty	3.8
Total dose calculation uncertainty	4.4
Expanded uncertainty (k=2)	8.7

These uncertainties increase markedly once other sources of dosimetric uncertainty are included from the clinical process of source implantation. In a joint ESTRO+AAPM report, Kirisits et al.[92] described the various uncertainty components. A standard uncertainty of 2% was associated with contouring structures using CT for permanent prostate brachytherapy for ^{125}I and postimplant day-0 CT. However, the largest uncertainty (i.e., 7%) was attributed to changes in anatomy between the implant and postimplant imaging due to edema. In combination with all other uncertainty components, a total dosimetric uncertainty (k=1) of 11% was estimated.

The 1985 ICRU Report 38[17] established criteria for reporting doses and volumes used in intracavitary brachytherapy for gynecological disease. This report was later updated to be generalized to other disease sites requiring interstitial brachytherapy in the 1997 ICRU Report 58.[93] The AAPM updated these recommendations by providing specifics for reporting criteria for permanent prostate brachytherapy in the TG-137 report.[94]

As part of its 2009 initiative to update all brachytherapy-related guidelines,[39] the American Brachytherapy Society (ABS) provided updated guidelines in 2012 on transrectal US-guided permanent prostate brachytherapy.[95] These guidelines included criteria for treatment with brachytherapy, contraindications for use, and an expansion of treatment options for patients stratified by risk grouping. Where patients were categorized as high risk, the ABS recommended use of brachytherapy in combination with EBRT and androgen deprivation therapy. Only the three radionuclides included in Table 29.1 were recommended for this treatment modality. Disappointingly, the report included recommendations for source strength in terms of apparent activity, requiring a leap of faith for the clinician to utilize an outdated conversion factor to correlate apparent activity with the brachytherapy dosimetry parameters. Prescription doses of 140–160 Gy were recommended for ^{125}I, not accounting for the prescription reset from 160 to 144 Gy due to traceable calibrations excluding titanium K-edge characteristic X-rays.[38,74,96] Similarly, prescription doses of 110–125 Gy were recommended for ^{103}Pd, not accounting for a prescription reset due to changes in source calibration standards.[38,62,97]

The ABS provided guidelines for LDR brachytherapy of cervical cancer in 2012.[98] These guidelines updated the prior ABS guidelines by Nag et al.[99,100] to expand the role of brachytherapy to include patients with disease stages IB2 to IVA of the International Federation of Gynaecology and Obstetrics known as FIGO.[101] For definitive treatments using temporary implants, a cumulative dose of 80–90 Gy was recommended, with two applications to allow for tumor reduction and improved tumor coverage with the second brachytherapy application about a week apart. Prescriptions require dose delivery to point A or to the 100% isodose line. The D_{90} and V_{100} for the high-risk clinical target volume should receive greater than 90% of the prescribed dose. Temporary implants using LDR ^{137}Cs are recommended for intracavitary treatments while LDR ^{192}Ir sources are also recommended for temporary interstitial treatments. LDR ^{131}Cs has also been used more recently for permanent implants.[102,103]

In 2013, the ABS provided new guidelines for brachytherapy of cancer of the penis[104] and for sarcomas.[105] The majority of patients for these two diseases have historically been treated with temporary LDR ^{192}Ir brachytherapy implants. As the use of HDR ^{192}Ir brachytherapy is becoming more prevalent, LDR brachytherapy for these diseases is not viewed as a procedure that will be common in the future.

While breast cancer was historically treated with LDR ^{192}Ir wires and ribbons, this practice has fallen out of favor given the dose modulation possibilities with HDR ^{192}Ir and its outpatient treatments. However, Pignol and colleagues have examined the feasibility of treating breast cancer with permanent implantation of LDR ^{103}Pd seeds.[106,107] Dose to breast tissue differed from dose to water by up to 36%.[108] They also examined the feasibility of permanent LDR ^{125}I brachytherapy for the breast but ruled it out due to concerns for radiation exposure from this high-energy, photon-emitting radionuclide.[109,110] However, Jansen and colleagues did not observe the same concerns for radiation exposure.[111]

Other sites of disease that may receive permanent LDR brachytherapy include the brain[112-114] and the lung.[115,116] Cancer of the head-and-neck region, anal canal, rectum, and skin are all regions where LDR brachytherapy is indicated and has shown favorable results but have been treated more recently with HDR ^{192}Ir brachytherapy. Ocular diseases are almost always treated with LDR brachytherapy instead of HDR brachytherapy, largely due to the dose conformity of low-energy seeds and the radiobiological advantage of a multiday temporary implant.[117] Here, the patient is often discharged following surgery to return to the hospital a few days later for surgical explant of the brachytherapy plaque.[118,119] Given the radiation shielding by the plaque,[120] there are radiological effects that prompt advancements in clinical practice so that radiation doses are more accurately known.[121-125]

FUTURE DEVELOPMENTS

While this chapter covers the current standards for LDR brachytherapy, it is also beneficial to the reader to know what lies around the corner as the field of brachytherapy will continue to advance dependably as it has over the last century.

In addition to the three radionuclides included in Table 29.1, several other radionuclides are being investigated for LDR brachytherapy. [169]Yb[126] has a 32-day half-life and has been considered as a source for both LDR and HDR applications. Radionuclides such as [170]Tm[127,128] with a 129-day half-life, [57]Co[129] with a 272-day half-life, and [153]Gd[130] with a 240-day half-life all have mean photon energies of <0.1 MeV. Some LDR brachytherapy sources have been considered to purposefully contain more than one radionuclide.[131,132] Improved understanding of radiobiology may indicate the optimal decay in dose (i.e., half-life) needed for a given disease site.[133,134]

In the past, there had been advancements with other novel radionuclides for LDR brachytherapy such as [252]Cf, which emits fission-energy neutrons and radium-like photons. Since its proposal as a clinical source in 1965,[135] a couple thousand patients have been treated worldwide with LDR [252]Cf brachytherapy.[136,137] However, concerns for radiation exposure to hospital personnel and increased controls for special by-product materials following the terrorist attacks in the United States on September 11, 2001 have prevented its use as a brachytherapy source.[138,140]

LDR brachytherapy sources have been designed to provide directional radiation,[139] without the azimuthal symmetry required by the TG-43 dose calculation formalism. However, this attribute would require a new approach to brachytherapy treatment planning and the ability to control and monitor the source orientation. Sources have also been designed[140,141] to be thinner (i.e., 0.5 mm outer diameter) than conventional 0.8 mm outer diameter seeds, more flexible through plastic encapsulation and elongated brachytherapy sources,[142-146] and even for the entire LDR source to be dissolvable within the patient and leave no radiographic trace after 1 year.

The scope of LDR brachytherapy is expanding through the development of new applicators such as for the treatment of disease within the brain.[147-149] For the GliaSite™ balloon brain brachytherapy applicator, a liquid solution of ^{125}I or [131]Cs is injected into the balloon for a temporary implant of cranial disease.

To remove the variability in human skills for interstitial implantation of brachytherapy sources, robotic means of delivery[150,151] are being developed. The AAPM TG-192 report provides an excellent review of the field.[152] Algorithms for automatic identification of LDR seeds are already available.[153] Further automation of the brachytherapy process has focused on the segmentation or contouring of structures[154] following image acquisition. This is important as structure contouring has been identified as being the most important contributor to the dosimetric uncertainties associated with clinical brachytherapy.[91,155] Given that brachytherapy is generally an invasive procedure and perturbs the natural state of human anatomy, algorithms are being developed in the field of deformable image registration[156-158] to alter the shape of the imaged anatomy and permit accurate dose summation of the brachytherapy dose distributions. These algorithms may also work in combination with results from EBRT treatment plans to estimate the total dose distribution.

While the current standard for specifying brachytherapy source strength is air-kerma strength, a more intuitive metric would be the dose rate at some distance in a reference medium.[159] One proposal that is gaining ground in Europe is to calibrate LDR brachytherapy source strength in terms of the dose rate to water at a specified time.[160-162] A potential advantage of this approach would be lower overall dosimetric uncertainties since there would be no need to measure the dose–rate constant.[151] However, there would need to be a significant change to the clinical TPSs and calibration traceability available to the clinical medical physicist. Changing to this new metric would require societal coordination and regulatory changes for this to go smoothly.

Another advancement in dose calculations for LDR brachytherapy sources is through improvements in the TG-43 dose calculation formalism.[163] Differences between liquid water and soft tissue can amount to more than 30%.[164-167] A simple approach is to replace the dosimetry parameters for liquid water with the dosimetry parameters for soft tissue, which can drastically improve the accuracy of dose determination. As a means to further adjust the means of dose calculation, precalculated Monte Carlo–based dose distributions may be used in conventional TPSs for a particular applicator type.[59] Again, these advancements would require societal coordination for widespread implementation, along with extensions to the current tasks used to commission brachytherapy dose calculation algorithms preceding clinical use.[168-169]

CONCLUSIONS

The field of LDR brachytherapy was established over a century ago, and there are established clinical practice standards for the safe and consistent delivery of this radiation-based treatment modality. The current standard for dose calculations is the TG-43 formalism, where dosimetry parameters and prescriptive criteria have dose to water as its foundation (due to its heritage of ^{226}Ra and ^{222}Rn dosimetry). Source strength is specified in terms of air-kerma strength, the only traceable quantity for clinical use as recommended by the AAPM. Brachytherapy has been applied to every disease site, and the clinical medical physicist should learn proficiency for this manual, multidisciplinary procedure where the dose gradients and clinical uncertainties are greater than for EBRT. There are many exciting developments underway to enhance and extend the field of brachytherapy.

KEY POINTS

- brachytherapy has been used since the early 1900s

- brachytherapy is typically an invasive treatment modality with the potential for more conformal dose distributions than other radiation treatment modalities

- the AAPM TG-43 dose calculation formalism has been adopted worldwide for consistent dose calculations

- air-kerma strength (S_K) is the preferred, traceable quantity of brachytherapy source strength

- clinical brachytherapy requires well-positioned sources for delivering the desired dose distribution

- advancements in brachytherapy will further enhance and extend the field

QUESTIONS

1. Which listing of radionuclide (and half-life) is correct?
   A. ^{125}I (59.4 days), ^{103}Pd (9.7 days), ^{131}Cs (17 days)
   B. ^{125}I (59.4 days), ^{103}Pd (17 days), ^{131}Cs (9.7 days)
   C. ^{125}I (17 days), ^{103}Pd (9.7 days), ^{131}Cs (59.4 days)
   D. ^{125}I (17 days), ^{103}Pd (59.4 days), ^{131}Cs (9.7 days)

2. Which is the correct format for the 1D format for the TG-43 dose calculation formalism?

   A. $\dot{D}(r) = S_K \cdot \Lambda \cdot \dfrac{G_L(r,\theta)}{G_L(r_0,\theta_0)}^2 \cdot g_P(r) \cdot \phi_{an}(r)$

   B. $\dot{D}(r) = S_K \cdot \Lambda \cdot \dfrac{G_L(r,\theta)}{G_L(r_0,\theta_0)}^2 \cdot g_L(r) \cdot \phi_{an}(r)$

   C. $\dot{D}(r) = S_K \cdot \Lambda \cdot \left(\dfrac{r_0}{r}\right)^2 \cdot g_P(r) \cdot \phi_{an}(r)$

   D. $\dot{D}(r) = S_K \cdot \Lambda \cdot \left(\dfrac{r_0}{r}\right)^2 \cdot g_L(r) \cdot \phi_{an}(r)$

3. Using the 1D dose calculation formalism, approximately what is the total dose delivered to the surface (r=0.04 cm) of a 1 U ^{125}I seed (L = 0.93 cGy/h^{-1}/U^{-1}) after 1 year?
   A. 11,949 Gy
   B. 5,741 Gy
   C. 498 Gy
   D. 120 Gy

4. Which metric for brachytherapy source strength is recommended for clinical use?
   A. apparent activity (A_{app})
   B. MBq
   C. mCi
   D. S_K
   E. dose rate to water at a distance of 1 cm from the source transverse plane

5. For which disease site is LDR brachytherapy most prevalent?
   A. eye
   B. breast
   C. prostate
   D. cervix
   E. lung

ANSWERS

1. **B** The other answers show incorrect half-lives, as can be found in Table 29.1. Section 29.2 covers this question.

2. **C** The other answers are incorrect since calculation of the dose rate would not replicate the original calculated or measured dose rate distribution since the dosimetry parameters are inconsistent. Section 29.3 covers this question.

3. **A** The half-life of ^{125}I is 59.4 days. After 1 year, this amounts to over 6 half-lives and the source may be assumed (within 1%) to have infinitely decayed. Using Eq. (29.1) with a dose–rate constant value of 0.93 cGy/h^{-1}/U^{-1} for ^{125}I, r=0.04 cm for the capsule radius, and assuming $g_P(0.04)$ equals unity, the initial dose rate in contact with a 1 U seed is about 581 cGy/h. After infinite decay,

this amounts to 1,194,946 cGy or 11,949 Gy. The other answers are incorrect, where (b) is low by a factor of 2.08 based on incorrectly inverting the ln(2) factor for deriving infinite decay, where (c) is low by a factor of 24 based on incorrectly converting the half-life for infinite decay, and where (d) is low by a factor of 100 for tricking the reader when converting dose to Gy. Sections 29.2 and 29.3 cover this question.

4. D The other answers are incorrect since only air-kerma strength (S_K) is a quantity traceable to NIST for determination of brachytherapy source strength. Answer a) should never be used since there are inconsistent correct factors. Answers b) and c) are often used for licensing and transportation purposes, but these refer to the contained activity. Answer e) remains a research project. Section 29.4 covers this question.

5. C LDR brachytherapy is most frequently performed for the prostate. The other disease sites have either lower incidence or are treated more frequently with HDR brachytherapy. Section 29.5 covers this question.

REFERENCES

1. Danlos H, Bloch P. Note sur le traitement du lupus erythematenx par des application de radium. *Ann Dermatol Syphil.* 1901;2:986–988.
2. Forssell G. La lutte social contre le cancer. *J Radiologie.* 1931;15:621–634.
3. Aronowitz JN. Benjamin Barringer: originator of the transperineal prostate implant. *Urology.* 2002;60:731–734.
4. Aronowitz JN. Dawn of prostate brachytherapy: 1915–1930. *Int J Radiat Oncol Biol Phys.* 2002;54:712–718.
5. Aronowitz JN. Buried emanation: the development of seeds for permanent implantation. *Brachytherapy.* 2002;1:167–178.
6. Aronowitz JN. Ethereal fire: antecedents of radiology and radiotherapy. *Am J Roentgenol.* 2007;188:904–912.
7. Aronowitz JN, Aronowitz SV, Robinson RF. Classics in brachytherapy: Margaret Cleaves introduces gynecologic brachytherapy. *Brachytherapy.* 2007;6:293–298.
8. Aronowitz JN. The golden age of prostate brachytherapy: a cautionary tale. *Brachytherapy.* 2008;7:55–59.
9. Aronowitz JN Robinson RF. Howard Kelly establishes gynecologic brachytherapy in the United States. *Brachytherapy.* 2010;9:178–184.
10. Aronowitz JN. Don Lawrence and the k-capture revolution. *Brachytherapy.* 2010;9:373–381.
11. Aronowitz JN. Partial breast irradiation by brachytherapy, 1927. *Brachytherapy.* 2011;10:427–431.
12. Aronowitz JN. Whitmore, Henschke, and Hilaris: The reorientation of prostate brachytherapy (1970–1987). *Brachytherapy.* 2012;11:157–162.
13. Aronowitz JN. Robert Abbe: Early American brachytherapist. Brachytherapy. 2012;11:421–428.
14. Aronowitz JN, Rivard MJ. The phylogeny of permanent prostate brachytherapy. *J Contemp Brachyther.* 2013;5:89–92.
15. Aronowitz JN, Rivard MJ The evolution of computerized treatment planning for brachytherapy: American contributions. *J Contemp Brachyther.* 2014;11:85–90.
16. Aronowitz JN. Introduction of transperineal image-guided prostate brachytherapy. *Int J Radiat Oncol Biol Phys.* 2014;89:907–915.
17. International Commission on Radiation Units and Measurements (ICRU). Dose and volume specification for reporting intracavitary therapy in gynecology, Report No. 38. Bethesda, MD: ICRU; 1985.
18. Bogdanich W. At V.A. hospital, a rogue cancer unit. *The New York Times*, June 20, 2009.
19. Venselaar J, Perez-Calatayud J. A practical guide to quality control of brachytherapy equipment. 1st ed. European Guidelines for Quality Assurance in Radiotherapy: Booklet No. 8; http://www.estro-education.org/publications/Documents/Booklet_n8.pdf Brussels, Belgium; 2004.
20. Nath R, Anderson LL, Meli JA, Olch AJ, Stitt JA, Williamson JF. Code of practice for brachytherapy physics: Report of the AAPM Radiation Therapy Committee Task Group No. 56. *Med Phys.* 1997;24:1557–1598.
21. Yu Y, Anderson LL, Li Z, Mellenberg DE, Nath R, Schell MC, Waterman FM, Wu A, Blasko JC. Permanent prostate seed implant brachytherapy: Report of the American Association of Physicists in Medicine Task Group No. 64. *Med Phys.* 1999;26:2054–2076.
22. Thomadsen BR. Achieving quality in brachytherapy. Medical Science Series, Institute of Physics Publishing. Bristol and Philadelphia; 2000.
23. Kennedy AS, et al. Pathologic response and microdosimetry of ^{90}Y microspheres in man: review of four explanted whole livers. *Int J Radiat Oncol Biol Phys.* 2004;60:1552–1563.
24. Dezarn WA, et al. Recommendations of the American Association of Physicists in Medicine on dosimetry, imaging, and quality assurance procedures for ^{90}Y microsphere brachytherapy in the treatment of hepatic malignancies. *Med Phys.* 2011;38:4824–4845.
25. Dinsmore M, Harte KJ, Sliski AP, Smith DO, Nomikos PM, Dalterio MJ, Boom AJ, Leonard WF, Oettinger PE, Yanch JC. A new miniature x-ray source for interstitial radiosurgery: Device description. *Med Phys.* 1996;23:45–52.
26. Rivard MJ, Davis SD, DeWerd LA, Rusch TW, Axelrod S. Calculated and measured brachytherapy dosimetry parameters in water for the Xoft Axxent X-Ray source: an electronic brachytherapy source. *Med. Phys.* 2006;33:4020–4032.
27. Garcia-Martinez T, Chan J-P, Perez-Calatayud J, Ballester F. Dosimetric characteristics of a new unit for electronic skin brachytherapy. *J Contemp Brachytherapy.* 2014;6:45–53.
28. Rivard MJ, Butler WM, DeWerd LA, Huq MS, Ibbott GS, Li Z, Mitch MG, Nath R, Williamson JF. Update of AAPM Task Group No. 43 Report: a revised AAPM protocol for brachytherapy dose calculations. *Med Phys.* 2004;31:633–674.
29. Rivard MJ, Butler WM, DeWerd LA, Huq MS, Ibbott GS, Meigooni AS, Melhus CS, Mitch MG, Nath R, Williamson JF. Supplement to the 2004 update of the AAPM Task Group No. 43 Report: A revised AAPM protocol for brachytherapy dose calculations. *Med. Phys.* 2007;34:2187–2205.
30. Ballester F, Granero D, Perez-Calatayud J, Melhus CS, Rivard MJ. Evaluation of high-energy brachytherapy source electronic disequilibrium and dose from emitted electrons. *Med. Phys.* 2009;36:4250–4256.
31. Anderson LL, Presser JE. Classical systems I for temporary interstitial implants. In: Williamson JF, Thomadsen BR, Nath R, eds. *Brachytherapy Physics, AAPM Summer School.* Madison, WI: Medical Physics Publishing; 1995.
32. Gillin MJ, Albano KS, Erickson B. Classical systems II for planar and volume temporary interstitial implants. In: Williamson JF, Thomadsen BR, Nath R, eds. *Brachytherapy Physics, AAPM Summer School.* Madison, WI: Medical Physics Publishing; 1995.
33. Gillin MJ, Mourtada F. Systems 1B: Manchester planar and volume implants and the Paris system. In: Thomadsen BR, Rivard MJ, Butler WM, eds. *Brachytherapy Physics.* 2nd ed. Joint AAPM/America Brachytherapy Society Summer School. Madison, WI: Medical Physics Publishing; 2005.

34. Zwicker RD. Quimby-based brachytherapy systems. In: Thomadsen BR, Rivard MJ, Butler WM, eds. *Brachytherapy Physics*. 2nd ed. Joint AAPM/American Brachytherapy Society Summer School. Madison, WI: Medical Physics Publishing; 2005.

35. Meisberger LL, Keller RJ, Shalek RJ. The effective attenuation in water of the gamma rays of gold-198, iridium-192, cesium-137, radium-226, and cobalt-60. *Radiology* 1968;90:953–957.

36. Rivard MJ, Venselaar JLM, Beaulieu L. The evolution of brachytherapy treatment planning. *Med. Phys.* 2009;36:2136–2153.

37. Failla G. Radium technique at the Memorial Hospital. *New York Arch Radiol Electrother*. 1920;25:3–19.

38. Davis BJ, et al. American Brachytherapy Society consensus guidelines for transrectal ultrasound-guided permanent prostate brachytherapy. *Brachytherapy*. 2012;11:6–19.

39. Nath R, et al. AAPM recommendations on dose prescription and reporting methods for permanent interstitial brachytherapy for prostate cancer: Report of Task Group 137. *Med. Phys.* 2009;36:5310–5322.

40. Nath R, et al. Dosimetry of interstitial brachytherapy sources: recommendations of the AAPM Radiation Therapy Committee Task Group No. 43. *Med. Phys.* 1995;22:209–234.

41. Eaton DJ, Highly cited papers in *Medical Physics*. *Med. Phys.* 2014;41:080401.

42. Paterson R, Parker HM. A dosage system for interstitial radium therapy. *Br J Radiol*. 1938;11:252–266.

43. Quimby EH, Castro V. The calculation of dosage in interstitial radium therapy. *Am J Roentgenol Radium Ther Nucl Med*. 1953;70:739–759.

44. Shalek RJ, Stovall M. The M. D. Anderson method for the computation of isodose curves around interstitial and intracavitary radiation sources. I. Dose from linear sources. *Am J Roentgenol Radium Ther Nucl Med*. 1968;102:662–672.

45. Dale RG. Some theoretical derivations relating to the tissue dosimetry of brachytherapy nuclides, with particular reference to iodine-125. *Med. Phys.* 1983;10:176–183 (1983).

46. Dale R. Revisions to radial dose function data for ^{125}I and ^{131}Cs. *Med Phys*. 1986;13:963–964.

47. Anderson LL, Nath R, Weaver KA. Interstitial Collaborative Working Group (ICWG). *Interstitial Brachytherapy: Physical, Biological, and Clinical Considerations*. New York: Raven; 1990.

48. Rivard MJ, et al. Comparison of dose calculation methods for brachytherapy of intraocular tumors. *Med Phys*. 2011;38:306–316.

49. Ibbott GS, et al. Fifty years of AAPM involvement in radiation dosimetry. *Med. Phys.* 2008;35:1418–1427.

50. Meigooni AS, et al. Instrumentation and dosimeter-size artifacts in quantitative thermoluminescence dosimetry of low-dose fields. *Med. Phys.* 1995;22:555–561.

51. Williamson JF, Rivard MJ. Quantitative dosimetry methods for brachytherapy. In: Thomadsen, BR, Rivard MJ, Butler WM, eds. *Brachytherapy Physics*. 2nd ed. Madison, WI: Medical Physics; 2005:233–294.

52. Williamson JF, Rivard MJ. Thermoluminescent detector and Monte Carlo techniques for reference-quality brachytherapy dosimetry. In: Rogers DWO, Cygler JE, eds. *Clinical Dosimetry for Radiotherapy: AAPM Summer School*. Madison, WI: Medical Physics; 2009: pp. 403–436, Chap. 13.

53. Stovall MA, Shalek RJ. Study of explicit distributions of radiation in interstitial implantations. I. Method of calculation with automatic digital computer. *Radiology*. 1962;78:950–954.

54. Rivard MJ, Granero D, Perez-Calatayud J Ballester F. Influence of photon energy spectra from brachytherapy sources on Monte Carlo simulations of kerma and dose rates in water and air. *Med. Phys.* 2010; 37:869–876.

55. Ellett WH, Brownell GL, Reddy AR. An assessment of Monte Carlo calculations to determine gamma ray dose from internal emitters. *Phys Med Biol*. 1968;13:219–230.

56. Krishnaswamy V. Calculation of the dose distribution about californium-252 needles in tissue. *Radiology*. 1971;98:155–160.

57. Williamson JF, Brachytherapy technology and physics practice since 1950: a half-century of progress. *Phys. Med. Biol*. 2006;51:R303–R325.

58. Thomadsen BR, Williamson JF, Rivard MJ, Meigooni AS. Anniversary paper: past and current issues, and trends in brachytherapy physics. *Med Phys*. 2008;35:4708–4723.

59. Rivard MJ, Butler WM, DeWerd LA, Huq MS, Ibbott GS, Li Z, Mitch MG, Nath R, Williamson JF. Erratum: update of AAPM Task Group No. 43 Report: a revised AAPM protocol for brachytherapy dose calculations [Med. Phys. 31, 633–674 (2004)]. *Med. Phys.* 2004;31:3532–3533.

60. Rivard MJ, Butler WM, DeWerd LA, Huq MS, Ibbott GS, Meigooni AS, Melhus CS, Mitch MG, Nath R, Williamson JF. Erratum: Supplement to the 2004 update of the AAPM Task Group No. 43 Report [Med. Phys. 34, 2187–2205 (2007)]. *Med. Phys.* 2010;37:2396.

61. Bice WS, Prestidge BR, Kurtzman S, Beriwal S, Moran B, Patel R, Rivard MJ, Recommendations for permanent prostate brachytherapy with ^{131}Cs: a consensus report from the Cesium Advisory Group. *Brachytherapy*. 2008;7:290–296.

62. Rivard MJ, Refinements to the geometry factor used in the AAPM Task Group Report No. 43 necessary for brachytherapy dosimetry calculations. *Med. Phys.* 1999;26:2445–2450.

63. Rivard MJ, Melhus CS, Granero D, Perez-Calatayud J, Ballester F. An approach to using conventional brachytherapy software for clinical treatment planning of complex, Monte Carlo-based brachytherapy dose distributions. *Med. Phys.* 2009;36:1968–1975.

64. Williamson JF, et al. Recommendations of the American Association of Physicists in Medicine on ^{103}Pd interstitial source calibration and dosimetry: implications for dose specification and prescription. *Med. Phys.* 2000;27:634–642.

65. Williamson JF, et al. Recommendations of the American Association of Physicists in Medicine regarding the impact of implementing the 2004 Task Group 43 report on dose specification for ^{103}Pd and ^{125}I interstitial brachytherapy. Med. Phys. 32, 1424–1439.

66. Rivard MJ, Nath R. Interstitial brachytherapy dosimetry update. *Rad Prot Dosim*. 2006;120:64–69.

67. DeWerd LA, Huq MS, Das IJ, Ibbott GS, Hanson WF, Slowey TW, Williamson JF, Coursey BM. Procedures for establishing and maintaining consistent air-kerma strength standards for low energy, photon-emitting brachytherapy sources: recommendations of the Calibration Laboratory Accreditation Subcommittee of the American Association of Physicists in Medicine. *Med. Phys.* 2004;31:675–681.

68. Butler WM, Bice WS, Jr., DeWerd LA, Hevezi JM, Huq MS, Ibbott GS, Palta JR, Rivard MJ, Seuntjens JP, Thomadsen BR, Third-party brachytherapy source calibrations and physicist responsibilities: report of the AAPM low energy brachytherapy source calibration working group. *Med. Phys.* 2008;35:3860–3865.

69. Williamson JF, Coursey BM, DeWerd LA, Hanson WF, Nath R. Dosimetric prerequisites for routine clinical use of new low energy photon interstitial brachytherapy sources. *Med. Phys.* 1998;25:2269–2270.

70. Rosenzweig DP, Schell MC, Yu Y. Toward a statistically relevant calibration end point for prostate seed implants. *Med. Phys.* 2000;27:144–150.

71. Ramos LI, Monge RM. Sampling size in the verification of manufacturer-supplied air kerma strengths. Med. Phys. 32, 3375–3378.

72. Wan S, Joshi CP, Carnes G, and Schreiner LJ. Evaluation of an automated seed loader for seed calibration in prostate brachytherapy. *J Appl Clin Med Phys* 2006;7:115–125.

73. Yue NJ, Haffty BG, Yue J, On the assay of brachytherapy sources. *Med Phys*. 2007;34:1975–1982.

74. Seltzer SM, Lamperti PJ, Loevinger R, Mitch MG, Weaver JT, Coursey BM. New national air-kerma-strength standards for ^{125}I and ^{103}Pd brachytherapy seeds. *J Res Natl Inst Stand Technol*. 2003;108:337–358.

75. Kubo H. Exposure contribution from Ti K x rays produced in the titanium capsule of the clinical ^{125}I seed. *Med Phys*. 1985;12:215–220.

76. Kubo HD, Coursey BM, Hanson WF, Kline RW, Seltzer SM, Shuping RE, Williamson JF. Report of the ad hoc committee of the AAPM Radiation Therapy Committee on ^{125}I sealed source dosimetry. *Int J Radiat Oncol Biol Phys*. 1998;40:697–702.

77. Williamson JF, et al. On the use of apparent activity (A_{app}) for treatment planning of ^{125}I and ^{103}Pd interstitial brachytherapy sources: recommendations of the American Association of Physicists in Medicine radiation therapy committee subcommittee on low-energy brachytherapy source dosimetry. *Med Phys*. 1999;26:2529–2530.

78. NRC Information Notice 2009–17: reportable medical events involving treatment delivery errors caused by confusion of units for the specification of brachytherapy sources. Nuclear Regulatory Commission, Washington, DC, August 28, 2009. http://pbadupws. nrc.gov/docs/ML0807/ML080710054.pdf

79. Nath R, et al., Specification of Brachytherapy Source Strength: Report of AAPM Task Group No. 32. Melville, NY: American Institute of Physics; 1987.

80. Pouliot J, Lessard E, Hsu I, Advanced 3D planning. In: Thomadsen BR, Rivard MJ, Butler WM, eds. *Brachytherapy Physics*. 2nd ed. Joint AAPM/America Brachytherapy Society Summer School. Madison, WI: Medical Physics Publishing; 2005.

81. Li Z. Quality review of brachytherapy treatment systems. In: Thomadsen BR, Rivard MJ, Butler WM, eds. *Brachytherapy Physics*. 2nd ed. Joint AAPM/America Brachytherapy Society Summer School. Madison, WI: Medical Physics Publishing; 2005.

82. Weeks KJ, Dennett JC. Dose calculations and measurements for a CT-compatible version of the Fletcher applicator. *Int J Radiat Oncol Biol Phys*. 1990;18:1191–1198.

83. Fellner C, et al. Comparison of radiography- and computed tomography-based treatment planning in cervix cancer in brachytherapy with specific attention to some quality assurance aspects. *Radiother Oncol*. 2001;5:53–62.

84. Harris T, et al. The variance of bladder and rectal doses calculated from orthogonal and simple stereo films in cervix high-dose-rate brachytherapy. *Brachytherapy*. 2007;6:304–310.

85. Kim RY, Pareek P. Radiography-based treatment planning compared with computed tomography (CT)-based treatment planning for intracavitary brachytherapy in cancer of the cervix: analysis of dose-volume histograms. *Brachytherapy* 2003;2:200–206.

86. Shin KH, et al., CT-guided intracavitary radiotherapy for cervical cancer: comparison of conventional point A plan with clinical target volume-based three-dimensional plan using dose-volume parameters. *Int J Radiat Oncol Biol Phys*. 2005;62:197–204.

87. Pötter R, et al. Recommendations from Gynaecological (GYN) GEC-ESTRO Working Group (II): concepts and terms in 3D image-based treatment planning in cervix cancer – 3D dose volume parameters and aspects of 3D image-based anatomy, radiation physics, radiobiology. *Radiother Oncol*. 2006;78:67–77.

88. Viswanathan AN, et al. Computed tomography versus magnetic resonance imaging-based contouring in cervical cancer brachytherapy: results of a prospective trial and preliminary guidelines for standardized contours. *Int J Radiat Oncol Biol Phys*. 2007;68:491–498.

89. Wachter-Gerstner N, et al. Bladder and rectum dose defined from MRI based treatment planning for cervix cancer brachytherapy: comparison of dose-volume histograms for organ contours and organ wall, comparison with ICRU rectum and bladder reference points. *Radiother Oncol*. 2003;68:269–276.

90. Haie-Meder C, et al. Recommendations from Gynaecological (GYN) GEC-ESTRO Working Group (I); concepts and terms in 3D image based 3D treatment planning in cervix cancer brachytherapy with emphasis on MRI assessment of GTV and CTV. *Radiother Oncol*. 2005;74:235–245.

91. Kirisits C, et al. Dose and volume parameters for MRI treatment planning in intracavitary brachytherapy for cervical cancer. *Int J Radiat Oncol Biol Phys*. 2005;62:901–911.

92. DeWerd LA, Ibbott GS, Meigooni AS, Mitch MG, Rivard MJ, Stump KE, Thomadsen BR, Venselaar JLM. A dosimetric uncertainty analysis for photon-emitting brachytherapy sources: report of AAPM Task Group No. 138 and GEC-ESTRO. *Med. Phys*. 2011;38:782–801.

93. Kirisits C, et al. Review of clinical brachytherapy uncertainties: analysis guidelines of GEC-ESTRO and the AAPM. *Radiother. Oncol*. 2014;110:199–212.

94. International Commission on Radiation Units and Measurements (ICRU). Dose and volume specification for reporting interstitial therapy, Report No. 58. Bethesda, MD: ICRU; 1997.

95. Horwitz EM. ABS brachytherapy consensus guidelines. *Brachytherapy*. 2012;11:4–5.

96. Williamson JF, et al. Guidance to users of Nycomed Amersham and North American Scientific, Inc. I-125 interstitial sources: recommendations of the American Association of Physicists in Medicine Radiation Therapy Committee Ad Hoc Subcommittee Low-Energy Seed Dosimetry. *Med. Phys*. 1999;26:570–573.

97. Rivard MJ, Butler WM, Devlin PM, Hayes JK, Jr., Hearn RA, Lief EP, Meigooni AS, Merrick GS, Williamson JF. American Brachytherapy Society recommends no change for prostate permanent implant dose prescriptions using iodine-125 or palladium-103. *Brachytherapy*. 2007;6:34–37.

98. Beyer D, et al. American Brachytherapy Society recommendations for clinical implementation of NIST-1999 standards for [103]palladium brachytherapy. *Int J Radiat Oncol Biol Phys*. 47, 273–275.

99. Lee LJ, et al. American Brachytherapy Society consensus guidelines for penile locally advanced carcinoma of the cervix. Part III: low-dose-rate and pulsed-dose-rate brachytherapy. *Brachytherapy*. 2012;11:53–57.

100. Nag S, et al. The American Brachytherapy Society survey of brachytherapy practice for carcinoma of the cervix in the United States. *Gynecol Oncol*. 1999;73:111–118.

101. Nag S, et al. Proposed guidelines for image-based intracavitary brachytherapy for cervical carcinoma: report from Image-Guided Brachytherapy Working Group. *Int J Radiat Oncol Biol Phys*. 2004;60:1160–1172.

102. International Federation of Gynaecology and Obstetrics, FIGO House, London SE1 8ST, UK. https://www.figo.org/

103. Wooten CE, Randall M, Edwards J, Aryal P, Luo W, Feddock J. Implementation and early clinical results utilizing Cs-131 permanent interstitial implants for gynecologic malignancies. *Gynecol Oncol*. 2014;133:268–273.

104. Feddock J, Cheek D, Steber C, Edwards J, Slone S, Luo W, Randall M. Reirradiation using permanent interstitial brachytherapy: a potentially durable technique for salvaging recurrent pelvic malignancies. *Int J Radiat Oncol Biol Phys*. 2017;99:1225–1233.

105. Crook JM, et al. American Brachytherapy Society–Groupe Européen de Curiethérapie–European Society of Therapeutic Radiation Oncology (ABS-GEC-ESTRO) consensus statement for penile brachytherapy. *Brachytherapy*. 2013;12:191–198.

106. Holloway CL, et al. American Brachytherapy Society (ABS) consensus statement for sarcoma brachytherapy. *Brachytherapy*. 2013;12:179–190.

107. Pignol J-P, Keller B, Rakovitch E, Sankreacha R, Easton H, Que W. First report of a permanent breast [103]Pd seed implant as adjuvant radiation treatment for early-stage breast cancer. *Int J Radiat Oncol Biol Phys*. 2006;64:176–181.

108. Pignol J-P, Rakovitch E, Keller BM, Sankreacha R, Chartier C. Tolerance and acceptance results of a palladium-103 permanent breast seed implant Phase I/II study. *Int J Radiat Oncol Biol Phys*. 2009;73:1482–1488.

109. Afsharpour H, et al. Influence of breast composition and interseed attenuation in dose calculations for post-implant assessment of permanent breast [103]Pd seed implant. *Phys Med Biol*. 2010;55:4547–4561.

110. Keller B, et al. A permanent breast seed implant as partial breast radiation therapy for early-stage patients: a comparison of palladium-103 and iodine-125 isotopes based on radiation safety considerations. *Int J Radiat Oncol Biol Phys*. 2005;62:358–365.

111. Keller BM, et al. A radiation badge survey for family members living with patients treated with a [103]Pd permanent breast seed implant. *Int J Radiat Oncol Biol Phys*. 2008;70:267–271.

112. Jansen N, Deneufbourg J-M, Nickers P. Adjuvant stereotactic permanent seed breast implant: a boost series in view of partial breast irradiation. *Int J Radiat Oncol Biol Phys*. 2007;67:1052–1058.

113. Ostertag CB, Kreth FW. Interstitial iodine-125 radiosurgery for cerebral metastases. *Br J Neurosurg*. 1995;9:593–604.

114. Schulder M, Black PM, Shrieve DC, Alexander E III, Loeffler JS. Permanent low-activity iodine-125 implants for cerebral metastases. *J Neurooncol*. 1997;33:213–221.

115. Bogart JA, et al. Resection and permanent I-125 brachytherapy without whole brain irradiation for solitary brain metastasis from nonsmall cell lung carcinoma. *J Neurooncol*. 1999;44:53–57.

116. Lee W, Daly BDT, DiPetrillo TA, Morelli DM, Neuschatz AC, Morr J, Rivard MJ, Limited resection for non-small cell lung cancer: Observed local control with implantation of I-125 brachytherapy seeds. *Ann Thorac Surg*. 2003;75:237–243.

117. Fernando HC, et al. Impact of brachytherapy on local recurrence rates after sublobar resection: results from ACOSOG Z4032 (alliance), a phase III randomized trial for high-risk operable non–small-cell lung cancer. *J Clin Oncol*. 2003;32:2456–2462.

118. Leonard KL, et al. A 17-year retrospective study of institutional results for eye plaque brachytherapy of uveal melanoma using ^{125}I, [103]Pd, and [131]Cs and historical perspective. *Brachytherapy*. 2011;10:331–339.

119. Nag S, Quivey JM, Earle JD, et al. The American Brachytherapy Society recommendations for brachytherapy of uveal melanomas. *Int J Radiat Oncol Biol Phys.* 2003;56:544–555.

120. Simpson ER, et al. The American Brachytherapy Society consensus guidelines for plaque brachytherapy of uveal melanoma and retinoblastoma. *Brachytherapy.* 2014;13:1–14.

121. Astrahan MA. Improved treatment planning for COMS eye plaques. *Int J Radiat Oncol Biol Phys.* 2005;61:1227–1242.

122. Rivard MJ, Melhus CS, Sioshansi S, Morr JB. The impact of prescription depth, dose rate, plaque size, and source loading on the central axis using ^{103}Pd, ^{125}I, and ^{131}Cs. *Brachytherapy.* 2008;7:327–335.

123. Rivard MJ, Chiu-Tsao S-T, Finger PT, Meigooni AS, Melhus CS, Mourtada F, Napolitano ME,. Rogers DWO, Thomson RM, Nath R. Comparison of dose calculation methods for brachytherapy of intraocular tumors. *Med Phys.* 2011;38:306–316.

124. Chiu-Tsao S-T, et al. Dosimetry of ^{125}I and ^{103}Pd COMS eye plaques for intraocular tumors: report of Task Group 129 by the AAPM and ABS. *Med Phys.* 2012;39:6161–6184.

125. Lesperance M, Martinov M, Thomson RM. Monte Carlo dosimetry for ^{103}Pd, ^{125}I, and ^{131}Cs ocular brachytherapy with various plaque models using an eye phantom. *Med Phys.* 2014;41:031706.

126. Aryal P, Molloy JA, Rivard MJ, Independent dosimetric assessment of the model EP917 episcleral brachytherapy plaque. *Med Phys.* 2014;41:092102.

127. Nath R, Gray L, Park CH, Dose distributions around cylindrical ^{241}Am sources for a clinical intracavitary applicator. *Med Phys.* 1987;14:809–817.

128. Ballester F, Granero D, Perez-Calatayud J, Venselaar JLM, Rivard MJ. Study of encapsulated ^{170}Tm sources for their potential use in brachytherapy. *Med Phys.* 2010;37:1629–1637.

129. Enger SA, D'Amours M, Beaulieu L. Modeling a hypothetical ^{170}Tm source for brachytherapy applications. *Med Phys.* 2011;38:5307–5310.

130. Enger SA, Lundqvist H, D'Amours M, Beaulieu L. Exploring ^{57}Co as a new isotope for brachytherapy applications. *Med Phys.* 2012;39:2342–2345.

131. Enger SA, Fisher DR, and Flynn RT. Gadolinium-153 as a brachytherapy isotope. *Phys Med Biol.* 2013;58:957–964.

132. Nuttens VE, Lucas S. AAPM TG-43U1 formalism adaptation and Monte Carlo dosimetry simulations of multiple-radionuclide brachytherapy sources. *Med Phys.* 2006;33:1101–1107.

133. Nuttens, VE, Lucas S. Determination of the prescription dose for biradionuclide permanent prostate brachytherapy. *Med Phys.* 2008;35:5451–5462.

134. Villeneuve M, et al. Relationship between isotope half-life and prostate edema for optimal prostate dose coverage in permanent seed implants. *Med Phys.* 2008;35:1970–1977.

135. Wang JZ, et al. Effect of edema, relative biological effectiveness, and dose heterogeneity on prostate brachytherapy. *Med Phys.* 2006;33:1025–1032.

136. Schlea CC, Stoddard DH. Californium isotopes proposed for intracavitary and interstitial radiation therapy with neutrons. *Nature.* 1965;206:1058–1059.

137. Liu H, et al. Californium-252 neutron brachytherapy combined with external beam radiotherapy for esophageal cancer: long-term treatment results. *Brachytherapy.* 2014;13:514–521.

138. Rivard MJ, Wierzbicki JG, Van den Heuvel F,Martin RC, McMahon RR. Clinical brachytherapy with neutron emitting 252Cf sources and adherence to AAPM TG-43 dosimetry protocol. *Med Phys.* 26, 87–96.

139. Melhus CS, et al. Shielding evaluation of a medical linear accelerator vault in preparation for installing a high dose rate ^{252}Cf remote afterloader. Rad. Prot. Dosim. 113, 428–437.

140. Lin L,Patel RR, Thomadsen BR, Henderson DL. The use of directional interstitial sources to improve dosimetry in breast brachytherapy. *Med Phys.* 2008;35:240–247.

141. Rivard MJ, Monte Carlo radiation dose simulations and dosimetric comparison of the model 6711 and 9011 ^{125}I brachytherapy sources. *Med Phys.* 2009;36:486–491.

142. Kennedy RM, Davis SD, Micka JA, DeWerd LA. Experimental and Monte Carlo determination of the TG-43 dosimetric parameters for the model 9011 THINSeed^{TM} brachytherapy source. *Med Phys.* 2010;37:1681–1688.

143. Meigooni AS, Awan SB, Rachabatthula V, Koona RA. Treatment-planning considerations for prostate implants with the new linear RadioCoil^{TM} ^{103}Pd brachytherapy source. *J Appl Clin Med Phys.* 2005;6:23–36.

144. Meigooni AS, Awan SB, Dou K, Feasibility of calibrating elongated brachytherapy sources using a well-type ionization chamber. *Med Phys.* 2006;33:4184–4189.

145. Bannon EA, Yang Y, Rivard MJ. Accuracy assessment of the superposition principle for evaluating dose distributions of elongated and curved ^{103}Pd and ^{192}Ir brachytherapy sources. *Med Phys.* 2011;38:2957–2963.

146. Rivard MJ, Reed JL, and DeWerd LA. ^{103}Pd strings: Monte Carlo assessment of a new approach to brachytherapy source design. *Med Phys.* 2017;41:011716.

147. Reed JL, Rivard MJ, Micka JA, Culberson WS, DeWerd LA. Experimental and Monte Carlo dosimetric characterization of a 1 cm ^{103}Pd brachytherapy source. *Brachytherapy.* 2014;13:657–667.

148. Dempsey JF, et al. Dosimetric properties of a novel brachytherapy balloon applicator for the treatment of malignant brain-tumor resection-cavity margins. *Int J Radiat Oncol Biol Phys.* 1998;42:421–429.

149. Monroe JI, et al. Experimental validation of dose calculation algorithms for the GliaSite^{TM} RTS, a novel ^{125}I liquid-filled balloon brachytherapy applicator. *Med Phys.* 2001;28:73–85.

150. Rogers LR, Rock JP, Sills AK, et al. Results of a phase II trial of the GliaSite radiation therapy system for the treatment of newly diagnosed, resected single brain metastases. *J Neurosurg.* 2006;105:375–384.

151. Rivard MJ, Evans D-AR, Kay I. A technical evaluation of the Nucletron FIRST* system: conformance of a remote afterloading brachytherapy seed implantation system to manufacturer specifications and AAPM Task Group report recommendations. *J Appl Clin Med Phys.* 2005;6:22–50.

152. Fichtinger G, et al. Robotically assisted prostate brachytherapy with transrectal ultrasound guidance – Phantom experiments. *Brachytherapy.* 2006;5:14–26.

153. Podder TK, et al. AAPM and GEC-ESTRO guidelines for image-guided robotic brachytherapy: report of Task Group 192. *Med Phys.* 2014;41:101501.

154. Holupka EJ, et al. An automatic seed finder for brachytherapy CT postplans based on the Hough transform. *Med Phys.* 2004;31:2672–2679.

155. Mahdavi SS, et al. Semiautomatic segmentation for prostate brachytherapy: Dosimetric evaluation. *Brachytherapy.* 2013;12:65–76.

156. De Brabandere M, Hoskin P, Haustermans K, Van den Heuvel F, Siebert F-A. Prostate postimplant dosimetry: Interobserver variability in seed localisation, contouring and fusion. *Radiother Oncol.* 2012;104:192–198.

157. Sabater S, et al. Dose accumulation during vaginal cuff brachytherapy based on rigid/deformable registration vs. single plan addition. *Brachytherapy.* 2014;13:343–351.

158. Kim H, Huq MS, Houser C, Beriwal S, Michalski D. Mapping of dose distribution from IMRT onto MRI-guided high dose rate brachytherapy using deformable image registration for cervical cancer treatments: preliminary study with commercially available software. *J Contemp Brachytherapy.* 2014;6:178–184.

159. Rivard MJ, Ghadyani HR, Bastien AD, Lutz NN, Hepel JT. Multi-axis dose accumulation of noninvasive image-guided breast brachytherapy through biomechanical modeling of tissue deformation using the finite element method. J. Contemp. *Brachytherapy.* 2015;7:55–71.

160. Siebert F-A, et al. Dose-rate to water calibrations for brachytherapy sources from the end-user perspective. *Metrologia.* 2012;49:S249–S252.

161. Aubineau-Lanièce I, Chauvenet B, Cutarella D, Gouriou J, Plagnard J, Aviles Lucas P. LNE–LNHB air-kerma and absorbed dose to water primary standards for low dose-rate ^{125}I brachytherapy sources. *Metrologia.* 2012;49:S189–S192.

162. Toni MP, Pimpinella M, Pinto M, Quini M, Cappadozzi G, Silvestri C, Bottauscio O. Direct determination of the absorbed dose to water from ^{125}I low dose-rate brachytherapy seeds using the new absorbed dose primary standard developed at ENEA-INMRI. *Metrologia.* 2012;49:S193–S197.

163. Schneider T. The PTB primary standard for the absorbed-dose to water for I-125 interstitial brachytherapy sources. *Metrologia* 2012;49:S198–S202.

164. Beaulieu L, et al. Report of the Task Group 186 on model-based dose calculation methods in brachytherapy beyond the TG-43 formalism: current status and recommendations for clinical implementation. *Med Phys.* 2012;39: 6208–6236.

165. Chibani O, Williamson JF. MCPI: a sub-minute Monte Carlo dose calculation engine for prostate implants. *Med Phys.* 2005;32:3688–3698.

166. Wang R, Sloboda RS, Brachytherapy scatter dose calculation in heterogeneous media: I. A microbeam ray-tracing method for the single-scatter contribution. *Phys Med Biol.* 2007;52: 5619–5636.

167. Landry G, Reniers B, Murrer L, Lutgens L, Gurp EB, Pignol J-P, Keller B, Beaulieu L, Verhaegen F. Sensitivity of low energy brachytherapy Monte Carlo dose calculations to uncertainties in human tissue composition. *Med Phys.* 2010;37:5188–5198.

168. Landry G, Reniers B, Pignol J-P, Beaulieu L, Verhaegen F. The difference of scoring dose to water or tissues in Monte Carlo dose calculations for low energy brachytherapy photon sources. *Med Phys.* 2011;38:1526–1533.

169. Rivard MJ, Beaulieu L, Mourtada F. Enhancements to commissioning techniques of brachytherapy treatment planning systems that use model-based dose calculation algorithms. *Med Phys.* 2010;37:2645–2658.Low Dose–Rate Brachytherapy

30 High-Dose-Rate Brachytherapy Treatment Planning

Bruce R. Thomadsen, Jessica Miller, Poonam Yadav, and Susan Richardson

GENERAL CONSIDERATIONS OF HIGH-DOSE-RATE BRACHYTHERAPY TREATMENTS

High-dose-rate (HDR) brachytherapy forms a special method of delivering brachytherapy where the treatment session lasts a short time. What constitutes "a short time" is considered in the following section, but in the overview, the treatment proper takes less than 30 minutes, as opposed to a day to several days for conventional, low-dose-rate (LDR) brachytherapy. Most of treatment planning for HDR brachytherapy remains identical to that for any form of brachytherapy, which is covered in Chapters 21 and 29. This chapter will consider only those aspects of treatment planning that are either unique for, or of much greater importance to, HDR planning.

Several methods have been used in the past to deliver the treatment in the short time, but all contemporary units use the same principle—a very intense radioactive source on computer-controlled cable steps through the target volume, pausing for specified periods at particular locations along the way. The pausing locations are referred to as *dwell positions*, and the duration for which the source pauses are *dwell times*. Often, the dwell times are normalized to a particular dwell-time location or the maximum, in which case the normalized values are called *dwell weights*. A unit that operates in such a manner is called a *stepping-source device*. The radioactive source for most contemporary units is ^{192}Ir, although ^{60}Co units are sometimes used outside of the United States. The operation of HDR units is discussed in detail in many texts.[1] Since this chapter deals with the treatment-planning aspect of HDR brachytherapy, further description of the units proper is left to the reader's initiative.

HDR brachytherapy offers several advantages over LDR brachytherapy.

1. **Improved dose optimization capability.** In an HDR brachytherapy application, the dwell positions perform the same role as the source positions do for LDR brachytherapy. For example, the same locations where individual iridium sources would fall in an LDR gynecological implant, the single HDR source would pause for a dwell position. Such an LDR implant could, and

should, be "optimized." "Optimization," in this context, means adjusting the strength or positions of the sources to obtain a dose distribution with specified, desired characteristics.[2] One optimization goal often is simply that a specified isodose surface covers a target volume. Other optimization criteria might include a specified required homogeneity for the dose through the target volume, or the maximum dose allowed to other anatomical structures. Optimization of a medium size LDR implants often requires 8 to 10 different discrete source strengths, which sometimes becomes difficult to obtain from a supplier. For an HDR unit, the dwell times at each dwell position, on the other hand, commonly may vary in increments of 0.1 or 0.2 s from 0 to 999 s. Thus, satisfying the optimization requirements becomes easier with the great flexibility in relative strength at each dwell position. Optimization plays such an important part in HDR treatment planning that a section of this chapter is devoted to this topic.

2. **More stable positioning.** For intracavitary insertions, HDR applicators usually lock into their treatment positions through fixation to the treatment couch. With the patient essentially immobilized (e.g., in stirrups), the applicator moves little with respect to the patient between imaging for dosimetry calculations and the completion of the treatment session. One series studying the movement of HDR tandem and ovoid applications reported an average movement based on skeletal anatomy of 2 mm.[3] This compares with an average of 2 cm movement for LDR tandem and ovoids.[4]

3. **Adding distance to normal tissue.** For some HDR treatments—notably gynecological intracavitary insertions, prostate, and head and neck interstitial implants—normal tissue structures can be pushed away from the path of the source during the treatment, reducing their dose. While not every treatment site can use this technique, in those for which it applies the dose reduction to normal structures can be marked. In general, the discomfort that similar tissue displacement would cause over the multiple-day treatments for LDR brachytherapy would be intolerable.

4. **Outpatient treatment.** The driving force that led to the wide use of HDR brachytherapy in the United States

was the economic shift in reimbursement it produced from the inpatient hospital to the clinical facility that delivers the HDR treatments. This occurs because most HDR treatments are delivered on an outpatient basis. In addition to changing the revenue patterns, outpatient treatments usually are much more convenient and comfortable for the patients than confinement in a hospital room in radiation isolation.

5. **Smaller applicators.** For gynecological intracavitary applications, the tandem used for HDR treatment of uterine cancer has only a 3-mm diameter compared with the 7-mm diameter tandem used for LDR brachytherapy, mostly due to the smaller size of an HDR source compared to the size of the older cesium sources. The dilation required to insert the LDR tandem forms the most painful part of the treatment procedure. By comparison, the sound used to measure the length of the uterine cavity before dilation takes place is also 3-mm in diameter and often requires no anesthesia.

6. **Intraoperative and perioperative treatments.** For interstitial cases, HDR brachytherapy treatment can commence immediately following insertion of the applicator or catheters, localization imaging, and dose calculations. LDR brachytherapy cases usually require ordering the sources, or if sources were ordered ahead, performing the implant as planned without the possibility of modifications based on new information noted during the operative procedure. This ability to treat immediately after placement, along with the short duration of treatment, opens the possibility of using HDR brachytherapy during operative cases (intraoperative) for irradiation of tumor beds during resection or for wider use of image-guided implants.[5]

7. **Reduction of radiation exposure to health care providers.** The final advantage of HDR brachytherapy is that all personnel leave the treatment room for the actual delivery of the radiation, and with adequately shielded walls and doors, the radiation exposure to staff should remain minimal.[a]

HDR brachytherapy also has disadvantages compared with LDR brachytherapy.

1. **Treatment unit complexity.** Compared with the usual LDR brachytherapy situation of sources manually inserted into an applicator, the HDR situation seems much more complicated. With the treatment unit, transfer tubes to guide the source between the unit and the applicator, and transferring treatment programs between the treatment-planning computer and the treatment unit computer, HDR brachytherapy entails a host of considerations not applicable to LDR brachytherapy.

2. **Compressed time frame.** Adding to the complexity of HDR brachytherapy, much of the action takes place in time frames short compared with LDR brachytherapy.

For example, after insertion of a tandem and ovoids for cervical cancer therapy, acquiring images and calculating the treatment program, the actual delivery of the treatment frequently takes 10 to 20 minutes. If there were an error in the treatment program, it would be easy for the error to be executed before detection. The longer time frame with LDR treatments provides some latitude for detecting errors. The long duration of the treatment gives more opportunity to spot and correct errors well before the end of treatment, when corrective actions could prevent serious injury.

3. **Radiobiological disadvantage.** The most serious disadvantage for HDR brachytherapy results from radiobiology. Radiobiology is also such an important aspect of HDR brachytherapy that it has its own section in this chapter. In the current discussion, it suffices to say that compared with LDR brachytherapy, radiation delivered at an HDR produces a greater damage to normal tissue compared to cancerous tissue.

4. **The potential for very high radiation doses resulting from mechanical failure.** The HDR source cable can become stuck or snagged, or the source can break free from the cable. In either case, the patient could receive an injurious amount of radiation in about 1 min. While the operator is unlikely to receive an injurious amount of radiation removing the stuck source from the patient, there is a real potential for receiving exposures in excess of allowed limits. While these accidents are extremely rare, this drawback cannot be neglected.

RADIOBIOLOGICAL CONSIDERATIONS

Accomplishing the goal of radiotherapy requires inflicting more damage to diseased cells than to normal tissue cells (the therapeutic ratio) The radiation dose rate, treatment fraction, delivery time, dose distribution, time between fractions, and treatment volume are important aspects of radiation biology. The success of radiation therapy is determined by the four R's of radiobiology, which are repair, reassortment, repopulation, and reoxygenation. Chapter 3 discusses the details of what makes them important radiobiological considerations for radiation therapy treatment.

Therapeutic Ratio

The therapeutic ratio is an important measure involved in the planning for the goal of uncomplicated cure of disease. The therapeutic ratio could be defined as the ratio of the damage to tumor cells to that to normal cells for the same delivered dose, or

$$\text{Therapeutic Ratio} = \left. \frac{\text{Damage to tumor cells}}{\text{Damage to normal cells}} \right|_{\text{Same dose}}$$

(30.1)

---

[a] The exception to this generalization is the use of a LDR remote afterloader—a device that moves LDR sources into applicators while the patient lies in a hospital bed. Since marketing of these units recently terminated, remote afterloading LDR brachytherapy will not be considered in this chapter.

Keeping the therapeutic ratio in mind helps to exploit the different responses of the normal tissues and tumor to the radiation dose. Since it becomes difficult to grade damage, and the damage to cells is not linear with dose, a more common equivalent expression often forms the basis for the calculation of this ratio, determining the ratio of the doses required for the same biological end point, for example, five logs of cell kill. The equation becomes

$$\text{Therapeutic Ratio} = \left.\frac{\text{Dose to normal cells}}{\text{Dose to tumor cells}}\right|_{\substack{\text{Same biological}\\\text{endpoint}}}$$

$$(30.2)$$

The more effective the radiation is at killing a certain type of cell, the lower the dose required to reduce a population of cells to a given level.

Figure 30.1 shows a typical cell-survival curve plotted as logarithmic function of the surviving fraction versus radiation dose. Simply, this curve relates the survival of cells to the radiation dose. Mathematically, the relationship between cell survival, S, and cell killing can be modeled as

$$S = e^{-\alpha D - \beta D^2} \qquad (30.3)$$

where D indicates the dose delivered, α and β are constants that characterize the slope of survival curve.

Equation 30.3 is just a model and should not be taken as the true description of the physical and biological process.

In the figure, the lines labeled "Normal acute" and "Tumor acute" indicate the response of typical normal tissue and typical tumor cells to a single dose of radiation. For any dose level, the tumor cells show an increased survival—not a desirable feature for radiotherapy. The other curves indicate responses for a conventional LDR treatment regimen, delivering the dose at approximately 0.5 Gy/h. For both tissue types, the survival increases due to repair of sublethal damage during the radiation delivery. However, the difference in survival between the two curves at any dose decreases compared with the acute curves. Looking at it the other way, compared to LDR delivery, the difference in response between normal tissue and tumor tissues becomes worse for HDR delivery.

Figure 30.2 illustrates the loss in therapeutic ratio with an increase in dose rate, and that loss in therapeutic ratio can be significant. Figure 30.2 also shows another interesting feature. The therapeutic ratio changes slowly with dose rate over the LDR portion of the curve (0.4–0.8 Gy/h, shown between green vertical lines in the figure), which accounts for historic LDR treatments giving similar results regardless of the exact dose rate. In that region, the therapeutic ratio does not change with absolute dose, only dose rate. At HDRs, above 20 Gy/h, the therapeutic ratio again varies little with the actual dose rate. Most HDR units deliver a dose at 1 cm at a rate of 100 to 500 Gy/h, but because much of an implant lies farther

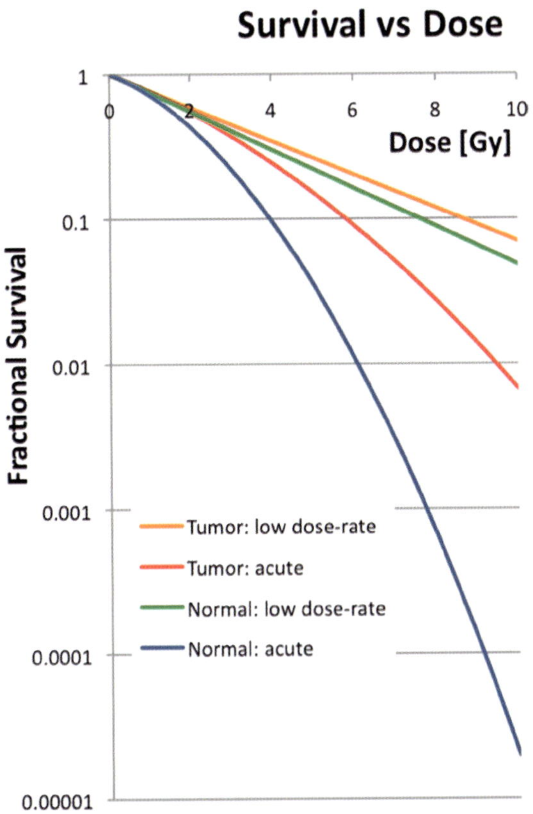

Survival vs Dose

FIGURE 30.1. A cell survival curve, plotting the fraction of cells surviving a single exposure to radiation as a function of the dose delivered. The curves are based on $\alpha = 0.25$ Gy^{-1}, $\beta_{\text{tumor}} = 0.025$ Gy^{-2}, $\beta_{\text{normal tissue}} = 0.083$ Gy^{-2}, $\mu_{\text{repair}} = 1.5$ h^{-1}. Cell proliferation has been ignored.

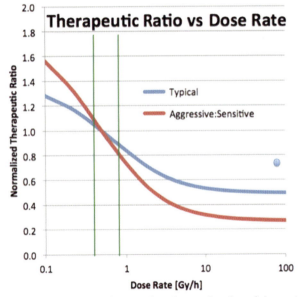

FIGURE 30.2. Relative therapeutic ratio as a function of dose rate, normalized to a dose rate of 0.5 Gy/h. Each line assumes a particular ratio for the a and b in Equation 16.3 for tumor cells and normal cells. The blue line represents a typical situation, with $\frac{\alpha}{\beta} = 10$ Gy for the tumor and 3 Gy for normal tissue. The red line applies to aggressive tumor, with an $\frac{\alpha}{\beta}$ of 20 Gy and normal tissue with $\frac{\alpha}{\beta}$ or 2 Gy. The vertical green lines indicate the LDR region. The blue dot indicates the normalized therapeutic ratio for fractionated HDR treatments for typical tumors.

away than 1 cm at least some of the treatment time, the dose rate can fall well below that, but seldom below 12 Gy/h. Over any realistic HDR application, the dose rates anywhere in a volume of interest remain in the flat region of the curve. However, the biological dose distribution for an HDR application depends on the absolute dose level, and so differs from the physical dose distribution.

A very different situation obtains in the middle, transition region. In this case, the biological effectiveness of the radiation varies greatly with the actual dose rate, and the biological effectiveness of a given amount of dose varies with position in the treated volume. Often, treatments using nominally LDR remote afterloaders actually deliver doses at this middle dose-rate range. High precision is required with these devices to avoid exceeding the tolerance of normal tissues.

The flat response in the HDR region of the curve traces back to the definition of "high dose-rate." In Equation 30.3, the term α in the exponent does not depend on the rate of dose delivery. This term is often associated with single-track killing, that is, one charged particle passing near the DNA strand produces sufficient ionization in the right location to break both sides of the DNA "ladder." Such a double-sided break can produce a biological effect, including cell death.[b] The term β can be thought of as representing the situation where the break on each side results from different charged particles. The cell can repair a single-sided break because the remaining side provides the template for the missing side. T_r, the half-time for repair of sublethal damage, characterizes this repair giving the time required to repair half of single-sided breaks. Measured values of T_r vary widely, but a typical value is 1 to 2 h for both normal and tumor cells. Some normal tissues exhibit repair with two components, one with a half-time of approximately the range of values given earlier but also a shorter component of about 20 minutes,[6] although other models of repair kinetics fit the data better.[7] Tumor cells seem not to have this faster component of repair, which gives another therapeutic advantage to the use of low dose rates. For the simple, single-component model for repair, the repair coefficient, μ, can be calculated as

$$\mu = 0.693/T_r \qquad (30.4)$$

Because the single-strand breaks repair over time, the probability for a second-sided break at the same location as the first but on the opposite side depends on how compact in time the radiation is delivered. When all the radiation passes through the DNA in a short period, the likelihood that the second side will break before the first side repairs increases compared with a long delivery. In this case, a "short" time relates to the half-time for repair of sublethal damage. Regardless of the actual dose rate, HDR treatment refers to a treatment where essentially all the breaks occur before any significant repair takes place.

In general, HDR treatments should be completed within half an hour of commencement.

Fractionation

While reducing the dose rate is one method to improve the therapeutic ratio, another is fractionation, in which treatment is split into a number of treatments, known as fractions, and is delivered over a course of time. Figure 30.3 shows survival curves for the same parameters as Figure 30.1 but includes the survival curves for delivering the doses in 2-Gy fractions. The fractionation reduces the effectiveness of the radiation at killing cells, but it also reduces the differences between the responses of the tumor and the normal tissues.

HDR brachytherapy generally fractionates the treatment course to mitigate the problem of loss of therapeutic ratio with the increase in dose rate. Figure 30.4 shows the improvement in the therapeutic ratio by adding one more fraction to the regimen. For example, if a plan is called for the use of three fractions, the therapeutic ratio would improve by 4.7% by using four fractions instead. If five fractions were used instead of four, the therapeutic ratio would improve another 4% above the 4.7% improvement from increasing from three to four. As can be seen, each additional fraction improves the therapeutic ratio, but by less than the addition of the fraction before. In external-beam treatment, which is delivered at dose rates similar to HDR, the number of fractions may be 35, which would

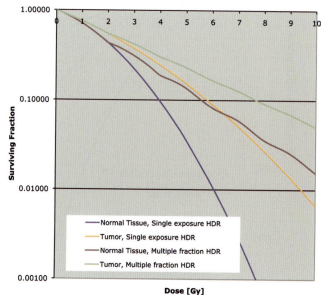

Cell Survival for Single and Multiple Fraction Exposures

FIGURE 30.3. Survival curves using the same parameters as in Figure 30.1 for acute (single fraction) exposures and for 2-Gy acute fractions.

[b] For more information, the reader may consult any basic radiobiology textbook, such as Hall EJ, Giaccia AJ. Radiobiology for radiologists, 8th ed. Philadelphia, PA: Wolters Kluwer, 2019.

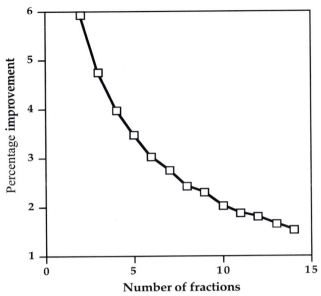

FIGURE 30.4. The percentage improvement in therapeutic ratio by the addition of one more fraction than the number on the abscissa. See the text for an example.

provide a great benefit in the therapeutic ratio, and the addition or deletion of one or two fractions would not make much a difference. Brachytherapy is both taxing on the patient and a drain on the personnel and resources of the facility, and, therefore, use of a high number of fractions, as common in external-beam therapy, is not an option. Thus, a compromise must be made between improved therapeutic ratio and practicality.

Depending on the tumor site, the dose-fractionation schedule for HDR brachytherapy treatment may change. Most often, users would find a treatment regimen from a protocol or guideline published by a professional organization. The number of fractions selected for curative cases depends on the amount of work involved and patient discomfort for each fraction, and these factors are taken into consideration when writing recommendations for a guidance document. For interstitial cases with rigid needle-like catheters in place, such as a prostate implant, three fractions are common for monotherapy or one or two in combination with external-beam treatments. On the opposite extreme, breast implants with flexible, soft catheters often use 10, twice-a-day fractions. Intracavitary insertions that involve the placement of a treatment applicator at each fraction often use three to six fractions. Tandem and ring applications using an indwelling Smit sleeve (a sheath for the tandem) in the uterine canal simplify the procedure to the point to which 12 fractions have been used.[8]

Prescription Doses

Because the biological effectiveness of radiation changes going from LDR treatments to fractionated HDR treatments, the absolute dose prescribed also has to change to

obtain the same therapeutic end point. As Equation 30.3 shows, cell survival has a more or less exponential relationship to dose, so dose proper is not the best variable to use when evaluating or predicting biological effects. Of several approaches, one of the most practical begins by taking the log of both sides of the dose–response curves from Equation 30.3,

$$Ln(S) = -\alpha D - \beta D^2 \qquad (30.5)$$

and then divided by $-\alpha$ to have at least the first term in dose alone, to give

$$BED = \frac{Ln(S)}{-\alpha} = D + \frac{\beta}{\alpha}D^2 = D\left(1 + \frac{D}{\alpha/\beta}\right) \qquad (30.6)$$

BED stands for biological equivalent dose. An equivalent term seen in the literature is the RDE, radiological dose equivalent. Equation 30.6 holds for acute, single exposures. The quantity $\left(1 + \frac{D}{\alpha/\beta}\right)$ is called the relative effectiveness, RF, which relates how the biological effectiveness of the radiation compares with physical dose, considering the biological factors and the delivery.

For multiple HDR exposures of n fractions of d Gy/fraction, the BED becomes

$$BED_{HDR} = n \cdot d\left(1 + \frac{d}{\alpha/\beta}\right) - \frac{0.693T}{\alpha T_{pot}} \qquad (30.7)$$

Equation 30.7 holds when each fraction is short compared with the half-time for repair for cellular sublethal damage, and the time between fractions is long compared with this same half-time. As discussed earlier, the duration of the treatment should be less than half an hour, and the time between should be about 4 half-times, or about 6 h. The newly included last term in Equation 30.7 gives the effect of cellular proliferation on the BED, where T is the total duration of the n fractions and T_{pot} is the potential doubling time for the cells. The equation shows that proliferation decreases the effectiveness of the radiation. This latter factor often is not known well; however, a compilation of values gleaned from the literature has been published by Bentzen et al.[9] Conventionally, due to the uncertainty in this parameter, the proliferation is often ignored. For interstitial cases, the total therapy duration often remains the same whether the therapy is HDR or LDR; and therefore, also the proliferation effect, whether the treatment chosen is HDR or LDR brachytherapy, as discussed later.

Protracted LDR therapy with some repair of sublethal damage taking place during treatment follows Equation 30.8,[10]

$$BED_{LDR} = D\left[1 + \left(\frac{2\dot{D}}{\frac{\alpha}{\beta}\mu}\right) \cdot \left(\frac{1 - e^{-\mu T}}{\mu T}\right)\right] - \frac{0.693T}{\alpha T_{pot}}, \qquad (30.8)$$

where $\dot{D}$ is the dose rate.

Assuming that the dose has been established for LDR treatments, the equation to produce the same biological effect with HDR brachytherapy can be calculated. The first step entails selecting the number of HDR fractions to use. As discussed earlier, this selection is an arbitrary compromise between improving the therapeutic ratio and practical utilization of resources. The next step sets the BED for each modality equal:

$$BED_{HDR} = BED_{LDR} \qquad (30.9)$$

or

$$
n \cdot d\left(1 + \frac{d}{\alpha/\beta}\right) - \frac{0.693T}{\alpha\, T_{pot}} \qquad (30.10)
$$
$$
= D\left[1 + \left(\frac{2\dot{D}}{\frac{\alpha}{\beta}\mu}\right) \cdot \left(\frac{1 - e^{-\mu T}}{\mu T}\right)\right] - \frac{0.693T}{\alpha\, T_{pot}}
$$

If the total times are similar, then the last terms on each side cancel. Even if they are not similar, since the values needed for their calculation are not well known, they often are simply ignored, giving

$$
n \cdot d\left(1 + \frac{d}{\alpha/\beta}\right) = D\left[1 + \left(\frac{2\dot{D}}{\frac{\alpha}{\beta}\mu}\right) \cdot \left(\frac{1 - e^{-\mu T}}{\mu T}\right)\right]
$$

$$(30.11)$$

The remaining unknown term in Equation 30.11 is the dose per fraction, d. Solving for d gives

$$
d = \frac{-(\alpha/\beta) + \sqrt{(\alpha/\beta)^2 + \left(\frac{4D}{n}\right)(\alpha/\beta) \cdot \left[1 + \left(\frac{2\dot{D}}{\mu}\right)\left(1 - \frac{1 - e^{-\mu T}}{\mu T}\right)\right]}}{2}
$$

$$(30.12)$$

BED depends on the tissue characteristics, as embodied in the values for α and β. Thus, the equivalence between LDR and HDR brachytherapy only applies to a single type of tissue—tumor or normal tissue. The dose cannot be equivalent for both simultaneously. An equivalent regimen must be selected to produce the same cure rate (equivalent for tumor) or the same normal-tissue reaction (equivalent for normal tissues). If the choice becomes too difficult, a compromise can be made—but at the cost of not being equivalent to the LDR regimen in any way. In general, making the HDR regimen equivalent to the LDR regimen for tumors tends to be the more common choice, since sacrificing the cure rate would argue strongly against performing HDR brachytherapy, and physical techniques often can mitigate the increased effects on the normal structures. Early in HDR brachytherapy experience, Orton suggested that doses should not exceed 7 Gy/fraction to avoid normal tissue complications.[11] The suggestion came from the review of a survey asking practitioners about their HDR experience. While the responses did indicate that complications increase with fraction sizes exceeding 7 Gy, the total doses for the cases in the survey were not controlled based on the linear-quadratic equations given here and commonly accepted in the present.

Despite earlier hesitation, current practice has embraced single fraction treatments for various anatomical sites including HDR and intraoperative brachytherapy procedures. For example, Kinj et al. performed a single fraction of multichannel breast brachytherapy in older patients with a dose of 16 Gy with reasonable toxicity and good clinical outcome.[12] First results of the TRIUMPH-T trial, which delivered 22.5 Gy in 3 fractions with breast brachytherapy applicators, were also successful.[13] Intraoperative radiation therapy (IORT) has also been used to treat breast cancer patients successfully with a single fraction dose of 20 Gy to the balloon surface.[14] A single 19 Gy fraction of HDR prostate brachytherapy study resulted in excellent results in terms of toxicity and patient satisfaction.[15] Improved imaging, immobilization and dosimetry may have allowed for these advances to treat in a single fraction beyond 7 Gy.

Complicating further the attempt to make an HDR brachytherapy treatment similar to one performed with LDR brachytherapy, notice that in Equation 30.12 the dose per HDR fraction, d, depends on the LDR dose to which it should be equivalent. This means that an HDR brachytherapy dose *distribution* can never be equivalent to an LDR brachytherapy dose *distribution*. Thus, to achieve a similar biological dose distribution, an HDR treatment should *not* duplicate the LDR physical dose distribution.

With interstitial implants, higher doses require more fractions to maintain normal tissues within tolerance doses due to proximity of tissues to the catheters. If the treatment catheters remain in place for the whole course of therapy, treatments frequently are given twice a day (BID). Table 30.1 relates LDR doses delivered at the rate of 0.5 Gy/h with the equivalent regimen with 2 HDR fractions per day. In general, the overall treatment duration—time with the catheters in place—remains about the same. The patient, however, need not be in radiation isolation with the HDR treatments. Due to prolonged treatment time and concerns such as edema and the resulting anatomical changes over the course of treatment that could alter the dose delivery, HDR brachytherapy allows reimaging, replanning and treatment at each fraction as

TABLE 30.1	Equivalent Treatments for Low-Dose-Rate and High-Dose-Rate Brachytherapy				
LDR Regimen (0.5 Gy/h)		**HDR Regimen (2 fractions/day)**			
Dose (Gy)	**Duration (day)**	**Number of fractions**	**Dose/ Fraction (Gy)**	**Total dose (Gy)**	
20	1.7	4	4.22	16.9	
30	2.5	6	4.25	12.5	
40	3.3	7	4.71	33.0	
50	4.2	8	5.03	40.2	
60	5.0	10	4.89	48.9	

necessary, which is not possible with the fixed source strengths in an LDR implant.

For intracavitary insertions, the prescribed dose often falls at an unambiguous (although often arbitrary) location, for example, the image-defined high-risk clinical target volume (CTV$_{HR}$, discussed in the section below on "Cervical Cancer Intracavitary Applications," and in International Commission on Radiation Units and Measurements [ICRU] report 87[16]) for cervical cancer, the surface of a cylinder for vaginal cancer, or 1 cm from the center of the applicator for esophageal applications. Interstitial implants are sometimes less well determined. Take, for example, a post-tylectomy breast implant with a seroma visible on computed tomography (CT). The CTV (see Chapter 1) might be the seroma plus a 1.5-cm margin, limited to remain 5 mm deep to the skin and not enter the pectoralis major. During the dosimetry-planning process, the prescription-dose (100%) isodose surface ideally is set at the CTV. All these seem very straightforward. However, depending on where the source tracks fall with respect to the CTV, the 100% isodose may lie on the edge of the more or less uniform dose plateau of the implant or in the rapidly decreasing gradient. (It should be assumed that the 100% isodose surface would never fall beyond the rapidly decreasing gradient to where the dose decreases more slowly; that would be a poor plan indeed.) Thus, in actual cases, some of the CTV may not receive the full dose and some of the prescription isodose surface may fall outside the CTV. Some guidelines for specifying the prescription dose are given in the section on "Evaluation."

Two-Gray-Fraction Equivalent Dose (EQD$_2$)

The concept of BED often seems abstract and vague to many of those working in radiotherapy clinics. This is because external-beam treatments using 2-Gy fractions constitute the great majority of treatments involving most radiation–oncology clinical staff. Expressing the BED in the equivalent dose, were the treatment delivered in 2-Gy fractions, helps make sense of the radiobiological effectiveness of a dose fraction regimen, referred to as the EQD$_2$. The conversion is actually very simple,

$$EQD_2 = \frac{BED}{1 + \frac{2}{\alpha/\beta}} \qquad (30.13)$$

The derivation can be found in Chapter 3.

One great advantage of working with "doses" in BED is that the total BED received to a tissue in the patient equals the sum of the BEDs for any treatments delivered, regardless of the fractionation schema. This advantage is shared by the EQD$_2$. As an example, consider a cervical cancer regimen delivering 45 Gy in 25 fractions of 1.8 Gy each of external-beam radiation, and 5 fractions of brachytherapy each delivering 6 Gy to the CTV$_{HR}$. Ignoring the final term in Equation 30.7, the BED for tumor with an $a/b = 10$

Gy is 53.1 Gy$_{10}$ for the external-beam treatments and 48 Gy$_{10}$ for the brachytherapy for a combined BED of 101.1 Gy$_{10}$.[c] Repeating the calculations for normal tissue with an $a/b = 3$ Gy gives 72 Gy$_3$ for the external-beam treatments and 90 Gy$_3$ for the brachytherapy for a combined BED of 162 Gy$_{13}$. These BED values mean little to most radiation oncologists or medical physicists, unless they work in radiobiology frequently. In terms of EQD$_2$, for tumor, the external-beam treatment becomes 44.3 Gy$_{2Eq}$ and the brachytherapy 40 Gy$_{2Eq}$, for a total of 84.3 Gy$_{2Eq}$. These numbers fall more into the realm of experience for the radiotherapy staff. The corresponding normal-tissue values are 43.2 Gy$_{2Eq}$ for the external-beam fractions and 54 Gy$_{2Eq}$, for the brachytherapy, giving a total of 97.2 Gy$_{2Eq}$.

EQD$_2$ has found its way into treatment planning. It often serves to look at the effective dose for organs at risk for a particular fraction, or for the summation of the doses for all treatments (including both external beam and brachytherapy) leading up to the fraction being treated. It also is used during the evaluation process as part of plan review. Figure 30.5 shows a spreadsheet used for guiding the treatment planning for cervical intracavitary brachytherapy that includes a conversion from doses to EQD$_2$ to simplify combining the effects of each fraction.

OPTIMIZATION

In brachytherapy, "optimization" generally connotes determination of some aspects of an application in order to achieve particular goals. For example, optimization may have the goal of delivering a minimum dose to a target volume with a specified homogeneity. With permanent implants of the prostate, optimization usually generates a pattern for locations of the sources to deliver 90% of the prescription dose to the entire CTV, limit the volume raised to 200% of the prescription dose and avoid doses to the rectum and urethra that exceed their respective tolerances. In HDR brachytherapy, the most common optimization process determines the dwell times that produce the desired dose distribution. In this chapter, determining and optimizing catheter location usually would be considered part of planning an application.

The optimization problem in HDR brachytherapy, with its single stepping source, tends to be simpler than for permanent implants and can usually come closer to achieving the goals of the optimization. While the permanent implant problem can only decide whether or not to place a source in a given location, the HDR brachytherapy problem can begin assuming activation of all possible dwell locations, and then simply determine each dwell time. Sometimes, the easiest approach determines the dwell times relative to either the maximum time or some specific time (dwell weights) for each

---

[c] Convention dictates that the units for BED indicate the α/β as a following subscript.

PRIOR RT

PRIOR RT COURSE PRESCRIPTIONS							
C1		C2		C3		C4	
Dose (Gy)	# Fx	Dose (Gy)	# Fx	Dose (Gy)	# Fx	Dose (Gy)	# Fx
1.8	25						

PRIOR RT COURSE EQD₂ DOSE CONTRIBUTION										
Summary	C1	C2	C3	C4	Weights	C1	C2	C3	C4
Rx a/b = 10	44.3	0	0	0	Rx	1	1	1	1
D90 a/b = 10	44.3	0	0	0	D90	1	1	1	1
Rectum D2cc a/b =	43.2	0	0	0	Rectum	1	1	1	1
Bladder D2cc a/b =	43.2	0	0	0	Bladder	1	1	1	1
Sigmoid D2cc a/b =	43.2	0	0	0	Sigmoid	1	1	1	1
Bowel D2cc a/b = 3	43.2	0	0	0	Bowel	1	1	1	1

BRACHY

BRACHYTHERAPY DOSES									
fx	1	2	3	4	5	6	7	8	9
Prescription	7.00	7.00	7.00	7.00					
D90	7.15	7.15	7.15	7.15					
Rectum D2cc	4.57	4.57	4.21	4.21					
Bladder D2cc	5.56	5.56	5.61	5.61					
Sigmoid D2cc	4.09	4.09	3.75	3.75					
Bowel D2cc	1.10	1.10	1.10	1.10					

BRACHY (EQD₂)

BRACHYTHERAPY COURSE EQD₂ DOSE CONTRIBUTION									
fx	1	2	3	4	5	6	7	8	9
Rx	9.9	9.9	9.9	9.9	0.0	0.0	0.0	0.0	0.0
D90	10.2	10.2	10.2	10.2	0.0	0.0	0.0	0.0	0.0
Rectum D2cc	6.9	6.9	6.1	6.1	0.0	0.0	0.0	0.0	0.0
Bladder D2cc	9.5	9.5	9.7	9.7	0.0	0.0	0.0	0.0	0.0
Sigmoid D2cc	5.8	5.8	5.1	5.1	0.0	0.0	0.0	0.0	0.0
Bowel D2cc	0.9	0.9	0.9	0.9	0.0	0.0	0.0	0.0	0.0

TOTAL EQD₂ (Gy)

CUMULATIVE EQD₂ DOSES					
	Pre	Brachy	Total	AIM	LIMIT
Rx	44.3	39.7	83.9	> 85 Gy	>85Gy
D90	44.3	40.9	85.1	> 85 Gy	>85Gy
Rectum	43.2	26.0	69.2	< 65 Gy	<75Gy
Bladder	43.2	38.4	81.6	< 80 Gy	<90Gy
Sigmoid	43.2	21.7	64.9	<70 Gy	<75Gy
Bowel	43.2	3.6	46.8	< 65 Gy	<75Gy

FIGURE 30.5. A spreadsheet used in planning cervical intracavitary brachytherapy. The dose for each brachytherapy fraction and the external-beam treatments are converted to EQD₂ and summed to give total effective doses. Guidelines and dose limits are from GEC-ESTRO recommendations.

dwell position in order to achieve some uniformity and then sets the times in proportion to the dwell weights required for the dose. If the solution for the problem does not require a particular dwell position, the optimization routine (optimizer) needs only set the weight to zero. There are several, very different approaches to optimization. Ezzell,[17] Ezzell and Luthmann,[18] and Libby et al.[19] present excellent discussion on optimization theory and characteristics.

The optimization problem usually specifies a goal. A simple goal might be to deliver a particular dose to a particular location. More specific goals might include delivering the same dose to a set of points or a surface. Even more complex goals not only specify the dose to a surface but also the homogeneity of the dose through the bounded volume and maximum doses allowed to neighboring sensitive normal structures. With the more involved goals, one of the features of the optimization

approach includes how to specify the problem and determine the importance of all the varied, and often conflicting, requirements. Many of the optimization approaches use an *objective function* (OF) to wrap all the goals into a single measure. An example of an OF for a prostate implant could be

$$
\begin{aligned}
OF = \ & w_t \sum_{\substack{all \\ target}} \left[(D_{prescribed} - D_t)^2 \text{ if}(D_t < D_{prescribed}) \right] \\
& + w_h \sum_{\substack{all \\ target}} \left[(2 D_{prescribed} - D_s)^2 \text{if}(D_t > 2 D_{prescribed}) \right] \\
& + w_r \sum_{\substack{all \\ rectum}} \left[\left(D_{rectal \atop limit} - D_r \right)^2 \text{if}(D_r > D_{rectal \atop limit}) \right] \\
& + w_u \sum_{\substack{all \\ urethra}} \left[\left(D_{urethra \atop limit} - D_u \right)^2 \text{if}(D_u > D_{urethra \atop limit}) \right]
\end{aligned}
$$

(30.14)

where D stands for doses and w for weighting for the term. The first term considers the target voxels, denoted by subscript t. The first goal would be to deliver the prescribed dose to the target. Any voxels falling below the prescribed dose would add to the OF. Homogeneity, indicated by the subscript h, also applies to the target voxels, and in the second term, voxels exceeding twice the prescribed dose add to the OF. The last two terms address dose to the rectum and urethra, and increase the OF for voxels that exceed a specified limit for the respective organ. The goal of an optimization could be to minimize this OF. OFs (sometimes called cost functions) can be simpler or more complicated and can be set such that the goal may be to minimize or maximize the function. The OF could also use the tumor control probability (TCP) and the normal-tissue complication probability (NTCP)[d] together, as a noncomplicated tumor-control probability.

Considering the function mentioned earlier, there may be many combinations of dwell times that satisfy all the requirements, so there would not be a unique solution. In the subset of all solutions, some may be better than others. If the differences in solutions make a difference in the perceived quality of the treatment plan, then the OF should be modified to reflect the additional requirements or tighten the specifications. If the differences in the solution remain unimportant, then the first solution found could be used.

While there are many approaches to optimization, they tend to fall into general categories. The actual distinctions between the categories seldom are as clear as it seems they should be, and into which category a given approach falls often remains debatable. Nevertheless, the discussion in the following section considers the characteristics of some of the major categories.

Over the last decade, there has been a great flurry of work published on optimization methods, approaches, and techniques. A few have worked their way into commercial treatment-planning systems and this chapter will mostly limit the discussion to those that have. While the concepts are not complicated, compared with earlier optimization algorithms, a thorough description of them becomes long and detailed, and the details are essential for an understanding of how they work and how they can fail. Such a discussion is beyond the scope of, and number of pages allotted to, this text. An article by Poulin et al. gives a useful summary of much of this topic.[20]

Deterministic Approaches

Deterministic approaches to optimization always find the same solution to the same problem, and generally solve equations to find the dwell times.

Heuristic Approaches

Heuristic approaches use pragmatic search techniques to construct solutions to the optimization problem. The search techniques may use surrogates for the optimized quantities if they are useful. Optimization purists might maintain that heuristics are not true optimization approaches because they tend not to produce a true optimum but merely a satisfactory result. For clinical problems, satisfactory results often serve the patient's needs well. In any case, the results of the optimization must be evaluated for appropriateness.

Several of the early HDR optimization approaches fell in this category, for example, Geometric Optimization, developed by Edmundson,[21] and Point-Dose Optimization, developed by van der Laarse.[22,23] Geometric optimization is not really an optimizer but an approach to approximate what a given geometry would need as far as relative dwell weights to deliver a more uniform dose than equal loading. Point-dose optimization solves algebraically to deliver as close as possible a uniform dose to a specified set of points. Both methods were breakthroughs when computer speeds limited what could be done with optimization. While still available in the commercial treatment-planning computers, neither is state of the art nor state of the practice now. For details about both of these, the reader is directed to the discussion in the 4th edition of this text.[24]

Convergent Searches

Also called "downhill searches," convergent searches minimize the OF iteratively.[25,26] At each iteration, the program decides which direction to make changes and how much change to make, based on the differential of the OF with respect to the parameter being optimized in that pass. These methods tend to get stuck in local minima if such occur between the starting condition and the true minimum. With large numbers of dwell positions and constraints, these searches tend not to be efficient and slow to converge.

Stochastic Approaches

A specialized form of downhill searching, stochastic approaches to optimization search for solutions by starting with a possible solution to the problem (in this case, the dwell times for all dwell positions), but not necessarily (or likely) the optimum solution. The OF is calculated for this solution. Then changes are made to the solution, and the OF calculated for the new solution. Another new solution would then be formed—guided by whether the value for the OF improved or degenerated. The nature of the search pattern differs for the various optimization programs, but all the stochastic approaches have some element of randomness in the search pattern. Because of this randomness, the programs may find different solutions with each run.

The only stochastic approach currently used in commercial HDR brachytherapy treatment planning is simulated annealing[27–30] and the genetic algorithm.[31,32] Ezzell[17] and Pouliot[33] present more detail on optimization techniques. For simulated annealing, the search

---

[d]For a discussion of TCP and NTCP, see Chapters 3 and 33.

makes somewhat random changes in the dwell times. The changes are not truly random, however. At first, the changes may be large. With each iteration, the sizes of the changes decrease. If after the change the OF improves, the next change pushes toward that same direction. On the other hand, if the OF becomes worse, a more random change is made. This process hones in on a "best" solution, but can get stuck in a local optimum, rather than the global optimum. To prevent a local trapping, occasionally, the program makes a very large change. If the new region of solutions does not seem promising after some tries, the program goes back to the place it left off before the big jump. Even though the process is computationally intensive because of the iterative nature of the search, as implemented commercially at the time of writing, optimization for an HDR prostate implant only takes a few seconds. With graphical processing units (GPUs), the times can be cut such the process seems live time.

The genetic algorithm takes a different approach to do the same thing as simulated annealing. Beginning with a random set of dwell weights for all the dwell positions in an implant (although, with any foreknowledge relevant to the implant, such as the optimal dwell-weight pattern that was found for a similar case, the time to convergence can be reduced), the dwell weights are lined up, such as simply by catheter number. In Figure 30.6, this would be the top line, Set A. Each color denotes a different dwell weight. Set B is a different, random set of dwell weights. Both sets are cut at the same location (i.e., between the same dwell positions) and the parts swapped, making two new sets, C and D that are the combinations of the two original sets. The OF for each of the four sets of dwell weights is calculated and the set with the best value is kept and becomes the new Set A' to become combined with a new, random Set B'. The process continues with the best of the four objection functions never being worse and eventually converging to a point where it stops improving.

The genetic algorithm is less likely to get caught in local minima than simulated annealing but at the cost of slower convergence.

Hybrid Optimization Approaches

While an improvement over the deterministic approaches, the statistical approaches tend to take a relatively long time to converge and seldom produce a dose distribution that completely satisfies a planner. The hybrid approaches usually start with a statistical optimization routine but with the modification of the OF to include information about OAR or the application geometry—a multiobjective optimization,[34] or combine the statistical optimization with other ways of controlling the outcome to be more like the planner desires. Equation 30.14 would be an example of a multiobjective function.

Simulated annealing often produces long dwell times at the ends of catheters and gives some catheters very long times while others are almost unused, which increases the inhomogeneity of the dose distribution.[35] Some hybrid optimizations control the wild unevenness of dwell weights.[35] One of the first approaches to fix the inhomogeneity issues with a statistical optimizer adds a modulation restriction factor. This factor is similar to van der Laarse's dwell-time gradient weighting factor used in point-dose optimization.[23] More recently, a dwell-time deviation constant (DTDC) was added to a commercial implementation of simulated annealing for HDR cases.[36] Lahanas et al. address this problem by using additional OF factors that specifically consider variation in the dose within a contour,

$$f_V = \frac{1}{N_V} \sum_{i=1}^{N_V} \frac{(d_i^V - m_V)}{m_V} \qquad (30.15)$$

where N_V is the number of sampling point in the volume, d is the dose at point i, and m_V is the average of the N_V points.[37,38] A similar equation can be used looking at points on the surface of the contour rather than through the volume if desired. This technique becomes the equivalent of optimizing on the dose-volume histogram (DVH) and can be applied for either a target volume or OARs.

The competition between target coverage and organ at-risk preservation forms one of the main conundrums encountered by the optimizers. Miliockovic et al. formed a multiobjective OF by adding as a criterion the inverse of the evaluation quantity, the conformal index, COIN,[39]

$$COIN = CN \prod_{i=1}^{n} \left[1 - \frac{OAR\ V_i(D_{OAR}\ D_{crit\,i})}{OAR\ V_i} \right] \qquad (30.16)$$

where CN is the Conformation Number, also an earlier version of COIN, which evaluates the conformance between the prescription isodose surface and CTV and relates to adequate dose coverage to the tumor.[40,41] This quantity is discussed in more detail in the section "Evaluation." Perfect correlation between the prescribed dose and the target gives a CN of unity. This value is then multiplied by the product for each of the OAR a measure of

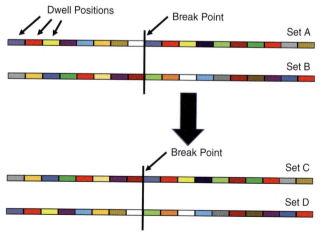

FIGURE 30.6. An illustration of the process used in the genetic optimization algorithm. See the text for explanation.

the volume of the OAR that is raised to a dose above its threshold tolerance, D_{crit}, as a fraction of the whole volume of the OAR. Ideally, COIN = 1. The further from one COIN is the worse the OF.

Comparing optimizations with the hybrid systems to just a statistic approach, Choi et al. looked at 20 tongue-cancer patients and found that the hybrid produced a slightly shorter treatment time but slightly more active dwell positions.[42] Clinically, either plan was adequate. Panettieri et al.[35] and Poulin et al.[20] had similar findings with prostate implants.[20,35] Intracavitary cervical brachytherapy following the GEC-ESTRO protocol presents a much greater challenge than the interstitial cases. Trnkova et al. compared manual planning for a tandem and ring applicator with supplemental needles with simulated annealing and a hybrid solver, finding the hybrid produced a better match with the treatment objectives than manual planning or straight simulated annealing while controlling the high-dose regions near the CTV_{HR}.[43] Of note, the simulated annealing produced serious high doses around the supplemental needles.

Manual Reoptimization

Optimization programs often satisfy the specified criteria but fail to produce the dose distribution that the operator had in mind. Manual reoptimization, also referred to as graphical optimization, remedies such a situation. In the study by Choi et al. cited earlier, after hybrid optimization, 40% of the patients required manual reoptimization.[42] Each commercial planning system for HDR includes a tool for adjusting the path of the isodose surfaces. With these tools, an isodose curve on a particular image slice can be grabbed by the cursor and moved to the desired position. The program then changes the dwell times to produce the change. The operator can choose to have the changes adjust just a single dwell position (local), all of the dwell positions (global), or any amount between. Global changes actually just renormalize the dose distribution to make a new dose as the prescription dose. Figure 30.7 shows manual optimization in action. Figure 30.7A shows the isodose distribution before adjustment, where the 100% isodose exceeds the target region of interest. Figure 30.7B shows the result of moving the 100% isodose curve to the target. For this example, the change level was set to "local." Even though the change is local, it still affects the dose distributions in other image cuts. Manual reoptimization must always be practiced iteratively, changing the dose distribution through a series of images and going back and adjusting them again, correcting the first cuts changes for the effects of the latter. At some point, the changes become small enough that further reoptimization becomes unnecessary.

Reoptimization requires caution. Increasing the size of the 100% isodose also increases the size of all the other isodose surfaces. In particular, the high-dose region can become large as a result. Manual reoptimization

should only be performed with the high-dose isodose lines visible on the images—following changes in one image, other images must be checked for unintended consequences.

Cervical Cancer Intracavitary Applications

While interstitial implants may vary in approach between facilities, for the most part, the optimization follows extremely similar criteria. Approaches to optimization for intracavitary gynecologic applications vary much more widely. Early work in HDR cervical applications attempted to duplicate the loading of LDR applications.[44] As noted in the discussion earlier on radiobiology, duplicating the *physical dose distribution* does not duplicate the *biologically effective dose distribution*.

Not only is duplicating the LDR physical distribution an incorrect way to approach the desired HDR dose distribution for the biological reason cited earlier, but the conceptual frameworks for the two types of treatments differ considerably. The first difference is most LDR treatments used the Manchester target of Point A for the prescription.[45] Point A was based on assumption of where the specification of the target should be (in the days before the target could be visualized) as well as the presumed location of critical normal tissues. The assumptions made in 1938 have been superseded by image-based information in the current era. Also important is that in the days of radium, and then cesium, the source capsules were large, about 2 cm in length or more. This size allowed only three sources in a uterine tandem. Most often there were only four strengths available: in mgRaeq, 25, 20, 15, and 10. With the sources available, in order to achieve a dose rate at point A of 55 R/h (the units of the time) typically required 10-mg sources in the tandem above and below point A, an additional 15-mg source in cephalad of the two 10-mg sources, and additional sources in the vaginal fornices. Related to the actual disease, the dose distribution under-treated larger tumors and over-treated small ones. The treatment doses also extended well superior and inferior to the disease.[16]

The current HDR approach follows the recommendations of the ICRU in defining the target based on disease demonstrated through MRI both at the time of diagnosis and at the beginning of brachytherapy.[16] The targets are defined as the High-Risk CTV (CTV_{HR}) and the Intermediate-Risk CTV (CTV_{IR}), and the doses to organs at risk are characterized as the minimum dose to the maximally exposed 2 cm^3 ($_{OAR}D_{2\,cm^3}$). In order to cover the disease adequately without overdosing the OARs, many cases require the use of supplemental interstitial needles. Some of the many applicators that facilitate these types of implants are shown in Figure 30.15. The details are important but too involved for discussion in this chapter; any facility performing cervical brachytherapy should become familiar with the report.

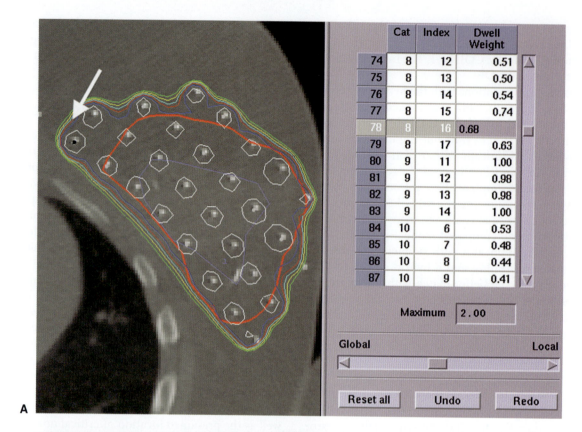

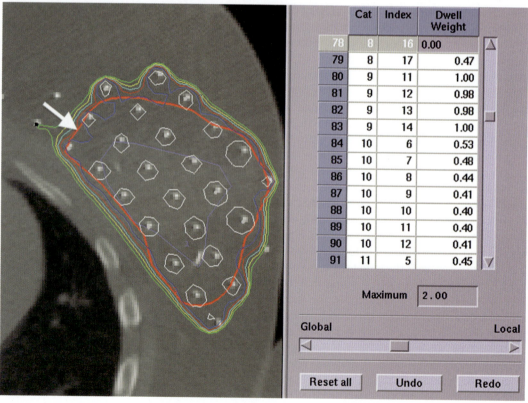

FIGURE 30.7. An example of manual optimization. **(A)** The isodose distribution before adjustment. **(B)** The result of the movement. The arrows follow the 100% isodose line (outer of the two darker, thin lines) as it moves to the edge of the target.

Inhomogeneity Correction

Until recently, the effect of inhomogeneities in brachytherapy had been ignored, mostly because the effectiveness of heterogeneity corrections in brachytherapy treatment planning has always lagged behind that of external beam radiotherapy. However, for several forms of intracavitary treatments, the effects of inhomogeneities have been shown to be important. Sometimes, the inhomogeneities result in erroneous dose calculations, such as from bone or resulting from the shields in vaginal ovoids.[46-48] In other cases, the inhomogeneity may perturb the geometry of the application, such as air pockets trapped on the surface of a vaginal applicator or on or within intracavitary breast applicator.[49-51] While for many years the hope had been for incorporation of full Monte Carlo simulations into brachytherapy treatment-planning systems, for various reasons this has not happened. However, each commercial treatment-planning system has incorporated a solver for the Boltzmann transport problem, and those solvers perform well compared with Monte Carlo simulations and differ importantly from calculations that ignore heterogeneities.[52,e] Figure 30.8 compares treatment plans with and without correction for heterogeneities. Such programs likely will become common in brachytherapy as they are in external-beam radiotherapy treatment planning. The use of correction software requires imaging with CT or magnetic resonance, which also has become more common.

A Final Word on Optimization

Optimization assists a planner in achieving the goals of treatment. The first step to achieving the goals is to place the treatment applicator in the ideal position. While optimization can sometimes compensate for a less-than-ideal placement, optimization cannot make a good treatment from a bad placement. Poor placement of an applicator results in poor homogeneity of the dose distribution, even with the best optimization.

EVALUATION

The generation of a treatment plan involves many steps—some fairly complicated—presenting many pathways and opportunities for plans to fail to achieve the treatment goals and the possibility for failures to propagate into a treatment error. Error prevention is addressed in the next section on "Quality Management." Evaluation of the quality of a treatment plan is part of the planning process proper as well as an important part of quality management (QM).

The inherent complexity of treatment planning often involves competing objectives, such as target coverage and OAR sparing. Choices often have to be made resulting in one or more aspects of the treatment plan being less than ideal. As noted in the section on "Optimization," the results of the optimization program may not be what was desired. Therefore, careful evaluation of an HDR treatment plan becomes very important. A fine line separates QM and treatment plan evaluation, and the evaluation serves as the first step in quality assurance (QA). The items to check do not have an unambiguous order. This section addresses the items from the more obvious to the more subtle.

Dose Prescription

The Absolute Dose to a Reference Location

Often, the dose distribution for brachytherapy shows isodose lines of a particular dose. In some cases, the isodose lines displayed by a treatment-planning computer may not correspond to the prescribed dose. Therefore, the first step of plan evaluation is to review isodose lines corresponding to the prescribed dose to a point or to a set of points. In most situations, the reference location should relate to the dose target, rather than regions of concern for normal tissues. Problems that can arise include the following:

1. Selecting the wrong point from among those entered for dose specification, for example, accidentally selecting the rectal point instead of Point A for a cervical treatment.
2. Having entered the specification point incorrectly, either through poor localization or through misinterpretation of the anatomy.
3. Specifying the dose to a set of points that have either large dose gradients in between or have widely varying realistic objectives.

While the first two problems represent errors, the last may be either a poor judgment or a complex patient presentation. A very simple example would be a treatment with a tandem and ovoids in a patient with a severely tipped uterus. The dose at Point A on the right and the left sides will be very different, and simply specifying the dose to the average of the two points could result in excessive dose on one side and too little dose on the other. A more involved situation would be specifying the dose to a set of points on the surface of a tumor with catheters running through. Depending on the geometry, the points may have too wide variation in doses to provide a good basis for the absolute dose specification.

Part of checking the prescribed dose includes review of the fractionation schema. The dose for the fraction should correspond to the total dose divided by the number of fractions. As part of this verification, the dose should also be checked against any relevant protocol that may change the dose based on concomitant external-beam therapy or

---

[e]For more about model-based dose calculations, see Chapter 21 and reference 44.

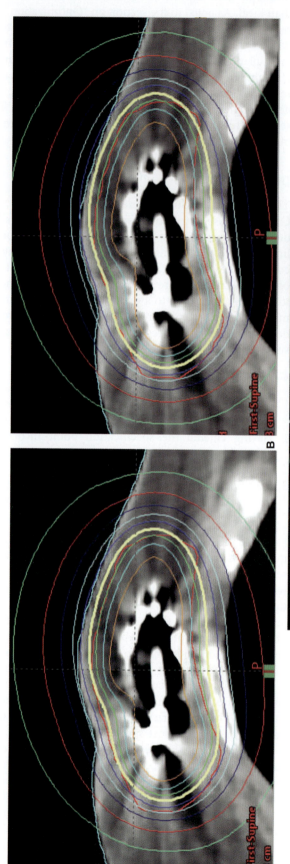

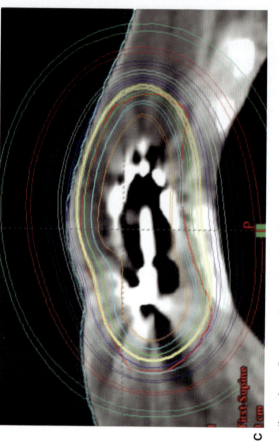

FIGURE 30.8. An illustration of inhomogeneity correction using a discrete-ordinates algorithm. **(A)** A treatment planning calculation performed assuming a homogeneous water medium. **(B)** The same plan with inhomogeneity corrections, taking into account the air inside the cavity and tissue-air interface at the body boundary, using the Acuros program. **(C)** The two plans superimposed [note difference near the skin surface due to lack of backscatter].

chemotherapy (in an era of satellite facilities and specialty referrals, such concomitant treatments may not be obvious to the treatment planner). Some treatment-planning systems encourage the use of planning for a single fraction and then delivering that plan multiple times to create a composite dose.

Relative Doses to Specified Volumes

The optimization process required some specification of locations that should receive some fraction of the prescription dose. In intracavitary cases, this may be a few points, for example, along an esophageal applicator or along a tandem and lateral to a vaginal ring. For a volume implant, it may be the target volume surface. In any case, these points define the goal for the treatment, and satisfaction of the prescription requires conformance of the dose distribution to these specifications. For the simpler cases, review of each optimization point may be performed, but volume implants probably require a DVH, as discussed later.

The dose to all the optimization points likely will not equal the specified dose, as noted earlier, but should be within some defined tolerance. Failure to adequately shape the dose distribution raises three planning options: accepting the results if compatible with the treatment objectives; changing the optimization parameters and trying to optimize the plan again; or manually intervening, as discussed in the section on "Optimization."

Limitations

The doses to limiting normal structures should be checked to assure that they remain below tolerance. Assessment of the doses to normal structures falls under the next section. The dose-calculation grid size plays a role in the accuracy of the treatment plan, albeit much less with modern treatment-planning systems than older systems. As an example, changing from a 0.25 × 0.25 × 0.125 cc reconstruction grid to a 0.125 × 0.125 × 0.0625 cc changes the CTV_{HR} mean dose from 8.7 to 8.8 Gy and the maximum dose from 40 to 72 Gy! With a protocol using a maximum dose, the dose grid can be an important factor.

Evaluation of Dose Distributions

Adequate coverage of the target usually involves visual inspection of the isodose lines throughout the 3D volume and review of DVH. While a DVH shows failure to include all targets within the prescription isodose surface, the DVH does not show where the failures occur or whether the volumes that fall below the prescription dose are contiguous (a potentially serious problem) or widely dispersed (often not significant). The same can be said for high-dose volumes (HDVs). The entire treatment region should be evaluated with consideration of dose-limiting structures.

Evaluation of the dose homogeneity is discussed in detail later in this section. However, two tools that assess the uniformity of the doses only apply when visually evaluating the isodose distribution for implants. The *maximum significant dose* (MSD) refers to the highest-level isodose surface that encompasses more than one needle track. The dose very near the source track can be very high, but the tissues tolerate these local HDVs. Figure 30.9 shows a gynecological interstitial implant with an MSD of 8 Gy.

The MSD provides a convenient criterion for when small HDVs become "significant" and likely to produce biological consequences. For an implant taken to normal tissue tolerance, the MSD corresponds to the tolerance dose. For what fraction of the prescription isodose surface, the MSD becomes limiting depends on several factors. The first is the volume of the implant—the tolerated level for the MSD decreases with volume. The second factor is where in the gradient around the implanted volume the prescription dose falls. Much of the modern experience with implants comes through the use of the Paris System (discussed later).[53–55] With that system, the prescription dose (Reference Dose [RD] in the System's parlance) equaled 85% of the Basal Dose (BD), that is, the mean of the local minima between needle tracks in the central plane. The Paris System further defined an HDV as that volume raised to 200% of the prescription dose (170% of the BD), and suggested that this dose tightly conforms to the needle tracks. Thus, for Paris System implants, the MSD would be somewhat less than 200% of the prescription dose. Translating this MSD to HDR treatments requires a few steps. First, assume an LDR treatment of 60 Gy delivered at 0.5 Gy/h. From Equation 30.8, the BED using an $\alpha/\beta = 10$ Gy^{-1}, appropriate for tumor cells, would be 72.8 Gy_{10}. The limitation on high doses in the target volume likely applies to normal tissue tolerances, since it is normal tissue breakdown that results in complications. Thus, the BED for the 200% dose, using $\alpha/\beta = 3$ Gy^{-1}, equals 290 Gy_3. Many HDR regimens could be used for this treatment, but this example assumes six fractions of 5.25 Gy each, which gives the same biological effect for the tumor. The physical dose that gives the same biological effectiveness for normal tissue as the MSD earlier is 8.45 Gy, or 160% of the prescription dose. This result highlights a general rule of HDR brachytherapy: *the variation in dose through the treated volume must remain markedly less than with LDR brachytherapy.* That rule just restates the relative increase in the sensitivity of normal tissue with the change to HDR treatments. The value of MSD of 160% matches well experience with breast implants that use the 150% isodose surface for the MSD, and that exceeding this level increases the probability of complications. This also agrees well with experience with large gynecological implants that the MSD should stay below 125% of the BD.[2,56] For small implants, the percentage of the prescription dose selected for the MSD can increase, but there is not as much data for small volume implant complications as for the large.

Another tool, developed by Neblett, considers the other boundary of the isodose distribution, finding the

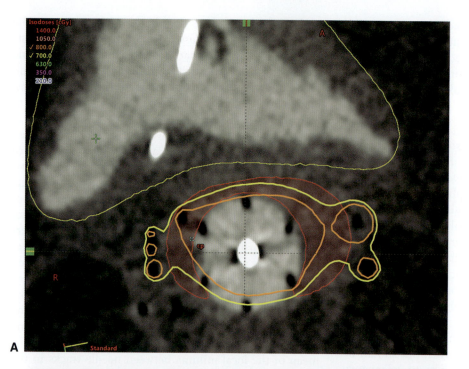

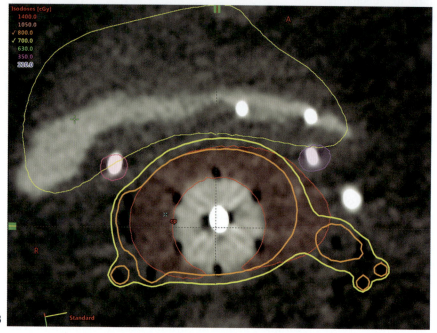

FIGURE 30.9. An illustration of the maximum significant dose, shown as an orange line, and maximum contiguous dose, as a yellow line. **(A)** and **(B)** show the dose distribution at two axial positions.

maximum contiguous dose (MCD), or the highest value for an isodose surface that completely surrounds the implanted needle tracks.[57] Isodose levels higher than the MCD break into small islands of high dose with lower doses separating volumes enclosed. The prescription dose should not exceed the MCD, but should not fall much outside the MCD isodose surface. Figure 30.9 also shows the MCD as 7 Gy.

Evaluation of dose distributions for intracavitary insertions, for the most part, remains to be visual inspection of isodose plots. The concepts that measure uniformity or

HDVs find little relevance in intracavitary applications because the dose always becomes high near the sources and falls continuously with distance. The question in evaluating the dose distribution becomes simply whether or not an adequate dose covers the target or targets and avoids excessive doses to limiting structures. One exception to this is intracavitary breast treatments with multi-lumen applicators. In these cases, tailoring the distribution to the patient often reduces the uniformity of the dose through the defined target volume, and measures of the homogeneity of the dose, as discussed later, provide insights into

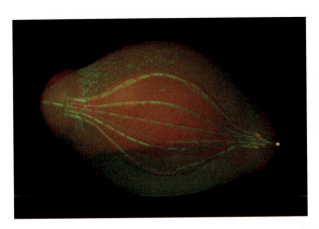

FIGURE 30.10. A three-dimensional view of the target and the 100% isodose surface for a breast implant using a strut-adjusted volume implant (SAVI) applicator. The PTV is shown as a red surface and the 3.4-Gy isodose surface in green. In this projection, the conformity looks very good.

the quality of the treatment. However, this can create a more optimal treatment and appropriate DVH.

For intracavitary and interstitial cases, target evaluation should be considered a three-dimensional process. However, three-dimensional views often become difficult to interpret. Figure 30.10 shows the target for a breast implant and the 100% isodose surface rendered around the target. In many cases, the three-dimensional images may seem confusing. Limiting the number of structures shown to a region of interest and one isodose surface helps during the interpretation. Another use of 3D rendering would involve the evaluation of skin dose for breast brachytherapy. Evaluation of skin dose is often complicated due to curving and steeply sloped surfaces. Point doses are also complicated due to determining what is actually included as the surface of the body. Rendering the body in a solid color as well as the limiting isodose surface (e.g., the prescription 4-Gy surface), one can see if the isodose line breaks through the skin rendering and where that may be located (e.g., in the breast fold).

Dose-Volume Histograms

The first step in quantitative evaluation involves review of the DVH. There are several different types of DVH, each presenting different information. The histograms in all cases display some function related to volume on the ordinate with dose (or a function of dose) on the abscissa.

Figure 30.11 shows a relative, cumulative DVH for an HDR prostate implant for a boost following external-beam therapy. The ordinate records the fraction of a structure that receives at least that dose shown on the abscissa. The normalization of the volume to the total volume of the region of interest makes the histogram "relative." Ideally, the curve labeled "prostate" would run along the top of the graph at 1.0 for all the doses until the prescription dose, indicating that the entire target receives at least the target dose, and then the curve rapidly falls. Of

course, the fall cannot be very sharp because there will always be HDVs around the needles. The entire prostate may not receive the prescription dose, either. Depending on the limitations on dose to the rectum, and potentially on the placement of the catheters due to the pelvic arch, some regions of the prostate may fall shy of the prescription dose.

Figure 30.11 also shows a curve for the rectum. Unlike the target, only part of the rectal contour usually is entered into the computer. Thus, the histogram actually shows the fraction of the *contoured* volume that receives the given dose. Some organs may be completely contoured during planning, and the fraction of the whole organ receiving particular doses may relate to complications or other treatment limitations. For long tube-like organs, complete contouring not only may be unlikely, but unnecessary. For volumes less than 5 cm^3, it makes little difference if the contour simply encircles the whole rectal cross section or specifically just outlines the wall. Some evidence indicates that rather than the fraction of the rectum being the critical variable, that the absolute volume may be important.

Various volumes have been proposed from 0.1 to 5 cm^3.[58-63] The GEC-ESTRO recommends evaluation of highest irradiated volumes of 0.1, 1, and 2 cm^3 for organs at risk. The value of interest for these volumes would be the minimum dose, since the maximum dose would be just a point, and not change for any of the volumes. While that may sound counterintuitive, consider Figure 30.12.

For the green OAR, the gray source delivers the highest dose at the black dot. The red isodose surface shows where the 2-cm^3 volume that contains the voxels with the highest doses. The union of that isodose surface and the OAR is shaded red, although you cannot see it all because it is covered by the blue isodose surface, which shows the 1 cm^3 volume of the OAR with the voxels with the highest doses. All of the blue-shaded volume is contained within the red volume, which is why it is shown in violet, except that part of the OAR that has the 0.1-cm^3 volume with the voxels with the highest doses. This last volume is shaded in gold, but because it is totally contained in both the blue and red volumes, it shows a mix of all the colors. In the red volume, the highest dose is the black dot and the lowest doses fall on the red circle. Therefore, the value of dose on the red circle is the minimum dose in the 2-cm^3 volume with the collectively highest doses. Similarly, with the blue and the gold circles, both have the highest value of dose at the black dot and the lowest on the circle, and each includes the collection of voxels with the highest dose for the total volume bounded by the circle.

The absolute maximum dose, found at the black dot, varies greatly based on the dose calculation grid and the accuracy by which the distance from the source to the dot is determined, making it a poor surrogate for the expected effect on the organ. Contrary to that, the minimum dose to that maximally irradiated 2-cm^3 volume is robust, changing little with minor changes in calculation techniques. It has also been found that the 2-cm^3 volume

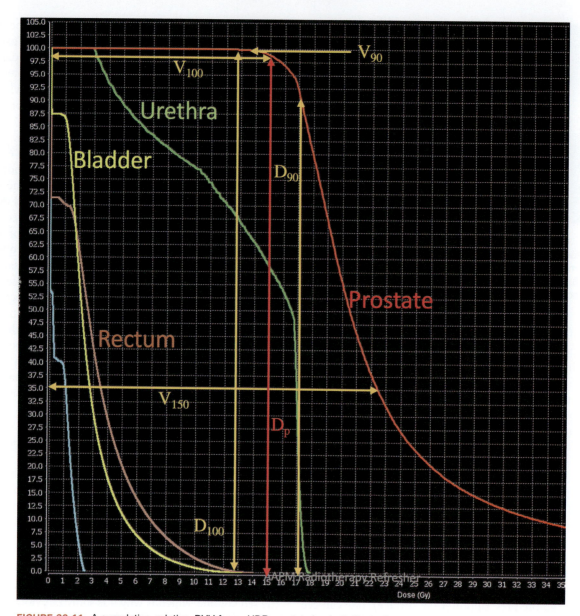

FIGURE 30.11. A cumulative, relative, DVH for an HDR prostate implant, illustrating some of the dose index quantities.

correlates much better to the toxicity in the rectum and bladder than the maximum point dose, the 0.1-cm^3 volume (which differs little from the maximum dose), or the 1-cm^3 volume.[61,64,65]

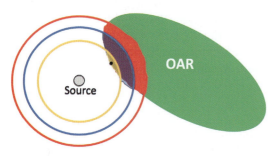

FIGURE 30.12. An illustration of the volume-dose concept for describing the dose to organs at risk.

DVH assists in evaluation of implants by calling attention to the fraction of the tumor that may receive less than the treatment dose or whether a neighboring structure exceeds tolerance. They can also help distinguish between plans that would better concentrate the dose in the target. However, as noted earlier, while presenting this information for rapid detection, DVH loses special information, such as *where* the target dose may be low.

Figures of Merit

The DVH distills the information from the isodose distributions in a two-dimensional format to simplify evaluations. *Figures of Merit* provide numerical values for particular aspects of implants, and can assist in evaluations and facilitate communication about the treatments. More detailed discussions can be found in Saw and

Suntharalingam, and Thomadsen.[66,67] While most of the quantities were developed for interstitial implants, mostly because intracavitary insertions concentrated on standardizing treatment geometries as much as possible. With the movement toward MR-guided cervical brachytherapy customizing the treatments for the individual patient, and the use of multichannel intracavitary breast applicators, interest in, and use of, figures of merit for intracavitary brachytherapy have increased. Some of the quantities apply quite directly from interstitial implants to intracavity insertions, while others require considerable modification and, at the time of writing, are in development. Following are some of the quantities most useful for HDR treatment planning.

Target Coverage

The first assessment should be whether the plan adequately covers the target. Several measures for that exist, each telling a slightly different story.

$D_{x\%}$ refers to the dose that covers $x\%$ of the target volume. Ideally, the prescription dose covers 100% of the target, although as mentioned before, that often cannot be the case. Recognizing this, many protocols call for the prescription dose to cover some particular fraction of the target volume, such as 95%. In such cases, $D_{95\%}$ becomes a value of great interest since it often defines the prescription. The companion quantity, V_x, gives the volume receiving a dose equal to or greater than x. This quantity assumes different forms depending on the conventions used for a treatment protocol. Most often the volume refers to the fraction of the CTV receiving at least the dose x, but at other times it is the absolute volume. The dose, x, may refer to the absolute dose, or it may be a fraction of the prescribed dose. The convention in use requires clarification. Again, ideally, $V_{100\%}$ should equal 1 in an ideal implant if V equals the fraction of the target volume with x normalized to the prescribed dose. For the remainder of this discussion, the convention will specify doses explicitly as either a percent of the prescription dose labeled with "%" or an absolute labeled with "Gy." Reference volumes will be percent, again labeled as "%" or absolute with units of cm³. Finally, the volume to which the quantity refers will be a leading subscript, to give quantities such as $_{CTV}D_{90\%}$ or $_{rectum}V_{60Gy}$.

The *Coverage index* (CI) specifies the fraction of the target volume receiving a dose equal to, or greater than, the target dose.[68] The CI corresponds to the value on the relative, cumulative DVH for the CTV at the prescription dose. Thus, CI = $_{CTV}V_{100\%}$.

Dose Uniformity

After assessing the adequacy of target coverage, the next question focuses on the uniformity of the dose through the target volume. As discussed earlier, the MSD must be controlled, but other measures also can help in this evaluation.

It has often been suggested that the delivery of doses well above the prescription dose to some of the treated

volume in brachytherapy may be responsible for the effectiveness of the treatment modality, particularly with respect to intracavitary applications. However, it has also been recognized that high doses to too large a volume can cause extreme toxicity. At the same time, those excessively high doses can be well tolerated as long as the volume remains low. Conceptually, because of the inverse-square law, doses very near sources can become extremely high. Quantification of high-dose region has been a focus of figures of merit for a long time, with one of the first systematic approaches coming from the HDV of the Paris System, which used a cut-off of 200% of the prescription dose.[54] Zwicker makes the factor a variable, p, used during optimization.[69] In the discussion earlier, converting from the LDR treatments to an HDR regimen, the Paris System's factor of 200% becomes 160%. Using an LDR factor of 150%, as suggested by the ICRU,[70] leads to an HDR factor of 123%. Limiting the MSD to 123% is seldom possible in a real implant. The rest of this discussion uses a value of 150% to define the HDV for HDR implants. Figure 30.13 shows a schematic of a section through the CTV, a prescription isodose surface as the $V_{100\%}$ and the surface corresponding to 1.5 times the prescription dose, $V_{150\%}$. In this figure, much of the $V_{100\%}$ and the CTV coincide, but some of the CTV remains below the prescribed dose while some of the prescribed dose falls outside the target. Some of the target and normal tissues receive in excess of 150%, which is very undesirable for the normal tissue and uselessly high for the tumor. Thus, the most desirable region has the CTV receiving doses between the 100% and the 150%. This figure may be helpful during the following discussion.

The *relative dose homogeneity index* (HI) measures the uniformity of the dose through the target volume as the fraction of the target volume receiving a dose between the target dose and the high dose level, or[71]

$$HI = _{CTV}V_{100\%} - _{CTV}V_{150\%} \qquad (30.17)$$

In Equation 30.17, both volumes are the fraction of the CTV raised to at least the percent of the prescription dose given. Originally, the HI referred only to the prescription

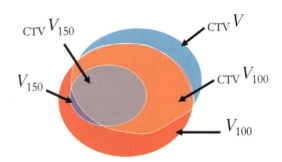

FIGURE 30.13. A schematic showing a section of a CTV (light blue) and surface corresponding to 100% of the prescribed dose (red) and the 150% in purple. The overlap (union) of the CTV and the 100% isodose volume is shown in orange, and 150% and the CTV in gray.

isodose volumes without regard to the target, dating from when target information usually was not available. Most often nowadays, Equation 30.17 is used.

A very similar index, the *dose nonuniformity ratio* (DNR) equals ratio of the HDV to that volume taken to at least the target dose,[72]

$$\text{DNR} = \frac{_{\text{CTV}}V_{150\%}}{_{\text{CTV}}V_{100\%}} \qquad (30.18)$$

This quantity indicates the price paid (in HDV) to set the prescription dose to cover the target. Obviously, the DNR and HI are related, so specification of both quantities becomes duplicative.

Dose Outside the Target

As a measure of the dose outside the target, the *external volume index* (EI) equals the volume of nontarget tissue receiving doses equal to or greater than the target dose, as a fraction of the target volume.[68,73] Thus,

$$\text{EI} = \frac{_{100\%}V - _{\text{CTV}}V_{100\%} \cdot _{\text{CTV}}V}{_{\text{CTV}}V} \qquad (30.19)$$

Here, $V_{100\%}$ indicates the entire volume enclosed by the prescription isodose surface and $_{\text{CTV}}V$ is the absolute volume of the CTV.

Since $_{\text{CTV}}V_{100\%}$ is the fraction of the CTV volume raised to at least 100% of the prescription dose, the product, gives the absolute volume of the CTV raised to at least 100% of the prescription dose.

For much of modern treatment planning, the dose to other structures, organs or other sensitive issues, are calculated to contoured surfaces and the doses to each contour compared with the dose limits for the particular tissues. The EI, rather than addressing the concept of tolerance, nowadays serves as a measure of precision of the application.

Conformity

The *conformation number* (CN) is the measures of the conformance of the prescription dose to the target,[40,41]

$$\text{CN} = \frac{_{\text{CTV}}V_{100\%}[\text{cm}]}{_{100\%}V[\text{cm}]} \frac{_{\text{CTV}}V_{100\%}[\text{cm}]}{_{\text{CTV}}V[\text{cm}]} \qquad (30.20)$$

The numerator of each factor gives the total volume of the CTV within the 100% isodose surface, as the volume of the CTV times the fraction of the CTV raised to the 100% dose. The first factor gives the dose within the CTV as a fraction of the whole 100% dose volume, a measure of the efficiency of the dose deposition. The second factor is related to the coverage of the target. Together they indicate how closely the prescription dose matches the target.

Figure of Merit Summary

Each of these figures of merit provides useful information about the implant. Several of them are redundant and which should be used becomes the user's preference. None of these quantities tells the entire story for a given implant. No single index or quantity perfectly characterizes any implant—evaluation requires consideration of many different aspects, not all of which optimize for the same conditions. Final decisions and the quality of an implant require consideration of the large overview of the implant.

Evaluation of Intracavitary Insertions

At this point it is useful to separate the discussion for intracavitary insertions and interstitial implants, first looking at the intracavitary cases. For intracavitary insertions, other than the general evaluation processes described earlier, the evaluation of plans differs for gynecological, breast, and intralumenal cases, each of which will be discussed later.

Plan Evaluation for Gynecological Insertions

The reader is directed to Chapter 11, which presents treatment planning for gynecological radiotherapy and presents concepts that are useful to understand before addressing plan evaluation.

The first check for cervical brachytherapy evaluates the prescription, mindful of any contribution from external-beam treatments. Early stage disease requires EQD_2 of ≥ 80 $\text{Gy}_{2\text{Eq}}$, while larger disease needs 85 to 90 $\text{Gy}_{2\text{Eq}}$.[74] The next check would compare the coverage of the CTV_{HR} with the prescription isodose surface. The $_{\text{CTV-HR}}D_{90\%}$ ideally should be no less than 95 Gy. However, for many large, irregularly shaped target volumes this becomes very difficult to achieve, even with supplemental interstitial needles and the planning may have to be satisfied with something on the order of $_{\text{CTV-HR}}D_{90\%} = 85$ Gy. Figure 30.14 shows a case that illustrates such a problem. The final piece of the evaluation reviews the doses to the bladder, rectum, sigmoid and other structures recommended by the ICRU in their Report 89.[16]

Plan Evaluation for Breast Applications

There are a variety of multichannel or multi-catheter breast applicators on the market for intracavitary breast brachytherapy treatments. Therefore, it is important to understand the applicator design prior to use and evaluate the reconstruction of the catheters accordingly. Different applicators rely on different visualization apparatus, as an example, the strut-adjusted volume implant (SAVI) applicator contains catheters adjacent to near metal in the struts. The metal struts can be easily visualized on CT and could lead to errors if, for example, the metal struts were assumed to be metal markers placed within the catheters. In a similar fashion for multichannel applicators, it's important to check that each catheter is indexed appropriately with accurate catheter lengths.

Contours should be reviewed to ensure all organs at risk are properly segmented and the doses to OARs, such as skin, chest wall, and ribs, are reasonable. In addition, the high-dose regions should be assessed by calculating the volume of the breast tissue receiving, 200% and 150% of the prescription dose. It is important that the applicator is not included in the calculation. If the dose to the applicator is not properly accounted for, DVH values will not represent the true dose to the breast tissue anvd this can propagate errors in uniformity calculations, such as the HI value.

Plan Evaluation for Intraluminal Insertions

Intraluminal insertions are just a special case of intracavitary brachytherapy where the cavity is long and narrow. Two examples that highlight the differences in this smallish class of brachytherapy are endobronchial and endoesophageal treatments. Endobronchial insertions usually have a single small-diameter (5 or 6 French[f]) catheter in a bronchus, although sometimes for a tumor between two branches, a catheter in each of the branches is used. Being a single catheter, or possibly two, optimization can only adjust the dwell times along the source track to have the dose follow the tumor contour.

Esophageal treatments often use specially designed applicators that expand to fill the esophagus to add distance from the source pathway, but also allow for several catheters positioned cylindrically around a central catheter. The central catheter provides a circumferential dose, and the multiple catheters closer to the surface can shape the dose distribution more locally.

In both cases, the applicator needs to extend beyond the target sufficiently so to inhibit motion along the lumen, and particularly for the endobronchial, to resist being coughed out of place.

The main items to check for these treatments include the following:

- As with all treatments, that the dose distribution follows the target appropriately, understanding in this case, the paucity of source pathways for optimization.

- That the first dwell position activated and the distance to the actual first dwell position was selected to move the dose distribution to the treatment site, and that the dose is not inadvertently at the end of the catheter.
- For esophageal applicators, that there is a method to ensure that the rotational orientation correctly places the circumferential catheters where they were with respect to the tumor during the optimization of the dose distribution during treatment planning.
- That the dwell times seem appropriate for the dose distribution using a consistency algorithm, such as that of Das et al. discusses in the section "Indicators of Reasonableness."

Evaluation of Interstitial Implants

Interstitial gynecological implants are usually extremely complex due to multiple factors: difficulty in accessing the treatment area, competing goals between tightly spaced targets and OARs, deep needle deflection and crossing, and potential movement of the implant between fractions. Additionally, some needles may actually penetrate bladder walls or be so close to the rectum they are unusable, even when placed by an experienced physician. A general evaluation strategy may be as follows:

Needles

Ensure all needles are numbered correctly. A difficult implant may have a tandem and more than 30 needles depending on target size. Accurate labeling and transmitting of labeling information to the planning system

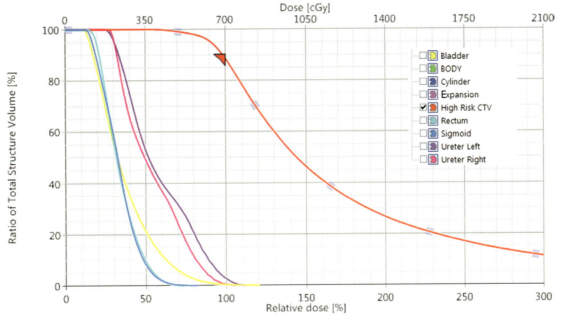

FIGURE 30.14. A treatment of a large, irregular cervical cancer using a Syed template. Even with the addition of needles, the $_{CTV-HR}D_{90\%}$ of 7 Gy fails to enclose the lobe of the disease on the patient's left side. The $_{HR}D_{100\%}$ is approximately 5 Gy.

---

[f]The French scale for catheter size numerically equals the diameter in millimeters times three, so is slightly less than, but approximately to, the circumference.

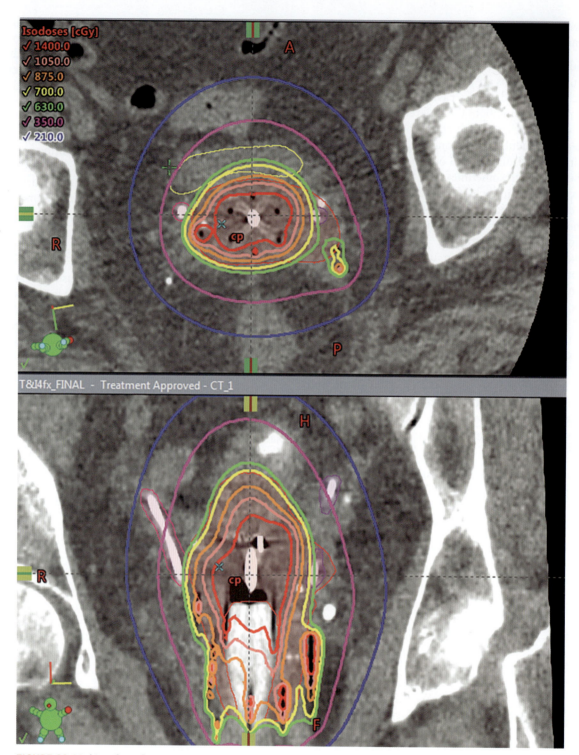

FIGURE 30.14. (*Continued*)

are imperative for correct delivery. This can be performed via a diagram that is checked by multiple individuals and standardization of planning routines (e.g., needle numbers increase clockwise in consecutive circles from inside to outside). Evaluate needles that penetrate or lie directly next to OARs. In such cases, they may be unused or minimally used—for example, the tip of a needle may be used when parallel and near the rectum where the rectal wall diverts away from the needle in the superior aspect of the patient. Another common situation is where the tip of a needle near the bladder may be unused but may be critical for coverage through the rest of the implant. Review of 2-cm^3 or smaller volumes of these structures can help find unwanted hot spots in the sensitive volumes as well as evaluating isodose levels of 200% or more.

Dwell Times

Dwell times should be evaluated for reasonableness—for a 10-Ci source, a dwell time in a needle of more than 5 s should be reviewed with a physician for criticality. Potentially, a different needle could be used to reduce some of that time or more dwell positions added within the needle. Dwell times within a single needle should vary smoothly so that any small offsets would not affect the robustness of the plan. A needle with 0.5-cm spacing is more robust with dwell times of 3, 3, and 3 s than a needle with 5, 0, and 5 s. When using inverse planning, the smoothing options in the optimizer may reduce unwanted significant dwell times in single dwells. Robustness of treatment plans is critical in interstitial implants due to potential single needle or entire implant motion—particularly if the patients will be keeping the implant in place overnight and treated multiple times.

Dose

As shown in Figure 30.5, the plan may have both aims and strict limits in evaluating the dose. The give and take between target dose and OAR dose may be shown with several iterations of a plan—one where all the target goals are met and one where all the OAR goals are met. Discussions with the brachytherapy team may help determine which (if any) are more appropriate for a particular patient. The physician may be more or less aggressive depending on patient's age or morbidities. Good communication between team members and managing expectations for complicated cases is extremely important.

QUALITY MANAGEMENT

QA for the treatment plan assesses first the adequacy of the generated treatment plan—the measures which were addressed in the section on "Plan Evaluation." The evaluation process includes verification that the plan delivers the intended dose to the correct location. The other purpose for QA is to detect and correct errors in the treatment plan before treatment delivery. QA, by definition, provides an indication that the plan contains no errors and is of the quality intended.

Before performing QA, quality control (QC) works to keep errors from happening in the first place. For HDR brachytherapy treatment planning, a useful and effective QC tool is a form for recording and transmitting necessary information. Such a form may serve as the prescription, since it should contain the information of the dose—fractionation and normal structure limitation—as well as a description of the application and any other relevant information. The form most likely would be electronic and may become part of the electronic health record. A treatment-planning protocol serves as the other very important QC tool. The protocol is a standard operating procedure that dictates routine planning decisions for various types of cases. Examples of information contained in a protocol include GEC-ESTRO guidelines for cervical intracavitary insertions and the step size for breast implants.[g]

"Independent verification" forms an invaluable part of QA. Having someone other than the person who generated a treatment plan check it greatly increases the probability of detecting errors. In addition, just as a form for recording and transmission of information helps prevent errors, forms to guide the plan evaluation also prevent omissions during the verification process. Guidance for developing forms can be found in Thomadsen.[67] If having an independent person check the plan is not an option at a facility, the use of forms and a fixed verification protocol becomes even more important, as do internal benchmarks and published nomograms.

Indicators of Reasonableness

One major challenge in QA is to judge whether the planner made a significant error. One approach to assess the plan for errors compares some value related to the plan with standards or expectations. The standards derive from previous experience or from the literature. The following sections consider some examples. For a more detailed discussion, again see Thomadsen.[67] It is important to note that secondary calculations using programs such as BrachyCheck (Oncology Data Systems, Oklahoma City, OK) or RadCalc (Lifeline Software, Inc., LAP GmbH Laser Applikationen, Schwarzenbruck Germany) will not find a *planning* error as the dose calculation is most likely correct but, most likely, at least one of the input values is incorrect (e.g., point A incorrectly identified).

Intraluminal Tests

Intraluminal cases generally use a single catheter, such as for endobronchial, endoesophageal, or biliary treatments. Some of the tests discussed later also apply for vaginal cylinder applications. Thomadsen reported an index[75]

$$\text{Index} = \frac{\text{Total dwell time [s]} \cdot \text{Source strength} [\text{Gy} \cdot \text{m}^2 \cdot \text{h}^{-1}]}{\text{Prescription dose [Gy]} \cdot \text{Lenth of prescription dose [cm]} \cdot \text{Distance to prescription dose [cm]}}$$

(30.21)

where the index should fall between 0.133 and 0.167 ([Gy m^2 s]/[Gy cm^2 h]). Obviously, the index actually has no true units since with multiplying by appropriate constants, the units cancel. However, for convenience, the equation keeps the units most likely used for each variable. This index increases above these limits for short treatment lengths compared to the prescription distance.

---

[g]The step size becomes very important in many implant cases. Large step sizes give a poorer ability to optimize the dose distribution. Small step sizes with very short dwell times may cause some units to render a treatment plan undeliverable following a source change if the automatically recalculated dwell times become shorter than the shortest time programmable.

Tandem and Ovoids

Indices similar to those discussed earlier have been used in gynecological applications, but because the constraints for optimization vary greatly between facilities, the actual values used with any such index must be developed locally. Two indices developed for use with the Madison System[3] assess whether a given tandem and ovoid application falls within the normal range[75]:

$$\text{Index 1} =$$

$$\frac{\text{Dwell time 1 cm from tip [s]} \cdot \text{Source strength} [\text{Gy} \cdot \text{m}^2 \cdot \text{h}^{-1}]}{\text{Prescription dose [Gy]}}$$

(30.22a)

and

$$\text{Index 2} =$$

$$\frac{\text{Total dwell time [s]} \cdot \text{Source strength} [\text{Gy} \cdot \text{m}^2 \cdot \text{h}^{-1}]}{\text{Prescription dose [Gy]} \cdot \text{Number of dwell poistions}}$$

(30.22b)

The location for the first index dwell falls far from the ovoids to consider mostly the loading of the tandem. The dwell times for the tip-most position vary greatly between patients and thus, do not serve well for measures of application consistency. The dwell 1 cm inferior to the first dwell position used becomes quite stable. Index 1 tells whether this one position falls within a normal range. Index 2 considers the application as a whole. The numerator simply gives the integrated reference air kerma (IRAK, which numerically equals the total reference air kerma, TRAK, of the ICRU).[76] The use of IRAK parallels the old mgRaeq·h used for evaluating the normalcy of LDR applications. Following the Madison System optimization pattern, the limits for the indices in units of $[\text{Gy m}^2 \text{ s}]/[\text{Gy h}]$ become as follows:

- Index 1—0.139 to 0.180
- Index 2
  - For small ovoids—0.098 to 0.123
  - For medium ovoids—0.123 to 0.147
  - For large ovoids—0.135 to 0.180

The indices also apply to applications using tandem with cylinders in the vagina, where Index 2 values become:

- For 2.0 cm diameter—0.098 to 0.139
- For 2.5 cm diameter—0.114 to 0.147
- For 3.0 cm diameter—0.109 to 0.160
- For 3.5 cm diameter—0.143 to 0.168

Interstitial Implants

Common optimized HDR implants conceptually tend to follow a cross between Manchester and Paris implants. The implants behave much like Manchester implants in that the differential source-strength distribution pattern varies much like in the Manchester rules. However, unlike the Manchester system, where the dose tends to correspond to the Paris System's BD, most practitioners specify the prescription to an RD outside the limits of the implant, similar to the Paris System. With this in mind, the

Manchester implant tables can be modified to apply to ^{192}Ir HDR implants by multiplication of the source strengths by 1.11 to set the RD to 90% of the BD, and converting from mgRaeq·h to ^{192}Ir IRAK. For a given treatment plan, the total duration of the treatment calculated by the planning computer can be compared with the time given by

$$\text{Time} = \frac{\text{Dose} [\text{Gy}] \cdot R_V [\text{Gy} \cdot \text{m}^2 \cdot \text{h}^{-1} \cdot \text{s/Gy}]}{\text{Source strength} [\text{Gy} \cdot \text{m}^2 \cdot \text{h}^{-1}]} \quad (30.23)$$

where in this equation $R_V = 0.00321 \, _{\text{Manchester}}R_V$, that is the R_V in the original Manchester tables, so

$$_{\text{Manchester}}R_V = 0.1091 \, V^{2/3} e^{0.007(E-1)} \quad (30.24)$$

where E is the longest dimension/shortest orthogonal dimension. Experience with breast implants shows that this formula generally agrees with the time calculated by the treatment-planning computer within 5%.

A similar approach holds for modifying the R_A values from the Manchester table to verify the calculations for planar implants.

Unified Index

Das et al. brought the check indices into modern approaches to brachytherapy dosimetry and considered predicting the treatment duration based on the volume of the prescription isodose surface, V_{100}.[77] Beginning with a point source approximation, they derived the equation

$$\text{Time} = \frac{\text{Prescribed dose} [\text{Gy}] \cdot K [\text{U} \cdot \text{s} \cdot \text{Gy}^{-1}] \cdot V_{100\%}^{2/3} [\text{cm}^2] \cdot EC}{\text{Air kerma strength} [\text{U}]}$$

(30.25)

where EC is the elongation correction, approximated as $1 + 0.06(E-1)^{1.26}$, and K is a constant depending on the number of catheters:

- 1 catheter, $K = 126,700$ U s/(Gy cm^2)
- 2 or 3 catheters, $K = 118,200$ U s/(Gy cm^2)
- More than three catheters, $K = 92,800$ U s/(Gy cm^2)

This approach and equation apply for intraluminal, intracavitary, and interstitial brachytherapy.

Treatment Unit Programming and Pretreatment Checks

Once the treatment plan passes the evaluation and QA tests, the treatment plan must be passed to the treatment unit in the form of a treatment program specifying all the treatment information: channel lengths (distance to the first dwell position), step size or sizes, and the dwell-time pattern for each channel. Verification of the program checks the items most likely to be in error.

The most likely error is selecting the wrong program for a given patient, if there is more than one program under the patient's identity. This situation frequently arises in regimens where new plans are generated at each fraction, such as gynecological intracavitary applications. Such plans may differ subtlety, so checking the plan entails verifying each dwell position. Fortunately, intracavitary plans generally contain few dwell positions. Large volume implants with more catheters than treatment unit channels form another common treatment with multiple files under a patient's identity. In this case, enough details of the file must be checked to assure selection of the correct file for the treatment underway. To prevent using the wrong patient's file for a treatment, the name on the program must be matched with the patient's identity.

Regardless of the number of files a patient has, the first fraction for any file must include a verification of the length for each catheter, particularly if the length differs from the default value. The most common error with HDR brachytherapy is unintended treatment with the default length when a customized length was intended. The step size also forms a simple, but very important parameter to check. Once these have been verified, and a sampling of the dwell-time pattern checked, the program can be approved. On subsequent treatment fractions, the checks to verify programming with the correct file suffice.

Developing a Quality Management Program

For thorough QM, the program should be based on a risk analysis of their HDR planning and delivery processes, as described in the report of Task Group 100 of the American Association of Physicists in Medicine.[78] This analysis is even more important if working in a solo environment. Wilkinson et al. performed an Failure Modes and Effects Analysis, FMEA, for brachytherapy treatment planning and found image sets, catheter reconstruction, indexer length, and incorrect dose points as the failures with the highest rankings in their analysis.[79] In a review of reported events from the Nuclear Regulatory Commission (NRC), one of the most frequently reported errors involved the treatment length being measured incorrectly or being entered into the treatment-planning system incorrectly.[80] Users should be familiar with standard lengths for applicators and reasonable tolerances. When implementing new applicators, conferring with colleagues or professional associates can prevent errors. And while using published risk analyses can be informative for users, each institution should perform its own site-specific evaluation.

TREATMENT PLANNING IMAGING

Imaging

A discussion of image guidance in radiotherapy treatment planning can be found in Chapter 17. This section specifically addresses imaging for brachytherapy, where it is often used to inform applicator placement pre-implant, guide applicator placement during implant, and in creation of the HDR treatment plan. Traditionally, brachytherapy procedures, such as cervical point A plans, were created using orthogonal, 2D radiographs. Fluoroscopy was sometimes used during applicator insertion. For the last two decades, ultrasound (US) imaging has been employed for image-guided brachytherapy to confirm proper applicator positioning.[81] US offers high spatial resolution without delivering additional imaging dose to the patient. While US is the most common imaging modality for image-guided brachytherapy, some institutions have begun implementing magnetic resonance imaging (MRI) and CT imaging to guide applicator placement. Each of these imaging modalities, as well as, positron emission tomography (PET) imaging, are often used pre-treatment to inform applicator placement and post-implant for treatment planning.

Volumetric treatment planning is widely implemented using MRI and CT imaging. CT is the most common imaging modality for treatment planning, due to scanner availability and the associated high spatial resolution and geometric accuracy. CT also allows for a wide range in applicator selection, as applicators are typically CT-compatible and easily visible on CT images allowing for an accurate applicator reconstruction. Often supplemental MR and PET images are registered to the CT image to aid in contouring disease and surrounding organs at risk. This process relies on an accurate image registration and can add uncertainty to the treatment-planning process.

The use of MRI in HDR brachytherapy, as the primary image set and as a supplemental data set for contouring, has increased significantly. MRI offers unparalleled soft-tissue contrast and functional imaging to allow for accurate tumor and surrounding soft tissue segmentation. A survey conducted by the American Brachytherapy Society found the use of MRI for target dose specification increased significantly from 2% to 38% from 2007 to 2014.[82] However, applicator compatibility must be carefully checked prior to use in an MRI scanner to avoid heating, mechanical tissue injuries, and prohibitive image artifacts. Applicator visibility may also be a challenge in MR images and care should be taken to include MR imaging sequences that optimize soft tissue contrast, geometric accuracy, and applicator visibility.

Imaging Compatibility

Care must be taken to ensure that applicators are safe for the imaging modality used. Applicator compatibility is necessary particularly with MR imaging. Applicators are either termed as MR safe, MR conditional or MR unsafe. MR safe applicators pose no known hazard in any MR environment, MR compatible applicators have been shown to pose no hazard in specific MR environments, and MR unsafe applicators are known to pose hazards in MR environments.[83] The American Society for Testing and Materials (ASTM) formed task group F04.30.11 dedicated to addressing the safety of implants and other medical devices in the MR environment.[h] They have

---

[h]The information from ASTM may change over time, particularly with new information added. The best way to find the reports on the particular material and situation in question is to do an internet search on ASTM F04.15.11 with the parameters needed.

published a series of reports describing measurements to ensure an applicator is MR compatible for a given environment. Tests include measurement of the displacement force, torque, RF heating, and image artifacts. The end users should verify with the manufacturer the specifications of a given applicator. These are typically distributed in the *Instructions for Use* documents included with the purchase of a new applicator.

Imaging Artifacts and Marker Wires

While only a few applicators are MR compatible, most applicators in brachytherapy are CT compatible. However, imaging requirements may differ based on the type and construction of the applicator itself. Scans that include applicators with thick metals may benefit from the use of metal artifact reduction algorithms. Applicators with shields may have dummy plastic holders for scanning with and without the shields in place. Certain marker wires can also add imaging artifacts into the CT scan. Evaluation of the wires and implants should be performed to determine if an implant is imaged better with or without marker wires in place. In some interstitial implants, it may be easier to recognize the empty needle voids rather than the marker wires themselves.

MR imaging carries different issues. Of particular concern is geometric distortion, which enters in many facets. The first, and obvious, is locating the positions of anatomy and the treatment applicators. Addressing the distortion requires working with a qualified magnetic-resonance medical physicist and a service engineer. Often the distortion that wreaks havoc in radiotherapy dosimetric imaging is unimportant in diagnostics. Another form of distortion occurs when using markers to indicate the source path in an applicator, and particularly when determining the first dwell position or end of the source wire, depending on the treatment unit used. The image of contrasting materials (i.e., anything that could be used for such markers) often extends beyond the physical boundaries of the object. This topic is discussed in the series of articles from GEC ESTRO on MRI-based cervical brachytherapy, in the AAPM Task Group Report 236 and in several articles.[84–86]

PLANNING AN IMPLANT

Planning, in general, is actually what goes before any intended action, or at least, what *should* go before. In the context of brachytherapy, before performing an implant or an insertion, planning entails determining the desired location of the treatment applicator—intracavitary or interstitial. During planning, such things are determined as where needles should be placed so that the dose distribution will be able to cover the target. After a procedure may come what is often referred to as "treatment planning," consisting of dose calculation and optimization.

The intention of optimization is to make the prescription isodose surface cover the target. Planning and executing the implant well increases the likelihood that the resultant dose distribution will achieve the treatment goals. In some cases, following a less-than-optimal implant, optimization can deliver the desired dose coverage to the target; however, the price paid becomes larger HDVs and higher doses to critical neighboring organs, increasing the probability of complication.

The initial steps for planning a brachytherapy procedure follow the same pattern as for any type of radiotherapy treatment: determining the target volumes. Earlier chapters discuss target delineation, so it will not be addressed here, other than to say that in brachytherapy the expansion margin from the CTV to form a planning target volume (PTV) usually remains small. Such an expansion needs to consider the ability to place the applicator in the desired location, and, for implants, the constraints placed on the location of needles by the implant pattern to conform to the CTV. As an example of the latter constraint, consider a template-guided implant where the edge of the CTV falls between needle rows. Covering the CTV may require an additional needle in the row outside of the CTV, thus effectively expanding the CTV to a PTV. For a cervical intracavitary application, depending on the quality of the fixation of the applicator, some practitioners add a small margin to the CTV_{HR} in the cephalocaudal direction, resulting in a PTV.

Applicator Selection and Placement

A variety of applicators exist for HDR brachytherapy applications. Applicators range from intracavity applicators, interstitial and intralumenal applicators. Applicators are selected to meet the need of the treatment. Planning while applicator to use and where to place the treatment applicator depends heavily on the form of the brachytherapy.

Intracavitary and Intralumenal Insertions

Intraluminal insertions allow little selection in the treatment applicator or location. For example, the only variable in endobronchial applications would be how far past the target to insert the tip of the treatment catheter. Possibly the diameter of the catheter may be selectable from two sizes, and in some cases the stiffness of the catheter. More applicators are available for endoesophageal applications because of the size of the lumen. These applicators have various thicknesses of the walls and number of channels, running from one in the center (giving a more penetrating dose distribution) to many around the periphery (allowing some tailoring of the dose distribution to the CTV). In any intralumenal treatment, attention must be given to covering the ends of the treatment volume, avoiding low doses.

Gynecological applications present a greater opportunity to select the applicator most appropriate to the patient.

For cervical cancer, the standard approach places a long tube (a tandem) in the uterus and channels for the source in the vagina, just as with the LDR treatments. While the tandem for all applicators remains mostly the same, the vaginal source channels differ greatly between applicators. The vaginal part of the applicator for four applicators will be compared for examples—ovoids, a ring, cylinders, and custom molds. Figure 30.15 shows examples of these applicators. The source travels through ovoids in a tube running axially through either ellipsoidal (from which the term ovoid—egg-shaped—derives) or cylindrical piece of plastic. Some ovoids contain shielding in the direction of the rectum and bladder and some do not. Ovoids come in three sizes, generally 1, 1.25, and 1.5 cm radius, sometimes with a "mini" size that maintains the 1-cm radius laterally but only a few millimeters medially to fit a smaller vagina. Some of these applicators have no fixed relationship between the tandems and ovoids, however some do.

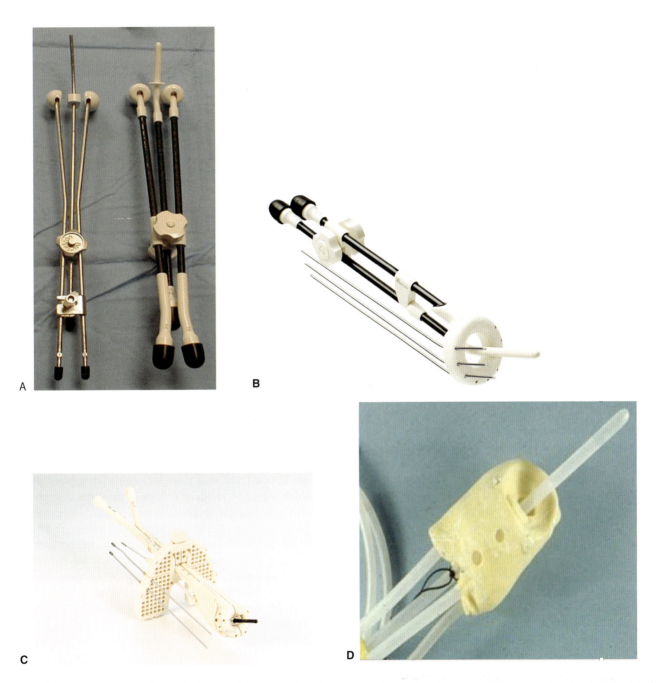

FIGURE 30.15. Applicators for cervical cancer intracavitary insertions: **(A)** Tandem and ovoid, on the left the conventional and on the right for CT or MR localization; **(B)** A tandem and ring with guide holes for needle catheters; **(C)** A Venezia applicator that supports most approaches needed in gynecological treatments; **(D)** A tandem and custom vaginal mold. (Pictures **B** and **C** courtesy of Elekta Brachytherapy, Waardgelder, Netherlands, subsidiary of Elekta AB, Inc., Stockholm, Sweden; Picture D courtesy Erik Van Limbergen).

The nonfixed applicators allow better conformance with the patient's anatomy, while the fixed systems maintain a standard geometry and allow vendor-provided digital applicator models (often called an applicator library filled with *solid* applicators) to be used during catheter reconstruction, as will be discussed in the following sections. The best dose distribution comes from using the largest size ovoids that fit in the vagina. This gives the greatest distance between the source track and the vaginal mucosa and thus, the greatest depth dose, just as increasing the source to surface distance in external-beam radiotherapy increases the fractional depth dose. Spreading the ovoids too far should be avoided because that leads to reduced doses to the cervix proper.

In the ring applicator, the vaginal source path follows a circle centered on the tandem. The ring comes in several diameters (26–34 cm). Typical cases only use the dwell positions in the lateral parts of the ring—somewhat simulating the dwell positions used in the ovoids. A plastic cap about 5-mm thick slips over the ring to provide spacing between the source track and the vaginal mucosa, reducing the local dose. Because the cap provides only half the spacing as the smallest ovoid, the ring projects the dose less deeply laterally. The smaller size of the ring applicator and the fixation to the tandem make insertion easier than ovoids. In addition to a tandem and ring applicator, different split-ring designs have been introduced which use two catheters to create dose distribution similar to that of a ring applicator.

Patients with very narrow vagina—not uncommon after high doses of external-beam radiation therapy—may not accommodate a tandem and ovoids or ring. One approach places plastic cylinders around the tandem where it passes through the vagina. While this approach allows for treatment, the dose distribution fails to provide the quality of coverage of tandems and ovoids. The difference results from constraining the source track to the tandem instead of spreading the tracks laterally, with a concomitant reduction in the coverage to the lateral aspects of the uterus.

Custom vaginal molds have been used to provide applications tailored to individual patients. These applicators use an impression of the patient's vagina with tracks drilled to accommodate catheters for the source tubes.[87–91] Figure 30.15D shows such a mold. In concept, these mold applicators should provide improved fit and stability for the applicators compared with standard ovoids or a ring. The advantage is more important with LDR gynecological applications and comes at the price of increased time commitments for construction of the mold.

Postoperative endometrial cancer treatments form one of the most common brachytherapy procedures in the United States. The treatment delivers radiation to the anastigmatic site at the superior end of the vagina following removal of the uterus, with the goal of preventing tumor recurrences in the surgical site. HDR treatments generally use either ovoids (without the tandem, since the uterus is gone) or cylinders. The ovoids tend to produce a dose distribution that conforms closely to the target at risk, while maintaining relatively low doses to the bladder and rectum. Cylinders give more dose to the rectum and the bladder than ovoids partially because the orientation of the source places these organs near the perpendicular bisector of the sources and the maximum of the anisotropy of the source. Using cylinders, the axis of the source, where the anisotropy function is relatively low, points toward the target at the end of the cylinder. For ovoids, the situation is reversed, with the low values of the anisotropy toward the bladder and the rectum and the maximum toward the target. However, Pearcey and Petereit report that relatively low doses (50 Gy_{10} or an LDR equivalent of 44 Gy) to the target produce control rates of greater than 98%, with complications not appearing until normal tissue doses of 100 Gy_3 (LDR equivalent of 60 Gy), and the Dutch PORTEC-2 study showed that 21 Gy in three fractions was as effective a 46 Gy of external-beam therapy with fewer gastrointestinal toxic events.[92,93] Uncomplicated control is the norm with this form of treatment. Thus, the differences between the applicators mean little with regard to the treatment outcome. There are, however, cylinders with source pathways forming a circle at the top, and rings without the tandem, that can combine the beneficial orientation of the source with the simplicity of the cylinder.

Interstitial Implants

Determining the needle pattern for an implant can be the most important decision for an implant. Many of the older systems developed rules for needle placement that still provide good guidance.[53,55,94–98] Most of the rules that apply for LDR implants also apply for HDR procedures.

Many of the conventional, LDR brachytherapy approaches give rules for implants with uniform source distribution, that is, source material not differentially distributed. The Manchester System forms the exception. It becomes more difficult to achieve relative dose uniformity when all sources have the same strength per centimeter along a needle track, and rules for needle track placement were developed to produce a dose as uniform in a plane of volume as possible given that constraint.[97,98] Beginning the planning for needle placement by following these rules generally requires less modulation of optimized dwell times to achieve the uniformity goals for the plan. Minimizing the required modulation of the dwell times reduces the likelihood of large high-dose regions. For most HDR multi-planar and volume implants, a needle separation of 1.5 cm results in a lower HDV than 1 cm, but increasing the separations more increases the HDV again.

Most commonly, an approach similar to the Paris System[53,55] is followed assuming that the prescription dose, as the Paris System's RD, falls outside of the actual implanted volume. The change to optimized HDR treatments carries also the need to adjust the Paris system's specifications a bit. Optimization reduced the higher doses that occur in the interior of the implant although increases the high doses near the ends of needle tracks. While the Paris System used an RD that surrounded the implanted volume and was equal to 85% of the Basal Dose (BD—mean of the local dose minima in the central plane), reducing the higher doses in the interior reduces the mean of the dose minima, and that means that the percentage relating the BD and the RD must increase to maintain the same location and value of the RD. Further, the change to HDR brachytherapy accentuates differences in dose, so the percentage must increase further. For a typical optimized HDR implant to give a similar biological RD as an LDR implant, the RD = 93% BD.[56] The higher ratio of BD to RD implies that the needles should be placed slightly closer to the edge of the target volume for HDR implants.

For planar implants or volumes made from planes, following a strict grid pattern with uniform loading often results in a region of low dose between the outlying needles and the rest of the implanted volume, essentially wasting the space implanted near the outliers, as demonstrated in Figure 30.16A, from Neblett.[99] Optimization can fill in

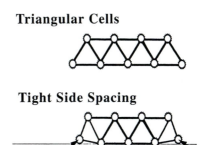

FIGURE 30.17. A demonstration of the process for tight-end loading. (From Neblett D. Clinical techniques and applicators available for interstitial implantation. In: Williamson JF, Thomadsen BR, Nath R, eds. *Brachytherapy Physics*. Madison, WI: Medical Physics Publishing; 1995, with permission from Medical Physics Publishing.)

this region but at the cost of increasing the HDV. Neblett recommends moving the corner needles closer to the main body of the implant than the regular spacing pattern would dictate, as demonstrated in Figure 30.17—a practice called tight-end loading.[99] Figure 30.16B shows the resultant dose distribution, with the prescription isodose surface encompassing the whole implant. Tight-end loading increases the MCD, reducing the HDV.

Unfortunately, some implants, particularly those with irregular shapes, require needles outside the target volume to assure adequate coverage. Figure 30.18 shows one CT image of a breast implant. This implant uses needles outside the target volume to boost the dose near the edge of the implant in several locations. Optimization would not need these needles to cover the target except for the restriction to hold the MSD to 150%. Without that restriction, the dwell times near the boundary would simply increase to extend the dose to the target edge. This case trades the extension of dose to tissue outside the implant for reducing the HDV inside the implant.

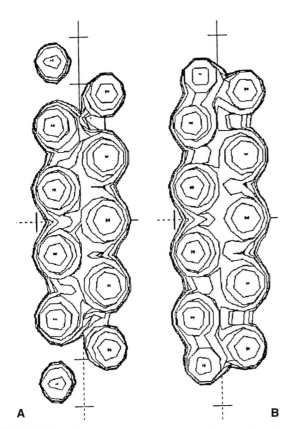

FIGURE 30.16. **(A)** A planar implant with evenly spaced, uniformly loaded needles showing the failure of the prescription isodose surface to include the volume between the main body of the implant and the corner needles. **(B)** The same implant as in **(A)** except with the corner needles moved inward slightly, eliminating the low-dose region. (From Neblett D. Clinical techniques and applicators available for interstitial implantation. In: Williamson JF, Thomadsen BR, Nath R, eds. *Brachytherapy Physics*. Madison, WI: Medical Physics Publishing; 1995, with permission from Medical Physics Publishing.)

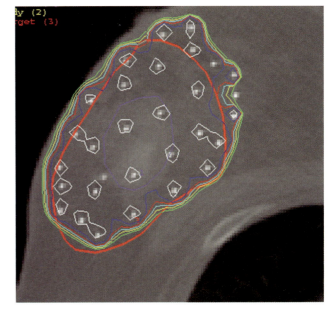

FIGURE 30.18. A breast implant, showing the necessity for needles outside the target volume in this image.

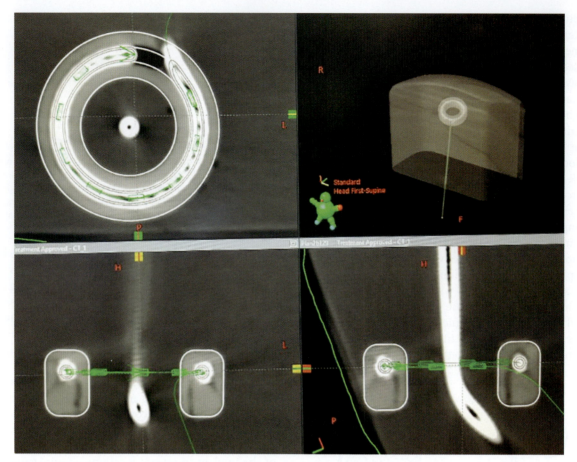

FIGURE 30.19. The superposition of a library model of an applicator on the CT images.

Recently applicators have been designed to facilitate concurrent intracavitary and interstitial implants for advanced gynecological disease. For advanced cervical disease, tandem and ovoid, tandem and ring, tandem and split-ring and tandem and cylinder applicators are manufactured with needles holes in the ovoids, ring, split-ring, and cylinder to allow access to tumors in the parametrium and virginal extensions. The needle hole can run parallel or oblique to the tandem to guide the needles to the desired location. Additional perennial templates are also offered which attach to some applicators to allow additional needle placement. These lateral needles are necessary to reach intermediate-risk disease for locally advanced cervical cancer.

Applicator Reconstruction

Applicator reconstruction is a critical step in any HDR treatment plan and care should be taken to ensure that accurate source paths are defined. Reconstruction of catheters is often done manually, using a marker with high contrast materials for identification of the source path. Metal wires typically serve as markers for CT imaging, while a variety of marker materials, such as saline, have been investigated for various MR sequences.[100–103] Markers are not always useful, as is the case with many needle applicators used for interstitial treatments. Reproducible and accurate needle reconstruction can be a challenge, particularly with MR imaging. Often registration with a CT image acquired post-implant can aid in needle reconstruction. Recently, several investigations have discussed electromagnetic 3D tracking and deep learning algorithms to efficiently and accurately reconstruct needles.[104–106]

Digital applicator models are also available for many intracavitary applications with rigid applicator geometry. These digital models rely on applicator landmarks and marker positions to create a consistent source path based on the applicator geometry. Applicator models can provide reduce variations in catheter reconstruction with respect to manual reconstruction techniques. Figure 30.19 demonstrates the overlay of a library model of an applicator on CT images.

Regardless of the reconstruction technique, care should be taken to ensure geometric accuracy and a lack of susceptibility artifacts in the treatment-planning images. Furthermore, the reconstructed source path should mimic that of the HDR source as it travels throughout the applicator. As an example, the path of an HDR source in ring and split-ring applicators has been found to deviate from centerline reconstructions and manual reconstructions that rely on a marker wire. Some vendor-provided applicator models account for these positional variations and some do not. The impact of these deviations may have a limited impact on the DVH, but a thorough understanding of the correct reconstruction technique for each applicator and the associated uncertainties should be well understood prior to treatment planning. Hellebust et al. provide very useful guidance for applicator reconstruction with MRI, which also applies well to CT.[84]

Dwell Position

Optimization often allows keeping the dwell positions all inside the target volume. The Paris system, and all the derivative systems for LDR treatments using uniform strength sources, requires that the sources extend beyond the target volume to assure adequate coverage. Optimization increases the relative dwell times on the ends of source tracks so the end dwell positions project the dose to the edge of the target. Increasing the dwell times at the ends of the tracks does require vigilance to prevent large HDV. This process simulates the crossing needles of the Manchester System.

As a general guidance for a starting point in planning dwell positions for an optimized implant, the distance from the surface of the target to the first dwell position in the target should be half the space between dwell positions.[56]

KEY POINTS

- Treatment delivery with HDR brachytherapy occurs over a very short time, with dose rates greater than 12 Gy/h. HDR brachytherapy offers several advantages over LDR brachytherapy including improved dose optimization capability, more stable positioning, ability to treat as an outpatient, and reduction in radiation exposure to health care providers. HDR brachytherapy also has disadvantages to LDR brachytherapy, including a reduction in the therapeutic ratio and the potential for very high radiation dose errors.

- The therapeutic ratio, defined as the ratio of the damage to tumor cells to that to normal tissue cells for the same dose, is lower for single-fraction HDR brachytherapy than for LDR brachytherapy. Fractioning the HDR treatment delivery will increase the therapeutic ratio. The optimum number of fractions for an HDR course of treatment is selected for practicality.

- HDR brachytherapy allows for improved treatment optimization in that source dwell times can be adjusted for all possible dwell positions. HDR dose distributions may also be manually optimized by moving an isodose curve to its desire location, causing the

planning system to adjust dwell time(s) accordingly to produce the change.

- The HDR plan should be evaluated to ensure it meets the treatment objectives. This evaluation should include verification of the dose prescription (both to the reference location and to other specified volumes) and of isodose coverage of the target. Additional quantitative evaluation tools include DVHs, dose uniformity metrics, conformity and external volume indices.

- QA is performed for HDR brachytherapy treatment plans to detect and correct errors in the treatment plan before delivery. Independent verification of the plan by someone other than the planner is an effective method of error detection. A number of indicators have been developed for simple single-catheter to more complex implants, to ensure the treatment plan is reasonable.

- Applicator selection and placement is an important component of a successful implant. This is particularly true for gynecological intercavitary implants, where a number of different applicators and sizes exist. For interstitial implants, many of the rules governing needle placement for LDR implants also apply to HDR procedures.

REVIEW QUESTIONS

1. High-dose-rate (HDR) brachytherapy typically involves dose rates greater than
   A. 100 Gy
   B. 0.5 Gy/h
   C. 0.5 cGy/h
   D. 12 Gy/h

2. Compared to LDR brachytherapy, HDR brachytherapy offers the advantage(s) of:
   A. Improved therapeutic ratio for a single-fraction treatment
   B. Higher energy radiation sources with better tissue penetration
   C. Less applicator movement over the course of the implant
   D. Reduction of radiation exposure to personnel

3. The cell survival curves for HDR brachytherapy
   A. Show a larger variation between tumor and normal tissues than those for a conventional LDR treatment regimen.
   B. Are substantially changed when considering normal tissue and tumor repair.
   C. Become closer to LDR cell survival curves when increasing fractionation
   D. Demonstrate a therapeutic ratio that is very dependent on dose rate.

4. Compute the biological equivalent dose (BED_{HDR}) to the CTV_{HR} for a five-fraction tandem and ovoid implant delivering 6 Gy/fraction over a period of

28 days. Assume $\alpha = 0.35$ Gy^{-1}, $\alpha/\beta = 10$ Gy, and T_{pot} = 7 days.
   A. 25 Gy$_{10}$
   B. 30 Gy$_{10}$
   C. 35 Gy$_{10}$
   D. 40 Gy$_{10}$

5. Calculate the EQD$_2$ for the treatment in question 4 following external-beam treatment of 45 Gy delivered in 1.8-Gy fractions:
   A. 27 Gy$_2$
   B. 75 Gy$_2$
   C. 84 Gy$_2$
   D. 101 Gy$_2$

6. Which of the following figures of merit may be used to evaluate the quality of an HDR implant?
   A. Relative dose homogeneity index
   B. Coverage index
   C. Conformation number
   D. Das's Unified Index

7. Which of the following QA measures should be performed prior to initiation of each HDR treatment delivery?
   A. Failure mode and effects analysis
   B. Independent verification of the plan, ideally by someone other than the planner
   C. Room shielding and barrier survey
   D. Verification of the treatment unit plan information

ANSWERS
1. D
2. C and D
3. A and C
4. D
5. C
6. A, B, and C
7. B and D

DISCUSSION

1. High-dose-rate (HDR) brachytherapy typically involves dose rates greater than
   A. 100 Gy—This is not a dose rate.
   B. 0.5 Gy/h—This is the typical dose rate for LDR treatment.
   C. 0.5 cGy/h—This is too low to be clinically useful.
   D. 12 Gy/h—The is in the range of HDR treatment.
2. Compared to LDR brachytherapy, HDR brachytherapy offers the advantage(s) of
   A. Improved therapeutic ratio for a single-fraction treatment—Quite the opposite, this is a disadvantage of HDR treatments.

   B. Higher energy radiation sources with better tissue penetration—The energy is not an issue since both LDR and HDR brachytherapy may use ^{192}Ir.
   C. Less applicator movement over the course of the implant—Definitely an advantage of HDR treatments because there is much less time for the applicator to move in the patient.
   D. Reduction of radiation exposure to personnel—This is an advantage of HDR brachytherapy but a minor one since modern LDR brachytherapy does not result in high doses to personnel.
3. The cell survival curves for HDR brachytherapy
   A. Show a larger variation between tumor and normal tissues than those for a conventional LDR treatment regimen—True.
   B. Are substantially changed when considering normal tissue and tumor repair—The change is not substantial.
   C. Become closer to LDR cell survival curves when increasing fractionation—True, and that is why

HDR brachytherapy (and external-beam treatment) are fractionated.

D. Demonstrate a therapeutic ratio that is very dependent on dose rate. —False. The therapeutic ratio remains mostly constant in the HDR brachytherapy range.

4. Compute the biological equivalent dose (BED_{HDR}) to the CTV_{HR} for a 5-fraction tandem and ovoid implant delivering 6 Gy/fraction over a period of 28 days. Assume $\alpha = 0.35$ Gy^{-1}, $\alpha/\beta = 10$ Gy, and $T_{pot} = 7$ days.

   A. 25 Gy$_{10}$
   B. 30 Gy$_{10}$
   C. 35 Gy$_{10}$
   D. 40 Gy$_{10}$—Using Equation 30.7, ignoring repopulation since no information is provided for that, gives this result.

5. Calculate the EQD_2 for the treatment in question 4 following external-beam treatment of 45 Gy delivered in 1.8-Gy fractions:

   A. 27 Gy$_2$
   B. 75 Gy$_2$
   C. 84 Gy$_2$—Using Equation 30.13 and summing the external-beam and brachytherapy contributions gives this result.
   D. 101 Gy$_2$

6. Which of the following figures of merit may be used to evaluate the quality of an HDR implant?

   A. Relative dose homogeneity index—This is a figure of merit.
   B. Coverage index—This is a figure of merit.
   C. Conformation number—This is a figure of merit.
   D. Das's Unified Index—This is not a figure of merit but a QA quantity.

7. Which of the following QA measures should be performed prior to initiation of each HDR treatment delivery?

   A. Failure mode and effects analysis—No, this is a process for designing quality management.
   B. Independent verification of the plan, ideally by someone other than the planner—This is a QA measure.
   C. Room shielding and barrier survey—This is not a QA measure but a procedure performed during design of a facility.
   D. Verification of the treatment unit plan information—This is a QA measure.

REFERENCES

1. Das RK, Thomadsen BR. High dose rate brachytherapy sources and delivery systems. In: Thomadsen BR, Rivard MJ, Butler WM, eds. *Brachytherapy.* 2nd ed. Madison, WI: Medical Physics Publishing; 2005.
2. Thomadsen BR, Shahabi S, Buchler DA. Differential loadings of brachytherapy templates. *Endocuriether/Hyperther Oncol.* 1990;6:197–202.
3. Thomadsen BR, Shahabi S, Stitt JA, et al. High dose rate intracavitary brachytherapy for carcinoma of the cervix: the Madison system: II. Procedural and physical considerations [published online ahead of print 1992/01/01]. *Int J Radiat Oncol Biol Phys.* 1992;24(2):349–357.
4. King CC, Stockstill TF, Bloomer WD, Kalnicki S. Point dose variations with time in brachytherapy for cervical carcinoma. *Med Phys.* 1992;19:777.
5. Gao S, Delclos ME, Tomas LC, Crane CH, Beddar S. High-dose-rate remote afterloaders for intraoperative radiation therapy [published online ahead of print 2007/12/07]. *AORN J.* 2007;86(5):827–836; quiz 837–840.
6. van den Aardweg GJ, Hopewell JW. The kinetics of repair for sublethal radiation-induced damage in the pig epidermis: an interpretation based on a fast and a slow component of repair. *Radiother Oncol.* 1992;23(2):94–104.
7. Fowler JF. Repair between dose fractions: a simpler method of analyzing and reporting apparently biexponential repair [published online ahead of print 2002/07/11]. *Radiat Res.* 2002;158(2):141–151.
8. Han I, Malviya V, Chuba P, et al. Multifractionated high-dose-rate brachytherapy with concomitant daily teletherapy for cervical cancer [published online ahead of print 1996/10/01]. *Gynecol Oncol.* 1996;63(1):71–77.
9. Bentzen SM, Constine LS, Deasy JO, et al. Quantitative analyses of normal tissue effects in the clinic (QUANTEC): an introduction to the scientific issues [published online ahead of print 2010/03/05]. *Int J Radiat Oncol Biol Phys.* 2010;76(3 Suppl):S3–S9.
10. Dale RG. The application of the linear-quadratic dose-effect equation to fractionated and protracted radiotherapy [published online ahead of print 1985/06/01]. *Br J Radiol.* 1985;58(690):515–528.
11. Orton CG, Seyedsadr M, Somnay A. Comparison of high and low dose rate remote afterloading for cervix cancer and the importance of fractionation [published online ahead of print 1991/11/01]. *Int J Radiat Oncol Biol Phys.* 1991;21(6):1425–1434.
12. Kinj R, Chand ME, Gal J, Gautier M, Lam Cham Kee D, Hannoun-Levi JM. Five-year oncological outcome after a single fraction of accelerated partial breast irradiation in the elderly [published online ahead of print 2019/12/23]. *Radiat Oncol.* 2019;14(1):234.
13. Khan AJ, Chen PY, Yashar C, et al. Three-fraction accelerated partial breast irradiation (APBI) delivered with brachytherapy applicators is feasible and safe: first results from the TRIUMPH-T trial [published online ahead of print 2019/01/07]. *Int J Radiat Oncol Biol Phys.* 2019;104(1):67–74.
14. Facer BD, Brett C, Morales_Paliza M, et al. A single-institution study of intraoperative radiation therapy (IORT) using electronic brachytherapy. *J Radiat Oncol.* 2020;9:59–65.
15. Gomez-Iturruaga A, Casquero F, Pijoan JI, et al. Health-related-quality-of-life and toxicity after single fraction 19 Gy high-dose-rate prostate brachytherapy: phase II trial. *Radiother Oncol.* 2018;126(2):278–282.
16. International Commission on Radiation Units and Measures. Prescribing, recording, and reporting brachytherapy for cancer of the cervix: ICRU Report 87 [published online ahead of print 2013/04/01]. *J ICRU.* 2013;13(1):2.
17. Ezzell G. Optimization in brachytherapy. In: Thomadsen BR, Rivard MJ, Butler WM, eds. *Brachytherapy Physics.* 2nd ed. Madison, WI: Medical Physics Publishing; 2005.

18. Ezzell G, Luthmann RW. Clinical implementation of dwell time optimization techniques. In: Williamson JF, Thomadsen BR, Nath R, eds. *Brachytherapy Physics*. 1st ed. Madison, WI: Medical Physics Publishing; 1995.

19. Libby B, Chen Z, (Jay), Thomadsen B, et al. General planning. In: Rivard MJ, Beaulieu L, Thomadsen B, eds. *Clinical Brachytherapy Physics: 2017 AAPM Summer School*. Madison WI: Medical Physics Publishing; 2017.

20. Poulin E, Varfalvy N, Aubin S, Beaulieu L. Comparison of dose and catheter optimization algorithms in prostate high-dose-rate brachytherapy [published online ahead of print 2015/11/13]. *Brachytherapy*. 2016;15(1):102–111.

21. Edmundson GK. Geometry based optimization for stepping source implants. In: Martinez AA, Orton CG, Mould RF, eds. *Brachytherapy HDR and LDR*. Columbia, MD: Nucletron Corporation; 1990:184–192.

22. van der Laarse R, Edmundson GK, Luthmann RW, Prins TPE. Optimization of HDR brachytherapy dose distributions. *Act Select User's Newsl*. 1991;5:94–101.

23. Thomadsen B, Houdek P, van der Laarse R. Treatment planning and optimization. In: Nag S, ed. *Textbook and High Dose Rate Brachytherapy*. Armonk, NY: Futura Publishing Co.; 1994.

24. Thomadsen B. High dose-rate brachytherapy treatment planning. In: Khan FM, Gibbons JP, Sperduto MD, eds. *Khan's Treatment Planning in Radiation Oncology*. 4th ed. Philadelphia, PA: Lippincott Wolters Kluwer; 2016:259–287.

25. Shewchuk JR. An introduction to the conjugate gradient method without the agonizing pain. http://www-2.cs.cmu.edu/~jrs/jrspapers.html. Accessed June 7, 2010, 2005.

26. Holmes T, Mackie TR, Simpkin D, Reckwerdt P. A unified approach to the optimization of brachytherapy and external beam dosimetry [published online ahead of print 1991/04/01]. *Int J Radiat Oncol Biol Phys*. 1991;20(4):859–873.

27. Lessard E, Pouliot J. Inverse planning anatomy-based dose optimization for HDR-brachytherapy of the prostate using fast simulated annealing algorithm and dedicated objective function [published online ahead of print 2001/06/08]. *Med Phys*. 2001;28(5):773–779.

28. Lessard E. Development and clinical introduction of an inverse planning dose optimization by simulated annealing (IPSA) for high dose rate brachytherapy [Thesis abstract]. *Med Phys*. 2004;31:2935.

29. Hsu IC, Lessard E, Weinberg V, Pouliot J. Comparison of inverse planning simulated annealing and geometrical optimization for prostate high-dose-rate brachytherapy. *Brachytherapy*. 2004;3:147–152.

30. Karabis A, Gelatt CD, Vecchi PM. Optimization by simulated annealing. *Science*. 1983;220:671–680.

31. Yu Y, Schell MC. A genetic algorithm for the optimization of prostate implants [published online ahead of print 1996/12/01]. *Med Phys*. 1996;23(12):2085–2091.

32. Yang G, Reinstein LE, Pai S, Xu Z, Carroll DL. A new genetic algorithm technique in optimization of permanent 125I prostate implants [published online ahead of print 1999/01/06]. *Med Phys*. 1998;25(12):2308–2315.

33. Pouliot J, Lessard E, Hsu I-C. Advanced 3D planning. In: Thomadsen BR, Rivard MJ, Butler W, eds. *Brachytherapy Physics*. 2nd ed. Madison, WI: Medical Physics Publishing; 2005.

34. Lahanas M, Baltas D, Giannouli S. Global convergence analysis of fast multiobjective gradient-based dose optimization algorithms for high-dose-rate brachytherapy [published online ahead of print 2003/04/17]. *Phys Med Biol*. 2003;48(5):599–617.

35. Panettieri V, Smith RL, Mason NJ, Millar JL. Comparison of IPSA and HIPO inverse planning optimization algorithms for prostate HDR brachytherapy [published online ahead of print 2014/12/11]. *J Appl Clin Med Phys*. 2014;15(6):5055.

36. Smith RL, Panettieri V, Lancaster C, Mason N, Franich RD, Millar JL. The influence of the dwell time deviation constraint (DTDC) parameter on dosimetry with IPSA optimisation for HDR prostate brachytherapy [published online ahead of print 2014/12/08]. *Aust Phys Eng Sci Med*. 2015;38(1):55–61.

37. Lahanas M, Baltas D, Zamboglou N. A hybrid evolutionary algorithm for multi-objective anatomy-based dose optimization in high-dose-rate brachytherapy [published online ahead of print 2003/03/01]. *Phys Med Biol*. 2003;48(3):399–415.

38. Karabis A, Giannouli S, Baltas D. HIPO: a hybrid inverse treatment planning optimization algorithm in HDR brachytherapy. *Radiother Oncol*. 2005;76:S29.

39. Milickovic N, Lahanas M, Papagiannopoulo M, Zamboglou N, Baltas D. Multiobjective anatomy-based dose optimization for HDR-brachytherapy with constraint free deterministic algorithms [published online ahead of print 2002/08/08]. *Phys Med Biol*. 2002;47(13):2263–2280.

40. van't Riet A, Mak AC, Moerland MA, Elders LH, van der Zee W. A conformation number to quantify the degree of conformality in brachytherapy and external beam irradiation: application to the prostate [published online ahead of print 1997/02/01]. *Int J Radiat Oncol Biol Phys*. 1997;37(3):731–736.

41. Baltas D, Kolotas C, Geramani K, et al. A conformal index (COIN) to evaluate implant quality and dose specification in brachytherapy [published online ahead of print 1998/02/11]. *Int J Radiat Oncol Biol Phys*. 1998;40(2):515–524.

42. Choi CH, Park SY, Park JM, Wu HG, Kim JH, Kim JI. Comparison of the IPSA and HIPO algorithms for interstitial tongue high-dose-rate brachytherapy [published online ahead of print 2018/10/05]. *PLoS One*. 2018;13(10):e0205229.

43. Trnková P, Baltas D, Karabis A, et al. A detailed dosimetric comparison between manual and inverse plans in HDR intracavitary interstitial cervical cancer brachytherapy. *J Contemp Brachyther*. 2010;2:163–170.

44. Houdek PV, Schwade JG, Abitbol AA, et al. Optimization of high dose-rate cervix brachytherapy; Part I: dose distribution [published online ahead of print 1991/11/01]. *Int J Radiat Oncol Biol Phys*. 1991;21(6):1621–1625.

45. Tod M, Meredith WJ. A dosage system for use in the treatment of cancer of the uterine cervix. *Br J Radiol*. 1938;11:809–824.

46. Mohan R, Ding IY, Martel MK, Anderson LL, Nori D. Measurements of radiation dose distributions for shielded cervical applicators [published online ahead of print 1985/04/01]. *Int J Radiat Oncol Biol Phys*. 1985;11(4):861–868.

47. Mohan R, Ding IY, Toraskar J, Chui C, Anderson LL, Nori D. Computation of radiation dose distributions for shielded cervical applicators [published online ahead of print 1985/04/01]. *Int J Radiat Oncol Biol Phys*. 1985;11(4):823–830.

48. Watanabe Y, Roy JN, Harrington PJ, Anderson LL. Three-dimensional lookup tables for Henschke applicator cervix treatment by HDR 192IR remote afterloading [published online ahead of print 1998/08/27]. *Int J Radiat Oncol Biol Phys*. 1998;41(5):1201–1207.

49. Richardson S, Palaniswaamy G, Grigsby PW. Dosimetric effects of air pockets around high–dose rate brachytherapy vaginal cylinders. *Int J Radiat Oncol Biol Phys*. 2010;78(1):276–279.

50. Huang YJ, Blough M. Dosimetric effects of air pocket sizes in MammoSite treatment as accelerated partial breast irradiation for early breast cancer [published online ahead of print 2010/02/18]. *J Appl Clin Med Phys*. 2009;11(1):2932.

51. Richardson S, Pino R. Dosimetric effects of an air cavity for the SAVITM partial breast irradiation applicator. *Med Phys*. 2010;3919–3926.

52. Beaulieu L, Tedgren AC, Carrier J-F, et al. Report of the Task Group 186 on model-based dose calculation methods in brachytherapy beyond the TG-43 formalism: current status and recommendations for clinical implementation. *Med Phys*. 2012;39(10):6208–6236.

53. Pierquin B, Dutreix A. For a new methodology in curietherapy: the system of Paris (endo- and plesioradiotherapy with non-radioactive preparation). A preliminary note]. *Ann Radiol (Paris)*. 1966;9:757–760.

54. Pierquin B, Dutreix A, Paine CH, Chassagne D, Marinello G, Ash D. The Paris system in interstitial radiation therapy [published online ahead of print 1978/01/01]. *Acta Radiol Oncol Radiat Phys Biol*. 1978;17(1):33–48.

55. Pierquin B, Marinello G. *A Practical Manual of Brachytherapy*. Madison, WI: Medical Physics Publishing; 1997.

56. Thomadsen BR. Clinical implementation of remote-after loading, interstitial brachytherapy. In: Williamson JF, Thomadsen BR, Nath R, eds. *Brachytherapy Physics*. Madison, WI: Medical Physics Publishing; 1995.

57. Neblett D, Syed AMN, Puthawala AA, et al. An interstitial implant technique evaluated by contiguous volume analysis. *Endocriether/Hyperthem.* 1985;1:213–221.

58. Schoeppel SL, LaVigne ML, Martel MK, McShan DL, Fraass BA, Roberts JA. Three-dimensional treatment planning of intracavitary gynecologic implants: analysis of ten cases and implications for dose specification [published online ahead of print 1994/01/01]. *Int J Radiat Oncol Biol Phys.* 1994;28(1):277–283.

59. Saarnak AE, Boersma M, van Bunningen BN, Wolterink R, Steggerda MJ. Inter-observer variation in delineation of bladder and rectum contours for brachytherapy of cervical cancer [published online ahead of print 2000/06/28]. *Radiother Oncol.* 2000;56(1):37–42.

60. Fellner C, Potter R, Knocke TH, Wambersie A. Comparison of radiography- and computed tomography-based treatment planning in cervix cancer in brachytherapy with specific attention to some quality assurance aspects [published online ahead of print 2001/02/13]. *Radiother Oncol.* 2001;58(1):53–62.

61. Wachter-Gerstner N, Wachter S, Reinstadler E, et al. Bladder and rectum dose defined from MRI based treatment planning for cervix cancer brachytherapy: comparison of dose-volume histograms for organ contours and organ wall, comparison with ICRU rectum and bladder reference point [published online ahead of print 2003/09/18]. *Radiother Oncol.* 2003;68(3):269–276.

62. Kirisits C, Potter R, Lang S, Dimopoulos J, Wachter-Gerstner N, Georg D. Dose and volume parameters for MRI-based treatment planning in intracavitary brachytherapy for cervical cancer [published online ahead of print 2005/06/07]. *Int J Radiat Oncol Biol Phys.* 2005;62(3):901–911.

63. Van den Berg F, Meertens H, Moonen L, Van Buningen BNFM, Blom A. The use of a transverse CT image for the estimation of the dose given to the rectum in intracavitary brachytherapy for carcinoma of the cervix. *Radiother Oncol.* 1998;47:85–90.

64. Kirisits C, Goldner G, Berger D, Georg D, Potter R. Critical discussion of different dose-volume parameters for rectum and urethra in prostate brachytherapy [published online ahead of print 2009/05/19]. *Brachytherapy.* 2009;8(4):353–360.

65. Georg P, Potter R, Georg D, et al. Dose effect relationship for late side effects of the rectum and urinary bladder in magnetic resonance image-guided adaptive cervix cancer brachytherapy [published online ahead of print 2011/02/25]. *Int J Radiat Oncol Biol Phys.* 2012;82(2):653–657.

66. Saw CB, Suntharalingam N. Quantitative assessment of interstitial implants [published online ahead of print 1991/01/01]. *Int J Radiat Oncol Biol Phys.* 1991;20(1):135–139.

67. Thomadsen BR. *Achieving Quality in Brachytherapy.* London: Taylor and Francis; 1999.

68. Saw CB, Waterman FM, Ayyangar K, Suntharalingam N. Quantitative evaluation of planar 192Ir implants [Abstract]. *Med Phys.* 1986;13:580.

69. Zwicker RD, Schmidt-Ullrich R. Dose uniformity in a planar interstitial implant system [published online ahead of print 1995/01/01]. *Int J Radiat Oncol Biol Phys.* 1995;31(1):149–155.

70. International Commission on Radiation Units and Measures. *Report 58: Dose and Volume Specification for Reporting Interstitial Therapy.* Bethesda, MD: International Commission on Radiation Units and Measures; 1997:58.

71. Wu A, Ulin K, Sternick ES. A dose homogeneity index for evaluating 192Ir interstitial breast implants [published online ahead of print 1988/01/01]. *Med Phys.* 1988;15(1):104–107.

72. Saw CB, Suntharalingam N, Wu A. Concept of dose nonuniformity in interstitial brachytherapy [published online ahead of print 1993/06/15]. *Int J Radiat Oncol Biol Phys.* 1993;26(3):519–527.

73. Saw CB, Suntharalingam N. Reference dose rates for single- and double-plane 192Ir implants [published online ahead of print 1988/05/01]. *Med Phys.* 1988;15(3):391–396.

74. Viswanathan AN, Beriwal S, Santos DL, et al. American Brachytherapy Society consensus guidelines for locally advanced carcinoma of the cervix. Part II: high-dose-rate brachytherapy. *Brachytherapy.* 2012;11(1):47–52.

75. Thomadsen BR. Clinical implementation of HDR intracavitary and transluminal brachytherapy. In: Williamson JF, Thomadsen BR, Nath R, eds. *Brachytherapy Physics.* Madison, WI: Medical Physics Publishing; 1995.

76. Measures ICoRUa. *Report 38: Dose and Volume Specification for Reporting Intracavitary Therapy in Gynecology.* Bethesda, MD: International Commission on Radiation Units and Measures; 1985.

77. Das RK, Bradley KA, Nelson IA, Patel R, Thomadsen BR. Quality assurance of treatment plans for interstitial and intracavitary high-dose-rate brachytherapy [published online ahead of print 2006/03/28]. *Brachytherapy.* 2006;5(1):56–60.

78. Huq MS, Fraass BA, Dunscombe PB, et al. The report of Task Group 100 of the AAPM: application of risk analysis methods to radiation therapy quality management [published online ahead of print 2016/07/03]. *Med Phys.* 2016;43(7):4209.

79. Wilkinson DA, Kolar MD. Failure modes and effects analysis applied to high-dose-rate brachytherapy treatment planning. *Brachytherapy.* 2013;12(4):382–386.

80. Richardson SL. A 2-year review of recent Nuclear Regulatory Commission events: what errors occur in the modern brachytherapy era? *Pract Radiat Oncol.* 2012;2.3:157–163.

81. Petereit DG, Sarkaria JN, Chappell RJ. Perioperative morbidity and mortality of high-dose-rate gynecologic brachytherapy [published online ahead of print 1998/12/30]. *Int J Radiat Oncol Biol Phys.* 1998;42(5):1025–1031.

82. Grover S, Harkenrider MM, Cho LP, et al. Image guided cervical brachytherapy: 2014 survey of the American Brachytherapy Society [published online ahead of print 2016/02/13]. *Int J Radiat Oncol Biol Phys.* 2016;94(3):598–604.

83. Woods TO. Standards for medical devices in MRI: present and future [published online ahead of print 2007/10/31]. *J Magn Reson Imaging.* 2007;26(5):1186–1189.

84. Hellebust TP, Kirisits C, Berger D, et al. Recommendations from Gynaecological (GYN) GEC-ESTRO Working Group: considerations and pitfalls in commissioning and applicator reconstruction in 3D image-based treatment planning of cervix cancer brachytherapy. *Radiother Oncol.* 2010;96(2):153–160.

85. Kim Y, Kim Y, Todor D, et al. Recommendations on volume-image-based treatment planning, dosimetry and quality management for HDR intracavitary brachytherapy: report of AAPM Task Group No. 236. *Med Phys.* 2021.

86. Kim Y, Muruganandham M, Modrick JM, Bayouth JE. Evaluation of artifacts and distortions of titanium applicators on 3.0-Tesla MRI: feasibility of titanium applicators in MRI-guided brachytherapy for gynecological cancer [published online ahead of print 2010/10/12]. *Int J Radiat Oncol Biol Phys.* 2011;80(3):947–955.

87. Twombly GH, Rosh R. A new method for applying radium in the vagina in cases of carcinoma of the uterine cervix. *Cancer.* 1955;8:1016–1020.

88. Chassagne D. La plesiocurietherapie des cancers du cavum avec support-moule et Yridium 192. *Ann Radiol.* 1963;6:719–726.

89. Lewis GC. Acrylic molds for vaginal radium application. *Radiology.* 1963;80:282–284.

90. Peracchia G, Salti C. A simple method of preparing custom molds for intracavitary treatment of gynecological cancer [published online ahead of print 1982/01/01]. *Int J Radiat Oncol Biol Phys.* 1982;8(1):141–143.

91. Bertoni F, Bertoni G, Bignardi M. Vaginal molds for intracavitary curietherapy: a new method of preparation [published online ahead of print 1983/10/01]. *Int J Radiat Oncol Biol Phys.* 1983;9(10):1579–1582.

92. Pearcey RG, Petereit DG. Post-operative high dose rate brachytherapy in patients with low to intermediate risk endometrial cancer [published online ahead of print 2000/06/28]. *Radiother Oncol.* 2000;56(1):17–22.

93. Nout RA, Smit VT, Putter H, et al. Vaginal brachytherapy versus pelvic external beam radiotherapy for patients with endometrial cancer of high-intermediate risk (PORTEC-2): an open-label, non-inferiority, randomised trial [published online ahead of print 2010/03/09]. *Lancet.* 2010;375(9717):816–823.

94. Paterson R, Parker H. A dosage system for gamma ray therapy: Part I [Clinical]. *Br J Radiol.* 1934;7:592–612.

95. Parker H. A dosage system for gamma ray therapy. Part II: physical aspects. *Br J Radiol.* 1934;7:612–632.

96. Meredith WJ. *Radium Dosage.* Edinburgh and London: E. & S. Livingstone; 1967.

97. Kwan DK, Kagan AR, Olch AJ, Chan PY, Hintz BL, Wollin M. Single- and double-plane iridium-192 interstitial implants: implantation guidelines and dosimetry. *Med Phys.* 1983;10(4):456–461.

98. Zwicker RD, Schmidt-Ullrich R, Schiller B. Planning of Ir-192 seed implants for boost irradiation to the breast. *Int J Radiat Oncol Biol Phys.* 1985;11(12):2163–2170.

99. Neblett D. Clinical techniques and applicators available for interstitial implantation. In: Williamson JF, Thomadsen BR, Nath R, eds. *Brachytherapy Physics.* 1st ed. Madison, WI: Medical Physics Publishing; 1995.

100. Haack S, Nielsen SK, Lindegaard JC, Gelineck J, Tanderup K. Applicator reconstruction in MRI 3D image-based dose planning of brachytherapy for cervical cancer [published online ahead of print 2008/11/04]. *Radiother Oncol.* 2009;91(2):187–193.

101. Hu Y, Esthappan J, Mutic S, et al. Improve definition of titanium tandems in MR-guided high dose rate brachytherapy for cervical cancer using proton density weighted MRI [published online ahead of print 2013/01/19]. *Radiat Oncol.* 2013;8:16.

102. Schindel J, Muruganandham M, Pigge FC, Anderson J, Kim Y. Magnetic resonance imaging (MRI) markers for MRI-guided high-dose-rate brachytherapy: novel marker-flange for cervical cancer and marker catheters for prostate cancer [published online ahead of print 2013/02/26]. *Int J Radiat Oncol Biol Phys.* 2013;86(2):387–393.

103. Tanderup K, Viswanathan AN, Kirisits C, Frank SJ. Magnetic resonance image guided brachytherapy [published online ahead of print 2014/06/17]. *Semin Radiat Oncol.* 2014;24(3):181–191.

104. Cunha JAM, Butler WM, Damato AL, Beaulieu L. Brachytherapy technologies in early clinical translation. In: Rivard MJ, Beaulieu L, Thomadsen B, eds. *Clinical Brachytherapy Physics.* Madison, WI: Medical Physics Publishing; 2017.

105. Cunha JAM, Flynn R, Belanger C, et al. Brachytherapy future directions [published online ahead of print 2019/11/16]. *Semin Radiat Oncol.* 2020;30(1):94–106.

106. van Heerden L, Schiphof-Godart J, Christianen M, et al. Accuracy of dwell position detection with a combined electromagnetic tracking brachytherapy system for treatment verification in pelvic brachytherapy [published online ahead of print 2020/10/11]. *Radiother Oncol.* 2021;154:249–254.

31 Electron Beam Treatment Planning

John A. Antolak

INTRODUCTION

High-energy electron beams first available for use in radiotherapy in the 1930s using Van de Graaff generators.[1] In the 1940s, the betatron became the machine of choice because higher energies allowed more than just the treatment of skin lesions.[1,2] Electron linear accelerators became commercially available in the 1950s but were not commonly used until about a decade after their introduction.[1,2] Adding electron beam capability to a medical linear accelerator added to the expense and complexity of the machine, and the use of electron beams for radiotherapy was not well understood for many years. Cobalt irradiators, which were used in the beginning of 1950s, were widely available and very reliable, so it took many years for the use of medical linear accelerators to gain traction in the radiotherapy clinic. It took even longer for groups such as the one at MD Anderson Hospital and Tumor Institute[3,4] to demonstrate the usefulness of megavoltage electron beams, which gradually led to their increased use in the general radiotherapy community. Currently, most medical linear accelerators are purchased with electron capabilities and it has become an expected capability in the modern radiotherapy clinic.

The most common energy range for electron beams in current medical linear accelerators is 6–20 MeV, which can treat tumors up to approximately 6 cm in depth. Primary clinical applications for electrons include skin cancers, chest wall irradiation for breast cancer, administration of boost treatments (i.e., breast, head, and neck), and intraoperative radiation therapy (IORT). All of these regions can be successfully treated with X-rays; however, electrons offer the distinct advantage of sparing dose to deeper, possibly critical, tissues, as well as delivering higher surface doses.

The purpose of this chapter is not to provide a comprehensive review, but to provide a practical understanding of the properties of electron beams used in radiation therapy so that the reader can confidently apply that knowledge in the clinic to plan electron beam treatments. In order to limit the scope of this chapter, it will be assumed that the reader has a modern 3D treatment-planning system (TPS) and uses it for electron beam treatment planning, or that they are considering making better use of the TPS for electron beam treatment planning. The next section on basic physics and beam properties provides an overview of the most important properties of electron beams as applied to patient treatments, because an understanding of electron beams is key to being able to apply them effectively in the clinic. The next section on treatment planning builds on that understanding to provide a qualitative description of how electron beams can be used to solve some basic treatment-planning problems. The next section on advanced treatment planning discusses techniques that may or may not be easily accomplished using most commercial planning systems. For a more comprehensive review of clinical electron beam dosimetry, the reader is encouraged to consult the two AAPM reports available on the subject,[5–7] and the excellent review article by Hogstrom and Almond.[1]

For a variety of reasons, electrons are arguably underutilized in the modern radiation therapy clinic.[8,9] Electron beam radiotherapy is a minority technology, and therefore some training programs give little thought to teaching about the utility of electron beams. In the 1990s, intensity-modulated radiation therapy (IMRT) and image-guided radiation therapy (IGRT) technology started to become readily available. Until then, one of the more common treatment sites for electron beams was treating the posterior neck region for head-and-neck tumors, after the spinal cord had received its tolerance dose from the lateral photon fields.

This created a dose distribution that wrapped around the spinal cord. Using IMRT, it was possible to create a similar dose distribution without the additional complexity of the added electron fields. The addition of IGRT technology contributes to even better accuracy and precision, so it is doubtful that older patched-field approaches will make a comeback.

BASIC PHYSICS AND BEAM PROPERTIES

Electrons are negatively charged fundamental particles with a small mass, approximately 2,000 times lighter than a nucleon (proton or neutron). Because of their electric charge, they readily interact with positively charged atomic nuclei and the negatively charged electrons that orbit the nuclei. The electric field of the nucleus can change the direction of the incident electron, which is called Coulomb scattering. Because this scattering occurs on a microscopic scale, it is not practical to try to follow each scattering event. If we look at this effect on a macroscopic scale, it is called multiple Coulomb scattering since we are including multiple scattering events at each step. The material that the electrons are passing through can be characterized by a scattering power, which is a measure of how easily a given material can change the angular distribution of the electrons passing through the material. Occasionally, the nuclear scattering interaction is strong enough that the incident electron loses energy in addition to scattering, and the lost energy is emitted as an X-ray. This is called bremsstrahlung production and is the primary process for producing X-rays in the anode of a diagnostic X-ray tube or in the target of a linear accelerator. Bremsstrahlung events remove energy from the beam, but this energy is not deposited locally and hence contributes very little to the deposited dose.

Incident electrons also interact with atomic electrons. This generates heat and causes ionization of the atoms in addition to scattering. This is where the majority of the energy deposition occurs. The material that the electrons are passing through can be characterized by a mass collisional stopping power, which is the energy lost to collisional interactions per unit length divided by the density of the material. The dose deposited is the product of the electron fluence (number of electrons per unit area) and the mass collisional stopping power. For biologic materials, the mass stopping power is relatively constant, so the energy deposition is determined primarily by the electron fluence, or the number of electrons passing through a given volume. The scattering power of the materials that the beam passes through determines how the electrons redistribute themselves, so calculating the dose deposition due to electron beams is primarily a problem of calculating the fluence distribution of the electrons in the material. While this is a somewhat simplified description of the electron interactions in matter, it is good enough to be able to qualitatively understand some of the basic properties of electron beams used in radiation therapy

Percent Depth Dose

Most of the energy loss for an incident electron beam involves the transfer of energy to orbital electrons in the medium (e.g., patient), and the rate of collisional energy loss depends primarily on the electron density of the material, which is closely related to the physical density for low-Z (biologic) materials. For the energy range used in electron radiation therapy, the energy loss is approximately 2.0 MeV per cm of water. Figure 31.1 shows percent depth dose (PDD) curves for a Varian TrueBeam™ linear accelerator (Varian Medical Systems, Palo Alto, CA). The practical range is at the depth of the intersection

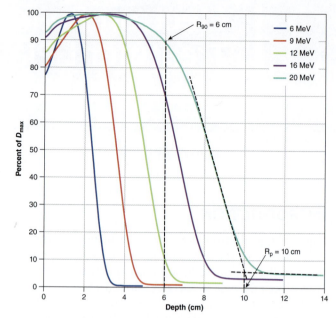

FIGURE 31.1. Electron central-axis percentage depth dose profiles for a Varian TrueBeam linear accelerator, 10 × 10 cm² applicator, 100-cm SSD. The practical range, R_p, and therapeutic depth, R_{90}, for the 20-MeV beam are illustrated.

of the linear portion of the distal dose falloff and the line representing the level of bremsstrahlung contamination. At depths shallower than the practical range, the dose is primarily due to the electrons, and it is readily apparent that the energy of the beam is approximately double the practical range. Very few electrons can reach the depth of the practical range due to multiple Coulomb scattering deflecting the electrons, and this gives rise to the distal slope of the electron PDD. The therapeutic depth of the electron beam increases with energy almost linearly, and a general rule of thumb is that the energy of the beam is approximately 3.3 times the depth of R_{90}.

Ideally, we would like to select the electron energy such that the target is shallower than R_{90}, and the critical structures are deeper than R_p. This implies that as the energy is increased, the separation between the target and critical structures also needs to increase if full sparing of the critical structures is to be maintained. Using the above rules of thumb for R_{90} and R_p, the optimal separation in depth (in cm) between the target and critical structures is approximately the beam energy (in MeV) divided by 5 (e.g., for the 20-MeV electron beam, this separation is about 4 cm). If the target to critical structure separation is less than that, an alternative might be to use IMRT with X-rays to get a sharper distal falloff. If heavier particle therapy (e.g., protons) is available, the distal falloff can be even sharper.

The central-axis depth dose curve, for the same nominal stated energy, may be different depending upon the equipment manufacturer. Factors contributing to these differences include, but are not limited to, differences in the materials used in the construction of scattering foils and ionization chambers, location of the scattering foils, and the geometry and materials of the tertiary collimation system (applicator or cone). Therefore, the depth dose curves and associated isodose distribution should be measured for each clinical treatment unit.

The surface dose for electron beams is higher than for X-ray beams, which can be an advantage for targets near the skin surface. The primary reason that the dose increases in the buildup region between the surface and R_{100} (d_{max}) is increased path length per unit depth caused by multiple Coulomb scattering. Since lower-energy electrons scatter more readily than higher-energy electrons, the slope in the buildup is steeper for lower energies and the surface dose is lower as well. This is contrary to the case for megavoltage X-rays, where the relative surface dose is lower for higher energies. As shown in Figure 31.1, the surface dose for the 6-MeV beam is less than 90%. If a full dose at the skin surface is desired, approximately 0.5 cm of additional bolus is needed to have a 90% dose at the surface. As a consequence, the therapeutic depth (in the patient) would be reduced, in this case to 1.2 cm.

The bremsstrahlung tail (or X-ray contamination) is what is left over after all of the electrons have stopped in the patient. In a modern medical linear accelerator, about half of the bremsstrahlung tail is due to X-rays generated in the high-Z components of the treatment head (e.g., scattering foils) and about half is due to X-rays generated in the patient. Because the relative dose in the bremsstrahlung tail is generally smaller than 5% of the maximum dose, it has little effect on how the electron beams are used clinically.

Isodose Distributions

Figure 31.2 shows isodose distributions for 9-MeV and 16-MeV beams at 100-cm source-to-surface distance (SSD) and 110-cm SSD. On the phantom surface, the penumbra width is proportional to the width of the angular distribution of the electrons at the level of the final collimation (cutout is at 95-cm SSD) multiplied by the gap between the final collimation and the phantom. Because lower-energy electrons are more readily scattered in the treatment head and air above the cutout, the width of the angular distribution of the 9-MeV electrons at this level is larger (more diffuse) than the 16-MeV electrons and hence the penumbra at the surface is larger for the 9-MeV beam. Comparing the 100-cm SSD isodose curves to the 110-cm SSD isodose curves, you can easily see that the penumbra at the surface is approximately three times larger because the gap between the final collimation and the surface is three times larger. However, there is less effect at R_{100} and R_{90} because the scattering in the phantom dominates relative to the contribution of scattering in the air gap.

Similar to X-ray beams, the beam edge in the lateral direction does not correspond to the therapeutic region (e.g., 90% isodose volume). When drawing the beam portal in the TPS, a good starting point is to add 1.0 cm to the planning target volume (PTV) in the beam's eye view. For a 12-MeV electron beam, Figure 31.3 shows that the distance between the 50% and 90% isodose lines at R_{100} is 0.8 cm. After computing the dose in the planning system, the difference between the prescription isodose line and the target volume can then be used to adjust the beam portal if needed for better conformality. For a clinical setup, where the TPS is not used, it is important to remember to include this dosimetric margin when creating the beam portal. For example, if the clinical target measures 8 cm in dimension on the skin surface, the beam portal should be a minimum of 10 cm, depending on what other structures might be present and must be avoided.

Field Shaping and Shielding

Field shaping on most modern medical linear accelerators is accomplished using a combination of an electron applicator (or cone) and a field-defining insert (or

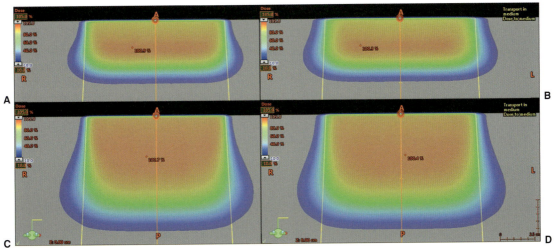

FIGURE 31.2. Isodose distributions for a 10 × 10 cm^2 applicator. (A) 9 MeV, 100-cm SSD. (B) 9 MeV, 110-cm SSD. (C) 16 MeV, 100-cm SSD. (D) 16 MeV, 110-cm SSD.

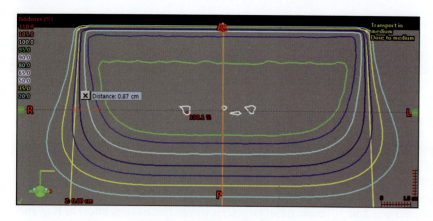

FIGURE 31.3. Isodose distribution for a 10×10 cm^2 applicator, 100-cm SSD, 12-MeV electron beam. Distance measurement is shown from the projected beam edge to the 90% isodose line.

cutout). Figure 31.4 shows an example of a 10×10 cm^2 applicator for a Varian 2100C linear accelerator (Varian Medical Systems, Palo Alto, CA) and a patient-specific insert. The applicator is usually constructed as a series of two to three scrapers with apertures that gradually shrink down to the size of the final collimation. The size of the opening of the photon jaws for each specific energy is integral to the proper functionality of the device, so specific jaw openings are automatically set when the applicator is inserted and a given energy is chosen. The thickness of the final insert must be enough to stop the highest-energy electrons. The AAPM Task Group #25 tabulated the thickness of lead required to stop various energy electrons and found a linear relationship with the minimum required thickness of lead in millimeters being equal to half of the energy in MeV.[5] They also recommended adding 20% to the thickness if a lead alloy was used instead. Adding 1 mm of lead for uncertainty is prudent, so the recommended thickness of lead as a function of energy is

$$t_{Pb}(mm) = 1 + E(MeV)/2 \qquad (31.1)$$

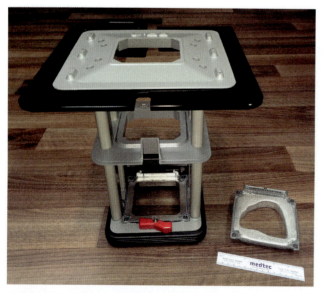

FIGURE 31.4. Electron applicator for cutouts up to 10×10 cm^2, and a patient insert made from low melting point alloy.

For a linear accelerator with a maximum energy of 20 MeV, the thickness required to stop the electrons is approximately 11 mm of lead or 13 mm of lead alloy. It is not an accident that the standard thickness of lead alloy electron inserts is approximately 13 mm. It is also possible to have these inserts commercially made to order from copper by sending the block outline from the treatment-planning computer to the vendor (.decimal, Inc., Sanford, FL), where they are manufactured using computerized machining and shipped to the customer In addition to being used for field shaping, lead and other high-density materials can be used for shielding normal tissues that need to be spared. For example, when treating a lesion near the eye, shielding the eye might be desirable. As shown in Figure 31.2, the penumbra of the beam is sharper when the applicator is placed closer to the patient. However, because of the size and shape of the applicator device, it is often necessary to treat at extended distances. In this case, shielding in the form of lead sheets can be placed on the patient surface. This usually requires making a positive mold of the patient so that the lead sheets can be formed to fit the patient surface. The required thickness is given by the above formula. Eye shields are commercially available (Civco Medical Solutions, Coralville, IA) that are fabricated from tungsten and coated with dental acrylic. The thickness of the tungsten is sufficient to shield up to 9-MeV electrons. The coating serves two purposes; one is to provide a smoother surface less prone to scratching sensitive tissues, and the other to absorb some of the backscattered electrons. Klevenhagen et al.[10] measured electron backscatter as a function of atomic number and showed that the amount of backscatter increases for higher atomic number materials and lower-energy electrons. These backscattered electrons generally have a spectrum of energies with a very low mean energy, and therefore, a relatively thin layer of lower atomic number material will absorb much of the backscattered energy. If the eye shields are placed under the eyelid, for example, the dental acrylic coating of the shield will greatly reduce the backscattered dose on the inside of the eyelid. Whenever shielding is placed inside the body to shield distal tissues, it is a good idea to place a layer of lower atomic number material upstream of the higher atomic number shielding.

Field Size Effects

When field sizes are smaller than the lateral scatter equilibrium field size, the percentage depth dose can change shape, and the dose output (dose per monitor unit) can change significantly. Understanding lateral scatter equilibrium is key to understanding how depth dose and dose output change as a function of field size and we will use a TPS to help understand this. The planning system allows us to create very accurate block openings, and to create complementary island blocks (even though they are not physically realizable). In this case, the treatment-planning algorithm being used is Eclipse Electron Monte Carlo (EMC 10.0.28, Varian Medical Systems, Palo Alto, CA), which has been shown to accurately calculate doses in heterogeneous materials under a variety of conditions.[11] Figure 31.5 shows the dose distributions for a 3×3 cm^2 field in a 10×10 cm^2 applicator, the same field with a central block (instead of an opening), and the summed

dose distribution. The summed dose distribution shows a dose distribution that looks very much like the normal open applicator dose distribution, other than a little bit of extra leakage dose through the block material (same number of electrons put into the phantom with double the monitor units).

Another way to look at the same data is shown in Figure 31.6, where the central-axis depth dose profiles are shown for the blocked fields and complementary central-blocked fields. Looking at the depth dose profiles for the 6×6 cm^2 field in a 10×10 cm^2 applicator and its complementary central-block field, you first see that the depth dose for the 6×6 cm^2 field is almost the same as the 10×10 cm^2 field. This is indicative of almost having lateral scatter equilibrium. Looking at the central-axis depth dose profile for the 6×6 cm^2 central-block field, the amount of dose on the central axis is very small, indicating that very few electrons from the outer part of the

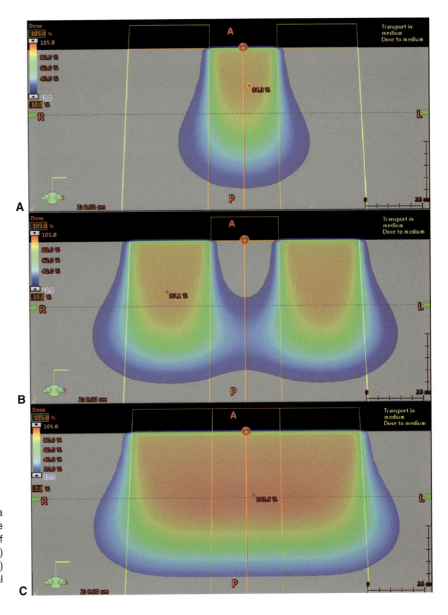

FIGURE 31.5. Isodose distribution for a 12-MeV electron beam at 100-cm SSD. The horizontal dashed line shows the location of R_{100} for the 10×10 cm^2 applicator field. (A) 3×3 cm^2 field in a 10×10 cm^2 applicator. (B) 10×10 cm^2 applicator with 3×3 cm^2 central block. (C) Sum of (A) and (B).

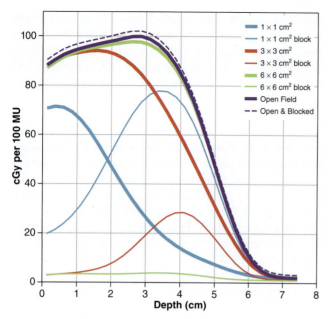

FIGURE 31.6. Calculated central-axis electron depth dose profiles for 12-MeV electron beams at 100-cm SSD. Thicker lines are for open-field sizes of 1 × 1, 3 × 3, 6 × 6, and 10 × 10 cm². Thin lines are for the corresponding open fields with central blocks, and the dashed line is the sum of the open field and centrally blocked field. All fields use the same monitor units and the dose axis is in cGy per MU.

field contribute to the dose on the central axis. Looking at the data for the 3 × 3 cm² field and the 3 × 3 cm² central-block field, the situation is not quite the same. The depth dose in the initial part of the buildup for the 3 × 3 cm² field follows the depth dose for the 10 × 10 cm² field for only about 1 cm before it starts deviating significantly. At shallow depths, electrons from outside the 3 × 3 cm² central area do not contribute dose on the central axis. As you go deeper, more of the dose on the central axis is due to electrons that started outside the 3 × 3 cm² central area. At 4-cm depth, which is past R_{100} for this energy, the contribution from electrons outside the 3 × 3 cm² central area reaches a maximum. It is easy to see that re-normalizing the depth dose for the 3 × 3 cm² field will give a depth dose that looks quite different from the original 10 × 10 cm² field. The surface dose will be higher relative to the maximum dose, and the therapeutic depth will be about 1-cm shallower. The curves for the 1 × 1 cm² field and the 1 × 1 cm² central-block field clearly show that lateral scatter equilibrium is not present at any depth.

Figure 31.7 shows the same open-field depth dose data normalized to the maximum dose on the central axis. Other than very small differences in the buildup region, there is very little difference between the 6 × 6 cm² field and the 10 × 10 cm² field. The output in dose per monitor unit is a little bit lower but using the same PDD for both fields would be very reasonable. For the 3 × 3 cm² field, the relative surface dose has increased, the depth of maximum dose has shifted toward the surface, and the therapeutic depth has decreased. In this case, we no longer have

lateral scatter equilibrium. It is very important to keep this in mind when deciding on the energy to use. If the field size is smaller than the lateral equilibrium field size, the therapeutic depth may shift far enough toward the surface that a higher energy may be needed to treat to the desired depth. For circular fields, the minimum radius for lateral scatter equilibrium is approximately $0.88\sqrt{E_{p,0}}$, where $E_{p,0}$ is the most probable energy of the electrons at the patient (phantom) surface.[12] If we approximate the most probable energy with the nominal energy, the minimum radius is approximately 3.0 cm for 12 MeV. This is approximately the same size as the 6 × 6 cm² field, which is consistent with the observations made about Figures 31.6 and 31.7.

For the 6 × 6 cm² field in the 10 × 10 cm² applicator (Fig. 31.7), the PDD is almost the same as the open 10 × 10 cm² field, so the depth coverage is about the same. However, as shown in Figure 31.6, the output (maximum dose per monitor unit) of the 6 × 6 cm² field is not the same. Figure 31.8 shows measured dose output (output factors) for cutouts in three different size applicators for the 12-MeV beam on a Varian TrueBeam™ linear accelerator (Varian Medical Systems, Palo Alto, CA). Each curve is in dose per monitor unit, so the difference in dose output of the open applicator is included in this graph. Because the 15 × 15 cm² applicator has larger openings, the X-ray jaw opening for this applicator is also larger to ensure that the electron field profile is uniform. Therefore, more electrons get through the X-ray jaws and larger applicators tend to have slightly greater dose output. Similarly, the jaw opening for the 6 × 6 cm² applicator is smaller, which tends to give less dose output. The actual magnitude of the output of the open applicator is a complicated function

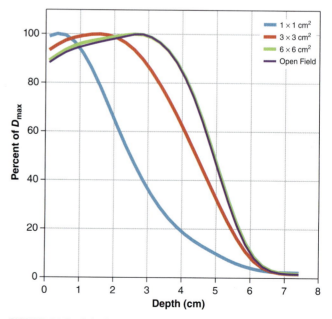

FIGURE 31.7. Calculated electron central-axis depth dose profiles for 12-MeV electron beams at 100-cm SSD, for open-field sizes of 1 × 1, 3 × 3, 6 × 6, and 10 × 10 cm² in a 10 × 10 cm² applicator.

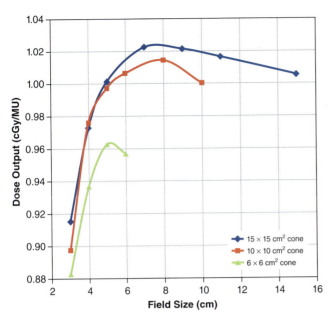

FIGURE 31.8. Measured output factors for 12-MeV electron beams at 100-cm SSD. For each electron cone, the dose output (cGy/MU) for the cutout field size is plotted.

output for a 5×5 cm^2 field in a 6×6 cm^2 applicator is approximately 3.5% smaller than the dose output for the same field size in a 10×10 cm^2 applicator. Most TPSs can model the change in depth dose as the field size changes, using either tables of PDD as a function of field size or an appropriate physics model. For the former (PDD tables), changes in dose output with different applicators may or may not be included and the radiotherapy team needs to be aware of how to convert the planning data to monitor units at the machine, if necessary. For the latter (physics model), the absolute dose output and PDD for each applicator are usually entered as part of the beam data, and the physics model takes care of modeling changes to the dose deposition as the field size is changed. While it is preferable for the TPS to provide the monitor units directly, it is not crucial as long as the radiotherapy team is aware of how the treatment-planning data need to be transferred to treatment and this is done correctly. In both cases, the formalism to calculate monitor units should be consistent with AAPM recommendations.[6,14] The AAPM also recommends that a second check of the monitor units is carried out prior to treatment (preferable) or before 10% of the treatment has elapsed.[15,16]

Extended SSD

In addition to changes in penumbra shown in Figure 31.2, increasing SSD can affect the shape of the depth dose distribution as well as the dose output (per monitor unit). To account for the change in the depth dose distribution, AAPM TG 25[5] recommended using a divergence factor to calculate the relative depth dose at extended SSD from the relative depth dose at the nominal SSD. As pointed out by Shiu et al.,[13] these changes in relative depth dose are expected to be relatively small because the electron penetration is small compared to the SSD. They evaluated this approach for a 20-MeV electron beam at 110-cm SSD for a 15×15 cm^2 field and a 6×6 cm^2 field. For the larger field size, they found the divergence factor worked well, but there were significant differences for the smaller field size. They hypothesized that these differences were due to a large number of low-energy electrons scattered from the edges of the final aperture. The number of scattered electrons depends on the design of the applicator. Modern applicators tend to simply remove electrons at the field edge, while older applicator designs had walls that contributed scattered electrons.

As shown in Figure 31.9, there are a few competing factors that affect the shape of the depth dose curve as the SSD is changed. For the 15×15 cm^2 field, the therapeutic depth (R_{90}) of the electron beam is hardly affected, but there is a deficit of electrons in the buildup region, which is consistent with the hypothesis of Shiu et al.[13] For the smaller 6×6 cm^2 field, we can see a few competing effects. First of all, the therapeutic depth of the 6×6 cm^2 field is smaller than the therapeutic depth of the 15×15 cm^2 field, as would be expected because of the loss of lateral scatter

of the design of the applicator, the energy of the beam, and the X-ray jaw opening. The X-ray jaw openings for each energy-applicator combination are usually fixed by the vendor to provide good dose uniformity for the open applicator and, in general, should not be changed by the end user. The dose output for each applicator should be measured and entered into the TPS.

Two features can be seen in Figure 31.8 that are consistently seen in measured output factor data. The first is the slight rise in dose output, as the field size gets slightly smaller than the open applicator field size. As the field size gets smaller, the field edges get closer to the central axis. Electrons scattering from the edges of the aperture can reach the central axis more easily and the dose output rises slightly. When the field size gets smaller than the field size required for lateral scatter equilibrium (about 6 cm for 12 MeV), the dose output drops quite dramatically as electrons that would normally contribute dose to central axis are removed from the beam. In addition, the shape of the depth dose is also changing, as seen in Figure 31.7. If planning clinical electron treatments (without the planning system), the change in dose output can be accounted for using tabulated output factors. However, the change in PDD is not so easy to deal with. Therefore, when dealing with field sizes smaller than the equilibrium field size, a good TPS is recommended to ensure that the treatment goals are met.

When delivering an electron beam, it is generally possible to deliver the same field shape using different applicators. The shape of the dose distribution primarily depends on the shape and size of the final collimation, as shown by Shiu et al.,[13] and the dose output depends on the chosen applicator. Referring to Figure 31.8, the dose

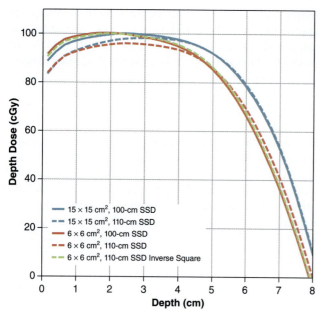

FIGURE 31.9. Calculated electron central-axis depth dose profiles for 20-MeV electron beams at 100- and 110-cm SSD, for open applicator field sizes of 6 × 6 and 15 × 15 cm². The vertical axis is absolute dose in cGy, and the monitor units for beams at 100-cm SSD were set to obtain 100 cGy maximum dose on central axis. For the beams at 110-cm SSD, the monitor units were increased using an inverse square factor and an effective source distance of 90 cm (scattering foil position for this linear accelerator). The curve labeled "inverse square" is the PDD for the 6 × 6 cm² field size at 110-cm SSD, calculated from the 100-cm SSD depth dose using just an inverse square correction.

equilibrium (discussed previously). If we do an inverse square (divergence) correction for the 6 × 6 cm² field to get to 110-cm SSD (as recommended by AAPM TG-25), then you can see that the depth dose does not change significantly. However, in reality, the shape of the depth dose and the magnitude of the dose output do change significantly. We no longer have side scatter equilibrium for the 6 × 6 cm² field, so the simple inverse square correction, which assumes side scatter equilibrium, is not sufficient to calculate the change in depth dose with SSD. In addition to the small reduction in dose output, we can see a small increase in the therapeutic depth, which is consistent with the slightly larger field size at the extended SSD. Similar to the case with X-ray beams, a simple divergence correction is inadequate for smaller fields because of differences in scattering conditions, and lateral scatter is arguably more important for electron beams.

Virtual Point Source

The virtual point source, as defined by AAPM TG-25,[5] is a useful concept for calculating the divergence of the electron beam. The basic idea is to determine the 50% width of the electron beam under conditions of lateral scatter equilibrium. The task group recommended a field size of 20 × 20 cm² or larger. For most linear accelerators, the virtual source position is close to the position of the primary scattering foil, which is not necessarily at the same

position as the X-ray target. While useful for calculating beam profiles using a pencil-beam algorithm (Hogstrom et al.[17]), it is less useful for calculating the dose variation with SSD.[5]

Effective Point Source

The effective SSD concept was introduced by Khan[18] to facilitate the calculation of the dose output as a function of SSD. There is no assumption of lateral scatter equilibrium in this case. The dose output is tabulated as a function of the air gap between the final collimation and the phantom surface. A plot of the inverse square root of the output as a function of the gap is fit to a straight line and extrapolated to an effective point source where the inverse square root of the output is zero (or the output is infinite). The range of air gaps used for the measurement should be representative of those used in the clinic. In practice, the effective point source is usually tabulated as a function of square or circular field size. The effective point source position and can vary systematically from 50 cm (for very small fields) to approximately the position of the primary scattering foil (90 cm for Varian, and 100 cm for Siemens). The output at the nominal SSD (100 cm) is corrected by an inverse square correction factor, ISC_{eff}, to give the output at the treatment SSD.

$$ISC_{eff}(r) = \left[\frac{SSD_{eff}(r) + d_0}{SSD_{eff}(r) + d_0 + g} \right]^2 \qquad (31.2)$$

where r is the field size, d_0 is the normalization depth for the electron beam, and g is the air gap difference between the nominal (calibration) SSD and the actual SSD. If the air gap is larger than what was used to determine the effective point source, a measurement of the dose output may be needed since the inverse square dependence of the dose output is only approximate and may not hold for larger air gaps.

Effective versus Virtual Point Source

For larger field sizes, where lateral scatter equilibrium exists, the effective point source and virtual point source are approximately the same. The electron beam appears to be emanating from a point near the primary scattering foil in the linear accelerator. As the size of the beam is reduced and lateral scatter equilibrium is lost, the effective source position of the electron beam appears to move toward isocenter. It is important to note that the effective source is not a true electron source position; it is only a result of the fact that the output of the beam is varying with distance as if the source was at a different location than the primary scattering foil. This is purely a product of the loss of lateral scatter equilibrium. In fact, one can show theoretically that the electrons in the middle of the beam are still diverging from a position near the primary scattering foil; it is just the output that is being reduced more quickly. In other words, the beam is geometrically diverging from the primary scattering foil, but the output is decreasing as if the source was closer to isocenter.

In Equation (31.2), g is the additional air gap between the nominal SSD (usually 100 cm) and the actual treatment SSD. It is not important how these effective source positions are measured, only that they exist and can be used for distance corrections. A drawback of this method is that finding (interpolating) the SSD_{eff} for an irregular field is not well defined.

Air Gap Factor

One of the more significant issues with the effective point source method of correcting the dose output is that the effective SSD quickly moves toward isocenter for small field sizes because of the loss of side scatter equilibrium. Small uncertainties in field size may lead to relatively large uncertainties in effective SSD and dose output. If the field shape is not the same as those used to measure the effective point source, then the field size used in the inverse square correction has even more uncertainty.

An alternative approach for determining the output of the electron beam at an extended distance is to use the virtual SSD method from AAPM TG-25, which uses the virtual SSD, SSD_{vir}, and an air gap factor, f_{air}, to calculate the output at extended SSD.

$$ISC_{\text{vir}}(r) = \left[\frac{SSD_{\text{vir}} + d_0}{SSD_{\text{vir}} + d_0 + g} \right]^2 f_{\text{air}}(r) \quad (31.3)$$

It is important to note that this is an alternative to the effective point source method and must not be used in addition to the effective point source method. The physical interpretation of this equation is that the electrons are diverging from the virtual point source (inverse square term), and the air gap factor, f_{air}, describes the deviation between inverse square dependence from the virtual point source and the true dose output. Note that the inverse square term no longer depends on field size, and that the field size dependence is fully contained in the air gap factor.

The effective point source and air gap factor methods have both been shown to give clinically acceptable results, provided the calculations are not made beyond the range of measured commissioning data. Either method is acceptable for determining electron beam monitor units in accordance with TG-71,[14] although the author prefers the air gap factor method.

Irregular Fields

In general, data for square or circular fields is collected when commissioning linear accelerators, but clinical electron fields are irregularly shaped. If data is collected for square fields, which is probably more common, it is useful to approximate the clinical irregular field by a rectangular field size.[14,19] Similar to what is done for X-ray beams, the basic idea is to find a rectangular field with approximately the same amount of scatter as the irregular field. Small portions of the irregular field that are more than $0.88\sqrt{E_{p,0}}$ cm from the point of interest (the minimum

radius for lateral scatter equilibrium as given by Khan et al.[12]) can be ignored. For a more detailed explanation of the rules for constructing equivalent rectangular fields for electrons and some examples, see the description by Hogstrom and Steadham,[20] which is reproduced by Gibbons et al.[14]

Multiple Coulomb scattering theory[17] gives several useful results that can be used to calculate dosimetric quantities for rectangular fields, given the same data for square fields. For PDD, the PDD for a rectangular X × Y cm^2 field is given by the geometric mean of the PDD for the square X × X cm^2 field and the square Y × Y cm^2 field.

$$PDD(X,Y,d) = \sqrt{PDD(X,X,d) \times PDD(Y,Y,d)} \quad (31.4)$$

Mills et al.[21] showed that a similar equation for output factors was more accurate than using $4A/P$ for the effective field size.

$$S_e(X,Y) = \sqrt{S_e(X,X) \times S_e(Y,Y)} \quad (31.5)$$

There is a similar equation for the air gap factor.[13]

$$f_{\text{air}}(X,Y) = \sqrt{f_{\text{air}}(X,X) \times f_{\text{air}}(Y,Y)} \quad (31.6)$$

There is no similar equation for the effective point source method. However, if you acknowledge that both methods should give the same result, the following equation can be derived for the effective source inverse square correction for the rectangular field

$$ISC_{\text{eff}}(r) = \frac{SSD_{\text{eff}}(X,X) + d_0}{SSD_{\text{eff}}(X,X) + d_0 + g} \times \frac{SSD_{\text{eff}}(Y,Y) + d_0}{SSD_{\text{eff}}(Y,Y) + d_0 + g}$$

$$(31.7)$$

Similar to sector integration methods for X-ray beams, Khan et al.[12,22–24] developed methods to be able to predict changes in depth dose and output factors for irregular fields. When applying these methods, it is more natural to use input data for circular fields, although square field sizes can be converted to equivalent circular field sizes to get the necessary input data. These methods are more suitable for computer implementation than for hand calculations and will not be discussed here.

Sloping Surfaces

When the electron beam is incident on a sloping surface, the isodose curves are affected in several ways. Figure 31.10 shows isodose curves for 12-MeV electron beams at normal incidence and 40° oblique incidence. The SSD along central axis and monitor units are the same for both beams. There are three main effects on the dose distribution as the beam angle is moved away from normal incidence. First, the penetration of the electron beam relative to the phantom surface is reduced, reducing the therapeutic depth. Second, the maximum dose along the central

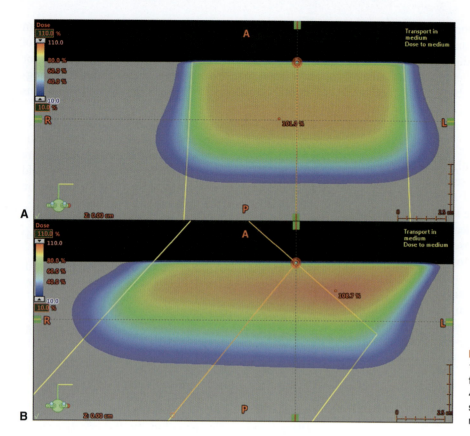

FIGURE 31.10. Calculated dose for 12-MeV 10 × 10 cm² fields at 110-cm SSD for (A) 0° incidence (perpendicular) and (B) 40° angulation. The beam weights were set to obtain 100% at the depth of maximum dose for the beam at 0° incidence.

axis is increased. This is due to electrons being scattering toward central axis by the phantom material upstream of the beam entry point (patient left in the figure). The last major effect is that the penumbra of the beam on the upstream side (patient left in the figure) is sharper (isodose lines are closer together) than the penumbra on the downstream side. The last effect is the same as what was shown previously in Figure 31.2 for normally incident beams with different source to surface distances.

Figure 31.11 shows calculated central-axis depth dose profiles for 12-MeV electron beams at different angles of incidence. The therapeutic depth along central axis is reduced, the maximum dose along the central axis is increased, and the practical range of the electron beam increases. On one side of the beam, we have phantom material upstream of the central-axis beam entry point, and on the other side, the phantom material is further away than the central-axis beam entry point. The upstream portions of the phantom scatter electrons toward the central axis that contribute more dose at shallower depths on the depth dose curve. The downstream portions are not scattered until farther distances (relative to central axis) and those scattered electrons contribute dose at deeper depths along the beam's central axis, which leads to what appears to be an increased range. Figure 31.12 shows depth dose data for the same beams, but in this case, the depth dose is perpendicular to the phantom surface. In this case, you see an increase in dose at shallower depths as the angle of incidence increases, as well as a decrease in the depth of

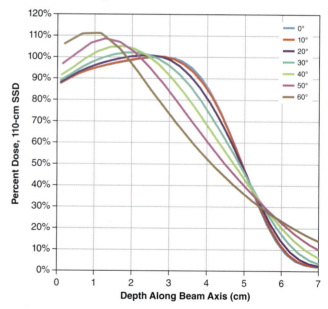

FIGURE 31.11. Calculated central-axis electron depth dose profiles for 12-MeV electron beams at 110-cm SSD. The beam weights were set to obtain 100% at the depth of maximum dose for the beam at 0° incidence. The entry point of the beam is fixed, and the depth dose is along the beam axis.

penetration relative to the skin surface. Because it maximizes the penetration of the electron beam, we generally try to place the electron beams at normal incidence relative to the skin surface.

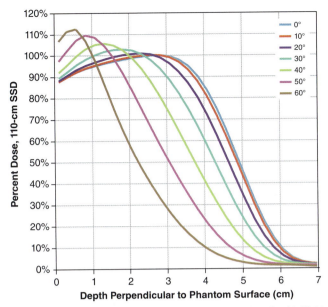

FIGURE 31.12. Calculated electron depth dose profiles for 12-MeV electron beams at 110-cm SSD. The beam weights were set to obtain 100% at the depth of maximum dose for the beam at 0° incidence. The entry point of the beam is fixed, and the depth dose is perpendicular to the phantom surface, or the depth from the phantom surface.

Surface Irregularities

Real patient surfaces are not flat. They can be rounded (e.g., extremities or skull) or very irregular (e.g., nose or surgical defect). The former is a more complicated sloping surface; the beam penetrates further where it has normal incidence, and less where the surface is sloping away from perpendicular incidence. The latter is perhaps more interesting in that it introduces us to heterogeneity effects.

Figure 31.13A shows the dose distribution for a nose phantom irradiated with an 8×8 cm^2 field of 16-MeV electrons at 100-cm SSD. The monitor units were set to deliver 100% maximum dose on central axis for the same field incident on a water phantom at the same SSD. The density of the external contour was set to unity to highlight the effect of the surface geometry. The resulting dose distribution looks very different compared to an open-field dose distribution (see Fig. 31.2), with hot spots of up to 120% of the dose for the open field on a water phantom. To explain why this is happening, let's look at the situation a small distance into the nose portion of the phantom. The electrons in the nose are scattered away from the nose. The electrons in the air tend to stay in the air, so the number of electrons just lateral to the nose increases as

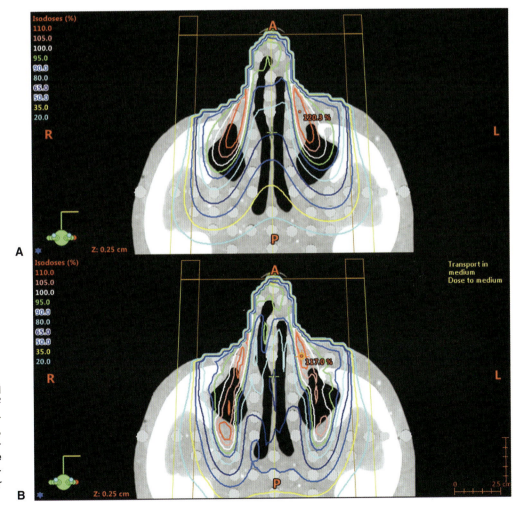

FIGURE 31.13. Calculated dose for 16-MeV 8×8 cm^2 field at 100-cm SSD incident on a nose phantom, (A) without and (B) with heterogeneity corrections. The monitor units were set to deliver 100% dose for a water phantom at the same SSD.

the electron beam penetrates the nose. As described earlier, more electrons imply more dose, which is the primary reason why there are significant hot spots just lateral to the nose. Because the electrons have been redistributed laterally from the nose, there are fewer electrons directly behind the nose, which leads to a cold spot. In general, any time there is a hot spot due to electron scattering, there will be a corresponding cold spot in the dose distribution.

Heterogeneities

Electron dose distributions can also be significantly affected by tissue heterogeneities such as bone, lung, and air cavities. Figure 31.13B shows the dose distribution for the same nose phantom as Figure 31.13A, except that the dose calculation now includes the effect of the CT densities (same electron field and monitor units). Compared to the homogeneous calculation, you can see that the hot spots just lateral to the nose are slightly reduced in magnitude. Inside the nose, we have air cavities and some of the electrons in the tissue portions of the nose are scattered into the internal air cavities and so fewer electrons scatter out of the nose and hence the hot spot lateral to the nose

is slightly reduced. Just behind those hot spots, there is another air cavity. The large number of electrons in the lateral hot spots can now penetrate deeper into the phantom because of the air, in addition to other electrons scattering into those air cavities. Directly behind the nose, the electrons tend to scatter into the long, narrow air cavities and hence can penetrate much further. Overall, the electron beam can penetrate much further into the phantom because of the air cavities.

It is not easy to see in Figure 31.13, but electrons in bone tend to scatter more readily (because of the higher density). Figure 31.14 shows the calculated dose distribution for cylindrical bone and air heterogeneities in a water phantom, and the hot spots streaming off the side of the bone are readily apparent. In most patient cases, the difference in density between the bone and normal tissue gives hot spots on the order of 3% to 5% as shown in the figure. For air cavities, the density difference is much larger, so hot spots of 10% or greater, as shown in the figure, are not uncommon.

Another common situation is shown in Figure 31.15, where we have an electron boost field on the chest wall. Without heterogeneity corrections, the dose appears to

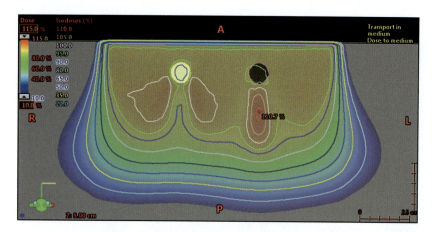

FIGURE 31.14. Calculated dose for 16-MeV 19 × 12 cm² field at 100-cm SSD incident on a water phantom with 1-cm cylindrical bone (patient right) and air (patient left) heterogeneities. The heterogeneities are at 1-cm depth and the monitor units were set to deliver 100 cGy at the depth of maximum dose for a uniform water phantom.

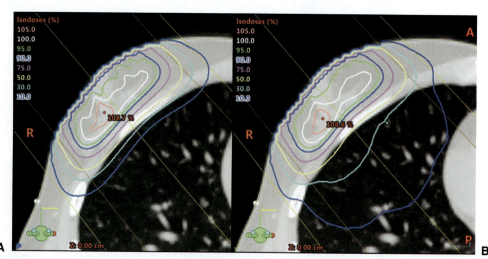

FIGURE 31.15. Dose for a 9-MeV chest wall boost field (A) calculated without heterogeneity corrections and (B) calculated with heterogeneity corrections.

not penetrate very far in the lung tissue. However, once the reduced density of the lung tissue is accounted for, it is readily apparent that the electron beam penetrates much farther into the lung tissue. Fortunately, this is just a boost field so relatively little of the total dose is given using this field.

Bolus

Bolus is a specifically shaped material, which is usually tissue equivalent and is normally placed either in direct contact with the patient's surface, close to the patient's surface, or inside a body cavity. In electron beam radiotherapy, the most common uses for bolus are to flatten out an irregular surface, reduce the penetration of the electrons in all or part of the field, and/or increase the surface dose.

A very common type of bolus material available in most clinics is superflab, which is a synthetic oil gel with a density very close to that of water. It is available in a variety of thicknesses from 0.2 to 3.0 cm in sheets that are typically 30×30 cm^2 in size. It can be easily cut using scissors or a utility knife and conforms reasonably well to patient surfaces. As seen in Figure 31.1, lower-energy electron beams may have a surface dose less than 90% of the maximum central-axis dose and this dose may be lower than desired, depending on the location of the target relative to the skin surface. In this case, adding superflab

(or equivalent) to the skin surface over the entire treatment field increases the surface dose. The desired bolus thickness depends on the desired skin dose and the energy of the beam being used for treatment. The penetration of the beam into the patient will be reduced by the thickness of the bolus, so higher electron energy may be needed depending on the depth of the target. Using a higher energy has the disadvantage that the slope of the distal dose falloff is not as steep, which gives more radiation dose to underlying normal tissues. Another reason to use constant thickness bolus is to reduce the range of the beam in the patient. For a typical linear accelerator, the energy spacing is such that the therapeutic depth spacing is approximately 1 cm. Combining these energies with 5-mm sheets of superflab bolus material, it is relatively easy to achieve 0.5-cm spacing in therapeutic depth.

When using superflab bolus to reduce the overall range of the beam or increase the skin dose, it is important that the bolus cover the entire electron field with some margin. Similar to what was seen with the nose phantom (Fig. 31.13), Figure 31.16 shows that sharp bolus edges within the field (or close to the field edge) will lead to significant hot and cold spots. If only partial coverage is desired (e.g., target depth variable across the field), then it is recommended that the edge of the bolus that is inside the electron field be tapered to not have a sharp edge as this will reduce the magnitude of the hot and cold spots. As shown in Figure 31.16, shallower angles (e.g., 30°) are

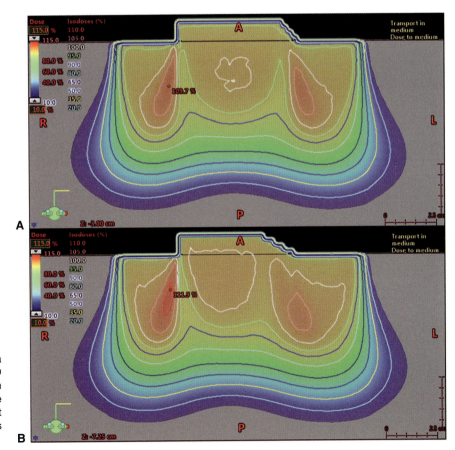

FIGURE 31.16. Calculated dose for a 16-MeV 19×12 cm^2 field at 100-cm SSD incident on a water phantom with 1-cm unit density bolus in only a portion of the field. The edge on the patient right is cut square, and the edge on the patient left is cut at a (A) 45° angle or (B) 30° angle.

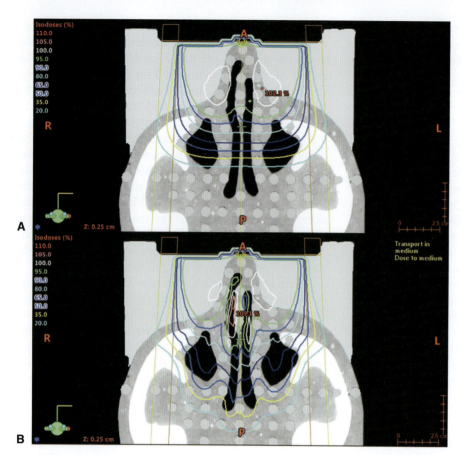

FIGURE 31.17. Calculated dose for a 16-MeV 8 × 8 cm² field at 100-cm SSD incident on a nose phantom with customized bolus, (A) without heterogeneity corrections and (B) with heterogeneity corrections. The monitor units were set to deliver 100% dose for a flat phantom at the same SSD.

preferable; the dose calculation shows almost no difference between cutting the bolus material square or at a 45° angle. As noted by Gerbi et al.,[6] the minimum width of the bolus for a scar boost treatment should be at least 2 cm to ensure dose buildup occurs instead of getting a cold spot due to out-scattering (e.g., as seen with the nose phantom).

Figure 31.17A shows the dose distribution for the same nose phantom as shown in Figure 31.13A, again with CT density set to unity. The bolus was shaped to conform to the shape of the nose and provide a flat surface for the electron beam using algorithms developed by Low et al.[25] In years past, similar results were achieved by molding beeswax (or similar material) around a positive impression of the patient. Some residual hot spots are remaining (<103%) as a result of an imperfect construction of the bolus material in the planning system, but the dose distribution for the 8 × 8 cm² field is almost restored to what would be expected for a flat phantom.

Unfortunately, the dose distribution in the phantom is changed significantly as a result of internal heterogeneities, as shown in Figure 31.17B, and it is obvious that a simple flat bolus may be inadequate if internal heterogeneities are significant. The dose distribution in the patient can be customized by changing the thickness of the bolus as a function of position in the field. Because of complex interplay between surface irregularities and internal heterogeneities, doing this by trial and error would be difficult at best. That was the motivation for Low et al.'s

bolus design investigations,[25] to provide a framework to systematically design an electron bolus to conformally treat the target volume and/or spare distal normal tissues. This technology has been further developed[26–28] and is now commercially available (BolusECT, .decimal, Inc., Sanford, FL, https://dotdecimal.com/). Clinically, the technology has been used in the treatment of paraspinal muscles,[29] postmastectomy chest walls,[30] and head and neck target volumes.[31] When using this technology, there is generally a tradeoff between target conformality and dose homogeneity. One way to decrease the impact of this tradeoff (improved dose homogeneity for the same conformality, or improved conformality for the same homogeneity) is to modulate the intensity of the electron beam within the field,[32] although the technology for intensity modulation of electron beams is not readily available.

Calibration and Monitor Units

In radiation therapy, calibration of the linear accelerator refers to the establishment of a relationship between the measured dose under reference conditions and the monitor units set on the treatment machine. The calibration protocol currently used in the United States and Canada is TG-51,[33] while the very similar TRS-398[34] is used almost everywhere else. While the calibration protocols are quite specific when describing how the measurements are to be performed, the measured dose at the reference depth

(d_{ref} in the protocol) is usually transferred to the R_{100} depth using the clinical percentage depth dose. A typical calibration statement for an electron beam might be 1 cGy per MU at a depth of R_{100} for a 10×10 cm^2 field size in a 10×10 cm^2 applicator at an SSD of 100 cm. The calibration and reference conditions are entered into the TPS by the physicist as part of the commissioning process. Other data, such as dose rates for other applicators, dose rates for different inserts, PDD, and virtual and/or effective SSDs for each energy may also be needed. The physicist needs to consult the documentation for the TPS to determine the required input data so that it can be measured at the time of machine commissioning.

Because surface irregularities and internal heterogeneities have a very significant effect on the dose distribution, the use of heterogeneity corrections in the TPS is highly recommended. Ideally, the treatment planner should be able to create the treatment plan to cover the target volume and have the TPS provide the monitor units required to deliver the treatment. If the planning system is capable of doing this, it is good practice to have an independent second check of the monitor units using either a hand calculation or another computer program.[14,16] If the planning system is not able to directly provide monitor units, the physicist will need to create a process to convert the *beam weight* in the TPS to monitor units that can be delivered on the treatment machine. The physicist will also need to determine the range of treatment over which the planning system provides adequate clinical accuracy (e.g., ±3%) by comparing it to measured commissioning data.

The ability of the TPS to adequately handle surface irregularities and internal heterogeneities is determined more by the algorithm implementation, although the quality of the input data may also affect the results. Shiu et al.[35] attempted to provide a standard set of measured data to test electron dose calculations, but there were some small but significant inconsistencies in the data due to measurements being carried out at different institutions on different machines. Boyd et al.[36] repeated the measurements on a single linear accelerator and validated the results using EGS4 Monte Carlo calculations,[37] creating a much more consistent and reliable dataset. The data is available from the authors and has been used to validate the accuracy of the pencil-beam redefinition algorithm[38] and the Varian Eclipse Electron Monte Carlo algorithm.[11]

BASIC TREATMENT PLANNING

Electron Dose Prescription

Recommendations for prescribing and reporting electron radiotherapy can be found in ICRU Report 71,[39] and the recommendations of the AAPM[5,6] are consistent with those recommendations. The basic concepts of gross tumor volume, clinical target volume, and PTV that are used for X-ray therapy and recommended by ICRU Reports 50 and 62[40,41] can be used for electron beam treatment planning. ICRU Report 71[39] recommends that dose be reported for a reference condition of the same beam incident on a homogeneous phantom. In general, this reference point should be in the center of the target volume; if not, then the reference dose in the center of the target volume should also be reported. In addition, the maximum and minimum dose to the PTV should be reported, as well as doses to organs at risk and/or dose–volume histograms.

Within the TPS, the treatment planner must enter a dose prescription for the electron treatment plan. While the precise details of how this is done in every TPS are beyond the scope of this work, there are a couple of general methods for accomplishing this task. Before the use of TPSs for electron beams became ubiquitous, a common *old-style* prescription would be something like a dose to 90% of the central-axis maximum dose. It is assumed that the central-axis maximum dose is in a water phantom at the same SSD as the patient's plan. If the beam weight in the TPS is directly related to the maximum dose in a water phantom for that beam at the same SSD, then it is possible to calculate the beam weight for the given prescription. However, it is more likely that the monitor units need to be calculated first and entered into the planning system. In other words, the second check is setting the beam weight, which is not the most desirable situation.

A more modern approach is to adjust the beam weight (or monitor units) until the prescription isodose line covers the target volume appropriately with the maximum dose inside the target volume approximately 10% higher than the prescription dose. In this case, the secondary monitor unit calculation or hand calculation is a true independent check. However, it is not entirely clear what dose should be entered into the second-check calculation. As described earlier, the dose in the electron beam is greatly affected by the patient surface and internal heterogeneities. There is no *easy* accurate heterogeneity correction method available for electron beams, so a method to estimate the dose for that same beam incident on a water phantom is needed. Similar to what is commonly done for IMRT verification, the treatment plan can be cast onto a water phantom to extract the desired dose. This removes the patient surface and internal heterogeneity effects, allowing the central-axis maximum dose to be obtained more reliably.

En-face Beams

The simplest situation to deal with is treatment planning for a single field (e.g., scar boost for a breast treatment), where target volumes are small enough to be treated with a single field cutout in a single applicator. All of the effects that were described earlier can come into play, which is why so much effort was put into describing how electron beams behave.

The first steps are to choose the energy, field size, and beam direction to use. The energy is primarily determined by the maximum depth of the target, with a good first approximation for the energy (in MeV) being 3.3 times the maximum depth of the target (in cm). The beam direction should be chosen to be approximately perpendicular to the skin surface that is nearest the target volume, because this maximizes the penetration of the electrons relative to the skin surface.

One strategy for choosing the SSD is to make it as close as possible to the skin surface to minimize the spreading of the electrons in the air gap between the final collimation and the skin surface. This allows the penumbra to be as sharp as possible, for sparing normal tissues lateral to the target volume. However, there is a risk to aggressively choosing a shorter SSD since potential collisions of the bulky applicator with the patient are not easily visualized in most TPSs. Therefore, another common strategy is to choose a *safe* SSD (e.g., 110 cm) that is very unlikely to cause a collision problem. The former strategy (choosing a shorter SSD) can give a slightly better lateral penumbra at the expense of having to occasionally replan the patient treatment if the shorter SSD can't be realized on the treatment machine. Proponents of the latter strategy would also argue that using the same SSD for all electron beams could potentially reduce setup errors that could occur if the norm was to use a different SSD for each patient. The author favors using a standard SSD that is slightly shorter than the *safe* SSD. Evaluating the plan for potential collision issues should be a standard part of the treatment-planning process, and the SSD could be extended for potential problem cases.

Once the beam direction, SSD, and energy are chosen, the beam aperture needs to be created in the TPS. As described above, the penumbra of the electron beam necessitates that there is a margin between the PTV and the beam portal, and a margin of 1 cm is a good starting point. This is very much like treatment planning for X-ray beams. The exact details of how these steps are accomplished differ from one system to another, so a step-by-step process will not be given, and it will be assumed that the treatment planner is familiar with the tools available for positioning beams, defining beam properties, and creating beam apertures. After setting the beam parameters, the dose can be calculated, and the beam weight set to get (or verify) the desired coverage.

The next task is for the treatment planner and/or physician to evaluate the dose distribution to determine if the goals of the treatment plan have been met. For example, the magnitude of hot and cold spots due to the external patient contour and internal heterogeneities should be compared to the planning objectives, and the conformality of the prescription isodose line should be compared to the PTV. It may be necessary to add a bolus to the patient surface, as described above, to make the dose more homogeneous and/or make the dose coverage more conformal. Field size effects may have reduced the depth dose of the electron beam and the electron beam energy may need to be increased. An understanding of all of the effects described above will allow the planner to determine if the

dose calculation results make sense and what can be done to improve the dose distribution to meet the treatment-planning goals.

Skin Collimation

In Figure 31.3, it was shown that the therapeutic portion of the beam can be on the order of 1 cm smaller than the field aperture, and the precise relationship between the therapeutic treatment volume and the total irradiated volume depends on the energy of the beam and the SSD. When the target is very small (e.g., 2–3 cm), the field size may need to be double the size of the target or greater to be able to give a uniform dose to the target. This means that the volume of significant dose extends well beyond the target. If a critical structure is located close (laterally) to the target volume, it is then very difficult to irradiate the target volume while sparing the critical structure.

For a given energy, the width of the penumbra depends on the distance between the final collimation and the patient surface, and the amount of scattering inside the patient. There isn't a lot that can be done about patient scattering. However, the component of the penumbra due to the collimator distance can be reduced if the patient can be moved closer to the final collimation. Unfortunately, that is often not possible, and one still has to consider setup uncertainty and its contribution to being able to spare the critical structure. Collimation, in the form of lead sheets, can also be placed on the skin surface. The required thickness of lead was given by AAPM TG-25 (see Field Shaping section) and the adequacy of the lead shielding should be verified before the skin collimation is used in the clinic. Lead shielding can be placed over a portion of the treated area, to shield a critical structure, or around the entire treated area to provide a more conformal treatment. The width of the lead shielding needs to be greater than the width of the penumbra. The projection of the aperture edge needs to be placed such that the edge of the lead is at approximately the 90% point on the beam profile if the lead were not there. The width of the lead needs to extend far enough to block the entire penumbra, extending out to the 5% level on the beam profile without the lead (for example).

Figure 31.18 illustrates some of the issues involved when using skin collimation. In Figure 31.18A, a high-density material is placed on the skin surface with a 4×4 cm^2 opening. It is relatively easy to see that using skin collimation in this way can give a nice sharp penumbra, and because placing it on the skin can be very reproducible, skin collimation can be used to shield structures that are quite close to the target region. Figure 31.18B shows the dose distribution for the 6×6 cm^2 electron field without the skin collimation. Note that the width of the 90% dose region is approximately the same size as the opening of the skin collimation. This is required so that the dose can be relatively uniform in the volume exposed by the skin collimation. The lateral extent of the

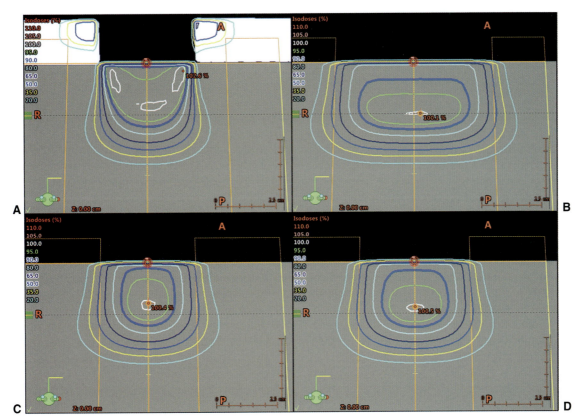

FIGURE 31.18. Calculated dose for a 9-MeV 6 × 6 cm² field at 110-cm SSD incident on a water phantom (A) with and (B) without skin collimation. The monitor units for each beam are the same and set to deliver 100% at the depth of maximum dose for the beam without skin collimation. The skin collimation was approximated by a bolus of density 5 g cm⁻³ and has an opening of 4 × 4 cm² on the skin surface. The lower panels show the calculated dose for a 9-MeV beam with (C) a field size of 4 × 4 cm² on the skin surface and (D) a field size of 4.6 × 4.6 cm² on the skin surface. The monitor units for the beams in the lower panels were set to deliver 100% at the depth of maximum dose for the blocked beam.

dose distribution without the skin collimation gives you an idea of how far the shielding needs to be extended. The dashed horizontal line is at the depth of R_{100}, and it is readily apparent that the depth penetration of the beam with skin collimation is less than the beam without skin collimation. It is also apparent that electrons scatter from the skin collimation and contribute to hot spots near the edge of the skin collimation. Because lateral scatter is the dominant factor determining the depth dose characteristics, the depth dose for the beam with skin collimation is primarily determined by the size of the opening. The dose output, however, is primarily determined by the size of the applicator insert. To illustrate this point, the same monitor units were used with and without skin collimation.

For comparison, Figure 31.18C shows the dose distribution if we used just an applicator insert that projected to 4 × 4 cm² on the skin surface (without skin collimation). The first observation about this dose distribution is that the size of the therapeutic region is significantly smaller than the dose distribution with skin collimation. In Figure 31.18D, the insert size was increased to 4.6 × 4.6 cm² to increase the size of the therapeutic region. In both of these cases, the therapeutic dose coverage is arguably inferior to the case with skin collimation, and the total volume of irradiated tissue is larger.

Currently, there are no commercially available TPSs that support skin collimation, which means that planning these treatments is not easy. Assuming that you have a way to fabricate the skin collimation in the first place, the planner will have to figure out a way to enter the skin collimation into the TPS, and then design the electron cutout to place the 90% point (or greater) of the beam profile at the edge of the lead collimation, keeping in mind that the outer edge of the lead collimation needs to block the rest of the penumbra. All of these *margins* depend on the beam energy and SSD, so if it is desired to do this on a regular basis, it might be worthwhile to tabulate some of these values in advance to assist in planning. Obviously, some tools available in the TPS could be potentially very useful, but we'll just have to keep our hopes up.

Electron–Electron Field Junctions

Electron field sizes using standard applicators are generally limited to 25 × 25 cm² by the size of the largest applicator. Rotating the collimator by 45° will allow for a slightly longer field that can be useful for treating the craniospinal axis.[42] Even then, it may be necessary to join multiple electron fields together to treat the entire spinal axis. There may also be scenarios where it may be desirable to treat different portions of the field with different energies because of the target depth differences. The scattering of the electrons complicates the dosimetry of the field junction.

Figure 31.19A shows the resulting dose distribution for two adjacent 12-MeV 10×10 cm² fields where the field junction is at the phantom surface, and it is obvious that this beam arrangement would not be desirable for a real patient case. The hot spot due to the field overlap at depth is greater than 25% of the delivered dose for each beam. This problem is not unique to electron beams, however, and a similar hot spot (different magnitude) would be seen if X-ray beams were used instead. Figure 31.19B shows the same fields, but with a slightly larger separation between the beams to create a smooth junction at the R_{100} depth. Unfortunately, it is pretty obvious that the dose near the surface is significantly colder than each electron beam, and if there were target tissue at that location, the dose would be inadequate.

A better geometry for field junctions (photon or electron) is to maintain a common source position for the fields and match the field edges at the junction. The simplest case is shown in Figure 31.20A, with two electron beams with half-beam blocks. Since the block is the only thing that is changed and the energy is the same, the dose in the junction is quite smooth. Another way to junction the fields is to angle the fields away from each other, as shown in Figure 31.20B, where the beams have been rotated by 2.9° such that the edges of the beams, as drawn by the TPS, are aligned with each other. Unfortunately, the field junction hot spot is almost 109%, so it is obvious that aligning the TPS field edge is not the correct way to do this. In this case, the TPS draws the field edge as if the source of the electrons was at the same position as the photon (or light-field) source. However, the actual source of the electron beam for this particular linear accelerator is approximately 90 cm from isocenter. Allowing for this difference in source position, the angle of the beam away from vertical and the separation of the beams both need to be increased slightly (3.2°) to create a smoother junction, as shown in Figure 31.20C. In this case, the magnitude of the hot spot is less than 103%, so this is quite close to aligning the actual edges of the electron beams. While not shown here, the virtual source position used by the dose calculation is approximately 82 cm from isocenter, so the ideal beam angulation is a little more than that shown in Figure 31.20C.

To further complicate matters, it is not uncommon for the energies of the electron beams to be different. Figure 31.20D shows the dose distribution for a junction between a 12-MeV and 16-MeV electron beam, using the same beam parameters as Figure 31.20C. Because the penumbra of the two beams is no longer matched, even though the beam edges are matched, there is a hot spot on the higher-energy side that is probably larger than we would like for a patient treatment. A fairly standard solution for this problem is to *feather* the junction, as shown in Figure 31.21A. In this case, we started by aligning the beams vertically as shown in Figure 31.19B (matching field edges at R_{100}) and

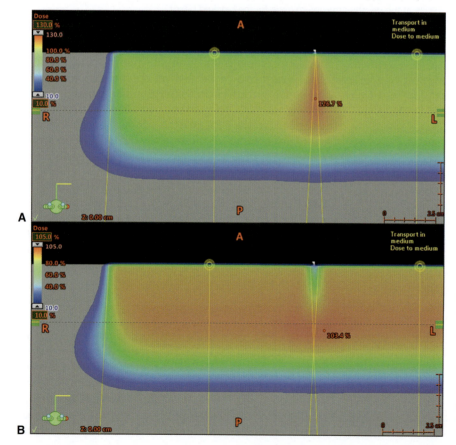

FIGURE 31.19. Calculated dose for two adjacent 12-MeV 10×10 cm² fields at 100-cm SSD incident on a water phantom. The monitor units for each field were set to deliver 100% dose at R_{100} for each field, and the central axes of the fields are separated by (A) 10 cm to junction the fields on the phantom surface and (B) 10.4 cm to junction the fields at the depth of R_{100}. Note that the dose scale for the colorwash is not the same in each panel.

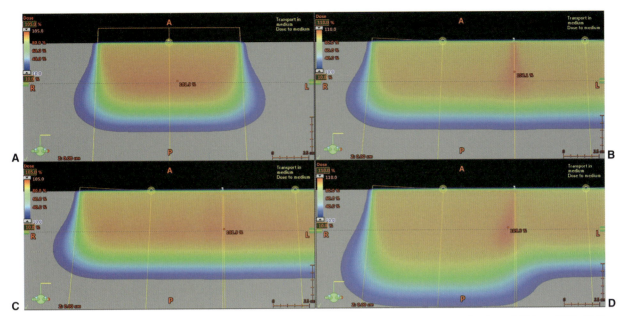

FIGURE 31.20. Calculated dose distributions for electron beam field junctions incident on a water phantom at 100-cm SSD. (A) Two adjacent 12-MeV 10 × 5 cm² fields, with monitor set to deliver 100% dose at R_{100} for a 10 × 10 cm² field. (B) Two adjacent 12-MeV 10 × 10 cm² fields, with monitor set to deliver 100% dose at R_{100}. The beam angles are 2.9° from vertical and the central axes of the fields on the phantom surface are separated by 9.99 cm to align the field edges (as drawn by the TPS) with each other. (C) Two adjacent 12-MeV 10 × 10 cm² fields, with monitor set to deliver 100% dose at R_{100}. The beam angles are 3.2° from vertical and the central axes of the fields are separated by 10.04 cm. (D) Adjacent 12- and 16-MeV 10 × 10 cm² fields, with monitor set to deliver 100% dose at R_{100}. The beam angles are 3.2° from vertical and the central axes of the fields are separated by 10.04 cm.

FIGURE 31.21. Calculated dose for two adjacent feathered 10 × 10 cm² fields (15 × 15 cm² applicator) incident on a water phantom. Each field has two additional subfields with the junction edge moved by 1 cm. The monitor units for each field are equally divided between the subfields, and the total number of monitor units for each field-set was set to deliver 100% dose at R_{100} for a single field. (A) Feathered field junction for 12-MeV fields at 100-cm SSD, where the central axes of the fields are separated by 10.4 cm to junction the fields at the depth of R_{100}. (B) Feathered field junction for 12-MeV and 16-MeV fields at 110-cm SSD, where the central axes of the fields are separated by 11.4 cm to junction the fields at the depth of 3 cm.

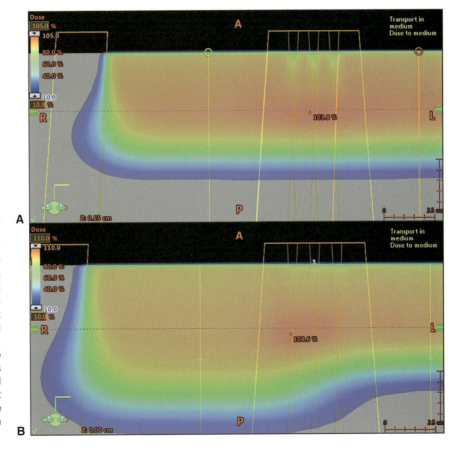

moving the junction edge by ±1 cm. The monitor units for each original field are equally divided into the subfields, and the resulting junction is quite smooth at all depths. There are still three fairly small low-dose regions near the skin surface. This could be improved further by starting with the beam arrangement with the virtual source at the same position (see Fig. 31.20C), but depending on the dosimetric requirements, the simpler method shown in Figure 31.21A is probably adequate. In many cases, using an extended SSD (e.g., 110 cm) is fairly common, and Figure 31.21B shows that this relatively simple approach works quite well even if the energies of the adjacent beams are not the same.

At this point it would be useful to review why this method works as well as it does. Figure 31.22 shows a dose profile at a depth of 3 cm for the junction as shown in Figure 31.21B. For each beam, the penumbra of the feathered edge is much wider than the nonfeathered edge and the width of the feathered penumbra is more dependent on the amount of feathering (±1 cm) than the penumbra width of the electron beam. With a wide penumbra, the summed dose profile does not change significantly for small changes in the junction position, which also explains why the junction is relatively smooth at all depths. A more practical problem is the number of cutouts and the sequence of treatment. One choice is to treat each subfield every day, dividing the monitor units equally as shown in the figure. However, this involves several trips into the treatment room to change the field cutout, which is inconvenient. It is also possible to change the cutouts once per week (for example), which reduces trips into the treatment room. However, there will be a cold spot near the patient surface daily. If the cold spot was a concern, the adjacent field could be matched on the patient surface before feathering the junction, or perhaps be matched at an intermediate depth. It would obviously be nice to have a device and algorithm to automate the edge feathering such as that proposed by Eley et al.[43]

Photon–Electron Field Junctions

It is also possible to have a junction between an electron field and a photon field, an example of which would be the junction between the whole-brain photon fields and the spinal electron field for the craniospinal technique described by Maor et al.[42] A more common example is the internal mammary chain (IMC) electron field commonly used with tangent photon fields for treating chest wall or whole breast. The traditional wisdom about the IMC electron field is that it should be angled a few degrees away from the anterior tangent field because of the bowing of the electron isodose lines. However, it should be angled away from the tangent because, even if the penumbra of the electron field was the same as the photon field, the angle is needed to match the divergence of the electron beam to the posterior edge of the tangent beams.

The difference in penumbra between the photon and electron beams makes a good junction very difficult to achieve. Figure 31.23 shows the result of blindly applying the feathering technique that worked well for electron–electron beam junctions. The resulting dose profile across the junction is not very homogeneous, and another approach is needed. Figure 31.24 shows a lateral dose profile at a depth of 2.8 cm for this junction, and it is a little clearer why this naive approach doesn't work as well as it did for the electron–electron junction. Feathering the junction for the electron beams produces a penumbra that is broad and fairly linear, while feathering the junction of the photon beam produces a stepped profile. While the hot and cold spots are reduced compared to a nonfeathered junction, it is clear that this is not an optimal solution.

The basic field junction problem boils down to matching the field edges and the penumbral profile. Because the photon beam has a very sharp penumbra relative to the electron beam, the amount of feathering (smoothing) required to match the penumbral shape is greater for the photon beam. Figure 31.25 shows one possible approach where the penumbra of the photon beam is feathered to try to match the penumbra of the single electron beam (without feathering). While not as smooth as the electron–electron junction, hot and cold spots in the junction are less than 10%. Further improvements could be made by feathering the electron field edge, and more feathering of the photon field edge to match that. In principle, IMRT optimization could be used to optimize the photon fluence to more accurately match the electron field edge with much less trial and error in planning.

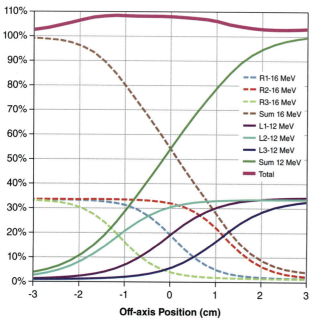

FIGURE 31.22. Calculated lateral dose profile for two adjacent feathered 10 × 10 cm² fields at 110-cm SSD incident on a water phantom (16-MeV on patient right, 12-MeV on patient left) at a depth of 3 cm (see Fig. 31.21B).

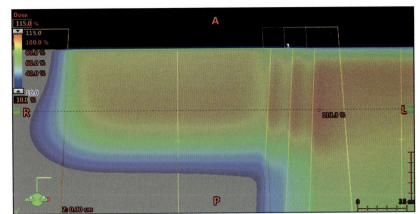

FIGURE 31.23. Calculated dose for two adjacent 10 × 10 cm² fields at 110-cm SSD incident on a water phantom (12-MeV electrons on patient right, 6 MV photons on patient left). Each field has two additional subfields with the junction edge moved by 1 cm. The monitor units for each field were set to deliver 100% dose at a depth of 2.8 cm, and the monitor units for each field were equally divided between the subfields.

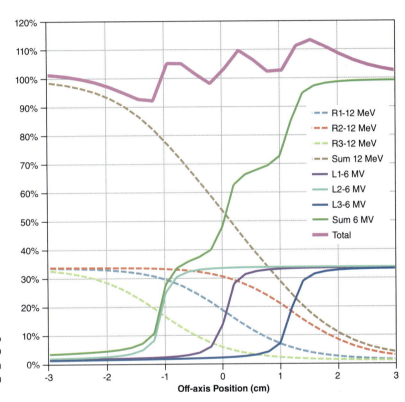

FIGURE 31.24. Calculated lateral dose profile for two adjacent feathered 10 × 10 cm² fields at 110-cm SSD incident on a water phantom (12-MeV electrons on patient right, 6 MV photons on patient left) at a depth of 2.8 cm (see Fig. 31.23).

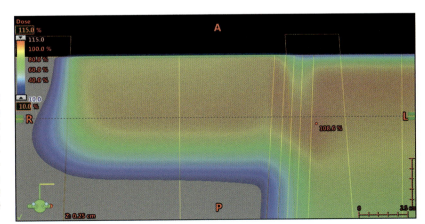

FIGURE 31.25. Calculated dose for two adjacent 10 × 10 cm² fields at 110-cm SSD incident on a water phantom (12-MeV electrons on patient right, 6 MV photons on patient left). The photon field has four additional subfields with the junction edge moved by 0.4 and 0.9 cm. The monitor units for each field were set to deliver 100% dose at a depth of 2.8 cm, and the monitor units for each field were equally divided between the subfields.

Energy Mixing

There are usually five to six choices for electron beam energy on a modern medical linear accelerator, and the typical energy range is 6 to 20 MeV. This gives a maximum therapeutic depth of approximately 6 cm and the spacing between beams is approximately 1 cm in therapeutic depth, as shown in Figure 31.1. There are a couple of ways to deal with target depths that are between the available therapeutic depths. The first method is to add bolus to the patient, either a constant thickness bolus such as superflab, or a commercially available customized electron bolus (BolusECT, .decimal, Inc., Sanford, FL, https:// dotdecimal.com/). A second method is to use a weighted mixture of two energies to get the desired depth coverage. Advantages of this technique are slightly lower surface dose (if that is desired) and not having to deal with a treatment accessory.

Mixing with Photon Beams

Given a situation where an electron beam provides adequate depth penetration but too much skin dose, combining an X-ray beam with an electron beam from the same direction provides a depth dose distribution that is similar to an electron beam with lower surface dose, transitioning to an X-ray depth dose after the electrons range out. Where this transition occurs depends on the electron and X-ray energies, and the beam weights. Modern TPSs should give a reasonable representation of the dose distribution for this situation, except for perhaps the immediate surface, which tends to be problematic for most TPSs. For a more accurate surface dose, measured surface doses are probably required.

MONITOR UNIT VERIFICATION

As mentioned earlier, it is recommended that the monitor units from the TPS be verified using an independent system, and most commonly this is done using a separate computer program. The current AAPM recommendations are contained in the TG-71 report[14] and the formalism used by the monitor unit verification system should be compatible with current recommendations. There are several different ways to accomplish this and it is beyond the scope of this chapter to provide an overview.

SPECIAL TECHNIQUES

Total Skin Electron Irradiation

Total skin electron irradiation (TSEI) was developed to treat the entire skin surface to a homogeneous dose (generally within ±10%) to treat mycosis fungoides, or cutaneous T-cell lymphoma. Once the treatment technique has been designed, there is generally very little treatment planning to be done. AAPM Report 23[44] describes the technique and dosimetry for this technique. Antolak and Hogstrom[45] provided more details on how TSEI beams can be designed for standard techniques, and the dosimetry that can be expected for such a technique was described by Antolak et al.[46] For patients that are unable to stand, a *lying-on-the-floor* technique, such as that described by Deufel and Antolak,[47] can be considered.

Electron Arc Therapy

As pointed out in the AAPM TG-70 report,[6] commercial TPSs do not implement the tools necessary to be able to do electron arc therapy. In particular, while some treatment machines are capable of delivering the treatment fields, there are no commercial TPSs that can calculate the dose distribution for those beams or deal appropriately with the skin collimation that is necessary for this technique. As such, the reader is referred to the AAPM report if they are interested in this historic technique.

Total Limb Irradiation

Wooden et al.[48] described a technique for treating the entire circumference of a limb. In their case, the patient had Kaposi sarcoma, although other indications for such a technique might include melanoma or lymphoma. In some ways, the treatment goal is similar to electron arc therapy in that the target volume is 2 cm or less around the circumference of an extremity. However, the technique that they described uses standard electron fields with a virtual isocenter in the center of the limb and six to eight fields around the limb. Similar to TSEI, the fields should be larger than the limb so that the electron beams can wrap around the limb and each point around the limb is irradiated by multiple beams. Wooden et al. described a methodology where the monitor units could be determined from the prescribed dose and output factor of the open field using a *body factor*, in their case 2.55, although the exact value will depend on the electron energy and the delivery equipment. Using a modern TPS, with the capability to accurately determine monitor units to deliver the required dose, planning becomes more straightforward, although it might be useful to do some sort of *in vivo* dosimetry to verify that the dose delivery is accurate. Using the TPS, it would also be possible to perhaps use different energies from different beam angles to vary the depth of the therapeutic dose region.

The most significant problem when delivering this type of treatment is the setup and immobilization of the patient. The extremity needs to be extended away from the body so that beams can be placed around the extremity. The immobilization can make it difficult or impossible to get the patient into the bore of the CT scanner to get images for treatment planning, so it might be necessary to resort to alternative methods of obtaining or estimating the patient contour for treatment planning, which will not be discussed here. To see how the immobilization might work for such a technique, the reader is referred to the original publication or the AAPM TG-70 report.[6]

THE FUTURE

After intensity-modulated techniques became available for high-energy X-ray beams, a natural progression for electron beams was the development of modulated electron radiation therapy (MERT) by several investigators.[49–54] Intensity modulation can be done with the X-ray *multi-leaf collimator* (MLC)[55–59] or an add-on electron MLC.[43,60,61] The former device is available on virtually every conventional linear accelerator in use today, while the latter device is only available as a research tool. Seuntjens et al. are developing a *few leaf electron collimator* (FLEC) as a simpler device that is capable of some degree of intensity modulation.[62–64] This device is less flexible than a dedicated electron MLC but has the advantage of being lighter

and simpler, which could make it easier to integrate with the treatment machine. Unfortunately, there are no commercial TPSs that are currently able to plan MERT treatments, so while promising, it will require more time before we start seeing MERT used routinely in the clinic.

Although electron beam radiotherapy has been around for many decades, its use in the clinic has been declining over the past several years. Competing technologies include conventional IMRT (including volumetric modulated arc therapy (VMAT)), helical tomotherapy, proton therapy, and HDR brachytherapy, and many of these technologies have seen major improvements in the last couple of decades. Delivery technology for electron beams is much the same as it was decades ago and has not seen the same kind of development. In order to be able to more fully utilize the unique advantages that electron beam radiotherapy offers, we need to convince commercial partners to make improvements to both electron delivery and planning systems.

KEY POINTS

- Megavoltage electron beams are useful for treating target volumes within a few centimeters of the patient surface.

- Understanding scatter effects, in-air and in-patient, is key to understanding the properties of electron beam dose distributions.

- Surface irregularities and heterogeneities scatter and redistribute electrons, giving rise to hot and cold spots in the dose distribution.

- Improved treatment-planning tools are needed to increase the clinical utility of electron beam radiotherapy, and treatment-planning vendors need to be made aware of this need.

- Improved electron delivery tools (e.g., electron MLC, and bolus ECT) are needed to allow electron beam radiotherapy to contribute to more effective delivery of conformal radiation therapy, and treatment machine vendors need to be made aware of this need.

REVIEW QUESTIONS

1. For an electron beam incident on a chest wall with rib heterogeneities, what is the approximate magnitude of the hot spots caused by the ribs?
   A. 3%
   B. 10%
   C. 15%
   D. 20%

2. A 9-MeV electron beam (R_p = 4.5 cm) is incident on a chest wall of thickness 2 cm. Assuming a lung density of 0.33, what is the total range of the electron beam (from the skin surface)?
   A. 2.5 cm
   B. 5.0 cm
   C. 7.5 cm
   D. 10.0 cm

3. What is the thickness of lead required for skin collimation in a 16-MeV electron beam?
   A. 3 mm
   B. 5 mm
   C. 7 mm
   D. 9 mm
   E. 11 mm

4. An electron beam is incident on the patient surface at an angle of 30° relative to perpendicular incidence. Compared to the same beam delivered at perpendicular incidence, the therapeutic depth of the electron beam is
   A. larger
   B. smaller
   C. the same
   D. not enough information

5. As the air gap between the final collimation and the patient increases, the output of an electron beam (dose per MU) decreases
   A. and follows the inverse square law
   B. more slowly than the inverse square law
   C. more rapidly than the inverse square law

ANSWERS

1. A
2. C
3. D
4. B
5. C

REFERENCES

1. Hogstrom KR, Almond PR. Review of electron beam therapy physics. *Phys Med Biol.* 2006;51(13):R455–R489.
2. Slater JM. From X-rays to ion beams: A short history of radiation therapy. In: Linz U, ed. *Ion Beam Therapy.* Berlin Heidelberg: Springer-Verlag; 2012:3–16.
3. Tapley N duV. *Clinical Applications of the Electron Beam.* New York, NY: John Wiley & Sons, Inc.; 1976.
4. Tapley N duV. Radiation therapy with the electron beam. *Semin Oncol.* 1981;8(1):49–58.
5. Khan FM, Doppke KP, Hogstrom KR, Kutcher GJ, Nath R, Prasad SC, et al. Clinical electron-beam dosimetry: report of AAPM Radiation Therapy Committee Task Group No. 25. *Med Phys.* 1991;18(1):73–109.
6. Gerbi BJ, Antolak JA, Deibel FC, Followill DS, Herman MG, Higgins PD, et al. Recommendations for clinical electron beam dosimetry: supplement to the recommendations of Task Group 25. *Med Phys.* 2009;36(7):3239–3279.
7. Gerbi BJ, Antolak JA, Deibel FC, Followill DS, Herman MG, Higgins PD, et al. Erratum: "Recommendations for clinical electron beam dosimetry: supplement to the recommendations of Task Group 25" [Med. Phys. 36, 3239–3279 (2009)]. *Med Phys.* 2010;38(1):548–548.
8. Karlsson M. SP-0110: Electrons, the lost particle: are they still in charge? For the motion! *Radiother Oncol.* 2013; 106:S42.
9. Mackie T. SP-0111: against the motion. *Radiother Oncol.* 2013;106:S42–S43.
10. Klevenhagen SC, Lambert GD, Arbabi A. Backscattering in electron beam therapy for energies between 3 and 35 MeV. *Phys Med Biol.* 1982;27(3):363–373.
11. Popple RA, Weinberg R, Antolak JA, Ye SJ, Pareek PN, Duan J, et al. Comprehensive evaluation of a commercial macro Monte Carlo electron dose calculation implementation using a standard verification data set. *Med Phys.* 2006;33(6):1540–1551.
12. Khan FM, Higgins PD, Gerbi BJ, Deibel FC, Sethi A, Mihailidis DN. Calculation of depth dose and dose per monitor unit for irregularly shaped electron fields. *Phys Med Biol.* 1998;43(10):2741–2754.
13. Shiu AS, Tung SS, Nyerick CE, Ochran TG, Otte VA, Boyer AL, et al. Comprehensive analysis of electron beam central axis dose for a radiotherapy linear accelerator. *Med Phys.* 1994;21(4):559–566.
14. Gibbons JP, Antolak JA, Followill DS, Huq MS, Klein EE, Lam KL, et al. Monitor unit calculations for external photon and electron beams: report of the AAPM Therapy Physics Committee Task Group No. 71. *Med Phys.* 2014;41(3):31501.
15. Fraass B, Doppke K, Hunt M, Kutcher G, Starkschall G, Stern R, et al. American Association of Physicists in Medicine Radiation Therapy Committee Task Group 53: quality assurance for clinical radiotherapy treatment planning. *Med Phys.* 1998;25(10):1773–1829.
16. Kutcher GJ, Coia L, Gillin MT, Hanson WF, Leibel S, Morton RJ, et al. Comprehensive QA for radiation oncology: report of AAPM Radiation Therapy Committee Task Group 40. *Med Phys.* 1994;21(4):581–618.
17. Hogstrom KR, Mills MD, Almond PR. Electron beam dose calculations. *Phys Med Biol.* 1981;26(3):445–459.
18. Khan FZ. *The Physics of Radiation Therapy.* Baltimore, MD: Williams & Wilkins; 1984:456 p.
19. Hogstrom KR, Steadham RE, Wong PF, Shiu AS. Monitor unit calculations for electron beams. In: Gibbons JP, ed. *Monitor Unit Calculations for External Photon and Electron Beams.* Middleton, WI: Advanced Medical Publishing, Inc.; 2000:113–125.
20. Hogstrom KR, Steadham RE. Electron beam dose computation. In: Palta J, Mackie TR, eds. *Teletherapy: Present and Future.* Madison, WI: Advanced Medical Publishing; 1996:137–174.
21. Mills MD, Hogstrom KR, Fields RS. Determination of electron beam output factors for a 20-MeV linear accelerator. *Med Phys.* 1985;12(4):473–476.
22. Khan FM, Higgins PD. Calculation of depth dose and dose per monitor unit for irregularly shaped electron fields: an addendum. *Phys Med Biol.* 1999;44(6):N77–N80.
23. Khan FM, Higgins PD. Field equivalence for clinical electron beams. *Phys Med Biol.* 2001;46(1):N9–N14.
24. Higgins PD, Gerbi BJ, Khan FM. Application of measured pencil beam parameters for electron beam model evaluation. *Med Phys.* 2003;30(4):514–520.
25. Low DA, Starkschall G, Bujnowski SW, Wang LL, Hogstrom KR. Electron bolus design for radiotherapy treatment planning: bolus design algorithms. *Med Phys.* 1992;19(1):115–124.
26. Antolak JA, Starkschall G, Bawiec Jr. ER, Ewton JR, Hogstrom KR. Clinical implementation of customized electron bolus. *Med Phys.* 1994;21(6):901.
27. Boyd RA, Hogstrom KR, Antolak JA, Rosenthal DI. Custom electron bolus treatment planning with skin collimation using the pencil-beam redefinition algorithm. *Int J Radiat Oncol Biol Phys.* 2003;57(2):S425.
28. Starkschall G, Antolak JA, Hogstrom KR. Electron-beam bolus for 3-D conformal radiation therapy. In: Purdy JA, Emami B, eds. *3D Radiation Treatment Planning and Conformal Therapy Symposium.* Madison, WI: St. Louis, MO: Medical Physics Publishing; 1993:265–282.
29. Low DA, Starkschall G, Sherman NE, Bujnowski SW, Ewton JR, Hogstrom KR. Computer-aided design and fabrication of an electron bolus for treatment of the paraspinal muscles. *Int J Radiat Oncol Biol Phys.* 1995;33(5):1127–1138.
30. Perkins GH, McNeese MD, Antolak JA, Buchholz TA, Strom EA, Hogstrom KR. A custom three-dimensional electron bolus technique for optimization of postmastectomy irradiation. *Int J Radiat Oncol Biol Phys.* 2001;51(4):1142–1151.
31. Kudchadker R, Antolak JA, Morrison WH, Hogstrom KR. Conformal head and neck radiotherapy using custom electron bolus. *Med Phys.* 2002;29(6):1337.
32. Kudchadker R, Hogstrom KR, Antolak JA. Electron conformal therapy combining bolus and intensity modulation. *Med Phys.* 2001;28(6):1227–1228.
33. Almond PR, Biggs PJ, Coursey BM, Hanson WF, Huq MS, Nath R, et al. AAPM's TG-51 protocol for clinical reference dosimetry of high-energy photon and electron beams. *Med Phys.* 1999;26(9):1847–1870.
34. IAEA. *Absorbed Dose Determination in External Beam Radiotherapy.* Technical Report Series. Vienna, Austria: IAEA; 2000.
35. Shiu AS, Tung SS, Hogstrom KR, Wong JW, Gerber RL, Harms WB, et al. Verification data for electron beam dose algorithms. *Med Phys.* 1992 May 1;19(3):623–636.

36. Boyd RA, Hogstrom KR, Antolak JA, Shiu AS. A measured data set for evaluating electron-beam dose algorithms. *Med Phys.* 2001;28(6):950–958.

37. Rogers DWO, Faddegon BA, Ding GX, Ma CM, We J, Mackie TR. BEAM: a Monte Carlo code to simulate radiotherapy treatment units. *Med Phys.* 1995;22(5):503–524.

38. Boyd RA, Hogstrom KR, Starkschall G. Electron pencil-beam redefinition algorithm dose calculations in the presence of heterogeneities. *Med Phys.* 2001;28(10):2096–2104.

39. ICRU. *Prescribing, Recording and Reporting Electron Beam Therapy.* Oxford: Oxford University Press; 2004.

40. ICRU. Prescribing, recording, and reporting photon beam therapy. Bethesda, MD: International Commission on Radiation Units and Measurements; 1993.

41. ICRU. ICRU Report 62 -1999 -Prescribing, Recording and Reporting Photon Beam Therapy (Supplement to ICRU Report 50). Journal of ICRU. Bethesda, MD: International Commission on Radiation Units and Measurements; 1999.

42. Maor MH, Fields RS, Hogstrom KR, van Eys J. Improving the therapeutic ratio of craniospinal irradiation in medulloblastoma. *Int J Radiat Oncol Biol Phys.* 1985;11(4):687–697.

43. Eley JG, Hogstrom KR, Matthews KL, Parker BC, Price MJ. Potential of discrete Gaussian edge feathering method for improving abutment dosimetry in eMLC-delivered segmented-field electron conformal therapy. *Med Phys.* 2011;38(12):6610–6622.

44. AAPM, American Institute of Physics I. *AAPM Report No. 23, Total Skin Electron Therapy: Technique and Dosimetry.* New York, NY: American Institute of Physics, Inc.; 1988.

45. Antolak JA, Hogstrom KR. Multiple scattering theory for total skin electron beam design. *Med Phys.* 1998;25(6):851–859.

46. Antolak JA, Cundiff JH, Ha CS. Utilization of thermoluminescent dosimetry in total skin electron beam radiotherapy of mycosis fungoides. *Int J Radiat Oncol Biol Phys.* 1998;40(1):101–108.

47. Deufel CL, Antolak JA. Total skin electron therapy in the lying-on-the-floor position using a customized flattening filter to eliminate field junctions. *J Appl Clin Med Phys.* 2013;14(5):115–126.

48. Wooden KK, Hogstrom KR, Blum P, Gastorf RJ, Cox JD. Whole-limb irradiation of the lower calf using a six-field electron technique. *Med Dosim.* 1996;21(4):211–218.

49. Lee MC, Jiang SB, Ma CM. Monte Carlo and experimental investigations of multileaf collimated electron beams for modulated electron radiation therapy. *Med Phys.* 2000;27(12):2708–2718.

50. Ma CM, Pawlicki T, Lee MC, Jiang SB, Li JS, Deng J, et al. Energy- and intensity-modulated electron beams for radiotherapy. *Phys Med Biol.* 2000;45(8):2293–2311.

51. Ma CM, Ding M, Li JS, Lee MC, Pawlicki T, Deng J. A comparative dosimetric study on tangential photon beams, intensity-modulated radiation therapy (IMRT) and modulated electron radiotherapy (MERT) for breast cancer treatment. *Phys Med Biol.* 2003;48(7):909–924.

52. Das SK, Bell M, Marks LB, Rosenman JG. A preliminary study of the role of modulated electron beams in intensity modulated radiotherapy, using automated beam orientation and modality selection. *Int J Radiat Oncol Biol Phys.* 2004;59(2):602–617.

53. Henzen D, Manser P, Frei D, Volken W, Neuenschwander H, Born EJ, et al. Forward treatment planning for modulated electron radiotherapy (MERT) employing Monte Carlo methods. *Med Phys.* 2014;41(3):1–10.

54. Eldib A, Jin L, Martin J, Fan J, Li J, Chibani O, et al. Investigating the dosimetric benefits of modulated electron radiation therapy (MERT) for partial scalp patients. *Biomed Phys Eng Express.* 2017;3(3):035013.

55. Klein EE, Li Z, Low DA. Feasibility study of multileaf collimated electrons with a scattering foil based accelerator. *Radiother Oncol.* 1996;41(2):189–196.

56. Klein EE. Modulated electron beams using multi-segmented multileaf collimation. *Radiother Oncol.* 1998;48(3):307–311.

57. Weinberg R, Antolak JA, Hogstrom KR, Starkschall G, Kudchadker RJ, White RA, et al. Electron intensity modulation with multileaf collimation for mixed-beam partial breast irradiation. *Int J Radiat Oncol Biol Phys.* 2008;72(1):S527.

58. Klein EE, Mamalui-Hunter M, Low DA. Delivery of modulated electron beams with conventional photon multi-leaf collimators. *Phys Med Biol.* 2009;54(2):327–339.

59. Míguez C, Jiménez-Ortega E, Palma BA, Miras H, Ureba A, Arráns R, et al. Clinical implementation of combined modulated electron and photon beams with conventional MLC for accelerated partial breast irradiation. *Radiother Oncol.* 2017;124(1):124–129.

60. Hogstrom KR, Boyd RA, Antolak JA, Svatos MM, Faddegon BA, Rosenman JG. Dosimetry of a prototype retractable eMLC for fixed-beam electron therapy. *Med Phys.* 2004;31(3):443–462.

61. Gauer T, Sokoll J, Cremers F, Harmansa R, Luzzara M, Schmidt R. Characterization of an add-on multileaf collimator for electron beam therapy. *Phys Med Biol.* 2008;53(4):1071–1085.

62. Al-Yahya K, Schwartz M, Shenouda G, Verhaegen F, Freeman C, Seuntjens JP. Energy modulated electron therapy using a few leaf electron collimator in combination with IMRT and 3D-CRT: Monte Carlo-based planning and dosimetric evaluation. *Med Phys.* 2005;32(9):2976–2986.

63. Al-Yahya K, Verhaegen F, Seuntjens JP. Design and dosimetry of a few leaf electron collimator for energy modulated electron therapy. *Med Phys.* 2007;34(12):4782–4791.

64. Connell T, Alexander A, Evans M, Seuntjens JP. An experimental feasibility study on the use of scattering foil free beams for modulated electron radiotherapy. *Phys Med Biol.* 2012;57(11):3259–3272.

32 Proton Beam Therapy

Hanne M. Kooy, Judith Adams, and Nicolas Depauw

HISTORY

Proton beam radiotherapy advances the central aim of radiation therapy: Reduce healthy tissue dose and increase malignant tissue dose. Proton beam radiotherapy was the first modality to demonstrate this axiom in hitherto untreatable disease.

Robert R Wilson at the Harvard Cyclotron Laboratory recognized the clinical potential of a proton beam in his article of 1947,[1] which proposed the use of the geometric and dosimetric localization properties of a monoenergetic proton beam to treat targets inside the body. The practicality was in doubt as available proton beams had insufficient penetrating energy: The first Harvard Cyclotron, built in 1937, had an energy of 12 MeV equal to 17 mm range! This cyclotron was moved to Los Alamos for the Manhattan project in 1943 and replaced in 1947 with the second Harvard Cyclotron with an initial energy of 90 MeV (6.4 cm range in water) and later upgraded to 160 MeV (17.7 cm range in water) in 1955. It was another 12 year before his vision became a reality.[2]

Proton beam radiotherapy has been used as a definitive modality as early as 60 years ago. Its recent emergence as a viable technology is a consequence of its historical success in treating otherwise incurable disease, the continued desire for increased conformal radiation therapy and the commercial availability of proton beam equipment. Proton radiotherapy was, ab initio, a conformal modality but only sparsely available; photon radiotherapy was a therapeutic analog to planar X-ray imaging and broadly available. Proton and photon radiotherapy, now, are competitive and the optimal use of either an important question.

Proton radiotherapy from its inception required careful attention to now standard-of-care detail because of the precision afforded by the proton beam even while the supporting technologies were minimal. The early adopters were neurosurgeons: Dr. Lars Leksell[3] in Stockholm Sweden and Dr. Raymond Kjellberg in Boston USA.[4] Neurosurgeons understand 3-dimensional (3D) cranial anatomy as visualized on X-rays at a time when computed tomography (CT) was not yet available. The early use was in abnormalities visible on those X-rays such as pituitary and arterio-venous abnormalities. Easy access to a proton beam at the Harvard Cyclotron Laboratory at Harvard University allowed Dr. Kjellberg to establish a proton radiosurgery program that continues to date. Dr. Leksell did not have this convenience and looked for alternatives culminating in the gamma knife.

Treatment of ocular melanomas also was an early adopter. The orbital anatomy and the use of x-ray opaque markers at the target margin provided sufficient information to apply proton beams.[5] Ocular melanoma treatments were a first application of 3D treatment planning with an emphasis on the 3D placement of the beam with respect to the target.[6] Consistent planning methodologies allowed for effective patient follow-up.[7]

Early adapters used existing post-nuclear research cyclotrons. Many, at Clatterbridge UK for example, were of low energy and could only be used for ocular targets. A few, at Harvard University (USA) and in Orsay (France) for example, had sufficient energy to treat internal targets. The treatment of those targets did not commence until the late 70s when CT volumetric imaging was available and the treatment planning tools were developed.[8,9] It is the treatment of those targets that introduced proton radiotherapy to the general practice of radiotherapy. Proton radiotherapy introduced many of the elements of "modern" conformal radiotherapy: attention to the details of imaging, setup, treatment planning, and delivery.

BASIC PROPERTIES OF A PROTON BEAM

A proton, as an ionizing particle, looses energy along its track as a function of the local stopping power (energy loss per length). The stopping power increases rapidly near the end of the track and results in a very large dose enhancement, the Bragg peak, at the end of the particle track. The large mass of the proton (938.3 MeV/c^2) results in near parallel tracks and all protons superimpose Bragg peaks at the same depth. The small mass of electrons (0.511 MeV/c^2) results in large scattered tracks, which smear the electron Bragg peak and only a distinct distal fall-off remains. A proton beam thus has 3D shaping features, in depth and laterally, compared to the 2D, lateral, controls in a photon beam.

The near-straight tracks of the protons produce a beam whose penumbral edge is intrinsically sharp. The individual protons undergo (primarily) multiple Coulomb scattering events, which result in a Gaussian-shaped broadening of an initially parallel proton beam. Safai et al.[10] describe the depth and energy properties of spread-out Bragg peak (SOBP) and pencil-beam scanning field penumbrae. They show (see Figure 5 there and adapted here as Fig. 32.1) that an aperture-collimated SOBP field offers a sharper penumbra below 150 mm at which the 80% to 20% penumbra is about 7 mm at depth. At higher ranges, the pencil-beam scanned (PBS) field penumbra changes little to about 9 mm at 300 mm range while the SOBP field increases to about 14 mm. The PBS field penumbra below 150 MeV can be improved through the use of apertures or Multi-Leaf Collimators.

The proton beam penumbra is also sharper compared to a single photon beam penumbra at depths below approximately 160 mm (in water). This single beam penumbra is relevant when one wishes to achieve the sharpest lateral fall-off of dose between a target and a critical structure. Proton beam treatments in the head-and-neck achieve, for example, a sharper lateral fall-off in a target around the brainstem compared to a photon beam treatment. A prostate or deep-seated targets, however, do not show a penumbral advantage for a proton beam but do show significant normal tissue sparing. Each site offers different opportunities.

In practice, it is the composite penumbra of multiple fields that determines the sharpest achievable penumbra and the integral dose "bath" in the patient. Photon beams have no localization ability along depth and "pass" through the target. Proton beams, in contrast, deposit no dose beyond the distal edge of the Bragg peak. This simple difference means that a composite of multiple proton beams will have approximately half the integral dose of a similarly arranged set of photon beams (see Fig. 32.2).

A single proton field is a composite of multiple individual dose-weighted Bragg peaks (see Fig. 8.1 in Chapter 8). A pencil-beam scanning field can deliver a modulated dose distribution to a target volume while scattered proton fields are constrained to deliver homogeneous dose. A single proton field can achieve superior dose shaping by virtue of the lateral penumbra and the distal fall-off that spares distal tissues (Fig. 32.3). The distal Bragg peak fall-off has the sharpest dose gradient (about half of the lateral penumbra) and would offer the best opportunity to achieve a dose differential between target and healthy tissues. In practice the range in patient has an uncertainty estimated on the order of 2.5% to 3.5%[11] (or ±5 mm for 160 mm range). One contribution is in the uncertainty in (relative) stopping power converted from CT Hounsfield Units to Relative (to water) Stopping Power.[12] The distal edge cannot be used to achieve a dose gradient between the target and a critical structure as this could result in a direct overshoot into the critical structure! Proton range

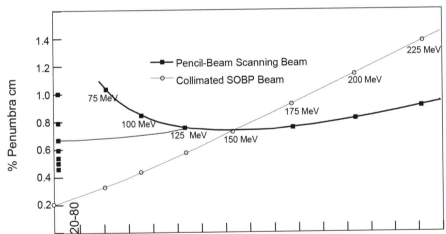

FIGURE 32.1. Adapted from Safai S, Bortfeld T, Engelsman M. Comparison between the lateral penumbra of a collimated double-scattered beam and uncollimated scanning beam in proton radiotherapy. *Phys Med Biol.* 2008;53:1729–1750, with permission of IOP Publishing. All rights reserved. The penumbra near the end of range for a PBS field (solid squares on the solid line and marked with the range-equivalent energy) and collimated SOBP field (open circles) as a function of range (depth) in water. The SOBP field has a continuously increasing penumbra as a function of depth. That is, a field of 150 mm range has a penumbra (20%–80%) of 2 mm at the entrance and increases (mostly along the dashed curve) to 7 mm at range-depth. The PBS field entrance penumbra is shown as solid-squares next to the y-axis (and emphasized for 125 MeV). The SOBP field penumbra is initially very sharp because of the aperture collimation the aperture placement as close as possible to the patient. The aperture effect decreases at increasing depth (range) and overtakes the intrinsic proton scatter penumbra above 150 MeV (or about 150 mm range). The PBS field penumbra varies little from the entrance penumbra to depth. The use of apertures, or MLC, in PBS field will improve this entrance penumbra essentially in line with the SOBP field results. The PBS field penumbra in-air (and on skin) is governed by the beamline optics that determine the beam emittance as it exits the nozzle. In the figure, the initial spread is taken as a constant over range as 3 mm.
MLC; PBS, pencil-beam scanning; SOBP, Spreadout Bragg Peak.

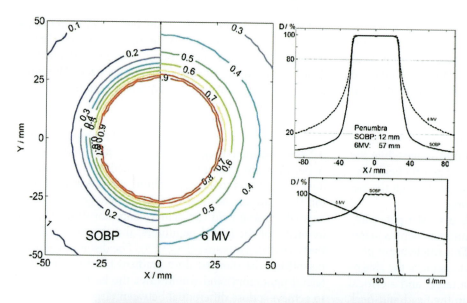

FIGURE 32.2. Consider a full arc of a proton SOBP field compared to a photon field whose depth doses are shown bottom-right. The resultant depth-doses are compared as profiles in the top-right and as isodoses (where the left half shows the SOBP isodoses and the right the photon isodoses). The volumetric reduction in dose is significant. SOBP, Spreadout Bragg Peak.

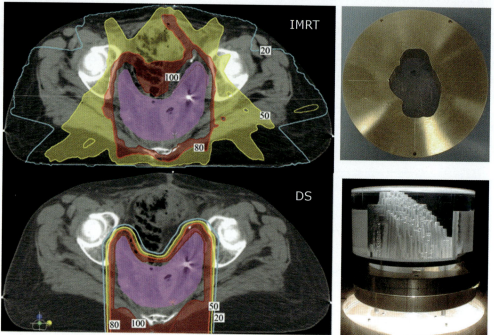

FIGURE 32.3. Treatment plans, IMRT and a single SOBP field, for endometrial nodal disease are compared. The IMRT plan uses seven fields and has an unavoidable dose bath (yellow between 50% and 80% isodose lines). The SOBP plan achieves coverage with a single posterior aperture and range-compensator field (examples of these devices [not those used for this treatment] are shown on the right). The aperture, as for a photon beam, achieves lateral Beam's Eye View conformance. The range-compensator shifts the proton penetration range in proportion to the local thickness to conform the dose to the distal surface of the target volume. Note that for an SOBP field, the entrance dose cannot be controlled and results for this case in near full skin dose.
IMRT; SOBP, Spreadout Bragg Peak.

imaging may allow sufficient improvement in location of the distal peak to increase the safe use of the distal edge.[13]

Proton dose distributions are biologically equivalent to photon dose distributions except for a constant radiological biological effect (RBE) factor of 1.1. That is, a photon dose of 54 Gy (Co60 equivalent) equals a physical, i.e., measured in an ionization chamber, proton dose of 54/1.1, or 49.1 Gy. Proton dose distributions are therefore stated as 54 Gy (RBE)[14] to indicate that the physical dose has been corrected by the RBE factor and

compares directly to a an equivalent photon dose distribution of 54 Gy. Dose-response knowledge from photon radiotherapy can thus be transferred to proton radiotherapy. This is a major advantage in the clinical application of proton radiotherapy. The RBE of heavier charged particles, Lithium and beyond, introduces significant complexities and unknowns in dose reporting. The calculation of differential biological effects is of great interest with the ability of pencil-beam scanning to modulate such effects.[15]

GENERATION OF CLINICAL PROTON FIELDS

A proton field is a composite of (1) SOBP fields, where each layer is of uniform intensity and superpositioned peaks form a flat dose plateau or (2) numerous individual scanned narrow pencil-beams, PBS fields, of arbitrary intensity that form an arbitrary dose profile. Both require an accelerator and its beam transport system to deliver a narrow mono-energetic beam of protons at the entrance of the field-creating nozzle. SOBP fields were the original mode of radiotherapy where mechanical means alone could be used to create a desired field. PBS fields utilize the full flexibility of a proton delivery system and have now replaced SOBP fields.

The generation of a clinical proton beam requires an accelerator to achieve a desirable clinical energy range of up to about 250 MeV. The latter corresponds to about 38 cm in water and is considered good maximum choice given the deepest seated targets. The lowest minimum range is about 3 to 4 cm (60 MeV) and is needed for orbital and other shallow targets.

Accelerator technology for radiotherapy is varied and complex.[16] Originally, cyclotrons were favored due to their historical availability and high current required for scattered fields. The use of scattered fields, however, has been now supplanted by pencil-beam scanning fields whose planning and treatment requirements now are the determinants of a particular technology for beam generation[17] and vendors offer various configurations and treatment delivery technologies.

Of particular relevance in any new proton system configuration is the integration of volumetric imaging technologies whose requirements in the proton setting exceed those in the photon setting to include volumetric imaging for in-patient stopping power[18] and in-patient range localication.[13]

SPREADOUT BRAGG PEAK FIELDS

SOBP fields are, primarily, produced by mechanical means but can also be produced by a combination of electromagnetical scanning and mechanical means. Here, we assume a scattered SOBP field. An initially narrow proton beam of a given energy, typically the highest in-patient desired range, is shifted to lower energies and spread in depth by different thickness absorbers, broadened and flattened laterally by carefully designed scatterers, and "stacked" with appropriate weights by synchronizing absorber insertion with monitor units or another integrated beam current measure.[19] SOBP fields produce homogeneous dose per field over a desired modulation width up to a maximum range.

An SOBP field is defined by two geometric parameters: (i) the range of its distal fall-off and (ii) the modulation width of the uniform plateau. In our practice, the range R of the SOBP field is the 90% fall-off of the deepest pristine Bragg peak and the modulation width is the distance between the range and the proximal 98% of the plateau dose. The third parameter is, of course, the prescription dose to the plateau as derived from treatment planning.

Field Shaping Devices

Scattered fields are shaped laterally by apertures and in depth by range-compensators.

Apertures are collimated to the beam's eye view projection of the target volume and require a distance of 7 to 12 mm (for prostate for example) between the target edge and aperture edge to account for the depth-dependent penumbra and setup uncertainties. The apertures thickness must suffice to fully absorb the incident range as a proton field changes little in intensity as it passes through an absorber. Insufficient thickness will result in full-dose to the patient!

The use of a range-compensator is unique to proton and heavy charged particles. The range-compensator adjusts the range across the lateral field profile such that the resultant distal dose surface closely matches the distal target volume surface. A range-compensator spares tissues distal to the target.

The thickness of the target volume, measured as the difference between the deepest and shallowest radiological pathlengths in the target volume, determine the desired maximum range of the SOBP field and the desired modulation width. The combination of an aperture and range-compensator thus achieves, for a single SOBP field, lateral and distal conformation and homogeneous dose in the target volume (see Fig. 32.3).

The aperture is placed as close as possible to the patient to reduce the effect of the large effective proton source, which has a spread on the order of 5 to 10 cm compared to 1 to 2 mm for a photon beam! The penumbra of this source can only be mitigated by, first, placing it as far as possible from the patient, i.e., at a source-to-axis distance (SAD) $\approx$ 3000 mm, and de-magnification by the aperture-patient distance over the aperture-source distance. Thus, in clinical practice, the effective source size is de-magnified 40-fold and its contribution to the penumbra for double scattered fields is on the order of 5%.

The design of the range-compensator considers individual radiological pathlengths from the source to the distal surface and sets the range-compensator thickness such that the distal fall-off of the SOBP is just beyond the target distal surface. Consider the "open" field maximum range R_d that reaches just beyond the deepest point P_d on the target distal surface. We wish to insert material for every other point P_i on the target distal surface equal to $T_i = R_d - R_i$, where R_i is radiological pathlength to point P_i. The range-compensator is constructed given the thicknesses T_i. The local range R_d shifts as it passes through the range-compensator along each ray from the source such that the distal edge of the proton composite dose distribution lies just beyond the target distal surface. The range-compensator is smeared to correct for setup uncertainties

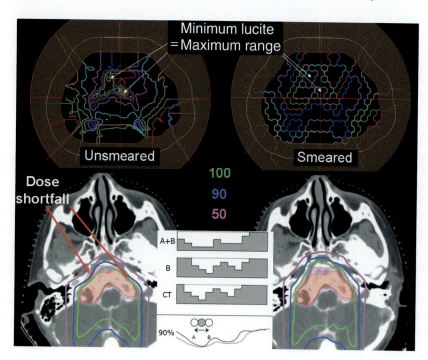

FIGURE 32.4. The use of range-compensators requires two steps, smearing and tapering, to achieve satisfactory target coverage. Smearing considers each point on the range compensator and replaces the thickness of that point with the minimum thickness found at other points within a smearing radius of the point under consideration. This has the effect to "throw" the dose deeper into the patient (see bottom-right compared to bottom-left). The middle insert illustrates the example where the CT represents the unsmeared compensator, while B (and similarly A) is the compensator if a shift were to occur. The composite compensator considers positions A and B. Smearing, originally, was introduced to compensate for geometric uncertainties by considering the "worst" case penetration range within a region. Tapering considers range-compensator gradients along the aperture edge and applies a smoothing to those gradients to remove scattering artifacts. In general, support for smearing and tapering is poor within existing treatment planning systems and requires considerable knowledge on the treatment planner to achieve a satisfactory result.

(see Figure 32.4). The ray-tracing method does not accurately consider the effect of proton scatter and a more accurate method uses dosimetric optimization of the range-compensator thickness such that the desired dose is achieved at the distal surface.

Known uncertainties in the patient or target position, caused by setup errors or otherwise, create variations in pathlengths that could lead to an underdose of the target or an overshoot into the healthy tissues. The range-compensator profile is, therefore, "smeared" where each point is assigned the largest range (or least thickness) from among the points in its neighborhood within a radius corresponding to the total expected variation (see Figure 32.4). This ensures worst-case coverage of the distal target surface in the presence of these variations. It does, however, push the distal fall-off dose further into the healthy tissues. This, and the inherent uncertainty in range stated earlier, means that the distal fall-off of the SOBP cannot be used to shape a gradient between the target volume and a critical structure.

Scattered fields can be mechanically dose-shaped in three dimensions with apertures and range-compensators, mechanically compensate for uncertainties and mechanically delivered with rotating modulation wheels. These were key features that allowed for the early use of proton radiotherapy and made proton radiotherapy the first conformal modality.

Absolute Dosimetry

The dose in the SOBP field is monitored by an upstream ionization chamber of finite size (for example $\phi = 20$ mm) in the uniform lateral area of the field. The relationship between physical dose (in Gy, converted to biological

effective dose by multiplying by RBE = 1.1) in the SOBP plateau and monitor unit (MU) is complicated. In principle, one could calibrate each pristine Bragg peak in units of Gy per MU or number of protons. This relationship for scattered fields is impractical even for the simplest beamlines. In general, the complex secondary interactions in a dual-scattering system and the variability of device settings preclude such a calibration or derivation.

One can establish an semi-theoretical relationship for the output factor Ψ (in Gy/MU) between MU and physical dose in water.[20] The SOBP output factor is the ratio between dose in the SOBP plateau and dose (i.e., MU) measured in the reference ionization chamber. The latter, in turn, is proportional to the entrance dose D0 of the SOBP. Thus Ψ is proportional to the ratio of DP/D0, which can be derived as described in and equals

$$\Psi(R,M) \;=\; \Psi_R \times \frac{D_0^R}{D_0(R,M)} \;=\; \Psi_R \times \frac{D_0^R}{100/(1+a\,r^b)}$$

(32.1)

where D_0^R is the SOBP entrance dose of the reference SOBP, which has an output factor Ψ_R, and the entrance dose $D_0(R,M)$ of the SOBP of interest (of range R and modulation M) is described by the two-parameter function $(1+ar^b)/100$ characterized by a form factor $r = (R-M)/M$ and the parameters, a and b have the theoretical values of 0.44 and 0.6 respectively.[21] In practice, a and b differ due to the secondary effects in the nozzle and are derived from measurement. Finally, the factor of 100 indicates our reference use of 100 for the open-field plateau dose.

In clinical practice, the applicability of eq. 32.1 depends on details of the delivery system. In our practice, the formula is successfully applied to both our radiosurgery single-scattering beamline and our dual-scattering large field gantry nozzle. The analytical model of eq. 32.1 removes the need for individual measurement of patient field output factors. The parameters *a* and *b* are obtained from calibration and are constant for each option. In general, eq. 32.1 will apply to a constant configuration of a nozzle where the SOBP shaping devices do not change, which is the case in the IBA[1] nozzle for each option.

Example Treatment Plan—Part 1

The example is a pediatric cervical chordoma, which has as critical structures the brainstem, cord, cochlea, and chiasm. The prescription dose is 50.4 Gy(RBE) to the clinical target volume (CTV) and 79.2 Gy (RBE) to the gross target volume (GTV). Dose constraints are chiasm below 62 Gy (RBE), brainstem and cord center (surface) below 55 (67) Gy (RBE), and cochlea below 60 Gy (RBE). The treatment approach reflects a long experience in sequencing the fields.

The first set of five fields to the CTV have gantry angles of 70, 100, 230, and 260 at a couch angle of 0 and a gantry angle of 155 at a couch angle of 90. The main objective of this field arrangement is to reduce the dose to the parotid glands with less consideration to the spinal cord. Each field, in the scattered field (DS) delivery, covers the CTV to homogeneous dose. The DS fields are not delivered in each treatment session; instead triplets of rotating combinations are used. Figure 32.5 shows the normalized dose distribution for a single field and the composite dose distributions for all five fields.

The GTV fields must avoid the brainstem and spinal cord, which were included in the CTV fields. For SOBP fields this can only be achieved by patch combinations. A patch combination is the proton equivalent of field edge matching. Given the finite range of the proton, one can now also patch the distal edge of one field to the penumbral edge of another field (Fig. 32.6). Each field delivers full dose within its sub-target volume and the combination of patch fields achieves full dose to the target volume. As noted before, however, the uncertainty in the distal range can lead to a cold or a hot spot. As a consequence, patch combinations are always "switched" around to feather this hot or cold spot. The construction of patch-field combinations for scattered SOBP fields is cumbersome in spite of some available support in treatment planning systems. Pencil-beam scanning with Intensity-Modulated Proton Therapy (IMPT) (where each field can assume arbitrary intensity-modulated dose) fields allows for automatic patching by specifying constraints for the overall dose in the target including the transitions regions. For illustrations purposes (Fig. 32.7) we use one of the three DS patch-field combination (in fact a "double" patch) and use the optimization engine to "auto-patch" the field without the use of an aperture and range-compensator. The results is (probably) more robust to cold or hot spots as the individual field dose distributions present a more gradual distal fall-off compared to the "true" pristine peak dose falloff.

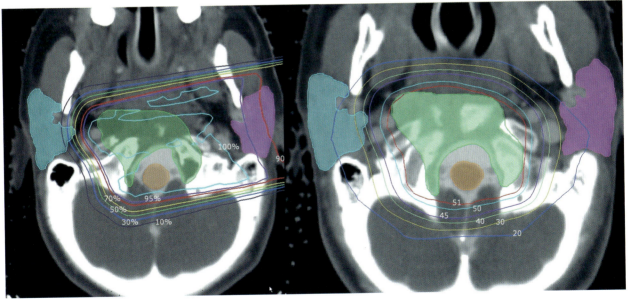

FIGURE 32.5. An example of a double-scattered field delivery to the CTV (green). Each of the five fields achieve full target coverage (>98% isodose line—not shown). Note how each field arrangement (one of which is shown on the left) spares the contralateral parotid. The full complement of five fields reduces the parotid dose to about 20% of 50 Gy (RBE) as only one field passes through each parotid. Note that the fixed modulation of the DS SOBP cannot control the entrance dose (as visible in left figure where the 95% isodose line crosses the parotid). The composite dose distribution (in Gy (RBE)) is on the right. The maximum dose to the CTV is 51 Gy (RBE) and indicates the high degree of homogeneity achievable with SOBP fields.
CTV, clinical target volume.

[1]IBA International, Louvain-la-Neuve Belgium

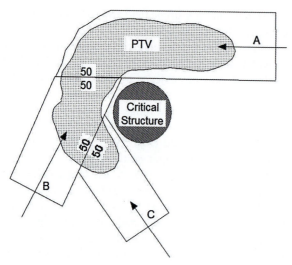

FIGURE 32.6. A Through-Patch combination can sculpt dose around a critical structure. The Through field (left) irradiates a subpart of the target (top-left) with an aperture and a compensator that treats to the distal surface of the subpart. A Patch (right-posterior) treats part of the subpart using an aperture and range-compensator, which now aims to achieve a dose match at the lateral edge of the Through field. A final second patch to the first patch treats the remainder. The Through-Patch match at the lateral edge is difficult as the distal edge of the Patch field is sharper compared to the lateral aperture edge of the Through field. In our practice, 35% of fields are patched achieved with an automated algorithm to create such fields.

Thus, any over- or undershoot effect is minimized by the lower gradient. We expect, in the clinical practice of pencil-beam scanning and subject to further validation, to continue to use the DS field approaches as these have inherent robust properties such as target avoidance with the penumbral edge and distal edges away from critical structures. Even with available robust optimization techniques, these DS field approaches retain their use.

Figure 32.8 shows the total, CTV + GTV, dose distributions for both the IMPT and DS plans. The IMPT plan does significantly improve on the parotid glands, which are primarily located in the integral dose region, which—as stated before—can be reduced on average by 50% with protons and even more with IMPT. In general, however, the DS plan is competitive with the IMPT plan and, in general, we do not expect as dramatic a change between IMPT and DS compared to IMRT and 3D conformal. Instead, PBS significantly reduces the treatment planning overhead to create the numerous DS fields (12 for this case) to achieve the patched dose distributions in patient.

SCANNED PROTON FIELDS

The PSI[2] team[22] demonstrated the technical and clinical effectiveness of scanned proton beam technology, which now is the standard in proton radiotherapy. Only scanned proton fields can support the level of automation and

complexity that now is expected in radiotherapy considering intensity-modulated radiotherapy (IMRT and PBS/IMPT), treatment planning optimization and adaptive radiotherapy.

Scanned proton fields use numerous narrow beams of protons of variable energy for depth control and variable magnetic fields for movement in the lateral dimensions. Thus, an almost arbitrary 3D dose distribution can be created inside the patient without the aid, per se, of field shaping devices such as apertures and range-compensators.

There are two (somewhat standard) clinical approaches for pencil-beam scanning (PBS) planning and delivery. The first, single-field optimized, (SFO),[23] mimics SOBP fields. In SFO, each PBS field is designed to deliver a homogeneous dose, like an SOBP field, to the target volume. The second mode, IMPT, uses two or more fields and optimizes the dose as a composite for all fields. This mode is analogous to IMRT field optimization, i.e., each individual field is inhomogeneous but all fields aggregate to the prescription dose.

SFO fields were favored because of their robustness against geometric and range uncertainties and in terms of spatial invariance of adding multiple homogeneous dose distributions. IMPT fields rely both on in-field reproducibility in patient of the planned inhomogeneous dose and the addition of multiple inhomogeneous dose distributions. Both are adversely affected by range and spatial uncertainties. The validation of IMPT robustness requires post-plan validation of the treatment plan or incorporation of the uncertainties in the optimization. These are discussed in the following section.

Pencil-Beam Scanned Optimization

The optimization problem in PBS is larger when compared to IMRT or even VMAT. The size of the problem is dictated by the large set of pencil-beams (1,000–10,000), the greater sensitivity to heterogeneities of the charged particle beam and the introduction of new clinical variables including biological effects (quantified by linear energy transfer (LET)) and error (robustness) consideration in the optimization.[15,24] The optimization algorithm should be able to partition these problems to allow, for example, robust optimization of a subset of objectives while optimizing LET for another subset.

The optimization solution yields the set of charges Q_j (or Monitor Units which are equipment dependent) assigned to each spot j. The optimization problem uses a spot-dose matrix D_{ij},[25] which is the dose from each spot of unit charge to every voxel. The D_{ij} allows for rapid computation of dose D_i to a voxel i in the optimization loop while changing the charges Q_j in the optimization convergence to a solution.

$$D_i = \sum_j Q_j D_{ij} \qquad (32.2)$$

The optimization problem is defined by a set of constraints and objectives where constraints cannot be

[2] Paul Scherrer Institute, Villigen, Switzerland.

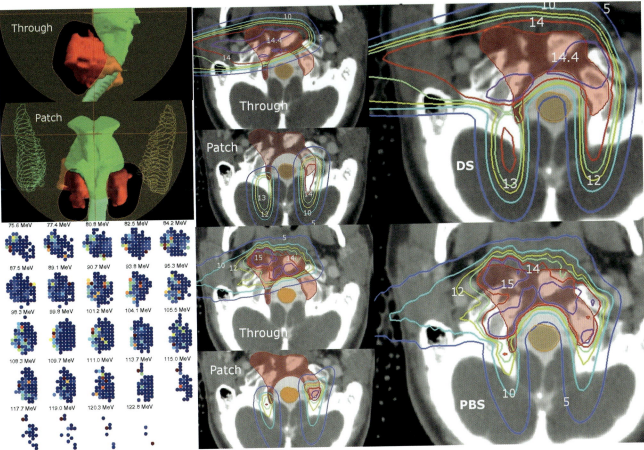

FIGURE 32.7. Patching of SOBP fields is a necessary technique to wrap the dose distributions around a target. As provided earlier, the Through field (left-top where the circle shows a 12 cm aperture) covers the anterior part of the GTV and the double-holed Patch field covers the posterior "horns." The top-right three figures show the dose distributions for the SOBP (DS) fields. The top row in the figure shows the (from left) the patch field construction in the BEV, the doses from the Through and Patch field and the composite dose for the SOBP field. The bottom row shows the same fields used in PBS optimization without the apertures or range-compensators. The desired prescription dose is 14.4 Gy (RBE). The construction of patching fields in DS is tedious as the field parameters—range, modulation and aperture size—must be carefully tweaked to achieve a dose distribution that covers the partial volumes to yield coverage of the total volume. For example, the Through field for the DS plan shows a distinct softening at its distal edge, which makes it harder for the Patch field to cover that volume. PBS with simultaneous optimization of all fields achieves a much more satisfactory result. The PBS Through field lateral edge is not as sharp compared to the SOBP Through field. The PBS gradient is defined by the varying pencil-beam intensities while the DS gradient is defined by the field edge. Thus, the PBS patch is probably less sensitive to errors. The PBS fields used a total of 1,600 pencil-beams with an initial spread of σ = 5 mm and with ranges between 4.5 and 14.5 cm (in water). The bottom-row right figure shows 1,103 spots for each of 24 energy layers for the Through PBS beam. The color indicates the number of Gigaprotons in each spot. Finally, apertures would achieve a sharper penumbra in as is our clinical practice.
BEV, beam's eye view; GTV, gross target volume; PBS, pencil-beam scanning; SOBP, Spreadout Bragg Peak.

FIGURE 32.8. The image shows a near symmetric chordoma wrapping around the spinal cord. The GTV is in red, the spinal cord in purple, and the parotid glands in cyan and purple. Isodose values are shown in Gy.RBE. The desired prescription dose for the GTV is 78 Gy.RBE. The left half shows an IMPT treatment plan and the right half shows a scattered field (DS) treatment plan. Both plans used the identical beam angles, as created for the DS plan. The choice of the DS beams inherently selects "robust" approaches (see text). Distinctive features in favor of the IMPT plan are (1) tighter and more complete coverage of the GTV especially into the posterior tails (see 78 Gy.RBE isodose), (2) better sparing of the parotid (see 30 Gy.RBE isodose), (3) significant less spinal cord dose (see 55 Gy.RBE isodose), and (4) lower integral dose as apparent from the 30 and 40 Gy.RBE isodose lines. Overall, however, the scattered field approach achieves a very comparable treatment plan.

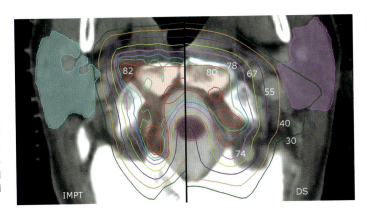

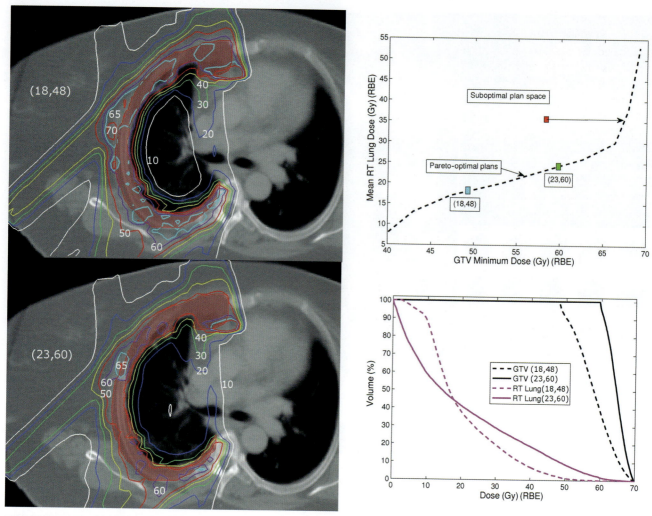

· **FIGURE 32.9.** Multi-criteria optimization (MCO) considers all constraints and objectives simultaneously. The constraints define the achievable solutions for the objectives. The set of optimal plans for this mesothelioma case lie on a Pareto-optimal line that shows the trade-off between lung sparing and target coverage. A non-MCO, nonoptimal, plan might lie somewhere above this line and its un-optimality is measured by the observation that it can achieve (arrow) much better target coverage for the same lung sparing. The left panels show two points (plans) on the Pareto-optimal line indicated by the trade-off pair of doses and the dose-volume histograms for each plan.

violated and objectives are to be optimized as an ensemble. The optimization might yield a single result that achieves the best values for the objectives or a Pareto-optimized set of plans[26] where a user can interactively navigate trade-offs between objectives (Fig. 32.9).

The quality of an optimizer can impact the quality of the achieved plan. It is a well-known problem in many single-plan optimizers that the achieved solution is not guaranteed to be the best (see Fig. 32.9) and requires a retweek of parameters to achieve a better solution. Pareto optimized solutions avoid this problem by providing optimal plans within the constraints and interactive evaluation. Breedveld et al. and Chen et al. describe optimization techniques well suited to radiotherapy problems that require performance, optimal convergence, multi-criteria and constraint immutability.[3]

The optimization problem may use one or more scenarios, each with its spot-dose matrix D_{ij}^{S}, where a scenario defines a particular physical or geometric state of the patient and may define a set of constraints and objectives. Uncertainty modeling, for example, may define a scenario for each of a set of isocenter position variations in the patient. The optimization algorithm uses all scenarios simultaneously to achieve a set of charges Q_j such that each scenario satisfied. The different scenarios easily increase the size of the optimization problem 10-fold further emphasizing the need for the highest performance optimizers.

Robustness in Pencil-Beam Scanned Treatment Planning

The robustness of a treatment plan measures its invariance against sets of uncertainties included in the optimization methodology as separate scenarios to achieve a single set of spot charges Q_j that satisfies the constraints

---

[3]Our proton planning system asteroid (.decimal Sanford FL) originally used the Chen method but now includes an efficient implementation of the Breedveld method (B. Gorissen NYMPH https://3142.nl/nymph/)

for all scenarios. For IMPT plans, each scenario is a sample in the range of range and positional uncertainties and quantified by the spot-dose matrix D_{ij}, which (again) describes the spot-dose to each point given the context of the scenario. Other scenarios can include those of target motion.[27] For the latter, motion of a target volume, i.e., in the lung, causes significant changes in radiological pathlengths and cannot be considered by a simple expansion of the CTV into a planning target volume (PTV). Such an expansion may be used for the lateral extent in the beam's eye view projection. Along the depth dimension, however, the final beam profile, managed with smeared range-compensator for SOBP fields and managed by differential pencil-beam intensities for IMPT, must ensure coverage of the target for all phases of motion. The correct consideration of these effects requires a computation over all phases instead of a geometric assumption such as the internal target volume (ITV) concept. Unkelbach et al.[28] provide an extensive review on this topic.

Robust optimization typically samples the extremes of the uncertainty phase space. It therefore results in a worst-case, albeit robust, plan. It is not clear, however, what robust optimization technology or technique would yield the best robust plan (as opposed to the worst case). Our practice, therefore, relies on site-specific post-planning robustness analysis of a given treatment approach (see Fig. 32.10).

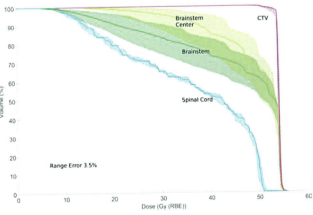

FIGURE 32.10. A proton treatment plan is sensitive to systematic and random errors. Random errors such as setup errors (which may have a systematic component) average to the mean whose variance can be reasonably understood given statistics. The range, however, is a systematic error with an expected magnitude on the order of 3%. Two general approaches are available. The first optimizes a plan considering only the nominal range followed by a recalculation of the plan on rescaled CT stopping power values. The second considers the range extents (3.5% in the figure) directly in the optimization and thus yields deliverable dose distributions given the range error. The previous figure shows the result for the first approach where the bands indicate possible DVH solutions. The band, however, is not a variance; the DVH will assume one line within the band of an organ. Thus, the target volumes seem reasonable within the systematic error in the range. The spinal cord, however, may change from 50 Gy.RBE to 55 Gy.RBE. A robust solution forces the spinal cord to remain at its hard limit of 50 Gy.RBE but will, as a consequence, degrade target coverage.

Multi-Criteria Optimization

Conventional optimization technologies in radiation therapy use a form of weighted objective functions that minimize the difference between the achieved dose and desired dose. Such optimization technologies yield, first, solutions that may not exactly meet desired limits and, second, are not guaranteed to be optimal. In the first case, a manual intervention is typically necessary to tweek the optimization parameters and achieve a better solution. The second case is not solvable with these technologies.

Both cases are addressed with multi-criteria optimization, Multicriteria optimization (MCO), which considers multiple trade-offs simultaneously.[29] The MCO approach, at least in our practice, computes all "possible" treatment plans, each of which is optimal within the choice of trade-offs. In MCO, the physician specifies a set of absolute constraints, such as minimum and maximum doses allowed to the target and or structures, and a set of objectives, such as "minimize the mean to the lung" or "minimize the maximum to the GTV." The MCO optimizer generates a set of plans, each of which meets the constraints, of sufficient number to sample all the possibilities of the stated objectives. These optimal treatment plans lie on the Pareto trade-off surface, which is a multidimensional surface (of dimension proportional to the number of objectives) formed by those points whose values are the optimal trade-offs (see Fig. 209). That is, changing one trade-off (such as increasing the target dose) will decrease another trade-off (such as higher critical structure dose). The user traverses this surface to select the desired set of trade-offs. Consider the example in Figure 32.9 that shows the Pareto surface (a curve in this case of two objectives) of a chest-wall target volume with a desired optimal dose of 70 Gy (RBE) but where a minimum of 40 Gy (RBE) was set to allow sufficient "room" to assess lung dose. The two objectives are "minimize the mean lung dose" and "maximize the minimum dose to the GTV." An optimal plan that lies on the curve means that improving lung dose will degrade target dose and vise versa.

Biological Optimization

The biological effectiveness of proton delivered dose is expressed in practice as a constant RBE=1.1. That is, a photon dose of 180 cGy equals a measured proton dose of 164 cGy. The RBE factor was chosen to ensure that the target dose delivered by protons would at least have the same biological effect as that of delivered by photons. Thus, the RBE=1.1 probably underestimates the biological dose. This, in turn, means that organ-at-risk doses are also underestimated and could be higher than assumed with RBE=1.1. Clinical site-specific experience has demonstrated near-equivalence but questions remain (see[30]).

The biological effectiveness, RBE, correlates with the dose-averaged LET (linear energy transfer; see Chapter 8 for definition and references and Grun et al.[31] here).

The correlation, albeit nonlinear, between RBE and LETD allows the latter to be used as a substitute to at least reduce RBE hot-spots out of organs-at-risk.

Unkelbach et al.[15] decompose the total, biological, dose into its physical dose component and biological-only component as

$$b_i = d_i + c\Sigma Q_j L_{ij} D_{ij} \qquad (32.3)$$

where Q_j is the charge of spot j, D_{ij} is the spot-dose matrix (as mentioned earlier) and L_{ij} is the spot-LETD matrix, which yields dose-averaged LET from spot j at the point i (c is an empirical scaling factor such that, on average, the RBE=1.1 given b_i). The quantity $c\Sigma j\ Q_j L_{ij} D_{ij}$ is amenable to optimization where the optimization uses objectives to minimize the quantity in organs-at-risk and allows for an increase (perhaps desirable) in the target. The optimization yields, again, the charges Q_j that satisfy the optimization criteria, which now include constraints on the LET. The RBE can be derived from the achieved dose and LETD through phenomenological models such as described by McNamara (see Chapter 8). Figure 32.11 shows an example LET optimization where the constraints achieved in a non-LET optimized plan are preserved while imposing additional LET constraints.

Absolute dosimetry

Pencil-beam scanning dosimetry only considers the interaction of the unmodified proton beam in medium. The proton pencil-beam parameters are the charge and lateral deflection defined in a reference plane. Figure 8.6 (Chapter 8)[32] shows a set of pristine Bragg peaks as a function of range and in units of Gy (RBE).mm²/Gp, which have been calibrated for treatment planning to match those delivered on the equipment. The Bragg peak specification allows the treatment planning system to relate dose in patient directly in terms of the delivery system control parameters. These parameters are also directly measured in the verification system.

The direct relationship between the plan parameters and dose in patient (see eq. 32–2) allows, in principle, for immediate assessment of dose during treatment delivery and offers unique opportunities for proton on-treatment adaptive therapy such as may be needed to treat moving targets.

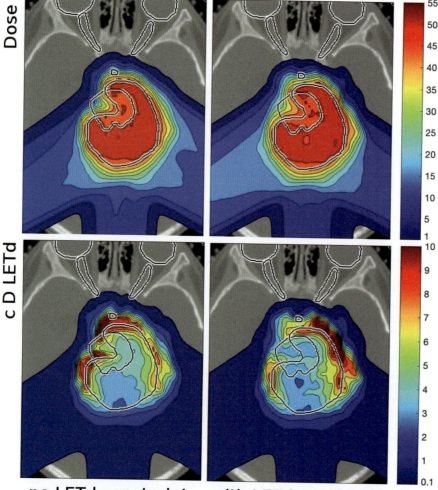

FIGURE 32.11. A treatment plan optimized given dose-only constraints is re-optimized to include LET constraints. The re-optimized plan maintains the original dose-only constraints (with an RBE = 1.1) while reducing regions of high LETd dose in the brainstem. These high regions are effectively moved into to the target volume. The original (left) and re-optimized (right) total doses are shown in the upper panels. The original (left) and re-optimized (right) LETd in the lower panels. The LETd is cast in the function $c \times D \times LETd$ whose units are [Gy.RBE] and can be interpreted as dose from high LETd regions. As visible, for this case and optimization algorithm, these regions correspond to the distal edge the three fields. Figure courtesy of Jan Unkelbach.

KEY POINTS

- A monoenergetic pristine narrow proton beam is modified by a double or single scattering system to produce a lateral flat field (within a desired diameter) and is modified by a set of range-shifters (either a set of individual shifters or mechanically constructed as a single device) to produce a depth-modulated SOBP such that the composite pristine peaks in the SOBP produce a flat depth-dose profile over a depth interval (labeled modulation width) up to the deepest pristine peak penetration.

- The SOBP field, either produced in a scattering system or by uniform scanning, is characterized by an open (within a maximum diameter) flat field and by a constant radiologic depth penetration set by the maximum energy of the SOBP pristine peak. An aperture conforms the flat open field to the BEV projection of the target— including a lateral margin. A variable thickness range-shifter or range-compensator (at high resolution in the beam-transverse plan) modulates the constant depth penetration (including patient heterogeneities) such that the penetration depth is adjusted across the field to conform the dose-distal penetration surface to the distal target surface and to reduce dose penetration distal to the target volume.

- Apertures in SOBP fields are characterized by a sharp penumbra due to the large SAD and close placement of the aperture to the patient. This geometry reduces the source size (on the order of centimeters) to a penumbra to a few millimeters. Pencil-beam scanning of narrow proton beams without an aperture may still have a large penumbra in comparison to the SOBP penumbra. Thus, the use of an aperture in a pencil-beam scanning field will yield a tenfold reduction in source penumbra. The total penumbra in patient, however, increases as a function of energy at depth of range due to multiple Coulomb scattering.

- The PTV concept in photon radiotherapy is valid because geometric perturbations in the patient have a negligible effect on the physical dose distribution. Thus, geometric alignment corresponds to dosimetric alignment. Proton radiotherapy dose distributions, however, are very sensitive to geometric perturbations

and the dose distributions can become a strong function of the geometric perturbation. Thus, a simple geometric expansion of the CTV will not suffice to a priori account for the dosimetric effect of these perturbations. PTV-like expansion maybe applied for site-specific field approaches (such as lateral fields for prostate or en-face single fields for breast chest-wall) if validated through variance (robust) simulation of the field arrangement.

- The number of optimization variables, the individual pencil-beam intensities, in pencil-beam scanning fields is very large and on the order of 1,000 to 10,000. One can therefore expect that given multiple clinical competing objectives, multiple plans should be considered to evaluate the best trade-off. Multi-criteria optimization (MCO) aims to provide a model where, instead of producing a single "optimal" plan, many optimal plans can be considered, each of which is optimal given an actual choice of objective values. The set of MCO plans (proportional to the number of objectives specified by the clinician) create a Pareto-optimal multidimensional surface where each point on the surface is a Pareto-optimal plan. The MCO interface allows interactive traversal over this surface to interactively visualize dose-objective trade-offs.

- Uncertainties in proton treatment plans include geometric setup errors, anatomical changes, and physical uncertainties in the stopping power determination in the patient and thus in the range penetration into the patient. Such uncertainties affect the dose distribution directly and cannot be mitigated by geometric solutions such as the PTV concept. Instead, uncertainties need to be considered in the treatment planning dosimetry directly to establish that, given the uncertainty extents, dose constraints remain clinically acceptable.

- Proton beams have a large increase in dose-averaged LET (the quantity most directly related to biological effect). LET – as dose – can be computed for each voxel. The product of voxel LET and voxel dose can be related to the biological effect dose and used to include LET as an optimization objective to minimize LET to critical structures. This method is currently the subject of clinical trials.

REVIEW QUESTIONS

1. A Pareto-optimal plan defines a set of objective and their values. If an objective value improves,
   A. all other objective values worsen
   B. some improve, some worsen
   C. some worsen, some remain the same
   D. some worsen, some reach a limit

2. Compared to an SOBP treatment plan, a PBS plan will always show (indicate all that are correct):
   A. Improved proximal dose reduction
   B. Better distal penumbra
   C. Worse distal penumbra
   D. Better lateral penumbra

3. Why do proton plans significantly reduce integral dose?
   A. Proton treatments use less fields
   B. Protons deposit no dose beyond the distal edge
   C. The proton Bragg peak deposits much more dose in the target compared to the rest of the tissues

ANSWERS

1. A   Every Pareto-optimal plan is a "point" on the Pareto surface whose dimensionality is determined from the plan objectives and where each point is a set of optimal objective values. Any change that improves one objective worsens all other objectives.

2. A   An SOBP field has a fixed modulation and therefore cannot control the dose proximal to the target (C), the SOBP field has a range-compensator that ensures that every proton "stops" at the distal surface and thus the distal penumbra is the distal penumbra from the pristine peak (which is at least two times sharper than the lateral penumbra). A PBS field whose spots are rather random with respect to the distal surface does not expose the pristine distal fall-off.

3. B   Protons deposit no dose beyond the distal edge. This (almost) reduces the integral dose by a factor of two.

REFERENCES

1. Robert R Wilson. Radiological Use of Fast Protons. *Radiology.* 1946;47:487–91.
2. Wilson R. *A brief history of the Harvard University cyclotrons.* Cambridge, Mass: Harvard University Dept. of Physics; 2004.
3. Leksell L, Larsson B, Andersson B, Rexed B, Sourander P, Mair W. Lesions in the depth of the brain produced by a beam of high energy protons. *Acta radiol.* 1960;54:251–64.
4. Kliman B, Kjellberg R N. Therapy of acromegaly. *N Engl J Med.* 1971;284:673.
5. Gragoudas E S, Goitein M, Verhey L, Munzenreider J, Suit H D, Koehler A. Proton beam irradiation. An alternative to enucleation for intraocular melanomas. *Ophthalmology.* 1980;87:571–81.
6. Goitein M, Miller T. Planning proton therapy of the eye. *Med Phys.* 1983;10:275–283.
7. Gragoudas 1 E S, Seddon J M, Egan K M, Glynn R J, Goitein M, Munzenrider J, Verhey L, Urie M. A Koehler Metastasis from uveal melanoma after proton beam irradiation. *Ophthalmology.* 1988;95:992–9.
8. Goitein M, Abrams M, Rowell D, Pollari H, Wiles J. Multi-dimensional treatment planning: II. Beam's eye-view, back projection, and projection through CT sections. *Int J Rad Onc Biol Phys.* 1983;9:789–797.
9. Suit H D, Goitein M, Tepper J, Koehler A M, Schmidt R A, Schneider R. Exploratory study of proton radiation therapy using large field techniques and fractionated dose schedules. *Cancer.* 1975;35:1646–57.
10. Safai S, Bortfeld T, Engelsman M. Comparison between the lateral penumbra of a collimated double-scattered beam and uncollimated scanning beam in proton radiotherapy. *Phys Med Biol.* 2008;53:1729–1750.
11. Paganetti H. Range uncertainties in proton therapy and the role of Monte Carlo simulations. *Phys Med Biol.* 2012;57:R99–R117.
12. Schneider U, Pedroni E, Lomax A. The calibration of CT Hounsfield units for radiotherapy treatment planning. *Phys Med Biol.* 1996; 41:111–124.
13. Verburg JM, Seco J. Proton range verification through prompt gamma-ray spectroscopy. *Phys Med Biol.* 2014;59:7089–106.
14. Deluca PM, Wambersie A, Whitmore G. Prescribing, Recording, and Reporting Proton-Beam Therapy (ICRU Report 78). *Journal of the ICRU.* 2007;7:(2)1–8.
15. Unkelbach J, Pablo Botas, et al. Reoptimization of Intensity Modulated Proton Therapy Plans Based on Linear Energy Transfer. *Int J Radiation Oncol Biol Phys.* 2016; 96:1097–1106.
16. Degiovanni A, Amaldi U. History of hadron therapy accelerators. *Physica Medica.* 2015;31:322e332.
17. Pedronia E, Meer D, Bula C, Safai S, Zenklusen S. Pencil beam characteristics of the next-generation proton scanning gantry of PSI: design issues and initial commissioning results. *Eur Phys J Plus.* 2011;126:66.
18. Poludniowski G, Allinson N M, Evans P M. Proton radiography and tomography with application to proton therapy. *Br J Radiol.* 2015;88(1053):20150134.
19. Gottschalk B. Passive Beam Spreading in Proton Radiation Therapy. https://gray.mgh.harvard.edu/attachments/article/212/pbs.pdf
20. Kooy H M, Schaefer M, Rosenthal S, Bortfeld T. Monitor Unit Calculations for Range Modulated Spread-Out Bragg Peak Fields. *Phys Med Biol.* 2003; 48:2797–2808.
21. Bortfeld T. An analytical approximation of the Bragg curve for therapeutic proton beams. *Med Phys.* 1997;24:2024–2033.
22. Lomax A J, Bohringer T, et al. Treatment planning and verification of proton therapy using spot scanning: Initial experiences. *Medical Physics.* 2004;31:3150–3157.
23. A Lomax Intensity modulation methods for proton radiotherapy. *Phys Med Biol.* 1999;44:185.

24. Chen W, Unkelbach J, Trofimov A, Madden T, Kooy H, Bortfeld T, Craft D. Robust Multi-Criteria IMPT Optimization. *Med Phys.* 2012;39:3981–3981.
25. Breedveld S, van den Berg B, Heijmen B. An interior-point implementation developed and tuned for radiation therapy treatment planning. *Comput Optim Appl.* 2017;68:209–242.
26. Chen W, Craft D, Madden T M, Zhang K, Kooy H M, Herman G T. A fast optimization algorithm for multicriteria intensity modulated proton therapy planning. *Med Phys.* 2010;37:4938–4945.
27. A J Lomax Intensity modulated proton therapy and its sensitivity to treatment uncertainties 2: the potential effects of inter-fraction and inter-field motions. *Phys Med Biol.* 2008;53:1043.
28. Unkelbach J, Albert M, et al. Robust radiotherapy planning. *Phys Med Biol.* 2018;63:22TR02.
29. Monz M, Kaefer K H, Bortfeld T R, Thieke C. Pareto navigation-algorithmic foundation of interactive multi-criteria IMRT planning. *Phys Med Biol.* 2008;53:985.
30. Haas-Kogan D, Indelicato D, et al. , National Cancer Institute Workshop on Proton Therapy for Children: Considerations Regarding Brainstem Injury. *Int J Radiat Oncol Biol Phys.* 2018 May 1;101(1):152–168.
31. Grun R, Friedrich T, Traneus E, Scholz M. Is the dose-averaged LET a reliable predictor for the relative biological effectiveness? *Med Phys.* 2019;46:1064–1074.
32. Clasie B, Depauw N, et al. Golden beam data for proton pencil-beam scanning. *Phys Med Biol.* 2012;57:1147–1158.

33 Treatment Plan Evaluation

Ellen D. Yorke, Andrew Jackson, and Gerald J. Kutcher

INTRODUCTION

Since the previous edition of this book, the basic tools of plan evaluation—dose–volume histograms (DVHs) and high-quality graphic dose displays—have not changed except for increase in calculation speed. These tools are available on all modern treatment planning systems and are almost universally used. A variety of dose–volume metrics that have been shown to correlate with outcomes are applied in daily clinical practice. "Biologic models," which condense the entire dose distribution into a single number that represents the probability of a specified outcome, are not widely used in clinical practice but are still of interest, and increasingly sophisticated statistical techniques are being used to extract model parameters and significant dose–volume points from clinical data.

The report of American Association of Physicists in Medicine's (AAPM's) Task Group 166, "The Use and QA of Biologically Related Models for Treatment Planning,"[1] includes a thorough review of current models and their implementations in commercial treatment planning systems for planning and plan evaluation.

What Is New?

Since the late 1990s, three-dimensional conformal radiation therapy (3DCRT) has gone from novel to passé, use of intensity-modulated radiation therapy (IMRT) has burgeoned, and other delivery techniques—volumetric-modulated arc therapy (VMAT), tomotherapy, "CyberKnife"—are now routinely used. Greatly increased computer speed and graphic capabilities make it possible to routinely plan these treatments in busy clinics—indeed, many planners find it easier to generate an IMRT or VMAT plan than a 3DCRT plan. Registered positron emission tomography (PET) and magnetic resonance imaging (MRI) studies are routinely used to supplement the planning computerized tomography (CT) scan. Treatment accuracy has been greatly increased by readily available tools for online image guidance. Partly thanks to this image-guided radiation therapy (IGRT), it is now possible to safely and effectively deliver highly hypofractionated treatment schedules to tumors anywhere in the body using stereotactic body radiotherapy

(SBRT) (also called stereotactic ablative body radiotherapy [SABR]). SBRT consists of a small number (1–10) of daily fractions, each delivering a high dose per fraction (5–30 Gy). SBRT is perhaps the greatest change in radiation therapy since the advent of IMRT, and its use has grown explosively (Fig. 33.1). It provides superior tumor control with a remarkably low rate of serious complications, although some new and unexpected complications have been observed.[2,3] There is incomplete mechanistic understanding of the excellent tumor control, but the rarity of serious complication is at least partly due to very accurate setup with online image guidance (IGRT) and the fact that many applications of SBRT are to small tumors (<100 cc). Thanks to the combination of 3D IGRT and increasing planning computer speed, clinicians are more seriously considering both online and offline "adaptive radiotherapy," where plans are changed during a treatment course to accommodate anatomical changes such as tumor shrinkage or growth.

Knowledge of relationships between dose distributions, medical variables, and normal tissue complications continues to grow as researchers take advantage of electronic medical records to more readily analyze outcomes from single- and multi-institutional patient cohorts. The systematic reviews of publications on normal tissue complications by the QUANTEC (Quantitative Analysis of Normal Tissue Effects in the Clinic) group have provided updated treatment planning dose–volume guidelines and impetus for new studies to address areas where information is lacking.[4] Members of the AAPM can access the QUANTEC reports through the AAPM website.

Not New but Necessary

Inspecting isodose distributions superimposed on a patient's planning CT scan (or on a registered PET or MRI scan) remains an important plan evaluation tool that can rapidly inform the planner of deficiencies in the dose distribution. The rapid volumetric dose calculations of modern planning systems allow users to rapidly scroll through the treated volume for a complete picture of the dose distribution in relation to anatomy and locate hot and cold spots with a single mouse click. For complex plans, this is a great improvement over the traditional "three principal planes

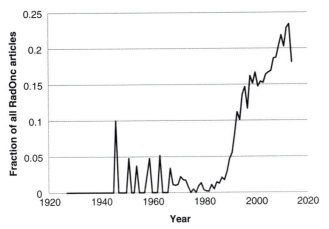

FIGURE 33.1. Growth in the number of Radiation Oncology articles dealing with stereotactic body radiotherapy and in PubMed. There were approximately 1,500 articles in 2014. Data from Dr. Jimm Grimm.

through isocenter" displays. Clinicians often prefer uniform target dose distributions unless there is a deliberate effort at nonuniform target coverage—called simultaneous integrated boost (SIB) or "dose painting."[5] The planner can deal with unintended high-dose regions by changing beam number or directions, using higher-energy beams and using dose-controlling "dummy structures" in optimization to arrive at a final plan. Graphic displays also provide useful geometric information such as whether a beam enters through a support device where attenuation must be considered or unnecessarily through an organ at risk (OAR), or whether the planning scan was acquired with an inadequate field of view such that a beam appears to traverse a shorter path length than it does in reality. However, for most people, graphic displays are hard to interpret in a comprehensive manner. For optimum plan evaluation, they should be used in parallel with the two general sets of tools described in the following section: DVHs, based on either physical or biologically equivalent doses, and metrics derived from biologic models of tumor control probability (TCP) and normal tissue complication probability (NTCP).

The questions posed in the previous edition of this book still plague clinicians: Conventional evaluation of treatment plans, which judges a "best treatment plan" using tradition, inspection of graphic isodoses and practical knowledge alone, is no longer adequate to answer the issues that continually arise in modern practice. For example, should we escalate the dose to the prostate to the highest nonuniform dose or to a lower, more uniform, target dose? Can the rectum and bladder tolerate a high localized dose to a small volume? If so, how small a volume and how high a dose? Finally, how should we balance tumor control and the risk of normal tissue complications?

Recent developments lead to new, unsolved questions in plan evaluation. Under what conditions might nonuniform target doses be more effective? When applying TCP models, should one look at the gross target volume (GTV), the clinical target volume (CTV) of suspected disease or the planning target volume (PTV) within which

the CTV might be found under conditions of setup error? What normal tissue evaluation metrics should be used for hypofractionated treatment?

In the following section, we describe briefly the basic structure and some applications of DVHs and modeling. We also describe some of the QUANTEC normal tissue guidelines and compare them with previous consensus recommendations.

Dose–Volume Histograms

DVHs may be represented in either differential or integral form. The former represents the volume of the organ receiving a dose within a specified dose interval, whereas the latter is defined as the volume receiving at least dose D as a function of D. The volume is represented either as the percent (or fraction) of the total volume of the organ or as the volume in cubic centimeters. The differential form lends itself well to rapid visual inspection of the range and uniformity of dose. This works well in finding cold spots in the target volume or hot spots in normal organs. The integral form facilitates the assessment of the total volume of tissue in such hot or cold spots and is the preferred format. A major deficiency of DVHs is that they give no information as to the anatomical location of hot or cold spots. In clinical plan evaluation, this is partly resolved by parallel inspection of the graphic dose distribution.

In traditional radiation therapy, the ideal target integral DVH is a step function—uniform dose to the entire target (Fig. 33.2). Since that is not physically achievable, a "good" target DVH is considered to be one where the bulk of the target receives prescription (e.g., D95 = prescription dose to 95% of the target receives prescription dose or higher) while restricting the minimum and maximum point doses (often to approximately 90% and 110% of prescription, respectively). For dose-painting treatments, the deliberate nonuniformity is reflected in the target DVH (Fig. 33.2B). The ideal DVH for a normal tissue is a delta-function at zero dose, which is also unachievable. OAR DVHs are analyzed in two ways. Most often, key dose–volume points on the integral DVH which are correlated with treatment outcome are evaluated (Fig. 33.3). For example, in conventionally fractionated therapy (1.5–2.5 Gy/treatment), the maximum spinal cord dose (D_{max}) is usually restricted to below 50 Gy in order to avoid the very serious complication of radiation myelitis. The limit is based on clinical experience and numerous publications: a 0.2% rate myelitis is estimated at $D_{max} = 50$ Gy in 2-Gy fractions.[6] The maximum organ dose is also significantly related to complication for the brainstem and optic nerves. The fraction of lung volume receiving over 20 Gy at standard fractionation (V20) is often held below 35% to limit the incidence of symptomatic radiation pneumonitis (RP). Similarly, intermediate DVH points are correlated with complication for other organs such as esophagus and rectum. Mean organ dose—the area under the integral DVH (with percent volume)—is another commonly used

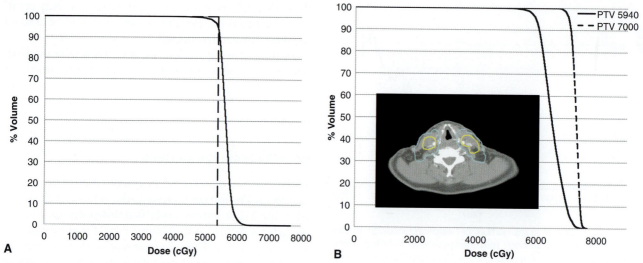

FIGURE 33.2. A: An ideal target dose–volume histogram (*dashed*) to treat target to 5,400 cGy with uniform dose and (*solid*) an actual target dose–volume histogram. **B:** Dose–volume histograms for a dose-painting case—planning target volume 7,000 (*dashed*) is inside planning target volume 5940 (*solid*).

evaluation criterion, as it is strongly related to symptomatic complications for organs such as lung, parotid, liver, and kidney.[4]

The second approach is to use the entire DVH of the OAR as input to a model that estimates NTCP. Several models are described in this chapter, as well as in an AAPM task group report[1] and many primary source papers. At present, despite their potential, use of models to evaluate treatment plans in routine clinical practice is largely confined to major academic centers where radiation oncologists and planners are sufficiently confident in models—sometimes ones developed at their center—to use them comfortably. An exception to this is the use of mean dose that is directly evaluated in many planning systems and with which there is known strong correlation with several complications (e.g., xerostomia or RP). Models are

sometimes used in treatment planning studies to evaluate possible effects of changes in treatment practice[7] or to compare proposed and existing techniques.[8] They also provide essential support for responsible extrapolation of treatments to new regimes (e.g., dose escalation) under phase I protocols.[9,10] In that context it is not necessary for the model to be correct in all details, provided it gives a reasonable estimate of how far the current treatment may be modified without excessive risk. Finally, models are used in advanced methods for optimization of treatment plans, where they enable quantification of tradeoffs.[11,12]

A robust model might determine the optimal DVH between two similar plans. For example, suppose an integral DVH for plan A lies to the left of one for plan B. If the organ is a nontarget tissue, then plan A is better; if the organ is the target, then plan B is better. A more complex comparison is given in Figure 33.4 where integral DVHs for a normal organ planned with a parallel-opposed (traditional) and multifield 3D plan are shown. Although the volume irradiated to any dose level can be used to quantitatively compare the treatment plans, the location of high-dose (or other) regions cannot be determined from the DVHs. Moreover, in the example shown, the DVHs cross one another so that it is not obvious which DVH is better.

Because SBRT is now widely used, it is necessary to be able to interpret both graphic distributions and DVHs of treatment plans for hypofractionated treatments and to rationally compare hypofractionated with conventionally fractionated plans. In order to do this, a detour to classical radiobiology is needed. Hypofractionation has a strong effect on biologic responses and using physical DVHs for SBRT may be misleading.

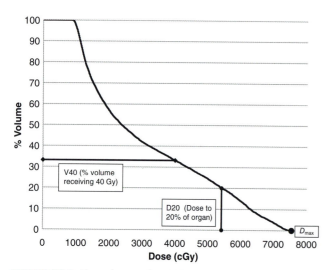

FIGURE 33.3. Normal organ (parotid) dose–volume histogram with different dose–volume points indicated. D_{max} ~7,500 cGy, V40 ~33%, D20 ~5,400 cGy.

Cell Survival Models

Decades of clinical and experimental experience show that the same dose delivered over a small number of daily

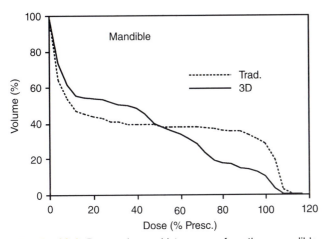

FIGURE 33.4. Dose–volume histograms for the mandible. (Reprinted from Kutcher GJ. Quantitative plan evaluation. In: Purdy JA, Simpson LR, eds. *Advances in Radiation Oncology Physics: Dosimetry, Treatment Planning, Brachytherapy.* New York, NY: American Institute of Physics; 1992:998–1021, with permission.)

fractions (e.g., 20 Gy × 3 fractions) has a greater cell-killing effect than if delivered over a large number of daily fractions (e.g., 2 Gy × 30 fractions). This is well known to radiation oncologists and medical physicists, for whom a course in radiobiology is a standard part of training.[13,14] Many mathematical models describe this behavior, but the Linear-quadratic (LQ) model is by far the most used because of its mathematical simplicity and because, over decades, its parameters have been measured for many cell types and under many conditions.[7–10] According to the LQ model, if a collection of identical cells receives a uniform dose D delivered in n acute fractions spaced several hours apart, the surviving fraction (SF) of cells is

$$SF = \exp - (\alpha D + \beta D^2/n) = \exp(-\alpha D(1 + (D/n)/(\alpha/\beta))) \quad (33.1)$$

α and β depend on the cell type and environment (e.g., oxic or hypoxic) and the type of radiation (e.g., heavy ions vs. megavoltage photons) but are independent of dose. Typical cell survival curves are found in many texts.[13,14] Because the range of SF over an experimentally achievable dose range covers five to six orders of magnitude, it is typical to use semilog plots.

The solid curve in Figure 33.5 shows the SF predicted by the LQ model for single acute doses to cells with α = 0.33 Gy^{-1} and α/β = 8.6 Gy (chosen to agree with α/β in a competing model[29]).

A mechanistic interpretation of the LQ model is that α describes irreparable DNA damage due to a single radiation "hit" while β describes the effect of two lesions, neither of which is lethal on its own but which can interact to produce lethal damage. Overall cell radiosensitivity is dominated by α, which is measured at low doses (when the quadratic term is negligible) or at low dose rates, when most double-hit lesions are repaired. Typical in vitro values of α range between about 0.05 Gy^{-1} (radioresistant, SF

due to single-hit alone at 2 Gy ~90%) and 1.5 Gy^{-1} (radiosensitive, single hit SF at 2 Gy = 5%).[15–17]

The parameter α/β is of particular clinical interest in clinical radiotherapy (and it is much easier to find tabulations of it) because it captures, with reasonable accuracy, changes in biologic response for different dose fractionation schedules. Knowing α/β allows clinicians to find treatment schedules with the same TCP or NTCP (isoeffective dose schedule) by assuming that isoeffective schedules result in the same SF of the relevant cells. From Equation 33.1, a total dose D given in n fractions and total dose D′ given in n′ fractions to an identical tissue are isoeffective if

$$D(1 + (D/n)/(\alpha/\beta)) = D'(1 + (D'/n')/(\alpha/\beta)) \quad (33.2)$$

The quantity $D(1 + (D/n)/(\alpha/\beta))$ is called the biologically effective dose (BED); it depends on the total dose, the number of fractions, the type of radiation, and the tissue of interest.[13,14] For clinical photon beams, many—but not all—tumors and "acutely responding" normal tissues, like skin, have high α/β of 10 Gy or more while "late responding tissues," where complications occur months to years after treatment, have low α/β, typically 1–5 Gy, depending on the tissue and the complication. Possible reasons for this difference are given by Thames and Hendry.[18]

For a tumor with α/β = 10 Gy, the BED of a typical fractionated schedule of 60 Gy in 30 fractions is 72 Gy while for a hypofractionated schedule of 60 Gy in 3 fractions, the tumor BED is 180 Gy. A nearby normal tissue with α/β = 3 Gy receives a BED of 100 Gy for conventional

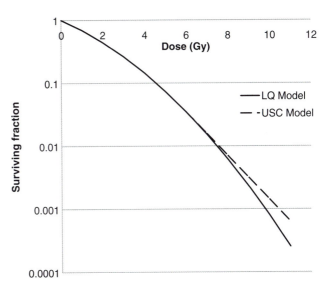

FIGURE 33.5. Semi-log plot of surviving fraction of cells predicted by the Linear-quadratic model (*solid*) and the Universal Survival Curve (*USC dotted*). At high doses the Linear-quadratic curve is "curvier" due to the effect of the β term. (Parameters were taken from Park C, Papiez L, Zhang S., et al. Universal survival curve and single fraction equivalent dose: useful tools in understanding potency of ablative radiotherapy. *Int J Radiat Oncol Biol Phys.* 2008;70:847–852.)

fractionation and 460 Gy for the hypofractionated schedule. In order to express LQ corrected doses on a scale that is more comparable to clinical experience, the LQ-corrected dose is often presented as the equivalent dose in 2-Gy fractions (EQD2)[19,20] where

$$EQD2 = BED/(1 + 2/(\alpha/\beta)) \qquad (33.3)$$

Regardless of α/β, EQD2 for dose delivered at 2 Gy/fraction must equal the physical dose. For dose/fraction less than 2 Gy, EQD2 is less than the physical dose and for dose/fraction above 2 Gy, EQD2 is greater. In the hypofractionation example provided earlier, the tumor EQD2 is 150 Gy while the normal tissue EQD2 is 276 Gy. It is very clear that hypofractionation calls for extreme protection of normal tissues.

In the interest of clarity, the International Commission on Radiation Units and Measurements (ICRU) recently introduced the symbol and term "Equieffective dose" = $EQDX_{\alpha/\beta}$ to describe the dose delivered at an arbitrary dose per fraction X to a tissue with a specified α/β that is equivalent to the dose D delivered to the same tissue in n fractions[21] (at dose per fraction $d = D/n$). Thus,

$$\begin{aligned} EQDX_{\alpha/\beta} &= D(d + \alpha/\beta)/(X + \alpha/\beta) \\ &= D(1 + d/\alpha/\beta)/(1 + X/\alpha/\beta) \end{aligned} \qquad (33.4)$$

The first equality is as stated in Bentzen et al.[21] while in the second, numerator and denominator are in more typical LQ model form. Until ICRU nomenclature is generally accepted, when reading publications, it is important to know whether the authors are reporting physical dose, BED, EQD2, or something else, and that for "biologically corrected" doses, they have specified α/β.

An important recent result of the isoeffective concept is the realization that α/β for prostate cancer is much lower than the generic $\alpha/\beta = 10$ Gy usually assumed for tumors. For prostate cancer, α/β is now considered to be ~ 1.5 Gy. This has important consequences for hypofractionated treatment of prostate cancer, the most common male cancer in the United States, with $\sim 221,000$ new cases per year. The initial discovery was prompted by work by Brenner and Hall and was motivated by the observation that prostate cancer cells—like many late-responding normal tissues—replicate slowly.[22] They started from the common hypothesis that the TCP of a uniformly irradiated tumor containing N clonogenic cells is achieved if zero clonogenic cells survive the treatment, that the SF, SF(D), is determined by the LQ model, and that cell killing is a random process that is well described by a Poisson distribution.[23]

Under these conditions,

$$\begin{aligned} TCP &= \exp(-NSF(D)) \\ &= \exp(-N\exp(-\alpha D(1 + (D/n)/(\alpha/\beta)))) \end{aligned} \qquad (33.5)$$

Brenner and Hall extracted the radiobiologic parameters from two large clinical studies of "biochemical failure"

after treatment for prostate cancer; one after a course of external beam therapy and the other after low dose-rate brachytherapy. Biochemical failure is a rise in the blood concentration of prostate-specific antigen (PSA) following a drop to a nadir in the months after therapy. PSA rise can be detected by a blood test long before clinical evidence of recurrence and freedom from biochemical failure (FFBF) is clinically equated with TCP at a chosen time point. In the external beam data set (233 patients), the dose per fraction was 2 Gy and the number of treatments was escalated from 30 to 40. For these patients, the LQ model was directly applied. The second data set consisted of 134 patients who had received I-125 brachytherapy with known peripheral dose D. Because of the extremely low dose rate of such implants (~ 6 cGy/hr), two-hit damage is completely repaired so the SF was exp-(αD). Each patient's initial PSA level and dosimetry (approximated as uniform tumor dose) were known, and the endpoint was FFBF at 3 years in both studies. The pretreatment PSA was taken as indicative of the initial number of cancer cells (N); N and α were determined by fitting the FFBF of groups of brachytherapy patients with the same initial PSA to their delivered doses. Knowing these parameters, β was determined from external beam patients with similar initial PSA. The study concluded that α/β was 1.5 Gy with 95% CI (0.8–2.2 Gy). There have since been numerous papers comparing PSA outcomes for prostate cancer patients treated under well-defined conditions with different fractionation schedules. Fowler et al.[24] summarized three large reviews (each involving thousands of patient records) that were all statistically consistent with $\alpha/\beta \sim 1.5$ Gy and concluded that "high fractionation sensitivity is an intrinsic property of prostate carcinomas."

The clinical impact of this realization is that SBRT is feasible for a large population of patients with prostate cancer because the tumor α/β is lower than that of the closest critical normal tissue—the rectum—for which α/β is believed to be ~ 3 Gy.[25] A major problem in prostate cancer treatment planning is that the prostate and the anterior rectal surface are in contact with each other and that rectal complications are associated with the high-dose region of the dose distribution. Therefore, tumor control and rectal sparing are strongly competing treatment goals. The minimum biologic target dose cannot be too low, yet it must be consistent with rectal sparing where the two organs are in contact. Given the excellent results and clinical efficiency of SBRT at other disease sites and the high prevalence of prostate cancer, it is desirable from medical and economic perspectives to safely treat prostate cancer with SBRT.

Figure 33.6 shows the physical DVHs for the PTV and the rectal wall from the dose distribution of a hypofractionated external beam prostate cancer treatment (8 Gy × 5 fractions). In Figure 33.6, the rectal maximum dose is clearly less than the physical dose to most of the PTV and, at conventional fractionation, would be well tolerated. However, at conventional fractionation, 40 Gy is totally

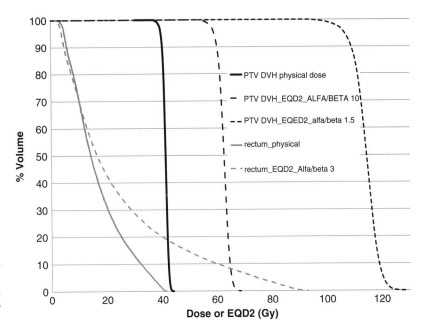

FIGURE 33.6. Dose–volume histograms and EQD2_VHs from a hypofractionated prostate plan of 8 Gy × 5 fractions. *Solid curves* are the planning target volume and rectal wall dose–volume histograms using physical dose. The *medium-dashed curve* is the rectal wall EQD2_VH taking α/β = 3 Gy, which is typical for a late-responding normal tissue. The *dark dashes* are the EQD2_VH for the planning target volume assuming that α/β = 10 Gy, a value often used for tumors. The *small-dash curve* is EQD2_VH for the planning target volume assuming that α/β = 1.5 Gy, as is currently believed to hold for prostate cancer. The dose distribution is the same for all the curves but their biologic effects are quite different.

inadequate to control prostate cancer; prescriptions for definitive conventionally fractionated prostate cancer treatments, which have both good tumor control and normal tissue sparing range from ~80 to 86 Gy. DVHs can be converted to EQD2$_{α/β}$_VHs by transforming the dose at the midpoint of each dose bin using Equation 33.3. The large dashes in Figure 33.6 show the PTV EQD2$_{α/β}$_VH assuming that the tumor α/β is 10 Gy and the smaller dashes are the PTV EQD2$_{α/β}$_VH for α/β = 1.5 Gy. The rectum EQD2$_{α/β}$_VH is calculated for α/β = 3 Gy (small, light dashes). If the tumor α/β were 10 Gy, SBRT would not be feasible because target equivalent dose (~60 Gy) is still much lower than what is curative at conventional fractionation while the high equivalent doses to the rectum far exceed those to the target. Increasing the target dose would raise the rectal maximum dose well beyond its tolerance level. But because it is well confirmed that prostate cancer has a low α/β, the EQD2$_{α/β}$-VHs for the same dose distribution with the prostate α/β = 1.5 Gy show a favorable therapeutic ratio because rectal complications are most correlated with maximum dose. Hypofractionated external beam treatment of prostate cancer is now widely and safely used,[26] although longer follow-up is needed to determine whether long-term TCP is comparable to conventionally fractionated treatment. The fractionation of Figure 33.6 is a realistic schedule, though some groups treat on alternate days to improve OAR sparing. As a general rule, hypofractionation is favored if the tumor has a smaller α/β than the most important adjacent critical normal structures and the dominant complications depend strongly on the structure maximum dose.

There is considerable controversy as to the validity of the LQ model for large fraction doses based on in vitro evidence that LQ overestimates cell killing for fraction doses above ~10 Gy.[27,28] The dotted curve in Figure 33.5

compares the SF predicted by the LQ model with predictions of one of the competing models, the Universal Survival Curve.[29] But to date, no model has replaced LQ, because of its mathematical simplicity, the availability of model parameters acquired over many decades and the lack of definitive evidence that it is wrong in cases of clinical interest.[16] Further investigations are needed for a definitive answer.

Biologic Models

Biologic models are an alternative method of evaluating treatment plans that use the complete DVH as well as other information to predict treatment outcomes. Although models are not currently in common use for plan evaluation, they may ultimately prove to be more effective than predictions based on single or a small number of dose–volume points. In general, TCP and NTCP are thought to increase sigmoidally from 0% to 100% as a function of dose or a combination of dose and other factors (e.g., smoking, age, chemotherapy, genetics[30]). The parameters that determine the midpoint and slope in the middle region of the curve are obtained from analyses of clinical outcomes. This section further describes some approaches to modeling TCP and NTCP.

TUMOR CONTROL PROBABILITY

The central assumption of most TCP models is that a tumor is destroyed if all viable clonogenic cells within it are killed.[23]

From this assumption, Brahme[31] and Goitein[32] derive TCP from the product of probabilities that individual clonogens (or tumorlets) are killed. The simplest form of these models assumes that clonogens in a tumor have identical radiosensitivities, respond independently to radiation damage, are uniformly distributed, and that the tumorlets are small enough so that the dose D in each tumorlet is homogeneous. Under these conditions, the TCP for a tumorlet with partial volume v can be inferred from the TCP for uniform irradiation of the whole tumor,

$$\text{TCP} = (v, D) = \text{TCP}(1, D)^v \qquad (33.6)$$

It then follows that the TCP of an inhomogeneously irradiated tumor is given by the product of tumorlet TCPs,

$$\text{TCP} = \prod_{i=1}^{N} \text{TCP}(v_i, D_i) = \prod_{i=1}^{N} [\text{TCP}(1, D_i)]^{v_i} \qquad (33.7)$$

where $\text{TCP}(v_i, D_i)$ is the TCP for the ith tumorlet receiving dose D_i and N is the number of tumorlets.

Several features of the model emerge immediately. The probability of controlling a tumor is dominated by any clonogens with low probability of being killed; thus, TCP is very sensitive to cold spots in the dose distribution. Given the large numbers of clonogens in a tumor, when the dose is uniform the probability of destroying any individual clonogen must be very close to one for TCP to be appreciable. Given reasonable values for radiosensitivities of tumor cells, the model implies a very sharp dose response not seen in clinical studies. This discrepancy is not explainable by variations in tumor size.[33,34] One way the observed shallow dose response might occur is if only a small number of clonogens can repopulate the tumor is small (approximately 200, which is many orders of magnitude less than the overall cell density of ~10^8/cc[35]). But definitive evidence for this hypothesis other than the shallow dose response, for which there are other explanations, has not been presented.

Goitein and others[36–40] propose that the radiosensitivity of tumors differs from patient to patient and that the averaging over this difference results in the relatively broad dose response seen in clinical studies of TCP that are always population averages. Site-, stage-, and grade-specific parameters that describe the radiosensitivity of individual tumors and their variation in the patient population have been collected from clinical studies and summarized by Okunieff et al.[41] Webb[42] adopted a similar approach, using it to fit four clinical tumor control data sets while assuming large (~10^7 cells/cc) clonogen density and Webb and Nahum[43] included the possibility of variations in clonogen density within a tumor. As a consequence of a distribution in radiosensitivities among patients, Zagars et al.[44] and Thames et al.[44] point out that an escalation in dose is most effective for patients with intermediate sensitivity. Those whose tumors are most sensitive do not require such a high prescribed dose, and those who are least sensitive rarely require a dose in excess of normal tissue constraints. This implies that assays predicting radiosensitivity would be useful in identifying patients who would benefit from dose escalation. Such a personalized approach is under investigation for Herpes papilloma virus (HPV) positive head and neck (H&N)

cancers, which have superior survival at the high-dose levels[45] possibly due to increased radiosensitivity.

As was shown by Brahme[31] for a tumor with identical clonogens, the highest TCP for a given mean dose is achieved by a uniform tumor dose distribution. Perhaps partly for this reason, a historical treatment planning goal is uniform PTV coverage. But there is mounting evidence for intratumoral heterogeneity due to both genetic[46] and environmental factors such as hypoxia.[17,47,48] Although this does not broaden the dose–response, it is increasingly important in treatment planning, as it suggests that non-uniform target coverage which places hot spots in regions that are known to be radioresistant or at high risk for failure for other reasons should be advantageous. IMRT can quite easily achieve such distributions and is instrumental to the now widely used technique of dose-painting (simultaneous integrated boost or SIB). Here the physician identifies tumor subvolumes at different degrees of risk and specifies the dose to be delivered to each by a single treatment plan. Usually the regions painted to higher or lower doses are determined by characteristics such as natural history of disease spread, surgical margins, and pretreatment[18] fluorodeoxyglucose (FDG) imaging. In theory, high-dose regions could also be identified by hypoxia imaging using the positron-emitting tracer 18F-misonidazole, though instability of hypoxic regions, which tend to reoxygenate during treatment, may be confounding.[49–52]

It is likely that clinical TCP observations are due to a combination of intratumoral and population distributions of tumor characteristics and that both dose painting and methods of predicting radiosensitivity within the patient population will be useful strategies.

The uncertainties in defining tumor boundaries, clonogenic tumor cell densities, the distribution of heterogeneous clonogen radiosensitivity, and the interaction between these uncertainties and the uncertainties in delivered dose distributions—setup error, physiologic motion, and anatomy changes over a treatment course—make it difficult to test model predictions of the effects of dose inhomogeneity against clinical TCP data. Nonetheless, a growing number of studies indicate effects of inadvertent target dose inhomogeneity on TCP. Terahara et al.[53] studied the effects of dose inhomogeneity on local control using DVH and outcome data from 115 patients treated for skull base chordomas with combined photons and protons. In these patients, with relatively small positional uncertainties and relatively large dose inhomogeneities in the target, a Cox multivariate analysis showed that models including gender and the minimum target dose were significantly associated with the outcome. A case report[54] described treatment failure near a parotid gland in three patients treated with parotid-sparing IMRT and suggested that future patients receive pretreatment PET imaging to assure that the parotid region is free of suspicious nodules. A study that reviewed records of 23 consecutive orbital lymphoma patients treated with 3DCRT, of whom 12 were treated to only the partial orbit, found that 4 of these had an intraorbital recurrence in volumes that had not been covered while no patient treated with whole orbit RT had such recurrence.[55] A study of the GTV dose distribution of 91 tumors (79 patients) treated with single-dose SBRT for paraspinal tumors reported 7 local failures. All were significantly correlated with the low-dose regions and no failures were observed if the minimum PTV dose exceeded 15 Gy.[56] The target dose distributions in paraspinal SBRT are deliberately nonuniform in order to protect the spinal cord which abuts the GTV. There were similar observations in a 332 paraspinal SBRT data set where 1-year local control was 88%. The minimum GTV BED was the only variable to remain correlated with local failure under multivariate Cox analysis and the authors recommended maintaining the minimum GTV dose above 14 Gy in 1 fraction and 21 Gy in 3 fractions.[57] In contrast, Levegrun et al.[58,59] found that the mean, but not the minimum, PTV dose was significantly correlated with biopsy outcome in a series of 132 patients treated with 3DCRT for prostate cancer. PTV coverage in this population was fairly homogeneous and the CTV was defined as the prostate gland and seminal vesicles, although it is likely that the tumor clonogens were confined to subvolumes of the prostate. Setup uncertainty was greater for these patients than those in the other studies, as they were treated before the era of image-guided RT. Random positional uncertainty on the order of 1 cm can be expected in the CTV location during treatment due to setup error and organ motion and the location of resulting underdoses with respect to tumor clonogens was unknown. The possible influence of setup uncertainty which may introduce tumor underdoses, on TCP of prostate cancer is suggested by a much later study from the same institution comparing outcomes for 186 patients treated with conventionally fractionated IMRT for prostate cancer using IGRT with 190 patients who also received IMRT to the same dose and the same planning and delivery technique but without IGRT. The image guidance consisted of setting the patients up by registering the images of radiopaque fiducials implanted in the prostate with their location at simulation using kilovoltage orthogonal radiographs. This assured that the planned high-dose region was delivered to the prostate rather than partially missing on some days due to physiologic changes such as bladder or rectal filling. The high-risk patients treated with IGRT had significantly better FFBF (PSA relapse-free survival) than those without IGRT (97% vs. 77.7%).[60]

Normal Tissue Complication Probability

The goal of NTCP models is to predict the probability of a complication as a function of the dose (or BED) distribution; more recently other factors such as smoking, comorbidities, and chemotherapy may also be included in the function. Intuitively, the modeled NTCP should increase in a roughly sigmoidal fashion (Fig. 33.7) as a function of the organ dose distribution, going from zero at no

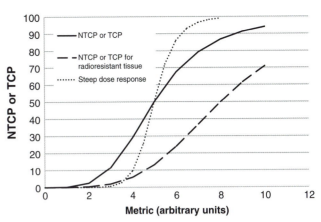

FIGURE 33.7. Sigmoidal dose responses that are expected for both tumor control probability and normal tissue complication probability. The "metric" might be purely dosimetric (e.g., mean dose or D_{max}) or might be a combination of dosimetric and other factors (smoker or nonsmoker). The location and shape of the curve is obtained by analysis of clinical data.

dose up to 100% with the model; the model parameters determine the location and shape of the curve. A given organ may have several different types of complications with different dose–volume parameters. For example, most organs have acute (during or within a few months of treatment) and late complications. Rectal complications include rectal bleeding (most analyzed complication), fecal incontinence, and stool frequency.[61]

All NTCP models must deal with the volume effect. Some complications are most sensitive to "hot spots" in the OAR, others to the mean organ dose, and yet others depend on the entire DVH in a more complex way. The phenomenologic model of Lyman[62] augmented by Kutcher and Burman (LKB model)[63,64] seeks to describe NTCP in terms of four parameters. They introduced the idea of "partial organ irradiation," where a fraction of an organ, v, receives a uniform dose D while the rest receives zero dose. This is not completely artificial—dose distributions of parallel opposed fields are good approximations to partial organ irradiation and such treatments were the clinical norm prior to 3DCRT. In the Lyman model, partial volume tolerance doses are related to each other through a power law in volume fraction. Specifically, if a complication rate c% is produced by uniform dose D to a whole organ, the same complication rate is produced by partial irradiation to a dose D' of a fraction v of the total organ or a chosen reference volume to a dose if

$$D' = D/v^n$$

where $n \geq 0$. If n is very small, v^n is approximately 1 and the complication has little volume dependence. The larger n, the stronger the volume dependence. A feature of the Lyman model is that there is always a partial volume dose for which complication will occur at a specific rate, no matter how small the irradiated partial volume is. The Lyman model is widely used in outcomes analysis, but much less so in clinical plan evaluation, though it is implemented on some planning systems.[1]

In the 1990s, there were efforts to develop other models based on the tissue architecture of organs. Withers[64] hypothesized that the work of an organ is carried out by "functional subunits" (FSUs) and that the volume effect of a complication is determined by how the FSUs combine to carry out the organ function. Nephrons in the kidney and alveoli in the lung are sometimes used as possible examples of FSUs. Architectural models are thoroughly described in the previous edition of this book, part of which is quoted here. Serial (critical element) models assume that certain organs are organized like chains; when one link (a functional subunit or FSU) is damaged the entire chain is broken.[65] A candidate for a serial organ is the spinal cord. Organs with this architecture have a small volume effect. For the parallel model (also called critical volume), a complication does not occur until a significant fraction of independent FSUs (functional reserve) have been incapacitated.[66–68] The volume effect in these tissues is large, because a complication does not occur if less than the functional reserve is irradiated. This behavior is not reflected in the LKB models unless augmented by an additional parameter such as a critical volume below which there is no complication.

The serial and parallel models are conceptually attractive and it was hoped that they might lead to mechanistic understanding of NTCP, but this goal has not been achieved. The models are seldom used in clinical plan evaluation although the names prevail. "Serial" is used for complications that depend mostly on the highest doses to the organ (small n in the Lyman model) and "parallel" for complications with a strong volume dependence (large n). However, a variant (also nonmechanistic), the "relative seriality" model,[69] is almost as widely used for NTCP calculation as the Lyman model, mostly in Europe. There is currently no definitive evidence that would lead users to prefer one of the three NTCP model types (Lyman, tissue architecture, relative seriality) in the clinic. For further discussion, see the references cited here and the earlier edition of this book.

Uniform Irradiation

Lyman[62] represents the NTCP for uniform partial volume irradiation of an organ with an error function of dose and volume.

$$\text{NTCP} = \left(1/\sqrt{2\pi}\right)\int_{-\infty}^{t}\exp\left(-t^2/2\right)dt \quad (33.8a)$$

$$v = V/V_{ref} \quad (33.8b)$$

$$t = [D - \text{TD}_{50}(v)]/[m \cdot \text{TD}_{50}(v)] \quad (33.8c)$$

$$\text{TD}_{50}(1) = \text{TD}_{50}(v) \cdot v^n \quad (33.8d)$$

The model contains four parameters: TD_{50},[62] the tolerance dose for whole organ irradiation; m, the steepness of the dose–response curve; V_{ref}, the reference volume, which in some cases may be the whole volume of the organ; n, which relates the tolerance doses for uniform whole and uniform partial organ irradiation. This latter parameter represents the volume effect. When n is near unity, the volume effect is large[1] and when it is near zero, the volume effect is small. A value of $n \sim 1$ implies that NTCP correlates with the mean dose, whereas a small volume effect implies a correlation with the peak organ dose. The NTCP for partial organ irradiation in the Lyman model was originally based on clinical estimates of partial organ tolerance doses. An early compilation by Emami et al.[70] was fitted to the model by Burman et al.[71] Although many of the parameter values he obtained are still in use, values resulting from maximum likelihood fits of DVH and complication data from 3D conformal dose escalation protocols are available for a growing list of organs. This will be described in more detail in the section "Current Supporting Data for NTCP."

Nonuniform Irradiation—Histogram Reduction and Equivalent Uniform Dose

The approach in the preceding text has been extended to inhomogeneous irradiation by converting the organ's DVH into an "equivalent" uniform one using the effective volume method.[63] The DVH is transformed into one in which the partial volume, v_{eff}, which is equal to or less than the whole organ volume, receives a dose equal to the peak organ dose. This effective volume transformation is self-consistent with the power law model for uniform irradiation in that it can be derived from just two hypotheses: The organ is homogeneous in response and each element of the organ obeys the same power law relationship as the whole organ. Moreover, there is a family of equivalent uniform DVHs with effective volume and dose related through the defining power law relationship. This method was extended to calculate the effective whole volume dose (d_{eff}) by Mohan et al.[72] More recently, use of the generalized equivalent uniform dose (gEUD, sometimes simply called EUD),[1,5,73] has become popular. This quantity is calculated in an identical fashion to d_{eff} (in the EUD formalism, the LKB model parameter n is replaced by the parameter a, they are related by $n = 1/a$).

While the LKB model was designed only for NTCP, gEUD is also used as a surrogate for TCP. Given the DVH for an organ or tumor, gEUD is calculated as

$$\text{gEUD} = \left(\sum_{i=1-N} D_i^a v_i\right)^{1/a} \quad (33.9)$$

where the sum runs over all the dose bins of the DVH, D_i is the dose at the center of the ith bin, and v_i is the fraction of the organ volume in that bin. To describe

---

[1]*Nothing prevents n being greater than 1, in which case greater emphasis is placed on large volumes exposed to lower doses.*

complications, $a \geq 0$ while to describe TCP, $a < 0$. Serial complications (small n or large a) depend strongly on the high-dose part of the DVH while the entire DVH affects the gEUD for small a (large n); for $n = 1$, gEUD is the mean dose. If a is large and negative, gEUD accentuates the low-dose portion of the DVH—the cold spots which are important for tumor control. gEUD is useful for relative ranking of treatment plans in regard to a chosen organ or target without the "judgmental" character of a full TCP or NTCP calculation.[2]

Although the original formulations of the Lyman model and gEUD used physical dose, $EQD2_{\alpha/\beta}$ (or a similar reduction to any desired reference dose) can replace physical dose if the DVH is converted to $EQD2_{\alpha/\beta}$-VH. Within the simplest form of the LQ model, this biologically equivalent EUD has only two parameters (a and α/β) and can potentially incorporate fractionation and volume dependence in a single number that can rank dose distributions delivered at nonstandard fractionation schedules in terms of their risk.

CURRENT SUPPORTING DATA FOR NORMAL TISSUE COMPLICATION PROBABILITY

Both models and dose–volume plan evaluation criteria are based on clinical data, although for many complications, data is still quite sparse and unreliable. This is due to several factors, including: treatments are designed to be "safe" so many reported series have low numbers of complications; publications use qualitatively different criteria for reporting complication severity; for some organs, publications use different definitions of the reference volume; doses are often not clearly specified—for example, a publication might report the number of complications and the prescription dose but give minimal details of an organ dose distribution. Developments such as computerized planning, accurate dose calculation algorithms, electronic record keeping, and prospective collection of dose distribution and complication data allow more opportunities for data collection, but radiation oncology still has a long way to go.[75]

The 1991 compilation of normal tissue tolerance doses and volume effects by Emami and eight co-authors[70] is one of the most cited articles in radiation oncology and its guidelines are still in use. It was the product of an NCI Collaborative Group charged with investigating the then-new tools and potentials of 3D, CT-based treatment planning. Most of the literature they reviewed was from the "2D" era when most treatments were simple (often parallel opposed), simulation images (if taken) were plane radiographs and, if patient-specific dose distributions were generated, they were often superimposed on a manually acquired, two-dimensional contour. In 2010, a group of physicists and physicians performed a systematic review that included more recent publications on dose and volume dependence of clinically reported normal tissue complications for 16 organs. They reviewed many studies that were published in the "3D" era, where patients were treated with the benefit of 3DCRT (and occasionally IMRT) and modern delivery tools (though most studies preceded IGRT). This group named itself QUANTEC. It received funding from both AAPM and American Society for Radiation Oncology (ASTRO), but was not a formal part of either organization. Its reports are published in a supplement to the *International Journal of Radiation Oncology, Biology and Physics*.[4] Surprisingly, QUANTEC found it difficult to extract dosimetric guidelines even from modern published literature for reasons summarized in Jackson et al.[75]

However, the QUANTEC groups were able to make recommendations and, for some complications, develop NTCP models for several organs. These are summarized in a large table in the QUANTEC issue.[4] These recommendations involve mean doses or one or a few DVH points and do not include more complex models. However, many of the organ-specific articles developed models based on the reviewed clinical data and in some cases recommended their use to limit toxicity. QUANTEC repeatedly urges caution in applying its guidelines to IMRT, since much of the reviewed literature described outcomes of 3DCRT, but not IMRT, treatment.

Here we briefly compare the QUANTEC and the 1991 guidance for several complications. For some organs, guidelines are similar although the modern complication endpoints may be less severe (perhaps thanks to guidance from the 1991 study as well as to improved dose conformality with 3DCRT).

Spinal cord:[6] The QUANTEC endpoint (grade 2 or greater myelopathy) includes complications that are less severe than "transverse myelitis," used in the 1991 study. The QUANTEC spinal cord group reviewed 16 publications covering 2,281 patients without prior irradiation, 14 papers with prior spinal radiation, and 10 papers reporting on patients who received SBRT. All reported complications were, understandably, at the low end of the dose–response curve—myelitis is the most feared radiation therapy complication and even slightly risky treatments are usually avoided. Using a logistic function model developed by Schultheiss[76] based on his earlier review of publications extending back into the 1970s, the QUANTEC group concluded that irradiation of the full cord cross section to a maximum dose of 50, 60, and 69 Gy was associated with 0.2%, 6%, and 50% rate of myelopathy. The spinal cord is narrow and visualizing it requires a myelogram or an MRI. Therefore, dosimetrists often contour the spinal canal and the dose distribution within the cord itself (or even the canal) is rarely closely examined in clinical plans. Also, many conventionally fractionated treatments have setup uncertainty that can blur the delivered dose

---

[2]Niemierko earlier introduced an "EUD" intended for TCP only and which used the LQ model directly (74).

distribution on the 0.5 to 1 cm scale of the cord diameter. Therefore, the QUANTEC guidelines[4] are to keep the cord point maximum dose ≤50 Gy, similar to the 1991 recommendation. For the increasingly common situation of retreatment of a volume that includes the spinal cord, QUANTEC found that when more than 6 months elapsed between two treatments, myelopathy was not seen for cumulative doses less than 60 Gy. For SBRT, they recommended that the point maximum be ≤13 Gy in a single fraction and 20 Gy in 3 fractions to keep the complication rate below 1%.

Lung:[77] For lung, the QUANTEC and the 1991 recommendations were again similar. Lung, regarding the complication of RP, is considered a "parallel" organ with a large volume effect. The 1991 paper[71] set the Lyman volume parameter $n = 0.87$ and TD50 = 24.5 Gy, $m = 0.18$. The QUANTEC group reviewed ~70 publications (all conventional fractionation), most of which had more statistically elegant analyses of institutional data than the "by eye" fits used in 1991. Their best estimate of n was 1.03, indicating that the mean lung dose is significantly correlated with RP. This correlation is robust across institutions, as shown in Figure 33.8. The QUANTEC team developed logistic and probit fits to the data in Figure 33.8, from which they recommended mean doses for keeping symptomatic RP between 5% and 40%.

Rectum:[25] Rectum is one of the organs that is defined differently in different studies: rectal wall, rectum including the lumen, anatomical rectum, and lengths determined by the high-dose region. The shape and volume of the rectum change between, and sometimes during, treatment fractions; thus the delivered rectal dose—which

determines the outcome—may differ in an unknown way from the planned dose. QUANTEC's preferred definition is the anatomical rectum on the planning scan, including the lumen. Most of the papers the QUANTEC team reviewed dealt with rectal complications following prostate external beam treatment (other cancers that give substantial rectal dose have a large brachytherapy component or are treating rectal disease). The QUANTEC endpoints were ≥ grade 2 and ≥ grade 3 late rectal toxicity, mostly bleeding and usually defined according to the Radiation Therapy Oncology Group (RTOG) grading scale.[78] These include milder complications than the 1991 study ("severe proctitis/necrosis/fistula") despite the higher doses used for modern prostate treatments. This reflects improvement in rectal protection with the use of 3DCRT. Both QUANTEC and the 1991 studies found that rectal complications have a weak volume dependence. In the 1991 Lyman model parameters, "n" is 0.12[71] while the QUANTEC n is 0.09 with 95% CI 0; 04–0.14. Both find rectum to be fairly radioresistant; the 1991 TD50 is 80 Gy, QUANTEC's is 76.9 or 78.5 Gy, depending on the publications they included in analysis. However, rather than simply specifying a maximum rectal point dose, QUANTEC recommends five intermediate DVH points, thus defining the upper limit of the DVH between 50 and 75 Gy.

Rectal complications other than bleeding may be better correlated with the dose distribution in specific parts of the rectum.[61] Because rectal dose distributions for IMRT treatment of prostate cancer look quite different from those from 3DCRT and the rectal complication rate following IMRT prostate treatment is much lower than for 3DCRT,[79] QUANTEC made no recommendations for

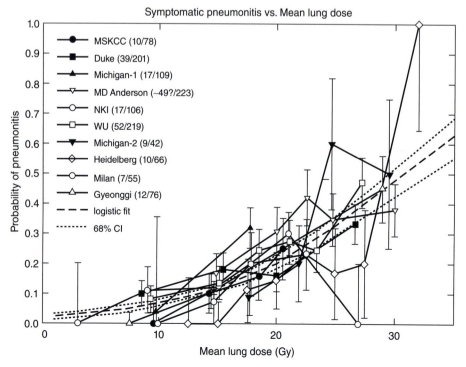

FIGURE 33.8. QUANTEC rate of symptomatic pneumonitis as a function of mean lung dose—comparison of data from 10 institutions. The *dashed line* is a logistic fit to the form $f/(1 + f)$ where $f = \exp(b0 + b1 \times$ mean lung dose). The best fit values (95% CI) are $b0 = -3.87$ (−3.33, −4.49), $b1 = 0.126$ (0.100, 0.153) corresponding to TD50 = 30.75 (28.7, 33.9) Gy and $\gamma50 = 0.969$ (0.833, 1.122), where $\gamma50$ represents the increase in response (measured as percentage) per 1% increase in dose near the 50% dose–response level. (Reprinted with permission from Marks LB, Bentzen SM, Deasy JO, et al. Radiation dose-volume effects in the lung. *Int J Radiat Oncol Biol Phys.* 2010;76(3):S70–S76.)

IMRT. However, a recent publication confirmed the QUANTEC Lyman parameters[7] as a secondary aspect of the research in that paper while another study on a large, different data set found a large discrepancy between Lyman parameters for rectal toxicity in 3DCRT versus IMRT.[80] Deciding whether or not the QUANTEC parameters describe rectal toxicity in IMRT and modeling rectal complications for SBRT prostate treatment remains to be done.

Optic structures (optic nerves and chiasm):[81] The endpoint for the 1991 study was blindness while QUANTEC included less severe complications as well (visual impairment or optic neuropathy). The optic structures are very small and both contouring and dose delivery accuracy confound efforts to find a volume effect. The 1991 guidelines are a 5% probability of blindness for a whole organ dose of 50 Gy and a 50% probability of blindness for 65 Gy. In general, QUANTEC finds that the optic structures are more radiation tolerant than suggested by the 1991 study, which may allow better target coverage in some brain and H&N cases.

QUANTEC's recommendations are for three point maximum values with the caveat that the D_{max} values are often very close to the dose to the whole organ. The QUANTEC maximum dose points are $D_{max} < 55$ Gy for NTCP < 3% (the 1991 model predicts 13.6%); D_{max} 55–60 Gy, NTCP 3%–7% (the 1991 model predicts up to 29%). The third D_{max} point involves only upper limits above 60 Gy (NTCP > 7%–20%), which doesn't allow comparisons.

1991 models more aggressive: For parotid, cochlea, kidneys, heart, and stomach, using the 1991 constraints is likely to lead to a higher complication rate than expected from subsequent literature; the QUANTEC recommendations are more conservative. For example, the parotids are key risk organs for H&N treatment: these cancers have a high cure rate and the nonlethal complication of xerostomia, with great impact on quality of life, is a concern. The parotids are "parallel" organs, with the 1991 Lyman model assigning an n of 0.7 while QUANTEC,[82] based on more recent information, focuses on the mean parotid dose. The 1991 Lyman model predicts <20% complication for mean parotid dose below 39 Gy, while today most H&N treatment protocols advise keeping the mean bilateral gland dose below 25 Gy if possible or, if high dose must be given to one parotid to achieve tumor control, keeping the spared parotid mean dose below 20 Gy.

Finally, for esophagitis and radiation-induced liver disease, the dose–volume behavior extracted by QUANTEC from modern studies is simply different than reported in the 1991 publication. And for the bladder, the quality of available data was inadequate to support guidelines. The 1991 report gives Lyman model parameters for several organs not included in QUANTEC (brachial plexus, external ear, rib cage, femoral head, thyroid, Temperomandibular (TM) joint, and mandible) while QUANTEC makes recommendations on the penile bulb.

For many organs, QUANTEC made no recommendations for hypofractionated treatment because literature at that time was scarce. Also, most of the literature reviewed by QUANTEC dealt with complications in adult patients. There are now two efforts patterned after QUANTEC— one to make literature-based recommendations for Pediatric normal tissue effects in clinic (PENTEC), and Working Group for Stereotactic Body Radiation Therapy (WGSBRT). These groups hope to make recommendations in the near future.

Fitting Clinical Complications Data to a Model: An Example

Thanks to the knowledge gained from over a century of radiation therapy and to advanced planning and delivery techniques, radiation-induced normal tissue complications are infrequent. Differences between patient populations, local preferences for certain treatment methods and dosing schedules, and local variations in accompanying therapies (surgery, chemotherapy) make the study of NTCP an exercise in extracting a weak signal from a noisy background. Controlled randomized clinical trials might provide high-quality data, but they are often cost-limited to small patient numbers and are aimed at answering a few specific questions that the funding organization deems important. Increasingly, sophisticated statistical methods are being applied to the problem of mining institutional databases or using peer-reviewed clinical data to develop and validate NTCP models.

Statistical Model of a Parallel Organ

In parallel element tissues, which have been modeled using binomial statistics,[66–68] a complication occurs if the fraction of eradicated FSUs exceeds a threshold fraction, the functional reserve of the organ. The kidney, liver, and lung are conjectured to behave as parallel organs. Because the number of FSUs is always large in these organs, the functional reserve can be defined by the fraction rather than the number of eradicated FSUs. Furthermore, as with TCP, the large number of FSUs leads to unrealistically large gradients of NTCP with dose in the region of NTCP = 50%. To remedy this, population averaging is invoked, which requires additional parameters. For example, if the functional reserve and the FSU radiosensitivity (defined by the dose required for 50% FSU death) vary among a population of patients, then two additional parameters are required to represent the widths of these distributions. In addition, intraorgan variation in radiosensitivity may also be considered. Fortunately, it can be demonstrated that intraorgan variability has a negligible effect on the slope of the local dose–response curve.[83]

A further simplification is possible if the width of the distribution of radiosensitivities is narrower than that of the functional reserve. In this limit the NTCP is given by the integral of the functional reserve up to the mean fraction of eradicated FSUs, that is, up to the fraction damaged.[83] This form is quite useful for fitting clinical complication data.

Fitting the Parallel Model to Clinical Complication Data

The method described here is now widely used in fitting biophysical models to clinical data. Such an approach is a starting point to suggest further developments in the collection and analysis of clinical data. We describe here one example in which a parallel model (described in preceding text) and the method of maximum likelihood is used to fit DVHs and complication data for radiation hepatitis of 93 patients treated for tumors of the liver.[83–85]

The method of maximum likelihood can be applied as follows. The DVH for each patient is used to calculate NTCP by first assigning a best guess for the model parameters. The predicted probability of a complication for each patient is then compared against the observed grade of complication in that patient. The overall likelihood L of the observations is then modeled according to

$$L(\gamma_1, \gamma_2, \ldots) = \prod_{\substack{m \\ \text{complication}}} O_m(t_m, \gamma_1, \gamma_2, \ldots)$$
$$\prod_{\substack{n \\ \text{no complican}}} [1 - O_n(t_n, \gamma_1, \gamma_2, \ldots)] \qquad (33.10)$$

where

$$O_m(t_m, \gamma_1, \gamma_2, \ldots) = O(t_m)\text{NTCP}_m(\gamma_1, \gamma_2, \ldots)$$

where L is the likelihood, $O(t_m)$ is the probability that a complication will manifest itself after the follow-up time t_m for the mth patient—calculated from complication and follow-up time data with the Kaplan–Meier method[86] and $\gamma_1, \gamma_2, \ldots$ indicates the model parameters. The likelihood function is then maximized with respect to the model parameters. Note that the likelihood is essentially the probability in the model of the observed complication pattern.

Furthermore, it is convenient to assume, as described earlier, that the organ has a functional reserve described with two parameters (whose values are to be obtained from the maximum likelihood fit) and that NTCP is given by the integral of the functional reserve up to the mean fraction of eradicated FSUs, that is, up to the fraction damaged.[83] For each patient, the fraction damaged is calculated by summing up the product of the fractional volume of each voxel of the organ and the probability of damage. The latter can be calculated using each patient's DVH and an assumed local response function with two parameters (whose values are to be obtained from the maximum likelihood fit).

The results of applying such an analysis to the hepatitis data is shown in Figure 33.9 for observed complication

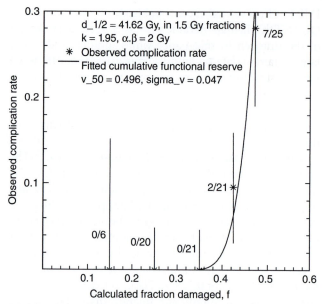

FIGURE 33.9. Observed complication rate for radiation hepatitis versus calculated fraction damaged. (Reprinted from Jackson A, Ten Haken RK, Robertson JM, et al. Analysis of clinical complication data for radiation hepatitis using a parallel architecture model. *Int J Radiat Oncol Biol Phys.* 1995;31:883–892, with permission.)

rate as a function of the calculated fraction of the liver that is damaged. The observed complications for this data set show a threshold effect with a steep response, which is described well with the parallel model. In this application, the best-fit functional reserve distribution and their confidence intervals predict that irradiation of less than one-third of the liver volume leads to negligible complications.[83] That is, the threshold volume is about one-third. A more detailed analysis of the fit revealed that the uncertainties in the width of the functional reserve distribution and radiosensitivity of FSUs were correlated. This arose because complications were seen only in the cohort of patients who received a whole liver irradiation as part of the treatment course. The lack of complications among patients given only partial volume irradiation suggested that an attempt to increase local control through dose escalation was feasible. After follow-up of subsequently treated patients, some of whom had received 90 Gy, Dawson et al. analyzed data from 138 patients, including 19 with radiation-induced liver disease (RILD). Observation of complications in patients with only partial volume irradiation helped to resolve the correlated uncertainties in the model parameters and the threshold limit was revised down from one-third to one-fourth.[87,88]

Current and Future Clinical Use of Normal Tissue Dose–Volume Criteria

Treatment plans are often designed to meet competing goals of target coverage and protection for nearby normal organs. These goals have been refined through experience so that they are relatively safe and effective ("acceptable" complication and control rates) and can be satisfied by plans that can be done by skilled planners (dosimetrists) within clinically reasonable times using acceptable beam arrangements (no mechanical collisions, not too many beams, none passing through strongly attenuating support structures). There are protection goals that must be satisfied (e.g., spinal cord) even if target coverage is compromised. For example, for conventionally fractionated treatments of patients without prior radiation, the maximum permitted spinal cord dose is below 50 Gy, which is often too low to achieve durable tumor control. A compromise for mediastinal tumors (devised long before the advent of 3DCRT, but still in use) is to treat to 40 to 45 Gy with Anterior/posterior (AP/PA) beams that cover the entire PTV and then "cone down" to "off cord" oblique beams that treat part of the PTV to 60 Gy but spare the spinal cord from further direct dose. IMRT often allows a plan that treats the tumor to 60 Gy in a single phase because intensity modulation decreases target dose from some beams to protect the cord but fills in target dose from other beam directions. In paraspinal SBRT, target coverage is usually compromised to achieve sufficient cord protection; with minor compromise, the treatments remain effective.[56,57] In some situations, it may be possible to make a clinical decision of priority between protection and coverage goals. In these cases, it is valuable for the planner to have guidance as to whether both can be satisfied before he starts. As an early example, Hunt et al.[89] retrospectively analyzed the treatment plans of 51 H&N cancer patients treated with dose-painting IMRT (PTVs for dose levels 54, 59.4, and 70 or 54–60 and 66 Gy). One or both parotid glands overlapped PTVs. To maintain a <25% risk of xerostomia, the mean parotid gland dose should be below 26 Gy but for tumor control, the plan should give each PTV full dose according to its level. The study derived the maximum fraction of parotid-PTV overlap and the necessary mean dose to the non-overlap region to achieve an overall mean parotid dose of 26 Gy without underdosing the PTV. These doses could be used as optimization goals for parotid portions outside the PTV. If a mean dose below 26 Gy cannot be achieved for a gland, a clinical decision must be made.

A more elaborate version of this approach is now being applied to "knowledge-based planning."[90,91] For a particular disease site and perhaps beam arrangement, a database of previous "good" plans is used as a training set to parameterize a treatment plan model. The "best" (as defined by the model) achievable OAR DVHs are then predicted for a new patient based on his anatomy. Of course users must agree on an appropriate training set. Knowledge-based planning is in its infancy, but in the future, it may reduce planning time, improve plan quality, and allow for more objective plan evaluation by comparison with high-quality reference plans that meet established treatment standards. On the down side, developing the plan model (commissioning the knowledge-based system) will require much work and institutions with different treatment goals would not be able to share models.

In a novel application of the knowledge-based approach,[7] treatment plans from an RTOG prostate IMRT treatment protocol were replanned using a knowledge-based model. The training set was 20 high-quality plans from one of the collaborating institutions. These plans satisfied all the RTOG protocol constraints and were selected for best OAR (rectum and bladder) sparing. The model was further tuned on the RTOG plans with the smallest difference between the plan rectal NTCP and that predicted by the knowledge-based program. Finally, for 30 RTOG plans (10 with the smallest NTCP difference from predicted, 10 with the largest difference, and 10 intermediate cases) model-predicted rectal DVHs were obtained. Each case was then replanned to give approximately the same PTV coverage as the original (in all cases meeting protocol requirements), to maintain or improve the bladder DVH and to use the rectal DVH predicted by the model as a guide for the new plan. The QUANTEC Lyman model parameters were confirmed as a separate part of the study and the improvement in plan quality was evaluated as the reduction in Lyman NTCP achieved by the new plan. Although all the original plans had met the protocol's constraints, they were not "optimal" in that the rectal NTCP was reduced in all the replanned cases without sacrificing coverage or other planning objectives. Should this or related methods become readily accessible and efficient, one would expect treatment complication rates, as well as planning time to decrease. Evaluation of individual plans would be partly based on their similarity to the plans in the model knowledge base. Models themselves might be evaluated by periodic institutional plan intercomparisons, though there would undoubtedly be debates about the gold standard. Of course with better quantitative understanding of plan outcome, plan quality metrics will change.

CONCLUSIONS

Dose–volume criteria are now widely used in planning and plan evaluation; models are available and interesting, but in order to come into general clinical use, proponents will have to demonstrate that they add something to the clinical process—more efficient planning or more efficient or objective plan evaluation. Especially, the latter will require stringent model validation and education of physicians, physicists, and dosimetrists as to their appropriate use. Clinical data is being mined to update evidence-based guidance, which is particularly needed to address new treatment paradigms. Currently, we are focused on hypofractionation but future developments may include combined modalities or molecular personalized medicine. Peer-reviewed clinical data should be presented in a format that allows "data pooling"[92] so that these efforts move forward more rapidly. Improved models and dose–volume constraints combined with knowledge-based planning may make it easier and more likely to arrive at superior plans to the benefit of future patients.

KEY POINTS

- Both volumetric graphic dose distributions and DVHs are required for evaluation of complex modern treatment plans. The quality of treatment plan dosimetry must achieve a balance between the probability of local tumor control (tumor control probability or TCP) and the probability of normal tissue complications (NTCP).

- The rapid growth of SBRT makes it necessary to account for the greater biologic potency of hypofractionated treatments in planning and plan evaluation. The LQ cell survival model is most often used for this purpose, although other models have been proposed.

- Some dose–volume metrics that can be read directly off a DVH (D_volume, V_dose) have been shown to correlate with outcomes but predictive models have also been devised. Both TCP and NTCP are approximately zero at low doses and rise to close to 100% at high doses but "low," "high," and the rate of increase with dose depend on the tissue. Ideally the key parameters that determine response are obtained and validated by analysis of clinical outcomes.

- Most TCP models are based on the hypothesis that a tumor is controlled only if the radiation course kills all clonogens (cells capable of regrowing the tumor). This approach, combined with the LQ cell survival model, led to recognition that SBRT can be safely delivered to prostate cancer.

- For NTCP, it is noted that different complications have different dependences on the radiation distribution in the organ. The two extremes are called "serial" and "parallel" responses. Serial responses depend on the highest dose in the organ while parallel responses depend on the overall organ dose, often approximated by the mean organ dose. NTCP models must account for these effects. A classical collection of NTCP dose–response information was published in 1991 (Emami et al.,[70] Burman et al.[71]). Recently, the QUANTEC group reviewed modern papers and provided guidelines and models for 16 organs. There is mixed agreement between QUANTEC and the 1991 studies.

- Models may be effectively used in comparing rival plans and delivery techniques, in dose–escalation trial design and in plan optimization and they are used in this way at large academic centers. However, for general use, they must be validated sufficiently for many clinicians to have confidence in them.

REVIEW QUESTIONS

1. Tumor type A has radiobiologic parameter $\alpha/\beta = 10$ Gy while tumor type B has $\alpha/\beta = 1.5$ Gy. Both tumors have 10^8 clonogens and have radiobiologic parameter $\alpha = 0.1$ Gy^{-1}. Which tumor type has the **larger change** in TCP when the treatment fractionation is changed from 60 Gy in 30 fractions to 60 Gy in 3 fractions?
   - **A.** A
   - **B.** B
   - **C.** Equal response
   - **D.** Neither tumor responds to such low doses

2. The complication probability for a normal tissue is said to be of "serial" type. What part of the dose distribution is most important in determining its NTCP?
   - **A.** The mean organ dose
   - **B.** The low-dose part of the distribution
   - **C.** The high-dose part of the distribution
   - **D.** The % volume receiving 20 Gy

3. The complication probability for a normal tissue is said to be of "serial" type. Which is most likely to be the Lyman model volume effect parameter, n?
   - **A.** $n = 0.05$
   - **B.** $n = 0.35$

   - **C.** $n = 0.75$
   - **D.** $n = 1.0$

4. A recent analysis of published NTCP data up to approximately 2010 was conducted by
   - **A.** Emami-Burman
   - **B.** QUANTEC
   - **C.** NRC
   - **D.** NTQABS

5. One way to use biologic models in treatment planning is
   - **A.** Comparing rival treatment plans
   - **B.** Reducing planning time
   - **C.** Reducing plan delivery time
   - **D.** All of the above

6. The gEUD is
   - **A.** The mean dose to an organ
   - **B.** The equivalent uniform dose that, when applied to the organ, has the same biologic (TCP or NTCP) effect as the actual dose distribution
   - **C.** The uniform radiation dose that has the same effect as a specified chemotherapy dose
   - **D.** Applicable only to parallel normal tissues

ANSWERS

1. B Tumor B: For Tumor A, the BED changes from 72 Gy to 180 Gy and TCP (Equation 33.4) changes from ~0 to 0.218 (approximately 21.8%). For Tumor B, the BED changes from 140 to 860 Gy and TCP changes from ~0 to 1 (or 100%).

2. C **(the high-dose part)** "Serial" is used for complications that depend mostly on the highest doses to the organ (small n in the Lyman model) and "parallel" for complications with a strong volume dependence (large n).

3. A ($n = 0.05$)—see explanation provided earlier.

4. B (QUANTEC) "In 2010, a group of physicists and physicians performed a systematic review that included more recent publications on dose and volume dependence of clinically reported normal tissue complications for 16 organs."

5. A (comparing rival treatment plans). Biologic models have no effect on plan delivery time and at present, there's no definitive evidence that they reduce planning time.

6. B (see section "Nonuniform Irradiation—Histogram Reduction and Equivalent Uniform Dose").

REFERENCES

1. Allen Li X, Alber M, Deasy JO, et al. The use and QA of biologically related models for treatment planning: short report of the TG-166 of the therapy physics committee of the AAPM. *Med Phys.* 2012;39:1386–1409. http://www.aapm.org/pubs/reports/RPT_166.pdf

2. Timmerman R, Bastasch M, Saha D, et al. Stereotactic body radiation therapy: normal tissue and tumor control effects with large dose per fraction. *Front Radiat Ther Oncol.* 2011;43:382–394.

3. Schultz DB, Diehn M, Loo BW Jr. To SABR or not to SABR? Indications and contraindications for stereotactic ablative radiotherapy in the treatment of early-stage, oligometastatic or oligoprogressive non-small cell lung cancer. *Semin Radiat OncSemin Radiat Oncol.* 2015;25:78–86.

4. Marks LB, Yorke ED, Jackson A, et al. Use of normal tissue complication probability models in the clinic. *Int J Radiat Oncol Biol Phys.* 2010;76(3 Suppl):S10–S19.

5. Wu Q, Mohan R, Morris M, et al. Simultaneous integrated boost intensity-modulated radiotherapy for locally advanced head-and-neck squamous cell carcinomas. I: dosimetric results. *Int J Radiat Oncol Biol Phys.* 2003;56:573–585.

6. Kirkpatrick JP, van der Kogel AJ, Schultheiss TE. Radiation dose-volume effects in the spinal cord. *Int J Radiat Oncol Biol Phys.* 2010;76(3 Suppl):S42–S49.

7. Moore KL, Schmidt R, Moiseenko V, et al. Quantifying unnecessary normal tissue complication risks due to suboptimal planning: a secondary study of RTOG 0126. *Int J Radiat Oncol Biol Phys.* 2015;92:228–235.

8. Widesott L, Pierelli A, Fiorino C, et al. Helical tomotherapy vs. intensity-modulated proton therapy for whole pelvis irradiation in high-risk prostate cancer patients: dosimetric, normal tissue complication probability, and generalized equivalent uniform dose analysis. *Int J Radiat Oncol Biol Phys.* 2011;80:1589–1600.

9. Kong FM, Ten Haken RK, Schipper MJ, et al., High-dose radiation improved local tumor control and overall survival in patients with inoperable/unresectable non-small –cell lung cancer: long term results of a radiation dose escalation study. *Int J Radiat Oncol Biol Phys.* 2005;63:324–333.

10. Rosenzweig KE, Fox JL, Yorke E, et al. Results of a phase I dose-escalation study using three-dimensional conformal radiation therapy in the treatment of inoperable nonsmall cell lung carcinoma. *Cancer.* 2005;103:2118–2127.

11. Long T, Matuszak M, Feng M, et al. Sensitivity analysis for lexicographic ordering in radiation therapy treatment planning. *Med Phys.* 2012;39:3445–3455.

12. Spalding AC, Jee KW, Vineberg K, et al. Potential for dose-escalation and reduction of risk in pancreatic cancer using IMRT optimization with lexicographic ordering and gEUD-based cost functions. *Med Phys.* 2007;34:521–529.

13. Hall EJ, Giaccia AJ. *Radiobiology for the Radiologist.* 7th ed. Philadelphia, PA: Lippincott, Williams and Wilkins; 2012.

14. Joiner M, van der Kogel A. *Basic Clinical Radiobiology.* 4th ed. London: Hodder Arnold; 2009.

15. Fowler JF. The linear-quadratic formula and progress in fractionated radiotherapy. *Br J Radiol.* 1989;62:679–694.

16. Nahum AE. The radiobiology of hypofractionation. *Clin Oncol (R Coll Radiol).* 2015;27:260–269.

17. Chapman JD. Can the two mechanisms of tumor cell killing by radiation be exploited for therapeutic gain? *J Radiat Res.* 2014;55:2–9.

18. Thames HD, Hendry JH. *Fractionation in Radiotherapy.* London: Taylor and Francis; 1987.

19. Bentzen SM, Joiner MC. Chapter 9: The linear-quadratic approach in clinical practice. In: Joiner M, van der Kogel A, eds. *Basic Clinical Radiobiology.* 4th ed. London: Hodder Arnold; 2009.

20. Joiner MC, Bentzen SM. Chapter 8: Fractionation: the linear-quadratic approach. In: Joiner M, van der Kogel A, eds. *Basic Clinical Radiobiology.* 4th ed. London: Hodder Arnold; 2009.

21. Bentzen SM, Dörr W, Gahbauer R, et al. Bioeffect modeling and equieffective dose concepts in radiation oncology – terminology, quantities and units. *Radiother Oncol.* 2012;105:266–268.

22. Brenner DJ, Hall EJ. Fractionation and protraction for radiotherapy of prostate carcinoma. *Int J Radiat Oncol Biol Phys.* 1999;43:1095–1101.

23. Munro TR, Gilbert CW. The relation between tumour lethal doses and the radiosensitivity of tumour cells. *Br J Radiol.* 1961;34:246–251.

24. Fowler JF, Toma-Dasu I, Dasu A. Is the α/β ratio for prostate tumours really low and does it vary with the level of risk at diagnosis? *AntiCancer Res.* 2013;33:1009–1011.

25. Michalski JM, Gay H, Jackson A, et al. Radiation dose-volume effects in radiation-induced rectal injury. *Int J Radiat Oncol Biol Phys.* 2010;76(3 Suppl):S123–S129.

26. Henderson DR, Tree AC, van As NJ. Stereotactic body radiotherapy for prostate cancer. *Clin Oncol.* 2015;27:270–279.

27. Brenner DJ. The linear-quadratic model is an appropriate methodology for determining isoeffective doses at large doses per fraction. *Semin Radiat Oncol.* 2008;18:234–239.

28. Kirkpatrick JP, Meyer JJ, Marks LB. The linear-quadratic model is inappropriate to model high dose per fraction effects in radiosurgery. *Semin Radiat Oncol.* 2008;18:240–243.

29. Park C, Papiez L, Zhang S, et al. Universal survival curve and single fraction equivalent dose: useful tools in understanding potency of ablative radiotherapy. *Int J Radiat Oncol Biol Phys.* 2008;70:847–852.

30. Tucker SL, Li M, Xu T, et al. Incorporating single-nucleotide polymorphisms into the Lyman model to improve prediction of radiation pneumonitis. *Int J Radiat Oncol Biol Phys.* 2013;85:251–257.

31. Brahme A. Dosimetric precision requirements in radiation therapy. *Acta Radiol Oncol.* 1984;23:379–391.

32. Goitein M. Causes and consequences of inhomogeneous dose distributions in radiation therapy. *Int J Radiat Oncol Biol Phys.* 1986;12:701–704.

33. Goitein M. The probability of controlling an inhomogeneously irradiated tumor. In Zink S ed. *Evaluation of Treatment Planning for Particle Beam Radiotherapy*, NCI Contract Report. Bethesday, MD: National Cancer Institute; 1987.

34. Bentzen SM, Thames HD. Tumor volume and local control probability: clinical data and radiobiological interpretations. *Int J Radiat Oncol Biol Phys.* 1996;36:247–251.

35. Zaider M, Minerbo GN. Tumour control probability: a formulation applicable to any temporal protocol of dose delivery. *Phys Med Biol.* 2000;45:279–293.

36. Niemierko A, Goitein M. Implementation of a model for estimating tumor control probability for an inhomogeneously irradiated tumor. *Radiother Oncol.* 1993;29:140–147.

37. Bentzen SM. Steepness of the clinical dose-control curve and variation in the in vitro radiosensitivity of head and neck squamous cell carcinoma. *Int J Radiat Biol.* 1992;62:417–423.

38. Suit H, Skates S, Taghian A, et al. Clinical implications of heterogeneity of tumor response to radiation therapy. *Radiother Oncol.* 1992;25:251–260.

39. Dutreix J, Tubiana M, Dutreix A. An approach to the interpretation of clinical data on the tumor control probability-dose relationship. *Radiother Oncol.* 1988;11:239–248.

40. Zagars GK, Schultheiss T, Peters LJ. Inter-tumor heterogeneity and radiation dose control curves. *Radiother Oncol.* 1987;8:353–361.

41. Okunieff P, Morgan D, Niemierko A, et al. Radiation dose-response of human tumors. *Int J Radiat Oncol Biol Phys.* 1995;32:1227–1237.

42. Webb S. Optimum parameters in a model for tumour control probability including interpatient heterogeneity. *Phys Med Biol.* 1994;39:1895–1914.

43. Webb S, Nahum AE. A model for calculating tumour control probability in radiotherapy including the effects of inhomogeneous distribution of dose and clonogenic cell density. *Phys Med Biol.* 1933;38:653–666.

44. Thames HD, Schultheiss TE, Hendry JH, et al. Can modest escalation of dose be detected as increased tumor control? *Int J Radiat Oncol Biol Phys.* 1991;22:241–246.

45. Kimple RJ, Harari PM. Is radiation dose reduction the right answer for HPV-positive head and neck cancer? *Oral Oncol.* 2014;50:560–564.

46. Swanton C. Intratumor heterogeneity: evolution through space and time. *Cancer Res.* 2012;72:4875–4882.

47. Horsman MR, Wouters BG, Joiner MC, et al. The oxygen effect and fractionated radiotherapy. In: Michael Joiner, Albert van derKogel, eds. *Basic Clinical Radiobiology*. 4th ed. London: Hodder Arnold; 2009:207–216.

48. Wouters BG, Koritzinsky M. The tumour microenvironment and cellular hypoxia responses In: Michael Joiner, Albert van derKogel, eds. *Basic Clinical Radiobiology*. 4th ed. London: Hodder Arnold; 2009:217–232.

49. Popple RA, Ove R, Shen S. Tumor control probability for selective boosting of hypoxic subvolumes, including the effect of reoxygenation. *Int J Radiat Oncol Biol Phys.* 2002;54:921–927.

50. Kim Y, Tome WA. Dose-painting IMRT optimization using biological parameters. *Acta Oncol.* 2010;49:1374–1384.

51. For an example, see RTOG protocol RTOG 0225, A phase II study of intensity modulated radiation therapy (IMRT) +/− chemotherapy for nasopharyngeal cancer; https://www.rtog.org/ClinicalTrials/ProtocolTable/StudyDetails.aspx?study=0225

52. Lin Z, Mechalakos J, Nehmeh S, et al. The influence of changes in tumor hypoxia on dose-painting treatment plans based on 18F-Miso positron emission tomography. *Int J Radiat Oncol Biol Phys.* 2008;70:1219–1228.

53. Terahara A, Niemierko A, Goitein M, et al. Analysis of the relationship between tumor dose inhomogeneity and local control in patients with skull base chordoma. *Int J Radiat Oncol Biol Phys.* 1999;45:351–358.

54. Cannon DM, Lee NY. Recurrence in region of spared parotid gland after definitive intensity-modulated radiotherapy for head and neck cancer. *Int J Radiat Oncol Biol Phys.* 2008;70:660–665.

55. Pfeffer MR, Rabin T, Tsvang L, et al. Orbital lymphoma: is it necessary to treat the entire orbit? *Int J Radiat Oncol Biol Phys.* 2004;60:527–530.

56. Lovelock DM, Zhang Z, Jackson A, et al. Correlation of local failure with measures of dose insufficiency in the high-dose single fraction treatment of bony metastases. *Int J Radiat Oncol Biol Phys.* 2010;77:1282–1287.

57. Bishop AJ, Tao R, Rebueno NC, et al. Outcomes for spine stereotactic body radiation therapy and an analysis of predictors of local recurrence *Int J Radiat Oncol Biol Phys.* 2015;92:1016–1026.

58. Levegrun S, Jackson A, Zelefsky MJ, et al. Analysis of biopsy outcome after three-dimensional conformal radiation therapy of prostate cancer using dose distribution variables and tumor control probability models. *Int J Radiat Oncol Biol Phys.* 2000;47:1245–1260.

59. Levegrun S, Jackson A, Zelefsky MJ, et al. Fitting tumor control probability models to biopsy outcome after three-dimensional conformal radiation therapy of prostate cancer: pitfalls in deducing radiobiologic parameters for tumors from clinical data. *Int J Radiat Oncol Biol Phys.* 2001;51:1064–1080.

60. Zelefsky MJ, Kollmeier M, Cox B, et al. Improved clinical outcomes with high-dose image guided radiotherapy compared with non-IGRT for the treatment of clinically localized prostate cancer. *Int J Radiat Oncol Biol Phys.* 2012;84:125–129.

61. Peeters ST, Lebesque JV, Heemsbergen WD. Localized volume effects for late rectal and anal toxicity after radiotherapy for prostate cancer. *Int J Radiat Oncol Biol Phys.* 2006;64:1151–1161.

62. Lyman JT. Complication probabilities as assessed from dose-volume histograms. *Radiat Res Suppl.* 1985;104:S13–S19.

63. Kutcher GJ, Burman C, Brewster L, et al. Histogram reduction method for calculating complication probabilities for three-dimensional treatment planning evaluations. *Int J Radiat Oncol Biol Phys.* 1991;21:137–146.

64. Withers HR, Taylor JM, Maciejewski B. Treatment volume and tissue tolerance. *Int J Radiat Oncol Biol Phys.* 1988;15:751–759.

65. Niemierko A, Goitein M. Calculation of normal tissue complication probability and dose-volume histogram reduction schemes for tissues with a critical element architecture. *Radiother Oncol.* 1991;20:166–176.

66. Niemierko A, Goitein M. Modeling of normal tissue response to radiation: the critical volume model. *Int J Radiat Oncol Biol Phys.* 1993;25:135–145.

67. Yorke ED, Kutcher GJ, Jackson A, et al. Probability of radiation-induced complications in normal tissues with parallel architecture under conditions of uniform whole or partial organ irradiation. *Radiother Oncol.* 1993;26:226–237.

68. Jackson A, Kutcher GJ, Yorke ED. Probability of radiation-induced complications for normal tissues with parallel architecture subject to non-uniform irradiation. *Med Phys.* 1993;20:613–625.

69. Källman P, Agren A, Brahme A. Tumor and normal tissue responses to fractionated non uniform dose delivery. *Int J Radiat Biol.* 1992;62:249–262.

70. Emami B, Lyman J, Brown A, et al. Tolerance of normal tissue to therapeutic irradiation. *Int J Radiat Oncol Biol Phys.* 1991;21:109–122.

71. Burman C, Kutcher GJ, Emami B, et al. Fitting normal tissue tolerance data to an analytic function. *Int Radiat Oncol Biol Phys.* 1991;21:123–135.

72. Mohan R, Mageras GS, Baldwin B. Clinically relevant optimization of 3D conformal treatments. *Med Phys.* 1992;19:933–944.

73. Niemierko A. A generalized concept of equivalent uniform dose (EUD). *Med Phys.* 1999;26;1101.

74. Niemierko A. Reporting and analyzing dose distributions: a concept of equivalent uniform dose. *Med Phys.* 1997;24;103–110.

75. Jackson A, Marks LB, Bentzen SM, et al. The lessons of Quantec: recommendations for reporting and gathering data on dose-volume dependencies of treatment outcome. *Int J Radiat Oncol Biol Phys.* 2010;76:S155–S160.

76. Schultheiss TE, Kun LE, Ang KK, et al. Radiation response of the central nervous system. *Int J Radiat Oncol Biol Phys.* 1995;31:1093–1112.

77. Marks LB, Bentzen SM, Deasy JO, et al. Radiation dose-volume effects in the lung. *Int J Radiat Oncol Biol Phys.* 2010;76:S70–S76.

78. Cox JD, Stetz J, Pajak TF. Toxicity criteria of the Radiation Therapy Oncology Group (RTOG) and the European Organization for Research and Treatment of Cancer (EORTC). *Int J Radiat Oncol Biol Phys.* 1995;31:1341–1346.

79. Zelefsky MJ, Levin EJ, Hunt M, et al. Incidence of late rectal and urinary toxicities after three-dimensional conformal radiotherapy and intensity-modulated radiotherapy for localized prostate cancer. *Int J Radiat Oncol Biol Phys.* 2008;70:1124–1129.

80. Troeller A, Yan D, Marina O, et al. Comparison and limitations of DVH-based NTCP models derived from 3D-CRT and IMRT data for prediction of gastrointestinal toxicities in prostate cancer patients by using propensity score matched pair analysis. *Int J Radiat Oncol Biol Phys.* 2015;91:435–443.

81. Mayo C, Martel MK, Marks LB, et al. Radiation dose-volume effects of optic nerves and chiasm. *Int J Radiat Oncol Biol Phys.* 2010;76:S28–S35.

82. Deasy JO, Moiseenko V, Marks L, et al. Radiotherapy dose-volume effects on salivary gland function. *Int J Radiat Oncol Biol Phys.* 2010;76:S58–S63.

83. Jackson A, Ten Haken RK, Robertson JM, et al. Analysis of clinical complication data for radiation hepatitis using a parallel architecture model. *Int J Radiat Oncol Biol Phys.* 1995;31:883–891.

84. Lawrence TS, Tesser RJ, ten Haken RK. An application of dose volume histograms to the treatment of intrahepatic malignancies with radiation therapy. *Int J Radiat Oncol Biol Phys.* 1990;19:1041–1047.

85. Lawrence TS, Ten Haken RK, Kessler ML, et al. The use of 3D dose volume analysis to predict radiation hepatitis. *Int J Radiat Oncol Biol Phys.* 1992;23:781–788.

86. Kaplan EL, Meier P. Nonparametric estimation from incomplete observations. *J Am Stat Assoc.* 1958;53:457–816.

87. Dawson LA, Ten Haken RK, Lawrence TS. Partial irradiation of the liver. *Semin Radiat Oncol.* 2001;11:240–246.

88. Dawson LA, Ten Haken RK. Partial volume tolerance of the liver to radiation. *Semin Radiat Oncol.* 2005;15:279–283.

89. Hunt MA, Jackson A, Narayana A, et al. Geometric factors influencing dosimetric sparing of the parotid glands using IMRT. *Int J Radiat Oncol Biol Phys.* 2006;66:296–304.

90. Wu B, Ricchetti F, Sanguineti G, et al. Patient geometry-driven information retrieval for IMRT treatment plan quality control. *Med Phys.* 2009;36:5497–5505.

91. Appenzoller LM, Michalski JM, Thorstad WL, et al. Predicting dose-volume histograms for organs-at-risk in IMRT planning. *Med Phys.* 2012;39:7446–7461.

92. Deasy JO, Bentzen SM, Jackson A, et al. Improving normal tissue complication probability models: the need to adopt a "data pooling" culture. *Int J Radiat Oncol Biol Phys.* 2010;76:S151–S154.

34 Knowledge-Based Treatment Planning

Todd R. McNutt, John P. Gibbons, and Binbin Wu

INTRODUCTION

Knowledge-based planning represents the next evolutionary step in the development of treatment planning. Initially, as experience in intensity-modulated radiotherapy (IMRT) treatment grew, treatment planners gained knowledge into what dose distributions were possible to both the planning target volume (PTV) and the relevant organs at risk (OAR). Out of this collective knowledge came standard protocols that planners use to control the optimal dose distribution through dose–volume objectives. These protocols are typically population based and reflect the objectives for a specific treatment technique and disease site. The concept of knowledge-based planning enables these optimization protocols to be specific to a patient, based on that patient's specific anatomy and target volumes. This is accomplished by capturing the knowledge of many treatment plans of geometrically similar patients and making predictions of the expected doses based on this set of prior planned patients. It is well published[1] that these methods can improve the efficiency of the treatment planning workflow while demonstrably improving the consistency and quality of treatment plans. This chapter focuses on current methods to store the prior knowledge, extract the relevant features that influence the dose and predict the expected doses that can drive optimization for intensity-modulated treatments.

INTRODUCTORY CONCEPTS

The basic concept of knowledge-based planning is to predict the expected dose distribution in a patient and use that prediction to formulate objectives to drive the optimization of IMRT. Figure 34.1 depicts the general algorithm flow for knowledge-based planning.

What Are We Predicting?

In knowledge-based planning, we are predicting the expected optimized dose for a given patient based on the anatomical geometry of the individual. The predicted dose must be in the appropriate form to be able to use in the objective functions that are used for optimization. These objective functions can be dose–volume based,

radiobiology based, and in some instances, the full predicted 3D dose distribution can be used to promote optimization. As an example, the predicted dose might be in the form of a typical dose–volume histogram (DVH) point such as the dose received by 50% of the volume of the particular region of interest (ROI). In general, the knowledge-based planning methods predict dose and use that dose prediction to formulate expected objective functions in various forms. It is possible in the future; however, that data-driven methods can predict biological outcomes directly.

How Are Predictions Used in Planning and Evaluation?

It is important to also recognize that when driving an optimization, it is most appropriate to use a prediction of the best achievable dose to avoid accepting a suboptimal dose prediction of the expected dose and generating a plan more akin to the average of prior patients. This concept of predicting the best achievable is critical for knowledge-based planning models to strive for continual improvement. Thus, the predictions should predict both the expected dose and the best achievable dose, so they can be used to assess plan quality and to drive optimization, respectively.

What Features Are Used for the Prediction?

To predict doses, the first step is to determine the set of features of the patient's geometry that impacts the optimized dose distribution. The features can represent the target shape, the spatial relationships between normal anatomical structures and the target volumes, or the full set of contours. This feature set will be the input to the prediction algorithms. It is critical to select those features that effect the particular aspects of the dose distribution that we are trying to predict.

What Methods Are Used for the Prediction?

Given a set of features, the goal of the prediction model is to predict the specific attributes of the dose distribution to drive optimization and evaluate patient-specific

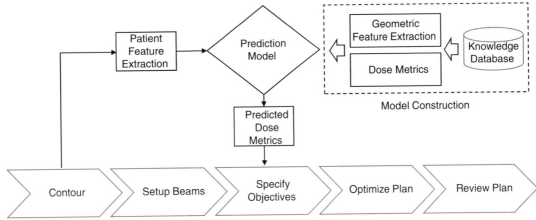

FIGURE 34.1. The basic treatment planning workflow introducing the knowledge-based planning predictions into the optimization objective.

plan quality. Models can be as simple as a fitted function of the dose based on a single dominant feature that effects the dose, or they can be complex machine-learning algorithms that sift through a large set of features in order to improve the prediction accuracy. The accuracy of these methods depends on several factors, including the available data in the knowledge base and the best selection of features to predict from. Another consideration for the models is how they learn and update as new knowledge becomes available.

A premise of knowledge-based planning is that current intensity-modulated treatment plans are not always optimal as the trial and error process and the clinical workflow does not always find the truly optimal plan since the desired objectives are not known.[2] Fundamentally, knowledge-based planning is about setting the appropriate objectives for a given patient's treatment plan that enable the optimization to generate the highest-quality solution. By using knowledge-based planning, the predictions can push the process to ensure the optimal plans are identified. For this reason, it is also important to continually capture new knowledge from new plans, thus improving the knowledge base of data and in turn updating and improving the prediction models over time.

THE KNOWLEDGE BASE

How to Aggregate and Curate? Where to Store?

The DICOM RT standard defines a format that supports most treatment plans in radiation therapy and is agnostic to, and supported by, most vendors. Some Vendor Neutral Archives (VNAs) also support query and retrieval of RT-specific objects. This format can provide a nice standard model for both transfer and archival of treatment plans, but may not be satisfactory for exploration with machine-learning algorithms. Several groups have developed structured query language (SQL) or no-SQL databases to

store the treatment planning data designed specifically to improve the efficiency of access to direct queries of various features of the data.[3]

In addition to the format of the data, it is also important to standardize naming conventions of the various entities. Most specific to knowledge-based planning is the standardized naming of regions of interest and target volumes present in the treatment plan. Standardizations such as those from American Association of Physicists in Medicine (AAPM) Task Group-263[4] allow users of the data to query information across large patient populations based on the standard names. As knowledge bases are used more, this is a critical step to the curation of data as it is entered into the databases. Treatment technique may be derived from the beam definitions in the DICOM RT Plan, but standardizing the technique naming is also critical if the knowledge-based planning utilizes predictions that consider the specific treatment technique such as gantry-static IMRT, tomotherapy, or volumetric-modulated arc therapy.

Updates and Refreshment?

Ideally, any knowledge base is set up to allow continuous updates with new data. These updates will reflect changes in practice such as prescription protocols and delivery techniques including target margin changes due to immobilization and localization of the patients. This promotes refined predictions based on more patient data with improved plan quality, as well as data reflecting the changes in practice used to update prediction models. In situations where the knowledge base is not continuously updated, the models used for the predictions should be evaluated and improved with newer data to reflect the improvements in plan quality or changes in clinical practice for a particular treatment protocol.

Conversely, it is important to remove old and obsolete knowledge from the database. Treatment protocols, margins change, and biologically driven dose goals may be updated to reflect new information from clinical trials. Treatment plans that no longer reflect the desired current practice may adversely impact prediction models and thus should be removed from the knowledge base or excluded from the prediction model training. Nakatsugawa[5] demonstrated how training models with varying timing strategies impact the accuracy of machine-learning models and one should balance the age of the data with the required sample size to maximize the accuracy of the predictions.

DOSE METRICS TO BE PREDICTED

The first step of building prediction models is to specify exactly what is to be predicted. For knowledge-based planning, these are the metrics of the dose distribution intended to drive optimization/inverse planning of IMRT.

Dose–Volume Metrics

The most common dose metrics are dose–volume objectives. These objectives are derived directly from the DVHs of the individual regions of interest defined in a treatment plan. Typical dose–volume metrics represent the minimum or maximum dose to a specified percent of volume of the region. These dose metrics can be extracted as points along a DVH and do not require knowledge of the 3D dose distribution.

In addition, metrics such as mean dose, equivalent uniform dose and other radiobiology-based objectives can be calculated from a full DVH for ROI rather than just a sample point along it. This also would only require prediction of DVH, not the full 3D dose distribution.

To drive optimization, the goal is to predict the full set of dose–volume objectives necessary to adequately drive the optimization of the treatment plan. This would typically be several volume levels for each organ at risk with selections based on clinical goals.

3D Dose

Alternatively, other systems may be designed to predict the full 3D dose distribution. Then, the objectives can be defined to reflect the difference between a planned dose and the predicted dose to drive optimization toward the predicted 3D dose distribution. This process is typically referred to as dose mimicking. Additionally, dose–volume metrics can also be computed from a predicted 3D dose and used for optimization.

Best Achievable vs. Expected

When aggregating data for predictions, it is important to recognize the difference between predicting an expected dose metric and a best achievable dose metric. For example, to predict the mean dose to an organ at risk for a patient with certain set of anatomical features, the average mean dose across all patients with similar characteristics may represent an expected mean dose that could be achieved for the new patient. However, to find the best achievable mean dose, it may be preferable to target at one or two standard deviations on the lower dose side, or perhaps even the minimum mean dose seen in that set of patients. The feature set and prediction models vary in how they handle this concept. It is important that the best achievable be practical for the given patient. The foundation of knowledge-based planning is to provide the optimization with a set of goals that are indeed achievable so the optimizer can find a reasonable solution automatically, but not overly compromised to result in a suboptimal plan.

Potential Patient Outcome/Toxicity

Perhaps the nirvana of knowledge-based planning is predicting actual patient outcomes based on the anatomy and predicted doses. It is possible to envision a prediction of treatment-related toxicities via predicted 3D dose or dose-volume metrics along with additional clinical factors that may exist in a knowledge base. These predictions could potentially be fed back into treatment optimization to personalize the treatment plan and reduce specific patient's risks of treatment-related complications. This is an active area of research, but outside the scope of this chapter.

WHAT FEATURES INFLUENCE THE PREDICTION?

Representation of Regions of Interest

The raw input data to knowledge-based planning is the patient's contoured anatomy and target volumes, usually in the form of a DICOM RT Structure Set. The typical format is a series of contours drawn on the planes making up an image volume such as a CT scan. These contours can be converted to the more primitive representation of a binary mask where each ROI is represented by a 0 or 1 in a volume having the same dimensions of the image volume. Thus, a voxel of the volume is either in the ROI or not.

In the purest sense, it is possible to treat each voxel of a binary mask as a feature of the ROI that can have a value of "in" or "out" of any specific ROI. Of course, this would represent a very large number of features to be used in a prediction model. Some methods of knowledge-based planning may be able to utilize this number of features. As with any mathematical models, the number of input variables and the number of predicted outputs impact the accuracy of prediction models. Therefore, most methods perform what is known as dimensionality reduction that generates features of the set of ROIs and targets that most heavily influence the output to be predicted, such as the dose metrics described in the prior section.

Individual Region of Interest Features: Shape and Volume

Several features may impact the dose–volume metric to be predicted for an individual ROI or target. For example, a large complex target may affect the ability to deliver a uniform dose to a target, whereas a very small spherical target may allow easier delivery of the desired dose. In this case, one could logically conclude that volume and surface area to volume ratio may be the two features that describe the size and complexity of a shape that could impact the predicted dose metrics. This would reduce the features of the binary mask to two specific features, thus reducing the number of features included in the prediction.

Another individual ROI feature may represent the concavity of an ROI. The more concave the target volume is, the more challenging it can be to spare normal anatomy in or around the concavity depending on the treatment beam arrangements.

As one can imagine, dimensionality reduction has the potential to filter out critical components that may adversely impact the ability to predict accurately. Several strategies of feature selection are available from manual selection based on understanding the physics of the problem, to full machine-learning methods that help to select the most relevant features for the given prediction.

Shape Relationships

Perhaps the most utilized features of the set of ROIs used in knowledge-based planning are the shape relationships between each organ at risk and the intended target volumes to be treated with radiation. This makes logical sense as the goal is to treat the target while sparing the OAR as much as possible. If the organ at risk is farther away from the target, logically, it should be easier to spare.

Commonly used features are derived from an overlap volume histogram[6] (OVH), or similarly a distance to target histogram (DTH), which represent the shape relationship between two shapes. The OVH represents the distance between some portion of an organ risk and the target. For example, one may say 50% of the bladder is at least 3 cm away from the PTV of the prostate. By expanding (and contracting) the target volume by a uniform distance d and calculating the percentage of overlap volume between the expanded target and the specific organ at risk, we can plot the OVH as a function of relative volume of overlap versus the expansion distance d. We can then determine what percentage of the organ at risk is d distance from the target. This particular feature can be directly related to the DVH in that they share the relative volume axis and thus can relate the distance to the relative volume of the OAR to the dose received to that relative volume.

Although the OVH can be generated by target expansion and overlap volume calculation, that process is very computationally expensive. Algorithmically, the calculation of OVH can be done using a Euclidean distance transform[7,8] on the target volume, then calculating the distance between each voxel in the OAR and the closest target surface. The histogram of these distances represents the differential OVH and then can be accumulated to form the OVH. The OVH calculation is depicted in Figure 34.2 in 2D and can be extrapolated to 3D.

The Euclidean distance transform takes advantage of the standard 3D Euclidean distance calculation of

$$d(x, y, z) = \sqrt{x^2 + y^2 + z^2}$$

The algorithm, shown graphically in Figure 34.2, accumulates the squared distance from the target binary mask volume in each primary direction and uses the square root to find the distance to the boundary. The process is to traverse each row of voxels in one direction, then traverse backwards to the start while accumulating the distance from the surface squared. Once a boundary of the target is encountered on the traversal, the squared voxel size is added to the next voxel and the cumulative squared distance is incremented for each voxel. If a second boundary is encountered, the cumulative distance is reset to 0, and the accumulation continues. When traversing the row in the opposite direction, the same accumulation of distance occurs, but the voxel value is replaced only if the current squared distance has either not been set or its current value is greater than the cumulative distance of the reverse traversal. Then to apply the y direction, each voxel is visited and the distance squared vector from that voxel is computed in the y direction. Finding the minimum value in the summed vector of the x^2 and y^2 distance provides the sum of the squared distance to that voxel from the nearest target boundary. To obtain the Signed Euclidean distance, the square root of the sum of each volume is computed and then, if inside the target mask, is set to a negative distance and outside positive.

Given the Euclidean distance volume of the target and the binary mask of a specific OAR, a histogram of the distance values in the OAR mask represents the volume of the OAR at each specific distance from the target. Normalizing the volume axis and accumulating the histogram results in the integral OVH.

The OVH is a primary feature of many knowledge-based planning methods. There are some variants of it that present valid features. For example, since treatment beams are typically arranged in a coplanar geometry around the patient, the shape relationship in the superior–inferior direction of the patient may have a different influence on the ability to spare the OAR and hence the prediction of dose. For this reason, it may be more appropriate to look at only the shape relationship in the anterior–posterior or lateral directions. Alternatively, a shape relationship feature that only considers the portion of the organ at risk that is within the extent of the treatment fields would be impacted by some portion of the beams. Such "in-beams" organ-at-risk OVHs have been shown to improve the predictions and hence the quality of

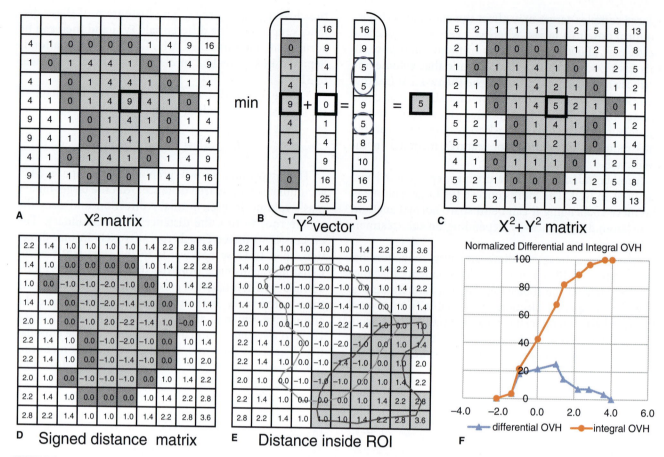

FIGURE 34.2. Calculation of Overlap Volume Histogram (in 2D) using the Euclidean Distance Transform. **(A)** Create a matrix of the x-distance squared by traversing right and then left filling in the minimum distance squared from the boundary voxel. **(B)** For each voxel find the minimum sum of the X2 distance and the Y2 distance from each voxel. **(C)** The resulting Euclidean Distance squared matrix. **(D)** Square root with negative assignment inside target gives the Signed Euclidean Distance from the target. **(E)** Calculate OVH from the distance values contained within the organ at risk. **(F)** Differential histogram showing the relative volume and the distance from the target and the integral OVH showing how far each percent of the volume is away from the target. (Ref Saito).

the knowledge-based treatment plans.[9] This "in-beams" concept is depicted in Figure 34.3.

In addition to the basic OAR-target OVH, advanced features may include the relationship of the OAR with other OARs of the patient, or possibly, the relationship of the target with the full composite set of OARs. Furthermore, one may derive more complex features that identify how much an OAR wraps around the target or limit the ability for radiation to reach the target without passing through it.

There are an infinite number of features that can be derived from the contoured anatomy and target volumes of the patient. Appropriate derivation and selection of the most influential features will ultimately result in better predictions of the dose metrics, and, provided they represent the best achievable dose metrics, should result in the highest-quality treatment plans possible for a given treatment technique.

Relating Overlap Volume Histogram Metrics to Dose Metrics

Figure 34.4 displays two fictional OAR and a target volume, each having the same amount of overlap with the target, with their associated OVHs. On the principle that the longer distance the volume has from the target, the easier it is to spare the OAR dosimetrically, we can see that the 50% volume level of OAR2 is more easily spared because 50% of OAR2 is 1.75 cm from the target whereas 50% of OAR1 is only a few millimeter from the target. Conversely, if it is a serial organ where we are concerned about the smallest volume receiving a high dose, then OAR1 may be more easily spared at the 1% level in that we have to compromise less of the target to achieve the lower dose (2 cm for OAR1 and 4 cm for OAR2 inside the target). In short, at any % volume level, the OVH to the left is harder to spare, and this

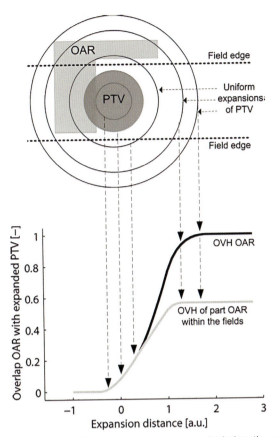

FIGURE 34.3. The OVH is constructed by calculating the overlap between the OAR and the expanded/contracted PTV for each expansion distance. The modified OVH can also be calculated for the part of the OAR that lies within the treatment fields (OARfields). The OVHs of both the entire OAR and of the OARfields are shown as function of the expansion distance in arbitrary units.

OAR, organ at risk; OVH, overlap volume histogram; PTV, planning target volume.

example shows how the OVH captures the relationship that can influence the eventual dose metrics at issue.

Principle Components of Dose–Volume Histogram

Principle components represent another method of dimensionality reduction whereby a DVH is represented by a few of its principle components.[10] This method establishes a set of principle component functions such that a DVH for any organ at risk can be represented as a weighted sum of the principle component functions and then the weights become the features.

METHODS USED TO MAKE PREDICTIONS?

There are many methods to predict the dose metrics with the selected features of the patient's anatomy, ranging from direct statistical models to full machine learning. The first fundamental part is to understand how a particular feature influences the dose metric. Ideally, this influence would be a monotonic relationship between the feature value and the dose metric.

Figure 34.5 shows the OVHs and DVHs for the bladder, left parotid gland, and mandible versus their target volumes in the back drop of many patients. You can see from the highlighted patient samples that, as the OVH moves to the left (where the organ at risk is closer to the target), the resulting DVH moves to the right indicating a higher dose. This relationship is perhaps obvious, but it very much depends on the quality of the treatment plans in the

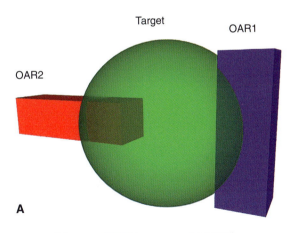

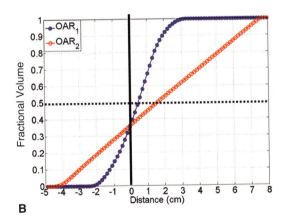

For parallel organs, OAR2 is more easily spared.

For serial organs, OAR1 is more easily spared.

FIGURE 34.4. Example geometrical shapes demonstrating the overlap volume histogram feature between organs at risk (red and blue) and a spherical target (green). The relationship shows how orientation effects the OVH and hence the different dose–volume features of the organs at risk based on the distance to the percent of volume of the two OARs. OAR, organ at risk; OVH, overlap volume histogram.

Bladder vs ptv_prostate_sv

Left parotid vs ptv_5810

Mandible vs ptv_7000

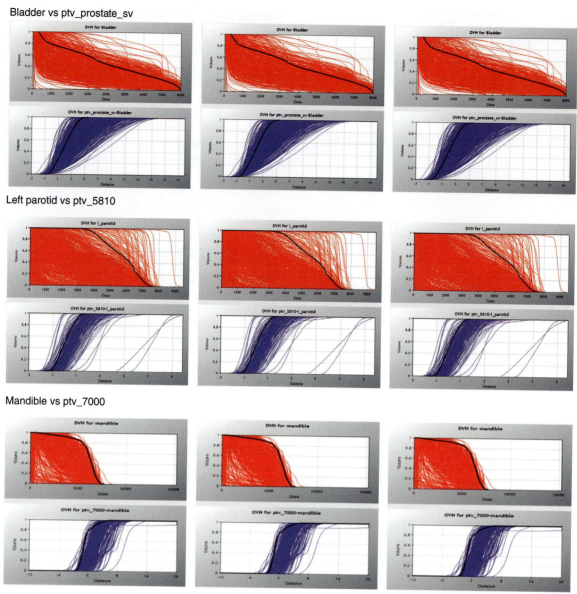

FIGURE 34.5. Overlap Volume Histograms and Dose Volume Histograms for select organs at risk versus their associated target volumes on the backdrop of many patients in a knowledge base. For each pair, as the OVH moves to the right (farther away), the DVH shows lower dose as can be seen in the selected patients (black) in the panels from left (closer) to right (farther). OVH, overlap volume histogram; DVH, dose–volume histogram.

database and that the specific organ at risk has roughly a similar shape across the many patients in the system.

The goal of knowledge-based planning is then to take this data and predict the specific points on the DVHs for each OAR in a treatment plan at volume levels selected to best drive the optimization. Several models have been proposed and are described in this section.

Issue of Accuracy and Input Knowledge? Needed Accuracy for Planning versus Evaluation

The accuracy of the knowledge in the database is critical to the prediction. A perfect prediction of the best

achievable dose for a given patient is more likely if every plan in the database would have to represent the best achievable dose. This is not realistic, and in most cases the treatment plans in the knowledge base represent what was treated clinically in the past and not necessarily the best that could possibly be achieved.[11] Alternatively, for plan evaluation, one may want to predict an expected dose metric. Perhaps it is reasonable to predict an expected dose from the knowledge base as represented by the database since the treatment plans were all used clinically and thus reached a level of quality that was deemed acceptable for clinical use. It is important for users to appreciate these differences, to understand what the input knowledge reflects.

Simple Lookup of Dose–Volume Points (Early Overlap Volume Histogram – Best of the Harder)

Given the relationship between OVH and DVH in Figure 34.5, a simple model for prediction of an expected dose–volume metric would be to find a subset of patients with similar OVH features and find a mean of a dose–volume metric from the subset as an estimate of the dose–volume metric for the new patient. If the goal was to find the best achievable dose, this model can be modified to look for the lowest dose achieved from the same subset of patients with the assumption that the lowest dose achieved in the knowledge base represents the best achievable dose among the subset. This describes the early work on OVH of Wu et al.[12] In the Wu model, to get the best achievable dose, the DVH value was queried at the specified percent–volume level for all patients harder to plan (i.e., patients with a target-OAR distance closer than the current patient) to find the lowest dose achieved in that group. Substantial improvement in plan quality and efficiency in head and neck (HN) cancer treatments was obtained.[13] This simple method took advantage of the OVH–DVH relationship and could be implemented quite fast with a simple database query.

Moore et al.[14] found that the mean dose to an OAR could be predicted from its overlap volume with the PTV with the following exponential relationship:

$$D_{pred} = D_{Rx} \cdot \left[0.2 + 0.8 \cdot \left(1 + e^{-3V_{overlap}/V_{OAR}} \right) \right]$$

where D_{pred} is the predicted mean OAR dose, and D_{Rx} is the prescribed dose to the PTV. $V_{overlap}$ and V_{OAR} are the overlap and OAR volumes, respectively.

An underlying assumption of these models is that adequate target volume coverage was obtained in all of the treatment plans used to make up the knowledge base. Therefore, target coverage requirements must be considered when identifying similar patients. This can be accomplished by limiting the data to be included in the lookup or model generation to those that meet the volume coverage requirement.

Models for Prediction of the Full-Dose Volume Histogram

Further advancement of the predictions seeks to predict the entire DVH for an OAR given the spatial relationship with the target volume(s). Predicting the entire DVH has the advantage of enabling the computation of other more complex dose metrics beyond dose–volume points such as mean doses or biologically effective dose and normal tissue complication probabilities.[15]

Appenzoller et al.[16] approached DVH prediction by formulating a set of skew normal basis functions that could be used to construct the differential DVH by assessing the dose found in sectors of the OAR at binned distances from the target for a large set of patients and finding the parameters of the basis functions to best model the differential DVH. Figure 34.6 displays an equidistance sector of an OAR from a target volume. In the Appenzoller model, the relative volume of each equidistant sector is the weight applied to the basis function of that specific sector. Figure 34.6 shows the set of basis functions and how they are accumulated to find the differential DVH. As expected, the sectors closest to the target reflect a distribution very close to the target dose skewing toward the higher dose closer to the target. As the sectors move farther from the target, they represent lower doses and skew more toward the lower dose side. Thus, for any patient, the differential DVH for an OAR can be predicted by first determining the fractional volume of each equidistance sector (which can be found from the Euclidean distance transform) and applying them as weights to the predetermined basis function set for that specific organ–target pair. Integral DVH can be determined from the differential DVH.

Principle Components Model

Another approach to DVH prediction uses principal component analysis to establish the set of functions used to make up the DVH.[17] The Rapid Plan™ Model,[18] commercialized in the Varian Eclipse™ treatment planning system (Varian Medical Systems, Palo Alto, CA) as a knowledge-based planning tool, was originally proposed by Yuan et al.[19] with the following anatomical features considered in their DVH estimating model: OAR volumes, PTV volumes, fraction of OAR volume overlapping with PTV (overlap volume), (DTH, equivalent to OVH defined by Wu et al.), and fraction of OAR volume outside the primary treatment fields (out-of-field volume). In their approach, principal component analysis is applied to DVHs and DTHs to reduce their dimensions. The two most significant components of principal component scores (PCS: PCS1 and PCS2) are used to represent the respective DVHs and DTHs. Stepwise multiple regression method is applied to identify the significant factors (R^2) among the proposed anatomical features in correlating DVHs' PCS1 and PCS2. For example, they found that the important anatomical features for predicting OAR doses in prostate and HN plans are DTH's median distance, gradient, and out-of-field OAR volume. In addition, the Rapid Plan™ Model estimates the whole OAR's DVH curve, rather than DVH points proposed by Wu et al.

Machine-learning Models—Random Forest

Machine-learning methods are well suited for cases of having many input features to predict a dose outcome. Various methods have been introduced in the

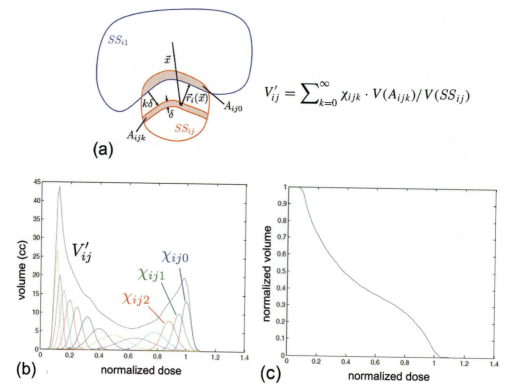

$$V'_{ij} = \sum_{k=0}^{\infty} \chi_{ijk} \cdot V(A_{ijk})/V(SS_{ij})$$

FIGURE 34.6. Graphical representation of predicting the differential DVH for an OAR from a set of skew normal basis functions representing the dose in sections of the OAR equidistant from the target volume. **(a)** diagrammatic representation of sector A_{ijk} a distance $\vec{r}_i(\vec{x})$ from structure SS_{i1}. **(b)** Graphical representation of jth OAR's differential DVH. **(c)** Cumulative DVH view. Reprinted from Appenzoller et al.[16]

literature.[17,20] They all follow a similar algorithmic development process that begins with feature selection and reduction, followed by algorithm training and validation. One of the benefits of machine learning is that it can include additional features beyond the OVH such as target volume and complexity.

Figure 34.7 shows the results of a two phase treatment for high-risk prostate cancer with an initial phase including the prostate and pelvic lymph nodes and a cone down to the prostate and seminal vesicles from a commercial system (Oncospace, Inc, Baltimore MD). Here, the predictions were performed based on a random forest prediction model. The displayed color bands represent the range of the 5th percentile representing the best achievable (left side) to the expected dose (right side) as predicted by the model. The individual points along the best achievable edge represent the dose metrics that are input as objectives to the treatment planning system to drive optimization for the initial and cone down. The composite dose prediction with the associated clinical dose goals are also shown for reference when evaluating plan quality. Figure 34.8 displays the resulting treatment plan DVHs on the backdrop of those same predictions resulting in DVHs that mostly fit into the predicted range, thus, indicating a treatment plan with a quality in the expected ranges for this specific patient based on their individual anatomy and targets. Interestingly, in this one, some of the overall protocol level dose goals were not met as the anatomy of

the patient made them very challenging and the method predicted this. This is another benefit of knowledge-based planning—knowing when it will be difficult to reach clinical dosimetric goals for a patient. Furthermore, the lack of objectives at the higher volumes of the femur heads resulted in no push toward a lower-dose level, demonstrating the selection of the volume levels to use can impact the results.

3D Predictions for Dose Mimicking

Predicting the 3D dose directly brings on different challenges. A few groups have deployed neural networks to predict the 3D dose.[21,22] These methods train neural networks by supplying contours and resulting dose distributions to teach the network what dose distribution to expect in a final treatment plan.

The predicted dose can be used as a reference dose target in an optimization strategy designed to mimic the predicted dose. In this case, the objective of optimization may be derived from the difference between the predicted 3D dose and the planned dose being optimized. This is referred to as a dose-mimicking approach, and can be used when a desired 3D dose is known beforehand. Alternatively, the dose volume-based objectives can be calculated from the predicted 3D dose, and be used in the more traditional plan optimization approach.

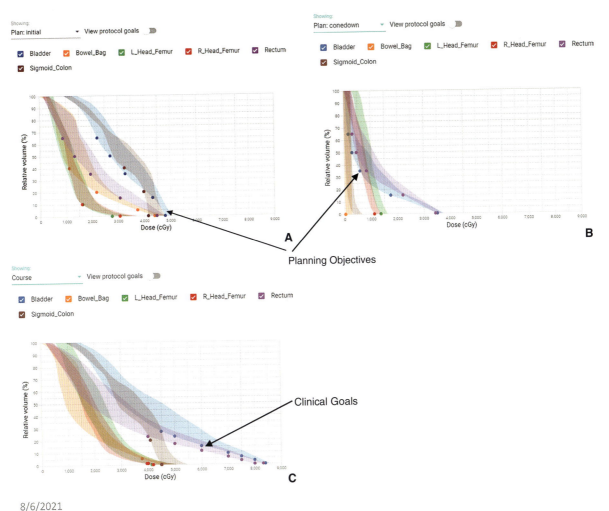

8/6/2021

FIGURE 34.7. Figure of DVHs predicted using a random forest algorithm to predict each DVH point for both initial **(A)** and cone down **(B)** treatment plans for a prostate treatment including the pelvic lymph nodes. The swath has the expected dose on the right side of the band, and the lowest achievable dose on the left. Also shown are selected points on the predicted DVHs to use for treatment plan optimization using dose–volume metrics. **(C)** Shows the prediction for the overall course (initial, cone down) with the associated clinical dose goals predicted. Courtesy of Oncospace Inc.

DVH, dose-volume histogram.

INFLUENCE OF TREATMENT DELIVERY TECHNIQUE

The delivery technique including beam energy also impacts the treatment plan quality. This introduces the question of how technique should be included in the prediction of dose for knowledge-based planning. One strategy would be to construct dose prediction models for each specific technique. This however may limit the number of treatment plans available for modeling, which in turn may limit the accuracy of the prediction. Alternatively, we could include a subset of similar techniques, which can increase the number of treatment plans but may add variability to the plan quality due to the limitations of the included techniques. A third possibility is to include the technique as a feature in the prediction model itself. Previous investigations[23] on the impact of technique on predictive modeling have found that it comes down to the data used in the model training and how the range of applicability of a model with regard to technique is applied. The more data are available for model training, the more refined the knowledge base planning can be for specific delivery techniques.

MODEL TRAINING

Model training is the process of curating the treatment planning data in the knowledge base and using that curated data to construct the prediction models. The number of cases needed and the quality of the included data depends on the specific algorithm used. They do all have some basic similarities in the quantity and quality of the data used.

The first step is to determine the appropriate patient grouping to use for your model. The data can be grouped at varying levels of target specificity as well as technique specificity. For example, for prostate, typical targets are

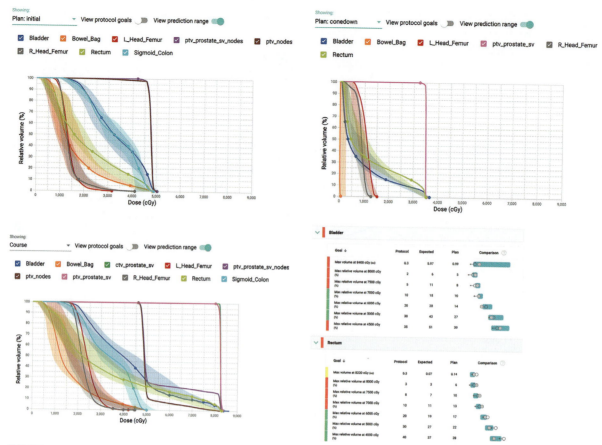

FIGURE 34.8. A display of the resulting automated treatment plan DVHs (lines) generated by the Pinnacle³ treatment planning system using the dose predictions with random forest and the selected object dose-volume points. The plan DVHs are displayed on the original predicted DVH bands from expected (right side) to lowest achievable (left side). The goal is to have the final plan DVHs within the bands of the prediction. Selecting the proper volume levels of the objectives for prediction play a role in the automation.

DVH, dose-volume histogram.

the intact prostate, the prostate plus seminal vesicles, the prostate plus pelvic lymph nodes, as well as the prostate bed and prostate bed plus pelvic lymph nodes for postprostatectomy cases. One could choose to model each target scenario separately, or to group a subset of the more similar ones into a single model based on the similarity in geometries. One could also include them all and then rely on the spatial relationship features used in the prediction model to discern the differences between patients within the whole spectrum of target scenarios. Other examples may include laterality as in unilateral versus bilateral HN treatment. When laterality is involved, it is possible to take advantage of symmetry of the patient to create a unilateral model as opposed to a separate left or right-side model.

Similarly, grouping by treatment technique can be done to make more technique specific models. When modeling, it is important to balance the number of plans in the knowledge base, as it is important to span the range of anatomical geometries within each group. When making these decisions, the available data and the impact on the accuracy of the model for the various scenarios should be considered.

Another consideration is the variation in dose prescriptions in the training set. If prescription doses are different but fall within a reasonable range, dose normalization can be used in the model construction to make all plans match. Then for the final predictions, the desired prescription for the new patient can be used to adjust the prediction to the specific prescription to be used.

An advantage of using a knowledge base of actually approved clinical treatment plans is that clinical decisions have been made on these plans. The clinical tradeoffs between targets and normal tissues[24] have been considered and those decisions are imbedded in the data. Though this is hard to quantify, the hope is that the knowledge base includes the proper tradeoffs and hence the predictions will reflect them. Knowing that the clinical plans may not be of the highest quality, we can be presented with the option to replan a case to improve the quality for inclusion in the knowledge base. If this is considered, one should make sure that the resulting plan receives the appropriate clinical review for those tradeoffs. This should be done with care, and in some cases it may be preferred to simply reject a low-quality plan rather than replan it.

Once the training data set is determined, the actual training depends on the specific model in use. They will all have a different process. Basically, they will calculate the spatial features of the anatomy and targets for each training plan and evaluate the features of the dose distribution that are to be predicted. During the modeling process, most methods will perform some type of cross-validation to provide an estimate of the accuracy of the model.

VALIDATION OF THE PREDICTION MODELS

During the modeling process, cross-validation can be used to assess the accuracy. One method is to leave out some of the training data set from the model building and then assesses the accuracy of the resulting predictions against the left-out data set. This process can be repeated by training a second model leaving out a different subset of the data. This is called folding, and is referred to as x-fold cross-validation where x is the number of subsets with the size of each subset as total/x cases. So, tenfold cross-validation would use 10% of the data for validation and would create 10 models. This method is primarily used to ensure the model itself is appropriate for the problem. The goal is to create a single model from the data for clinical use.

When constructing the single model, we simply want to have a training data set and a separate validation data set. If we train and validate with data from the same clinic or same physician, then we only are validating the model internally knowing the environment that the data represents. To expand the use of the model beyond the known environment, it should be externally validated against additional cases where the model may be applied, prior to any clinical use.

SETTING OBJECTIVE PROTOCOLS

Now that we can predict the doses from our knowledge base, we still need to identify the objectives to use for our patients. What volume levels and how many should be used for DVH-based planning? This part remains in the hands of the expert user until we can incorporate best volume levels to choose from the knowledge base. Typically, this is done by setting protocol templates that may list a set of dose–volume objectives and their associated relative volumes. Then, the models can predict the expected doses for each to drive the optimization.

OVERALL QUALITY IMPROVEMENT

A promise of knowledge-based planning is to improve the quality of treatment for patients. In a study by Moore et al.[25] of the RTOG 0126 clinical trial, the quality of the treatment plans was evaluated retrospectively using a knowledge-based prediction model of Normal Tissue Complication Probability (NTCP) for the rectum. Figure 34.9 shows the results, indicating that use of knowledge-based planning could have reduced the risk for some patients by as much as 15% and on average by 4.7%.

Wu et al.[13] performed a prospective study of HN patient and showed that the use of knowledge-based planning reduces max doses to the cord and brainstem by 1.68 Gy and 2.77 Gy, respectively, compared to the plans manually created by human planners.

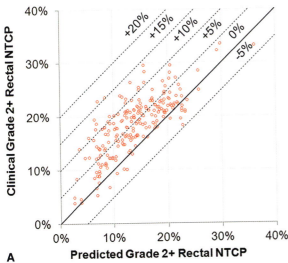

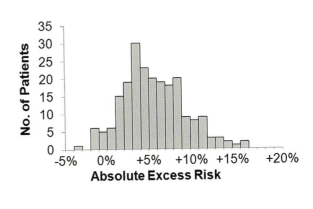

A   **B**

FIGURE 34.9. A secondary study on RTOG 0126 quantified excess risk of late rectal complication due to suboptimal IMRT planning. **(A)** Data-driven prediction of NTCP versus the actual treated plans' NTCP. **(B)** Frequency histogram showed a mean excess risk of 4.7% ± 3.9%.
NTCP, normal tissue complication probability; IMRT, intensity-modulated radiotherapy; RTOG, Radiation Therapy Oncology Group.

CONCLUSION

Knowledge-based planning is relatively new to radiation therapy. In its current form, planning in radiation therapy in many respects repeats the processes over and over again for many patients. This is ripe for automation, but the automation must maintain the personalization of treatment we expect for each individual patient. As we gain more clinical experience and are able to capture the details of our treatment plans in large knowledge bases, it is inevitable that knowledge-based planning will become the norm. The selection of anatomical features that maintain the personalized treatment and ensure the highest treatment plan quality will result in broader implementation of knowledge-based planning. Cloud-based implementations of software systems will facilitate larger-scale accumulation of digital knowledge to further advance these methods and make them available broadly and globally. The examples in this chapter represent just a few of those studies and the field is likely to see more refinement approaches as automation reaches more diseases sites and treatment delivery techniques.

REFERENCES

1. Moore KL. Automated radiotherapy treatment planning. *Semin Radiat Oncol.* 2019;29:209–218. doi:10.1016/j.semradonc.2019.02.003.
2. Nelms BE, Robinson G, Markham J, et al. Variation in external beam treatment plan quality: an inter-institutional study of planners and planning systems. *Pract Radiat Oncol.* 2012;2:296–305.
3. Robertson S, Quon H, Kiess, A, et al. A data-mining framework for large scale analysis of dose-outcome relationships in a database of irradiated head and neck (HN) cancer patients. *Med Phys.* 2015 Sep;42(7):4329.
4. Mayo CS, Moran JM, Bosch W, et al. AAPM task group 263: standardizing nomenclatures in radiation oncology AAPM TG 263. *Int J Radiat Oncol Biol Phys.* 2018;100(4):1057e1066.
5. Nakatsugawa M, Cheng Z, Kiess A, et al. The needs and benefits of continuous model updates on the accuracy of RT-induced toxicity prediction models within a learning health system. *Int J Radiat Oncol Biol Phys.* 2019 Feb;103(2,1):460–467.
6. Wu B, Ricchetti F, Sanguineti G, et al. Patient geometry-driven information retrieval for IMRT treatment plan quality control. *Med Phys.* 2009 Dec;36(12):5497–5505.
7. Kazhdan M, Simari P, McNutt T, et al. A shape relationship descriptor for radiation therapy planning. *Medical Image Computing and Computer-Assisted Intervention.* 2009;5762/2009(12):100–108.
8. Saito, T, Toriwaki, J. New algorithms for euclidean distance transformation of an n-dimensional digitized picture with applications. *Pattern Recognit.* 1994;27(11):1551–1565.
9. Petit SF, Wu B, Kazhdan M, et al. Increased organ sparing using shape-based treatment plan optimization for intensity modulated radiation therapy of pancreatic adenocarcinoma. *Radiother Oncol.* 2012;102:38–44.
10. Sohn M, Alber M, Yan D. Principal component analysis-based pattern analysis of dose-volume histograms and influence on rectal toxicity. *Int J Radiat Oncol Biol Phys.* 2007;69:230–239.
11. Das IJ, Cheng CW, Chopra KL, et al. Intensity-modulated radiation therapy dose prescription, recording, and delivery: patterns of variability among institutions and treatment planning systems. *J Natl Cancer Inst.* 2008;100(5):300–307.
12. Wu B, Ricchetti F, Sanguineti G, et al. Data-driven approach to generating achievable dose-volume histogram objectives in intensity modulated radiotherapy planning. *Int J Radiat Oncol Biol Phys.* 2011 Mar 15;79(4):1241–1247. Epub 2010 Aug.
13. Wu B, McNutt T, Zahurak M, et al. Fully automated simultaneous integrated boosted-intensity modulated radiation therapy treatment planning is feasible for head-and-neck cancer: a prospective clinical study. *Int J Radiat Oncol Biol Phys.* 2012 Dec 1;84(5):e647–53.
14. Moore KL, Brame RS, Low DA, et al. Experience-based quality control of clinical intensity-modulated radiotherapy planning. *Int J Radiat Oncol Biol Phys.* 2011;81:545–551.
15. Marks LB. Use of normal tissue complication probability models in the clinic. *Int J Radiat Oncol Biol Phys.* 2010;76(3 suppl):S10–S19.
16. Appenzoller L, et al. Predicting dose-volume histograms for organs-at-risk in IMRT planning. *Med Phys.* 2012 Dec;39(12):7446–7461.
17. Zhu X, Ge Y, Li T, et al. A planning quality evaluation tool for prostate adaptive IMRT based on machine learning. *Med Phys.* 2011;38:719–726.
18. Varian Medical Systems, Inc. *Eclipse Photon and Electron Algorithms Reference Guide.* Palo Alto, CA: Varian Medical Systems; 2017:209–220.
19. Yuan L, et al. Quantitative analysis of the factors which affect the interpatient organ-at-risk dose sparing variation in IMRT plans. *Med Phys.* 2012 Nov;39(11):6868–6878.
20. Naqa IE, Li R, Murphy MJ, eds. *Machine Learning in Radiation Oncology: Theory and Applications.* Cham, Switzerland: Springer International Publishing; 2015.
21. Berlin A, Conroy L, Tjong MC, et al. Clinical application of a novel voxel- and machine learning-based automated planning method for prostate volumetric arc radiation therapy. *Int J Radiat Oncol Biol Phys.* 2018 Nov 01;102:e533. doi:10.1016/j.ijrobp.2018.07.1495
22. McIntosh C, Welch M, McNiven A, et al. Fully automated treatment planning for head and neck radiotherapy using a voxel-based dose prediction and dose mimicking method. *Phys Med Biol.* 2017 July 6;62:15.
23. Lian J, Yuan L, Ge Y, et al. Modeling the dosimetry of organ at-risk in head and neck IMRT planning: an intertechnique and interinstitutional study. *Med Phys.* 2013;40:121704.
24. Craft D, Halabi T, Bortfeld T. Exploration of tradeoffs in intensity-modulated radiotherapy. *Phys Med Biol.* 2005;50:5857–5868.
25. Moore KL, Schmidt R, Moiseenko V, et al. Quantifying unnecessary normal tissue complication risks due to suboptimal planning: a secondary study of RTOG 0126. *Int J Radiat Oncol Biol Phys.* 2015;92(2):228–235. doi:10.1016/j.ijrobp.2015.01.046.

Index

Note: Page numbers followed by f indicate figures; those followed by t indicate tables.